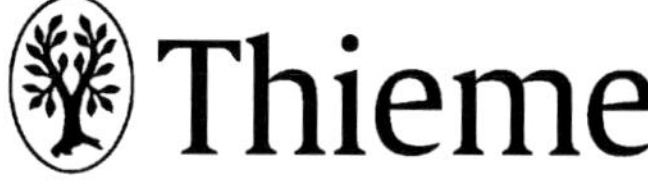

Differential Diagnosis in Musculoskeletal MRI

Gary M. Hollenberg, MD, FACR
Associate Professor of Radiology and Imaging Sciences
University of Rochester Medical Center
Director
Advanced Fellowship in Magnetic Resonance Imaging
University of Rochester School of Medicine and Dentistry
Rochester, New York

Eric P. Weinberg, MD
Associate Professor of Radiology and Imaging Sciences
University of Rochester Medical Center
Medical Director of University Medical Imaging
University of Rochester School of Medicine and Dentistry
Rochester, New York

Steven P. Meyers, MD, PhD, FACR
Professor of Radiology, Imaging Sciences, and Neurosurgery
University of Rochester Medical Center
Director
Radiology Residency Program
University of Rochester School of Medicine and Dentistry
Rochester, New York

Thieme
New York • Stuttgart • Delhi • Rio de Janeiro

Thieme Medical Publishers, Inc.
333 Seventh Ave.
New York, NY 10001

Executive Editor: William Lamsback
Managing Editor: J. Owen Zurhellen IV
Senior Vice President, Editorial and Electronic Product Development: Cornelia Schulze
Production Editor: Sean Woznicki
International Production Director: Andreas Schabert
International Marketing Director: Fiona Henderson
Director of Sales, North America: Mike Roseman
International Sales Director: Louisa Turrell
Vice President, Finance and Accounts: Sarah Vanderbilt
President: Brian D. Scanlan
Printer: Everbest Printing Co Ltd.

Library of Congress Cataloging-in-Publication Data

Hollenberg, Gary M., author.
Differential diagnosis in musculoskeletal MRI / Gary M. Hollenberg, Eric P. Weinberg, Steven P. Meyers.
p. ; cm.
Includes bibliographical references.
ISBN 978-1-60406-683-8 (hardcover) –
ISBN 978-1-60406-684-5 (ebook)
I. Weinberg, Eric P., author. II. Meyers, Steven P., author. III. Title.
[DNLM: 1. Musculoskeletal Diseases–diagnosis–Atlases.
2. Diagnosis, Differential–Atlases. 3. Magnetic Resonance Imaging–Atlases. WE 17]
RC925.7
616.7'07548–dc23
2014016257

Thieme Publishers New York
333 Seventh Avenue, New York, NY 10001 USA
1-800-782-3488, customerservice@thieme.com

Thieme Publishers Stuttgart
Rüdigerstrasse 14, 70469 Stuttgart, Germany
+49 [0]711 8931 421, customerservice@thieme.de

Thieme Publishers Delhi
A-12, Second Floor, Sector -2, NOIDA -201301
Uttar Pradesh, India
+91 120 45 566 00, customerservice@thieme.in

Thieme Publishers Rio, Thieme Publicações Ltda.
Argentina Building 16th floor, Ala A, 228 Praia do Botafogo
Rio de Janeiro 22250-040 Brazil
+55 21 3736-3631

Printed in China 5 4 3 2 1

ISBN 978-1-60406-683-8

eISBN 978-1-60406-684-5

Important note: Medicine is an ever-changing science undergoing continual development. Research and clinical experience are continually expanding our knowledge, in particular our knowledge of proper treatment and drug therapy. Insofar as this book mentions any dosage or application, readers may rest assured that the authors, editors, and publishers have made every effort to ensure that such references are in accordance with **the state of knowledge at the time of production of the book**.

Nevertheless, this does not involve, imply, or express any guarantee or responsibility on the part of the publishers in respect to any dosage instructions and forms of applications stated in the book. **Every user is requested to examine carefully** the manufacturers' leaflets accompanying each drug and to check, if necessary in consultation with a physician or specialist, whether the dosage schedules mentioned therein or the contraindications stated by the manufacturers differ from the statements made in the present book. Such examination is particularly important with drugs that are either rarely used or have been newly released on the market. Every dosage schedule or every form of application used is entirely at the user's own risk and responsibility. The authors and publishers request every user to report to the publishers any discrepancies or inaccuracies noticed. If errors in this work are found after publication, errata will be posted at www.thieme.com on the product description page.

Some of the product names, patents, and registered designs referred to in this book are in fact registered trademarks or proprietary names even though specific reference to this fact is not always made in the text. Therefore, the appearance of a name without designation as proprietary is not to be construed as a representation by the publisher that it is in the public domain.

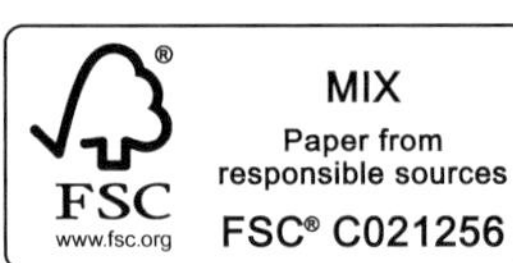

Dedicated to my parents, Nancy and Dr. Murray Hollenberg, for teaching me the value of hard work and perseverance; and to my wife Susan, and children Alex, Michelle, and Ronnie, for their love, support, and humor that helped bring this project to completion. – *GMH*

I dedicate this book to my teachers for sharing their knowledge and enthusiasm, to my colleagues for their help and encouragement, and to my wife Margot, and children Sam, Amelia and Julia, for their love and support. – *EPW*

Dedicated to my wife Barbara, and son Noah; for their continuous patience, love, and support during this project. I am also very grateful to all of my former teachers and mentors who have helped me before and during my career in Medicine. – *SPM*

Contents

Foreword

Diagnostic imaging is continually changing. The introduction of magnetic resonance imaging (MRI) approximately three decades ago revolutionized musculoskeletal imaging with the importance of MRI growing exponentially since its inception. Most of this growth is not related to the discovery of new pathologic conditions in the musculoskeletal system but, rather, to the continuous development and refinement of the MRI technology including both new imaging sequences and the description of new diagnostic signs. Because of its unmatched high soft tissue contrast resolution, MRI is particularly useful in the evaluation of the soft tissue components in both joints and tumors where it has replaced other imaging modalities or created a large number of new imaging indications.

This book is composed of an introductory chapter followed by a total of 49 tables describing the MRI findings of various diseases complemented by the findings of other imaging modalities and pertinent clinical findings. The introduction focuses in a succinct manner on the MRI physics and techniques including pulse sequences relevant for musculoskeletal imaging followed by a condensed description of bone formation and the MRI features of physiologic and pathologic components of both normal and pathologic conditions involving the musculoskeletal system. The gist of the book consists of differential diagnostic tables. Each table lists all important pathologic conditions for a specific anatomic location, and by providing both characteristic MRI presentation and pertinent pathologic and clinical data that help the reader to arrive at a likely diagnosis and reasonable differential diagnosis. Since most disorders present in many different locations, some overlap in the text is unavoidable. The chosen tabular format minimizes repetition. High quality images are enclosed to visually demonstrate the MRI findings under discussion. The tabular format offers a contrast to other musculoskeletal MRI textbooks which are disease oriented. This book includes all the relevant information contained in other standard texts but, besides an extensive description of the MRI findings, only the most essential etiologic, clinical and pathologic information is included.

This book is intended for radiologists, orthopedists and physicians with interest in musculoskeletal imaging who interpret MRI examinations. The book is a comprehensive outline of musculoskeletal MRI findings and appears to be particularly useful to radiology residents who wish to strengthen their diagnostic acumen and prepare for their specialty examination. Any physician involved in the interpretation of musculoskeletal MRI studies should find this text helpful in direct proportion to his or her curiosity. Drs. Hollenberg, Weinberg, and Meyers are to be congratulated for their original approach to this text, the excellent and complete coverage of musculoskeletal MRI, and their succinct presentation of the material. I believe this book will be an invaluable resource for residents, fellows, radiologists, orthopedists, physiatrists and other clinicians with interest in this topic. There is no doubt in my mind that this book will receive extraordinary acceptance in the medical community.

Francis A. Burgener, MD
Professor of Radiology
University of Rochester Medical Center
Rochester, New York

Preface

Imaging of musculoskeletal injuries and lesions is a broad subject encompassing multiple imaging modalities. Traditionally, this included conventional radiography, which has been well-described by many authors over the years. Radiography has been supplemented by CT and nuclear medicine, and continues to serve an important role in the evaluation of these abnormalities. Magnetic Resonance Imaging (MRI) has become progressively more accessible, and now often plays a crucial role along with conventional radiography and CT, in the evaluation of various abnormalities involving joints, soft-tissue and bones. It is estimated that there are over 50,000 MRI scanners worldwide performing approximately 150 million MRI exams per year. MRI has the unique ability to demonstrate subtle soft tissue abnormalities given its exceptional high soft-tissue contrast resolution. In addition, MRI can often detect cortical and bone marrow signal abnormalities not visible with conventional radiography or CT.

As Academic Radiologists, we have been directly involved in the education of Radiology Residents and Fellows in the realm of Musculoskeletal MRI for many years. We have been fortunate to have access to state-of-the-art MRI scanners as well as the benefit of our association with and referrals from outstanding Orthopedic surgeons, Physiatrists, Neurosurgeons, and Neurologists at the University of Rochester in New York.

The main purpose of this book is provide a single, easy-to-use image-rich text on the MRI appearance of various musculoskeletal injuries, inflammatory, infectious and arthritic diseases, as well as benign and malignant lesions of bone and soft tissue. The book is organized into lists of differential diagnoses based on locations (Shoulder, Elbow, Wrist and Hand, Hip, Knee, and Ankle and Foot, and involving different sites of bone and soft tissue) as well as specific MRI features in a tabular format. Each of the musculoskeletal lesions and abnormalities listed in the tables has a column summarizing the **MRI Findings** and pertinent radiographic and/or CT findings with associated images for illustration, and a **Comments** column summarizing key clinical and pathologic data. The book's organization into these sections of differential diagnosis helps the reader obtain desired information efficiently and quickly.

We hope this text provides a valuable resource for practicing radiologists, fellowship trainees, and residents who encounter the multitude of musculoskeletal injuries, their mimics, and lesions involving bones, joints and surrounding structures. This book will be also useful to orthopedic and sport medicine specialists and trainees. This book is intended to become a "well-thumbed" text at the PACS station, and in the orthopedic and sports medicine clinics. It will also serve as a useful review and teaching guide for radiology trainees.

Acknowledgments

We wish to thank the staff at Thieme Medical Publishers for their dedication, hard work, and attention to detail with the manuscript of this book. We also thank Ms. Colleen Cottrell for her outstanding secretarial work, and Ms. Margaret Kowaluk and Ms. Sarah Peangatelli for their excellent work with formatting the numerous figures for this book.

In addition, we wish to acknowledge the following for their contribution of interesting cases: Francis A. Burgener, MD; James J. Lester, MD; Richard White, DO; Steven Weiss, MD; Peter Rosella, MD; Andrea Zynda-Weiss, MD; Valeriy Kheyfits, MD; Allan Bernstein, MD; David Shrier, MD; Charlene Varnis, MD; and Timothy Braatz, MD.

We extend our special thanks to all of our coworkers and physician colleagues at University Medical Imaging at Clinton Crossings, the Outpatient Diagnostic Imaging Facility of the University of Rochester Medical Center. We could not ask for a greater group of dedicated people to work with in the clinical practice of Diagnostic Radiology.

List of Abbreviations

ABC	aneurysmal bone cyst
aBME	acute bone marrow edema
AC	acromioclavicular
ACL	anterior cruciate ligament
ADC	apparent diffusion coefficient
AIDS	acquired immune deficiency syndrome
AITF	anteroinferior tibiofibular ligament
ALL	acute lymphoblastic leukemia
ALPSA	anterior labrum periosteal sleeve avulsion
AML	acute myelogenous leukemia
ANA	antinuclear antibodies
AP	anteroposterior
APL	abductor pollicus longus
ATFL	anterior talofibular ligament
AVN	avascular necrosis
Ca	calcium
CF	calcaneofibular ligament
CLL	chronic lymphocytic leukemia
CML	chronic myelogenous leukemia
CMPD	chronic myeloproliferative disease
CNL	calcaneonavicular ligament
CNS	central nervous system
CPPD	calcium pyrophosphate dihydrate deposition
CSF	cerebrospinal fluid
CT	computed tomography
3DFT	three-dimensional Fourier transform
DDH	developmental dysplasia of the hip
DEH	dysplasia epiphysealis hemimelica
DFS	dermatofibrosarcoma
DFSP	dermatofibrosarcoma protuberans
DISH	diffuse idiopathic skeletal hyperostosis
DISI	dorsal intercalated instability
DTPA	diethylene triamine pentacetic acid
DWI	diffusion-weighted imaging
ECU	extensor carpi ulnaris
EG	eosinophilic granuloma
EPB	extensor pollicus brevis
FAI	femoral acetabular impingement
FCD	fibrous cortical defect
FHL	flexor hallucis longus tendon
FLAIR	fluid attenuated inversion recovery
FS	frequency selective fat signal suppression
FSE	fast spin echo
FS PDWI	fat-suppressed proton density-weighted imaging
FSPGR	fast spoiled gradient-recalled echo
FS T1WI	fat-suppressed T1-weighted imaging
FS T2WI	fat-suppressed T2-weighted imaging
GCSF	granulocyte colony-stimulating factor
Gd-contrast	gadolinium chelate contrast

GLAD	glenoid labrum articular cartilage disruption
GRE	gradient-refocused echo pulse sequence
HADD	calcium hydroxyapatite deposition disease
HAGL	humeral avulsion of the glenohumeral ligament
HD	Hodgkin disease
HMB-45	human melanoma black monoclonal antibody
HPF	high power field
HU	Hounsfield unit
IT band	iliotibial band
JIA	juvenile idiopathic arthritis
JRA	juvenile rheumatoid arthritis
LCH	Langerhans cell histiocytosis
LCL	lateral collateral ligament
LCP	Legg Calve Perthes disease
LFC	lateral femoral condyle
LUCL	lateral ulnar collateral ligament
MCL	medial collateral ligament
MCP	metacarpal phalangeal joint
MDP	methylene diphosphonate
MDS	myelodysplastic syndrome
MFC	medial femoral condyle
MFH	malignant fibrous histiocytoma
MGL	middle glenohumeral ligament
MIP	maximum intensity projection
MPNST	malignant peripheral nerve sheath tumor
MR	magnetic resonance
MRA	magnetic resonance angiography
MRI	magnetic resonance imaging
NF1	neurofibromatosis type 1
NF2	neurofibromatosis type 2
NHL	non-Hodgkin lymphoma
NOF	nonossifying fibroma
NSAID	non-steroid anti-inflammatory drugs
OA	osteoarthritis
OCD	osteochondritis dissecans
PB	peroneus brevis tendon
PCL	posterior cruciate ligament
PCV	polycythemia vera
PDWI	proton density weighted imaging
PET	positron emission tomography
PHAT	pleomorphic hyalinizing angiectatic tumor
PIN	posterior interosseus nerve
PIP	proximal interphalangeal joint
PITF	posteroinferior tibiofibular ligament
PL	peroneus longus tendon
PNET	primitive neuroectodermal tumor
POPS	painful os peroneum syndrome
PTH	parathyroid hormone
PTT	posterior tibial tendon
PVNS	pigmented villonodular synovitis
RA	rheumatoid arthritis
RBC	red blood cell
RCL	radial collateral ligament
RF	radio frequency

RF	rheumatoid factor
RSD	reflex sympathetic dystrophy
SCFE	slipped capital femoral epiphysis
SE	spin echo
SFT	solitary fibrous tumor
SLAC	scapholunate advanced collapse
SMA	smooth muscle actin antibodies
SLAP	superior labrum anterior to posterior
STIR	short tau (T1) inversion recovery
S-100	cellular calcium binding protein in cytoplasm and/or nucleus
T1	spin-lattice or longitudinal relaxation time
T2	spin-spin or transverse relaxation time
T2*	effective spin-spin relaxation time using GRE
T1WI	T1-weighted imaging
T2WI	T2-weighted imaging
TA	tibialis anterior tendon
TB	tuberculosis
TE	echo time
TFC	triangular fibrocartilage
TFCC	triangular fibrocartilage complex
TI	inversion time
TOF	time-of-flight
TR	repetition time
UBC	unicameral bone cyst
UCL	ulnar collateral ligament
VISI	volar intercalated instability
WHO	World Health Organization

Chapter 1

Introduction to Magnetic Resonance Imaging for Evaluation of Musculoskeletal Abnormalities

1

1 Introduction to Magnetic Resonance Imaging for Evaluation of Musculoskeletal Abnormalities

Steven P. Meyers

Magnetic resonance imaging (MRI) is a powerful medical imaging method that has been used extensively in the evaluation of musculoskeletal disorders, including congenital, developmental, metabolic, inflammatory/infectious, and hematologic abnormalities as well as neoplastic and tumor-like lesions.[1–25] MRI can provide "in vivo" anatomical images of the human body with high soft tissue contrast resolution. The magnetic resonance (MR) images can be obtained in multiple planes (i.e., sagittal, axial, coronal, or various oblique combinations). The "signal" used to generate an MR image comes from hydrogen nuclei (protons) within a human body. In essence, MRI is basically a hydrogen scan.

The hydrogen nucleus has a net charge of +1 and spins at a frequency that is dependent on the ambient magnetic field and its particular physical characteristic known as its gyromagnetic ratio. The spinning charge of each hydrogen nucleus gives off a tiny magnetic field perpendicular to the axis of spin, thus acting like a tiny bar magnet. Outside the bore of a magnet, the net magnetic properties (magnetic moment) of a person will be zero because the spinning hydrogen nuclei will be oriented randomly resulting in an overall cancellation of the sum total of tiny magnetic fields. Once placed into a high field strength magnet, spinning hydrogen nuclei within the human body become aligned or magnetized along the magnetic field of the magnet. This net magnetization of hydrogen nuclei is oriented in a low energy alignment (ground state) that is parallel to the magnetic field of the magnet. The hydrogen nuclei spin (precess) at a frequency proportional to their specific gyromagnetic ratio and the magnetic field, in a relationship known as the Larmor equation. The precessional frequency of hydrogen nuclei at 1.5 Tesla (T) is 64 MHz.

To generate an MR signal, energy is transferred to the hydrogen nuclei within the magnet by using a radio frequency (RF) pulse at the Larmor frequency. The Larmor frequency is dependent on the field strength of the magnetic device and the gyromagnetic ratio, which is specific for the element or molecule of interest. For MRI, that element is the hydrogen nucleus. The hydrogen nuclei absorb this energy and move out of their ground-state alignment. When the RF pulse is turned off, the energy absorbed by the hydrogen nuclei is emitted at the same frequency. This emitted energy, or MR signal, can be detected by the receiver coils (which act like antennae) in the magnet, and used to produce an MR image. Soft tissue contrast results from (1) the densities of protons (hydrogen nuclei) within different tissues; (2) the different rates at which the protons in various tissues realign themselves with the magnetic field of the magnet (also referred to as T1 relaxation, longitudinal relaxation, or spin-lattice relaxation); and (3) rates of signal decay or dephasing (also referred to as T2 relaxation, transverse relaxation, or spin-spin relaxation). Using these biophysical properties of different normal and abnormal tissues allows MRI to have greater soft tissue contrast than computed tomography (CT).

The main components of a typical MRI scanner include (1) a large-bore magnet with high field strength (0.3 to 3 T); (2) RF coils within the magnet that can transmit and receive properly tuned RF pulses, as well as set spatially dependent magnetic fields (gradients) that allow localization of specific regions of anatomical interest; and (3) a computer that operates the device as well as processes the RF signal data received from the patient to form an anatomical image. To generate an MR image, a person is placed onto a table that can move into specific locations within the bore of the magnet. Once in the magnet, the operator selects programs that include the RF pulse sequences necessary to generate images with the desired contrast parameters based on the proton densities and the T1 and T2 values of the various tissues. The data received from the subject or patient are processed by the computer using computer algorithms (two- or three-dimensional Fourier transformation). The images are displayed on the monitor console and can be transferred to other computers (Picture Archival Communications System [PACS]), as well as DVDs, CD-ROMS, and film.

Not all patients can have MRI examinations. Intracranial aneurysm clips not documented and verified to be safe for MRI, cardiac pacemakers, and metallic foreign bodies in the eyes are absolute contraindications for MRI. In addition, the presence of surgical clips, metallic rods, wires, and other orthopedic hardware can produce artifacts obscuring visualization of the anatomical structures in the region of interest.

Major advantages of MRI for musculoskeletal imaging include excellent soft tissue contrast resolution, multiplanar imaging capabilities, dynamic rapid data acquisition, and various available contrast agents. MRI has proven to be a powerful imaging modality for abnormalities involving fat, muscles, ligaments, tendons, nerves, bone, and bone marrow, and has been used in the evaluation of the following:

1. Congenital and developmental musculoskeletal anomalies
2. Disorders of histogenesis
3. Metabolic and genetic disorders
4. Infectious and noninfectious inflammatory diseases
5. Traumatic lesions
6. Degenerative abnormalities
7. Ischemia and infarction of muscles, fat, and bone marrow
8. Hemorrhage
9. Neoplasms of the bone, muscles, fat, and nerves
10. Tumor-like lesions of bone and soft tissue
11. Response of neoplasms to neoadjuvant (preoperative chemotherapy) and postoperative chemotherapy or radiation treatment
12. Residual or recurrent tumor after surgery

MR data can also be used to generate images of arteries and veins (MR angiography) in displays similar to those of conventional angiography. The appearance of blood vessels on MR images depends on various factors such as the type of MRI pulse sequence; pulsatility and range of velocities in the vessels of interest; and size, shape, and orientation of the vessels relative to the image plane. Useful anatomical information regarding blood vessels can be gained by using spin echo pulse sequences, which can display patent vessels as zones of signal void (black-blood images), or gradient recall echo (GRE) pulse sequences, which display the moving hydrogen atomic-nuclei (protons) in blood as zones of high signal (bright-blood images). Other options with clinical MRI scanners include magnetic resonance spectroscopy (acquisition of spectral data to characterize the biochemical properties of selected regions of interest in the soft tissues), diffusion-weighted imaging (evaluation of different rates of proton diffusion between normal and abnormal tissue), and perfusion imaging (evaluation of the differences in rates of contrast enhancement between normal and abnormal tissue).

The appearance of muscle, fascia, tendons, ligaments, and bone cortex and marrow depends on the MRI pulse sequence used as well as the age of the patient imaged. In addition to the commonly used standard spin echo or fast spin echo sequences for evaluation of the musculoskeletal system, other MRI pulse sequences or imaging options are sometimes used, such as inversion recovery (short TI inversion recovery [STIR] used for fat signal suppression, fluid-attenuated inversion recovery [FLAIR] used for fluid signal suppression, etc.), GRE imaging with or without MR angiography, magnetic transfer, diffusion/perfusion MRI, and frequency-selective chemical saturation. Detailed discussions of these sequences and options can be found elsewhere. Contrast-enhanced MRI using gadolinium-chelate agents administered intravenously often provides useful information in the evaluation of musculoskeletal lesions such as neoplasms, tumor-like lesions, inflammation, infection, and ischemia.[7,8,11–13,15–17,19–24,26] With these diseases and disorders, abnormal gadolinium-contrast enhancement is typically seen. For evaluation of musculoskeletal neoplasms, dynamic MRI after bolus intravenous administration of gadolinium-chelate contrast can sometimes be useful in distinguishing between rapidly enhancing tumor from initially nonenhancing perineoplastic edema or necrosis.[7]

Another use of these gadolinium-chelate contrast agents is MR arthrography. MR arthrography is performed after the intra-articular injection of gadolinium-chelate contrast using fluoroscopic or ultrasonographic guidance. MR arthrography has been used in the evaluation of abnormalities involving the shoulder, hip, knee, and wrist.[27–33] Newer MRI techniques, such as diffusion-weighted imaging and MR spectroscopy, have been used in clinical research studies for the evaluation of musculoskeletal neoplasms and other lesions, although their clinical relevance requires further study.[34–37]

Bone formation occurs by either endochondral or membranous ossification. Longitudinal growth occurs by endochondral bone formation in which a calcified cartilaginous matrix at the growth (physeal) plates is remodeled into bone.[16,38,41] The physeal plate contains four parallel zones oriented perpendicular to the long axis of bone.[16,38–41] The four zones from peripheral (nearest the epiphysis) to proximal (nearest the metaphysis) are (1) resting zone; (2) proliferating zone; (3) hypertrophic zone; and (4) calcifying zone. Active cartilage cell division and maturation occur in the proliferating and hypertrophic zones.[16,38,41] Osteoid matrix formation and mineralization occur in the calcifying zone (also referred to as the zone of provisional calcification). The resting, proliferating, and hypertrophic zones are radiolucent and on MRI have slightly high to high signal on T2-weighted imaging (T2WI) and fat-suppressed (FS) T2WI and show gadolinium-contrast enhancement; whereas the zone of provisional calcification has attenuation similar to mature mineralized bone on radiographs and CT, and has low signal on T2WI and FS T2WI.[16,38,39,41] At the adjacent metaphyseal region (primary spongiosa) just proximal to the calcifying zone, remodeling of bone occurs with osteoclastic activity, which appears as a thin zone with slightly high to high signal on FS T2WI.[41] With membranous bone formation, bone cells form directly from the periosteum (long bones, facial bones, clavicle) for axial growth, or dura (calvarium) without intervening growth plates.

The periosteum has low signal on T1WI and T2WI and is attached to the outer surface of the bone cortex in the metadiaphyseal regions by collagen fibers (fibers of Sharpey). The periosteum is composed of an outer fibrous layer and an inner cellular layer referred to as the cambrium.[25,41] The periosteum is absent at the articular ends of bones. Osteoblastic activity occurs in the cambrium and is responsible for increasing the diameter of bone during growth in childhood. The periosteum is loosely attached to the cortex in children, whereas it is firmly attached in adults. Reactivation of the periosteum in adults can occur as a result of trauma, infection, or tumors. Periosteal membranous bone formation occurs with induction of fibroblasts (in the fibrous layer or adjacent soft tissues) into osteogenic precursor cells that eventually develop into active osteogenic cells in the cambrium.[25,41] Hyperemia from fracture, infection, or tumor can accelerate new periosteal bone formation, which can be seen as a radiodense line superificial to the cortex on radiographs or CT.[11,25] Periosteal reaction can have variable configurations related to the disease process.[25] MRI can demonstrate periosteal elevation from diseases as well as subperiosteal abnormalities such as hemorrhage, pus, or tumor.[11,25]

Within the medullary portion of bone, MRI signal is related to the presence of hematopoietic (red) marrow that contains 40% fat, 40% water, and 20% protein, or hematopoietically inactive fatty (yellow) marrow containing 80% fat, 15% water, and 5% protein. Fatty marrow usually has signal similar to subcutaneous fat on T1WI and FS T2WI. Red marrow typically has intermediate signal on T1WI that is slightly lower than fat and has intermediate signal on FS T2WI that is often similar to muscle. In infants and young children, bone marrow is predominantly composed of red (hematopoietic) marrow.[10,16,39,41,42] In the normally developing child, progressive conversion of red to yellow marrow occurs in the hands and feet followed by the distal long bones.[10,16,39,41] In long bones, progressive red to yellow marrow conversion occurs in the diaphyseal regions during the first decade.[10,16,39,41] The marrow of ossified epiphyses and trochanters is typically fatty.[10,16,39,41]

In adults, red marrow is typically found in the spine, flat bones, skull, and proximal portions of the femora and humeri. MRI can demonstrate the process of red to yellow marrow because of the slightly differing signal characteristics on T1WI and FS T2WI. In adults over the age of 20 years, no appreciable gadolinium-contrast enhancement is seen in normal marrow. This situation differs from that with infants and young children.[38,39,41] Gadolinium-contrast enhancement can be normally seen in the physeal cartilage as well as involving the vascular canals of epiphyseal cartilage in infants and toddlers.[38–41] With progressive skeletal maturation and epiphyseal ossification, contrast enhancement of the epiphyseal cartilage decreases relative to physeal cartilage.[38,40,41] Slightly high to high signal on T2WI and FS T2WI, as well as contrast enhancement of the physeal cartilage, eventually evolve into a low signal physeal scar with no contrast enhancement at skeletal maturation.[38,41] In children, hematopoietic red marrow is richly vascularized and typically shows contrast enhancement.[39,41] Contrast enhancement of metaphyseal red marrow in children progressively decreases with age and is typically absent after the age of 20 years.[39,41] Contrast enhancement in epiphyseal marrow is typically lesser in degree compared with metaphyseal marrow and is not usually seen after the age of 2 years.[39]

Most pathological processes increase the T1 and T2 relaxation coefficients of the involved tissues resulting in decreased signal on T1WI and increased signal on T2WI relative to adjacent normal tissue. Such processes include ischemia, infarction, inflammation, infection, metabolic or toxic disorders, trauma, neoplasms, and radiation injury. Hemorrhage, however, can have variable appearances depending on the age of the hematoma, oxidation states of the iron in hemoglobin, hematocrit, protein concentration, clot formation and retraction, location, and size.[5] Oxyhemoglobin in a hyperacute blood clot has ferrous iron and is diamagnetic. Oxyhemoglobin does not significantly alter the T1 and T2 values of the tissue environment other than causing possible localized edema. After a few hours during the acute phase of the hematoma, the oxyhemoglobin loses its oxygen to form deoxyhemoglobin. Deoxyhemoglobin also has ferrous iron, although it has unpaired electrons and becomes paramagnetic. As a result, deoxyhemoglobin shortens the T2 value of the acute clot but does not significantly change the T1 value. On MRI, deoxyhemoglobin in the clot will have intermediate T1 signal and low signal on T2-weighted spin echo or gradient echo images. Later in the early subacute phase of the hematoma, deoyxhemoglobin becomes oxidized to the ferric state, methemoglobin, which is strongly paramagnetic. Methemoglobin shortens the T1 value of hydrogen nuclei resulting in high signal on T1WI. While the red blood cells in the clot are intact-intracellular methemoglobin, the T2 values will also be decreased resulting in low signal on T2WI. In the late subacute phase, breakdown of the membranes of the red blood cells results in extracellular methemoglobin, which now results in high signal on both T1WI and T2WI. In the chronic phase, methemoglobin becomes further oxidized and broken down by macrophages into hemosiderin, which has prominent low signal on T2WI and low-intermediate signal on T1WI.

Other processes that can result in zones of high signal on T1WI are fat, dermoids (intact or ruptured), teratomas, lipomas, cystic structures with high protein concentration or cholesterol, and pantopaque. Lesions or structures with low signal on T1WI and T2WI can result from calcifications, very high protein or gadolinium-chelate concentrations, magnetic susceptibility effects—especially from metal fragments or surgical clips, and artifacts.

The first portion of this book is focused on the differential diagnosis, description, and categorization of the MRI features of abnormalities involving the joints of the musculoskeletal system by grouping them into lists of differential diagnoses based on anatomical locations (shoulder, elbow, wrist and hand, hip, knee, and ankle and foot). This approach is similar to one of the coauthors' prior collaborations for the following books: *Differential Diagnosis in Magnetic Resonance Imaging* by Frances A. Burgener, Steven P. Meyers, Raymond K. Tan, and Wolfgang Zaubauer, Thieme, 2002; *MRI of Bone and Soft Tissue Tumors and Tumor-like Lesions: Differential Diagnosis and Atlas* by Steven P. Meyers, Thieme, 2008; and *Differential Diagnosis in Computed Tomography, 2nd edition,* by Frances A. Burgerner, Christopher Herzog, Steven P. Meyers, and Wolfgang Zaunbauer, Thieme, 2011. The other portion is focused on the differential diagnosis, description, and categorization of the MRI features of both benign and malignant bone and soft tissue tumors and tumor-like lesions of the musculoskeletal system using a similar tabular format.

For this book, MRI signal of the various entities will be described as low, intermediate, high, or mixed on T1WI, proton density-weighted imaging (PDWI), or intermediate weighted imaging, and T2WI, and whether there is gadolinium-contrast (Gd-contrast) enhancement or not. When available, comments and examples will be given regarding MRI features with fat-suppression techniques such as frequency-selective fat-presaturation (FS) applied on T1WI, PDWI, T2WI, or use of the STIR sequence. Both techniques enable distinction of pathological processes (e.g., neoplasm, infection, inflammation, edema) from normal anatomical structures with high signal from intrinsic fat, such as marrow and subcutaneous soft tissues.

1.1 References

[1] Aboulafia AJ, Monson DK, Kennon RE. Clinical and radiological aspects of idiopathic diabetic muscle infarction: rational approach to diagnosis and treatment. J Bone Joint Surg Br 1999; 81: 323–326

[2] Arndt CA, Crist WM. Common musculoskeletal tumors of childhood and adolescence. N Engl J Med 1999; 341: 342–352

[3] Berquist TH, Ehman RL, King BF, Hodgman CG, Ilstrup DM. Value of MR imaging in differentiating benign from malignant soft-tissue masses: study of 95 lesions. AJR Am J Roentgenol 1990; 155: 1251–1255

[4] Biondetti PR, Ehman RL. Soft-tissue sarcomas: use of textural patterns in skeletal muscle as a diagnostic feature in postoperative MR imaging. Radiology 1992; 183: 845–848

[5] Bush CH. The magnetic resonance imaging of musculoskeletal hemorrhage. Skeletal Radiol 2000; 29: 1–9

[6] Choi H, Varma DG, Fornage BD, Kim EE, Johnston DA. Soft-tissue sarcoma: MR imaging vs sonography for detection of local recurrence after surgery. AJR Am J Roentgenol 1991; 157: 353–358

[7] Dyke JP, Panicek DM, Healey JH, et al. Osteogenic and Ewing sarcomas: estimation of necrotic fraction during induction chemotherapy with dynamic contrast-enhanced MR imaging. Radiology 2003; 228: 271–278

[8] Ejindu VC, Hine AL, Mashayekhi M, Shorvon PJ, Misra RR. Musculoskeletal manifestations of sickle cell disease. Radiographics 2007; 27: 1005–1021

[9] Grigoriadis E, Fam AG, Starok M, Ang LC. Skeletal muscle infarction in diabetes mellitus. J Rheumatol 2000; 27: 1063–1068

[10] Hanrahan CJ, Shah LM. MRI of spinal bone marrow, II: T1-weighted imaging-based differential diagnosis. AJR Am J Roentgenol 2011; 197: 1309–1321

[11] Jaramillo D. Infection: musculoskeletal. Pediatr Radiol 2011; 41 Suppl 1: S127–S134

[12] Miller SL, Hoffer FA. Malignant and benign bone tumors. Radiol Clin North Am 2001; 39: 673–699

[13] Murphey MD, Smith WS, Smith SE, Kransdorf MJ, Temple HT. From the archives of the AFIP. Imaging of musculoskeletal neurogenic tumors: radiologic-pathologic correlation. Radiographics 1999; 19: 1253–1280

[14] Shuman WP, Patten RM, Baron RL, Liddell RM, Conrad EU, Richardson ML. Comparison of STIR and spin-echo MR imaging at 1.5 T in 45 suspected extremity tumors: lesion conspicuity and extent. Radiology 1991; 179: 247–252

[15] Stacy GS, Heck RK, Peabody TD, Dixon LB. Neoplastic and tumorlike lesions detected on MR imaging of the knee in patients with suspected internal derangement, I: Intraosseous entities. AJR Am J Roentgenol 2002; 178: 589–594

[16] States LJ. Imaging of metabolic bone disease and marrow disorders in children. Radiol Clin North Am 2001; 39: 749–772

[17] Turecki MB, Taljanovic MS, Stubbs AY, et al. Imaging of musculoskeletal soft tissue infections. Skeletal Radiol 2010; 39: 957–971

[18] Vade A, Eissenstadt R, Schaff HB. MRI of aggressive bone lesions of childhood. Magn Reson Imaging 1992; 10: 89–96

[19] van der Woude HJ, Bloem JL, Pope TL. Magnetic resonance imaging of the musculoskeletal system, IX: Primary tumors. Clin Orthop Relat Res 1998; 347: 272–286

[20] van der Woude HJ, Verstraete KL, Hogendoorn PC, Taminiau AHM, Hermans J, Bloem JL. Musculoskeletal tumors: does fast dynamic contrast-enhanced subtraction MR imaging contribute to the characterization? Radiology 1998; 208: 821–828

[21] van Rijswijk CSP, Geirnaerdt MJA, Hogendoorn PCW, et al. Soft-tissue tumors: value of static and dynamic gadopentetate dimeglumine-enhanced MR imaging in prediction of malignancy. Radiology 2004; 233: 493–502

[22] Vanel D, Shapeero LG, De Baere T, et al. MR imaging in the follow-up of malignant and aggressive soft-tissue tumors: results of 511 examinations. Radiology 1994; 190: 263–268

[23] Walker EA, Fenton ME, Salesky JS, Murphey MD. Magnetic resonance imaging of benign soft tissue neoplasms in adults. Radiol Clin North Am 2011; 49: 1197–1217, vi

[24] Walker EA, Salesky JS, Fenton ME, Murphey MD. Magnetic resonance imaging of malignant soft tissue neoplasms in the adult. Radiol Clin North Am 2011; 49: 1219–1234, vi

[25] Wenaden AET, Szyszko TA, Saifuddin A. Imaging of periosteal reactions associated with focal lesions of bone. Clin Radiol 2005; 60: 439–456

[26] Kattapuram TM, Suri R, Rosol MS, Rosenberg AE, Kattapuram SV. Idiopathic and diabetic skeletal muscle necrosis: evaluation by magnetic resonance imaging. Skeletal Radiol 2005; 34: 203–209

[27] Acid S, Le Corroller T, Aswad R, Pauly V, Champsaur P. Preoperative imaging of anterior shoulder instability: diagnostic effectiveness of MDCT arthrography and comparison with MR arthrography and arthroscopy. AJR Am J Roentgenol 2012; 198: 661–667

[28] Choo HJ, Lee SJ, Kim OH, Seo SS, Kim JH. Comparison of three-dimensional isotropic T1-weighted fast spin-echo MR arthrography with two-dimensional MR arthrography of the shoulder. Radiology 2012; 262: 921–93110.1148/radiol.11111261

[29] Ciliz D, Ciliz A, Elverici E, Sakman B, Yüksel E, Akbulut O. Evaluation of postoperative menisci with MR arthrography and routine conventional MRI. Clin Imaging 2008; 32: 212–219

[30] Jung JY, Jee WH, Park MY, Lee SY, Kim YS. Supraspinatus tendon tears at 3.0T shoulder MR arthrography: diagnosis with 3D isotropic turbo spin-echo SPACE sequence versus 2D conventional sequences. Skeletal Radiol 2012; 41: 1401–1410

[31] Magee T. Comparison of 3-T MRI and arthroscopy of intrinsic wrist ligament and TFCC tears. AJR Am J Roentgenol 2009; 192: 80–85

[32] Mathieu L, Bouchard A, Marchaland JP, et al. Knee MR-arthrography in assessment of meniscal and chondral lesions. Orthop Traumatol Surg Res 2009; 95: 40–47

[33] Schaeffeler C, Eiber M, Holzapfel K, Gollwitzer H, Rummeny EJ, Woertler K. The epiphyseal torsion angle in MR arthrography of the hip: diagnostic utility in patients with femoroacetabular impingement syndrome. AJR Am J Roentgenol 2012; 198: W237--W243

[34] Costa FM, Canella C, Gasparetto E. Advanced magnetic resonance imaging techniques in the evaluation of musculoskeletal tumors. Radiol Clin North Am 2011; 49: 1325–1358, vii–viii

[35] Fayad LM, Barker PB, Jacobs MA, et al. Characterization of musculoskeletal lesions on 3-T proton MR spectroscopy. AJR Am J Roentgenol 2007; 188: 1513–1520

[36] Sostman HD, Prescott DM, Dewhirst MW, et al. MR imaging and spectroscopy for prognostic evaluation in soft-tissue sarcomas. Radiology 1994; 190: 269–275

[37] Wang CK, Li CW, Hsieh TJ, Chien SH, Liu GC, Tsai KB. Characterization of bone and soft-tissue tumors with in vivo 1 H MR spectroscopy: initial results. Radiology 2004; 232: 599–605

[38] Barnewolt CE, Shapiro F, Jaramillo D. Normal gadolinium-enhanced MR images of the developing appendicular skeleton, I: Cartilaginous epiphysis and physis. AJR Am J Roentgenol 1997; 169: 183–189

[39] Dwek JR, Shapiro F, Laor T, Barnewolt CE, Jaramillo D. Normal gadolinium-enhanced MR images of the developing appendicular skeleton, II: Epiphyseal and metaphyseal marrow. AJR Am J Roentgenol 1997; 169: 191–196

[40] Jaramillo D, Villegas-Medina OL, Doty DK, et al. Age-related vascular changes in the epiphysis, physis, and metaphysis: normal findings on gadolinium-enhanced MRI of piglets. AJR Am J Roentgenol 2004; 182: 353–360

[41] Laor T, Jaramillo D. MR imaging insights into skeletal maturation: what is normal? Radiology 2009; 250: 28–38

[42] Zawin JK, Jaramillo D. Conversion of bone marrow in the humerus, sternum, and clavicle: changes with age on MR images. Radiology 1993; 188: 159–164

Chapter 2

The Shoulder

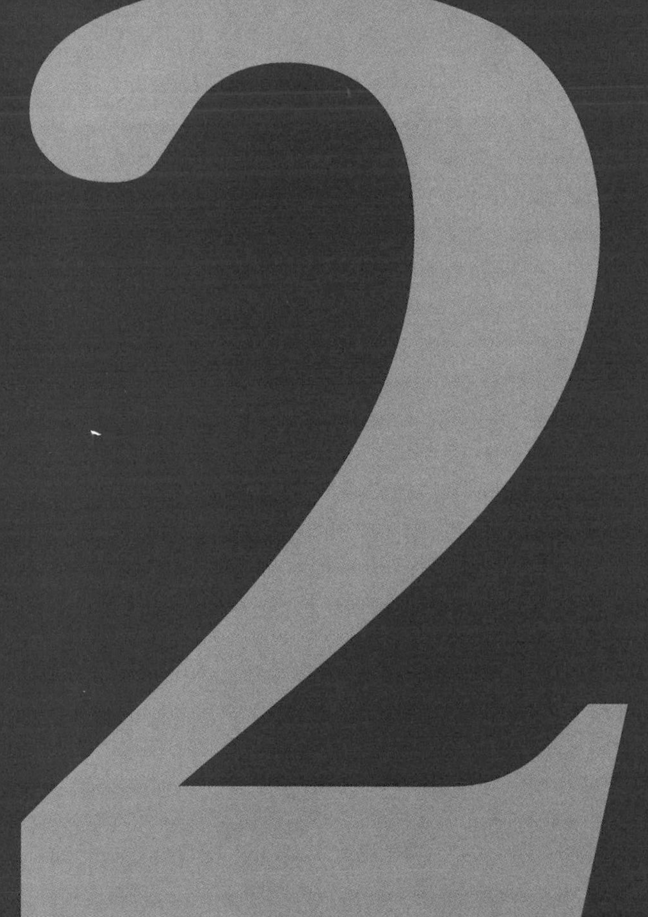

2 The Shoulder

Gary M. Hollenberg

2.1 Lesions of the Rotator Cuff

- Tendinopathy/tendinosis
- Partial-thickness tendon tears
- Full-thickness tendon tears
- Subscapularis tears
- Calcific tendonitis/bursitis: calcium hydroxyapatite deposition disease (HADD)
- Adhesive capsulitis
- Pectoralis muscle tears/strain

Table 2.1 Lesions of the rotator cuff

Abnormalities	MRI findings	Comments
Tendinopathy/ tendinosis (▶ Fig. 2.1)	Thickening and abnormal intermediate signal within the tendon substance on proton density–weighted imaging (PDWI) or T1-weighted imaging (T1WI) is typical for tendinosis. Abnormal tendons demonstrate heterogeneous signal, irregularity, thickening, and abnormal morphology. Fat-suppressed T2-weighted imaging (FS T2WI) and short TI inversion recovery (STIR) images are abnormal as well with heterogeneous increased signal, not, however, reaching fluid signal. May also see distal thinning of atrophic tendons. Tendinopathy can be distinguished from an articular side rotator cuff tear by the lack of a contrast-filled defect on magnetic resonance (MR) arthrography, using FS T1-weighted imaging (T1WI).	Tendinopathy reflects collagen degeneration, typically involving the supraspinatus, infraspinatus, and subscapularis tendons. Causes include impingement syndrome or degeneration secondary to overuse. Tendinopathy and partial tears are often seen together and may be difficult to distinguish. Typically involves anterior margin of supraspinatus with thickening, heterogeneity and increased signal on most pulse sequences. Signal changes of tendinopathy persist on FS T2WI. Signal abnormalities in magic angle phenomenon are not associated with morphological changes of the tendon. Check for associated findings, including subacromial/subdeltoid fluid/bursitis, acromioclavicular degeneration and acromial spurs.

(continued on page 10)

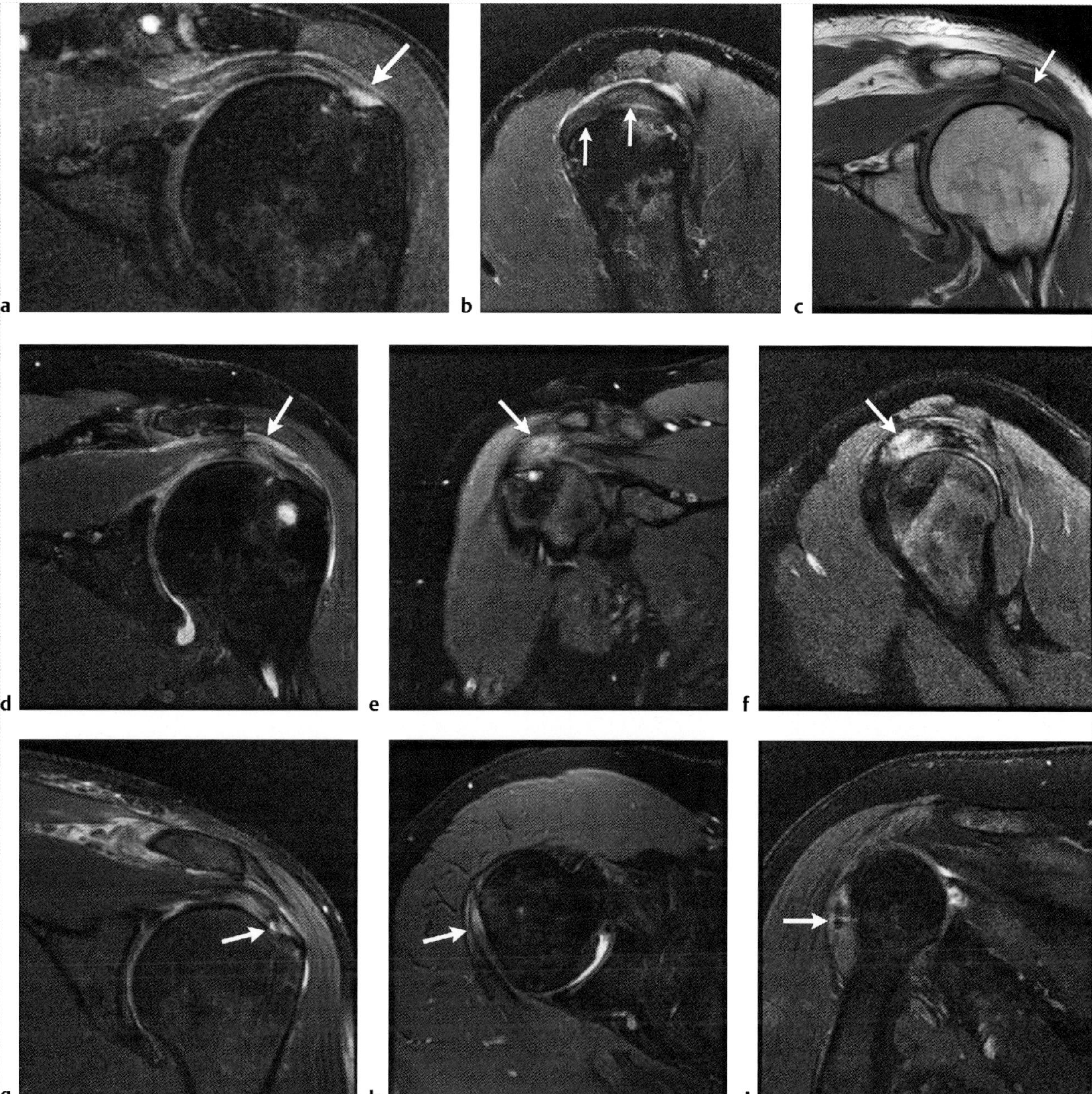

Fig. 2.1 (a) Tendinopathy is seen with mildly increased T2 signal of the distal supraspinatus tendon (arrow) on oblique coronal fat-suppressed T2-weighted imaging (FS T2WI), and (b) similarly abnormal signal involving the distal supraspinatus and infraspinatus tendons (arrows) on oblique sagittal FS T2WI. Note crescent of high signal fluid in the subdeltoid bursa. (c) In a different patient, more severe tendinopathy of the distal supraspinatus and infraspinatus tendons with loss of normal tendon architecture and abnormally increased signal (arrow) on oblique coronal proton density–weighted imaging (PDWI). (d) Abnormally increased signal in the distal tendons (arrow) is also seen on oblique coronal FS T2WI. The abnormal signal does not reach that of fluid, indicating that tendinopathy, rather than tearing, is the predominant abnormality. (e) In a different patient, severe distal supraspinatus tendinopathy of the anterior tendon margin (arrows) on oblique coronal FS T2WI and (f) oblique sagittal FS T2WI with increased signal, tendon thickening, and loss of normal tendon architecture. (g) In a different patient, supraspinatus tendinopathy with a superimposed distal articular-sided partial tear (arrow) on oblique coronal FS T2WI. (h) Mild tendinopathy of the teres minor, with abnormally increased signal about the musculotendinous junction (arrows) on axial FS T2WI and (i) on oblique coronal FS T2WI. It is unusual to encounter teres minor tendinopathy on routine shoulder magnetic resonance scans.

Table 2.1 (Cont.) Lesions of the rotator cuff

Abnormalities	MRI findings	Comments
Partial-thickness tendon tears (▶ Fig. 2.2)	Partial tears may be articular sided, bursal sided, or interstitial in location. Interstitial tears will not communicate with the joint or subacromial bursa. Assess for abnormal tendon shape, including a thickened or thinned tendon and irregular tendon morphology. A spectrum of abnormalities from tendon fraying to tendon retraction may be seen. Partial tears and tendinopathy may appear similar, particularly when small partial tears are present. Partial tears demonstrate abnormal intermediate signal on T1WI and PDWI. On FS T2WI and STIR images a partial tear demonstrates high signal in the tear site representing either fluid or granulation tissue. Assess for fluid within the torn or frayed portion of the tendon on fluid-sensitive sequences. Partial tears show gadolinium (Gd)-contrast enhancement if granulation tissue has developed at the tear site. MR arthrography may show high signal contrast within an articular-sided tear on FS T1WI.	Rim-rent tears are believed to be the most common partial-thickness tendon tear. A rim-rent tear is an insertional tear at the greater tuberosity, typically articular, involving either the supraspinatus anteriorly or the infraspinatus more posteriorly. Tendons are prone to tearing at this location due to the 90-degree curvature of the tendon as it inserts on the greater tuberosity. Cuff tears, while multifactorial, are typically associated with subacromial impingement–decreased size of the coracoacromial arch, or wear and tear/overuse followed by tendon degeneration and tearing. Various theories are proposed regarding the etiology of cuff tears. In addition to subacromial impingement proposed by Neer, other theories exist. Codman developed the concept of the "critical zone" involving the distal portion of the tendon as the location for tendon degeneration. Look for associated labral tears and intratendinous cysts. The clinical differential diagnosis for partial tears includes full-thickness tear, calcific tendonitis, and adhesive capsulitis. Early treatment of rotator cuff tears may prevent progression.

(continued on page 12)

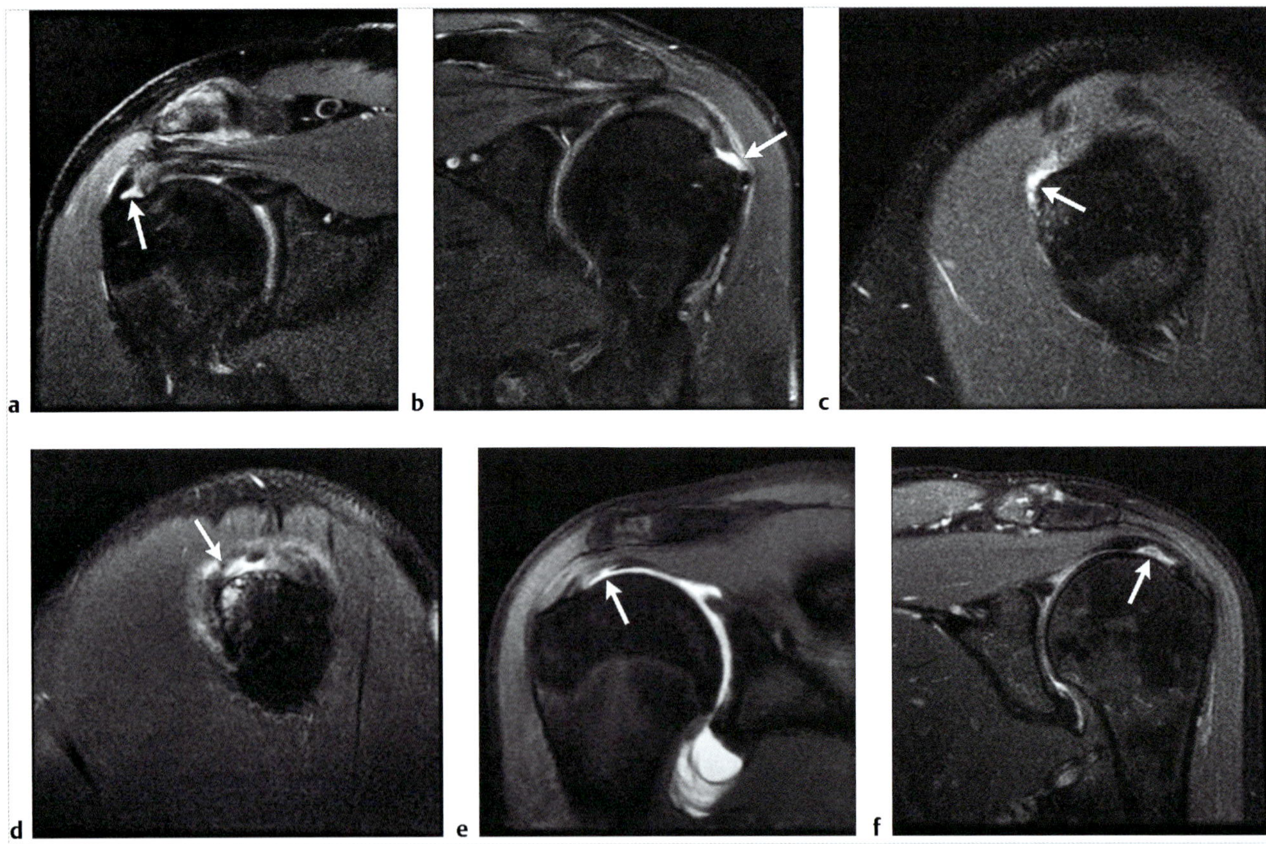

Fig. 2.2 (a) Note abnormally increased T2 signal of a partial-thickness, articular-sided "rim–rent" tear of the supraspinatus tendon (arrow). Superimposed tendinopathy is seen more proximally on oblique coronal fat-suppressed T2-weighted imaging (FS T2WI). (b) In a different patient note a thin preserved rim of overlying supraspinatus tendon (arrow) on oblique coronal FS T2WI. (c) In a different patient, note a high signal rim–rent tear (arrow) at the anterior margin of the supraspinatus tendon on oblique sagittal FS T2WI. (d) Example in a different patient of a larger rim–rent tear (arrow) with associated humeral head geodes and reactive marrow edema on oblique sagittal FS T2WI. (e) In a different patient, note contrast extending into a focal articular surface tear of the more proximal infraspinatus tendon (arrow) on oblique coronal FS T1 arthrogram. (f) A larger articular-sided tear of the more proximal supraspinatus tendon in a different patient (arrow) on oblique coronal FS T2WI. (*continued*)

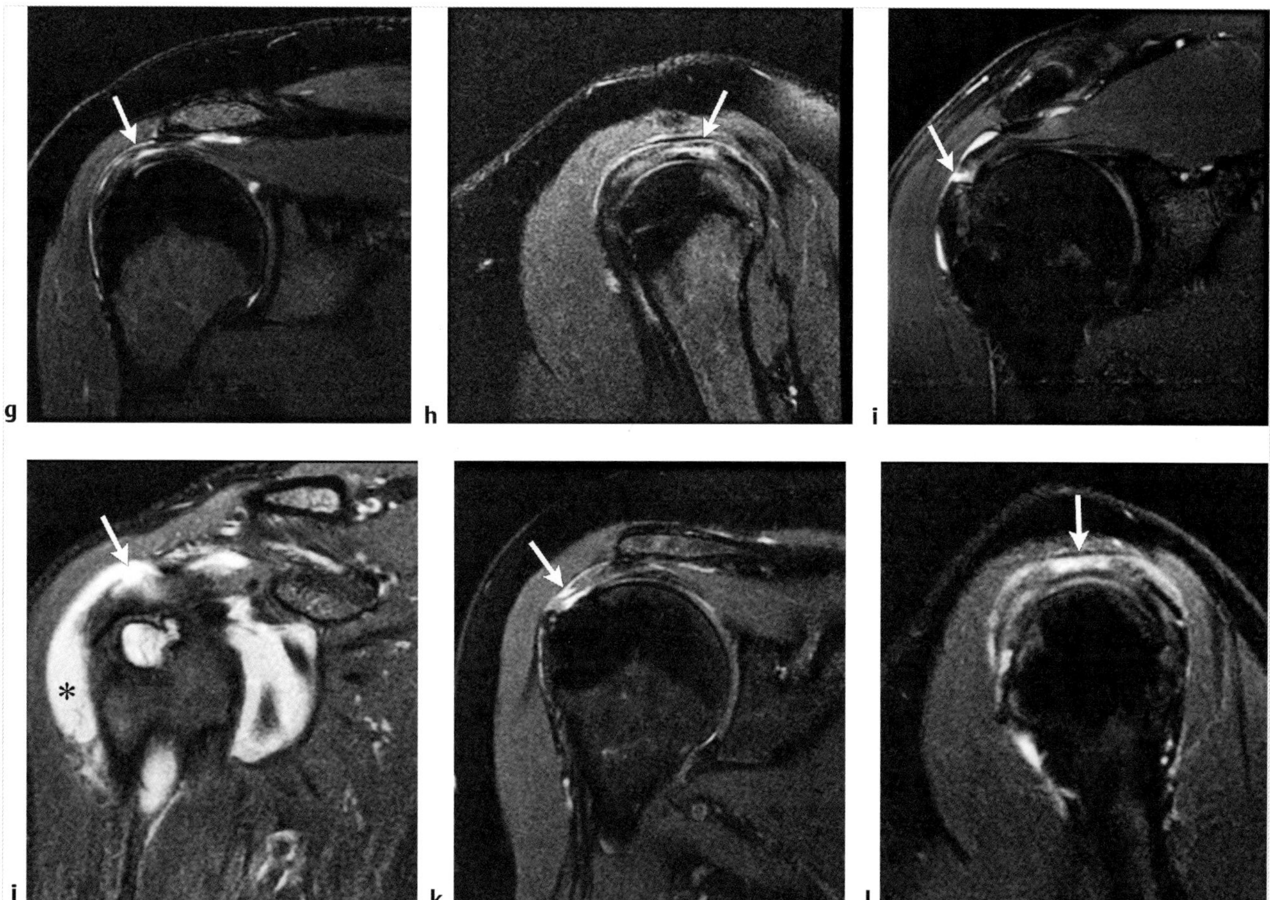

Fig. 2.2 (*continued*) (g) Interstitial tear within the substance of the more proximal supraspinatus tendon (arrows) on oblique coronal FS T2WI and (h) on corresponding oblique sagittal FS T2WI. (i) Bursal-sided large partial cuff tear (arrow) on oblique coronal FS T2WI. Note fluid in the subacromial/subdeltoid bursa, due to bursitis. (j) Severe bursal-sided cuff tear (arrow) with a large amount of fluid in the subacromial/subdeltoid bursa (asterisk) on oblique coronal FS T2WI. (k) Note bursal and articular-sided tears (arrow) with a thin remaining tendon on oblique coronal FS T2WI. (l) Irregular bursal-sided tear (arrow) on oblique sagittal FS T2WI.

Table 2.1 (Cont.) Lesions of the rotator cuff

Abnormalities	MRI findings	Comments
Full-thickness tendon tears (▶ Fig. 2.3)	A full-thickness tendon tear, involving the supraspinatus tendon for example, is defined as a defect in the tendon resulting in communication between the glenohumeral joint and subacromial subdeltoid bursa. On PDWI, look for an indistinct tendon with thickened or discontinuous tendon ends. On FS T2WI and other fluid-sensitive sequences, the key finding is fluid signal at the tear site. Fluid may extend along the tear continuously from the bursa to the articular region. With a tendon gap or retracted tendon, fluid may outline the torn tendon ends. Full-thickness tears are best seen on oblique sagittal and oblique coronal FS T2WI. On axial images look for a fluid-filled zone replacing the tendon on fluid-sensitive sequences. In some cases full-thickness tears may not demonstrate intervening fluid signal due to the development of scar or granulation tissue at the tear site. MR arthrography improves visualization of tears. Gd-contrast may also be identified in the subacromial/subdeltoid bursa on MR arthrography using FS T1WI, confirming the diagnosis of a full-thickness tear.	Causes of full-thickness tears include acute trauma, overuse with underlying tendinopathy, and as a sequela of impingement. Full-thickness tears are better seen with MRI than partial-thickness tears. Findings suggestive of full-thickness tendon tears include fluid in the subacromial/subdeltoid bursa or peribursal fat replaced by granulation tissue. Check for fatty replacement/atrophy of the involved muscles in chronic tears. Assess for the degree of retraction and involvement of the supraspinatus and/or infraspinatus tendons. Tears may range from a full-thickness tendon perforation to a complete tendon tear with retraction. Isolated infraspinatus tendon tears are unusual. Massive tears of the cuff usually involve full-thickness supraspinatus and infraspinatus tears with retraction and a high-riding humeral head. Look for associated glenohumeral degeneration, geodes of the humeral head, and a concave articular surface to the acromion in massive cuff tears. Assess biceps and subscapularis tendons in the setting of cuff tears. The teres minor tendon is rarely torn.

(continued on page 14)

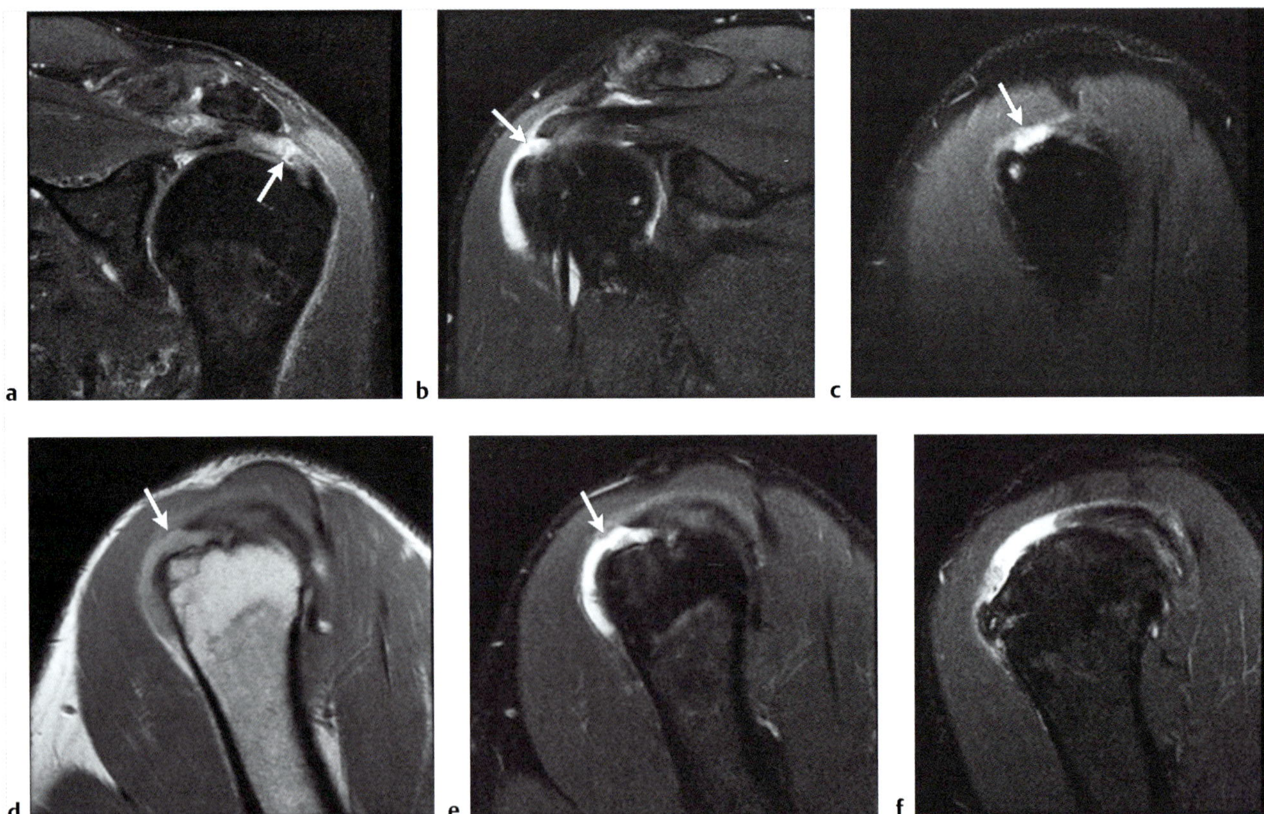

Fig. 2.3 Examples of progressively larger full-thickness tears of the distal supraspinatus tendon. (a) Focal linear tear (arrow) on oblique coronal fat-suppressed T2-weighted imaging (FS T2WI). (b) Tear with a small gap (arrow) on oblique coronal FS T2WI and (c) on oblique sagittal FS T2WI. (d) Anterior margin supraspinatus tear (arrow) with infraspinatus tendinopathy noted more posteriorly on oblique sagittal proton density–weighted imaging (PDWI) and (e) on corresponding oblique sagittal FS T2WI. (f) Larger tendon tear retracted beyond the field of view on oblique sagittal FS T2WI and (*continued*)

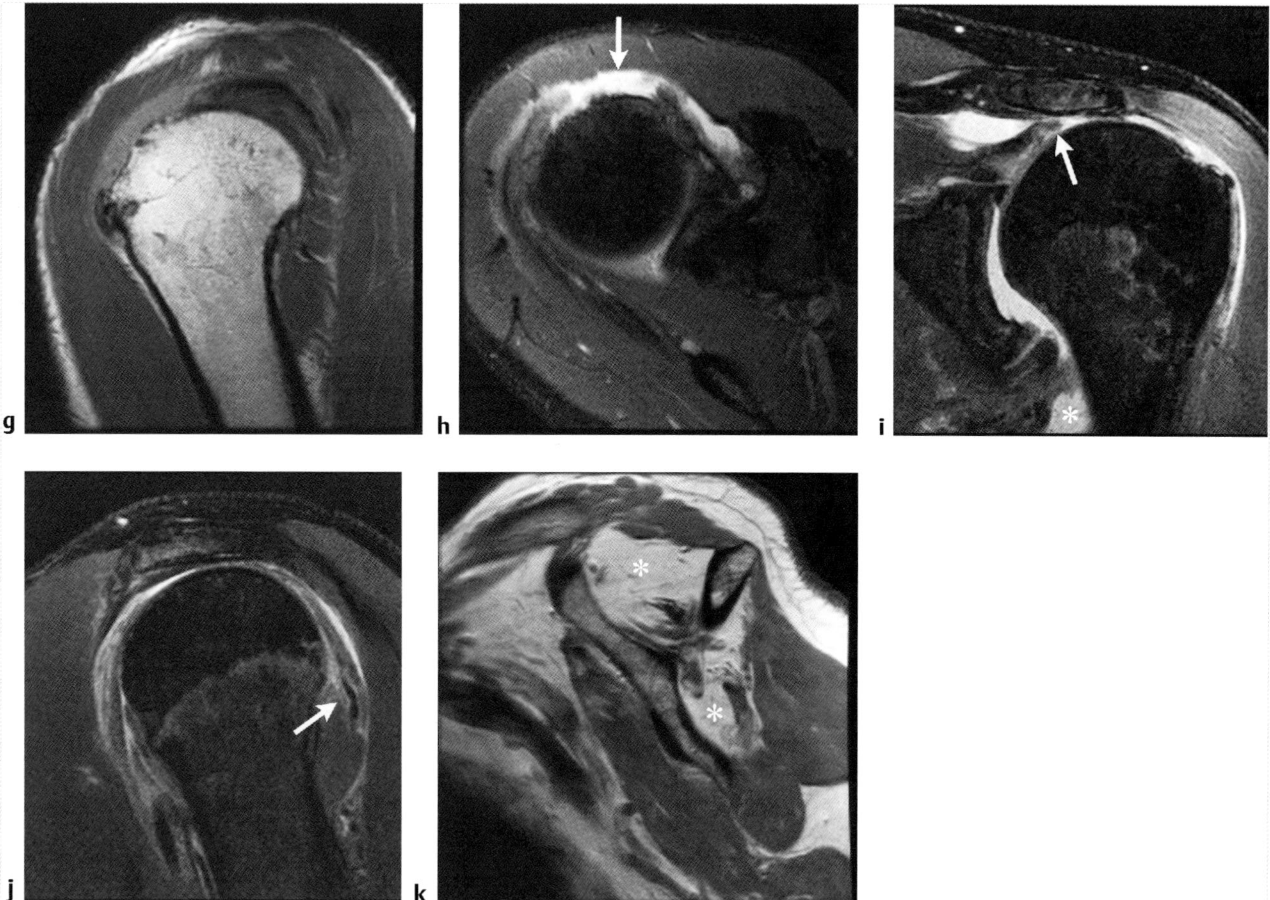

Fig. 2.3 (*continued*) (g) on oblique sagittal PDWI. (h) Corresponding tear site is seen anteriorly (arrow) on axial FS T2WI. (i) High-riding humeral head due to massive cuff tear with the retracted torn supraspinatus tendon (arrow) seen on oblique coronal FS T2WI. Fluid is seen dissecting inferior to the axillary pouch (asterisk) representing a tear of the axillary pouch/inferior glenohumeral ligament. (j) In the same patient there is superimposed teres minor tendinopathy/muscle sprain (arrow) seen on oblique sagittal FS T2WI. (k) Sequela of long-standing rotator cuff tear. Chronic muscle atrophy with fatty replacement (asterisks) of the torn supraspinatus and infraspinatus (torn ends not shown) on oblique sagittal PDWI.

Table 2.1 (Cont.) Lesions of the rotator cuff

Abnormalities	MRI findings	Comments
Subscapularis tears (▶ Fig. 2.4)	The subscapularis tendon attaches normally to the lesser tuberosity. The adjacent transverse humeral ligament crosses the lesser tuberosity maintaining the biceps tendon in the bicipital groove. Subscapularis tears are best seen on axial and sagittal images. Check for tearing or irregularity of the subscapularis tendon as it approaches the lesser tuberosity. T1WI and PDWI will show abnormal tendon thinning or thickening or morphological change of the tendon. On axial T2WI look for fluid in a tendon gap or discontinuity seen with a complete tear. Tendinopathy and small tears may initially be seen in the more superior portion of the tendon.	A spectrum of subscapularis abnormalities from mild tendinopathy to complete tendon tears with retraction can be seen. Typically these abnormalities are seen in patients over age 40. Subscapularis tears are usually partial-thickness articular-surface tears, involve the superior fibers, and are associated with biceps tendon abnormalities and supraspinatus tendon tears. They may be associated with massive cuff tears. Causes of subscapularis tendon abnormalities include anterior dislocation, subcoracoid impingement, or prior tendon degeneration. Medial subluxation or dislocation of the biceps tendon is often seen with subscapularis tears. If posterior shoulder dislocation has occurred, check for subscapularis tendon tears and lesser tuberosity avulsion fracture. Subcoracoid impingement has been suggested as a cause for subscapularis tears but is controversial. The "roller-wringer" phenomenon has been suggested as a cause–whereby the tendon is put under increased tension as it passes between the lesser tuberosity and coracoid process, resulting in articular-surface tears.

(continued on page 16)

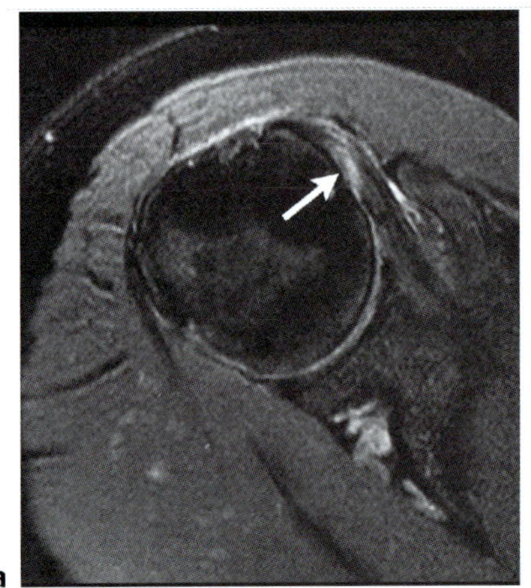
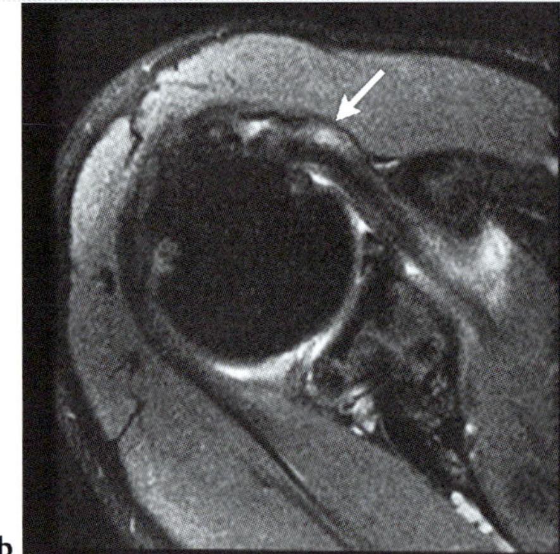
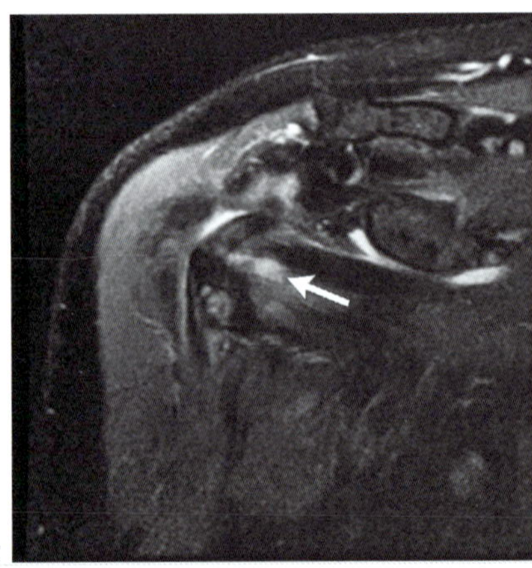
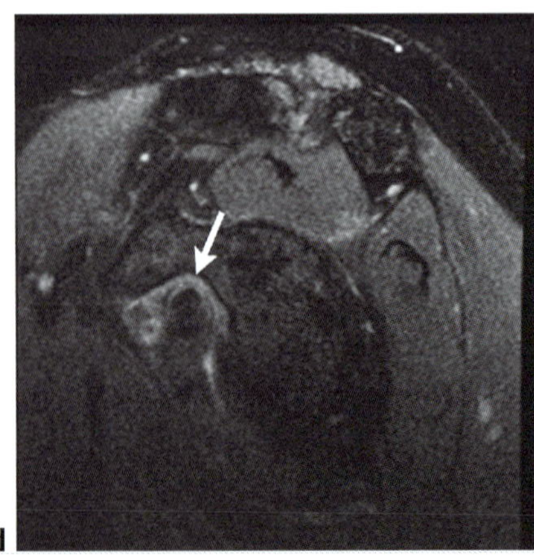

Fig. 2.4 (a) Mild tendinopathy of the distal subscapularis tendon with abnormal increased signal of the distal tendon worse along the articular side (arrow) on axial fat-suppressed T2-weighted imaging (FS T2WI). (b) Examples of tendinopathy (arrow) along the bursal side of the tendon on axial FS T2WI and (c) on oblique coronal FS T2WI (arrow). (d) Note abnormal signal of tendinopathy often seen in the superior portion of the tendon (arrow) on sagittal FS T2WI. *(continued)*

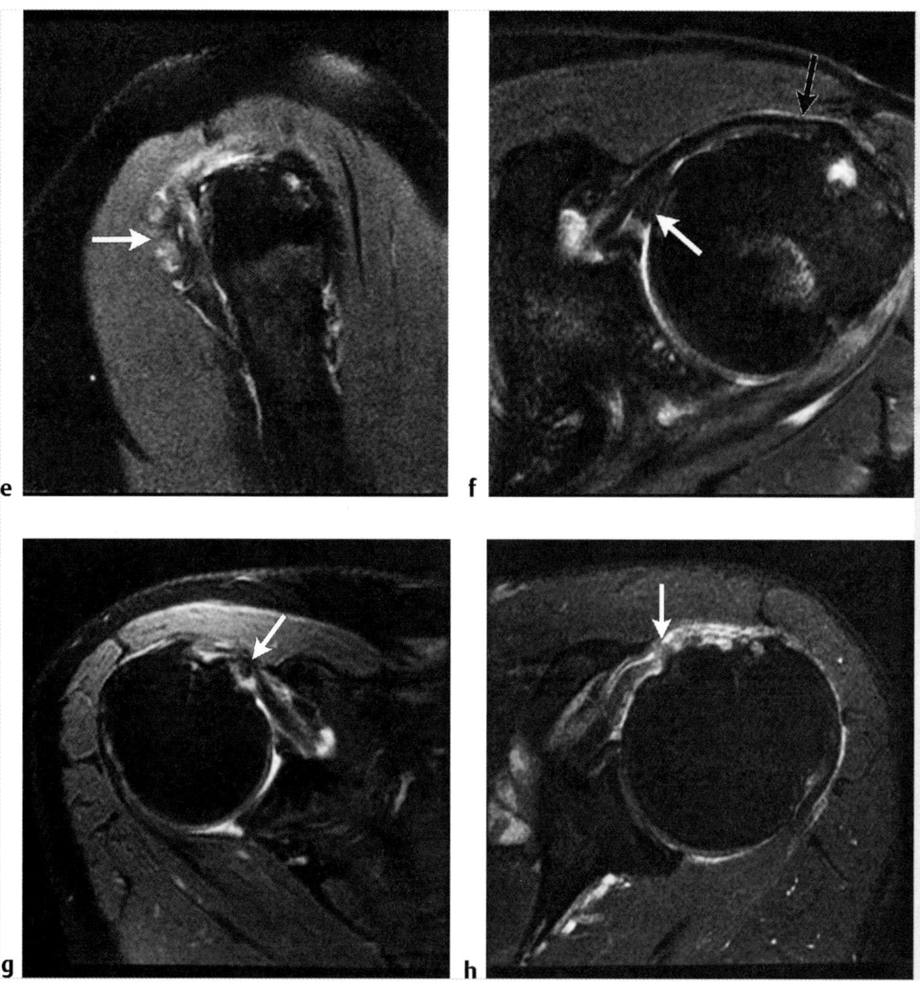

Fig. 2.4 (*continued*) (e) Note abnormal signal of tendinopathy often seen in the superior portion of the tendon (arrow) on sagittal FS T2WI. (f) Thinned, partly torn subscapularis tendon (black arrow) with medial subluxation of the biceps tendon (white arrow) on axial FS T2WI. (g) Thinned and partly torn subscapularis tendon with medial subluxation of the biceps tendon abutting the torn undersurface of the tendon (arrow) on axial FS T2WI. Debris is seen within the bicipital groove. (h) Different patient with a complete subscapularis tendon tear with wavy fibers (arrow) retracted from the lesser tuberosity on axial FS T2WI.

Table 2.1 (Cont.) Lesions of the rotator cuff

Abnormalities	MRI findings	Comments
Calcific tendonitis/ bursitis: calcium hydroxyapatite deposition disease (HADD) (▸ Fig. 2.5)	Focal low signal zones on gradient recall echo (GRE), T1WI, and T2WI. However, if calcium hydroxyapatite is in a thick liquid form, it may be of increased signal on FS PDWI. Deposits are often of lower signal than normal tendon, and interrupt the normal fibrillar architecture of the tendon. Surrounding Gd-contrast enhancement reflects inflammation. This condition spares the articular cartilage. Correlate for homogeneous focal to diffuse calcific deposits on radiographs. May be associated with rotator cuff partial tears.	Most commonly involved tendons: supraspinatus > infraspinatus > teres minor > subscapularis. Patients 30 to 50 years of age, either asymptomatic or with symptoms similar to impingement. Differential includes degenerative calcifications within a torn tendon, which are usually smaller and seen in older patients. Loose bodies are usually not identified within a tendon, whereas HADD is usually located within the tendon substance. Assess for loose body donor site or associated osteoarthritis. Also consider synovial osteochondromatosis (multiple loose chondral or osseous articular bodies) in the differential diagnosis.
Adhesive capsulitis (▸ Fig. 2.6)	Thickening (> 3 to 4 mm), of the inferior joint capsule (the axillary pouch) formed by the inferior glenohumeral ligaments seen on coronal PDWI or T2WI. Check for associated edema of the axillary pouch on fluid-sensitive sequences in more acute cases. On oblique sagittal images look for replacement of normal fat in the rotator interval by inflammatory or scar tissue that may also surround the superior and middle glenohumeral ligaments.	Also known as frozen shoulder, adhesive capsulitis is a disorder of painful decreased range of motion at the shoulder joint. There may be a history of trauma/surgery, or this condition may occur with unknown etiology. Impingement may present in a similar pattern. Increased capsular signal and synovial proliferation in the axillary pouch on FS T2WI is seen with more active cases of adhesive capsulitis, whereas the lack of T2 hyperintensity is consistent with scarring.

(continued on page 18)

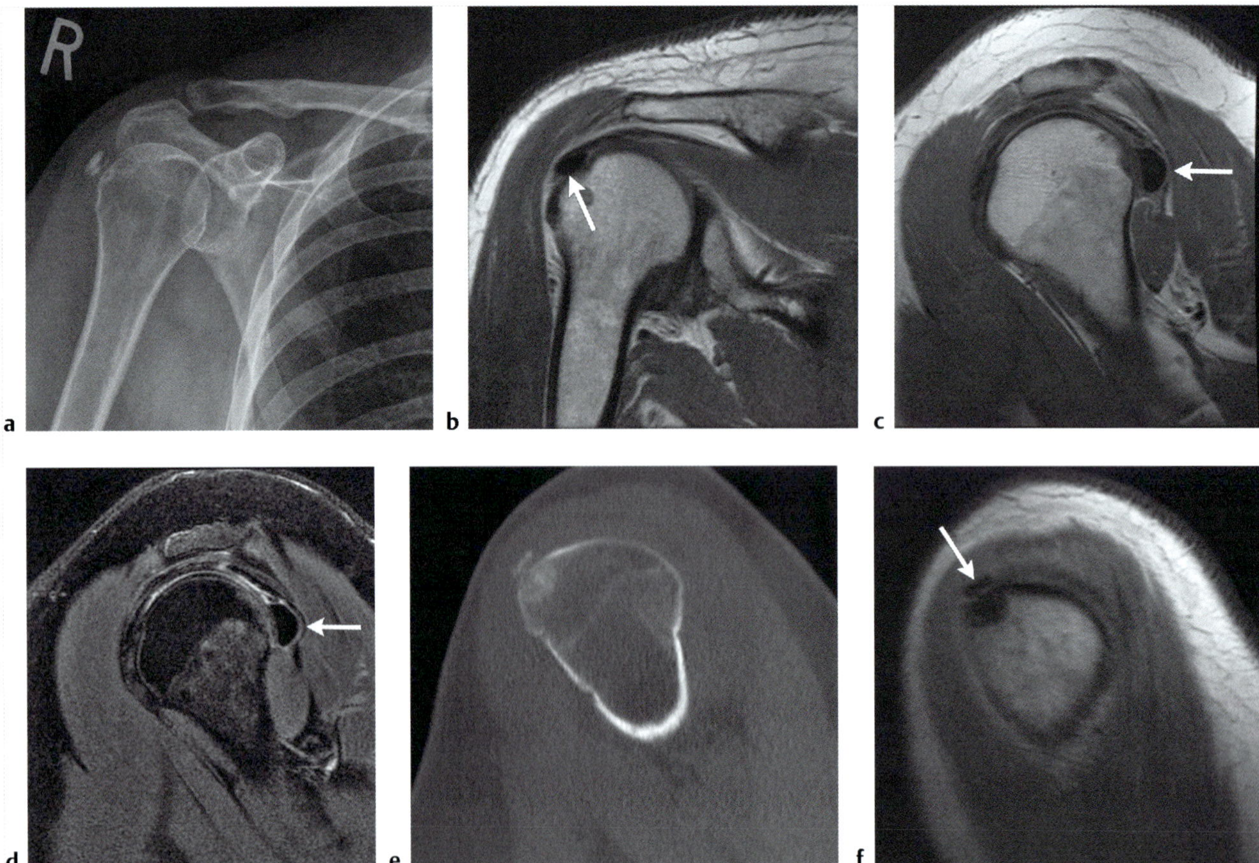

Fig. 2.5 (a) Calcific tendonitis with hydroxyapatite crystal deposition in the distal rotator cuff on anteroposterior radiograph. (b) Deposits are of lower signal than the tendon (arrow) on oblique coronal proton density–weighted imaging (PDWI). (c) Larger low signal focus of calcific tendonitis (arrow) in a different patient involving the infraspinatus tendon on oblique sagittal PDWI (arrow) and (d) on oblique sagittal fat-suppressed T2-weighted imaging (FS T2WI) (arrow). (e) Intraosseus calcific tendonitis with calcification in the distal supraspinatus tendon and intraosseus extension through a small cortical defect in the humeral head on sagittal computed tomographic image. (f) Note corresponding low signal (arrow) on oblique sagittal PDWI.

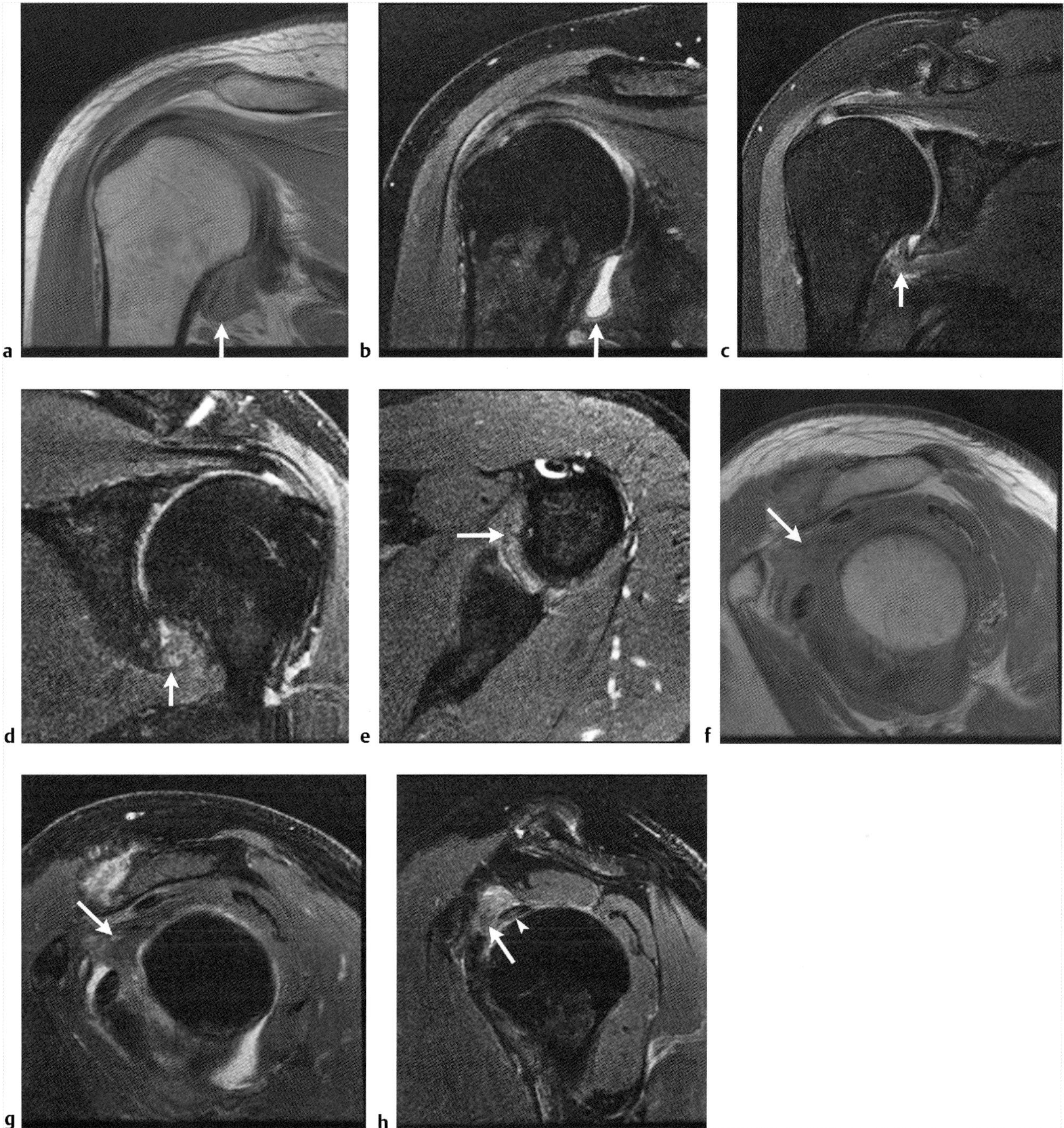

Fig. 2.6 (a) Thickened axillary pouch (arrows) in chronic adhesive capsulitis with low signal on both oblique coronal proton density–weighted imaging (PDWI) and (b) oblique coronal fat-suppressed T2-weighted imaging (FS T2WI). (c,d) Examples of acute adhesive capsulitis with increased signal and thickening of the axillary pouch, on oblique coronal FS T2WI and (e) thickening of the inferior capsule on axial FS T2WI. (f) Associated finding of obliteration of fat and replacement with soft tissue signal material in the subcoracoid region/rotator interval on oblique sagittal PDWI and (g) on oblique sagittal FS T2WI. In a different patient (h), note increased signal synovitis (arrow) along the superior margin of the subscapularis tendon abutting the proximal biceps tendon (arrowhead) on sagittal FS T2WI.

Table 2.1 (Cont.) Lesions of the rotator cuff

Abnormalities	MRI findings	Comments
Pectoralis muscle tears/strain (► Fig. 2.7)	Key finding of muscle edema/hemorrhage seen on fluid-sensitive sequences along the humeral insertion of the pectoralis major. Also assess the chest wall for muscle edema/hemorrhage. T1WI and PDWI may show hematoma or loss of muscle architecture indicating injury. Consider including the patient's contralateral side to help identify the normal-appearing distal tendon.	Most pectoralis muscle tears are partial tears and involve the musculotendinous junction or the tendon insertion distally at the lateral margin of the bicipital groove along the humeral shaft. Note that the tendon arises from both a sternal head and a clavicular head. Injury is typically seen in weightlifters performing benchpresses.

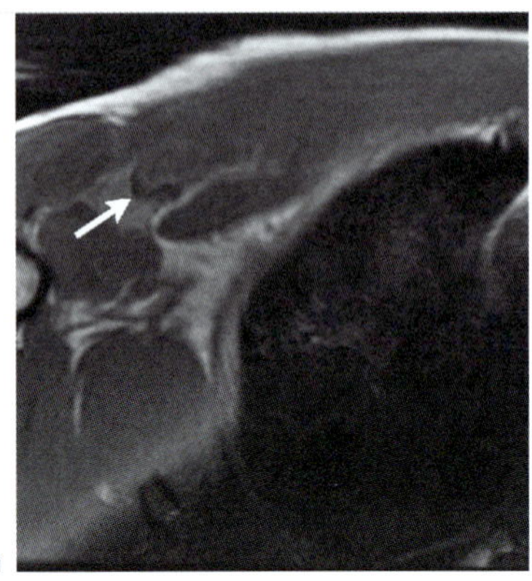
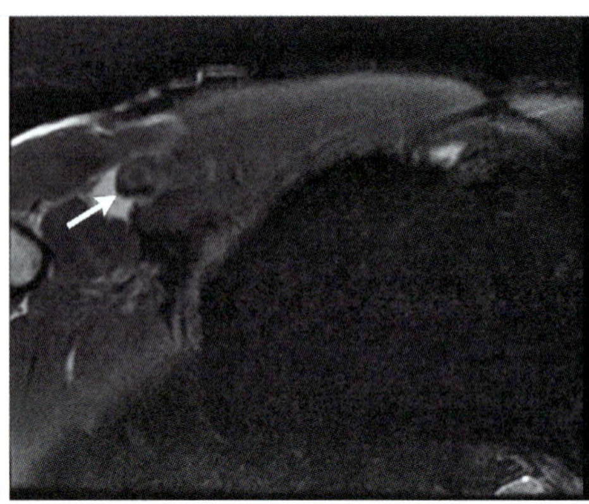
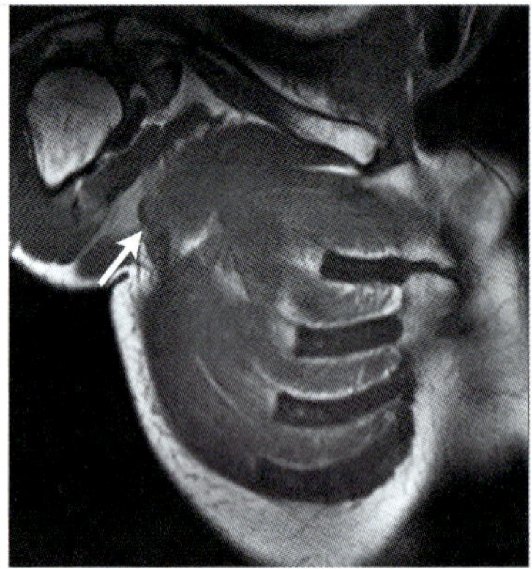

Fig. 2.7 (a) Torn and retracted low signal tendon of the pectoralis major muscle. Note irregular wavy fibers of the retracted tendon (arrow) on axial proton density–weighted imaging (PDWI). (b) The retracted tendon is of low signal (arrow) with surrounding edema/hemorrhage on axial fat-suppressed T2-weighted imaging. (c) Coronal PDWI demonstrates the degree of tendon retraction (arrow).

2.1.1 Lesions of the Rotator Cuff Suggested Reading

[1] Chundru U, Riley GM, Steinbach LS. Magnetic resonance arthrography. Radiol Clin North Am 2009; 47: 471–494

[2] Flemming DJ, Murphey MD, Shekitka KM, Temple HT, Jelinek JJ, Kransdorf MJ. Osseous involvement in calcific tendinitis: a retrospective review of 50 cases. AJR Am J Roentgenol 2003; 181: 965–972

[3] Mohana-Borges AV, Chung CB, Resnick D. MR imaging and MR arthrography of the postoperative shoulder: spectrum of normal and abnormal findings. Radiographics 2004; 24: 69–85

[4] Morag Y, Jacobson JA, Miller B, De Maeseneer M, Girish G, Jamadar D. MR imaging of rotator cuff injury: what the clinician needs to know. Radiographics 2006; 26: 1045–1065

[5] Morag Y, Jamadar DA, Miller B, Dong Q, Jacobson JA. The subscapularis: anatomy, injury, and imaging. Skeletal Radiol 2011; 40: 255–269

2.2 Lesions Associated with Impingement

- Subacromial bone spur
- Acromioclavicular (AC) joint degeneration
- Other suggested osseous contributors to subacromial impingement: acromial shape, slope, orientation, and os acromiale
- Internal/posterosuperior glenoid impingement

Table 2.2 Lesions associated with impingement

Abnormalities	MRI findings	Comments
Subacromial bone spur (▶ Fig. 2.8)	While small subacromial spurs are commonly seen in older patients, spurs equal to or greater than 5 mm have been associated with supraspinatus tendon tears. Spurs are seen along the anterior margin of the acromion on oblique sagittal proton density–weighted imaging (PDWI) or fat-suppressed T2-weighted imaging (FS T2WI). When looking for a subacromial spur, do not confuse a normal deltoid insertion on the acromion with a true subacromial spur that usually contains abnormal marrow signal on FS T2WI.	Subacromial impingement was originally described by Neer in 1972. Several entities result in a decreased space beneath the coracoacromial arch causing impingement and subsequent supraspinatus tendon degeneration and tears. Impingement syndrome is a clinical diagnosis believed to result from compression of the supraspinatus and biceps tendons and subacromial bursa. This results in clinical symptoms of shoulder pain, particularly with abduction and external rotation or elevation and internal rotation. Decrease in the subacromial space to less than 7 mm places the patient at risk for subacromial impingement. Controversy exists as to whether tears are due to intrinsic tendinopathy/degeneration or mechanical impingement.

(continued on page 22)

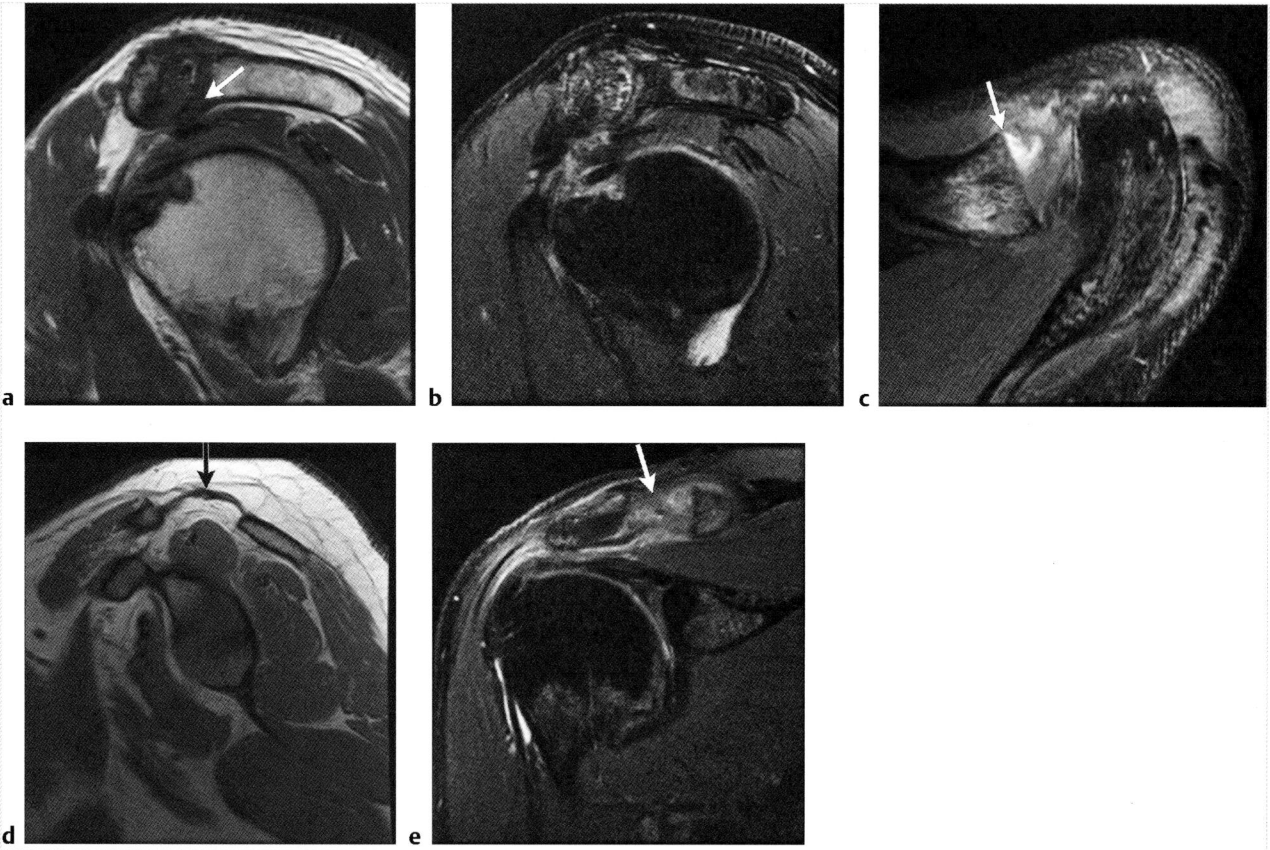

Fig. 2.8 (a) Note a subacromial osteophyte (arrow) impressing on the musculotendinous junction of the supraspinatus with associated moderate degenerative changes of the acromioclavicular joint on oblique sagittal proton density–weighted imaging (PDWI) and (b) oblique sagittal fat-suppressed T2-weighted imaging (FS T2WI). (c) Surgical treatment of impingement syndrome may include subacromial decompression and resection of the distal clavicle (arrow) seen on axial FS T2WI or (d) acromioclavicular (AC) joint resection (arrow) on oblique sagittal PDWI and (e) on oblique coronal FS T2WI (arrow).

Table 2.2 (Cont.) Lesions associated with impingement

Abnormalities	MRI findings	Comments
Acromioclavicular (AC) joint degeneration (▶ Fig. 2.9)	Degenerative changes including inferiorly positioned osteophytes and capsular hypertrophic changes are commonly seen. Degenerative changes may also result in an impression on the underlying supraspinatus with obscuration of the subacromial fat on PDWI. These findings are suggestive of impingement in the correct clinical setting. Assess for irregularities of the articular surfaces; osteophyte formation, particularly inferiorly; AC joint capsular thickening; and effaced subacromial fat in suspected impingement. The finding of marrow edema on either side of the AC joint has been associated with symptomatic disease.	AC joint arthritic changes are very common and may not result in impingement, particularly if spurring extends cephalad away from the joint. With chronic rotator cuff tear, arthrogram contrast may be seen to extend into the AC joint and into the subcutaneous tissues cephalad to the AC joint, the "geyser lesion." A synovial cyst may also develop superior to the AC joint and present clinically as a palpable mass. In younger patients with similar-appearing arthritic changes, consider posttraumatic osteolysis of the AC joint. This condition is seen in athletes or after an episode of acute trauma. With osteolysis there will be a greater degree of articular irregularity and surrounding marrow edema than is seen in cases of osteoarthritis. Additional findings include loss of cortical definition and synovitis.

(continued on page 24)

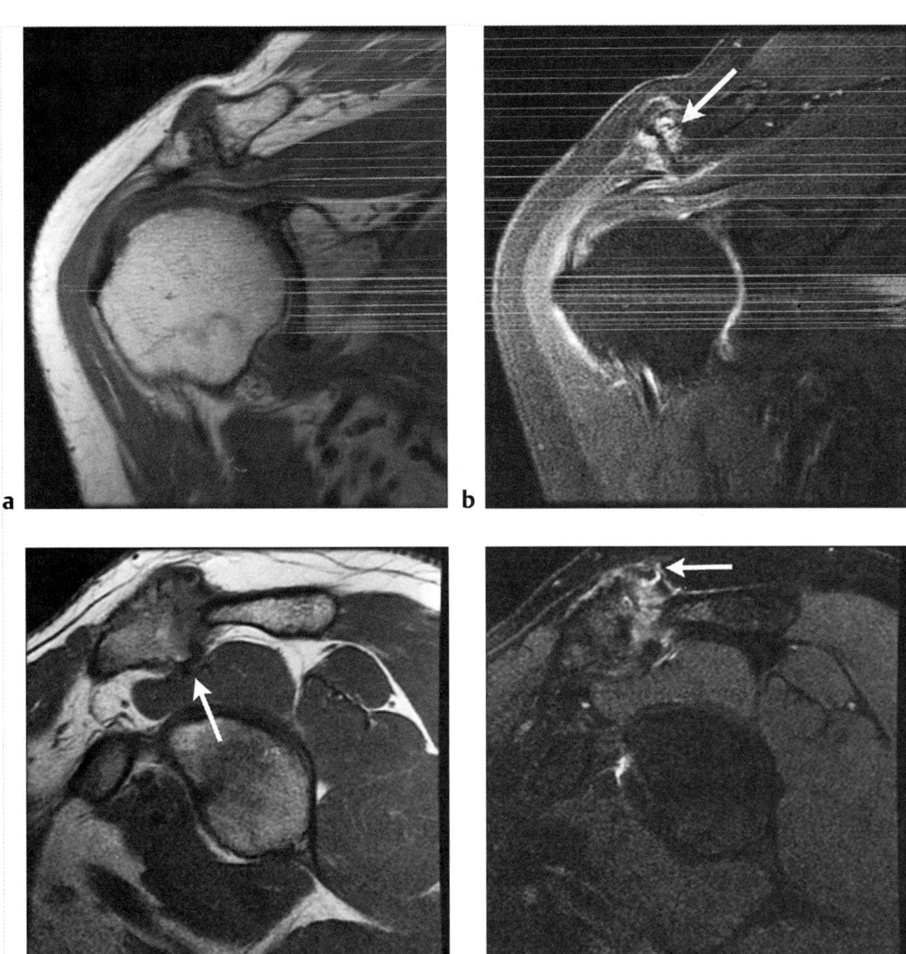

Fig. 2.9 (a) Acromioclavicular (AC) joint osteoarthritis is a common finding in asymptomatic patients; however, the presence of marrow edema may be seen in symptomatic patients. Typical findings include osteophytosis, articular irregularity, capsular hypertrophy, and loss of the subacromial fat plane and an impression on the underlying musculotendinous junction of the supraspinatus on oblique coronal proton density–weighted imaging (PDWI) and on (b) oblique coronal fat-suppressed T2-weighted imaging (FS T2WI). Note reactive marrow edema (arrow). (c) Additional case of AC joint osteoarthritis with more pronounced changes, including a prominent impression on the supraspinatus (arrow) on oblique sagittal PDWI. (d) On oblique sagittal FS T2WI note a similar impression on the supraspinatus and magnetic susceptibility artifact with characteristic curvilinear foci of adjacent high and low signal (arrow) due to tiny metallic fragments related to prior AC joint injection.

Table 2.2 (Cont.) Lesions associated with impingement

Abnormalities	MRI findings	Comments
Other suggested osseous contributors to subacromial impingement: acromial shape, slope, orientation, and os acromiale (▶ Fig. 2.10)	Although controversial, the following acromial findings have been associated with impingement. An inferolateral-tilting, down-sloping, or low-lying acromion can be identified on oblique coronal and oblique sagittal images. A type II acromion with a concave inferior surface and a type III acromion with anteroinferior hooking can be seen on sagittal images. An os acromiale may be identified on axial and coronal images.	Acromial shape has been previously implicated in impingement but is controversial. Acromial slope and position have also been associated with impingement. Os acromiale is an accessory center of ossification usually fused by 25 to 30 years of age. When the os is mobile, it may cause impingement due to a decrease in the coracoacromial space. Meso os acromiale is the most common type. An os acromiale may be a confusing finding on coronal magnetic resonance (MR) images if it is mistaken for the AC joint. Check axial images to identify the os acromiale separate from the AC joint.
Internal/posterosuperior glenoid impingement (▶ Fig. 2.11)	Look for three key associated findings: partial undersurface tear at the junction of the supraspinatus and infraspinatus tendons, geodes along the posterosuperior humeral head, and labral tears/degeneration along the posterosuperior labrum. Cuff abnormalities are typically best seen on oblique sagittal FS T2WI and oblique coronal FS T2WI. Labral findings are often best seen on FS T1 arthrogram images.	Typically seen in overhead-throwing athletes and in occupations requiring overhead work. Impingement occurs in abduction, external rotation. In the late cocking phase of throwing there is impingement between the junction of the posterior supraspinatus/anterior infraspinatus with the humeral head and between the posterosuperior glenoid and the labrum.

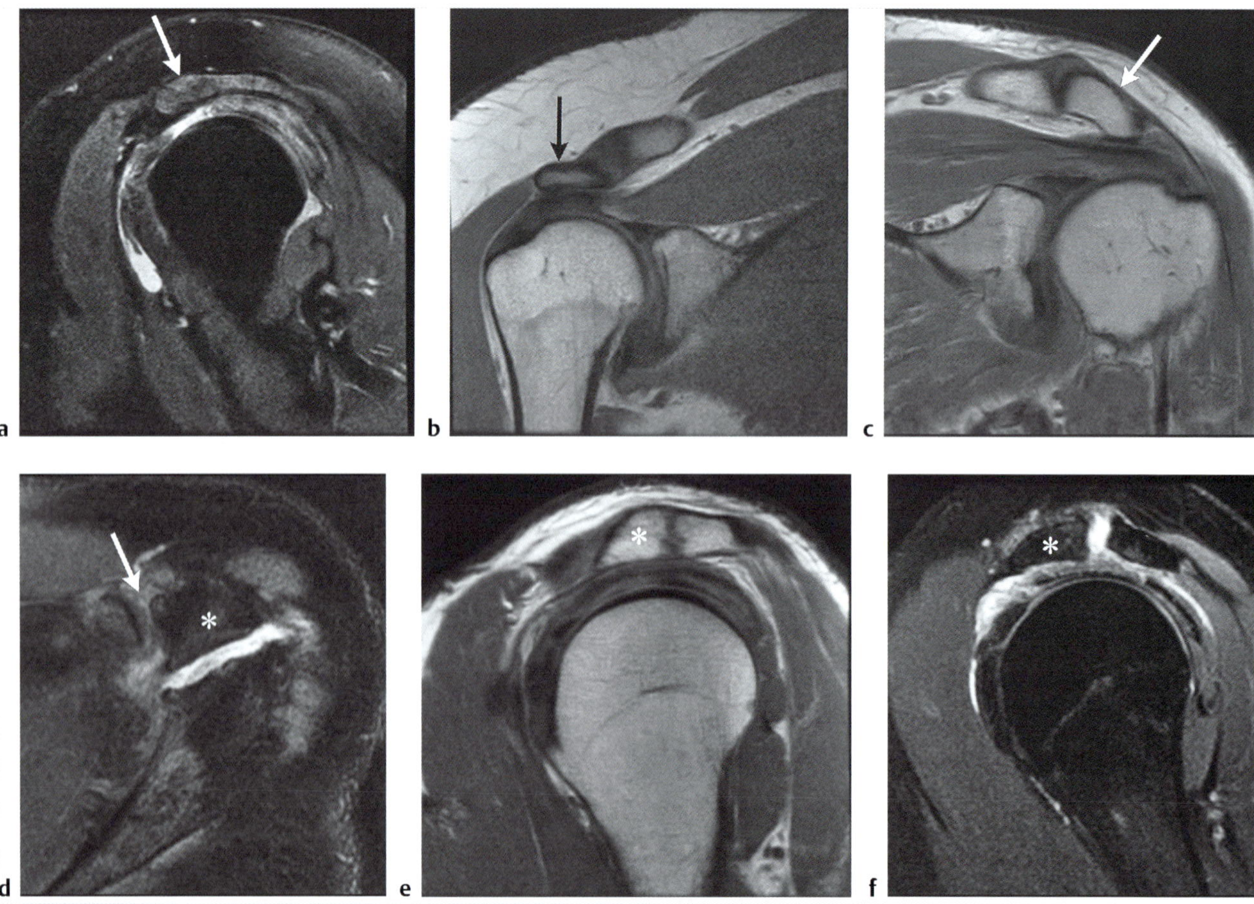

Fig. 2.10 Other osseous contributors to subacromial impingement. Although controversial, type II and III acromial variants and abnormal acromial position, tilt, and slope have been associated with impingement. (a) Note a type II anteriorly curved acromion (arrow) and underlying full-thickness supraspinatus tear on oblique sagittal fat-suppressed T2-weighted imaging (FS T2WI). (b) A low-lying acromion (arrow) relative to the distal clavicle is seen on oblique coronal proton density–weighted imaging (PDWI). (c) Inferolateral tilt to the acromion (arrow) is seen on oblique coronal PDWI. (d) Os acromiale (asterisk) is an accessory ossification center of the distal acromion as seen on axial FS T2WI. Note the adjacent acromioclavicular joint (arrow). (e,f) Two additional examples of os acromiale (asterisks) identified on oblique sagittal PDWI and on oblique sagittal FS T2WI.

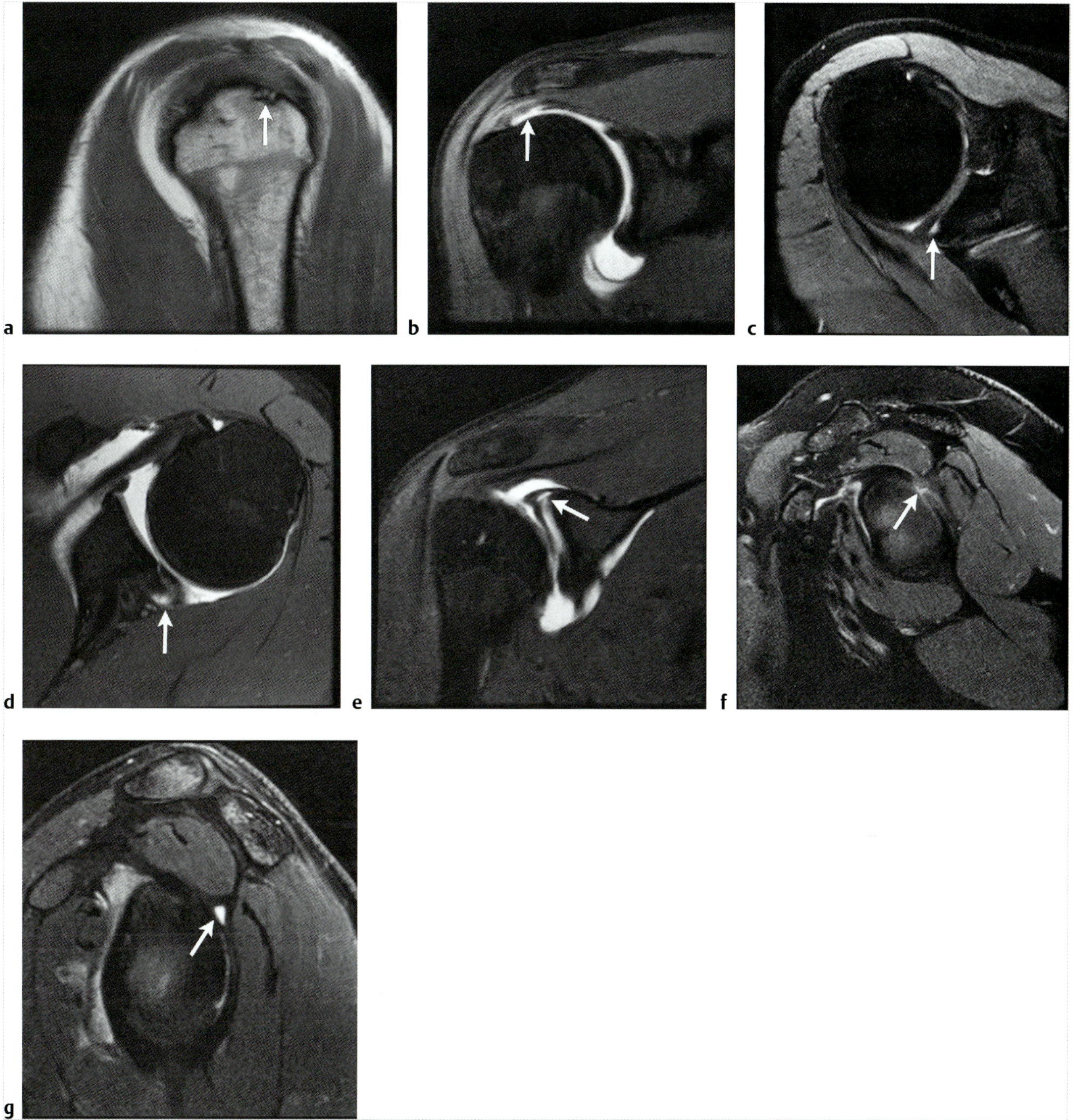

Fig. 2.11 Internal/posterosuperior glenoid impingement may be suspected in overhead-throwing athletes and overhead workers with posterior shoulder pain. (a) The following combination of findings is often seen in this condition: geodes (arrow) near the humeral head insertion of the infraspinatus on oblique sagittal proton density–weighted imaging (PDWI), (b) infraspinatus/supraspinatus junction undersurface tears on oblique coronal fat-suppressed (FS) T1 arthrogram, and (c) posterosuperior labral tears (arrows) on axial arthrogram images. (d) Posterosuperior labral tears (arrows) on axial, (e) oblique coronal, and (f,g) oblique sagittal FS T1 arthrogram images.

2.2.1 Lesions Associated with Impingement Suggested Reading

[1] Borrero CG, Casagranda BU, Towers JD, Bradley JP. Magnetic resonance appearance of posterosuperior labral peel back during humeral abduction and external rotation. Skeletal Radiol 2010; 39: 19–26

[2] Giaroli EL, Major NM, Higgins LD. MRI of internal impingement of the shoulder. AJR Am J Roentgenol 2005; 185: 925–929

[3] Tshering Vogel DW, Steinbach LS, Hertel R, Bernhard J, Stauffer E, Anderson SE. Acromioclavicular joint cyst: nine cases of a pseudotumor of the shoulder. Skeletal Radiol 2005; 34: 260–265

2.3 Lesions Associated with Shoulder Instability

- Bankart lesion
- Bankart fracture
- Perthes lesion
- Anterior labrum periosteal sleeve avulsion (ALPSA) lesion
- Glenoid labrum articular cartilage disruption (GLAD) lesion
- Posterior instability/posterior labral tears
- Posterosuperior labral tears/paralabral cysts
- Humeral avulsion of the glenohumeral ligament (HAGL) lesion

Table 2.3 Lesions associated with shoulder instability

Abnormalities	MRI findings	Comments
Bankart lesion (▶ Fig. 2.12)	An anteroinferior labral detachment seen between the 3 o'clock and 6 o'clock anterior portions of the glenoid with an associated tear of the adjacent periosteum. Best seen on axial fat-suppressed (FS) T1 arthrogram. High signal contrast extends between the low signal labrum and intermediate signal glenoid articular cartilage. Imaging may or may not demonstrate an associated labral tear, which will demonstrate abnormal signal or morphology of the labrum. A labral tear may extend cephalad to the level of the subscapularis tendon. Findings may also be seen on axial, oblique coronal, and oblique sagittal, FS T2-weighted imaging (T2WI). Look for associated Hill-Sachs impaction fracture of the posterolateral humeral head or bony Bankart lesion of the glenoid.	In patients with anterior instability following anterior shoulder dislocation, a Bankart lesion is the most common labral abnormality. The spectrum of injury includes a partial labral tear or labral crush injury, an abnormally small and torn anterior labrum, or a detached/displaced labrum torn from the anterior scapular periosteum. During anterior dislocation, the humeral head impacts the anterior bony glenoid and results in an associated Bankart fracture in a minority of patients. Anterior labral tears may occur without a history of anterior dislocation or instability.

(continued on page 28)

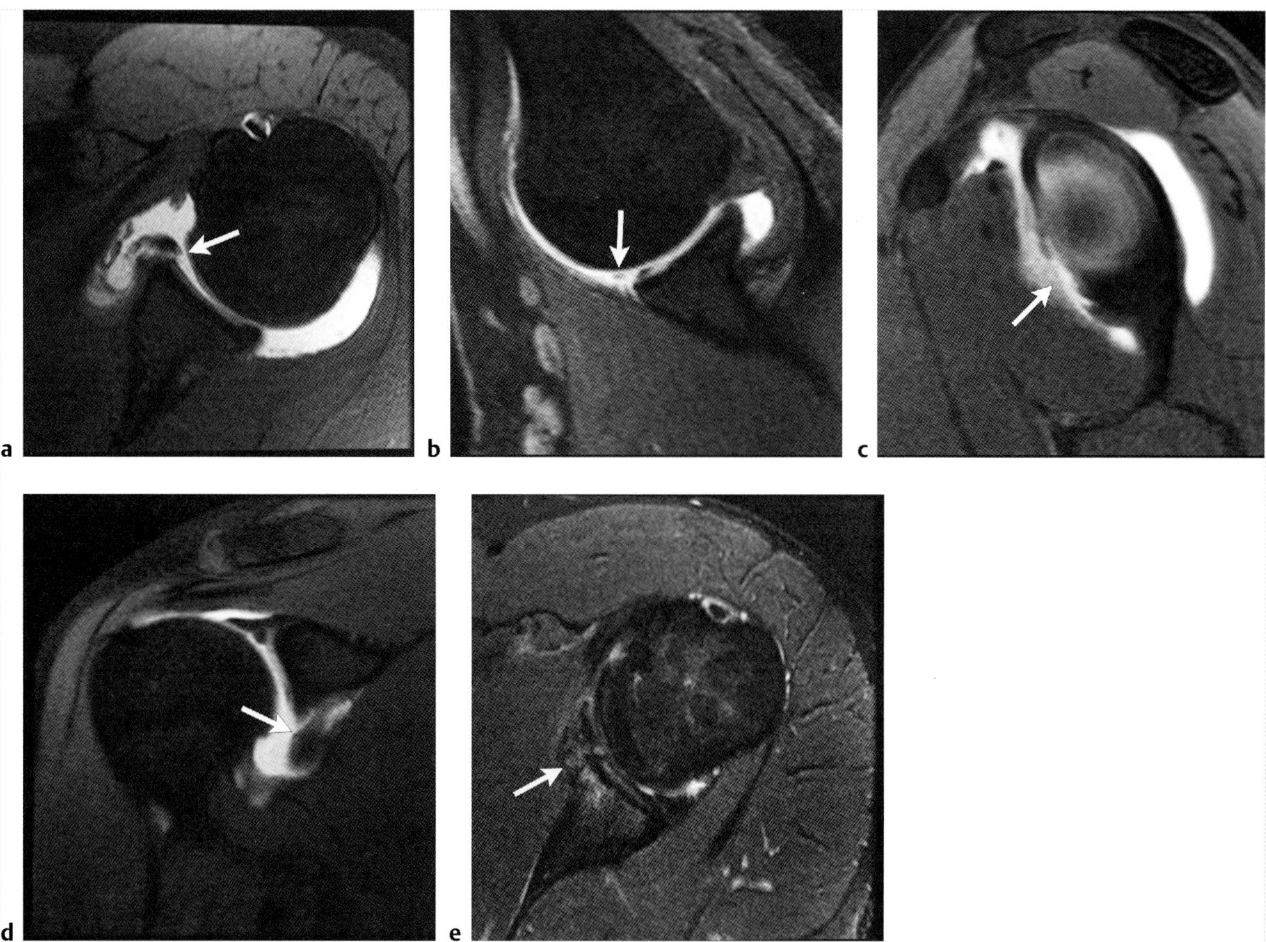

Fig. 2.12 (a) Bankart lesion, note detachment and tear/irregularity of the anteroinferior labrum (arrow) on axial fat-suppressed (FS) T1 arthrogram. (b) A smaller Bankart lesion (arrow) is seen in another patient on the abduction internal rotation (ABER) view on FS T1 arthrogram. (c) The extent of the labral tear (arrows) is seen on oblique sagittal FS T1 arthrogram and (d) on oblique coronal FS T1 arthrogram. (e) A chronic Bankart tear (arrow) is seen on axial FS T2WI. Note glenoid marrow edema from recurrent injury.

Table 2.3 (Cont.) Lesions associated with shoulder instability

Abnormalities	MRI findings	Comments
Bankart fracture (▶ Fig. 2.13)	Seen as a cortical fracture along the anterior or anteroinferior glenoid rim following anterior glenohumeral dislocation. Look for high signal marrow edema surrounding the fracture lines and bone fragments on FS T2WI. In our experience, oblique sagittal proton density–weighted imaging (PDWI) is the most useful sequence to detect a Bankart fracture as a discontinuity or irregularity of the anterior glenoid. The shoulder capsule may obscure the fragment on other planes.	Bankart fractures are seen in association with a Hill-Sachs impaction fracture or humeral head bone bruise. Recurrent dislocations may worsen a Hill-Sachs lesion and further deform the anterior glenoid rim.
Perthes lesion (▶ Fig. 2.14)	Less severe Bankart variant with intact scapular periosteum. Focal linear abnormal signal is seen on axial FS T2WI between an avulsed anteroinferior labrum and bony glenoid. Perthes lesions may be best seen on FS T1 arthrogram using the abduction external rotation (ABER) position. Labrum is usually not displaced.	The ABER position is useful for detecting subtle anteroinferior labral tears as this technique places the inferior glenohumeral ligament and capsule under tension. Tears not seen on routine axial imaging are often displayed using the ABER position.

(continued on page 30)

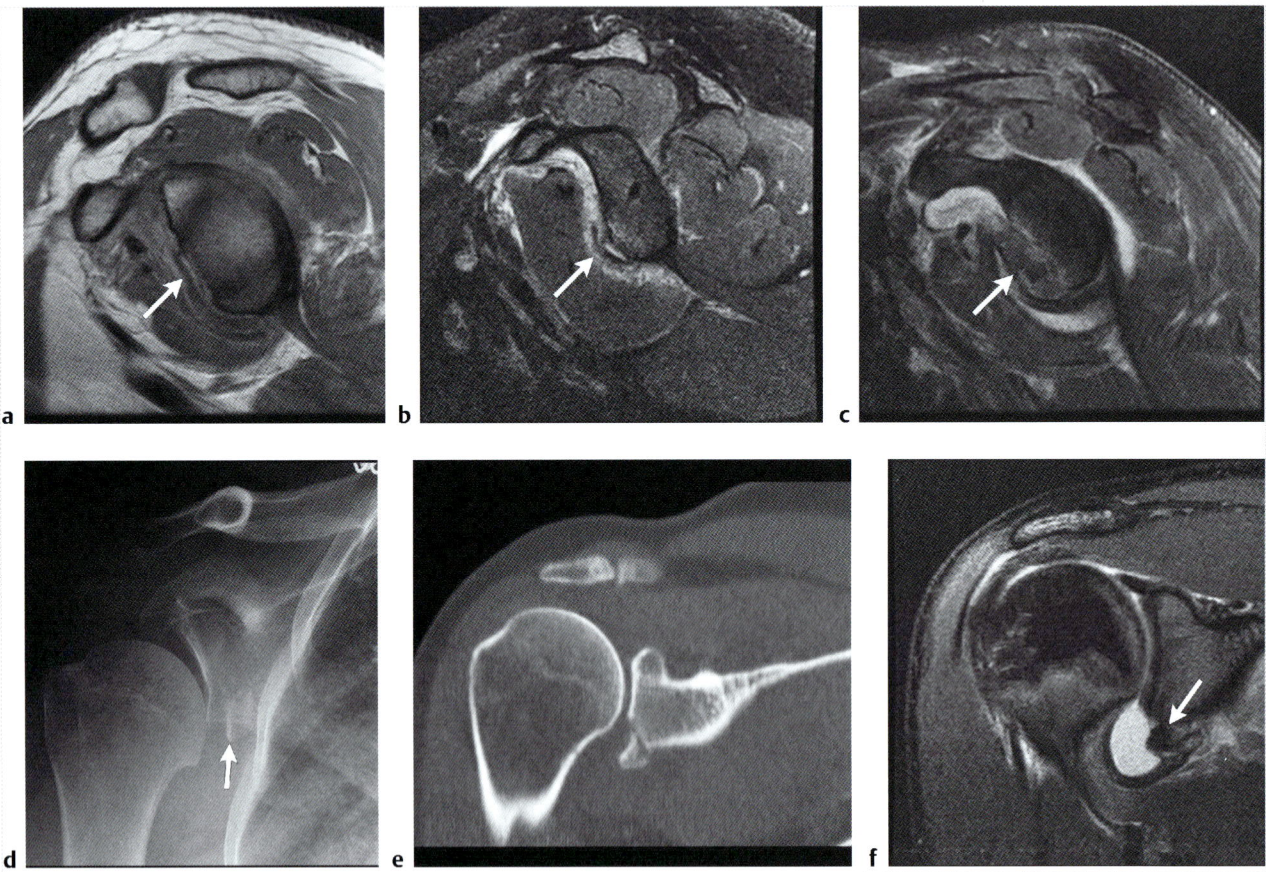

Fig. 2.13 (a) Bankart fracture in three patients with history of prior anterior dislocation. Note curvilinear fracture fragments (arrows) from the anteroinferior glenoid on oblique sagittal proton density–weighted imaging (PDWI) and (b,c) oblique sagittal fat-suppressed T2-weighted imaging (FS T2WI). (d) Three additional patients with Bankart fractures: a medially displaced fracture fragment (arrow) on anteroposterior shoulder radiograph, (e) coronal computed tomographic reconstruction of an oblique fracture, and (f) a medially displaced Bankart fracture (arrow) on coronal FS T2WI. *(continued)*

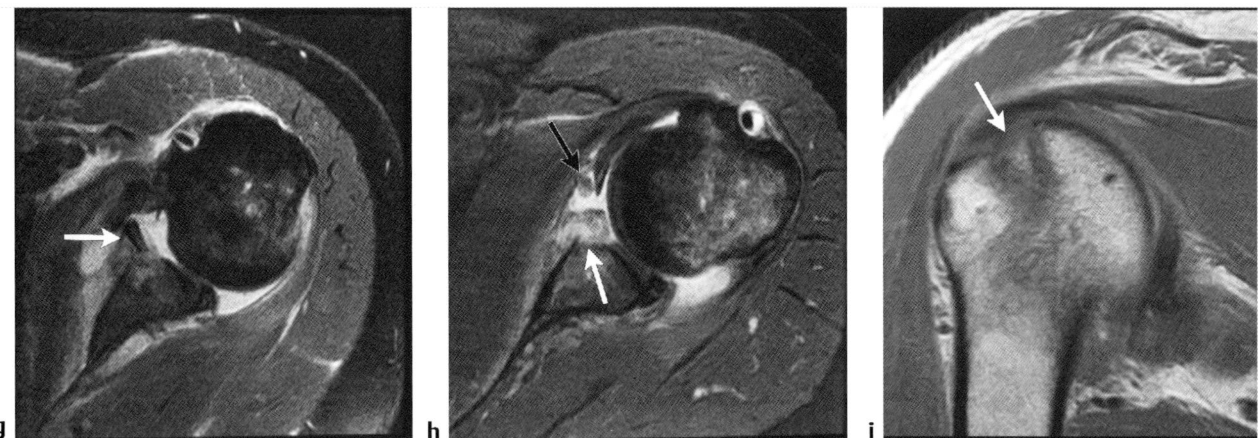

Fig. 2.13 (*continued*) Axial images through the inferior portion of the glenoid in different patients with Bankart fractures. (g) Note the displaced fragment and marrow edema (arrow) on axial FS T2WI. (h) Note cortical irregularity indicating a fracture (white arrow) and adjacent deformed torn labrum with a loose body (black arrow), on axial FS T2WI. (i) A Hills-Sachs fracture of the posterolateral humeral head is the sequela of anteroinferior dislocation of the humeral head. Note notch defect on coronal PDWI (arrow).

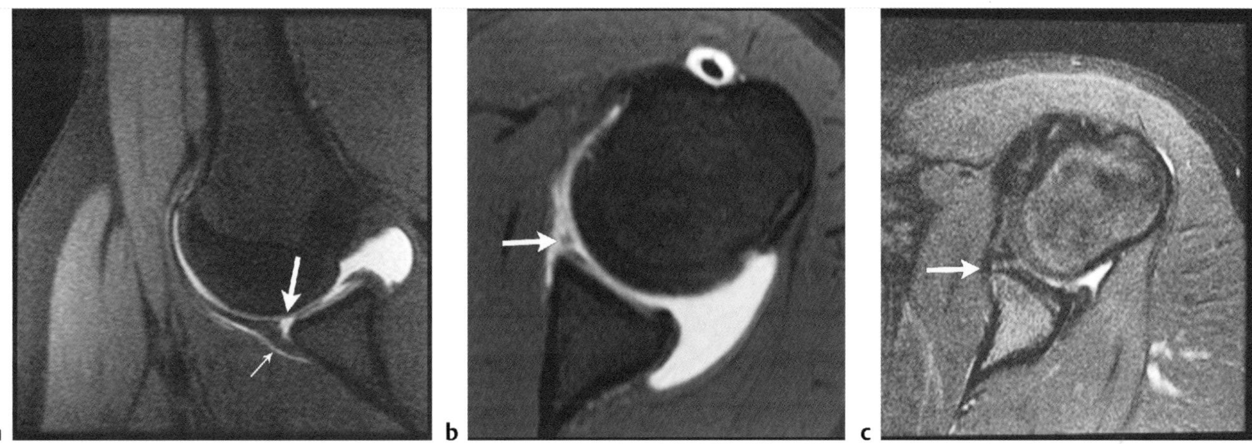

Fig. 2.14 (a) A Perthes lesion with an anterior labral tear (large arrow) with slight labral displacement and intact scapular periosteum (small arrow) on abduction external rotation (ABER) fat-suppressed (FS) T1 arthrogram. (b) In a different patient note abnormal signal separating a slightly displaced anterior labrum from the glenoid (arrow) on axial FS T1 arthrogram. (c) In a third case, note a nondisplaced torn and diminutive anteroinferior labrum (arrow) on axial FS T2WI. The lack of increased T2 signal within the tear suggests an old scarred down lesion.

Table 2.3 (Cont.) Lesions associated with shoulder instability

Abnormalities	MRI findings	Comments
Anterior labrum periosteal sleeve avulsion (ALPSA) lesion (▶ Fig. 2.15)	A Bankart variant with detachment of the anterior labrum from the anteroinferior labrum with an intact scapular periosteum. The key finding is labroligamentous complex displacement inferiorly and/or medially. The sleeve of the avulsed periosteum remains intact and in continuity with the detached and displaced labrum. This may be associated with a glenoid (Bankart) fracture. Best sequence to define this lesion is either axial or ABER FS T1 arthrogram or axial FS T2WI. Check for a displaced labrum and edema or thickening of the adjacent capsule. A greater degree of edema is identified with acute injuries.	Medial labral displacement, if chronic, may result in a malpositioned labral fragment along the anterior glenoid with fibrosis. Follow the course of the glenohumeral ligaments on magnetic resonance (MR) arthrogram to distinguish an ALPSA from a prominent middle glenohumeral ligament. ALPSA and Bankart lesions are associated with shoulder instability.
Glenoid labrum articular cartilage disruption (GLAD) lesion (▶ Fig. 2.16)	An articular cartilage flap or chondral defect associated with a partial tear of the anterior labrum. Well seen on axial or ABER FS T1 arthrogram or axial FS T2WI as abnormally increased signal of a partial labral tear associated with a chondral abnormality. The partial labral tear in a GLAD lesion is typically nondisplaced.	GLAD lesions are typically identified without a history of anterior dislocation or injury to the capsule. There may be a history of pain without instability. MR findings are more subtle than with other types of labral pathology.

(continued on page 32)

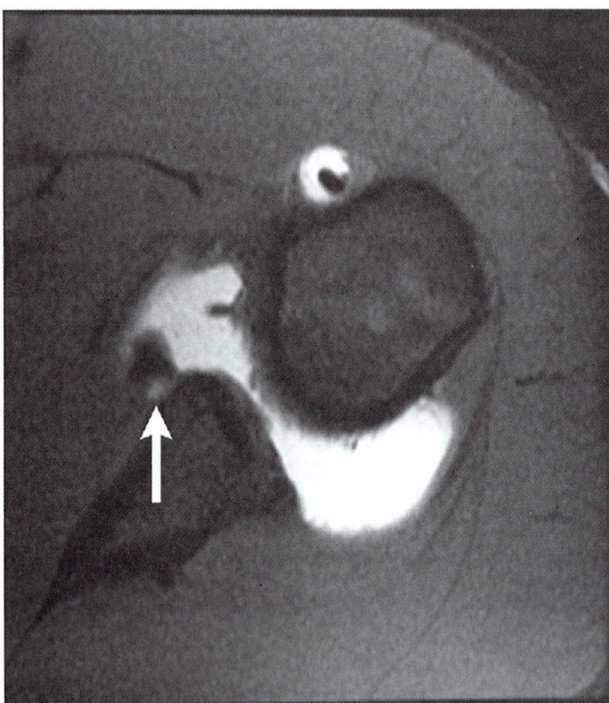

Fig. 2.15 Anterior labrum periosteal sleeve avulsion (ALPSA) lesion. The labrum is detached from the anterior glenoid and displaced medially (arrow) on axial fat-suppressed (FS) T1 arthrogram. The stripped scapular periosteum permits the labroligamentous complex to displace medially.

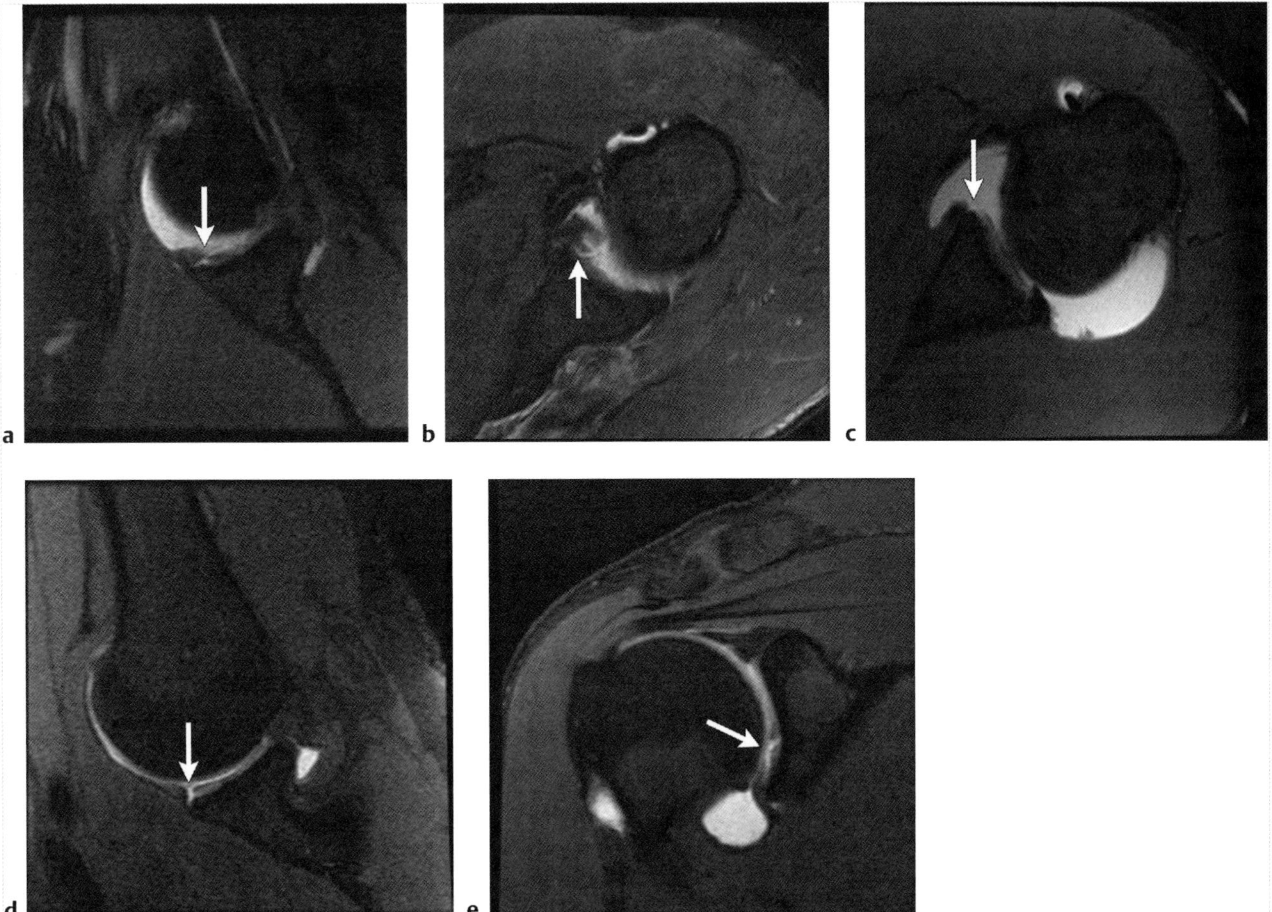

Fig. 2.16 Glenoid labrum articular cartilage disruption (GLAD) lesion in different patients. Arrows show anteroinferior labral tears with involvement of the adjacent glenoid articular cartilage on (a) abduction external rotation (ABER) fat-suppressed (FS) T1 arthrogram and (b) axial FS T2-weighted imaging (T2WI). (c) Note a gap with irregular signal and fraying of the anterior glenoid cartilage and torn labrum (arrow) on axial FS T1 arthrogram. (d) Note increased signal fluid demarcating the chondrolabral separation on ABER FS T1 arthrogram. (e) An elongated chondral defect is well seen on coronal FS T1 arthrogram.

Table 2.3 (Cont.) Lesions associated with shoulder instability

Abnormalities	MRI findings	Comments
Posterior instability/ posterior labral tears (▶ Fig. 2.17)	Look for abnormal linear signal within the posterior labrum on FS T2WI or FS T1 arthrogram. Tears may be partial labral tears or posterior Bankart lesions with labral detachment. Tears may be focal linear signal abnormalities or more complex appearing lesions with tearing and superimposed degeneration with intermediate signal changes on fluid-sensitive sequences. The posterior labral lesions are associated with reverse bony Bankart and reverse Hills-Sachs fracture. Look for cortical bone indentation on PDWI and marrow edema on FS T2WI. On X-ray, the reverse Hills-Sachs presents as the "trough sign" seen along the anteromedial humeral head. Posterior labral tears may be associated with injury to the posterior band of the inferior glenohumeral ligament injury (posterior HAGL [PHAGL]). A posterior labral periosteal sleeve avulsion (POLPSA) lesion is analogous to the ALPSA lesion described earlier. A POLPSA lesion is a posterior labral tear in which the torn labrum remains attached to the glenoid via a sleeve of stripped periosteum. A shallow/hypoplastic glenoid fossa is seen with atraumatic posterior dislocations and may be associated with posterior labral tears.	Posterior instability and associated posterior labral tears may be atraumatic due to a developmentally hypoplastic glenoid. Alternatively, blunting of the posterior glenoid may be the sequela of prior posterior subluxation as seen with repetitive trauma in athletes. This may lead to posterior labral tears. Posterior dislocation, although uncommon, may be post-traumatic or due to a seizure. Differential for posterior labral tear includes the Bennett lesion–heterotopic ossification/ calcification adjacent to the posterior glenoid/posterior labral injury. This is seen in throwing athletes.

(continued on page 34)

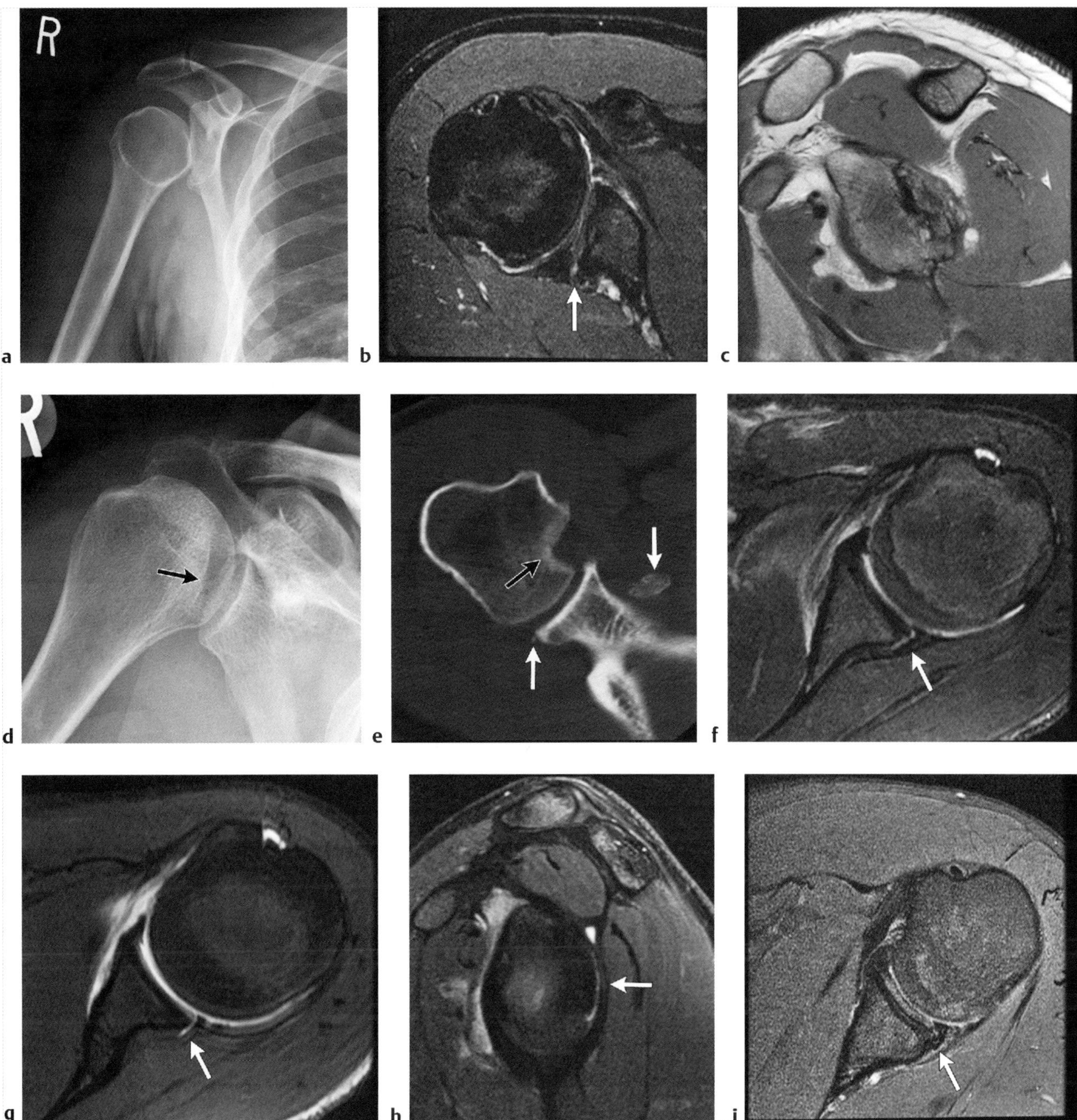

Fig. 2.17 Posterior instability/posterior labral tears. (a) Glenoid dysplasia with abnormally shallow and lobulated glenoid allowing for atraumatic posterior dislocation on radiograph. (b) Another case of glenoid dysplasia with a reverse Bankart lesion and abnormal signal through the labrum and posterior glenoid, (arrow) on axial fat-suppressed T2-weighted imaging (FS T2WI). (c) Sequelae of multiple episodes of posterior dislocation with posttraumatic arthritic changes of the posterior glenoid on oblique sagittal proton density–weighted imaging (PDWI). (d) Trough sign of prior posterior dislocation on radiograph and (e) axial computed tomographic image (black arrow). Note small fracture fragment at the posterior glenoid and larger displaced fragment anterior to the glenoid (white arrows). (f) Example of posterior labral pathology with posterior labral detachment and high signal fluid deep to the stripped glenoid periosteum (arrow) on axial FS T2WI. (g) High signal Gd-contrast defines posterior labral detachment in a different patient on axial FS T1 arthrogram and (h) sagittal FS T1 arthrogram (arrows). (i) Complex tears of the posterior labrum (arrow) in a different patient on axial FS T2WI.

Table 2.3 (Cont.) Lesions associated with shoulder instability

Abnormalities	MRI findings	Comments
Posterosuperior labral tears/paralabral cysts (▶ Fig. 2.18)	Paralabral cysts are most commonly seen posterosuperiorly accompanied by a tear of the posterosuperior or posterior labrum. Cysts are easily identified by their rounded or oval appearance and fluid signal–low signal on T1WI and PDWI and increased signal on FS T2WI or other fluid-sensitive sequence such as short TI inversion recovery (STIR). Septations within paralabral cysts are common. Cysts are often seen in the spinoglenoid or suprascapular notch. MR arthrogram contrast may fill the cyst.	Paralabral cysts are the result of joint fluid extending through a labral tear with subsequent development of a cyst. The presence of a paralabral cyst is presumptive of a labral tear, although the tear may not be visible. Larger cysts may result in compression of the suprascapular nerve and resultant muscle edema or atrophy of the supraspinatus or infraspinatus muscle. Superior labrum anterior to posterior (SLAP) lesions may also demonstrate a posterosuperior paralabral cyst. Throwers with posterosuperior/internal impingement may demonstrate labral tears/degeneration of the posterosuperior labrum–a subtype of a SLAP II tear.
Humeral avulsion of the glenohumeral ligament (HAGL) lesion (▶ Fig. 2.19)	Usually identified on oblique coronal FS T2WI or on FS T1 arthrogram. Look for discontinuity of the inferior glenohumeral ligament, which will be avulsed from its humeral attachment and result in a J-shaped inferior margin of the joint capsule. There may be a secondary sign of edema or extravasation of contrast beyond the expected margin of the capsule on fluid-sensitive sequences. This finding will be visible at the inferior margin of the capsule/axillary pouch. Note that arthrogram contrast may also be seen beyond the capsule due to iatrogenic causes in cases without a HAGL lesion.	The inferior glenohumeral ligaments are key stabilizers of the glenohumeral joint. HAGL lesions are associated with anterior instability. In addition to the above MR findings, also check for avulsion of a bone fragment with the torn inferior glenohumeral ligament, a bony HAGL (BHAGL) lesion. Look for sequelae of shoulder dislocation/instability and associated tears of the subscapularis tendon. Variants of a HAGL include a sprain of the axillary pouch with a discontinuity of the midportion of the capsule. A HAGL lesion is less common than a Bankart lesion after anterior dislocation. Still less common is the reverse or posterior HAGL lesion (PHAGL lesion) following posterior subluxation.

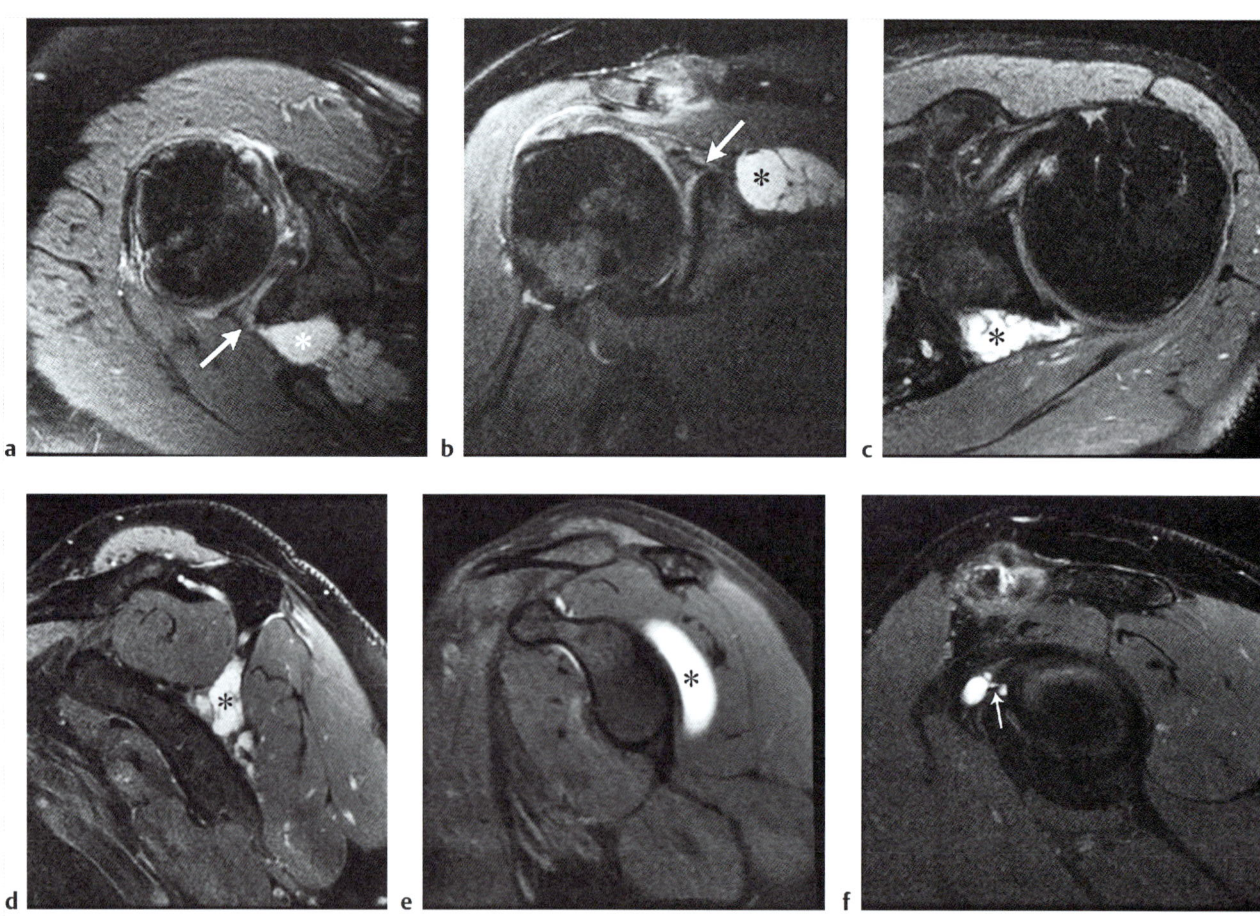

Fig. 2.18 Posterosuperior labral tears/paralabral cysts. (a) Posterosuperior paralabral cyst (asterisks) associated with a superior labrum anterior to posterior (SLAP) tear (arrows) on axial fat-suppressed T2-weighted imaging (FS T2WI) and (b) coronal FS T2WI. (c) A septated paralabral cyst (asterisk) arising from a posterior labral tear on axial FS T2WI. (d) The paralabral cyst (asterisk) extends between the muscle bellies of the supraspinatus and infraspinatus muscles on sagittal FS T2WI. (e) A different patient with a paralabral cyst (asterisk) posterior to the glenoid filling with contrast on oblique sagittal FS T1 arthrogram. (f) A smaller anterosuperior paralabral cyst with a thin neck (arrow) associated with a SLAP tear (not shown) on oblique sagittal FS T2WI.

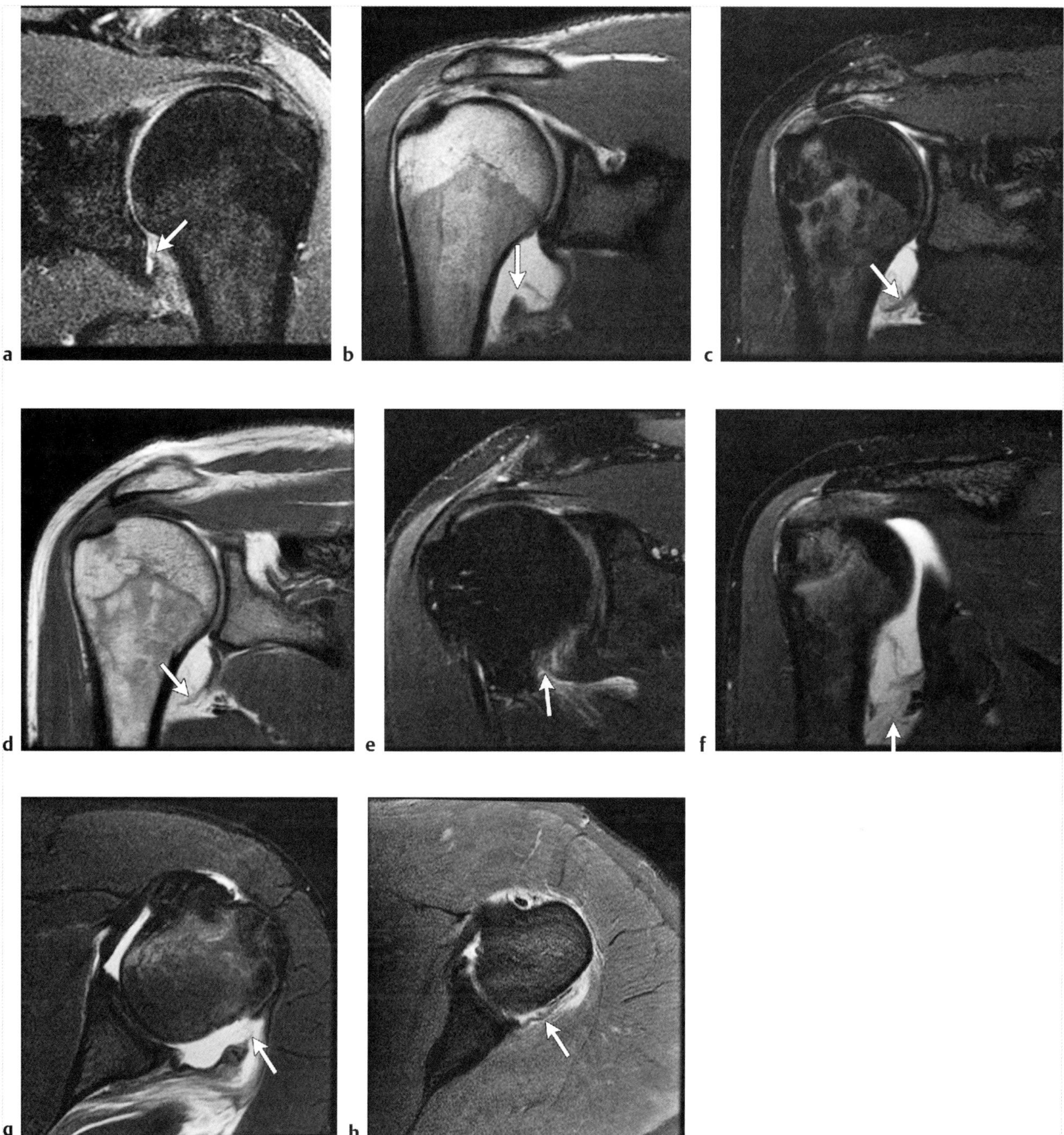

Fig. 2.19 Humeral avulsion of the glenohumeral ligament (HAGL). (a) Note avulsion of the inferior glenohumeral ligament from its humeral attachment (arrow) with high signal fluid/edema inferior to the capsule on oblique coronal fat-suppressed T2-weighted imaging (FS T2WI) and (b) in a different patient on oblique coronal proton density–weighted imaging (PDWI) (arrow). Note high signal arthrogram contrast inferior to the capsule along the humeral shaft. (c) A different patient with an ill-defined torn inferior glenohumeral ligament (arrow) on oblique coronal FS T2WI and (d) on oblique coronal PDWI. (e) An axillary pouch sprain on oblique coronal FS T2WI. Note ill-defined and partly torn capsule (arrow) with fluid extending inferiorly. (f) In a different patient a complete mid substance disruption of the capsule is seen on oblique coronal FS T1 arthrogram (arrow). (g) A posterior HAGL (arrow) on axial FS T1 arthrogram as a result of a posterior dislocation with tearing of the posterior capsule/glenohumeral ligament. Note high signal arthrogram contrast outlining the tear. (h) Additional example of a posterior capsule injury with wavy torn fibers (arrow) seen on axial FS T1 arthrogram.

2.3.1 Lesions Associated with Shoulder Instability Suggested Reading

[1] Harish S, Nagar A, Moro J, Pugh D, Rebello R, O'Neill J. Imaging findings in posterior instability of the shoulder. Skeletal Radiol 2008; 37: 693–707

[2] Omoumi P, Teixeira P, Lecouvet F, Chung CB. Glenohumeral joint instability. J Magn Reson Imaging 2011; 33: 2–16

[3] Saleem AM, Lee JK, Novak LM. Usefulness of the abduction and external rotation views in shoulder MR arthrography. AJR Am J Roentgenol 2008; 191: 1024–1030

[4] Yu JS, Ashman CJ, Jones G. The POLPSA lesion: MR imaging findings with arthroscopic correlation in patients with posterior instability. Skeletal Radiol 2002; 31: 396–399

2.4 SLAP Lesions and Biceps Tendon Abnormalities

- Normal labral findings/variants: sublabral sulcus or recess
- Normal labral findings/variants: sublabral foramen/hole
- Normal labral findings/variants: Buford complex
- Superior labrum anterior to posterior (SLAP) tear/lesion
- Long head biceps: tendinosis/partial/complete tears
- Biceps tendon subluxation/dislocation

Table 2.4 SLAP lesions and biceps tendon abnormalities

Abnormalities	MRI findings	Comments
Normal labral findings/variants: sublabral sulcus or recess (▶ Fig. 2.20)	Well seen on magnetic resonance (MR) arthrogram or fluid-sensitive sequences, a sublabral sulcus/recess is a high signal cleft at the interface between the superior labrum and the glenoid articular cartilage. The sublabral sulcus will be smooth in contour and will not extend completely through the junction between the labrum and articular cartilage. The sulcus will follow the contour of the articular cartilage coursing medially toward the glenoid. Do not mistake this common finding for a superior labrum anterior to posterior (SLAP) tear that is irregular and extends laterally to involve the labral substance, rather than medially along the articular cartilage.	The most common labral variants to be aware of include the sublabral sulcus/recess, the sublabral foramen/hole, and the Buford complex. A sublabral sulcus will be found between the eleven and one o'clock positions, while the sublabral foramen/hole and the Buford complex will be seen in the anterior quadrant of the labrum between the one and three o'clock positions.
Normal labral findings/variants: sublabral foramen/hole (▶ Fig. 2.21)	Look for the anterosuperior labrum smoothly separated from the adjacent glenoid articular cartilage on axial FS T2WI and on axial FS T1 arthrogram. More inferiorly, the labrum will reattach to the glenoid at the level of the "equator" – the superior third of the anterior glenoid near the level of the subscapularis tendon.	The sublabral foramen will communicate with the subscapularis bursa. Do not confuse fluid in the foramen for a paralabral cyst.
Normal labral findings/variants: Buford complex (▶ Fig. 2.22)	Cordlike middle glenohumeral ligament (MGL) and absence of the anterosuperior labrum. The thickened MGL will be well seen as a low signal, thick band on axial and sagittal images posterior to the subscapularis tendon and anterior to the labrum. This finding is located in the anterosuperior quadrant superior to the level of the subscapularis tendon. Look for fluid around the MGL on MR arthrogram images.	To distinguish a Buford complex from a sublabral foramen, on axial images look for the MGL to sweep anteriorly to join the capsule on subsequent inferior axial images. The sublabral foramen will disappear on more inferior axial images as the labrum fuses normally to the glenoid.

(continued on page 38)

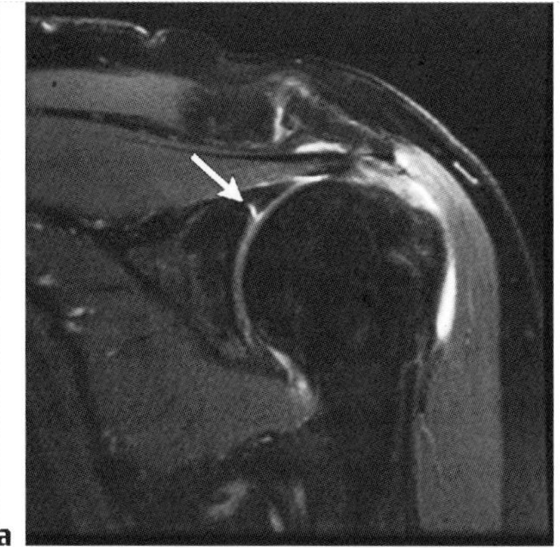
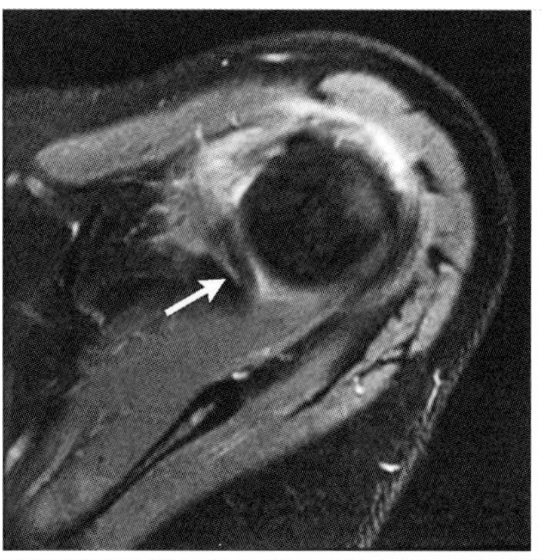
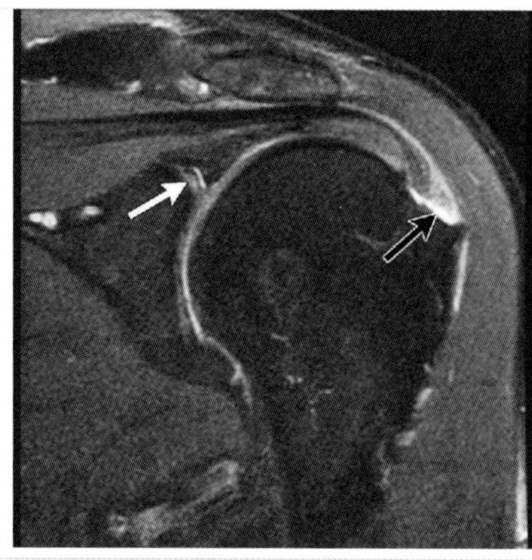

Fig. 2.20 Normal labral findings/variants: sublabral sulcus/recess. (a) Note an increased signal recess extending medially separating the hyaline articular cartilage of the glenoid from the fibrocartilage of the superior labrum (arrow), on oblique coronal fat-suppressed (FS) T1 arthrogram. (b) Corresponding axial image demonstrates the sublabral recess (arrow) extending anterior to posterior on axial FS T1 arthrogram. This should not be confused with a superior labrum anterior to posteror (SLAP) tear. (c) Another patient demonstrating a larger sublabral recess (white arrow) as well as a full-thickness insertional tear of the supraspinatus (black arrow) on oblique coronal FS T2-weighted imaging post arthrography.

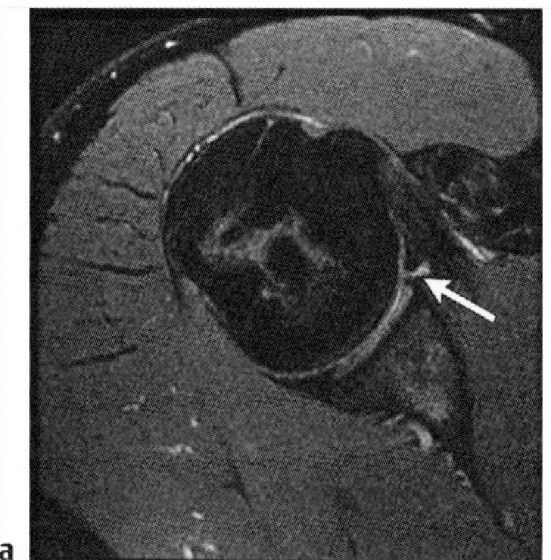
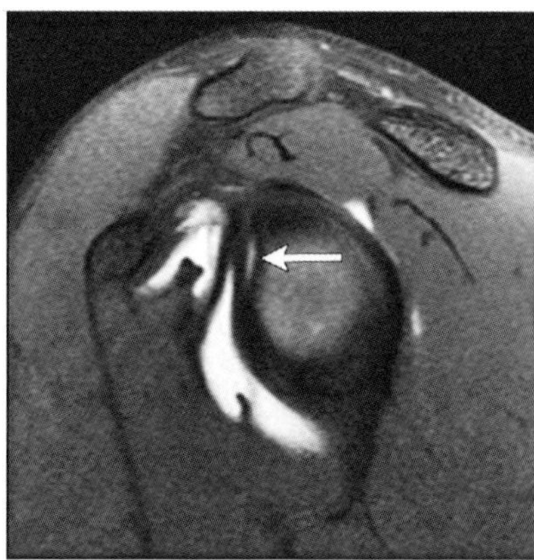

Fig. 2.21 Normal labral variant: sublabral foramen/hole. (a) Note a sublabral foramen (arrows) separating the anterior labrum from the glenoid on axial fat-suppressed T2-weighted imaging (FS T2WI) and (b) on oblique sagittal FS T1 arthrogram. More inferiorly the labrum reattaches to the glenoid shown on the oblique sagittal image.

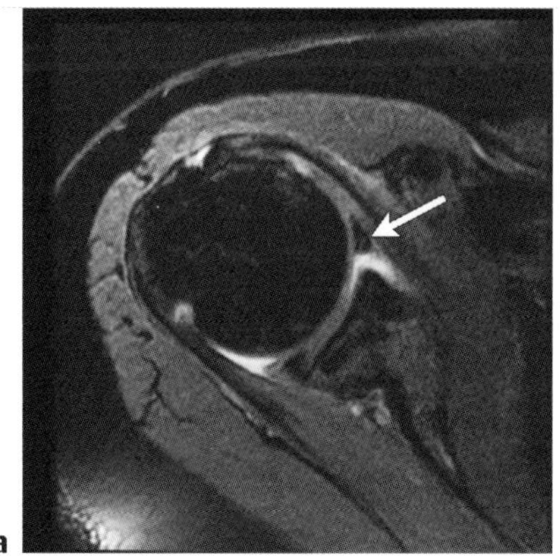
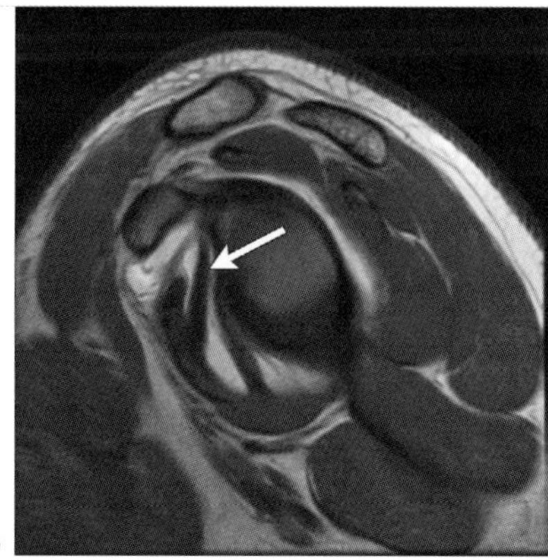

Fig. 2.22 Normal labral variant: Buford complex. (a) A thickened middle glenohumeral ligament (arrow) positioned anterior to the glenoid with absence of the anterosuperior labrum on axial fat-suppressed (FS) T1 arthrogram. (b) Note the thickened cordlike middle glenohumeral ligament (MGL) (arrow) between the superior and inferior glenohumeral ligaments on sagittal proton density–weighted imaging postarthrography.

Table 2.4 (Cont.) SLAP lesions and biceps tendon abnormalities

Abnormalities	MRI findings	Comments
Superior labrum anterior to posterior (SLAP) tear/lesion (▶ Fig. 2.23)	Common types: type I–fraying/degeneration of the superior labrum demonstrating increased signal on proton density–weighted imaging (PDWI) and fat-suppressed T2-weighted imaging (FS T2WI), type II–either tearing of the superior labrum from anterior to posterior or detachment of the superior labrum from its superior glenoid attachment. Abnormal signal on FS T2WI or FS T1 arthrogram within the superior labrum may be seen in any plane, often best identified on coronal images. A type III SLAP is a superior labral tear with a "bucket handle" component. A type IV lesion is a bucket handle tear with involvement of the long head biceps tendon. Other types of SLAP tears involve different portions of the labrum and surrounding structures.	SLAP tears include a spectrum of labral abnormalities, with many types described. A key imaging distinction is to determine the condition of the biceps tendon anchor and the proximal biceps tendon. Look for abnormal signal replacing the normally low signal biceps anchor and proximal biceps tendon. Oblique coronal images are useful to determine if the labral abnormality is "degenerative" (type I SLAP lesion often seen in older patients), a partial- or full-thickness SLAP tear, or a labral detachment. Increased signal due to a normal sublabral sulcus will extend medially and follow the contour of the glenoid, well seen on coronal images. SLAP tears will appear more irregular with abnormal signal extending laterally away from the glenoid. Labral detachment will demonstrate abnormal fluid signal separating the labrum and glenoid. A finding of complete glenolabral separation may help distinguish labral detachment from a sublabral sulcus where a degree of glenolabral attachment is maintained.

(continued on page 40)

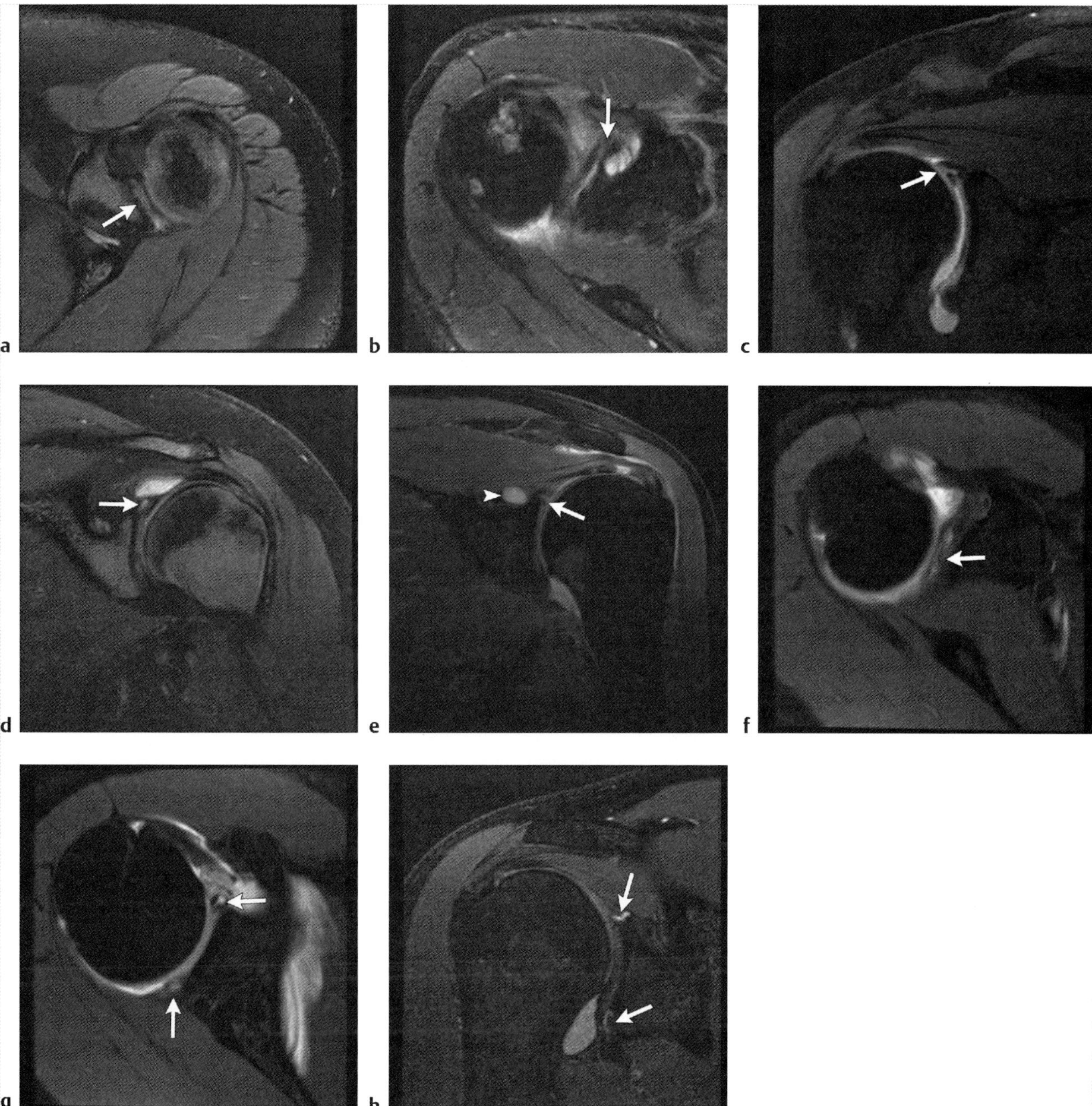

Fig. 2.23 Superior labrum anterior to posterior (SLAP) tear/lesion. (a) Irregular linear zone of high signal contrast material (arrow) extends across the superior labrum from anterior to posterior, a SLAP lesion, representing a detachment of the superior labrum from the glenoid on axial fat-suppressed (FS) T1 arthrogram. (b) SLAP lesion with abnormal increased signal extending into the biceps anchor (arrow) on axial FS T1 arthrogram. (c) SLAP tears with abnormal high signal contrast within a torn superior labrum (arrow) on oblique coronal FS T1 arthrogram and (d) in a different patient on oblique coronal FS T2-weighted imaging (T2WI) (arrow). (e) More subtle SLAP tear (arrow) with an adjacent paralabral cyst (arrowhead) and an articular-side partial-thickness supraspinatus tear on oblique coronal FS T1 arthrogram. (f,g) Extensive SLAP tear involving the entire labrum: superior, anterior, and posterior tears seen on axial FS T1 arthrogram (arrows). (h) Superior and inferior components of the tear are seen on oblique coronal FS T2WI. Biceps anchor was also involved, not shown.

Table 2.4 (Cont.) SLAP lesions and biceps tendon abnormalities

Abnormalities	MRI findings	Comments
Long head biceps: tendinosis/partial/complete tears (▶ Fig. 2.24)	PDWI and FS T2WI demonstrate proximal abnormal increased signal in the biceps tendon with thickening or thinning if associated with partial tear or longitudinal split tear. Abnormal biceps tendon signal proximally at the attachment on the supraglenoid tubercle/superior labrum is seen with some SLAP lesions. Check the rotator interval and bicipital groove for abnormal signal or absent tendon on oblique sagittal and coronal images.	Proximal biceps tendon abnormalities are associated with supraspinatus tendon and labral pathology. With a cuff tear, the acromion impinges upon the biceps tendon resulting in tendinopathy and tearing. Complete biceps tears occur commonly in the rotator interval or more proximally near the supraglenoid tubercle. If a thinned biceps tendon is seen, it is likely a partial tear. Acute tears may also occur at the musculotendinous junction. Look for an empty bicipital groove in complete or retracted tears.
Biceps tendon subluxation/dislocation (▶ Fig. 2.25)	Look for an empty bicipital groove on axial and coronal images in cases of suspected biceps tendon dislocation. The tendon may be seen medial to the humeral head in dislocation. In subluxation, the tendon may displace anteromedially relative to the bicipital groove. Either condition may be associated with a tear of the subscapularis tendon. On MR arthrogram, assess for contrast extending along the lesser tuberosity as a sign of subscapularis tear.	Long head biceps subluxation and dislocation implies a tear of the transverse humeral ligament, which helps to maintain the location of the biceps tendon. The biceps tendon may also displace within or anterior/posterior to a torn subscapularis tendon. Note partial subscapularis tears are more common than complete tears. Subscapularis tears are also typically associated with supraspinatus tears.

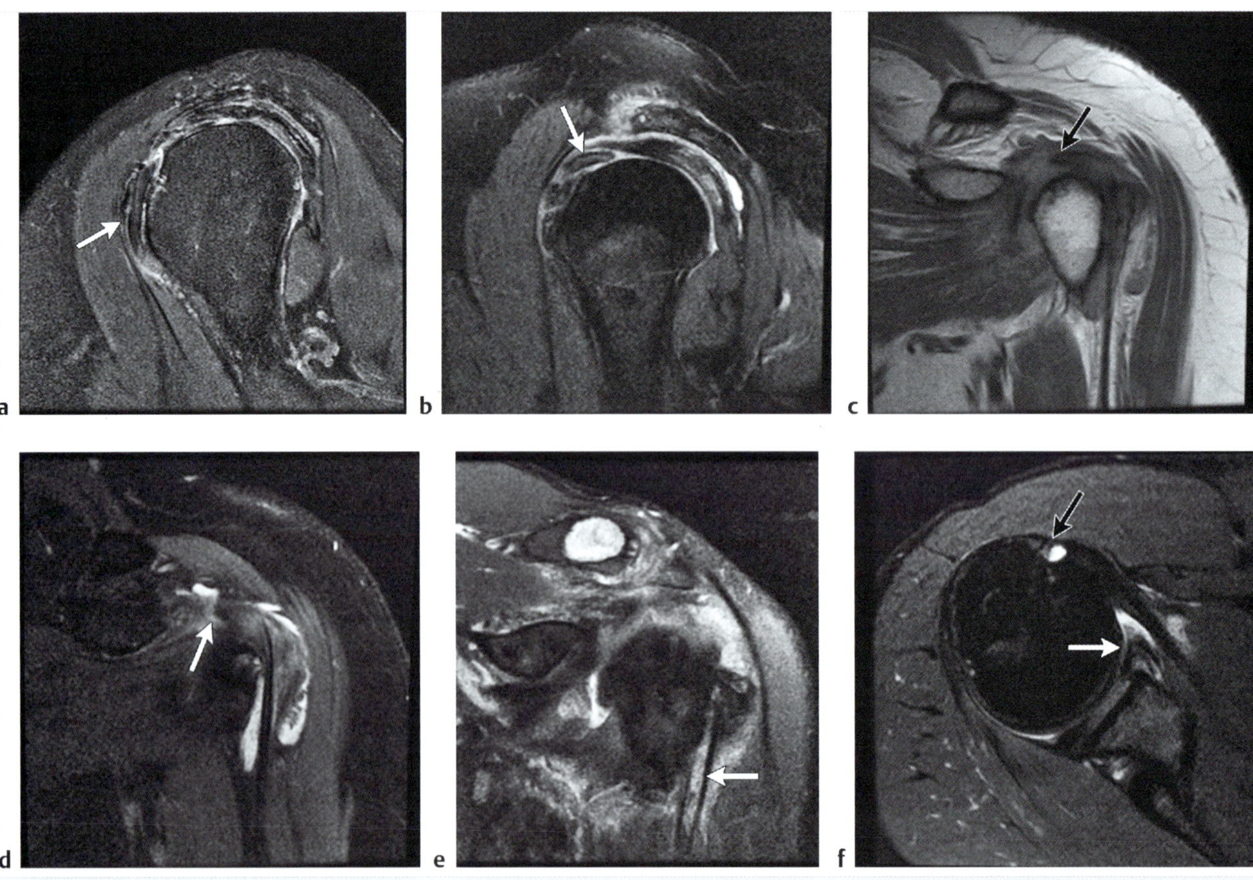

Fig. 2.24 Long head biceps tendon: tendinosis/tears. (a,b) Proximal biceps tendinopathy with increased intratendinous signal on oblique sagittal fat-suppressed T2-weighted imaging (FS T2WI) (arrows). (c) Torn proximal biceps tendon with the torn irregular end retracted from its anchor (arrows) on oblique coronal proton density–weighted imaging and (d) on oblique coronal FS T2WI. (e) Split tear of the biceps tendon (arrow) within the bicipital groove in a patient with rheumatoid arthritis on oblique coronal FS T2WI. Note high signal pannus within the tendon split. (f) Patient with a known retracted torn biceps tendon (not shown). Note an empty bicipital groove (black arrow) and an associated anterior labral tear (white arrow) on axial FS T2WI.

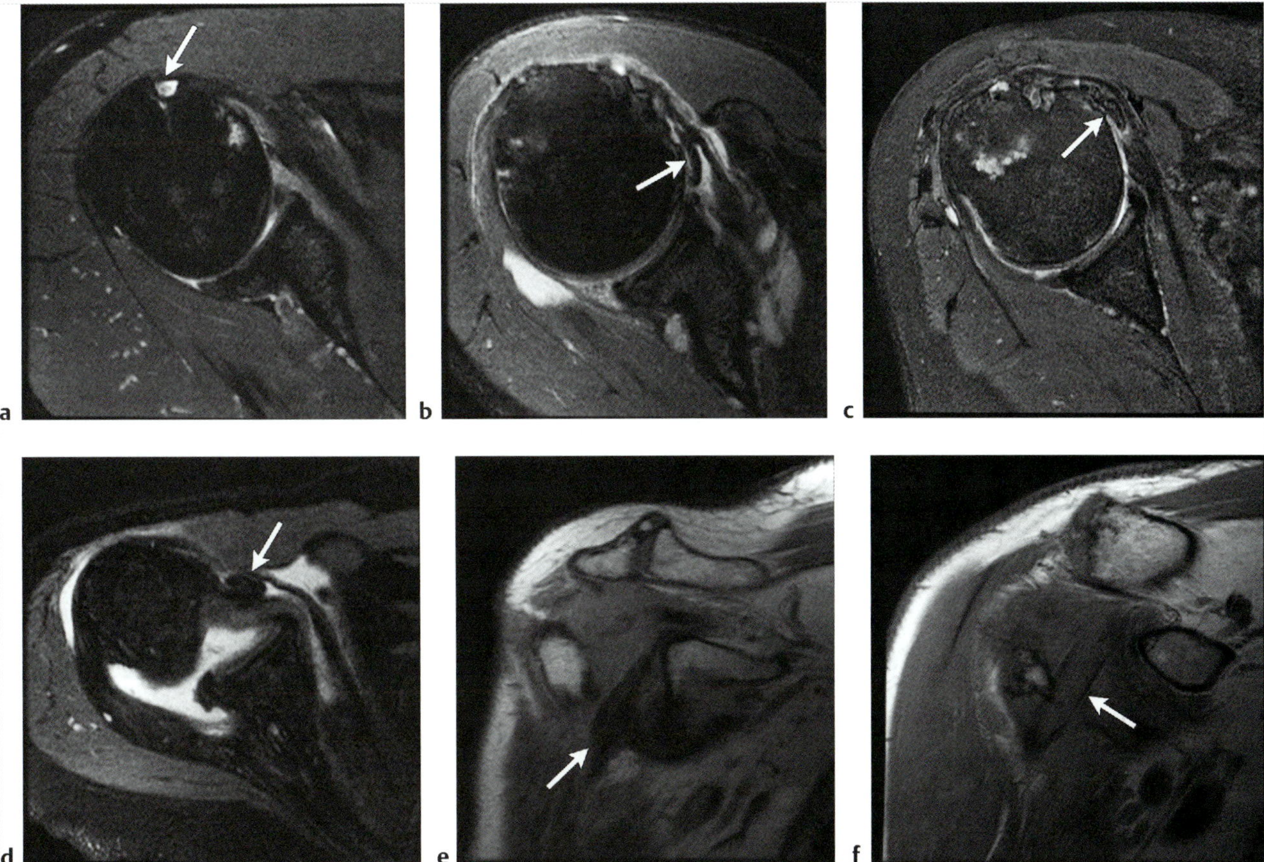

Fig. 2.25 Biceps tendon dislocation. (a) An empty bicipital groove containing only debris (arrow) should initiate a search for either a torn or dislocated biceps tendon on axial fat-suppressed (FS) T1 arthrogram. Examples of dislocated biceps tendons in different patients. (b) Note intra-articular long head biceps tendon dislocation (arrow) posterior to a thinned, wavy, partly torn subscapularis tendon on axial FS T1 arthrogram. (c) Biceps tendon dislocation (arrow) into a delamination tear of the subscapularis tendon on axial FS T2WI. (d) Dislocation of the biceps tendon (arrow) medial to the humeral shaft in a patient with a subscapularis tendon tear on axial FS T1 arthrogram. (e) Patient with medial biceps tendon dislocation (arrow) on oblique coronal PDWI. (f) Note a similar case of medial biceps tendon dislocation with severe biceps tendinopathy and medial angulation of the proximal tendon (arrow) on oblique coronal PDWI.

2.4.1 SLAP Lesions and Biceps Tendon Abnormalities Suggested Reading

[1] Chang EY, Fliszar E, Chung CB. Superior labrum anterior and posterior lesions and microinstability. Magn Reson Imaging Clin N Am 2012; 20: 277–294

[2] Modarresi S, Motamedi D, Jude CM. Superior labral anteroposterior lesions of the shoulder, I:Anatomy and anatomic variants. AJR Am J Roentgenol 2011; 197: 596–603

[3] Modarresi S, Motamedi D, Jude CM. Superior labral anteroposterior lesions of the shoulder, II: Mechanisms and classification. AJR Am J Roentgenol 2011; 197: 604–611

[4] Nakata W, Katou S, Fujita A, Nakata M, Lefor AT, Sugimoto H. Biceps pulley: normal anatomy and associated lesions at MR arthrography. Radiographics 2011; 31: 791–810

[5] Robinson G, Ho Y, Finlay K, Friedman L, Harish S. Normal anatomy and common labral lesions at MR arthrography of the shoulder. Clin Radiol 2006; 61: 805–821

[6] Tuite MJ, Rutkowski A, Enright T, Kaplan L, Fine JP, Orwin J. Width of high signal and extension posterior to biceps tendon as signs of superior labrum anterior to posterior tears on MRI and MR arthrography. AJR Am J Roentgenol 2005; 185: 1422–1428

2.5 Neural Abnormalities of the Shoulder

- Quadrilateral space syndrome
- Parsonage-Turner syndrome (acute brachial neuritis)
- Entrapment of the suprascapular nerve

Table 2.5 Neural abnormalities of the shoulder

Abnormalities	MRI findings	Comments
Quadrilateral space syndrome (▶ Fig. 2.26)	Fatty replacement of the teres minor muscle well seen on sagittal oblique T1 or proton density–weighted imaging (PDWI), typically without acute muscle edema. Check for a mass in the quadrilateral space, which is defined by the humerus laterally, the long head biceps medially, the teres minor superiorly, and the teres major inferiorly.	Etiology of the quadrilateral space syndrome is entrapment or compression of the axillary nerve posteriorly. The offending lesion is rarely identified; however, fibrous strands are often implicated. Other causes include dissecting paralabral cyst, mass (i.e., lipoma), or fracture. Patients may present with pain, weakness, or paresthesias.
Parsonage-Turner syndrome (acute brachial neuritis) (▶ Fig. 2.27)	Key imaging finding is abnormal signal on fat-suppressed T2-weighted imaging (FS T2WI) or short TI inversion recovery (STIR) (fluid-sensitive sequences) indicating muscle edema. Typically this condition involves the supraspinatus and infraspinatus muscles but may involve the deltoid and other muscles. The abnormal muscle signal is best identified on sagittal fluid-sensitive sequences where affected muscles can be compared with adjacent normal muscles.	Intramuscular denervation involving muscles of the shoulder girdle. Etiology is unknown, possibly viral. This painful disorder is not associated with trauma, thus allowing distinction from a brachial plexus injury.
Entrapment of the suprascapular nerve	Muscle edema implies an acute or subacute process. Atrophy with fatty infiltration implies a chronic process. Signal changes of the supraspinatus and infraspinatus muscles imply proximal nerve entrapment at the level of the suprascapular notch. Isolated signal changes of the infraspinatus imply distal nerve entrapment at the level of the spinoglenoid notch posteriorly and inferiorly. Look for possible offending ganglion/paralabral cyst as the cause of entrapment. Cyst will follow fluid signal: low on T1/PDWI and increased on FS T2WI.	Patients present with pain and muscle weakness. Look for a paralabral cyst and labral tear associated with muscle findings. Consider other masses impressing on the suprascapular nerve or sequela of trauma. Another cause for compression of the suprascapular nerve is the spinoglenoid ligament. The suprascapular nerve is a branch of the brachial plexus (C5–C6); therefore consider more proximal cervical spine pathology.

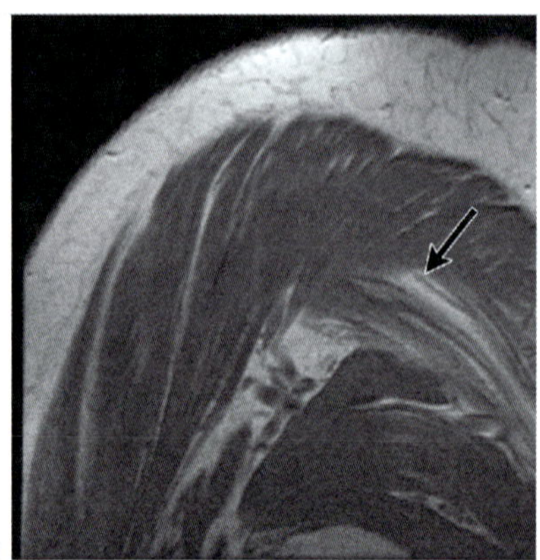

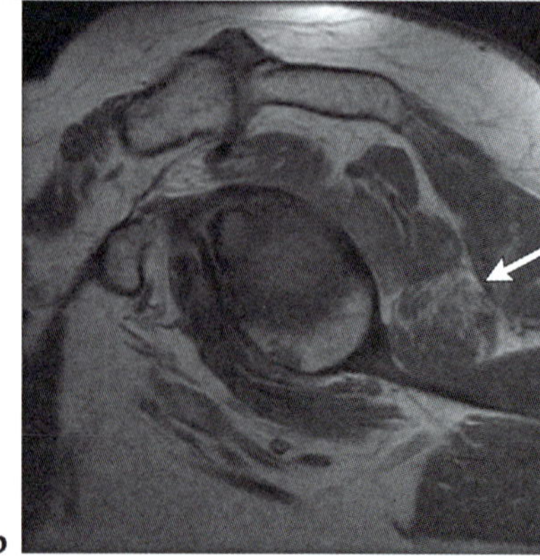

Fig. 2.26 Quadrilateral space syndrome. (a) Bands of fatty replacement (arrows) representing fatty atrophy involving the teres minor muscle are seen posteriorly on oblique coronal proton density–weighted imaging (PDWI) and (b) on oblique sagittal PDWI. Note difference when compared with surrounding normal muscles. No muscle edema was present on fluid-sensitive sequences.

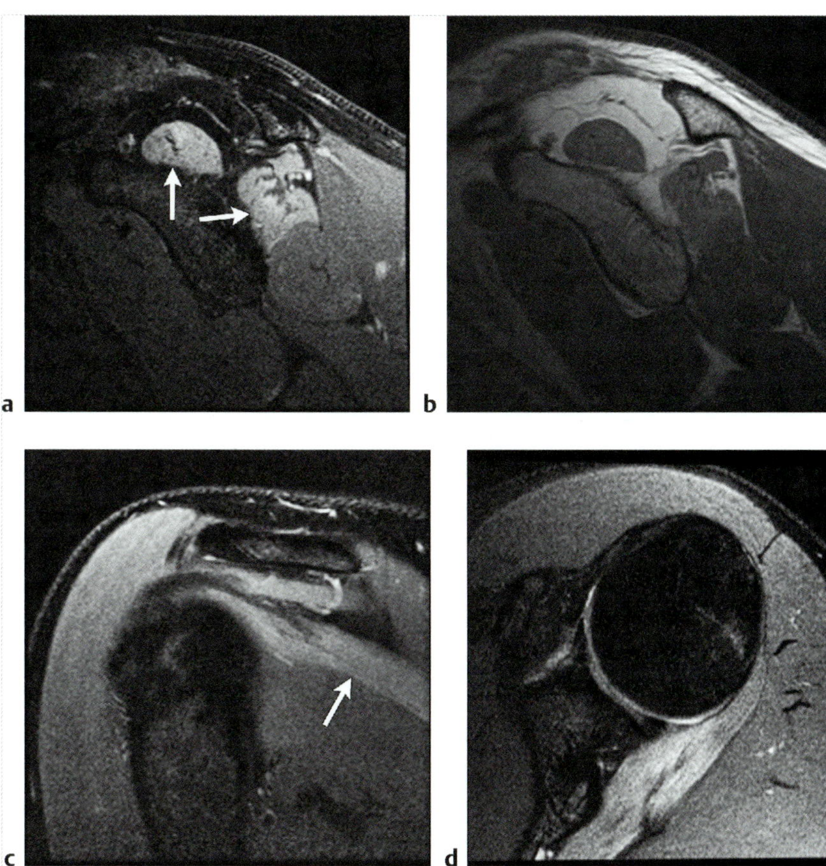

Fig. 2.27 Parsonage-Turner syndrome. (a) In this patient with acute pain without injury, note muscle edema of the supraspinatus and infraspinatus muscles (arrows) indicating acute or subacute involvement of the suprascapular nerve on oblique sagittal fat-suppressed T2-weighted imaging (FS T2WI). (b) Comparison oblique sagittal PDWI demonstrates subtle increased signal in the muscles. (c) Muscle edema can also be seen on oblique coronal FS T2WI (arrow) and (d) on axial FS T2WI.

2.5.1 Neural Abnormalities of the Shoulder Suggested Reading

[1] Scalf RE, Wenger DE, Frick MA, Mandrekar JN, Adkins MC. MRI findings of 26 patients with Parsonage-Turner syndrome. AJR Am J Roentgenol 2007; 189: W39–44

[2] Sofka CM, Lin J, Feinberg J, Potter HG. Teres minor denervation on routine magnetic resonance imaging of the shoulder. Skeletal Radiol 2004; 33: 514–518

2.6 Osseous Lesions and Arthritis of the Shoulder

- Little Leaguer's shoulder: proximal humeral epiphyseal overuse syndrome
- Avascular necrosis (AVN) of the humeral head
- Fracture of the greater tuberosity
- Osteoarthritis/degenerative joint disease
- Rheumatoid arthritis
- Synovial osteochondromatosis

Table 2.6 Osseous lesions and arthritis of the shoulder

Abnormalities	MRI findings	Comments
Little Leaguer's shoulder: proximal humeral epiphyseal overuse syndrome (▶ Fig. 2.28)	A Salter-Harris I fracture or epiphysiolysis of the proximal humeral growth plate. Look for widening of the lateral humeral physis on radiographs and on coronal or sagittal magnetic resonance (MR) images.	An injury most typically seen in 13- to 16-year-old baseball pitchers who undergo humeral rotational stress during throwing. Lateral involvement of the physis is more common due to the thicker periosteum of the posteromedial proximal humerus.
Avascular necrosis (AVN) of the humeral head (▶ Fig. 2.29)	On T1-weighted imaging (T1WI) and proton density–weighted imaging (PDWI) look for a low signal serpiginous line in the subchondral marrow and preservation of marrow fat centrally. On fat-suppressed T2-weighted imaging (FS T2WI) look for a low signal outer rim with a higher signal inner rim, the "double line sign." Diffuse marrow edema is seen on fluid-sensitive sequences. In later stages, subchondral collapse will result in a flattened portion of the humeral head or interruption of the normal curvature of the head. Cystic degenerative change may be seen later in the disease.	Check for history of predisposing factors, including steroid use and sickle cell disease. Although a humeral head fracture may appear similar to AVN of the humeral head, these usually occur in different locations. AVN often involves the superomedial margin of the humeral head, an uncommon location for fracture. Distinguish AVN from tumor by the preservation of marrow fat with AVN, although edema may be superimposed on marrow fat. With negative radiographs, magnetic resonance imaging (MRI) is a useful test to detect early AVN, which will present as marrow edema.

(continued on page 46)

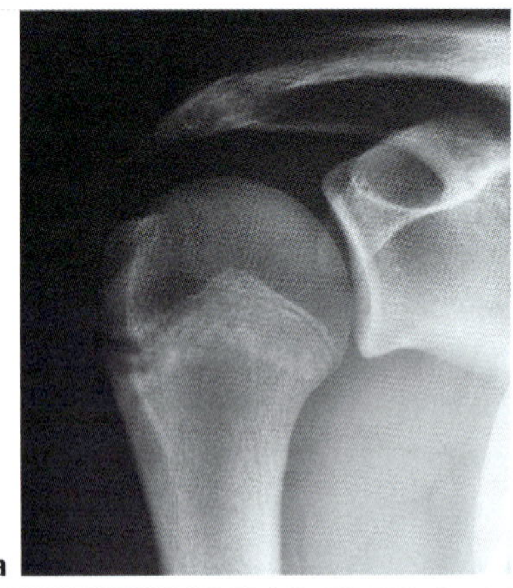

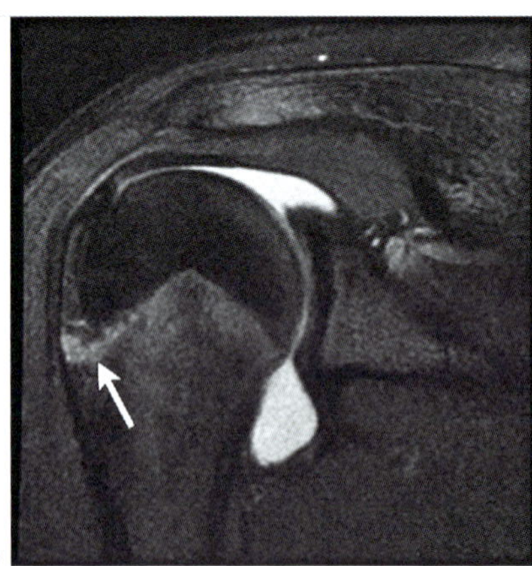

Fig. 2.28 Little Leaguer's shoulder. (a) Note widening of the lateral humeral physis on anteroposterior radiograph and (b) corresponding edema along the lateral physeal margin (arrow) on oblique coronal fat-suppressed T2-weighted imaging.

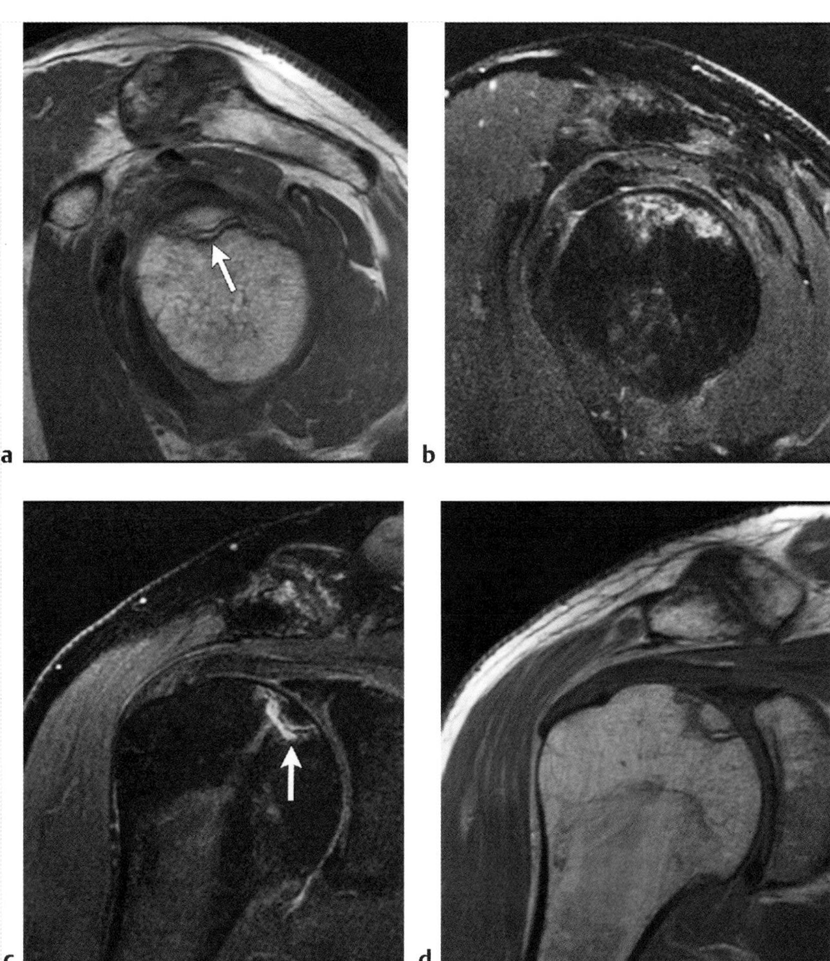

Fig. 2.29 Avascular necrosis (AVN) of the humeral head. (a) A serpiginous zone of low signal (arrow) in the superomedial margin of the humeral head is seen in AVN on oblique sagittal proton density–weighted imaging (PDWI). (b) There is corresponding marrow edema on oblique sagittal fat-suppressed T2-weighted imaging (FS T2WI). (c) In a different patient the "double line sign" of AVN with a low signal outer margin and an increased signal inner margin is seen (arrow) on oblique coronal FS T2WI. (d) Note preserved marrow fat centrally within the lesion on corresponding oblique coronal PDWI.

Table 2.6 (Cont.) Osseous lesions and arthritis of the shoulder

Abnormalities	MRI findings	Comments
Fracture of the greater tuberosity (▶ Fig. 2.30)	The common imaging finding on MRI is marrow edema at the greater tuberosity on fluid-sensitive sequences. Look for associated subtle cortical interruption and trabecular fracture on T1WI or PDWI. Marrow edema seen on FS T2WI will outline the fracture site. Fractures may not be displaced and often are not easily visible on radiographs. There may be only bone bruising without fracture fragment identification on MRI.	Greater tuberosity fractures are most commonly seen secondary to direct trauma or following anterior dislocation. Assess the condition of rotator cuff tendons attaching to the greater tuberosity fracture fragment. The Hills-Sachs lesion is considered a variant of the greater tuberosity fracture.
Osteoarthritis/degenerative joint disease (▶ Fig. 2.31)	The main benefit of MRI in evaluating osteoarthritis (OA) is to detect early cartilage degeneration before radiographic findings are evident. In early OA look for cartilage thinning, irregularities, fissures, and defects presenting as increased or fluid signal foci on FS T2WI within the normally intermediate signal cartilage. Findings are often seen centrally within the humeral head and along the posterior margin of the glenoid. Later findings of OA include osteophytosis, subchondral cyst formation, and synovial inflammation (SI). Subchondral cysts will typically be marginated by a low signal rim on PDWI. Synovitis typically presents as heterogeneous increased SI material within the glenohumeral joint on fluid-sensitive sequences.	Patients presenting with OA of the shoulder are typically older than those patients presenting with acute rotator cuff tears and instability. It is important to differentiate OA from septic arthritis, inflammatory arthropathy, and neuropathic changes.

(continued on page 48)

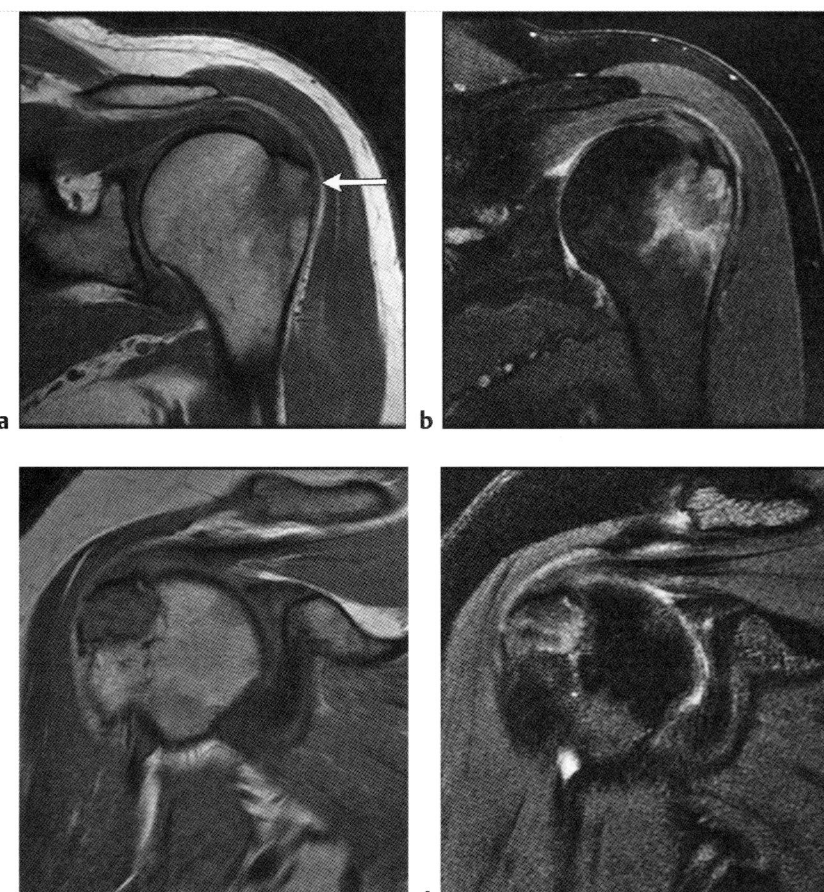

Fig. 2.30 Fracture of the greater tuberosity. (a) A radiographically occult, slightly displaced acute fracture of the greater tuberosity following trauma. Note the supraspinatus tendon remains attached to the fracture fragment (arrow) on oblique coronal proton density–weighted imaging (PDWI). (b) There is associated extensive marrow edema on oblique coronal fat-suppressed T2-weighted imaging (FS T2WI). (c) A larger example of a greater tuberosity fracture with displacement of the fragment on oblique coronal PDWI. (d) Because this injury was subacute, lesser marrow edema is found on oblique coronal FS T2WI.

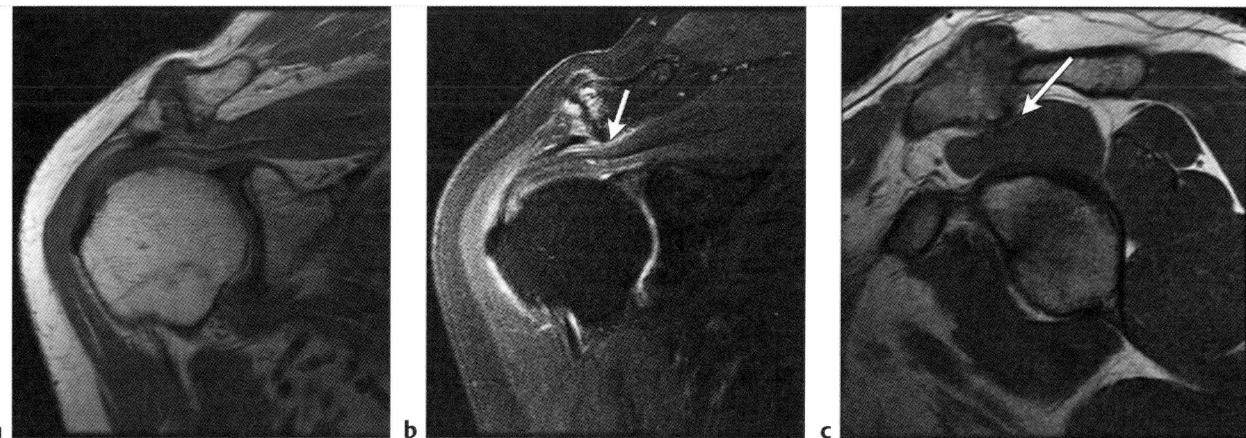

Fig. 2.31 Osteoarthritis/degenerative joint disease. (a) Acromioclavicular joint degeneration with spur/osteophyte formation at the joint, capsular fibrous hypertrophy, and subchondral cyst formation on oblique coronal proton density–weighted imaging (PDWI). (b) An associated impression on the supraspinatus musculotendinous junction (arrow) is seen on oblique coronal fat-suppressed T2-weighted imaging (FS T2WI). (c) More advanced example of acromioclavicular joint degeneration with marked hypertrophic changes and impression on the supraspinatus muscle (arrow) on oblique sagittal PDWI. (*continued*)

Table 2.6 (Cont.) Osseous lesions and arthritis of the shoulder

Abnormalities	MRI findings	Comments
Rheumatoid arthritis (▸ Fig. 2.32)	Findings of prominent synovitis, erosions, cartilage degeneration and loose bodies (rice bodies), and uniform joint space narrowing distinguish this entity from the osteophytosis and nonuniform joint space narrowing seen with OA. On T1WI and PDWI hypertrophied synovium will be of low to intermediate signal. On T2WI hypertrophied synovium will be of varied signal depending on the degree of fibrin, fibrotic material, and hemosiderin. Thickened synovium may demonstrate nodular or frondlike enhancement. Look for marginal bone erosions, joint effusion, bursal collections, and osseous and extra-articular cysts. Assess for possible resorption of the distal clavicle and involvement of other joints.	Rheumatoid arthritis is a chronic arthritic disease with symmetric involvement of peripheral joints. Joint destruction may occur as the disease progresses. Consider other inflammatory arthropathies.
Synovial osteochondromatosis (▸ Fig. 2.33)	Often recognized as multiple loose bodies within a joint. MR findings in osteochondromatosis vary depending on the degree of osseous tissue and cartilage within the nodular lesions. Low signal is characteristic of calcifications on routine MR sequences. Signal void may be seen in densely calcified lesions. Those portions of the lesions without calcification will show low/intermediate signal on T1WI and relatively increased signal on T2WI. Larger or more mature ossific foci may demonstrate a fatty marrow center and low signal rim. Postcontrast images demonstrate peripheral or septal enhancement.	Primary synovial osteochondromatosis occurs with metaplastic proliferation of cartilaginous and osseous elements within the synovial lining of joints. The resulting osteochondral nodules may detach and become loose bodies. Secondary synovial osteochondromatosis occurs in the setting of arthropathy such as OA or trauma. The loose bodies are formed as a result of avulsion of hyaline cartilage fragments. These loose bodies increase in size with nutrient supply from synovial fluid. Differential includes other inflammatory arthropathies including rheumatoid arthritis, PVNS, gout, and infectious arthritis.

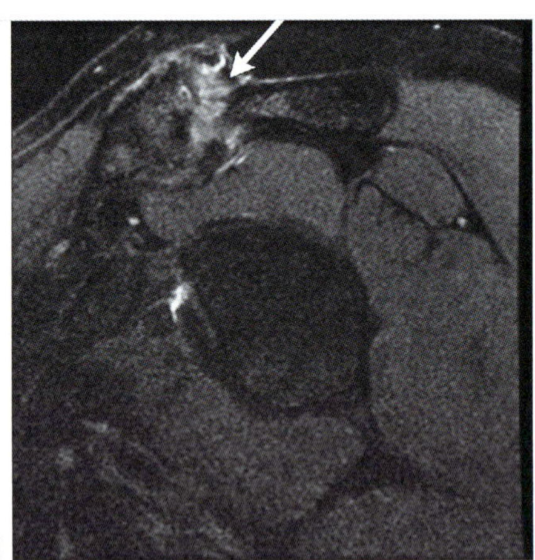

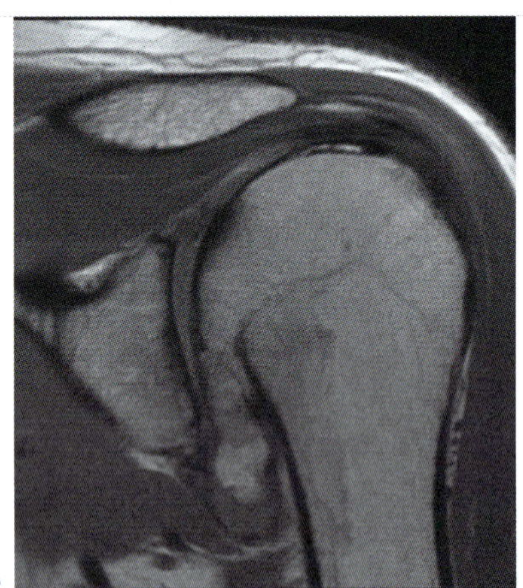

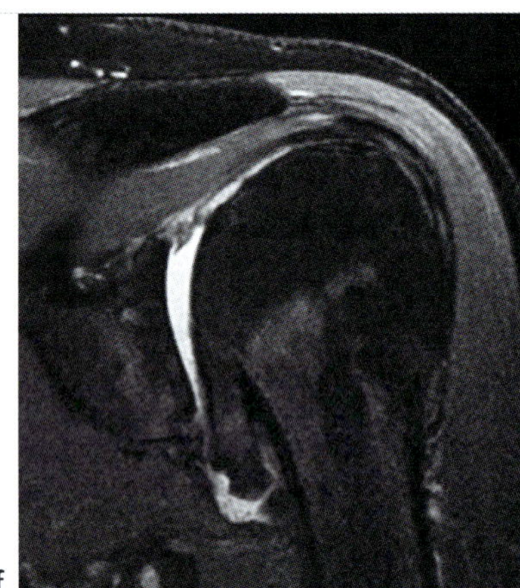

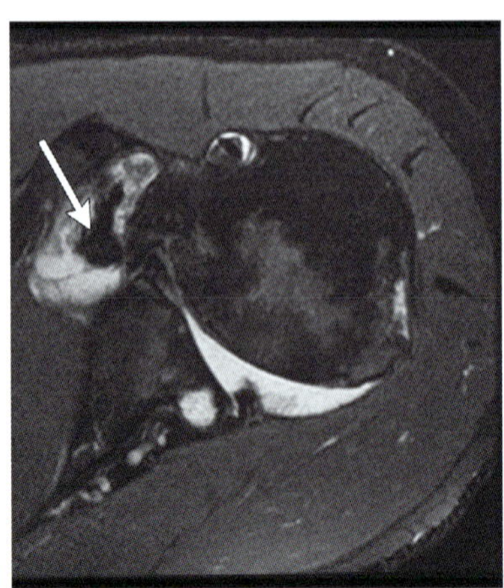

Fig. 2.31 (*continued*) (d) Note edema and fluid within and surrounding the acromioclavicular joint on oblique sagittal FS T2WI. (e) Severe glenohumeral osteoarthritis with marked osteophyte formation, full-thickness cartilage loss at the glenohumeral joint, and sclerosis on oblique coronal PDWI and (f) on corresponding oblique coronal FS T2WI. (g) Note low signal loose body anterior to the glenohumeral joint (arrow) on axial FS T2WI.

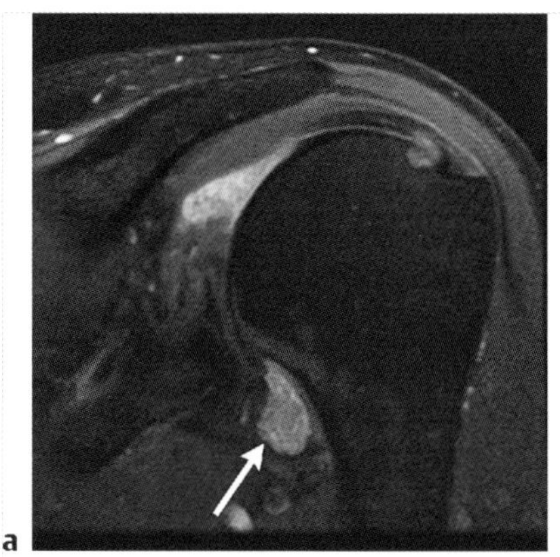

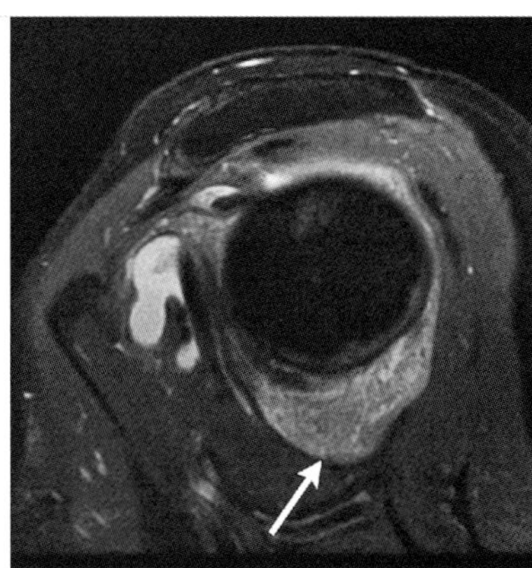

Fig. 2.32 Rheumatoid arthritis. (a) Proliferative synovium (pannus) with rice bodies and irregular intermediate signal foci within the shoulder joint (arrows) on oblique coronal fat-suppressed T2-weighted imaging (FS T2WI) and (b) on oblique sagittal FS T2WI.

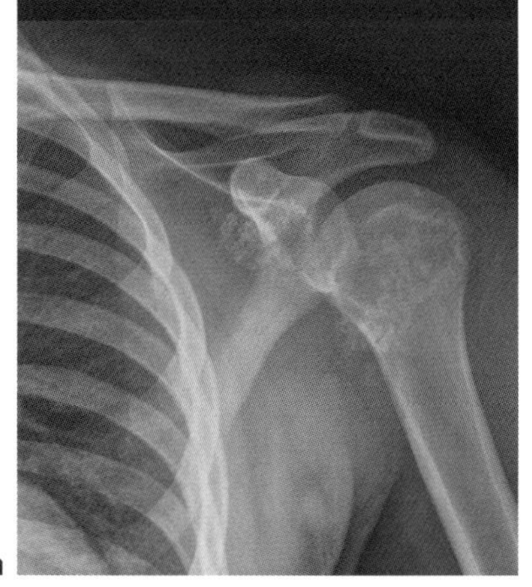

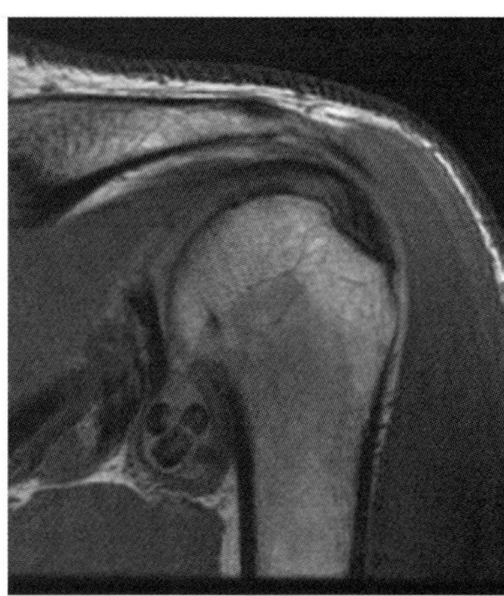

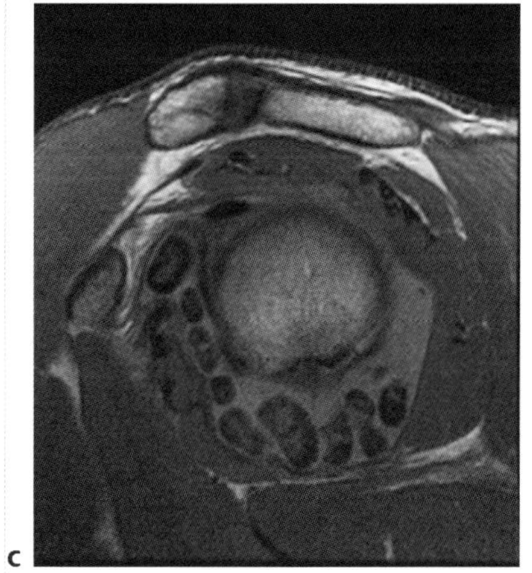

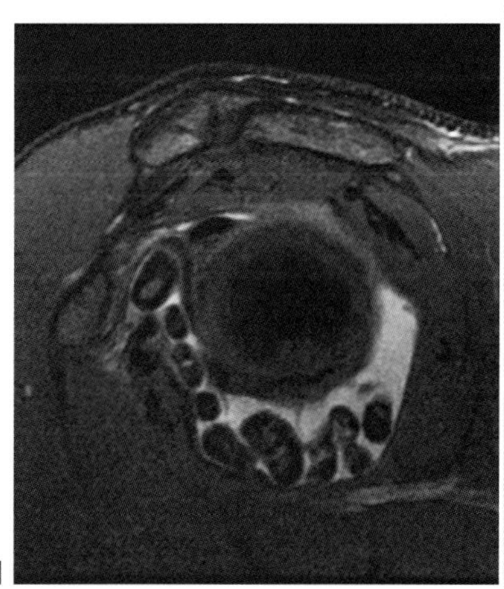

Fig. 2.33 Synovial osteochondromatosis. (a) Note multiple rim calcified nodular foci of varying size overlying the left shoulder joint on anteroposterior radiograph. (b) Variably sized foci of low signal correspond to radiographic finding on oblique coronal proton density–weighted imaging (PDWI), (c) oblique sagittal PDWI, and (d) oblique sagittal fat-suppressed T2-weighted imaging.

2.6.1 Osseous Lesions and Arthritis of the Shoulder Suggested Reading

[1] Emery KH. MR imaging in congenital and acquired disorders of the pediatric upper extremity. Magn Reson Imaging Clin N Am 2009; 17: 549–570

[2] Emery KH. Imaging of sports injuries of the upper extremity in children. Clin Sports Med 2006; 25: 543–568

[3] Rosas HG, Tuite MJ. The current state of imaging the articular cartilage of the upper extremity. Magn Reson Imaging Clin N Am 2011; 19: 407–423

2.7 Suggested Reading: The Shoulder

[1] Cook TS, Stein JM, Simonson S, Kim W. Normal and variant anatomy of the shoulder on MRI. Magn Reson Imaging Clin N Am 2011; 19: 581–594

[2] Fitzpatrick D, Walz DM. Shoulder MR imaging normal variants and imaging artifacts. Magn Reson Imaging Clin N Am 2010; 18: 615–632

[3] Stoller DW, Wolf EM, Li AE, Nottage WM, Tirman PFJ. The shoulder. In: Stoller DW, ed. Magnetic Resonance Imaging in Orthopaedics and Sports Medicine. 3rd ed. Baltimore, MD: Lippincott Williams & Wilkins; 2007:1131–1462

[4] Stoller DW, Tirman PFJ, Bredella MA, Beltran S, Branstetter RM, Blease SCP. Shoulder. In: Diagnostic Imaging Orthopaedics. Vol 1. Salt Lake City, UT: Amirsys; 2004:2–153

[5] Helms CA, Major NM, Anderson MW, Kaplan PA, Dussault R. Shoulder. In: Musculoskeletal MRI. 2nd ed. Philadelphia, PA: Saunders; 2009:177–223

[6] Chen Q, Miller TT, Pardon M, Beltran J. Normal shoulder. In: Pope TL, Bloem HL, Beltran J, Morrison WB, Wilson DJ, eds. Imaging of the Musculoskeletal System. Philadelphia, PA: Saunders; 2008:101–125

[7] Nomikos GC, Rafi M. Shoulder impingement syndromes. In: Pope TL, Bloem HL, Beltran J, Morrison WB, Wilson DJ, eds. Imaging of the Musculoskeletal System. Philadelphia, PA: Saunders; 2008:150–198

[8] Tuite MJ. Glenohumeral instability. In: Pope TL, Bloem HL, Beltran J, Morrison WB, Wilson DJ, eds. Imaging of the Musculoskeletal System. Philadelphia, PA: Saunders; 2008:199–220

[9] Farber AJ, Khanna AJ, Fayad LM, Johnson TS, McFarland EG. The shoulder. In: Khanna AJ, ed. MRI for Orthopaedic Surgeons. New York, NY: Thieme; 2010:97–117

Chapter 3

The Elbow

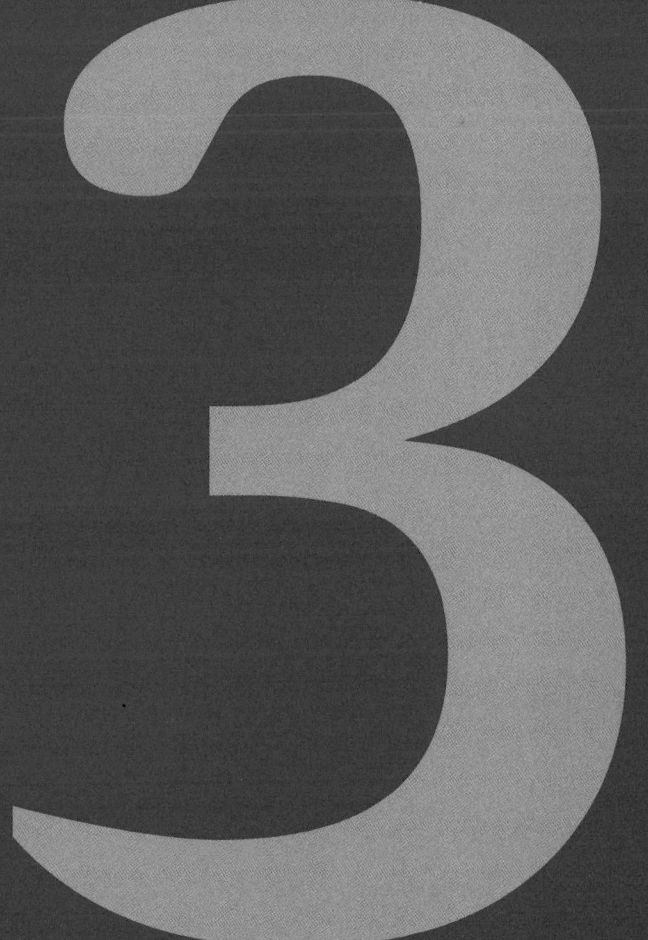

3 The Elbow

Gary M. Hollenberg

3.1 Lesions of the Elbow Ligaments

- Ulnar collateral ligament (UCL) partial and complete tears
- Radial collateral ligament (RCL) complex tears

Table 3.1 Lesions of the elbow ligaments

Abnormalities	MRI findings	Comments
Ulnar collateral ligament (UCL) partial and complete tears (▶ Fig. 3.1)	Injury to the ulnar collateral ligament is best seen on coronal magnetic resonance (MR) images. MR imaging findings include edema surrounding and within the UCL, lack of definition, and irregularity or discontinuity of the normally low signal ligament on fat-suppressed T2-weighted imaging (FS T2WI). Partial tears are typically seen distally at the ligament insertion on the sublime tubercle of the proximal ulna. Look for the "T" sign on fluid-sensitive sequences or on arthrography. High signal fluid will be seen wrapping around the sublime tubercle forming a "T" between the partially torn deep fibers of the anterior band and the tubercle. Partial tears will spare the more superficial UCL fibers. Check for associated sprain or partial tear of the common flexor tendon.	The anterior bundle of the UCL is the most important stabilizer to valgus stresses at the elbow. The ligament demonstrates a fanlike attachment to the medial epicondyle proximally, and tapers distally to the sublime tubercle. UCL injury is often seen in overhead throwers due to repetitive valgus stress seen in the late cocking phase and early acceleration phase of pitching. Similar injury is also seen in other overhead throwing activities. Partial tears are best diagnosed with arthrography. Note that there are also transverse and posterior bundles as part of the UCL complex, but not seen routinely.

(continued on page 54)

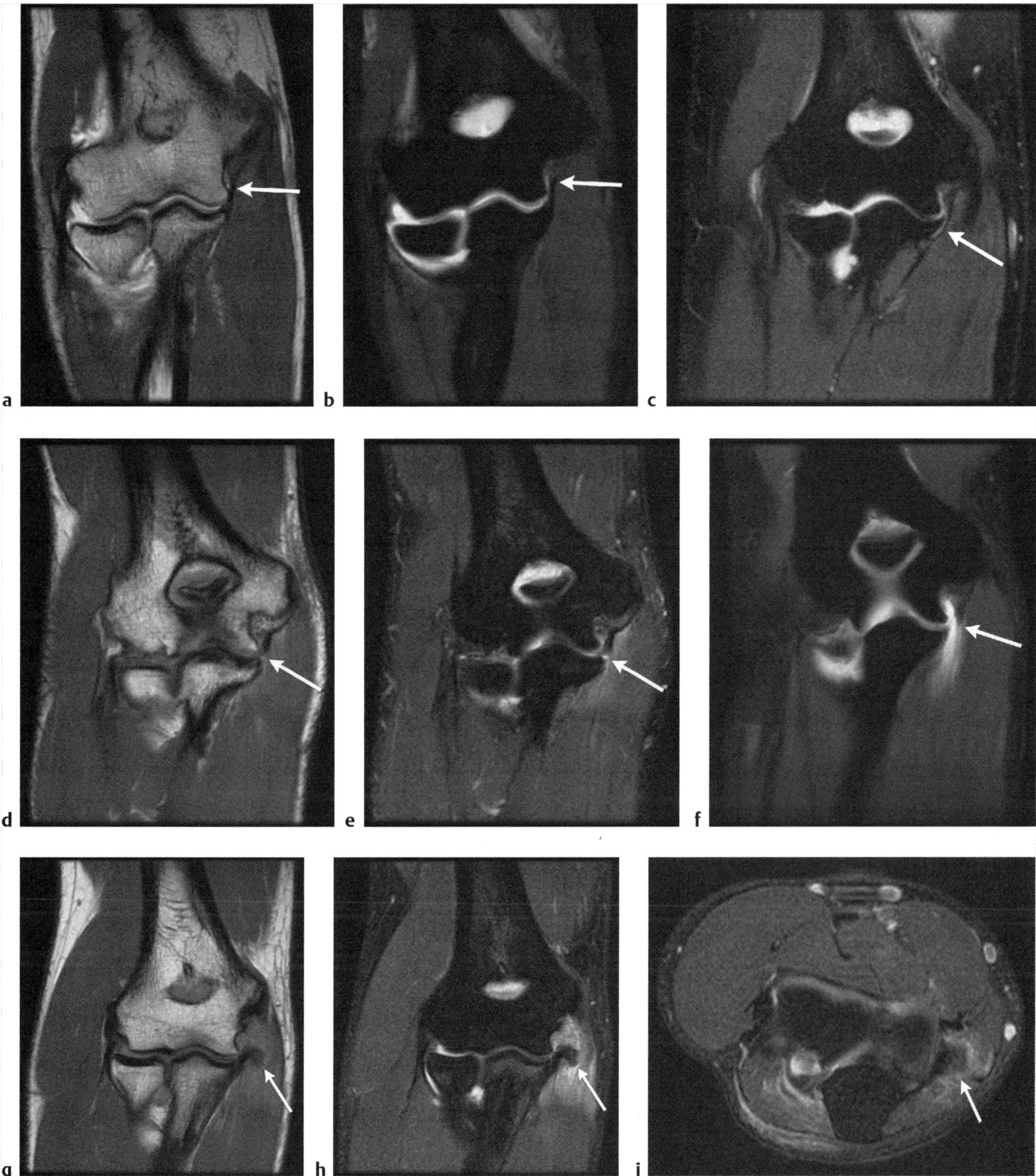

Fig. 3.1 (a) A normal ulnar collateral ligament (UCL) (anterior band) (arrow) demonstrating a thin low signal ligament extending from the medial epicondyle to the medial coronoid process/sublime tubercle on coronal proton density–weighted imaging (PDWI), and (b) coronal fat-suppressed (FS) T1 arthrogram (arrow). Note the proximal ligament fanning out normally at its attachment. (c) A partial tear of the UCL with a "T" sign formed by high signal joint fluid extending between the sublime tubercle and the UCL (arrow) on coronal FS T2-weighted imaging (T2WI) post–saline arthrogram. (d) Example of a larger partial tear of the UCL with separation between the UCL and sublime tubercle on coronal PDWI (arrow). (e) Note high signal fluid at the tear site (arrow) and edema representing a muscle strain in the flexor pronator group on coronal FS T2WI. (f) A complete tear of the UCL (arrow) with contrast material extending through the tear and into the flexor pronator group on FS T1 arthrogram. (g) Complete UCL tear from the medial epicondyle with medial angulation of the ligament (arrow) on coronal PDWI. (h) Note extensive edema in the flexor pronator group and bulbous appearance to the torn UCL on coronal FS T2WI and (i) axial FS T2WI (arrows).

Table 3.1 (Cont.) Lesions of the elbow ligaments

Abnormalities	MRI findings	Comments
Radial collateral ligament (RCL) complex tears (▶ Fig. 3.2)	Sprains of the normally low signal radial collateral complex will demonstrate edema within and surrounding the ligament, which may also be of abnormal caliber. With partial tears, the ligament will demonstrate an irregular contour. Ligament discontinuity with intervening fluid will be seen with complete tears. These findings are best demonstrated on coronal FS T2WI or on FS T1 arthrogram. Most injuries will occur near the lateral epicondylar attachment of the RCL and the lateral ulnar collateral ligament (LUCL). Check for associated tears of the common extensor tendon.	The most important components of the RCL complex are the RCL proper and the LUCL. The RCL complex lies immediately deep to the common extensor tendon. Note that the distal RCL attaches to the annular ligament, allowing fluid to normally dissect between these structures. The more posteriorly positioned LUCL may be seen coursing obliquely across the radial head to its insertion on the proximal ulna. Injuries can occur due to chronic varus stress or acute injury such as posterior dislocation. Patients with RCL complex injuries are predisposed to posterolateral rotary instability of the elbow, which can progress from subluxation to dislocation.

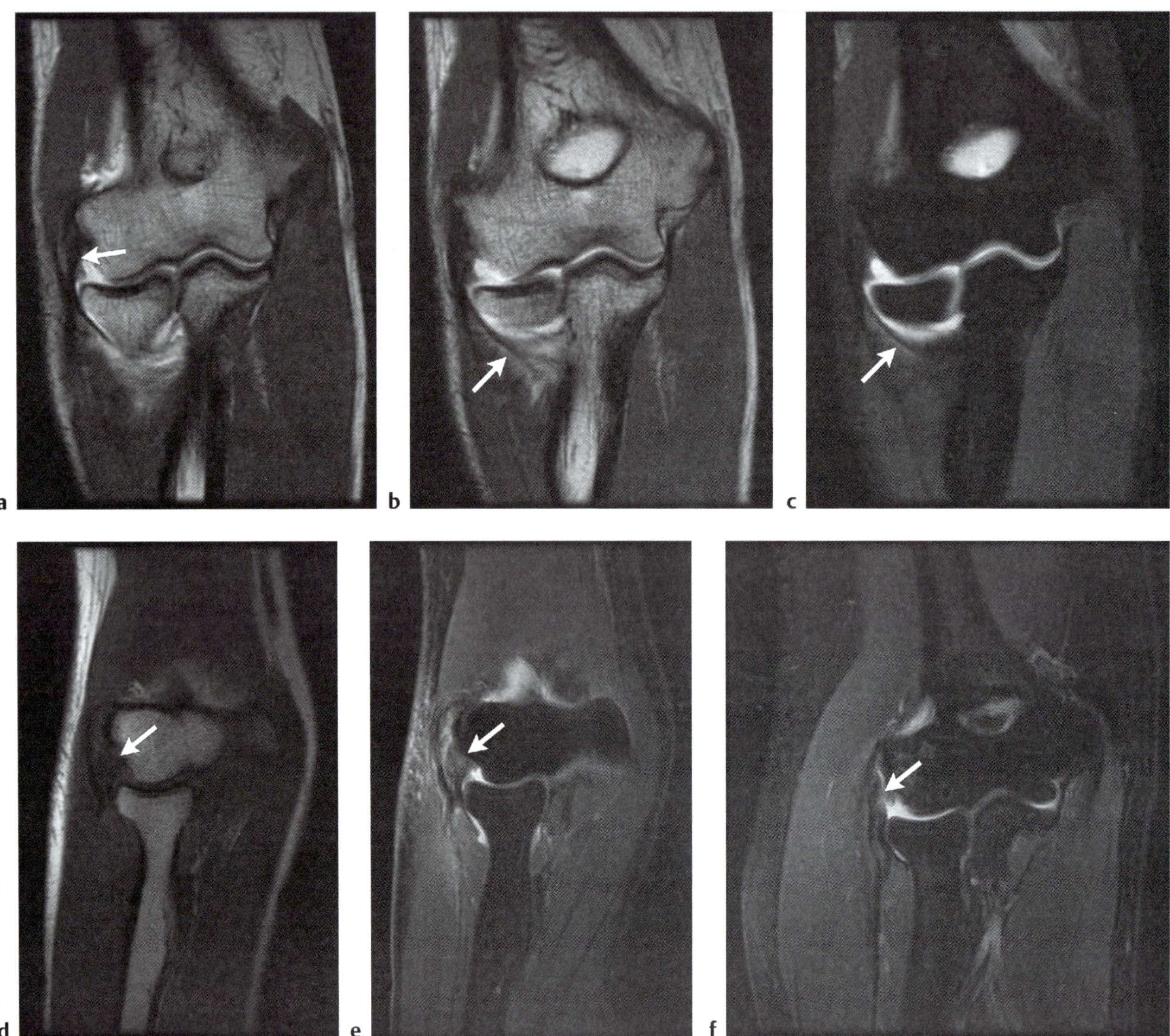

Fig. 3.2 (a) A normally thin low signal radial collateral ligament (RCL) proper (arrow) is seen deep to the common extensor origin coursing from the lateral epicondyle to the annular ligament on coronal proton density–weighted imaging (PDWI). (b) A slightly more posterior image demonstrates the lateral ulnar collateral ligament (LUCL) portion of the RCL complex coursing from the more posterior aspect of the lateral epicondyle to the lateral ulna (arrows) on coronal PDWI and on (c) coronal fat-suppressed (FS) T1 arthrogram. (d) A partial tear of the proximal RCL (arrow) with ligament thickening and increased signal proximally. Note adjacent tearing and tendinopathy of the common extensor tendon on coronal PDWI. (e) The corresponding FS T2-weighted imaging (T2WI) demonstrates increased proximal RCL signal and thickening (arrow) with associated muscle sprain at the common extensor origin. (f) In a different patient, a large partial tear of the proximal RCL (arrow) with mild underlying marrow edema of the lateral epicondyle. Waviness of the adjacent common extensor tendon indicating partial tear on coronal FS T2WI post–saline arthrogram. (*continued*)

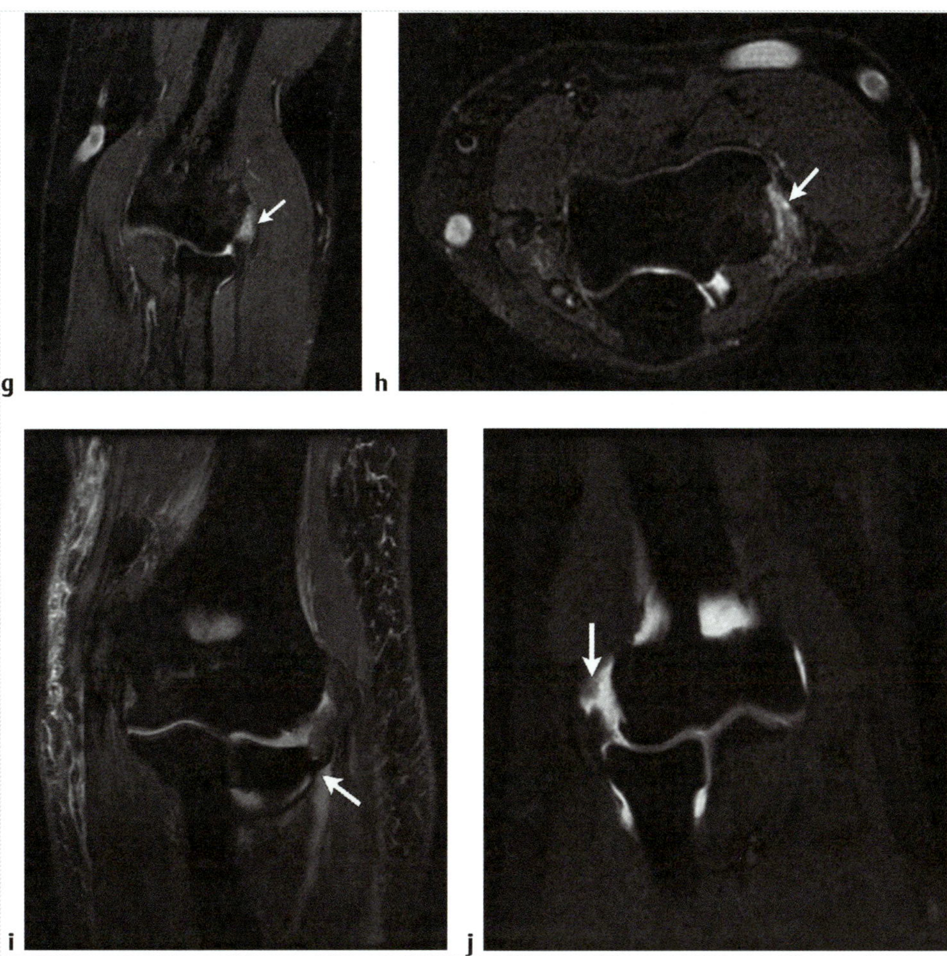

Fig. 3.2 (*continued*) (g) Full-thickness tear of the RCL and adjacent partial tear of the common extensor tendon (arrow). Note the lack of definition between these two structures on coronal FS T2WI. (h) Fluid signal within the RCL tear site is seen on corresponding axial FS T2WI (arrow). (i) Avulsion of the lateral ulnar collateral ligament (LUCL) from the lateral epicondyle. Edema extends along the thickened LUCL (arrow). Note overlying common extensor tendinopathy and muscle sprain on coronal FS T2WI. (j) Avulsion with lateral displacement of the radial collateral ligament (arrow) on coronal FS T1 arthrogram.

3.1.1 Lesions of the Elbow Ligaments Suggested Reading

[1] Sampaio ML, Schweitzer ME. Elbow magnetic resonance imaging variants and pitfalls. Magn Reson Imaging Clin N Am 2010; 18: 633–642

[2] Stein JM, Cook TS, Simonson S, Kim W. Normal and variant anatomy of the elbow on magnetic resonance imaging. Magn Reson Imaging Clin N Am 2011; 19: 609–619

3.2 Lesions of the Elbow Tendons

- Common extensor tendinopathy/lateral epicondylitis: "tennis elbow"
- Common flexor tendinopathy/medial epicondylitis: "pitcher's (or golfer's) elbow"
- Biceps tendinopathy and tears
- Brachialis muscle strain/tendinopathy
- Triceps tendon tear

Table 3.2 Lesions of the elbow tendons

Abnormalities	MRI findings	Comments
Common extensor tendinopathy/lateral epicondylitis: "tennis elbow" (▶ Fig. 3.3)	Increased signal within the normally low signal common extensor tendon attachment on the lateral epicondyle is seen with tendinopathy. Signal changes are visible on routine sequences but are best seen on fat-suppressed T2-weighted imaging (FS T2WI). Changes may be seen on coronal, axial, and sagittal images. Morphological changes to the tendon include proximal thickening and blurring of tendon fibers in cases of tendinopathy. Assess for fluid-filled gaps representing the site of partial or complete tears. Chronic tears may not demonstrate fluid due to the presence of intermediate signal scar. Look for associated tears of the underlying radial collateral ligament complex. Marrow signal changes in the underlying lateral epicondyle are unusual in our experience.	Lateral epicondylitis is the most common cause of lateral elbow pain. This condition is a chronic tendinopathy of the extensor/supinator group arising from the lateral epicondyle. This abnormality results from repetitive microtrauma, repair, and degeneration with scar and partial tearing. It is seen with chronic repetitive varus stress on the common extensor tendon most commonly involving the extensor carpi radialis brevis tendon. Evaluate for entrapment of the posterior interosseous nerve in patients with lateral elbow pain but without common extensor tendon abnormalities.

(continued on page 58)

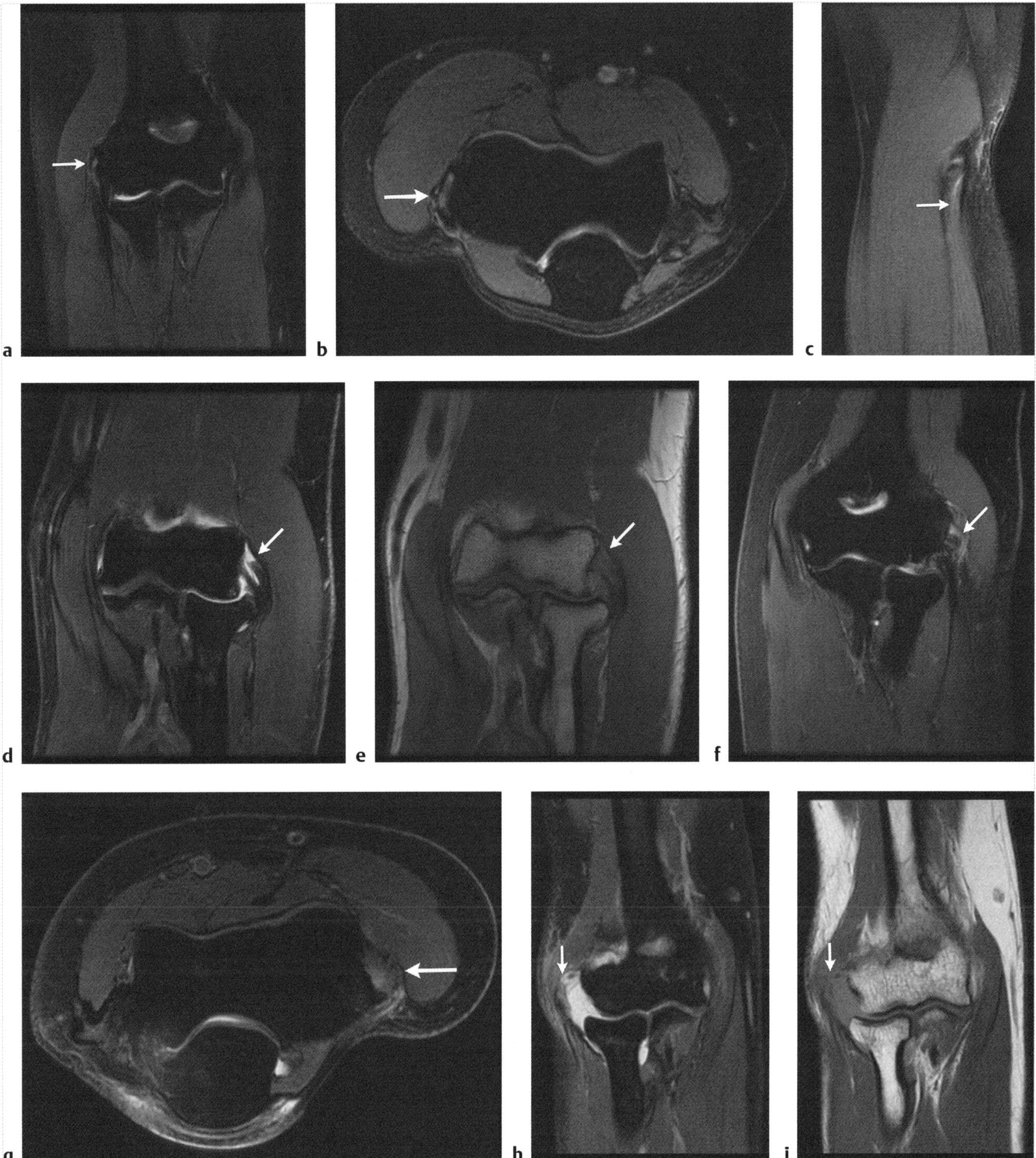

Fig. 3.3 (a) Partial tear of the normally low signal common extensor tendon origin (arrow) with increased signal noted at the tear site on coronal fat-suppressed T2-weighted imaging (FS T2WI). Note low signal intact radial collateral ligament (RCL) deep to the common extensor tendon. (b) Corresponding axial FS T2WI demonstrates linear increased T2 signal at the tear site (arrow). (c) On sagittal FS T2WI, linear high signal in the common extensor tendon tear extends into the musculotendinous junction, representing a superimposed muscle strain (arrow). (d) Partial tears of the RCL and common extensor tendon in a tennis player with lateral elbow pain. High T2 signal fluid surrounds the RCL and partly torn common extensor tendon on coronal FS T2WI post–saline arthrogram (arrow). Note chondral wear and geode formation at the radiocapitellar joint. (e) The corresponding coronal proton density–weighted imaging (PDWI) demonstrates intermediate signal fluid surrounding the partly torn RCL and common extensor tendon (arrow). (f) Complete tear of the common extensor tendon with waviness and retraction of fibers (arrow) on coronal FS T2WI. Note associated abnormal morphology and partial tear of the RCL. (g) Corresponding axial FS T2WI demonstrates edema at the site of tear (arrow). (h) Complete tear of the common extensor tendon with lateral displacement, and associated avulsion of the lateral ulnar collateral ligament on coronal FS T2WI (arrow). (i) Corresponding coronal PDWI demonstrates intermediate signal fluid between the torn tendon and ligament (arrow) and the lateral epicondyle.

Table 3.2 (Cont.) Lesions of the elbow tendons

Abnormalities	MRI findings	Comments
Common flexor tendinopathy/medial epicondylitis: "pitcher's (or golfer's) elbow" (▶ Fig. 3.4)	Increased signal within the normally low signal common flexor tendon attachment on the medial epicondyle. Signal changes are visible on routine sequences but are best seen on FS T2WI. Tendinopathy will demonstrate abnormal intermediate signal on FS T2WI, commonly seen with tendon thickening, although thinning may be seen in other cases. With partial and complete tears, fluid signal will be identified at the tear site. There may be adjacent muscle edema in the flexor pronator group, which coalesces to form the common flexor tendon. Look for associated tears of the ulnar collateral ligament (UCL) complex and ulnar nerve abnormalities.	Medial epicondylitis (also known as "medial tennis elbow") is the result of repetitive valgus stress resulting in tendinopathy of the flexor pronator group. The pronator teres and flexor carpi radialis are usually the involved muscles. Tendinopathy and tears of the common flexor tendon are associated with UCL injuries and ulnar neuritis. Note the importance of true coronal images bisecting the epicondyles to adequately profile the common flexor and extensor tendons and collateral ligaments.

(continued on page 60)

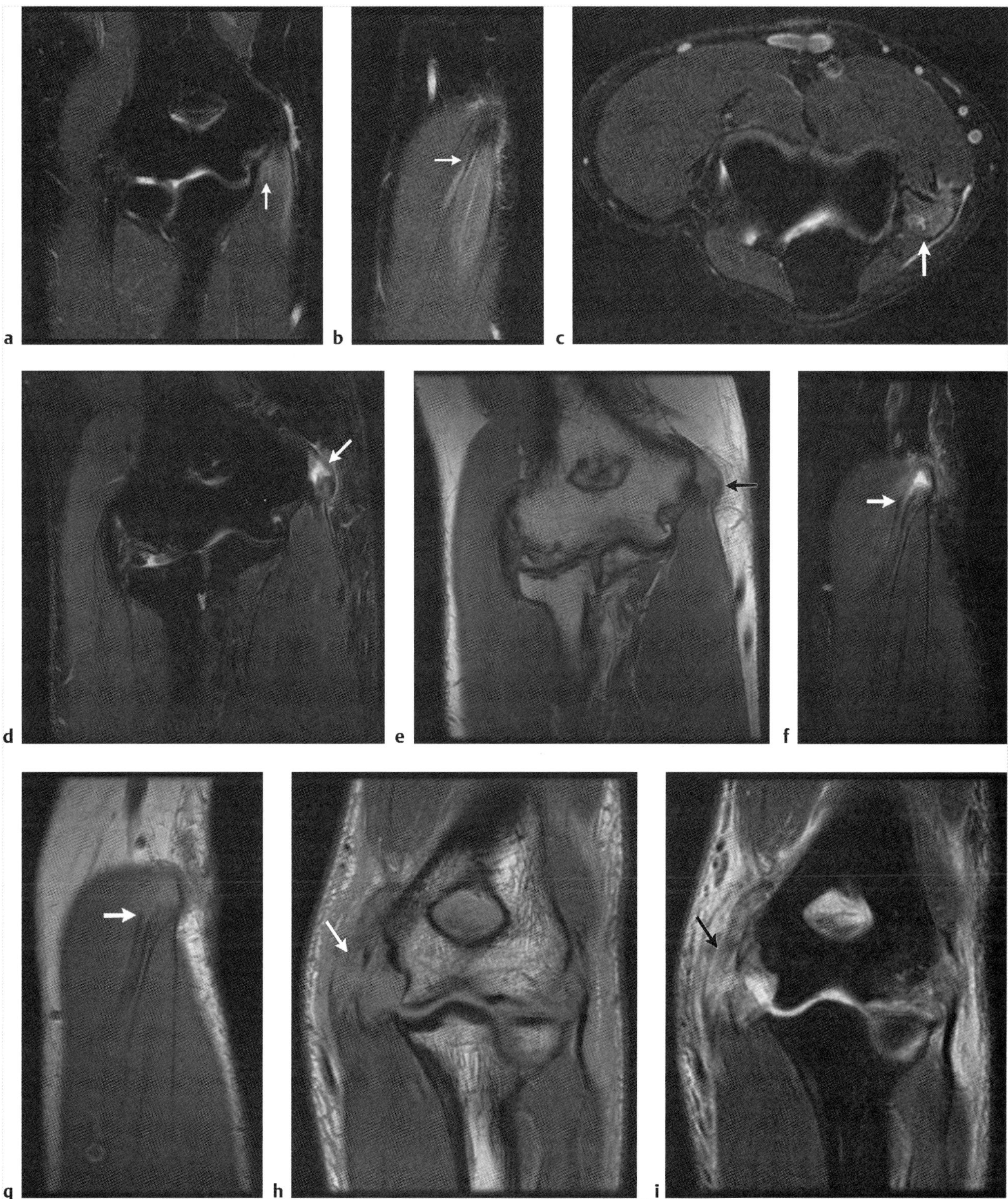

Fig. 3.4 (a) Strain of the flexor pronator group and common flexor tendinopathy in a patient with medial elbow pain. Note increased signal muscle edema in the flexor pronator group on coronal fat-suppressed T2-weighted imaging (FS T2WI) (arrow). (b) Corresponding sagittal FS T2WI demonstrates feathery appearance of muscle edema extending to the flexor pronator origin on the medial epicondyle (arrow). (c) Muscle edema is noted adjacent to the intact ulnar collateral ligament on axial FS T2WI (arrow). (d) Large partial tear of the normally low signal common flexor tendon with tendon retraction and fluid (arrow) at the tear site on coronal FS T2WI. (e) Note the intermediate signal retracted tendon (arrow) on coronal proton density–weighted imaging (PDWI). (f) On sagittal FS T2WI, note high signal fluid at the tear site and the wavy appearance of the torn common flexor tendon (arrow). (g) Corresponding sagittal PDWI demonstrates wavy retracted tendon fibers (arrow) distal to the intermediate signal fluid. (h) Complete tears of the common flexor tendon and ulnar collateral ligament (arrow) following posterior elbow dislocation. In addition, note tear of the RCL and partial tear of the common extensor tendon on coronal PDWI. (i) Extensive soft tissue edema is seen about the site of the torn common flexor tendon and flexor pronator muscles (arrow). Also note high signal edema due to tearing of the lateral structures on coronal FS T2WI.

Table 3.2 (Cont.) Lesions of the elbow tendons

Abnormalities	MRI findings	Comments
Biceps tendinopathy and tears (▶ Fig. 3.5)	Abnormal signal within the distal biceps tendon is best seen on axial images obtained to include the radial tuberosity. Tendinopathy and partial tears may appear similar with increased signal within the distal tendon on routine proton density–weighted imaging (PDWI) and FS T2WI. Partial tears may be distinguished by the presence of fluid signal within a thinned distal tendon. The partly torn fibers may be bulbous and retracted. Bicipitoradial bursitis, radial tubercle marrow edema, or edematous changes in more proximal soft tissues may help confirm a partial tear. Complete tears are easier to detect by the absence of an intact tendon along its expected course. More proximal images in the axial and sagittal plane will help determine the size of the tendon gap. The proximal biceps tendon will often be thickened, wavy, or bulbous in appearance. Edema in the antecubital fossa often surrounding the torn proximal end is well seen on FS T2WI.	The biceps muscle is positioned superficial to the brachialis muscle. A single tendon is usually seen extending to the radial tubercle; however, a bifid tendon can be seen. Most biceps tendon ruptures are complete and occur with a single traumatic event involving forced extension from a flexed elbow. The bicipital aponeurosis (lacertus fibrosus) arises from the distal biceps muscle and courses medially. The aponeurosis serves to maintain the location of the normal biceps tendon and may prevent retraction of a completely torn tendon and mask the diagnosis on exam. Magnetic resonance imaging (MRI) is useful in the diagnosis of tendon rupture because it allows for surgical planning. With suspected biceps tears, be sure to extend imaging proximally to allow identification of the torn tendon end or to visualize injury to the musculotendinous junction. Sagittal images will often demonstrate the retracted torn tendon.

(continued on page 62)

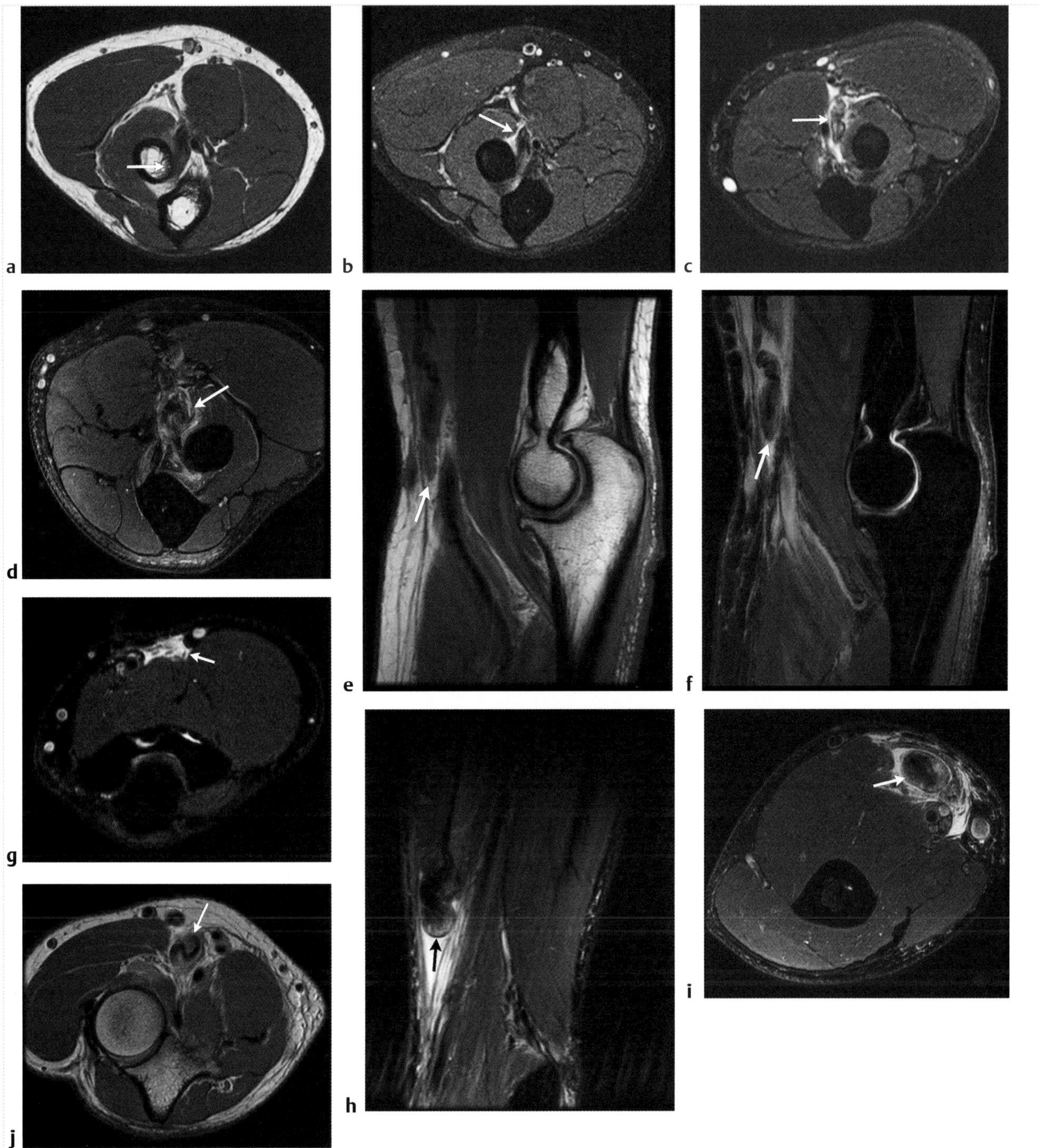

Fig. 3.5 (a) Biceps tendinopathy with increased signal within the normally low signal biceps tendon (arrow) is seen at the attachment on the radial tuberosity on axial proton density–weighted imaging (PDWI). (b) Corresponding axial fat-suppressed T2-weighted imaging (FS T2WI) demonstrating increased tendon signal and a small amount of fluid signal within the bicipitoradial bursa (arrow) between the tendon and radial tuberosity. (c) In a different patient, biceps tendinopathy and partial tearing of the distal biceps tendon (arrow) with increased T2 signal and a lobulated tendon contour on axial FS T2WI. (d) A more severe example of a distal tendon partial tear with a thinned intact distal tendon remnant. There is enlargement, a bulbous appearance, and retraction of the partly torn tendon (arrow) on axial FS T2WI. (e) Distal biceps tendon tear with retraction from the radial tuberosity. Note wavy retracted tendon (arrow) on sagittal PDWI. (f) Corresponding sagittal FS T2WI demonstrates the torn retracted tendon (arrow) surrounded by high signal fluid/hemorrhage. (g) A high signal fluid-filled gap (arrow) is seen in a different patient at the expected location of a torn and retracted biceps tendon on axial FS T2WI. (h) Additional example of a torn and retracted biceps tendon with the torn and retracted thickened end demonstrating a bulbous appearance (arrows) on sagittal FS T2WI and (i) axial FS T2WI. (j) Note the serpiginous appearance of a torn and retracted biceps tendon (arrow) in a different patient on axial PDWI.

Table 3.2 (Cont.) Lesions of the elbow tendons

Abnormalities	MRI findings	Comments
Brachialis muscle strain/tendinopathy (▸ Fig. 3.6)	Look for muscle edema visible on FS T2WI with brachialis muscle strains. Hematomas will be of variable signal on T1 and PDWI depending on age, but are often of increased signal on FS T2WI. Increased tendon signal on both PDWI and FS T2WI indicates tendinopathy.	The brachialis muscle lies deep to the biceps muscle. The brachialis tendon can be followed to its attachment on the coronoid process and ulnar tuberosity. Brachialis tendon injuries are seen with activities such as climbing and multiple pull-ups. In patients with anterior elbow pain, check both the biceps and the brachialis tendon attachments.

(continued on page 64)

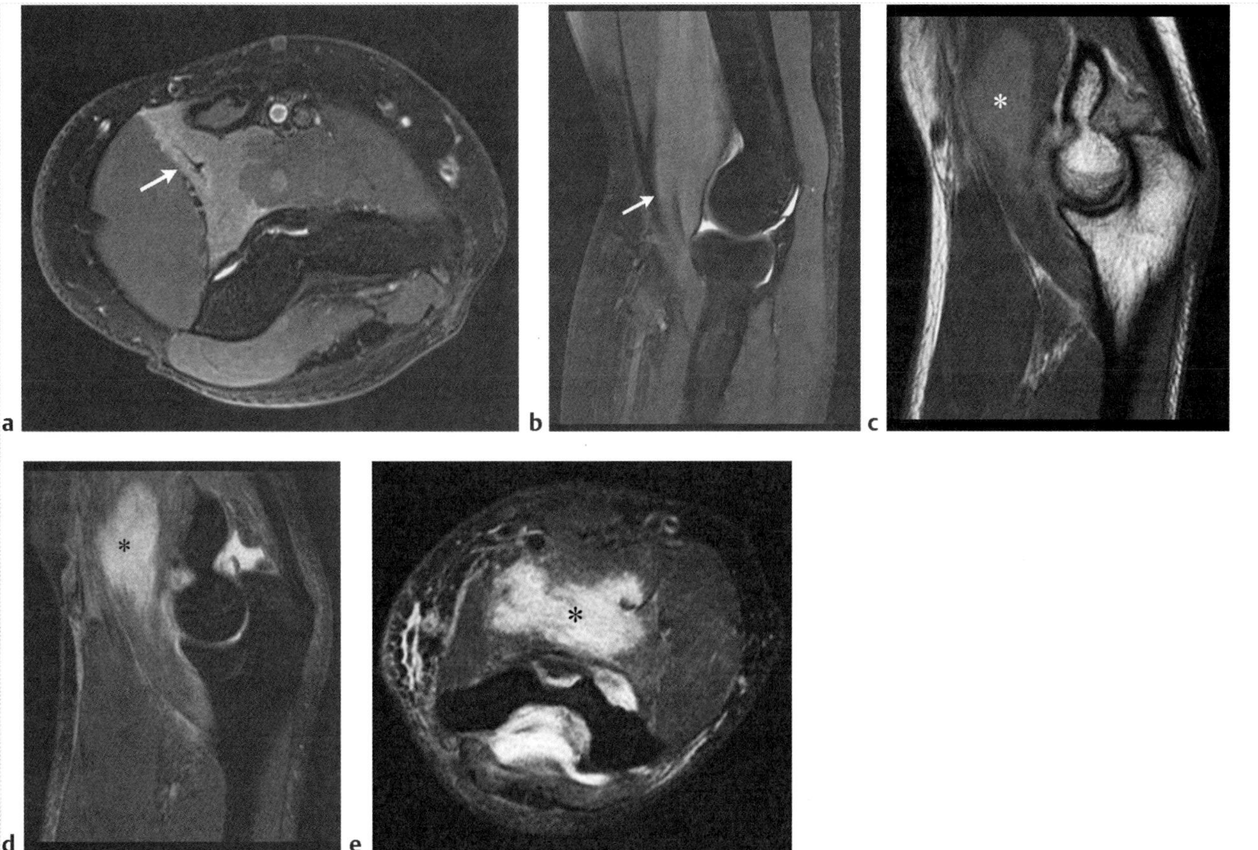

Fig. 3.6 (a) Muscle strain at the musculotendinous junction of the brachialis with focally increased signal surrounding the tendon (arrow) and surrounding edema within the muscle on axial fat-suppressed T2-weighted imaging (FS T2WI). (b) Muscle strain at the musculotendinous junction of the brachialis with focally increased signal surrounding the tendon (arrow) and surrounding edema within the muscle on sagittal FS T2WI. (c) Example of a brachialis hematoma following acute injury. Note intermediate signal muscle hematoma (asterisk) on sagittal proton density-weighted imaging (PDWI). (d) On sagittal FS T2WI the high signal hematoma (asterisk) is seen along with edema extending distally toward the ulnar insertion of the brachialis tendon. (e) Corresponding axial FS T2WI demonstrates an intact biceps muscle and tendon anterior to the brachialis hematoma (asterisk). Note high signal joint effusion more posteriorly.

Table 3.2 (Cont.) Lesions of the elbow tendons

Abnormalities	MRI findings	Comments
Triceps tendon tear (▶ Fig. 3.7)	Triceps tendinopathy will demonstrate increased signal within the abnormal portion of tendon with associated tendon thickening. Partial or complete rupture of the triceps tendon from its insertion on the olecranon will demonstrate increased signal on PDWI and FS T2WI. Axial and sagittal images are most useful in diagnosis. Sagittal images best demonstrate the degree of retraction. A variable fluid-filled gap may be seen best on FS T2WI depending on the size of the tear. Bony avulsion fragments or calcifications related to tendinopathy may also be seen. Look for associated fluid in the overlying olecranon bursa reflecting olecranon bursitis.	A normal triceps tendon demonstrates a distally striated appearance. Injury to the triceps tendon may occur due to direct trauma or deceleration stress on a contracted muscle. MR is useful to distinguish tendinopathy from tears and to assess the degree of tendon retraction. Common differential considerations include a muscle hematoma, olecranon fracture, olecranon bursitis, or mass.

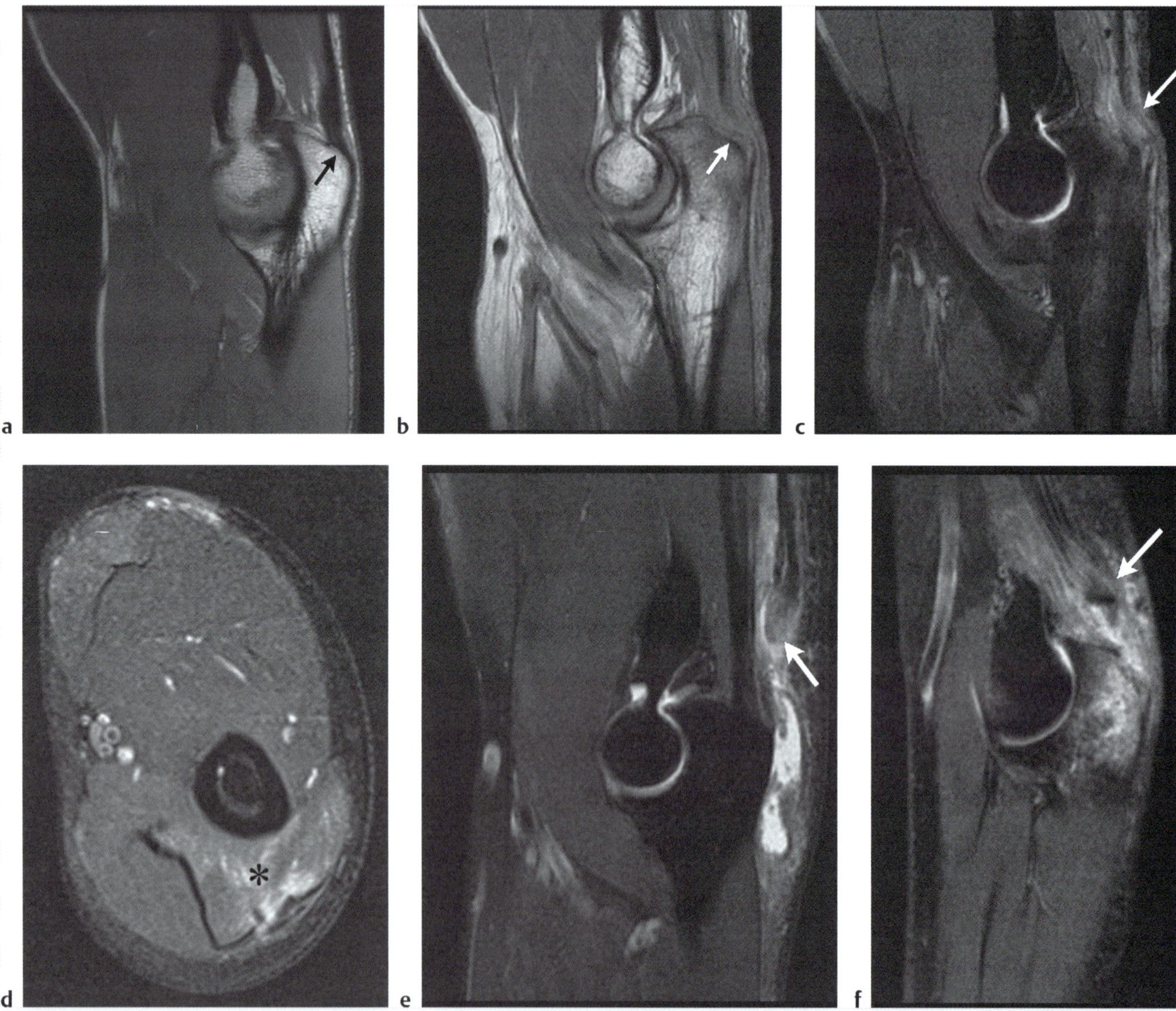

Fig. 3.7 (a) Note a normal low signal distal triceps tendon inserting distally on the olecranon (arrow) on sagittal proton density–weighted imaging (PDWI). (b) Partial tear of the distal triceps tendon (arrow) with intermediate signal within the more proximal remaining intact fibers representing superimposed tendinopathy on sagittal PDWI. (c) Corresponding sagittal fat-suppressed T2-weighted imaging (FS T2WI) demonstrates a few intact distal triceps tendon fibers (arrow) and surrounding edema at the olecranon. Note low signal calcifications more proximally indicative of chronic underlying tendinopathy. (d) Axial FS T2WI demonstrates high signal edema of the more proximal musculotendinous junction strain (asterisk). (e) Another example of a partial triceps tendon tear with retraction of the torn posterior tendon fibers (arrow). Note high signal fluid in the olecranon bursa more distally on sagittal FS T2WI. (f) Complete tear and retraction of the triceps tendon including a low signal ossific fragment (arrow) from the olecranon. Note extensive olecranon marrow edema on sagittal FS T2WI. *(continued)*

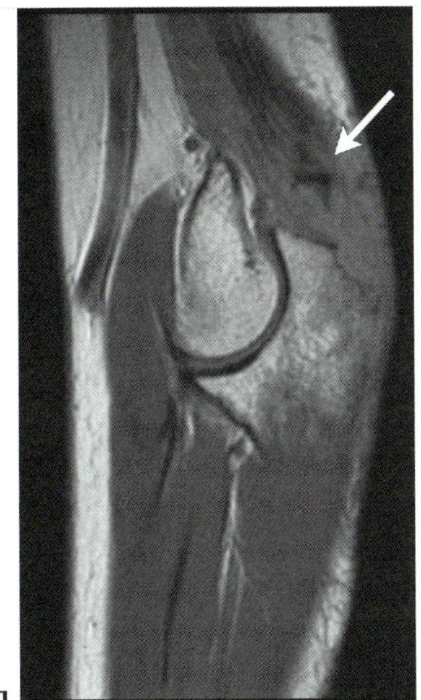

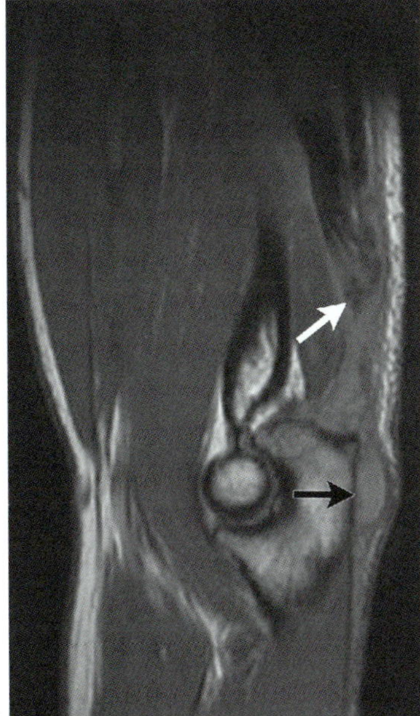

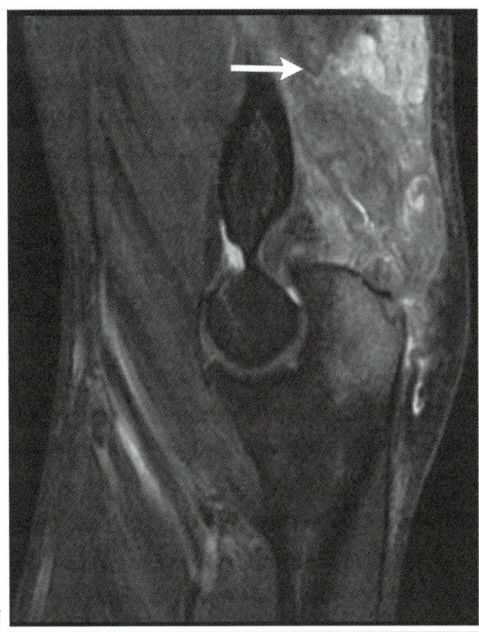

Fig. 3.7 *(continued)* (g) Corresponding sagittal PDWI demonstrates thickening and abnormally increased signal of the retracted tendon (arrow) as well as the low signal cortical fragment. (h) Example of a complete triceps tendon tear with a greater degree of tendon retraction (white arrow), and intermediate signal olecranon bursa fluid more distally (black arrow) on sagittal PDWI. (i) Extensive hematoma in a different patient due to an acute triceps tendon avulsion with a heterogeneous hematoma and marrow edema at the olecranon. Proximally retracted tendon is seen (arrow) on sagittal FS T2WI.

3.2.1 Lesions of the Elbow Tendons Suggested Reading

[1] Belentani C, Pastore D, Wangwinyuvirat M, et al. Triceps brachii tendon: anatomic-MR imaging study in cadavers with histologic correlation. Skeletal Radiol 2009; 38: 171–175

[2] Chew ML, Giuffrè BM. Disorders of the distal biceps brachii tendon. Radiographics 2005; 25: 1227–1237

[3] Dirim B, Brouha SS, Pretterklieber ML, et al. Terminal bifurcation of the biceps brachii muscle and tendon: anatomic considerations and clinical implications. AJR Am J Roentgenol 2008; 191: W248–55

[4] Hayter CL, Adler RS. Injuries of the elbow and the current treatment of tendon disease. AJR Am J Roentgenol 2012; 199: 546–557

[5] Stevens KJ. Magnetic resonance imaging of the elbow. J Magn Reson Imaging 2010; 31: 1036–1053

[6] Walz DM, Newman JS, Konin GP, Ross G. Epicondylitis: pathogenesis, imaging, and treatment. Radiographics 2010; 30: 167–184

3.3 Bursitis and Arthritis of the Elbow

- Bicipitoradial bursitis
- Olecranon bursitis
- Osteoarthritis
- Rheumatoid arthritis

Table 3.3 Bursitis and arthritis of the elbow

Abnormalities	MRI findings	Comments
Bicipitoradial bursitis (▶ Fig. 3.8)	When distended with fluid, the bursa will be low to intermediate signal on axial T1-weighted imaging (T1WI) and proton density–weighted imaging (PDWI), and high signal on fat-suppressed T2-weighted imaging (FS T2WI). Intermediate signal material within a distended bursa indicates hemorrhage, hypertrophied synovium, or loose bodies. Look for associated biceps tendinopathy or partial tear.	The bicipitoradial bursa separates the distal biceps tendon from the anterior margin of the radial tuberosity. The distended bursa may surround the distal biceps tendon, which does not have a true tendon sheath but is covered by a paratenon. Look for radial tuberosity bony hypertrophy, which has been associated with this condition. A distended bursa may be mistaken for an antecubital mass. Use of contrast-enhanced images will help make this distinction if needed.

(continued on page 68)

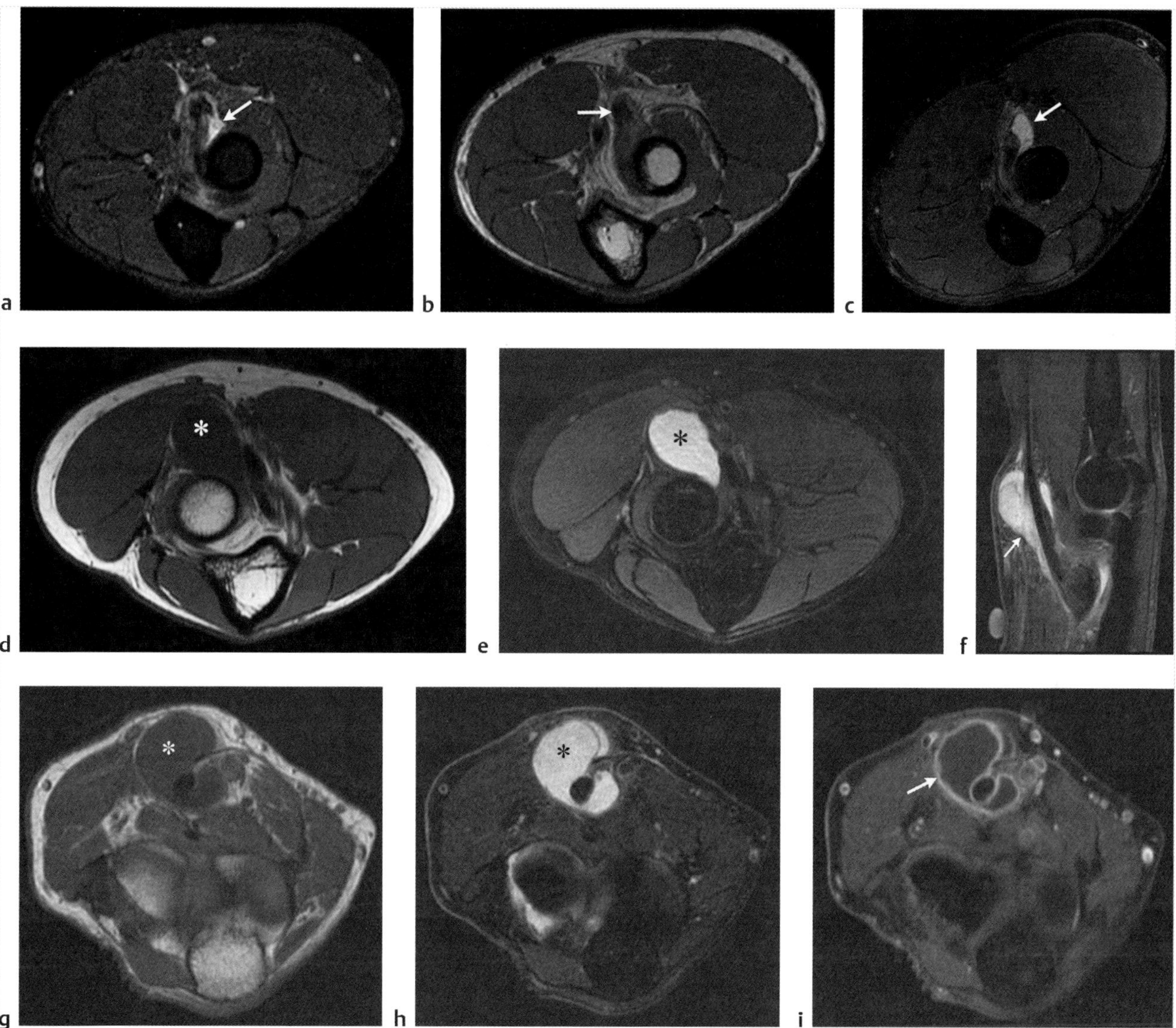

Fig. 3.8 (a) Small amount of fluid in the bicipitoradial bursa in this patient with tendinosis and partial tearing of the distal biceps tendon at its insertion. Note a small amount of high signal bursal fluid (arrow) on axial fat-suppressed T2-weighted imaging (FS T2WI). (b) There is tendon irregularity and increased signal due to partial tearing and tendinosis (arrow) on axial proton density–weighted imaging (PDWI). (c) A different patient also demonstrating distal biceps tendinosis, and a larger amount of fluid distending the bicipitoradial bursa (arrow) on axial FS T2WI. (d) A large, distended bicipitoradial bursa adjacent to an intact low signal biceps tendon. The fluid demonstrates low signal on axial PDWI, and (e) increased signal on axial FS T2WI (asterisks). (f) Large amount of fluid fills the bicipitoradial bursa and extends proximally along the tendon in a different patient. Fluid (arrow) surrounds the distal biceps tendon on sagittal FS T2WI. (g) Note the low to intermediate signal bursal fluid (asterisk) on axial PDWI and (h) corresponding high signal fluid (asterisk) on axial FS T2WI. (i) Because the bursa is a synovial lined sac, a thin rim of contrast enhancement (arrow) is seen peripherally on gadolinium (Gd)-contrast enhanced axial FS T1WI.

Table 3.3 (Cont.) Bursitis and arthritis of the elbow

Abnormalities	MRI findings	Comments
Olecranon bursitis (▶ Fig. 3.9)	On magnetic resonance imaging (MRI) look for a fluid signal collection in the bursa between the skin and triceps tendon and olecranon posteriorly. Bursal fluid will demonstrate low to intermediate signal on T1-weighted imaging (T1WI) and proton density–weighted imaging (PDWI), and increased signal on fat-suppressed T2-weighted imaging (FS T2WI). Postcontrast imaging demonstrates a thin rim of synovial enhancement, which may be seen along the periphery of the bursa. If bursitis is complicated by hemorrhage or infection, fluid/debris will be of mixed signal.	The olecranon bursa overlies the olecranon process of the ulna superficial to the insertion of the triceps tendon. Normally the bursa is not distended and therefore not seen on magnetic resonance imaging (MRI). Inflammation of the olecranon bursa, leading to bursitis, may be seen with causes including trauma, gout, or infection. Look for associated triceps tendon injuries.

(continued on page 70)

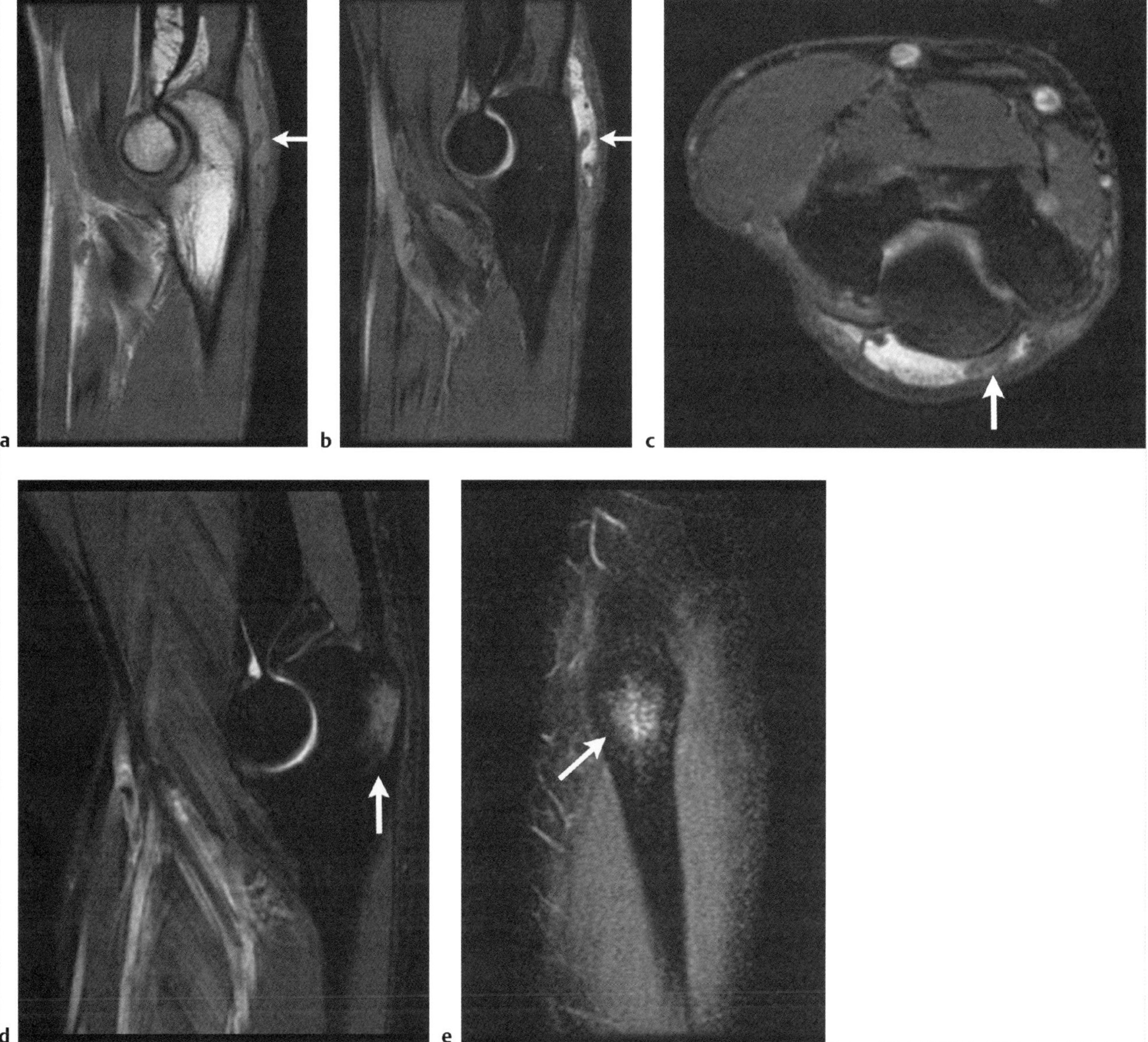

Fig. 3.9 (a) Patient with painful swelling over the olecranon. Intermediate signal fluid (arrow) is seen within the olecranon bursa adjacent to an intact triceps tendon on sagittal proton density–weighted imaging (PDWI). (b) Fluid within the bursa (arrow) is of high signal with a peripheral thickened, low signal, synovial lining (arrows) on corresponding sagittal fat-suppressed T2-weighted imaging (FS T2WI) and (c) axial FS T2WI. (d) Differential considerations include an olecranon bone bruise (arrows) as seen on sagittal FS T2WI and (e) coronal FS T2WI.

Table 3.3 (Cont.) Bursitis and arthritis of the elbow

Abnormalities	MRI findings	Comments
Osteoarthritis (▶ Fig. 3.10)	As with osteoarthritis in other joints, typical findings include osteophytes, cartilage thinning with joint space narrowing, subchondral low signal/sclerosis, and subchondral cysts well seen on T1WI or PDWI. Loose bodies typically will follow marrow signal on PDWI and FS T2WI and will demonstrate a low signal calcified/ossified rim, which distinguishes them from lobules of fat. Joint effusions will follow fluid signal; high signal on FS T2WI and lower signal on PDWI and T1WI.	Be sure to always check radiographs and clinical history before interpreting MRIs. Osteoarthritis may be primary, due to repeated episodes of microtrauma with involvement of multiple regions of the elbow joint. Secondary osteoarthritis is seen after an episode of significant trauma or due to other underlying arthropathy, and usually involves only a portion of the joint. Synovitis may be seen in osteoarthritis and with inflammatory arthropathy. Loose bodies may impinge upon and restrict flexion and extension of the elbow, resulting in symptoms of locking. Also consider inflammatory arthropathy (rheumatoid arthritis [RA]) and crystal arthropathy (gout and calcium pyrophosphate dihydrate [CPPD] crystal arthropathy) in the differential diagnosis.

(continued on page 72)

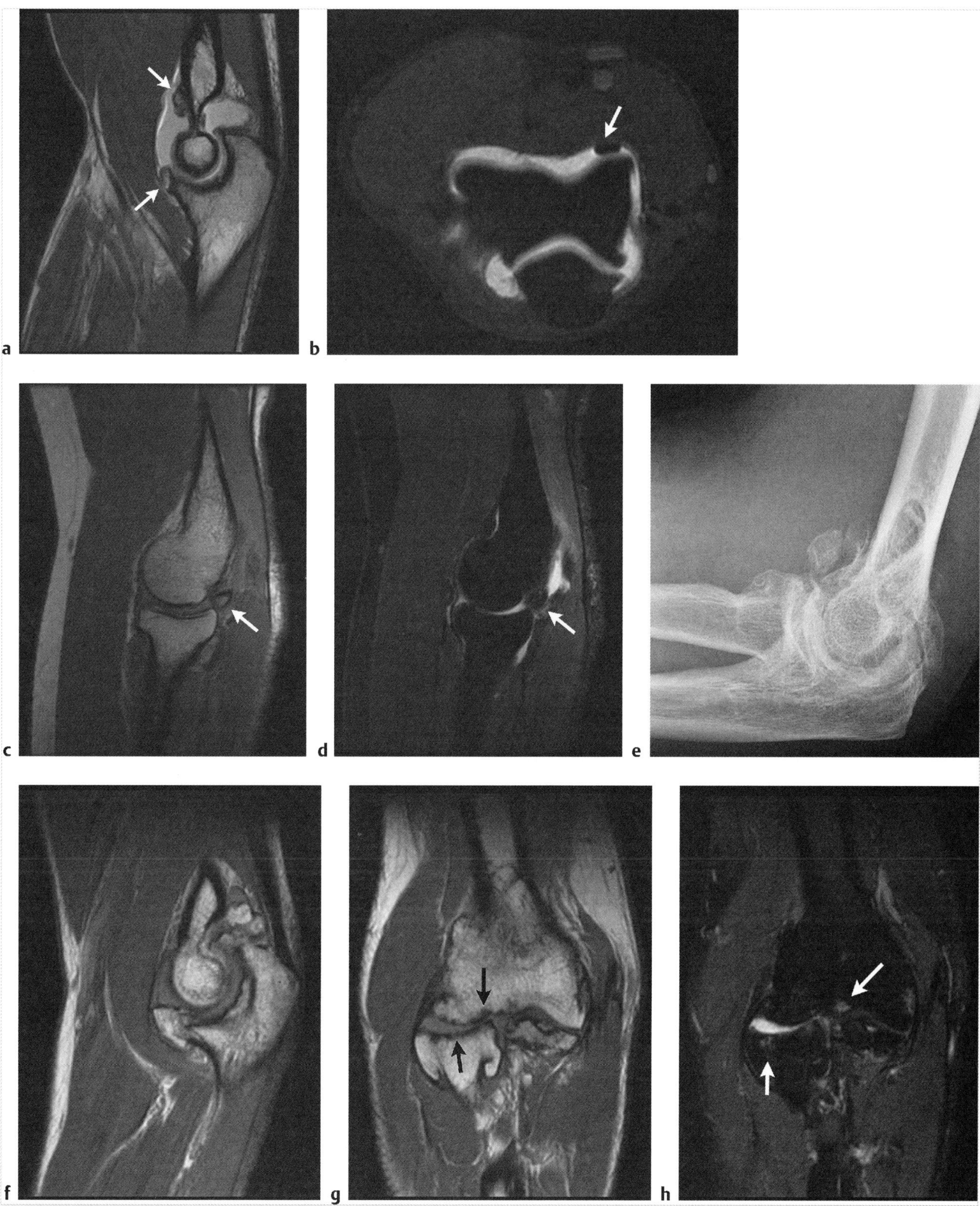

Fig. 3.10 (a) Osteoarthritic changes about the ulnohumeral joint with osteophyte formation (arrows) along the anterior margin of the distal humerus and at the coronoid process of the ulna on sagittal proton density–weighted imaging (PDWI) arthrogram. (b) Note low signal air bubble (arrow) anteriorly within the elbow joint on axial fat-suppressed (FS) T1 arthrogram. This should not be confused with a loose body. (c) Comparison case of a true loose body (arrow) posterior to the radiocapitellar joint demonstrating a low signal rim and central marrow fat signal on sagittal PDWI. (d) Note the loose body follows marrow signal (arrow) on corresponding sagittal FS T2-weighted imaging (T2WI). (e) Case of severe posttraumatic osteoarthritis with extensive osteophyte formation, remodeling, and joint space narrowing on lateral elbow radiograph. (f) Corresponding sagittal PDWI demonstrates extensive osteophytosis. (g) Degenerative subchondral foci of low signal (arrows), osteophytes, and joint space narrowing are seen on coronal PDWI. (h) Corresponding coronal FS T2WI demonstrates joint space narrowing with chondral thinning, and subchondral foci of increased signal representing small geodes (arrows).

Table 3.3 (Cont.) Bursitis and arthritis of the elbow

Abnormalities	MRI findings	Comments
Rheumatoid arthritis (RA) (► Fig. 3.11)	Look for hypertrophied synovium/pannus, which may have a varied appearance including diffuse, nodular, and villous. This is usually seen associated with varying amounts of joint fluid. On routine MR sequences look for complex joint fluid as a clue to the presence of synovitis. Synovitis demonstrates varying signal intensity; low to intermediate on T1WI and PDWI and low to intermediate to higher signal on FS T2WI. Postcontrast imaging is helpful to differentiate enhancing synovium/pannus from joint fluid.	Subchondral edema and marginal erosions are seen with RA. The presence of enhancing synovium alone is not diagnostic of RA, and clinical criteria must be met for diagnosis. Usual RA involvement is seen about the smaller joints–hands and wrists. Note MRI may be useful for monitoring therapy.

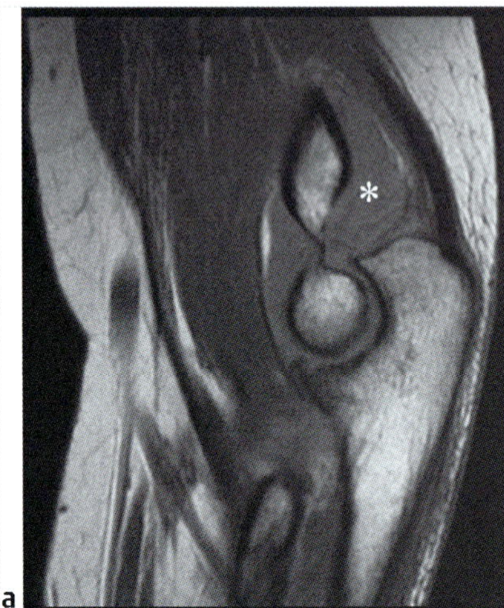

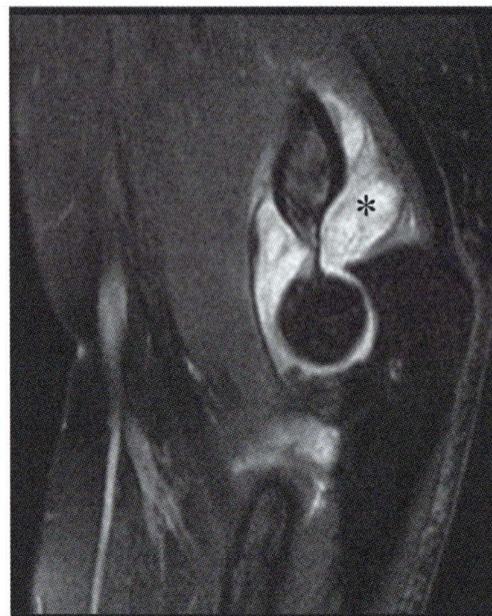

Fig. 3.11 (a) Patient with known rheumatoid arthritis (RA) demonstrates heterogeneous synovial proliferation (asterisk) about the distal humerus and ulnohumeral joint on sagittal proton density–weighted imaging (PDWI). (b) Corresponding heterogeneous high signal of the pannus (asterisk) is appreciated on sagittal fat-suppressed T2-weighted imaging (FS T2WI).

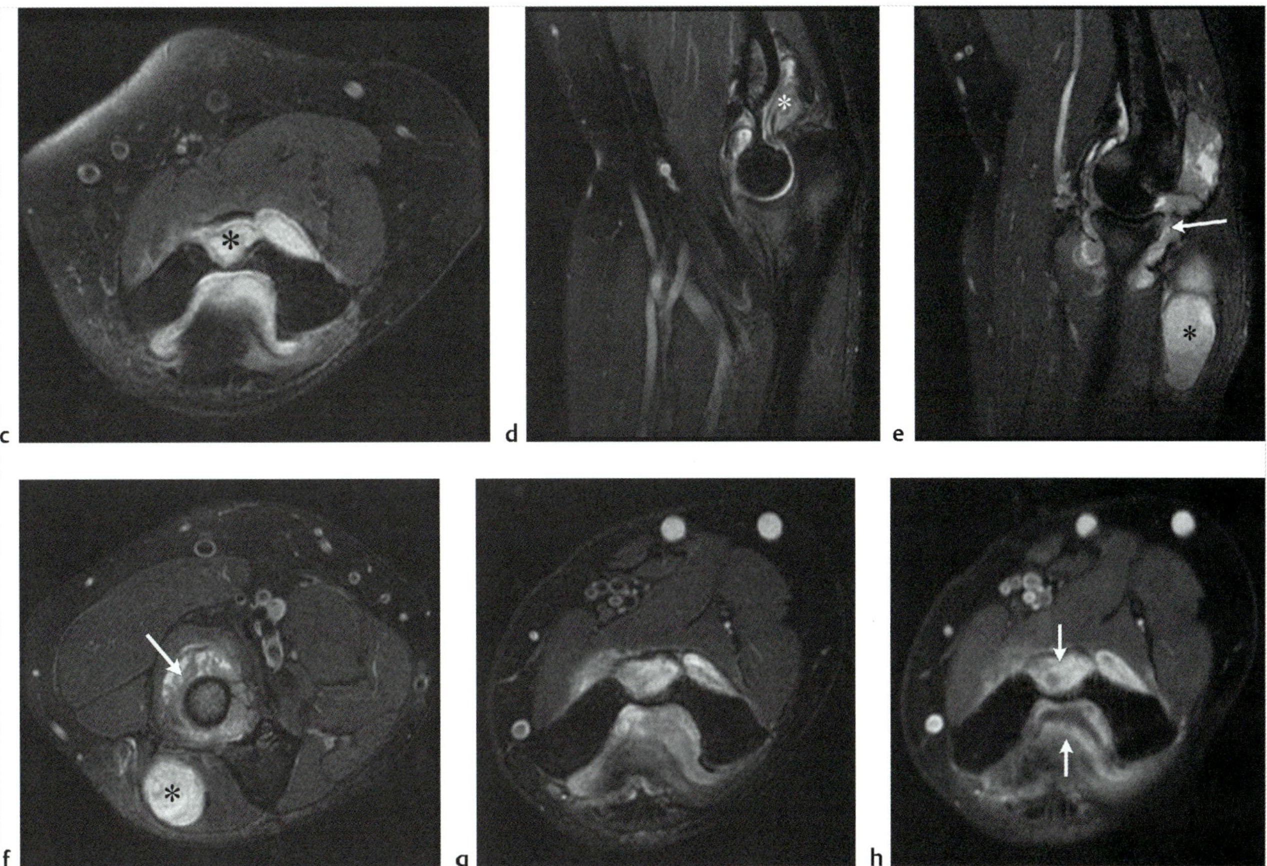

Fig. 3.11 *(continued)* (c) Corresponding heterogeneous high signal of the pannus (asterisk) is appreciated on axial FS T2WI. (d) More extensive synovial proliferation in a different case of RA. On sagittal FS T2WI, note extensive heterogeneous increased signal pannus (asterisk). (e) Pannus herniates beyond the joint distally into the extensor carpi ulnaris (ECU), resulting in a soft tissue "mass" posteriorly (asterisk). Note joint space narrowing at the radiocapitellar joint and erosion of the dorsal margin of the radial head (arrow) on sagittal FS T2WI. (f) Corresponding axial FS T2WI demonstrates the frond-like synovial proliferation (arrow) about the proximal radius with surrounding joint fluid. Note herniation of the pannus extending posteriorly (asterisk). (g) Additional case of RA demonstrating the ability of Gd-contrast to distinguish between a complex joint effusion and synovitis. On axial FS T2WI, it is difficult to distinguish synovial hypertrophy from joint fluid. (h) Gd-contrast enhanced axial FS T1WI demonstrates enhancing synovium (arrows). This surrounds a curved band of low signal joint fluid posterior to the humerus.

3.3.1 Bursitis and Arthritis of the Elbow Suggested Reading

[1] Petscavage JM, Ha AS, Chew FS. Radiologic review of total elbow, radial head, and capitellar resurfacing arthroplasty. Radiographics 2012; 32: 129–149

[2] Rosas HG, Tuite MJ. The current state of imaging the articular cartilage of the upper extremity. Magn Reson Imaging Clin N Am 2011; 19: 407–423

3.4 Elbow Trauma

- Osteochondral lesions of the capitellum
- Little Leaguer's elbow
- Olecranon fracture

Table 3.4 Elbow trauma

Abnormalities	MRI findings	Comments
Osteochondral lesions of the capitellum (▶ Fig. 3.12)	Osteochondral lesions typically occur along the anterior margin of the capitellum well seen on sagittal sequences, including T1-weighted imaging (T1WI), proton density–weighted imaging (PDWI), and fat-suppressed T2-weighted imaging (FS T2WI). The osteochondral fragment may demonstrate low signal on T1WI or PDWI and increased signal on FS T2WI. Fragment signal is variable, however, depending on the degree of sclerosis. Unstable lesions are often larger and demonstrate a fluid signal rim surrounding the fragment or cystic foci within the adjacent capitellum. Assess overlying cartilage for continuity. Stable lesions demonstrate intact overlying cartilage. Look for fragmentation and chondral discontinuity with unstable lesions. Variable signal loose bodies may be found adjacent to the olecranon and coronoid fossae. The presence of a joint effusion or the use of magnetic resonance (MR) arthrography is helpful for identifying loose bodies and evaluating lesion stability. Imaging may demonstrate residual capitellar irregularity following healing. Always correlate the MR findings with radiographs.	This condition is believed to occur due to chronic impaction at the radiocapitellar joint and a relatively poor blood supply leading to osteonecrosis. Osteochondral lesions of the capitellum are seen in young athletes, including throwers and gymnasts 12 to 16 years of age. Differentiate from Panner disease seen in 5- to 11-year-old patients in which loose fragments are not seen. In Panner disease diffuse signal changes of the capitellum tend to resolve over time. The pseudodefect of the capitellum is a posteriorly located normal irregularity of the capitellum often well seen on coronal PDWI. This is not associated with marrow edema or loose fragments.

(continued on page 76)

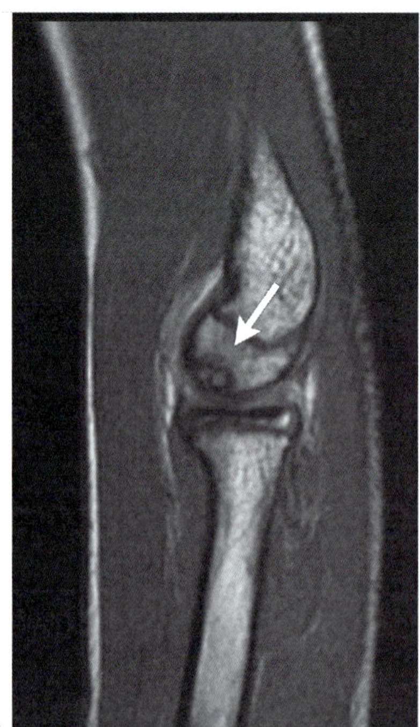
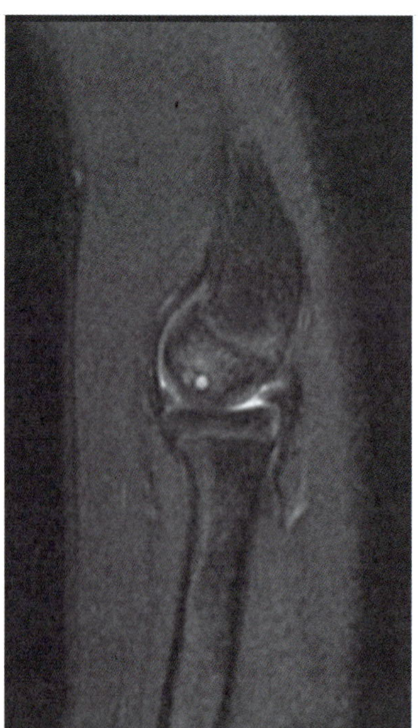
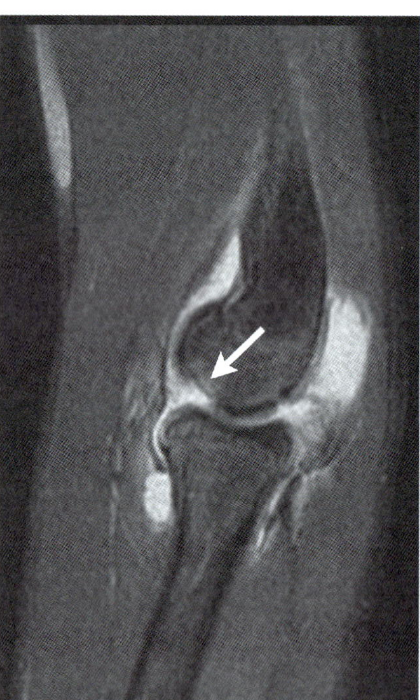

Fig. 3.12 (a) Osteochondrosis (Panner disease) of the capitellum in an 11-year-old male baseball pitcher with long-standing elbow pain. Note subchondral cystic change (arrow) surrounded by a sclerotic margin on sagittal proton density–weighted imaging (PDWI). (b) On fat-suppressed T2-weighted imaging (FS T2WI), the overlying cartilage is intact as is the contour of the cortex. A loose body was not identified. (c) Osteochondral lesion of the capitellum in a 13-year-old male with a focal chondral defect along the anterior margin of the capitellum. Note fluid filling the gap at the site of the lesion (arrow) on sagittal FS T2WI, saline arthrogram. (*continued*)

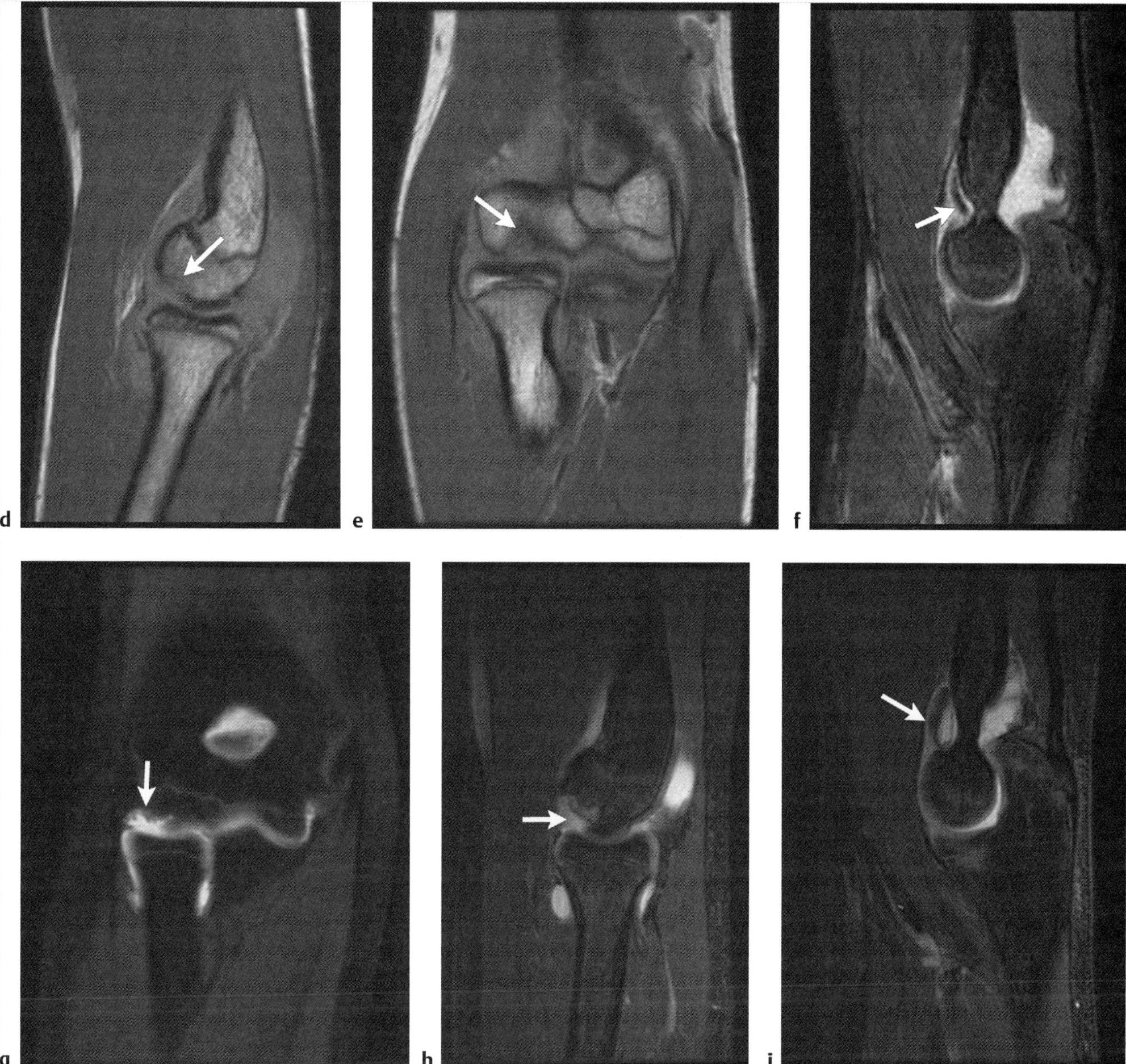

Fig. 3.12 (*continued*) (d) Corresponding sagittal PDWI demonstrates interruption of the low signal cortex and subtle flattening of the anterior cortical margin of the capitellum (arrow). (e) The lesion is also seen on coronal PDWI (arrow). (f) The low signal loose osteochondral fragment (arrow) is seen medially in the coronoid fossa on sagittal FS T2WI. (g) Osteochondral lesions should not be confused with the pseudodefect of the capitellum seen more posteriorly in a different patient on coronal FS T1 arthrogram. (h) Large osteochondral lesion in a patient with a fluid-filled gap (arrow) and mild capitellar marrow edema on sagittal FS T2WI. (i) The osteochondral fragment (arrow) is identified anteriorly in the coronoid fossa on sagittal FS T2WI.

Table 3.4 (Cont.) Elbow trauma

Abnormalities	MRI findings	Comments
Little Leaguer's elbow (▶ Fig. 3.13)	Variable degrees of medial epicondyle avulsion will be seen with separation of the medial epicondylar apophysis from the humerus. Marrow edema on FS T2WI is typically seen adjacent to the area of widening. T1WI and PDWI may also show the zone of separation and potential fragmentation of the apophysis. Assess condition of the ulnar collateral ligament and flexor/pronator group.	An overuse/valgus overload with repetitive throwing motion seen most commonly in 5- to 14-year-old patients. This may present as the sequela of repetitive injury or as an acute injury. Edema in the flexor pronator group adjacent to the apophysis is an associated finding. Adolescents and adults may also present with medial epicondyle avulsions.
Olecranon fracture (▶ Fig. 3.14)	Look for abnormal linear low signal fracture line on T1, PDWI, and FS T2WI traversing the middle third of the olecranon process of the ulna. On FS T2WI acute fractures will demonstrate olecranon marrow edema surrounding the fracture site. Fractures may be radiographically occult, but may demonstrate a positive fat pad sign indicating an elbow joint effusion. Look for associated fractures of the coronoid process of the ulna. Assess for triceps tendon tear or avulsion injury at the olecranon.	While radial head fractures are most common, olecranon fractures account for 20% of elbow fractures in adults. A type I Mayo classification fracture of the olecranon involves an undisplaced fracture, which may be best seen with magnetic resonance imaging (MRI). Displaced fractures (Mayo types II and III) of the olecranon are more common. These may present as a stress injury in throwers. Although often an isolated injury, there is a need to assess for other elbow fractures. It is important to distinguish an olecranon fracture from the normal ossification center of the olecranon seen more proximally along the olecranon. The ossification center of the olecranon normally fuses by 16 to 18 years of age. Do not mistake the cortical notch of the olecranon for a fracture.

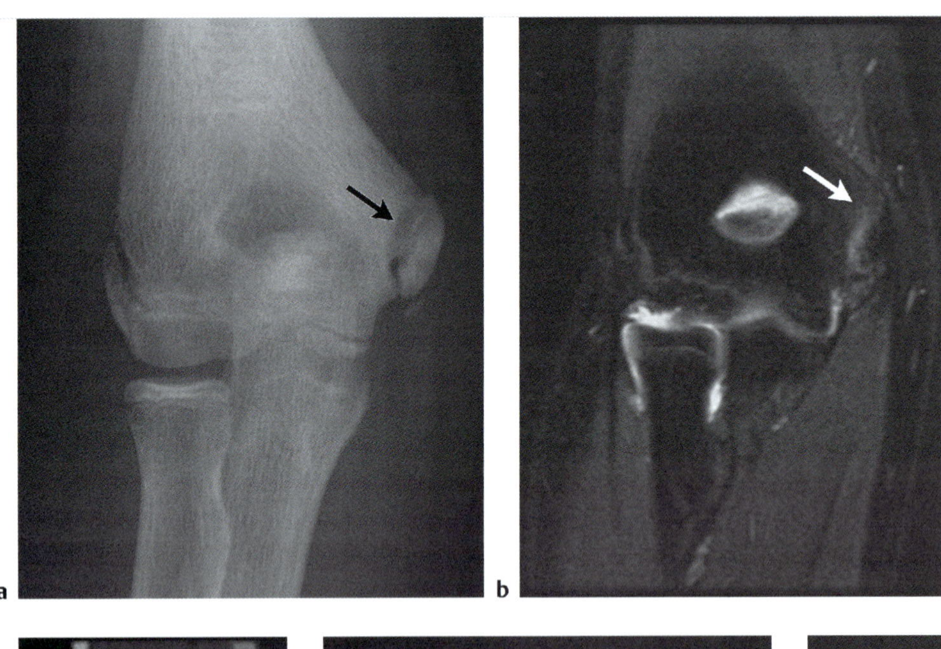

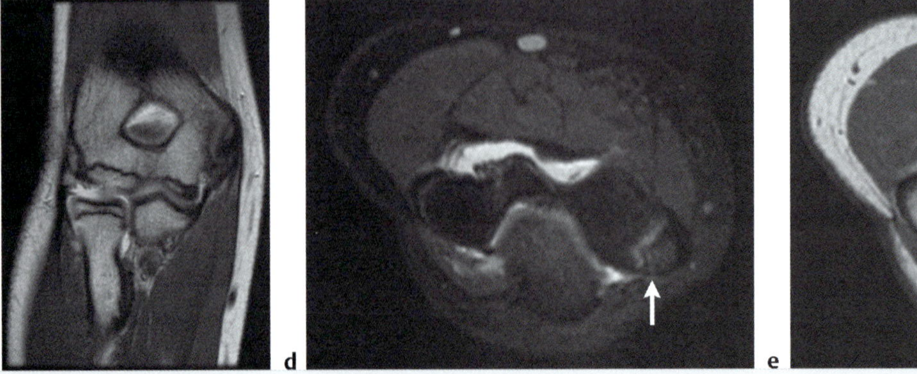

Fig. 3.13 (a) Pediatric baseball pitcher with pain over the medial epicondyle demonstrating widening of the medial epicondyle physis (arrow) and a small distal avulsion fragment on anteroposterior radiograph of the elbow. (b) Corresponding coronal fat-suppressed T2-weighted imaging (FS T2WI) demonstrates increased signal and widening of the medial epicondyle physis (arrow). (c) Sclerosis and irregularity are seen at the apophysis on coronal proton density–weighted imaging (PDWI). (d) Corresponding axial FS T2WI demonstrates the widened medial physis with marrow edema in the apophysis (arrow). (e) Subchondral low signal reactive changes are noted in the apophysis (arrow) on corresponding axial PDWI.

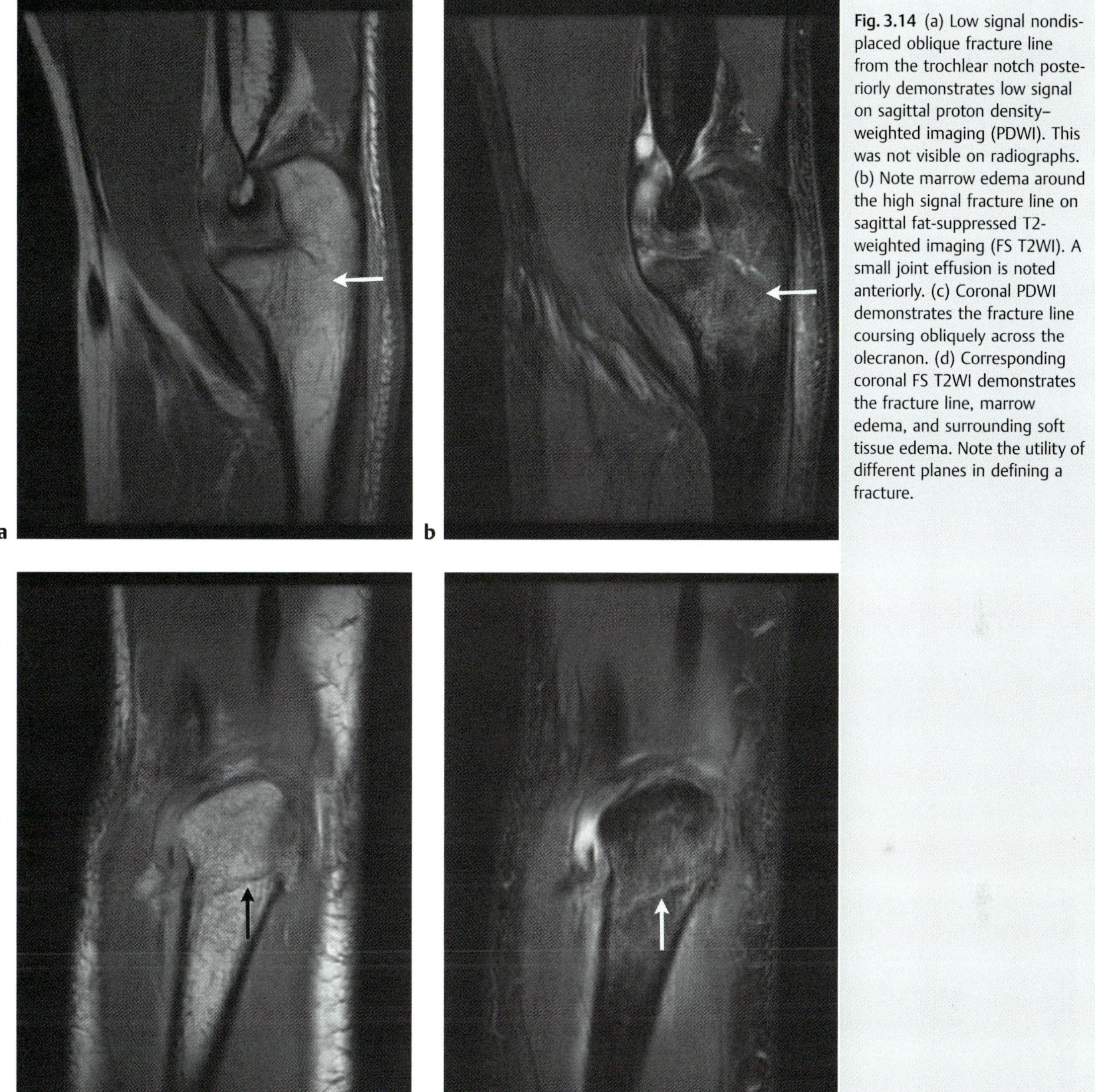

Fig. 3.14 (a) Low signal nondisplaced oblique fracture line from the trochlear notch posteriorly demonstrates low signal on sagittal proton density–weighted imaging (PDWI). This was not visible on radiographs. (b) Note marrow edema around the high signal fracture line on sagittal fat-suppressed T2-weighted imaging (FS T2WI). A small joint effusion is noted anteriorly. (c) Coronal PDWI demonstrates the fracture line coursing obliquely across the olecranon. (d) Corresponding coronal FS T2WI demonstrates the fracture line, marrow edema, and surrounding soft tissue edema. Note the utility of different planes in defining a fracture.

3.4.1 Elbow Trauma Suggested Reading

[1] Davis KW. Imaging pediatric sports injuries: upper extremity. Radiol Clin North Am 2010; 48: 1199–1211

[2] Hayter CL, Giuffre BM. Overuse and traumatic injuries of the elbow. Magn Reson Imaging Clin N Am 2009; 17: 617–638

[3] Jaimes C, Jimenez M, Shabshin N, Laor T, Jaramillo D. Taking the stress out of evaluating stress injuries in children. Radiographics 2012; 32: 537–555

3.5 Nerve Abnormalities of the Elbow

- Ulnar neuropathy
- Anconeus epitrochlearis
- Radial nerve branch: posterior interosseous nerve (PIN) injury

Table 3.5 Nerve abnormalities of the elbow

Abnormalities	MRI findings	Comments
Ulnar neuropathy (▶ Fig. 3.15)	The ulnar nerve is normally located in the cubital tunnel surrounded by a retinaculum. With ulnar neuropathy, the nerve may demonstrate thickening and loss of definition on T1-weighted imaging (T1WI) and proton density–weighted imaging (PDWI). Edematous changes of the nerve will be seen on fat-suppressed T2-weighted imaging (FS T2WI). Look for thickening of the cubital tunnel retinaculum on T1WI and PDWI resulting in ulnar nerve compression. An accessory muscle, the anconeus epitrochlearis, may also result in nerve compression (see below).	Other causes of ulnar nerve entrapment/compression at the elbow include prior trauma, bone spurs, ganglia, or masses. With congenital absence of the cubital retinaculum the nerve is more susceptible to subluxation and injury. Ulnar neuropathy may be seen in patients with medial epicondylitis or ulnar collateral ligament injury. Note that the ulnar nerve may be compressed proximal to the cubital tunnel at the arcade of Struthers or distally as it passes through the heads of the flexor carpi ulnaris.
Anconeus epitrochlearis (▶ Fig. 3.16)	The anconeus epitrochlearis muscle follows normal muscle signal on all sequences: intermediate on T1WI, PDWI, and FS T2WI. The muscle follows the expected course of the cubital retinaculum from the medial olecranon to the inferior portion of the medial epicondyle. When present, this muscle replaces the cubital tunnel retinaculum and can result in compression and abnormally increased T2 signal and enlargement of the ulnar nerve.	The cubital retinaculum is thought to be a remnant of the anconeus epitrochlearis. When the muscle is present it forms the roof of the cubital tunnel and may result in compression of the ulnar nerve. Patients will present with ulnar neuritis if the muscle is causing compression. Other causes of ulnar nerve compression include callus formation following fractures, dislocation, masses, and arthritic processes.

(continued on page 80)

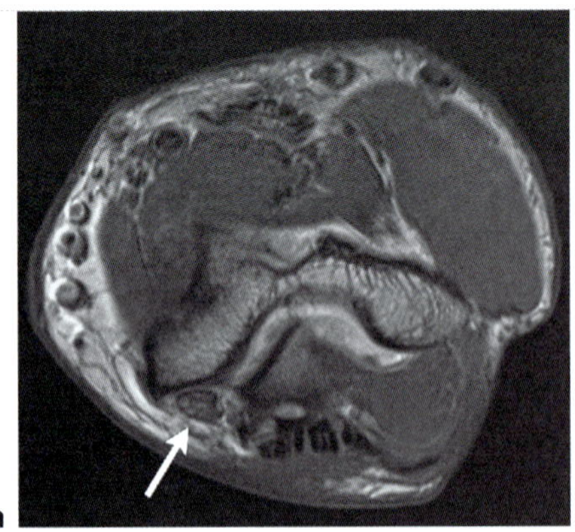
a

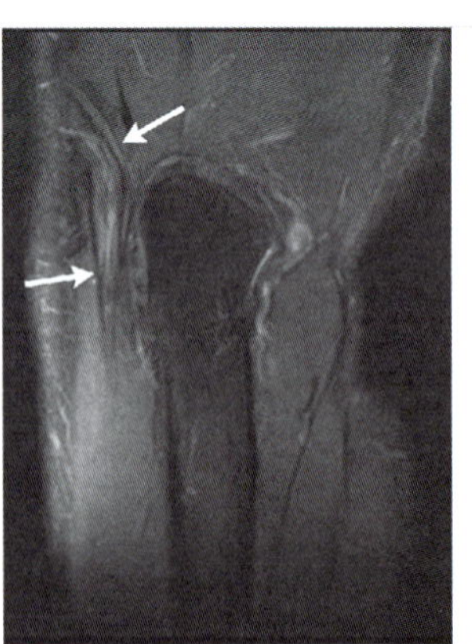
b

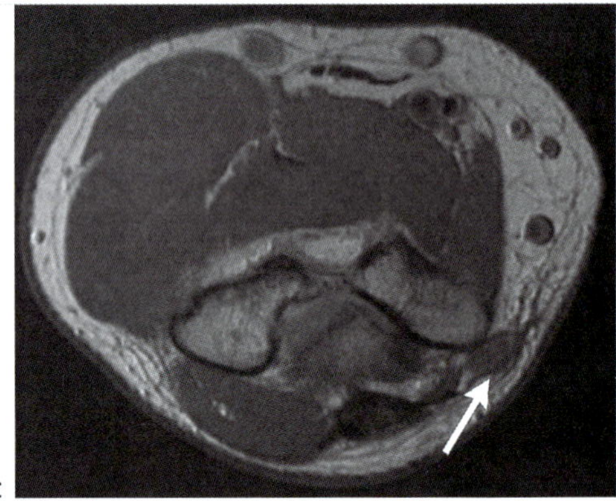
c

Fig. 3.15 (a) Patient with ulnar neuritis and common flexor tendinopathy (not shown) demonstrates an enlarged ulnar nerve (arrow) on axial proton density–weighted imaging (PDWI). (b) Note increased signal and enlargement of the ulnar nerve (arrows) on corresponding coronal fat-suppressed T2-weighted imaging (FS T2WI). (c) A different patient with an absent cubital retinaculum leading to chronic anterior subluxation and neuritis of the ulnar nerve. Note thickening of the subluxed nerve (arrow) on axial PDWI. (*continued*)

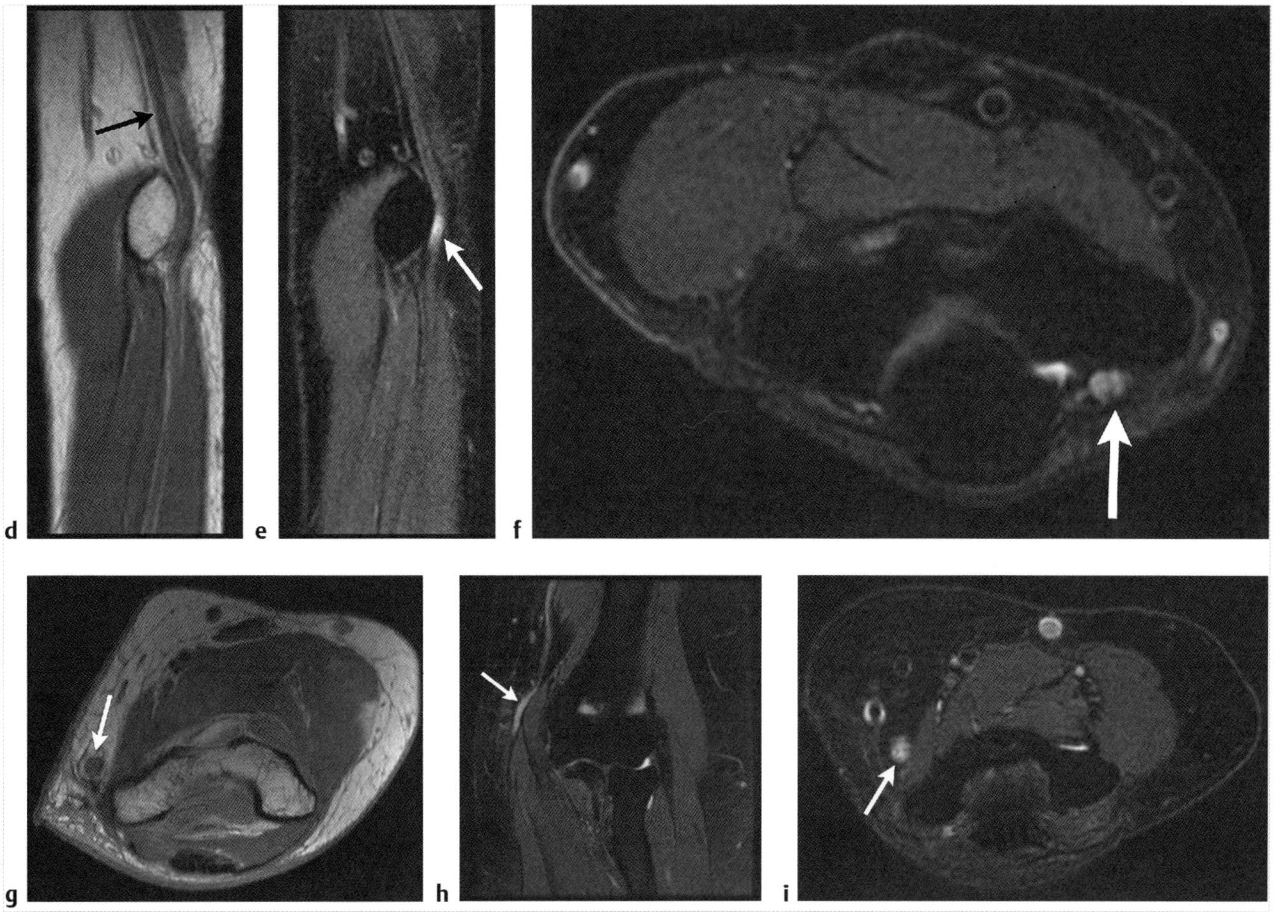

Fig. 3.15 (*continued*) (d) A different patient with symptoms of ulnar neuritis. The normally positioned ulnar nerve is well seen on sagittal PDWI, but in (e) reveals focal abnormal increased signal on sagittal FS T2WI and (f) axial FS T2WI (arrows). (g) Postoperative appearance of ulnar nerve anterior transposition following failed conservative treatment. Note the anterior subcutaneous position of the transposed nerve (arrow) on axial PDWI.
(h) Increased signal in the ulnar nerve (arrows) on coronal FS T2WI and (i) axial FS T2WI may persist after surgery, and does not necessarily imply persistent neuritis in the postoperative setting.

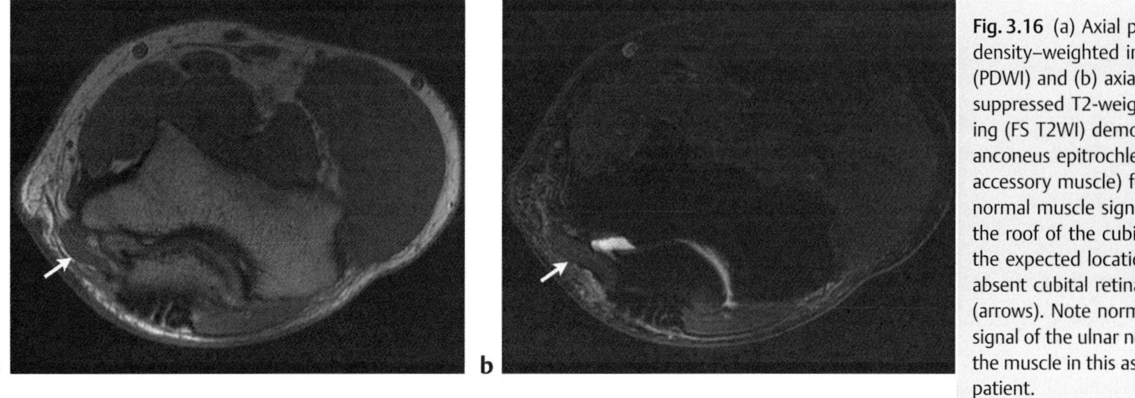

Fig. 3.16 (a) Axial proton density–weighted imaging (PDWI) and (b) axial fat-suppressed T2-weighted imaging (FS T2WI) demonstrate the anconeus epitrochlearis (an accessory muscle) following normal muscle signal. It forms the roof of the cubital tunnel in the expected location of the absent cubital retinaculum (arrows). Note normal size and signal of the ulnar nerve deep to the muscle in this asymptomatic patient.

Table 3.5 (Cont.) Nerve abnormalities of the elbow

Abnormalities	MRI findings	Comments
Radial nerve branch: posterior interosseous nerve (PIN) injury ▸ Fig. 3.17	Denervation muscle edema following injury to the posterior interosseous nerve branch of the radial nerve is best seen on FS T2WI most commonly involving the extensor muscles and the supinator. If muscle atrophy has occurred, increased signal due to fatty replacement will be seen on T1WI or PDWI.	The PIN is a deep branch of the radial nerve that may be entrapped at several locations, most commonly at the tendinous origin of the supinator muscle known as the arcade of Fröhse. Injury may also occur following distal biceps tendon repair. Injury results in a painless motor deficit involving several extensor muscles, including the extensor carpi ulnaris, extensor digitorum, extensor digiti minimi, extensor indicis, extensor pollicis longus and brevis, abductor pollicis longus, and variably the supinator muscle. PIN syndrome may be difficult to distinguish clinically from lateral epicondylitis. These conditions may coexist, making magnetic resonance imaging (MRI) useful for diagnosis. Note a lack of sensory abnormalities with PIN compression.

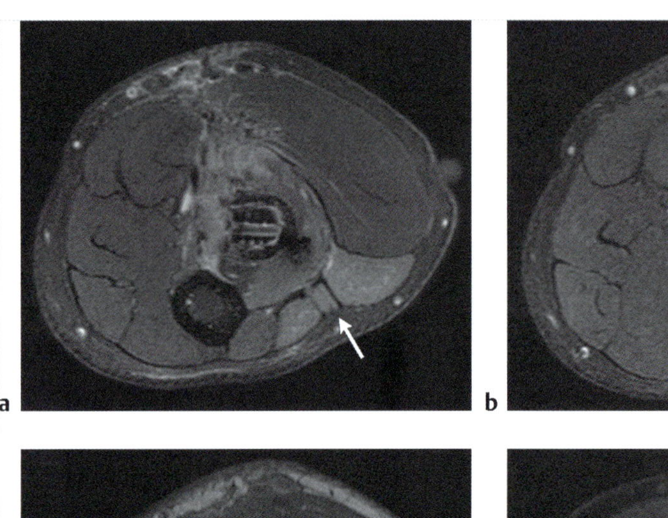
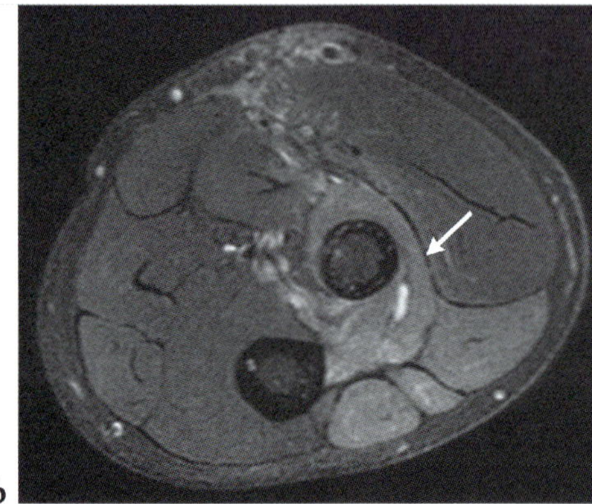
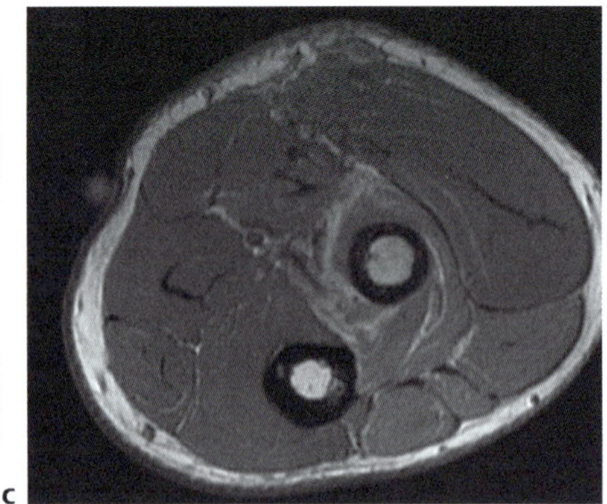
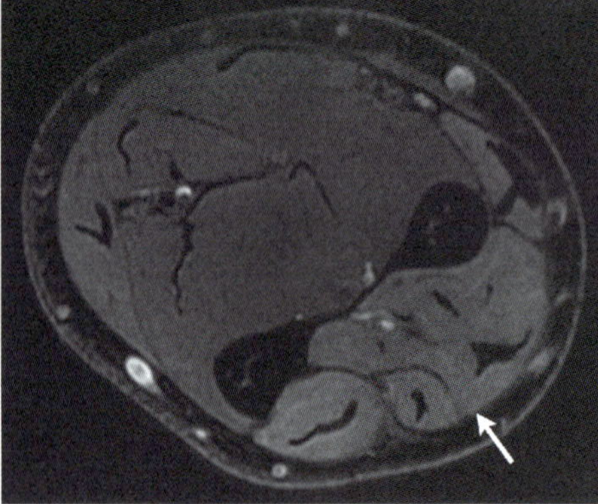

Fig. 3.17 (a, b) Patient with posterior interosseous nerve (PIN) syndrome with a surgical anchor in the proximal radius and increased T2 signal at the expected biceps tendon attachment site following biceps tendon repair. Note muscle edema (arrows) involving the extensor and supinator muscles posteriorly on axial fat-suppressed T2-weighted imaging (FS T2WI) in this patient with postoperative extensor neuropathy. (c) Corresponding axial proton density–weighted imaging (PDWI) also demonstrates mild signal changes of the extensor muscles. (d) Extensor muscle edema (arrow) is also seen more distally in the forearm on axial FS T2WI.

3.5.1 Nerve Abnormalities of the Elbow Suggested Reading

[1] Kim SJ, Hong SH, Jun WS, et al. MR imaging mapping of skeletal muscle denervation in entrapment and compressive neuropathies. Radiographics 2011; 31: 319–332

[2] Miller TT, Reinus WR. Nerve entrapment syndromes of the elbow, forearm, and wrist. AJR Am J Roentgenol 2010; 195: 585–594

[3] Sookur PA, Naraghi AM, Bleakney RR, Jalan R, Chan O, White LM. Accessory muscles: anatomy, symptoms, and radiologic evaluation. Radiographics 2008; 28: 481–499

3.6 Suggested Reading: The Elbow

[1] Bencardino JT, Beltran J. Soft tissue injury to the elbow. In: Pope TL, Bloem HL, Beltran J, Morrison WB, Wilson DJ, eds. Imaging of the Musculoskeletal System. Philadelphia, PA: Saunders; 2008:254–271

[2] Blease S, Stoller DW, Safran MR, Li AE, Fritz RC. The elbow: In: Stoller DW, ed. Magnetic Resonance Imaging in Orthopaedics and Sports Medicine. 3rd ed. Baltimore, MD: Lippincott Williams & Wilkins; 2007:1463–1626

[3] Helms CA, Major NM, Anderson MW, Kaplan PA, Dussault R. Elbow. In: Musculoskeletal MRI. 2nd ed. Philadelphia, PA: Saunders; 2009:224–243

[4] Shankman S, Liu B. Acute osseous injury of the elbow and forearm. In: Pope TL, Bloem HL, Beltran J, Morrison WB, Wilson DJ, eds. Imaging of the Musculoskeletal System. Philadelphia, PA: Saunders; 2008:241–253

[5] Stoller DW, Tirman PFJ, Bredella MA, Beltran S, Branstetter RM, Blease SCP. Elbow. In: Diagnostic Imaging Orthopaedics. Vol 2. Salt Lake City, UT: Amirsys; 2004:2–101

[6] Yacoub E, Beltran J, Miller TT. Normal elbow. In: Pope TL, Bloem HL, Beltran J, Morrison WB, Wilson DJ, eds. Imaging of the Musculoskeletal System. Philadelphia, PA: Saunders; 2008:221–240

Chapter 4

The Wrist

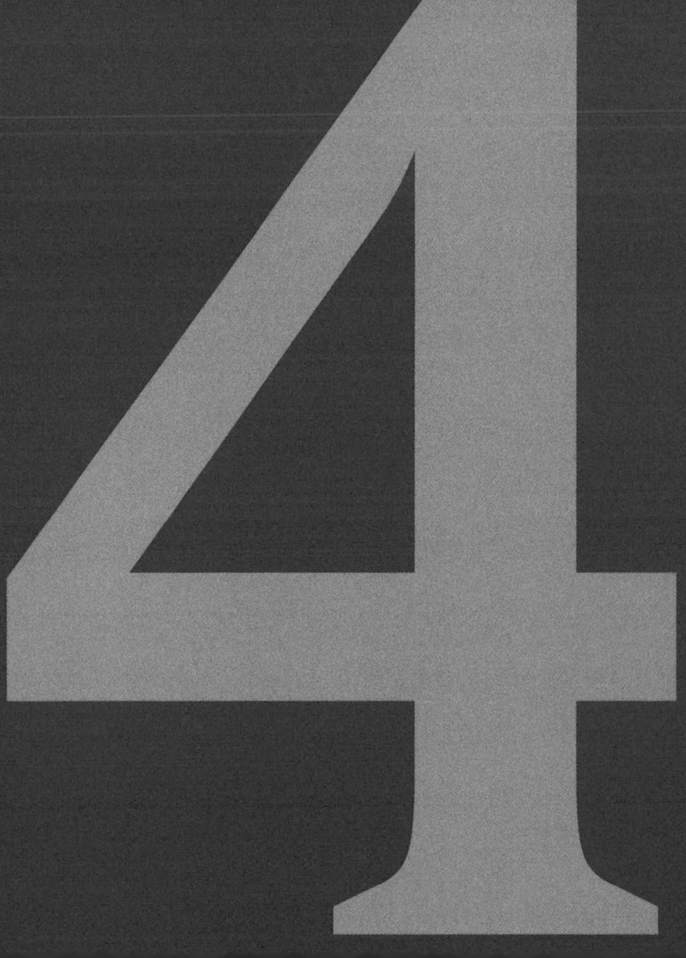

4 The Wrist

Eric P. Weinberg

4.1 Triangular Fibrocartilage Complex Tears

- Normal triangular fibrocartilage complex (TFCC)
- Thinning and degeneration of the TFCC disk
- Perforation of the TFCC disk
- Ulnar-sided TFCC tears

Table 4.1 Triangular fibrocartilage complex tears

Abnormalities	MRI findings	Comments
Normal triangular fibrocartilage complex (TFCC) (▶ Fig. 4.1)	The normal TFCC is low signal on proton density–weighted imaging (PDWI) and fat-suppressed T2-weighted imaging (FS T2WI). There is normally heterogeneous increased signal seen on FS T2WI in the region between the ulnar fovea and styloid attachments of the TFCC.	The normal TFCC consists of a fibrocartilagenous disk combined with several different ligaments, which together form a complex. The elements of this complex are not agreed upon by all authors. Most authors include the following components in the complex; triangular fibro-cartilage (TFC), meniscus homologue, ulnar collateral ligament, dorsal and volar radioulnar ligaments, and sheath of the extensor carpi ulnaris. There are two ulnar attachments of the TFC disk, the ulnar styloid tip and the ulnar fovea; there is one radial attachment, which joins to the cartilage of the distal radius at the sigmoid notch.
Thinning and degeneration of the TFCC disk (▶ Fig. 4.2)	Degenerative changes of the TFCC are usually seen as regions of increased signal intensity in the TFC disk. This abnormal increased signal does not extend to the articular surfaces of the TFC. Thinning of the disk is often seen in combination with disk degeneration. These findings are best seen on coronal images, particularly T2 intermediate-weighted fast spin echo images with fat suppression	Thinning and degeneration of the TFC disk are often seen with advancing age and may be asymptomatic. These findings can also be seen in the setting of ulnar positive variance. In this case the TFC disk is often thinned, and early degenerative changes in the adjacent distal ulna and proximal lunate can be seen. This situation can result in ulnolunate impaction syndrome. These patients often do have ulnar-sided wrist pain.

(continued on page 86)

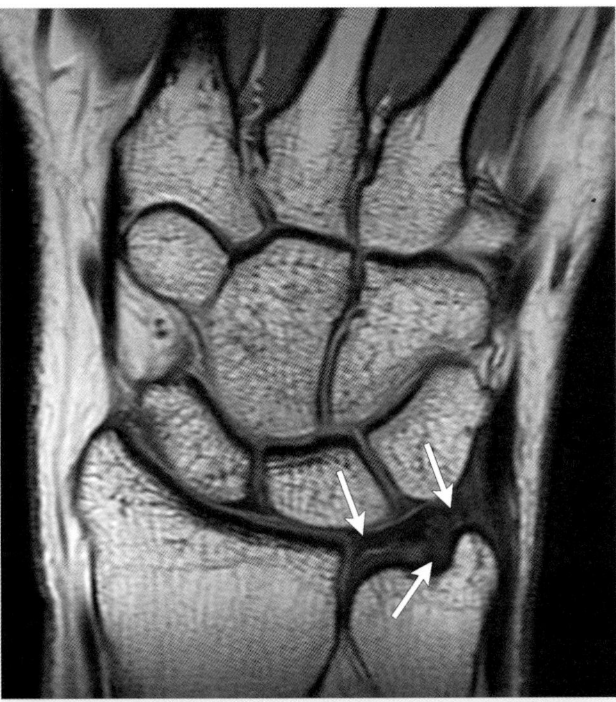

Fig. 4.1 Coronal proton density–weighted imaging shows normal triangular fibrocartilage complex (TFCC) with normal radial and ulnar attachments. The radial attachment of the TFCC is to the sigmoid notch of the distal radius (arrow), the ulnar attachments are to the ulnar styloid (arrow) and to the fovea of the distal ulna (arrow).

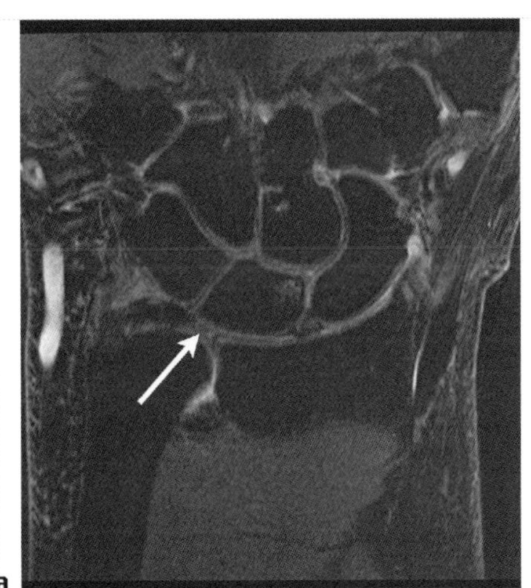

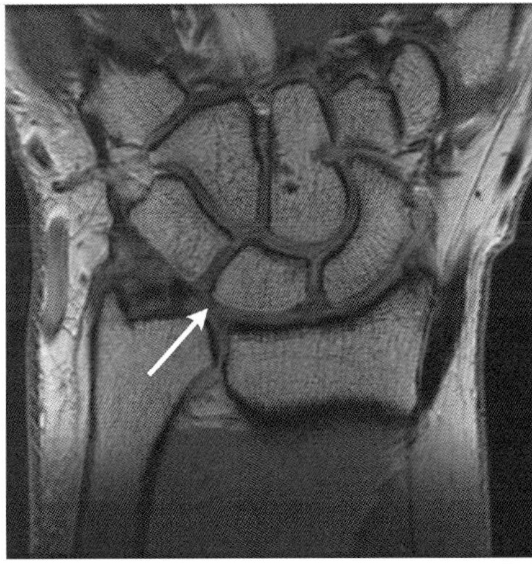

Fig. 4.2 (a) Coronal fat-suppressed T2-weighted imaging shows heterogeneous increased signal in the disk of the triangular fibrocartilage (arrow). (b) Coronal proton density–weighted imaging shows heterogeneous increased signal in the disk of the triangular fibrocartilage (arrow).

Table 4.1 (Cont.) Triangular fibrocartilage complex tears

Abnormalities	MRI findings	Comments
Perforation of the TFCC disk (▶ Fig. 4.3; ▶ Fig. 4.4; ▶ Fig. 4.5)	Perforation of the TFCC disk may be traumatic or degenerative. The imaging characteristics of both types of tear are similar. Both types of tears may be partial or full thickness. Coronal FS T2WI typically reveals a thin linear band of increased signal extending from one articular surface to the other. Usually degenerative tears will be more centrally located within the TFCC disk, and traumatic tears will be nearer the radial attachment. Partial-thickness tears are more difficult to see on conventional magnetic resonance imaging (MRI) examinations and are seen as linear high signal extending from an articular surface partway through the TFCC disk. Magnetic resonance (MR) arthrography can often better define these lesions. On coronal FS T1-weighted imaging (T1WI) contrast-laden injected saline traverses the disk perforation and is seen as a well-defined linear band of bright signal that is isointense to other injected fluid seen within the injected compartment of the wrist. MR arthrography is ideal for highlighting partial-thickness tears, which are seen as a bright, small focus of signal extending from one articular surface to partway through the TFCC disk. It should be noted that MR arthrography may not reveal all partial-thickness tears because usually only one wrist compartment is injected, typically the radiocarpal joint. If the partial-thickness tear is on the proximal surface of the disk then a distal radioulnar joint injection would be needed.	Degenerative and traumatic perforations (tears) of the TFCC disk are difficult to distinguish by MRI criteria alone. Degenerative tears are more common than traumatic tears and occur with increasing frequency as patient age increases. Degenerative tears are more common in the central portion of the TFCC disk because this is the thinnest part of the disk. This type of tear is uncommon before the third decade of life. Traumatic tears are often symptomatic, whereas degenerative tears may not be. The combination of tear location, patient history, symptoms, and age can help determine if a tear is traumatic or degenerative. The location of the tear will also help determine the treatment choice. The TFCC disk does not have a uniform blood supply, with the central portion being avascular and the periphery having a blood supply.

(continued on page 88)

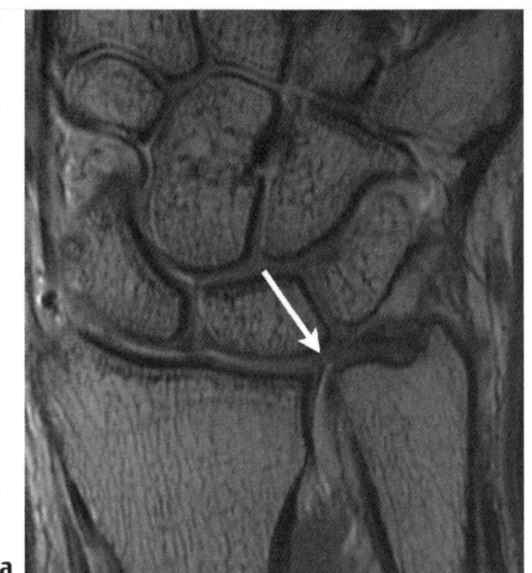

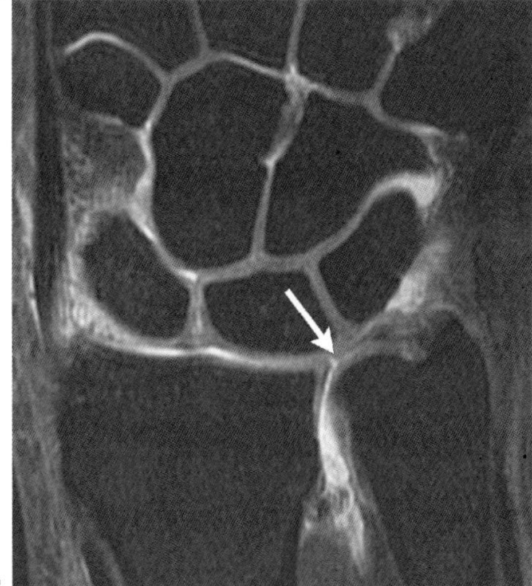

Fig. 4.3 (a) Coronal proton density–weighted imaging shows a small perforation of the triangular fibrocartilage complex (TFCC) near the radial attachment (arrow). (b) Coronal fat-suppressed T2-weighted imaging from a magnetic resonance arthrogram shows a small perforation of the TFCC near the radial attachment (arrow).

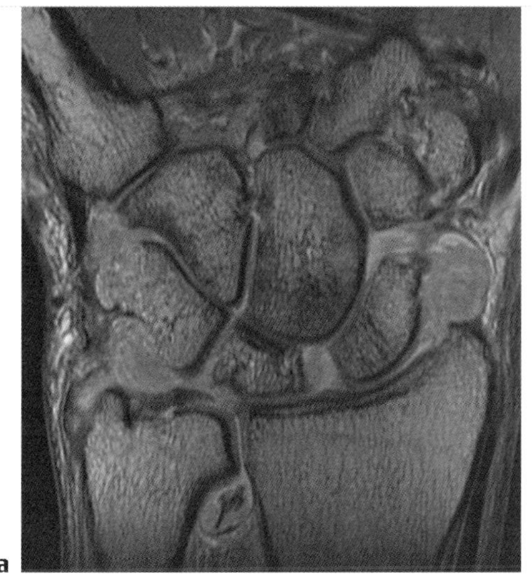

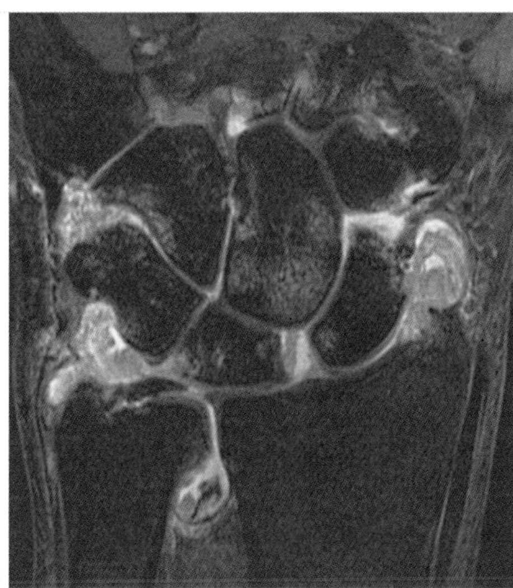

Fig. 4.4 (a) Coronal proton density–weighted imaging shows a large tear of the triangular fibrocartilage complex (TFCC) at the radial attachment. There is also heterogeneous joint effusion representing synovial hypertrophy. A large tear of the scapholunate (SL) ligament is also seen. (b) Coronal fat-suppressed T2-weighted imaging (FS T2WI) shows a large tear of the TFCC at the radial attachment. There is also a joint effusion with heterogeneous signal fluid and debris representing synovial hypertrophy. There is also a large tear of the SL ligament and marrow edema in the capitate.

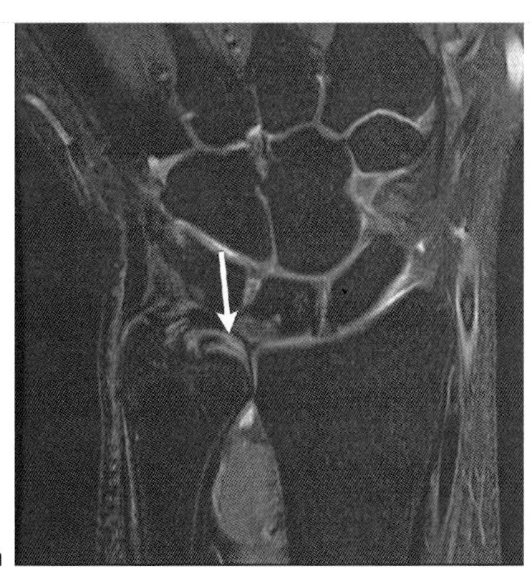

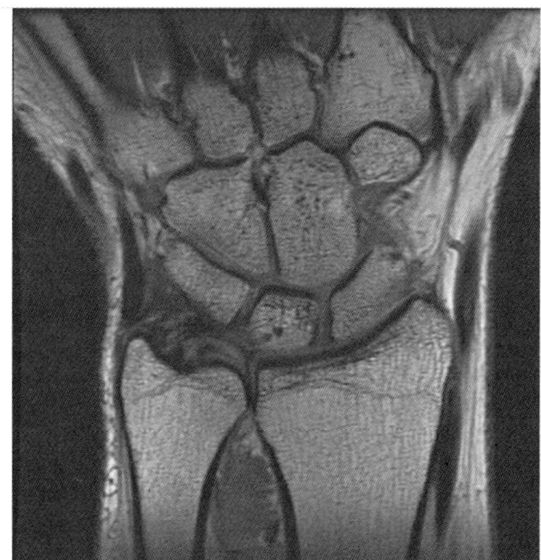

Fig. 4.5 (a) Coronal fat-suppressed T2-weighted imaging from a second patient shows a large longitudinal tear of the disk of the triangular fibrocartilage complex (TFCC) (arrow). (b) Coronal proton density–weighted imaging from the same patient also shows a large longitudinal tear of the disk of the TFCC.

Table 4.1 (Cont.) Triangular fibrocartilage complex tears

Abnormalities	MRI findings	Comments
Ulnar-sided TFCC tears (▶ Fig. 4.6)	Ulnar-sided tears and avulsions are difficult to diagnose, especially when there is increased fluid in the ulnar side of the wrist. On conventional MRI scans it may not be possible to determine if there is focal synovitis or ulnar-sided tear. On coronal FS T2WI ulnar-sided tears may appear as an altered shape of the ulnar attachment of the TFC, increased fluid, or avulsed ulnar attachments, either foveal or styloid or both. MR arthrography can be used to better define ulnar-sided tears. On coronal FS T1WI contrast can be seen to directly enter the site of tear even in the presence of increased ulnar-sided joint fluid. The joint fluid will be low signal, whereas the contrast will be high signal on FS T1WI.	Ulnar-sided tears are diagnosed less frequently than central or radial-sided tears. This is likely due to decreased incidence of these tears combined with decreased detection of these tears with conventional MRI. The anatomy of the ulnar side of the TFC is complex, and its normal appearance on MRI can lead to false-positive interpretations. There is normally fibrovascular connective tissue seen between the ulnar and foveal attachments of the TFCC disk. This region is known as ligmentum subcruentum and is high in signal on intermediate fat-saturated images. This is not a tear. Adding to the difficulty in determining if there is a tear is the common occurrence of degenerative and inflammatory changes in and around the ulnar attachments of the TFCC. Ulnar-sided tears are often symptomatic with significant ulnar-sided wrist pain. Patient history combined with MRI can help distinguish between traumatic injury and chronic inflammatory or degenerative changes.

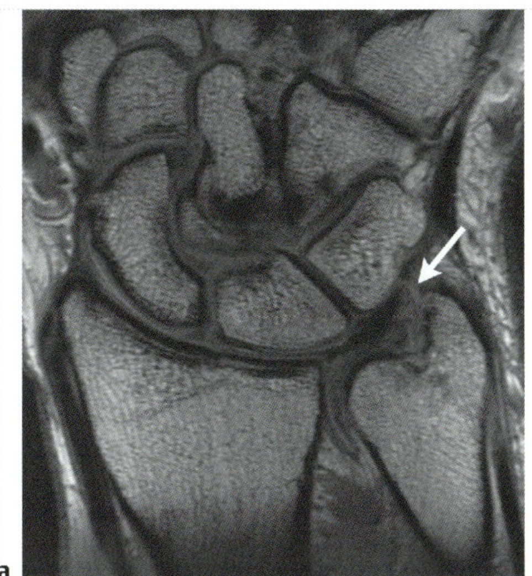

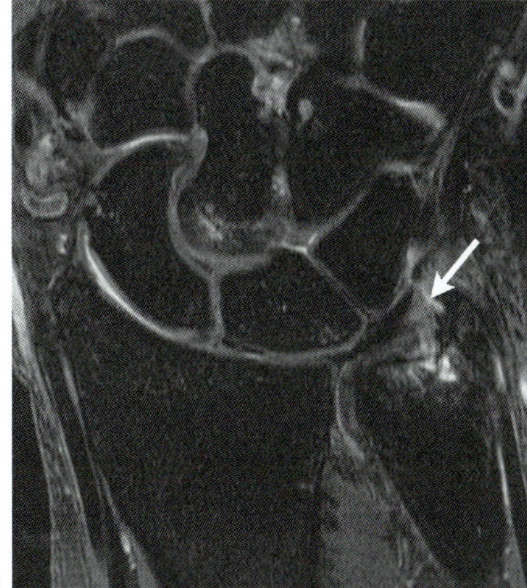

Fig. 4.6 (a) Coronal proton density–weighted imaging shows discontinuity of the ulnar styloid attachment of the triangular fibrocartilage complex (TFCC) (arrow). (b) Coronal fat-suppressed T2-weighted imaging shows discontinuity of the ulnar styloid attachment of the TFCC and degenerative marrow edema with small geodes in the distal ulna (arrow).

4.1.1 Triangular Fibrocartilage Complex Tears Suggested Reading

[1] Burns JE, Tanaka T, Ueno T, Nakamura T, Yoshioka H. Pitfalls that may mimic injuries of the triangular fibrocartilage and proximal intrinsic wrist ligaments at MR imaging. Radiographics 2011; 31: 63–78

[2] Maizlin ZV, Brown JA, Clement JJ, et al. MR arthrography of the wrist: controversies and concepts. Hand (NY) 2009; 4: 66–73

[3] Smith TO, Drew B, Toms AP, Jerosch-Herold C, Chojnowski AJ. Diagnostic accuracy of magnetic resonance imaging and magnetic resonance arthrography for triangular fibrocartilaginous complex injury: a systematic review and meta-analysis. J Bone Joint Surg Am 2012; 94: 824–832

[4] Weinberg EP, Hollenberg GM, Adams MJ, Tan RK, Lechner MJ. High-resolution outpatient imaging of the wrist. Semin Musculoskelet Radiol 2001; 5: 227–234

[5] Zlatkin MB, Rosner J. MR imaging of ligaments and triangular fibrocartilage complex of the wrist. Radiol Clin North Am 2006; 44: 595–623, ix

4.2 Extrinsic and Intrinsic Ligaments of the Wrist

- Scapholunate ligament tear
- Lunotriquetral ligament tear
- Normal extrinsic wrist ligaments
- Extrinsic wrist ligament tear

Table 4.2 Extrinsic and intrinsic ligaments of the wrist

Abnormalities	MRI findings	Comments
Scapholunate ligament tear (▶ Fig. 4.7)	The normal MRI appearance of the scapholunate ligament is a dark band of low signal on all pulse sequences traversing the proximal aspect of the scaphoid and lunate carpal bones. The scapholunate ligament may have a linear or triangular configuration. In most cases the ligament will be homogeneous low signal; however, a central linear zone of intermediate signal may be seen within the scapholunate. The scapholunate ligament may be partially torn or completely torn. In addition, degenerative tears may also occur. Partial tears typically involve the volar portion of the ligament. MRI shows focal irregularity or fluid signal in a portion of the ligament. Magnetic resonance (MR) arthrography shows contrast leak into a portion of the ligament. MRI of complete scapholunate ligament tears shows extensive fluid signal extending between the scaphoid and lunate carpal bones. There is often widening of the scapholunate space. MRI of degenerative tears typically reveals focal fluid signal only within the central or membranous portion of the scapholunate ligament.	The scapholunate ligament is an intrinsic wrist ligament with volar, membranous central, and dorsal components. The dorsal component is thought to be the most important in stabilizing the wrist. When there is radiographically apparent scapholunate widening the volar and dorsal components are usually torn as well as the radioscaphoid extrinsic ligament. Degenerative tears of the central membranous portion may be symptomatic though are unlikely to result in instability. Complete tears of the scapholunate may result in dorsal intercalated instability (DISI). The capitate can then migrate into the gap between the scaphoid and lunate. The scapholunate ligament is a small, complex structure that is seen to better advantage with 3-T MRI scanners. High spatial resolution, thin sections, and excellent signal to noise are required to accurately evaluate this ligament. The scapholunate ligament is best seen on coronal images. 3-T MRI arthrography is often needed to diagnose partial tears.

(continued on page 92)

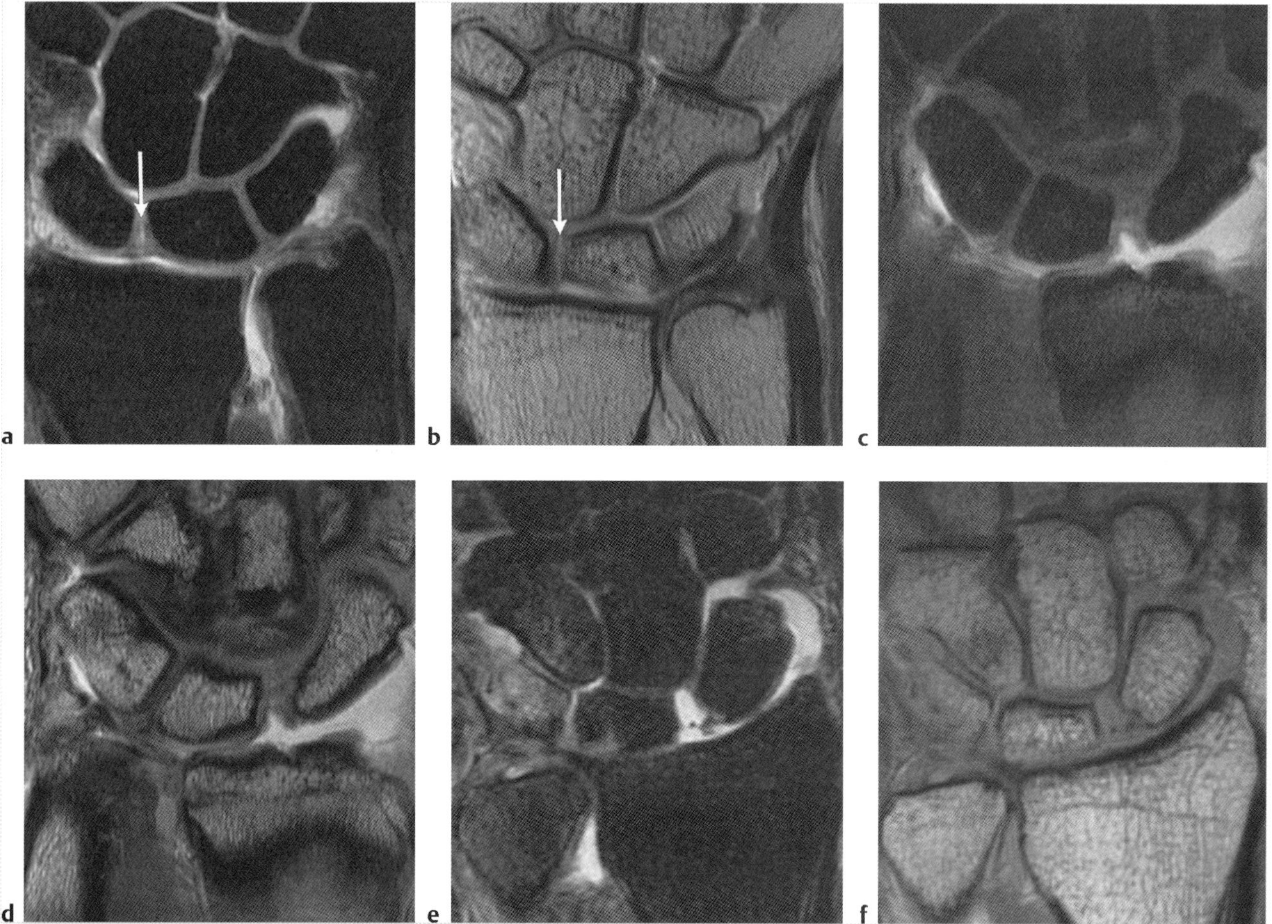

Fig. 4.7 (a) Coronal fat-suppressed T2-weighted imaging (FS T2WI) from an magnetic resonance (MR) arthrogram shows membranous perforation of the scapholunate ligament (arrow). (b) Coronal proton density–weighted imaging (PDWI) shows membranous perforation of the scapholunate ligament (arrow). (c) Coronal FS T2WI from a wrist MR arthrogram in a second patient shows a partial tear of the volar portion of the scapholunate ligament. (d) Coronal PDWI from a wrist MR arthrogram from the same patient shows a partial tear of the volar portion of the scapholunate ligament. (e) Coronal FS T2WI from a third patient shows a complete tear of the scapholunate ligament. (f) Coronal PDWI from the same patient shows a complete tear of the scapholunate ligament.

Table 4.2 (Cont.) Extrinsic and intrinsic ligaments of the wrist

Abnormalities	MRI findings	Comments
Lunotriquetral ligament tear (▸ Fig. 4.8)	The lunotriquetral ligament connects the proximal portions of the lunate and triquetral carpal bones. The lunotriquetral ligament has a variable appearance on MRI. Usually the ligament has a delta shape and is a thin, low signal band on all imaging sequences. The ligament is composed of volar, membranous or central portion and dorsal component. Tears of the lunotriquetral ligament may be partial or full thickness. Chronic degenerative tears also occur. To date MRI has had low sensitivity and specificity in the accurate diagnosis of these tears. On fat-suppressed T2-weighted imaging (FS T2WI) partial and complete tears are seen as increased signal between the lunate and triquetral bones. With complete tears there may be nonvisualization of the ligament. There may also be widening of the space between the lunate and triquetral carpal bones. MRI arthrography is likely more accurate in identifying all types of lunotriquetral ligament tears and in particular partial tears.	Tears of the lunotriquetral ligament are often clinically significant. This is true for both partial and complete tears. Patients with tears both partial and complete may complain of wrist pain, loss of grip strength, and decreased wrist range of motion. Wrist instability may also be present. Chronic lunotriquetral tears, including partial tears, can result in osteoarthritis. Some lunotriquetral tears are asymptomatic.
Normal extrinsic wrist ligaments (▸ Fig. 4.9)	The dorsal and volar extrinsic wrist ligaments are uniformly low signal on all MRI sequences.	The extrinsic ligaments of the wrist are important for overall wrist stability. They are thought to be weaker than the intrinsic ligaments. Currently most authors believe there is insufficient evidence regarding the efficacy of MRI in the imaging diagnosis of tears of these ligaments. The extrinsic ligaments are divided into volar and dorsal groups. There are more and stronger volar extrinsic wrist ligaments. The volar group consists of radioscaphocapitate, radiolunotriquetral, and short radiolunate ligaments. The dorsal group consists of radiocarpal (composed of radioscaphoid, radiolunate, and radiotriquetral segments) and dorsal intercarpal ligaments.
Lesions of the extrinsic wrist ligaments (▸ Fig. 4.10)	Extrinsic wrist ligaments are usually dark signal bands on all MRI pulse sequences. When they are torn there may be visible discontinuity and focally increased signal. These tears can be partial or full thickness. In the experience of this author there may also be associated ganglion cysts.	Tears of the extrinsic wrist ligaments are difficult to identify with MRI and are best seen with 3-T MRI using small field of view, thin slices, and high matrix. As a result many radiologists choose not to comment on these ligaments in their reports.

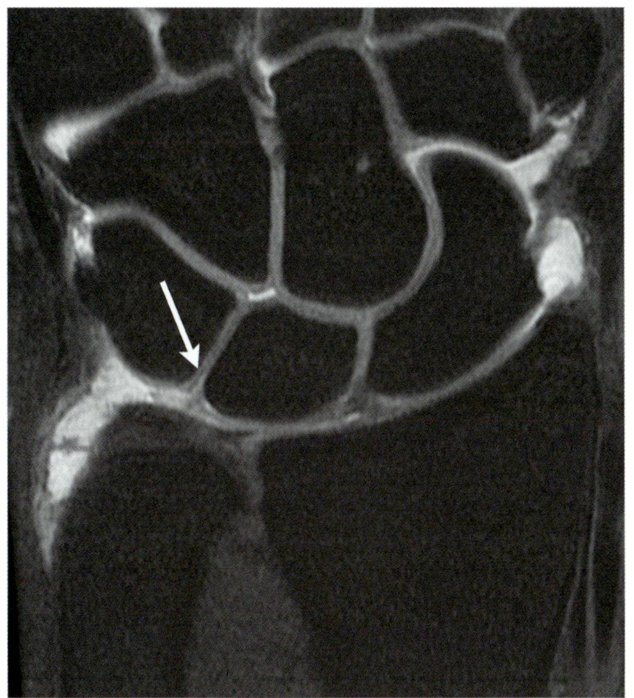

Fig. 4.8 Coronal fat-suppressed T1-weighted imaging from a magnetic resonance arthrogram shows a partial tear of the lunotriquetral ligament (arrow).

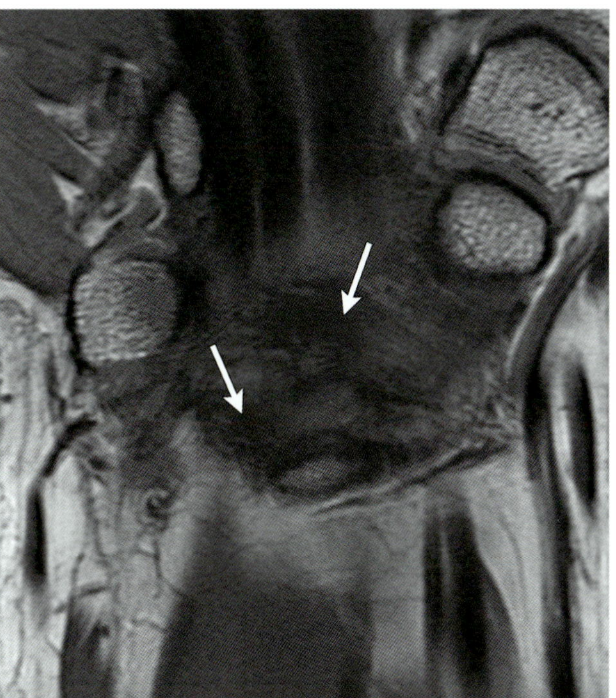

Fig. 4.9 Coronal proton density–weighted imaging shows normal low signal volar extrinsic wrist ligaments (arrows).

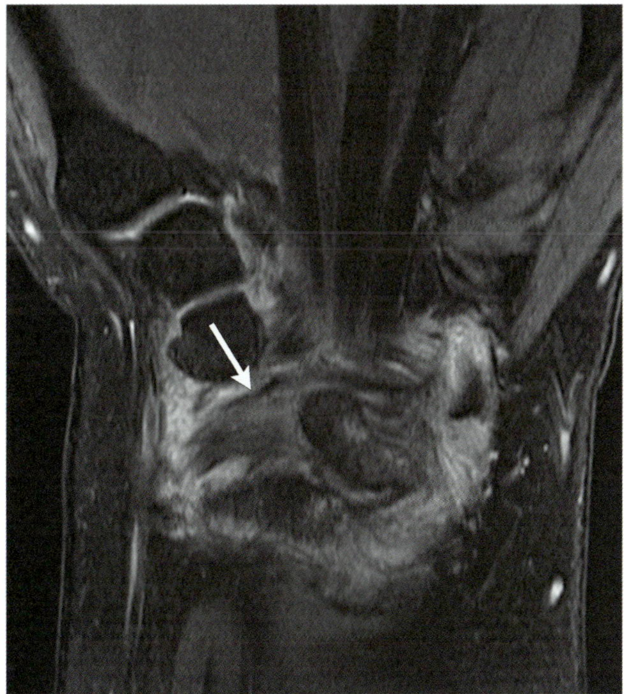

Fig. 4.10 Coronal fat-suppressed T2-weighted imaging shows partially torn volar extrinsic wrist ligaments, which are thickened with increased signal (arrow).

4.2.1 Extrinsic and Intrinsic Ligaments of the Wrist Suggested Reading

[1] Chhabra A, Soldatos T, Thawait GK, et al. Current perspectives on the advantages of 3-T MR imaging of the wrist. Radiographics 2012; 32: 879–896

[2] Mak WH, Szabo RM, Myo GK. Assessment of volar radiocarpal ligaments: MR arthrographic and arthroscopic correlation. AJR Am J Roentgenol 2012; 198: 423–427

[3] Shahabpour M, Van Overstraeten L, Ceuterick P, et al. Pathology of extrinsic ligaments: a pictorial essay. Semin Musculoskelet Radiol 2012; 16: 115–128

[4] Taljanovic MS, Malan JJ, Sheppard JE. Normal anatomy of the extrinsic capsular wrist ligaments by 3-T MRI and high-resolution ultrasonography. Semin Musculoskelet Radiol 2012; 16: 104–114

[5] Weinberg EP, Hollenberg GM, Adams MJ, Tan RK, Lechner MJ. High-resolution outpatient imaging of the wrist. Semin Musculoskelet Radiol 2001; 5: 227–234

[6] Zlatkin MB, Rosner J. MR imaging of ligaments and triangular fibrocartilage complex of the wrist. Radiol Clin North Am 2006; 44: 595–623, ix

4.3 Congenital and Acquired Lesions of the Wrist

- Carpal boss
- Type II lunate
- Carpal coalition
- Madelung deformity
- Ulnolunate impaction
- Ganglion cyst
- Synovial cyst

Table 4.3 Congenital and acquired lesions of the wrist

Abnormalities	MRI findings	Comments
Carpal boss (▶ Fig. 4.11)	The carpal boss is located on the dorsum of the wrist at the base of the second or third metacarpal. This accessory ossicle typically has a triangular shape and is isointense to other bones on all sequences obtained. Occasionally there can be marrow edema seen in this ossicle on fat-suppressed T2-weighted imaging (FS T2WI). The carpal boss is best seen on axial and sagittal planes.	A carpal boss is a bony protuberance caused by an accessory ossification center and is also known as an os styloideum. This ossicle may or may not be fused with its adjacent metacarpal. The patient may or may not be symptomatic. When symptoms are present they are usually a combination of pain and decreased range of motion. Differential diagnostic considerations include ganglion cysts, bursitis, and localized osteoarthritis.

(continued on page 96)

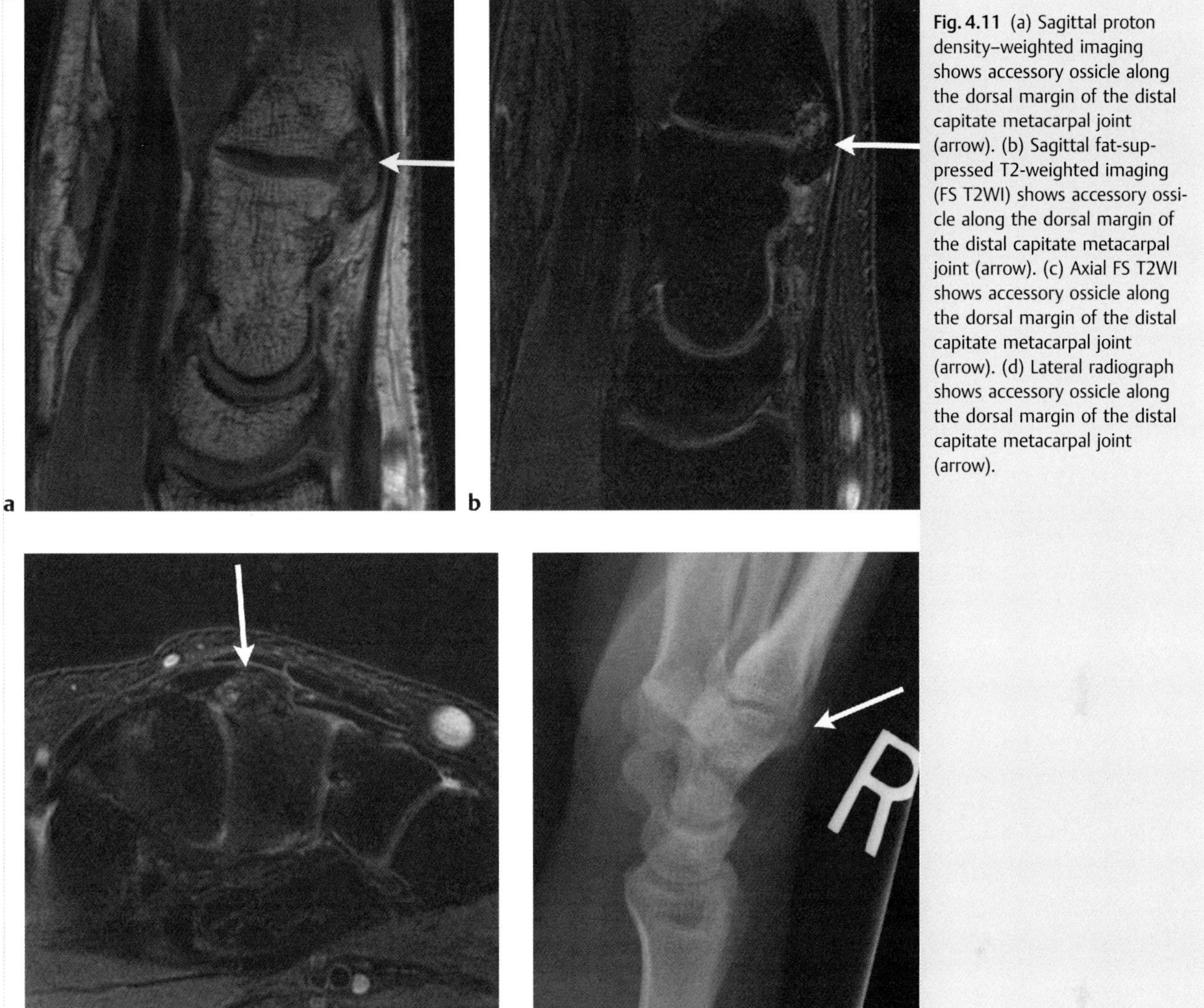

Fig. 4.11 (a) Sagittal proton density–weighted imaging shows accessory ossicle along the dorsal margin of the distal capitate metacarpal joint (arrow). (b) Sagittal fat-suppressed T2-weighted imaging (FS T2WI) shows accessory ossicle along the dorsal margin of the distal capitate metacarpal joint (arrow). (c) Axial FS T2WI shows accessory ossicle along the dorsal margin of the distal capitate metacarpal joint (arrow). (d) Lateral radiograph shows accessory ossicle along the dorsal margin of the distal capitate metacarpal joint (arrow).

Table 4.3 (Cont.) Congenital and acquired lesions of the wrist

Abnormalities	MRI findings	Comments
Type II lunate (▶ Fig. 4.12)	The type II lunate has an articulation with the hamate. There are often osteoarthritic changes at the hamatolunate articulation. On 3-T coronal FS T2WI significant cartilage damage can be seen in the proximal pole of the hamate. There may also be geodes and reactive marrow edema at the hamatolunate articulation. The coronal plane is the best for identifying this abnormality.	A type I lunate articulates distally only with the capitate, and the type II lunate has an extra-articular facet that articulates with the proximal hamate. The type II lunate is common. There is often advanced cartilage damage seen in the proximal pole of the hamate. Type II lunate can be an unidentified cause of ulnar-sided wrist pain.
Carpal coalition (▶ Fig. 4.13)	Coronal images show bony coalition between the triquetrum and lunate. Coalitions may be osseous, fibrous, or cartilaginous. Some cases may be associated with marrow edema and cystic changes in the coalescent carpal bones, which can mimic osteoarthritic disease.	Lunotriquetral carpal coalition is the most common, with capitohamate the next most frequent coalition of the carpal bones. Carpal coalition is a rare occurrence with female predominance. Carpal coalitions are frequently bilateral. There is a reported association with widened scapholunate joint space, which is a normal variant; a normal scapholunate ligament is seen at arthrography.

(continued on page 98)

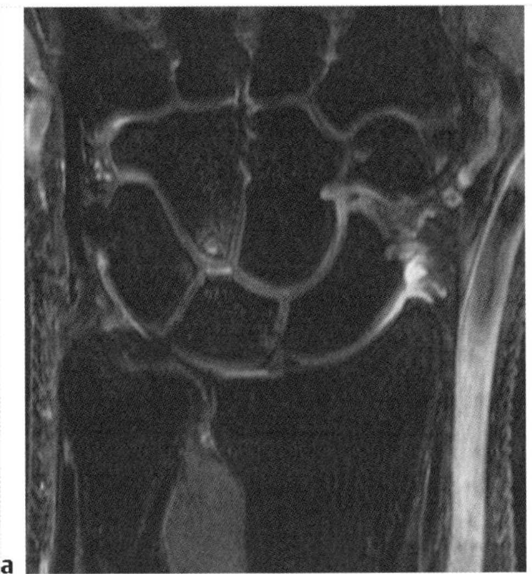

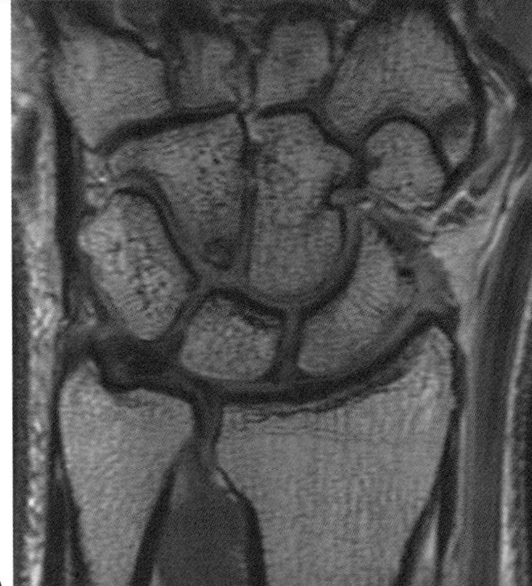

Fig. 4.12 (a) Coronal fat-suppressed T2-weighted imaging (FS T2WI) shows an extra-articular facet along the distal aspect of the lunate, which articulates with the hamate. Small subcortical geode is seen in the proximal hamate along with mild reactive degenerative marrow edema. (b) Coronal proton density–weighted imaging shows an extra-articular facet along the distal aspect of the lunate, which articulates with the hamate. A small, low signal subcortical geode is seen in the proximal pole of the hamate.

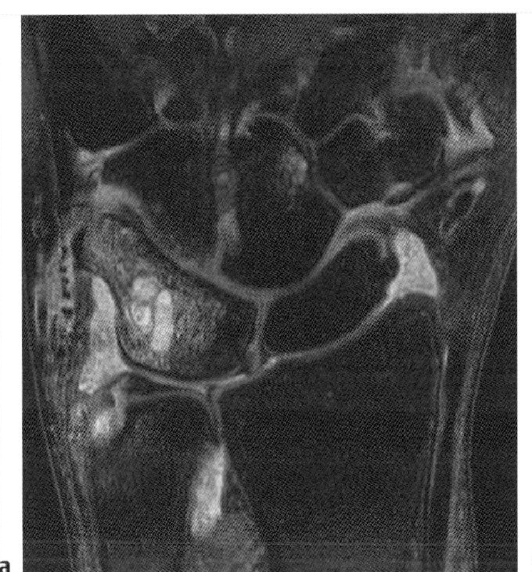

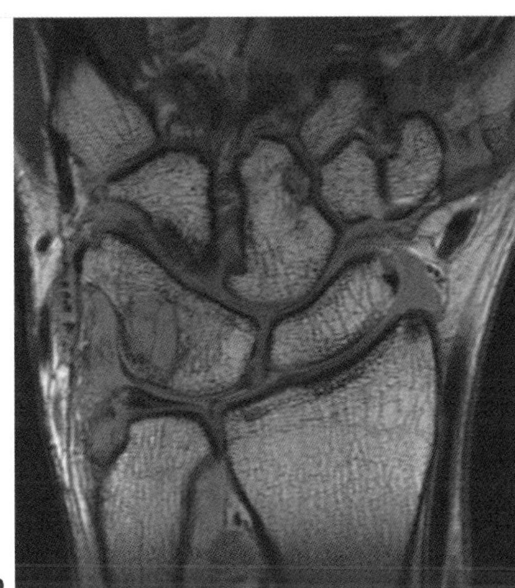

Fig. 4.13 (a) Coronal fat-suppressed T2-weighted imaging shows a lunotriquetral coalition with large degenerative intraosseous cysts and heterogeneous signal joint fluid, likely synovitis. (b) Coronal proton density–weighted imaging shows a lunotriquetral coalition.

Table 4.3 (Cont.) Congenital and acquired lesions of the wrist

Abnormalities	MRI findings	Comments
Madelung deformity (▸ Fig. 4.14)	MRI shows ulnar tilting of the radius and radial tilting of the ulna. There is volar tilting of the distal articular surface of the radius and a triangular shape of the epiphysis. A physeal bar bridging the distal radius metaphysis and epiphysis is usually seen. There is often a hypertrophied anomalous radiotriquetral ligament. The proximal carpal row has a pyramidal shape.	This deformity can be caused in several ways. Prior trauma to the distal radial growth plate can result in a bony bar causing the deformity. Congenital causes include dyschondrosteosis, multiple hereditary exostosis, gonadal dysgenesis, Turner syndrome, and sickle cell disease. Madelung deformity is more common in females, is more often bilateral, and usually presents between the ages of 6 and 13. Patients may have wrist pain and decreased range of motion.
Ulnolunate impaction (▸ Fig. 4.15)	MRI shows ulnar positive variance. There is marrow edema, subchondral cyst formation, and cartilage destruction in the proximal lunate and distal ulna. Triangular fibrocartilage tears are also usually seen. Coronal MRI scans best demonstrate this abnormality.	Patients with ulnolunate impaction usually complain of ulnar-sided wrist pain. Most patients will have ulnar positive variance, which can be congenital or acquired and which usually occurs secondary to an impacted distal radius fracture. Ulnar positive variance causes repetitive impaction on the proximal lunate with resulting loss of cartilage and often tearing of the triangular fibrocartilage (TFC).
Ganglion cyst (▸ Fig. 4.16)	On FS T2WI ganglion cysts are high signal, often with multiple thin septations. On proton density–weighted imaging (PDWI) ganglion cysts are usually low signal. On postcontrast FS T1-weighted imaging (T1WI) there is a very thin rim of peripheral enhancement with no internal enhancement. The postcontrast appearance of ganglion cysts is often helpful in distinguishing this lesion from a solid mass or enhancing venous structure.	Ganglion cysts are the most common soft tissue mass in the wrist and hand. They may be symptomatic or asymptomatic. They are more common in women. These lesions are often seen in close association with wrist ligaments, particularly dorsal extrinsic ligaments of the wrist. On histological examination there is a lining of pseudosynovial cells with a mucinous fluid-filled cavity. Ganglion cysts can erode adjacent bone such that they become partially intraosseous and communicate with the adjacent joint. Ganglion cysts may be entirely intraosseous, particularly in the carpal bones. Intraosseous ganglion cysts may be radiographically occult.
Synovial cyst	On FS T2WI synovial cysts are high signal, often without internal septations. On PDWI they are low signal. On postcontrast FS T1WI there is usually thin peripheral enhancement with no internal enhancement.	Synovial cysts communicate with the joint. These cysts have a true lining of mesothelial cells. The cyst cavity is filled with mucinous fluid.

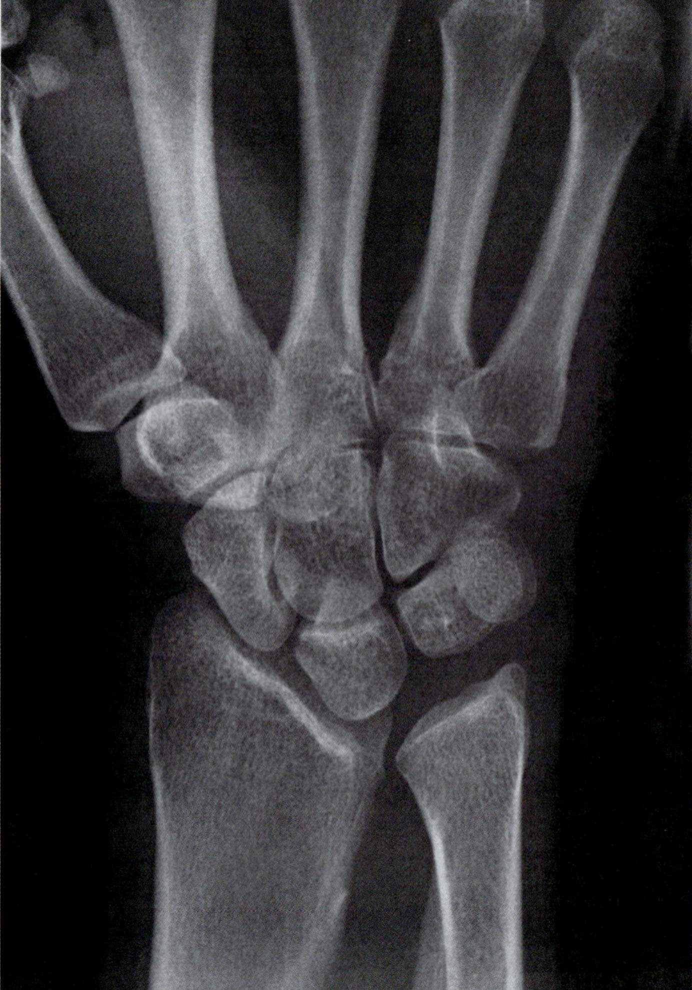

Fig. 4.14 Madelung deformity. Anteroposterior radiograph shows characteristic angulation of the distal radius and ulna so that there is an overall V-shaped appearance.

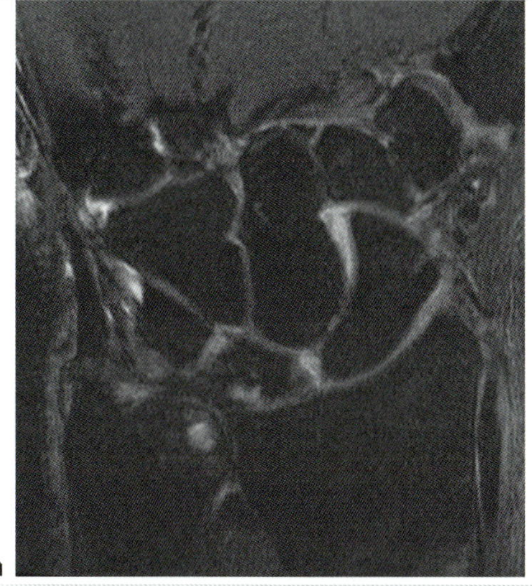

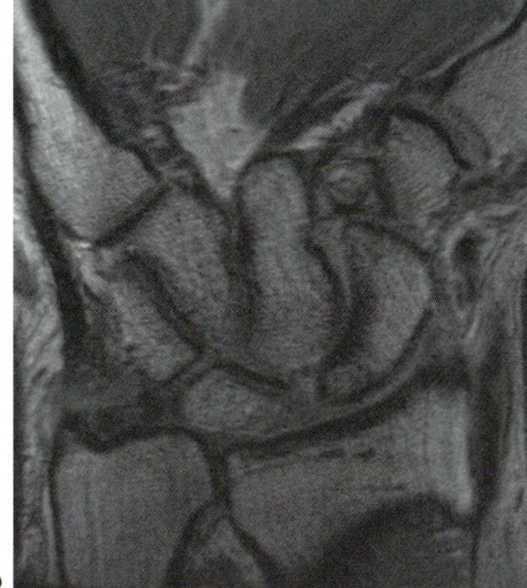

Fig. 4.15 (a) Coronal fat-suppressed T2-weighted imaging shows ulnar positive variance with degenerative marrow edema in the distal ulna and opposite lunate. There is a subcortical geode seen in the distal ulna. (b) Coronal proton density-weighted imaging shows ulnar positive variance of the distal ulna with marked narrowing of the ulnolunate space.

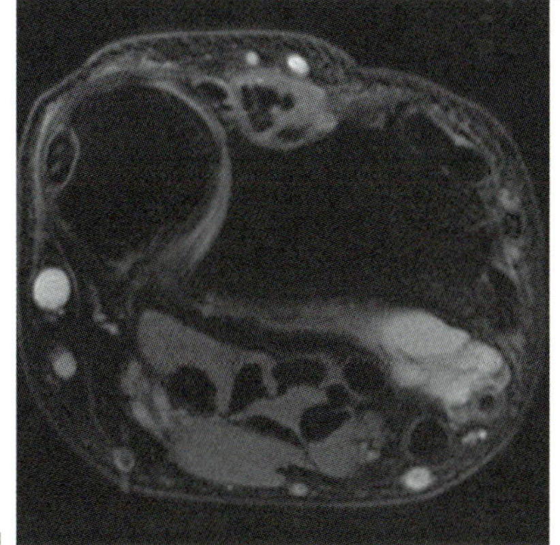

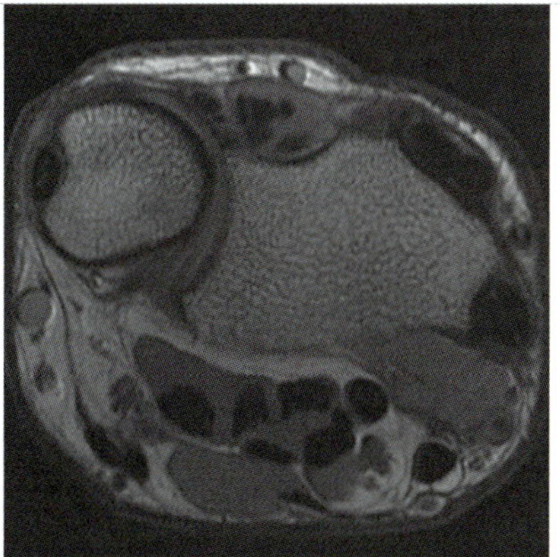

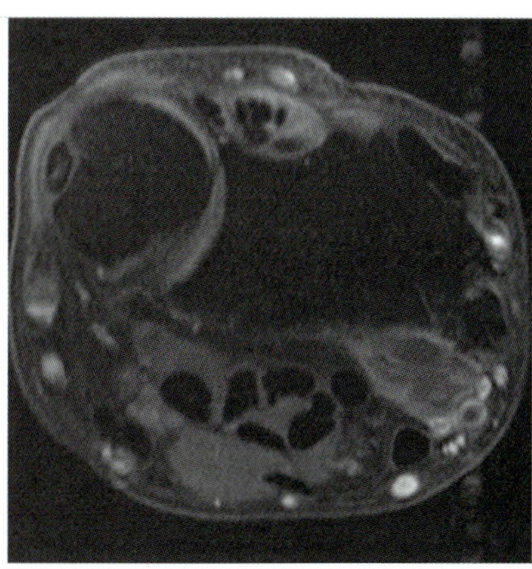

Fig. 4.16 (a) Axial fat-suppressed (FS) T2-weighted imaging shows a large, high signal septated ganglion cyst along the volar aspect of the distal radius. (b) Axial proton density-weighted imaging shows a large, intermediate signal septated cyst. (c) Axial FS T1-weighted imaging postcontrast shows a septated cyst along the volar aspect of the distal radius with only minimal peripheral enhancement.

4.3.1 Congenital and Acquired Lesions of the Wrist Suggested Reading

[1] Cerezal L, del Piñal F, Abascal F, García-Valtuille R, Pereda T, Canga A. Imaging findings in ulnar-sided wrist impaction syndromes. Radiographics 2002; 22: 105–121

[2] Cook PA, Yu JS, Wiand W, et al. Madelung deformity in skeletally immature patients: morphologic assessment using radiography, CT, and MRI. J Comput Assist Tomogr 1996; 20: 505–511

[3] Freire V, Guérini H, Campagna R, et al. Imaging of hand and wrist cysts: a clinical approach. AJR Am J Roentgenol 2012; 199: W618–28

[4] Malik AM, Schweitzer ME, Culp RW, Osterman LA, Manton G. MR imaging of the type II lunate bone: frequency, extent, and associated findings. AJR Am J Roentgenol 1999; 173: 335–338

[5] Pfirrmann CWA, Zanetti M. Variants, pitfalls and asymptomatic findings in wrist and hand imaging. Eur J Radiol 2005; 56: 286–295

[6] Timins ME. Osseous anatomic variants of the wrist: findings on MR imaging. AJR Am J Roentgenol 1999; 173: 339–344

4.4 Bone Lesions of the Wrist

- Scaphoid fractures
- Hamate fractures
- Triquetral fractures
- Incomplete fractures of the wrist
- Avascular necrosis (AVN)/scaphoid AVN
- Kienböck disease
- Physeal injuries
- Carpal instability

Table 4.4 Bone lesions of the wrist

Abnormalities	MRI findings	Comments
Scaphoid fractures (▶ Fig. 4.17)	On T1-weighted imaging (T1WI) or proton density–weighted imaging (PDWI) there is a transverse low signal line across the scaphoid waist or middle third of the scaphoid, which is best seen in the coronal plane. On fat-suppressed T2-weighted imaging (FS T2WI) there is a low signal line in the same position with high signal marrow edema on one or both sides of the fracture. Low signal fracture line usually extends to involve the cortex, and there may be displacement of proximal and distal scaphoid poles. If the fracture does not extend to the cortex this could represent an incomplete acute fracture (fracture line limited to medullary bone) or a chronic fracture.	Most scaphoid fractures occur secondary to a fall, with 80% occurring in the scaphoid waist or middle third of the scaphoid. The remaining 20% of scaphoid fractures occur in the proximal and distal poles with equal frequency. Patients with scaphoid fractures typically present with pain in the anatomical snuffbox, decreased range of motion, and decreased grip strength. When the fracture results in displacement of the proximal and distal poles there is often resultant wrist instability. Proximal pole scaphoid avascular necrosis is an important complication. This can occur in the setting of delayed diagnosis and treatment secondary to radiographically occult nondisplaced scaphoid fractures. Other complications include nonunion or malunion, osteoarthritis, and wrist instability.

(continued on page 102)

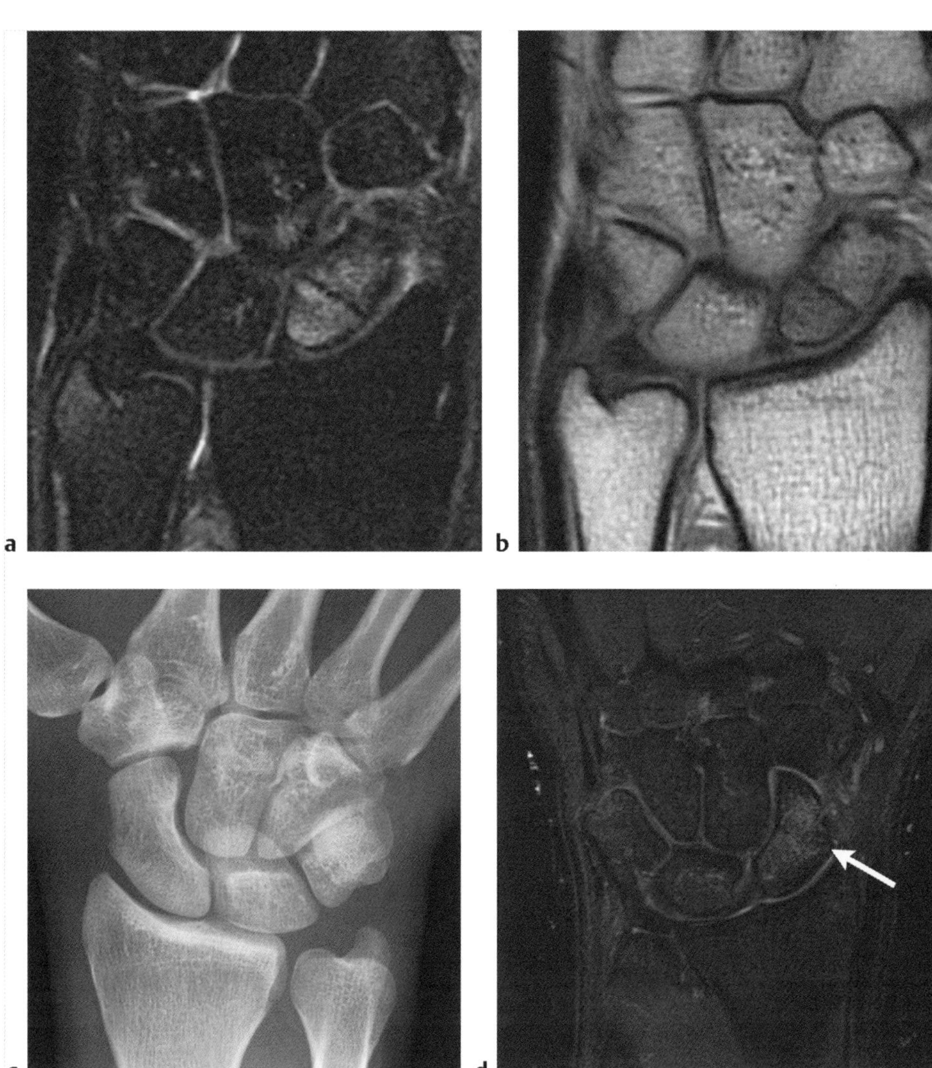

Fig. 4.17 (a) Coronal fat-suppressed T2-weighted imaging (FS T2WI) shows diffuse edema in the scaphoid with a well-defined low signal fracture across the scaphoid waist. (b) Coronal proton density–weighted imaging (PDWI) shows diffuse edema in the scaphoid with a well-defined low signal fracture across the scaphoid waist. (c) Anteroposterior radiograph from a second patient is normal with no evidence of scaphoid fracture. (d) Coronal FS T2WI from the same patient shows a low signal fracture line at the scaphoid waist (arrow) with marrow contusion on either side. This is a radiographically occult scaphoid fracture.

Table 4.4 (Cont.) Bone lesions of the wrist

Abnormalities	MRI findings	Comments
Hamate fractures (▶ Fig. 4.18)	Hamate fractures typically involve the hook or body of the bone, either the proximal or distal pole. On PDWI and FS T2WI they are seen as a hypointense line. On FS T2WI there is often hyperintense marrow edema on both sides of the fracture line. Body fractures may involve the articular surface. Hook fractures are oriented horizontally on axial images and vertically on sagittal images. They may not be seen in the coronal plane. Some hook fractures may cause mass effect on the ulnar aspect of the carpal tunnel.	Most hamate fractures occur secondary to a fall on an outstretched wrist or direct trauma. Patients often complain of ulnar-sided wrist pain, soreness in the palm, decreased grip strength, and sometimes ulnar nerve palsy. Most patients are young, active athletes, with males more frequently seen than females. These fractures may be seen in specific sports, including baseball, hockey, golf, and tennis. Most hamate body fractures will heal; however, some hook fractures will go on to nonunion. On occasion an incompletely fused ossification center of the hook of hamate may be confused with a fracture.
Triquetral fractures (▶ Fig. 4.19)	Most fractures of the triquetral carpal bone are avulsion fractures involving the dorsal cortex. On FS T2WI there is edema adjacent to the fracture site. PDWI shows low signal adjacent to the fracture site and will more often demonstrate discontinuity of the thin, black, cortical line. The displaced cortical fragment may be small and difficult to see with MRI. Sagittal and axial planes are more likely to optimally show this fracture.	Fractures of the triquetrum often occur when there is a fall on the outstretched hand. Patients often complain of pain and swelling at the dorsum of the wrist along its ulnar aspect. These fractures can be difficult to see with radiography. Computed tomography may be the best modality for evaluating triquetral fractures. Fractures of other carpal bones are uncommon. All carpal fractures should be detected with MRI, with FS T2WI showing marrow edema.

(continued on page 104)

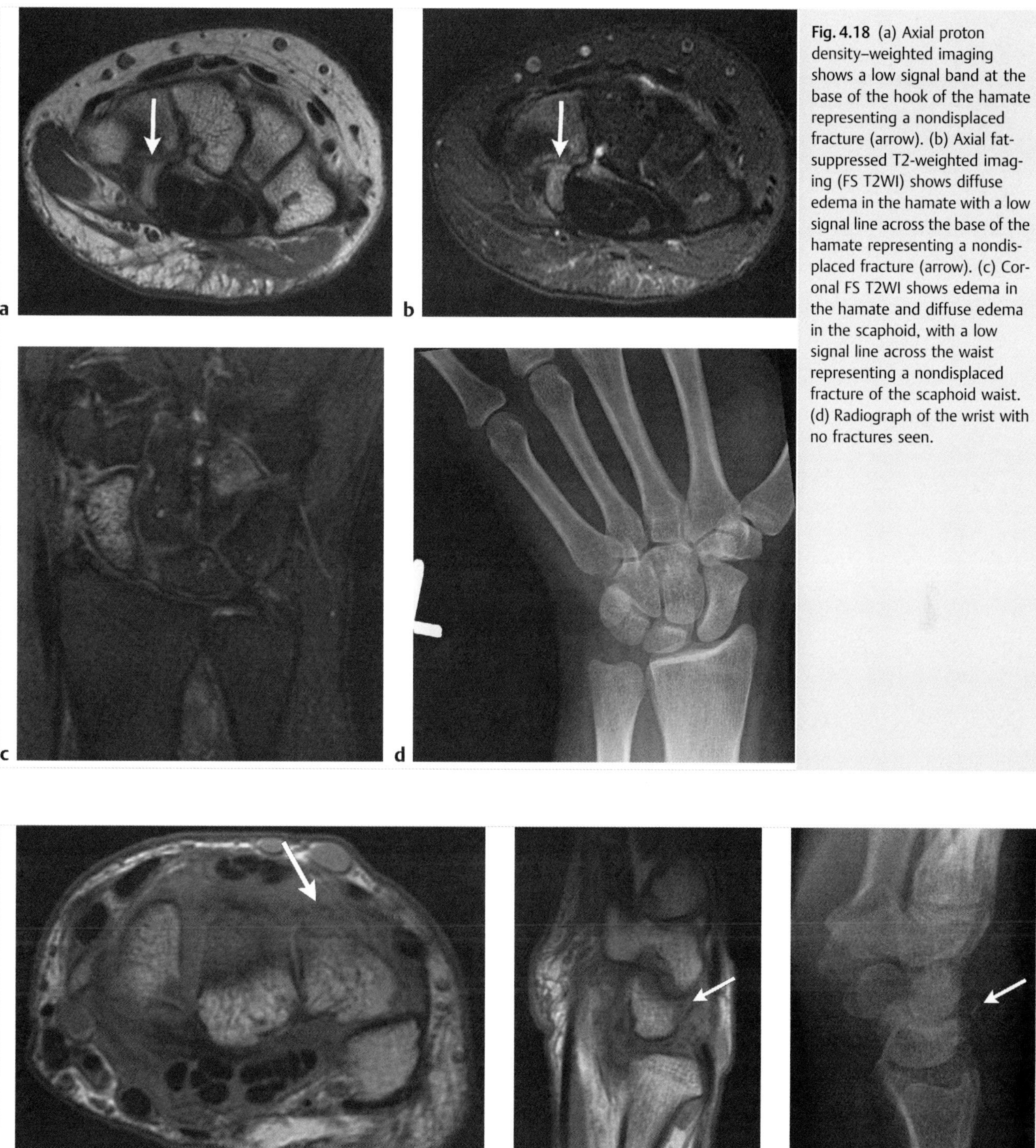

Fig. 4.18 (a) Axial proton density–weighted imaging shows a low signal band at the base of the hook of the hamate representing a nondisplaced fracture (arrow). (b) Axial fat-suppressed T2-weighted imaging (FS T2WI) shows diffuse edema in the hamate with a low signal line across the base of the hamate representing a nondisplaced fracture (arrow). (c) Coronal FS T2WI shows edema in the hamate and diffuse edema in the scaphoid, with a low signal line across the waist representing a nondisplaced fracture of the scaphoid waist. (d) Radiograph of the wrist with no fractures seen.

Fig. 4.19 (a) Axial proton density–weighted imaging (PDWI) shows cortical fracture with fragment along the dorsal margin of the triquetrum (arrow). (b) Sagittal PDWI shows cortical fracture along the dorsal margin of the triquetrum (arrow). (c) Lateral radiograph shows fracture along the dorsal cortex of the triquetrum (arrow).

Table 4.4 (Cont.) Bone lesions of the wrist

Abnormalities	MRI findings	Comments
Incomplete fractures of the wrist (▶ Fig. 4.20)	Incomplete fractures can occur in any bone. Incomplete fractures are intramedullary fractures, which do not extend to the cortical bone. A well-defined linear zone of low signal is seen on PDWI in the medullary portion of the bone, usually surrounded on both sides by high signal marrow edema on FS T2WI. The presence of marrow edema alone can indicate an occult fracture, which on follow-up may eventually demonstrate a fracture line. In the wrist the distal radius and scaphoid are typical locations for incomplete fractures. These fractures are radiographically occult.	Patients with incomplete wrist fractures present with wrist pain. If these fractures are detected a perfect treatment outcome can be expected. However, if these fractures are not identified they can go on to involve the nearest cortical surface, resulting in a complete fracture. In the scaphoid carpal bone avascular necrosis can occur when incomplete fractures are not detected.

(continued on page 106)

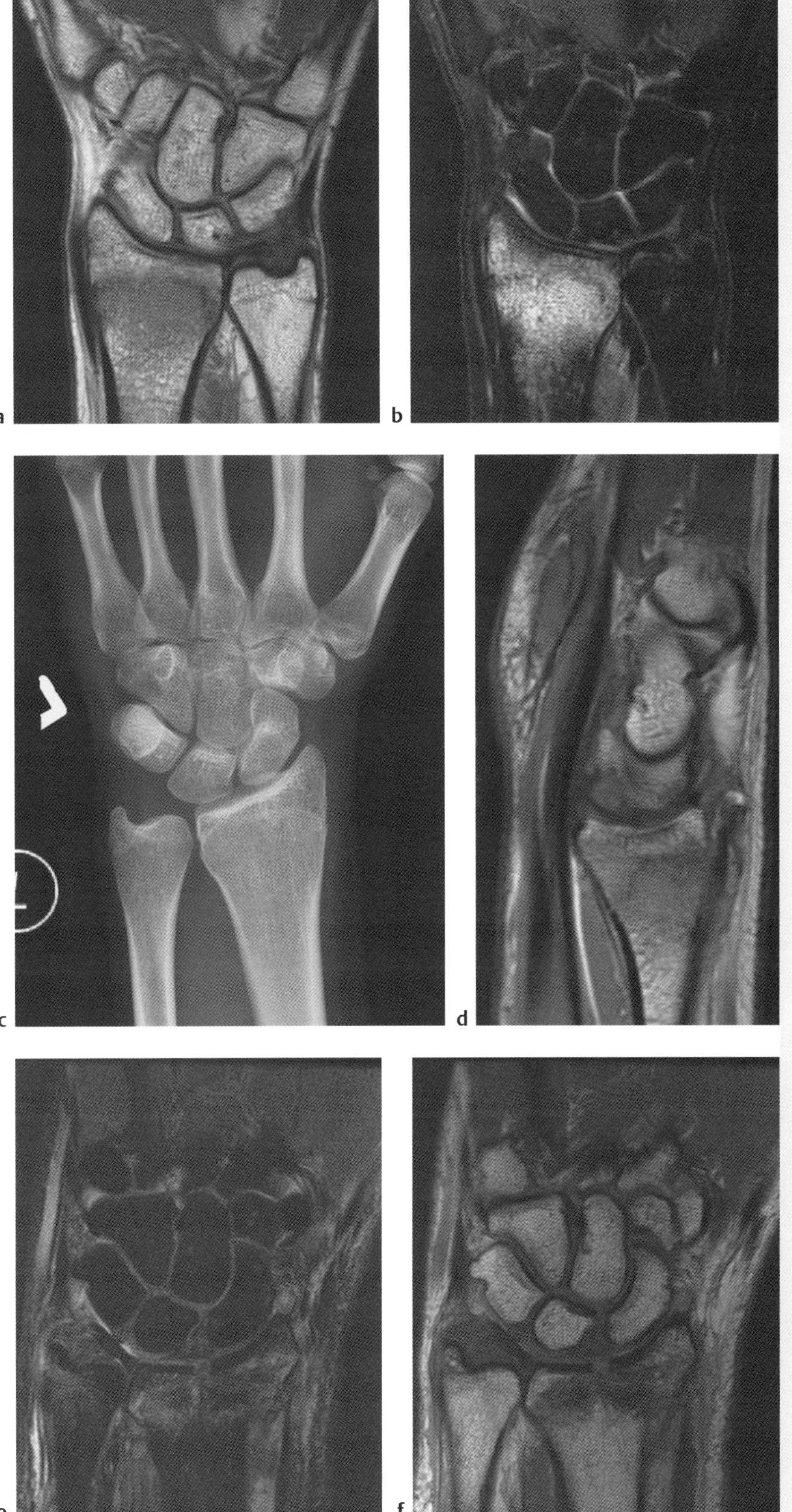

Fig. 4.20 (a) Coronal proton density–weighted imaging (PDWI) shows low signal edema in the distal radius. (b) Coronal fat-suppressed T2-weighted imaging (FS T2WI) shows diffuse high signal edema in the distal radius with a curvilinear line across the distal radius representing a nondisplaced fracture. (c) Wrist radiograph with no fracture seen. (d) Sagittal PDWI shows a low signal nondisplaced fracture line in the distal radius, which does not involve cortical bone. (e) Coronal FS T2WI from a second patient shows a displaced fracture with cortical disruption of the distal radius. (f) Corresponding coronal PDWI from the same patient also shows a displaced fracture of the distal radius.

Table 4.4 (Cont.) Bone lesions of the wrist

Abnormalities	MRI findings	Comments
Avascular necrosis (AVN)/scaphoid AVN (▶ Fig. 4.21)	On PDWI images marrow signal is normally high, indicating the presence of normal fatty marrow. Low signal in the scaphoid marrow on both PDWI and FS T2WI is highly suspicious for AVN. These findings usually occur in the proximal pole. High signal marrow on FS T2WI images and corresponding low signal on PDWI indicate several possibilities, including marrow edema, granulation tissue, and early AVN. In later stages of AVN there is cortical disruption and fragmentation.	The most common location for AVN of the scaphoid is the proximal pole. The blood supply to this location is easily disrupted by trauma. Disruption of this blood supply is a major cause of scaphoid waist fractures going on to nonunion.
Kienböck disease (▶ Fig. 4.22)	On PDWI normal bright signal marrow is entirely replaced with low signal. Low signal marrow in the lunate on both PDWI and FS T2WI is highly suspicious for AVN. When only a portion of the lunate is involved or there is high signal on FS T2WI other possible diagnoses need to be considered, including bone contusion, granulation tissue related to healing AVN, early-stage AVN, or degenerative reactive marrow edema. The sagittal plane is essential in evaluating the lunate because some fractures are seen only in this plane.	Lunate osteonecrosis may occur as a result of acute fracture, ulnar minus variation, and repetitive microtrauma. Patients complain of pain that is worse with activity, loss of grip strength, decreased range of motion, and diffuse swelling. The blood supply of the lunate is more easily disrupted in patients with variant anatomy in which there is a single nutrient vessel.

(continued on page 108)

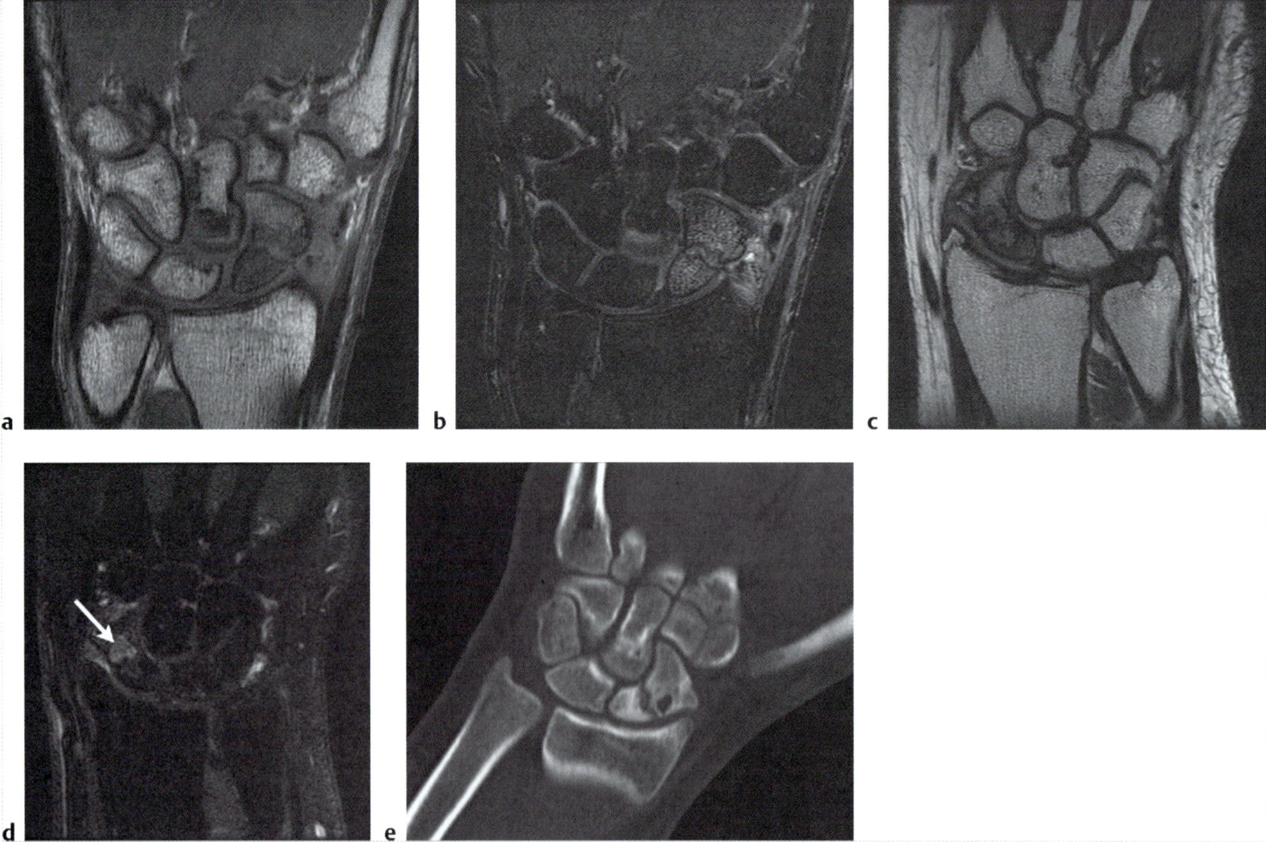

Fig. 4.21 (a) Coronal proton density–weighted imaging (PDWI) shows low signal proximal pole of scaphoid and scaphoid waist fracture with nonunion. There is no evidence for collapse of the proximal pole. (b) Coronal fat-suppressed T2-weighted imaging (FS T2WI) shows increased signal in both proximal and distal poles of the scaphoid carpal bone. There is also a scaphoid waist fracture with nonunion. The presence of high signal in the proximal pole on FS T2WI and corresponding low signal on PDWI indicates early avascular necrosis (AVN). (c) Coronal PDWI from a second patient shows low signal in the proximal pole of the scaphoid. (d) Coronal FS T2WI from the same patient also shows low signal in the in the proximal pole of the scaphoid, indicating more advanced AVN. Note a large posttraumatic cyst at the site of previous fracture (arrow). (e) Coronal two-dimensional reformat from a CT scan of the wrist shows proximal pole scaphoid increased sclerotic density seen in AVN.

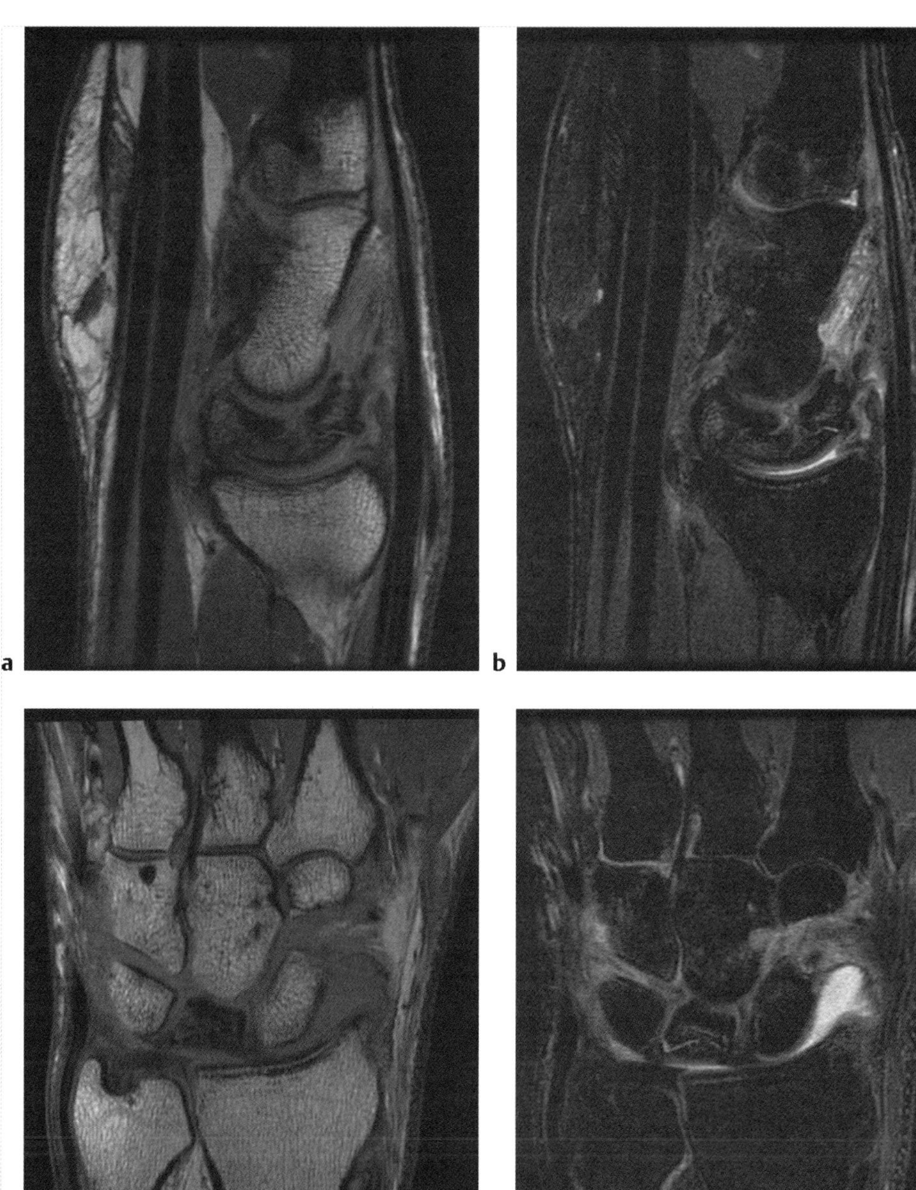

Fig. 4.22 (a) Sagittal proton density–weighted imaging (PDWI) shows diffuse low signal in the lunate with comminuted fracture and collapse. Findings are consistent with lunate avascular necrosis (AVN) (Kienböck disease) with collapse. (b) Sagittal fat-suppressed T2-weighted imaging (FS T2WI) shows patchy increased signal in the lunate with comminuted fracture and collapse. Findings are consistent with lunate AVN (Kienböck disease) with collapse. (c) Coronal PDWI shows diffuse low signal in the lunate with comminuted fracture and collapse. (d) Coronal FS T2WI shows patchy increased signal with high signal at fracture site.

Table 4.4 (Cont.) Bone lesions of the wrist

Abnormalities	MRI findings	Comments
Physeal injuries (▶ Fig. 4.23)	Acute physeal injuries of the wrist occur in the distal radius and ulna and are low signal on PDWI and high signal on FS T2WI. MRI can identify the mildest to the most severe cases of physeal injury. Many mild physeal injuries will be radiographically occult. The major complication of physeal injury is formation of a bar, bony or fibrous. These bars are well seen on coronal and sagittal plane images as low signal on both PDWI and FS T2WI.	These injuries are most commonly seen in young athletes. Some physeal injuries will go on to form a bony or fibrous bar traversing the physis, which will result in growth disturbance with eventual limb length discrepancy.

(continued on page 110)

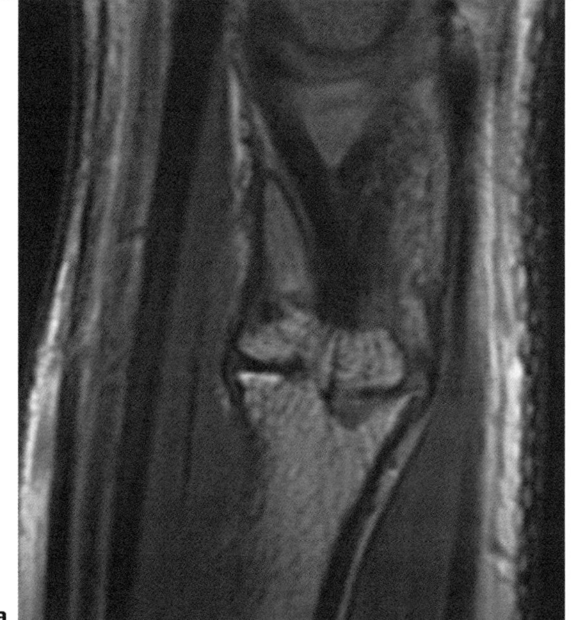

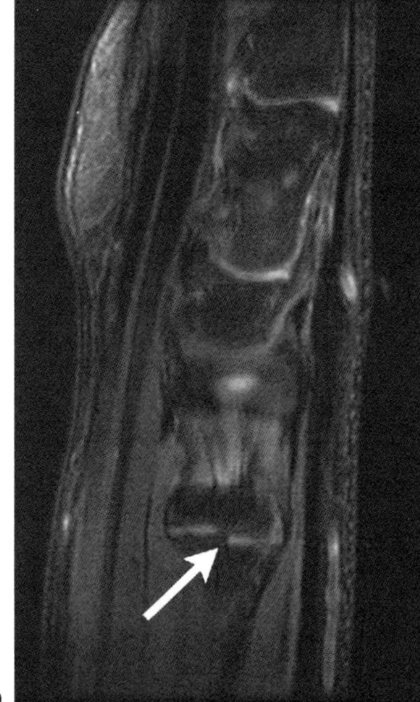

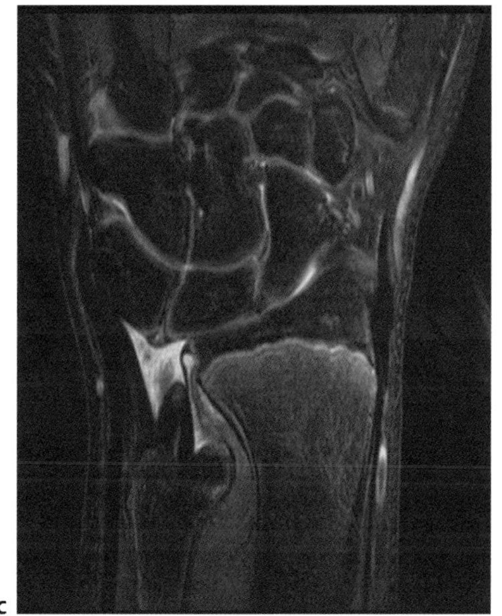

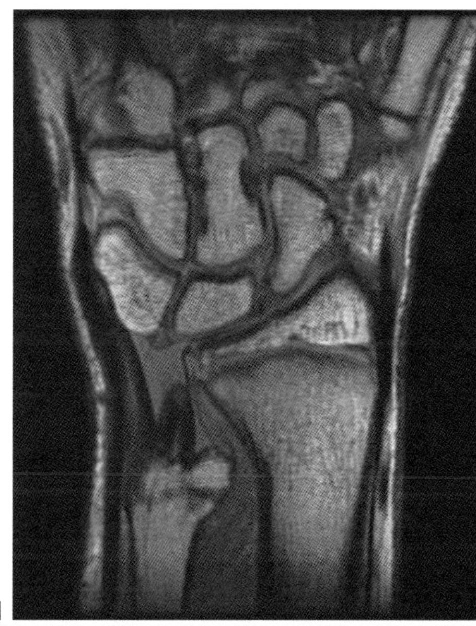

Fig. 4.23 (a) Sagittal proton density–weighted imaging (PDWI) shows a short ulna with bony bar across the distal physis. (b) Sagittal fat-suppressed T2-weighted imaging (FS T2WI) shows a low signal posttraumatic bony bar across the distal ulna, which is shortened (arrow). (c) Coronal FS T2WI shows a short ulna with severe distortion of the triangular fibrocartilage complex (TFCC) and ulnar angulation of the distal radius. (d) Coronal PDWI shows a short ulna with severe distortion of the TFCC and ulnar angulation of the distal radius.

Table 4.4 (Cont.) Bone lesions of the wrist

Abnormalities	MRI findings	Comments
Carpal instability (► Fig. 4.24)	There are several patterns of carpal instability, including dorsal intercalated instability (DISI), volar intercalated instability (VISI), and scapholunate advanced collapse (SLAC). SLAC and DISI are usually seen in association with rupture of the scapholunate ligament. This ligament tear can be directly visualized on conventional wrist MRI and is also well seen on wrist MRI arthrography. There is usually associated widening of the scapholunate space. In DISI there is dorsal tilting of the lunate with respect to the capitate, which is best seen on sagittal images. In SLAC there is widened scapholunate space, proximal migration of the capitate, and degenerative changes at the radioscaphoid articulation. In VISI there is usually a tear of the lunotriquetral ligament and volar tilting of the lunate with respect to the capitate, best seen on sagittal images.	Carpal instability is a complex subject. The different patterns of carpal instability can often be seen on radiographs of the wrist. MRI is useful to further define the ligamentous abnormalities associated with these instability patterns. Patients with carpal instability often complain of wrist pain, decreased range of motion, and loss of grip strength.

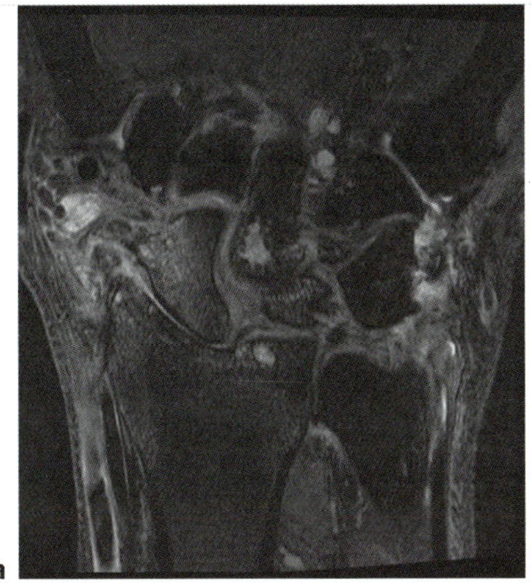
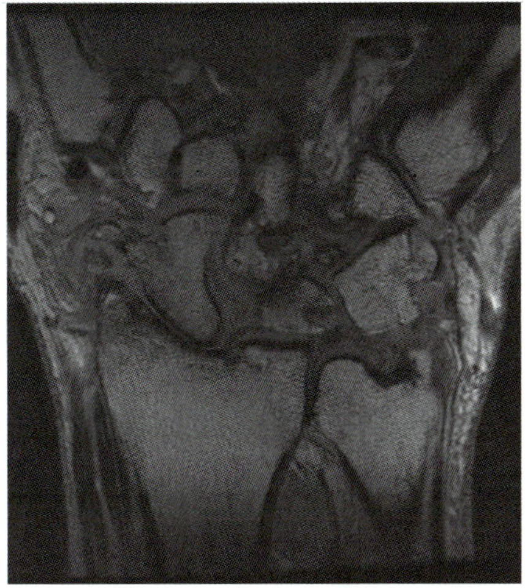
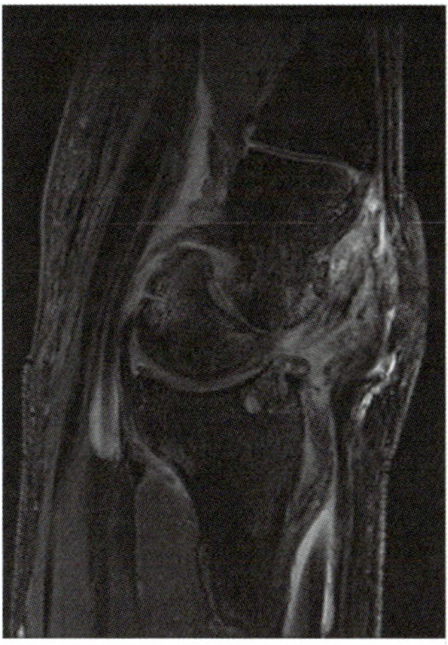

Fig. 4.24 (a) Coronal fat-suppressed T2-weighted imaging (FS T2WI) shows carpal instability with widened scapholunate space and proximal carpal migration. There is also reactive degenerative marrow edema seen in multiple carpal bones along with geodes in several carpal bones. (b) Coronal proton density–weighted imaging (PDWI) shows carpal instability with widened scapholunate space and proximal carpal migration. (c) Sagittal FS T2WI shows dorsal tilt of the lunate and degenerative reactive marrow edema.

4.4.1 Bone Lesions of the Wrist Suggested Reading

[1] Blum AG, Zabel JP, Kohlmann R, et al. Pathologic conditions of the hypothenar eminence: evaluation with multidetector CT and MR imaging. Radiographics 2006; 26: 1021–1044

[2] Fotiadou A, Patel A, Morgan T, Karantanas AH. Wrist injuries in young adults: the diagnostic impact of CT and MRI. Eur J Radiol 2011; 77: 235–239

[3] Fox MG, Gaskin CM, Chhabra AB, Anderson MW. Assessment of scaphoid viability with MRI: a reassessment of findings on unenhanced MR images. AJR Am J Roentgenol 2010; 195: W281-W286

[4] Mallee W, Doornberg JN, Ring D, van Dijk CN, Maas M, Goslings JC. Comparison of CT and MRI for diagnosis of suspected scaphoid fractures. J Bone Joint Surg Am 2011; 93: 20–28

[5] Schmitt R, Christopoulos G, Wagner M, et al. Avascular necrosis (AVN) of the proximal fragment in scaphoid nonunion: is intravenous contrast agent necessary in MRI? Eur J Radiol 2011; 77: 222–227

[6] Schmitt R, Froehner S, Coblenz G, Christopoulos G. Carpal instability. Eur Radiol 2006; 16: 2161–2178

[7] Schuind F, Eslami S, Ledoux P. Kienbock's disease. J Bone Joint Surg Br 2008; 90: 133–139

4.5 Tendon Lesions of the Wrist

- Traumatic injuries of the tendons
  - Partial tendon tears
  - Complete tendon tears
- Inflammatory lesions of the tendons
  - Extensor carpi ulnaris (ECU) tendonopathy
  - De Quervain syndrome
  - Flexor tendon tenosynovitis

Table 4.5 Tendon lesions of the wrist

Abnormalities	MRI findings	Comments
Traumatic injuries of the tendons		
Partial tendon tears (▶ Fig. 4.25)	The normal MRI appearance of tendons is a low signal, rounded structure on all sequences. Some wrist tendons have mild heterogeneously increased signal on fat-suppressed T2-weighted imaging (FS T2WI). The normal extensor carpi ulnaris may have this appearance. Partial wrist tendon tears are seen as focal zones of increased signal on proton density–weighted imaging (PDWI) and on FS T2WI. There may also be obvious partial discontinuity of the tendon. Sagittal and axial planes are best for wrist tendon evaluation.	Partial tears of the wrist tendons can arise secondary to penetrating trauma such as knife wounds or may occur after wrist fracture. If there is less than 50% tendon thickness transection conservative nonsurgical treatment may be sufficient.
Complete tendon tears (▶ Fig. 4.26)	Complete tendon tears may have a variable MRI appearance depending on the nature of the injury. Complete tendon tears are seen as areas of tendon discontinuity, which can be best appreciated on sagittal images. On FS T2WI there is high signal in the region of the gap between the torn tendon ends. The tendon ends may be sharply defined, typically after acute knife injuries. The tendon ends may alternatively be frayed and irregular, or in the case of a more chronic injury there may be ill-defined blurring of the torn tendon ends.	Complete tendon tears more commonly occur over the dorsum of the wrist and involve the extensor tendons. The length of the gap between the torn tendon ends needs to be determined in each case. This will determine the type of surgical treatment employed. Shorter gaps can be primarily repaired by suturing the torn ends together. Longer gaps often require a tendon graft to bridge the torn ends of the native tendon.
Inflammatory lesions of the tendons		
Extensor carpi ulnaris (ECU) tendonopathy (▶ Fig. 4.27)	On FS T2WI fluid may be seen surrounding the tendon (tensosynovial effusion). There may also be increased signal in the tendon and tendon thickening. The tendon may also be displaced from its groove on the ulna. These findings are best seen in the axial plane. On FS T2WI stippled increased signal within the tendon with no thickening or pertindinous fluid is often asymptomatic.	ECU tendinopathy occurs commonly and is usually located near or at the level of the ulnar head. Patients usually complain of pain and swelling at the level of the ulnar head. ECU tendon sheath disruption can occur in association with triangular fibrocartilage complex (TFCC) tears. Disruption of the ECU tendon sheath can result in ECU tendon subluxation.

(continued on page 114)

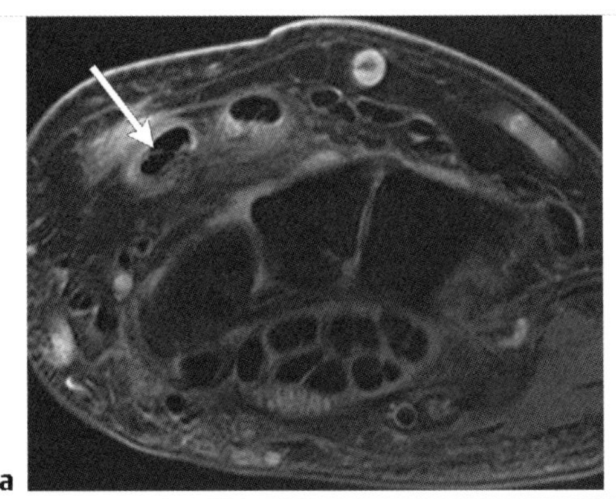

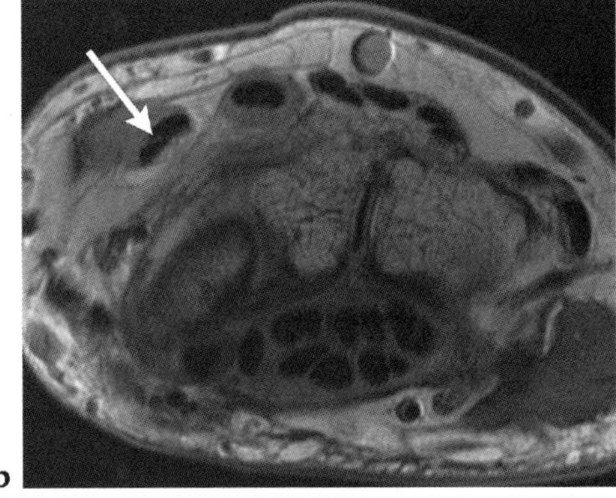

Fig. 4.25 (a) Axial fat-suppressed T2-weighted imaging shows a partial split tear of the extensor carpi radialis longus (arrow). There is also tenosynovitis of the extensor carpi radialis longus and adjacent extensor pollicis longus. (b) Axial proton density–weighted imaging (PDWI) shows partial split tear of the extensor carpi radialis longus (arrow).

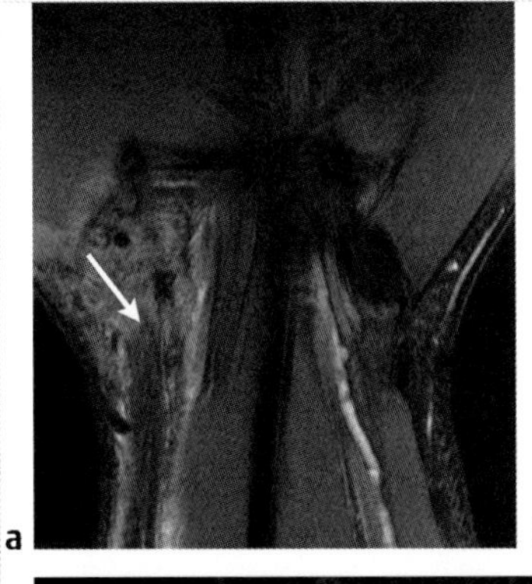

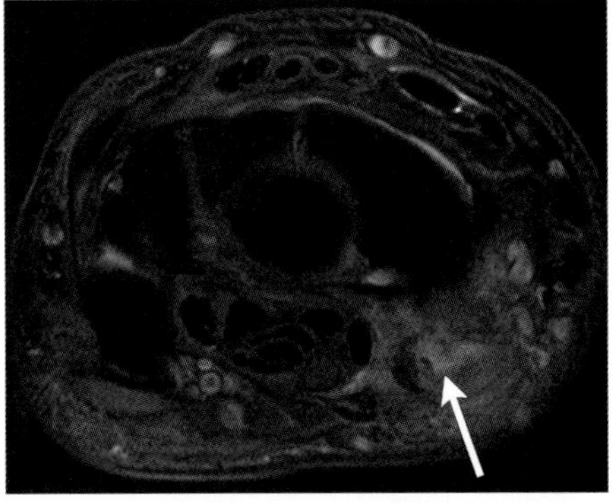

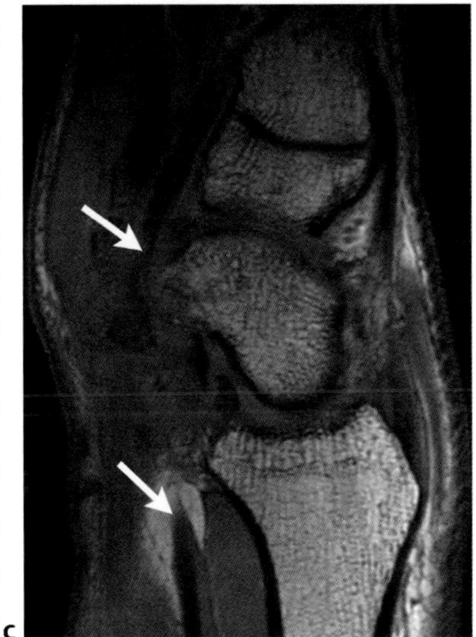

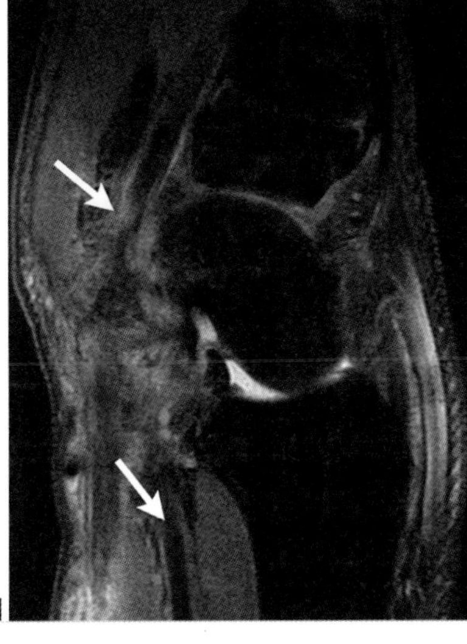

Fig. 4.26 (a) Coronal fat-suppressed T2-weighted imaging (FS T2WI) shows a complete tear of the flexor carpi radialis tendon (arrow). (b) Axial FS T2WI shows a complete tear of the flexor carpi radialis tendon (arrow). (c) Sagittal proton density–weighted imaging shows a complete tear of the flexor carpi radialis tendon (arrows). (d) Sagittal FS T2WI shows a complete tear of the flexor carpi radialis tendon (arrows).

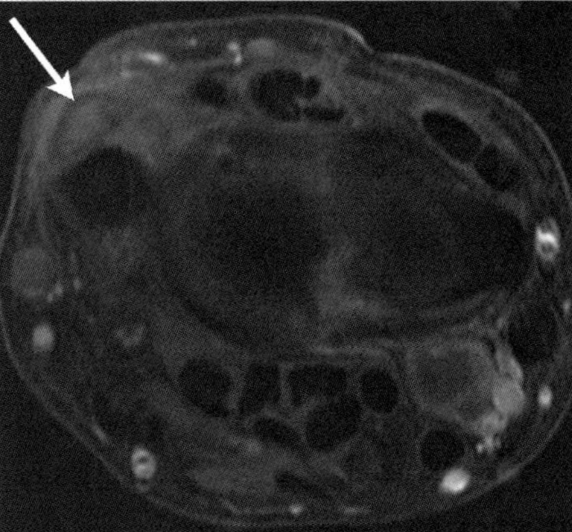

Fig. 4.27 (a) Axial fat-suppressed (FS) T2-weighted imaging shows thickened extensor carpi ulnaris (ECU) with increased signal (arrow). Incidental note is made of a large ganglion cyst adjacent to the volar aspect of the distal radius. (b) Axial FS T1-weighted imaging after intravenous contrast shows mild enhancement of the ECU (arrow).

Table 4.5 (Cont.) Tendon lesions of the wrist

Abnormalities	MRI findings	Comments
De Quervain syndrome (▶ Fig. 4.28)	Early findings of tenosynovitis on FS T2WI include increased bright signal fluid within the tendon sheath surrounding the abductor pollicis longus (APL) and extensor pollicis brevis (EPB). As severity progresses there may be increased signal on FS T2WI in the surrounding soft tissues with distortion of the adjacent fat planes. With continued progression of severity there is thickening of the tendon and increased bright signal on FS T2WI in the substance of the tendons (tendinosis).	The APL and EPB tendons are in the first dorsal extensor compartment. The tendons are commonly inflamed secondary to overuse. Patients present with pain and swelling in the region of the radial styloid. Both wrists can be affected. In some patients surgical decompression is required.
Flexor tendon tenosynovitis (▶ Fig. 4.29)	Increased bright signal on FS T2WI is seen surrounding the tendons and within the tendons. The flexor tendons may be thickened, and after intravenous contrast administration there is often enhancement seen on FS T1-weighted imaging (T1WI) within the tendons and throughout the flexor compartment. The axial plane is best for evaluating the flexor tendons.	Flexor compartment tenosynovitis can result in compression of the median nerve, resulting in carpal tunnel syndrome. The flexor retinaculum may be bowed. The MRI appearance of the median nerve is unreliable in the diagnosis of carpal tunnel syndrome. There may be increased signal with the nerve on FS T2WI and thickening of the nerve.

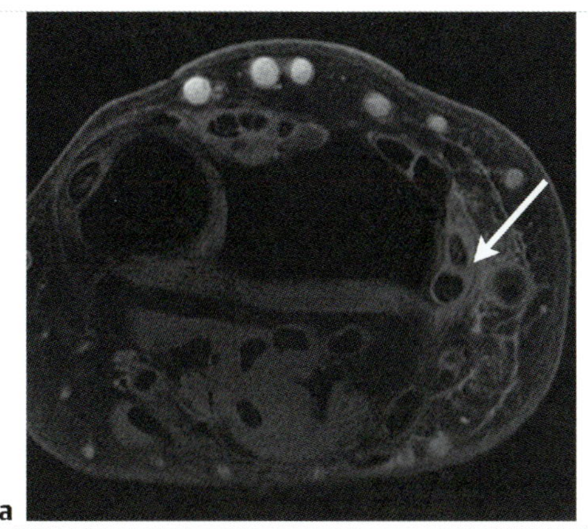

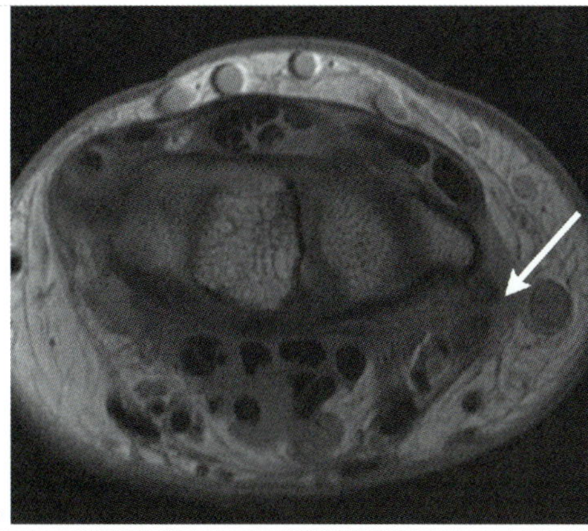

Fig. 4.28 (a) Axial fat-suppressed T2-weighted imaging shows increased signal in the first dorsal compartment of the wrist (arrow). The first dorsal compartment includes the abductor pollicis longus and extensor pollicis brevis. (b) Axial proton density–weighted imaging shows diffusely increased signal in the first dorsal compartment of the wrist (arrow).

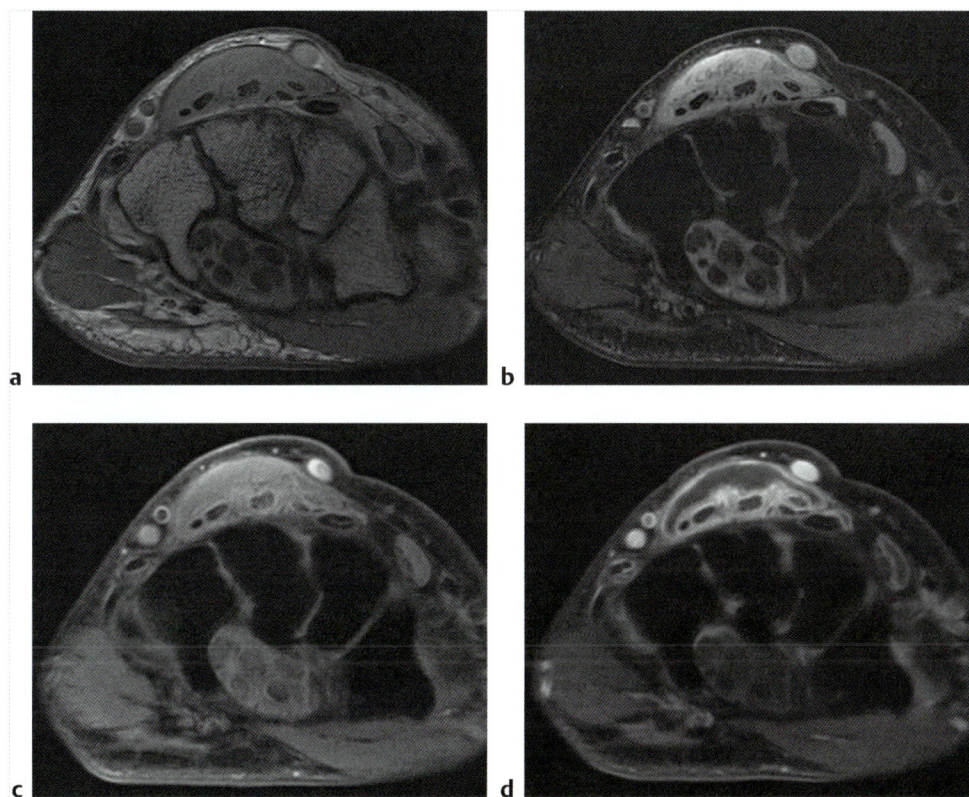

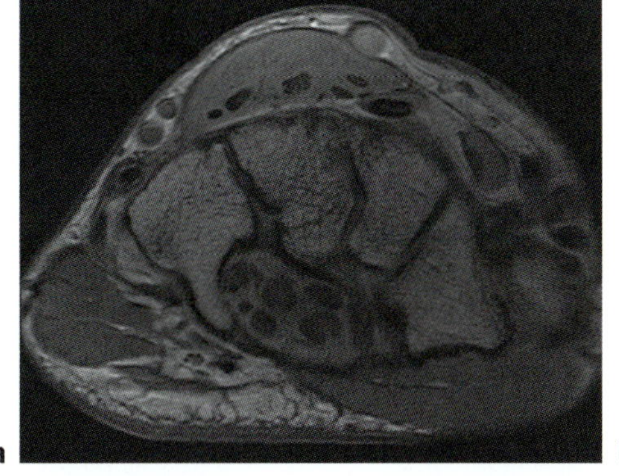

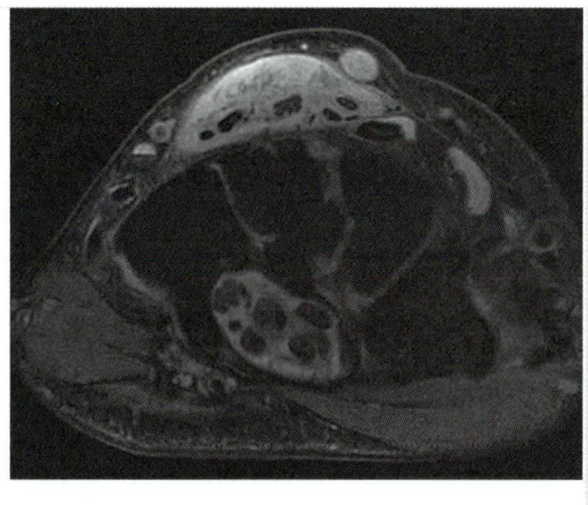

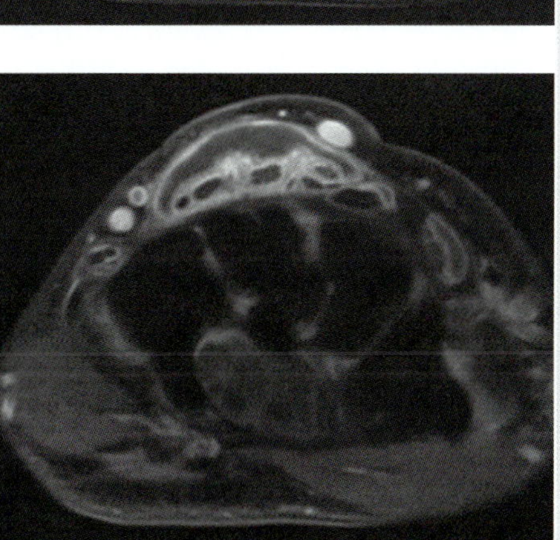

Fig. 4.29 (a) Axial proton density–weighted imaging shows increased heterogeneous signal fluid surrounding the flexor and extensor tendons. (b) Axial fat-suppressed (FS) T2-weighted imaging shows increased high signal fluid with debris surrounding the flexor and extensor tendons. There is likely some synovial proliferation. (c) Axial FS T1-weighted imaging (T1WI) shows increased fluid in the flexor and extensor compartments. (d) Axial FS T1WI post-contrast shows synovial enhancement in the extensor compartment greater than the flexor compartment.

4.5.1 Tendon Lesions of the Wrist Suggested Reading

[1] Chhabra A, Soldatos T, Thawait GK, et al. Current perspectives on the advantages of 3-T MR imaging of the wrist. Radiographics 2012; 32: 879–896

[2] Glajchen N, Schweitzer M. MRI features in de Quervain's tenosynovitis of the wrist. Skeletal Radiol 1996; 25: 63–65

[3] Lee YH, Choi YR, Kim S, Song HT, Suh JS. Intrinsic ligament and triangular fibrocartilage complex (TFCC) tears of the wrist: comparison of isovolumetric 3D-THRIVE sequence MR arthrography and conventional MR image of 3 T. Mag Reson Imaging 2013;31(2):221–226.

4.6 Arthritis of the Wrist

- Normal wrist cartilage
- Osteoarthritis (OA)
- Rheumatoid arthritis (RA)

Table 4.6 Arthritis of the wrist

Abnormalities	MRI findings	Comments
Normal wrist cartilage (▶ Fig. 4.30)	MRI is the best modality for the noninvasive evaluation of wrist cartilage. Normal wrist cartilage is thin, which results in technical challenges in accurate MRI evaluation. Successful MRI of cartilage requires high field strength, 3 T, powerful gradients, and dedicated multichannel small field of view surface coils. In addition imaging parameters need to be optimized to maximize the potential for accurate evaluation. Thin 1- to 1.5-mm coronal sections using fat-suppressed T2-weighted imaging (FS T2WI) with intermediate TR/TE allow for proper distinction between cartilage, cortical bone, and fluid while maintaining sufficient signal to noise so that anatomical details are not lost. On optimized MRI thinning, signal heterogeneity and ultimately focal and diffuse defects in the articular cartilage can be seen. Often indirect signs of cartilage damage must suffice. These include marrow edema and subcortical cystic changes.	The current gold standard for evaluation of wrist cartilage is arthroscopy. The reported sensitivity and specificity of MRI in detecting wrist articular cartilage pathology currently vary widely. Wrist cartilage may be abnormal for a variety of reasons, including osteoarthritis, inflammatory arthropathy, and trauma. Patients with abnormal wrist cartilage may complain of wrist pain.
Osteoarthritis (OA) (▶ Fig. 4.31; ▶ Fig. 4.32)	In early-stage osteoarthritis MRI findings are limited to alteration in cartilage signal. Typical early findings include heterogeneous increased cartilage signal on FS T2WI. In the wrist the coronal plane is best for evaluating cartilage. As the disease progresses there are additional findings on MRI, including cartilage fissures and eventually full-thickness defects. Concurrently, as cartilage abnormalities increase in severity, changes in the underlying subcortical bone develop. This begins as mild subcortical marrow edema seen on FS T2WI, often in a roughly symmetric pattern across both sides of the joint line. Later stages of OA result in subcortical geode formation, subchondral sclerosis, and marginal osteophyte formation.	OA is a disease characterized by loss of joint function and increased joint pain, all secondary to cartilage destruction with changes in the underlying bone. OA is generally a progressive disease strongly associated with increased prevalence with increased age. Many factors contribute to the development of OA, including normal aging, diet, physical activity, obesity, and heredity. Unusual activity such as may be seen in certain occupations can result in early OA. Traumatic joint injuries will also often result in early OA.

(continued on page 118)

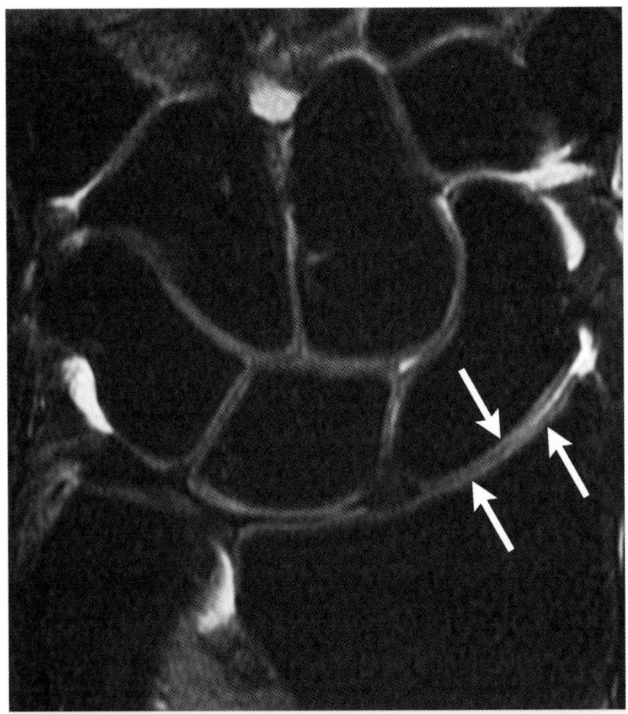

Fig. 4.30 Coronal fat-suppressed T2-weighted imaging shows normal gray signal cartilage along cortical articular surface of the wrist. Arrows are at the cartilage surfaces of the distal radius and opposite the scaphoid carpal bone.

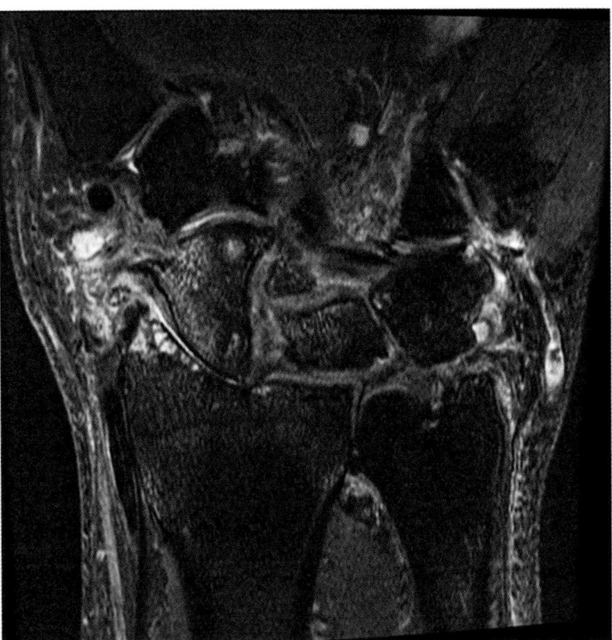

Fig. 4.31 Coronal fat-suppressed T2-weighted imaging shows severe radiocarpal joint space narrowing, small subcortical geodes in the distal radius, and degenerative reactive marrow edema in the distal radius and scaphoid.

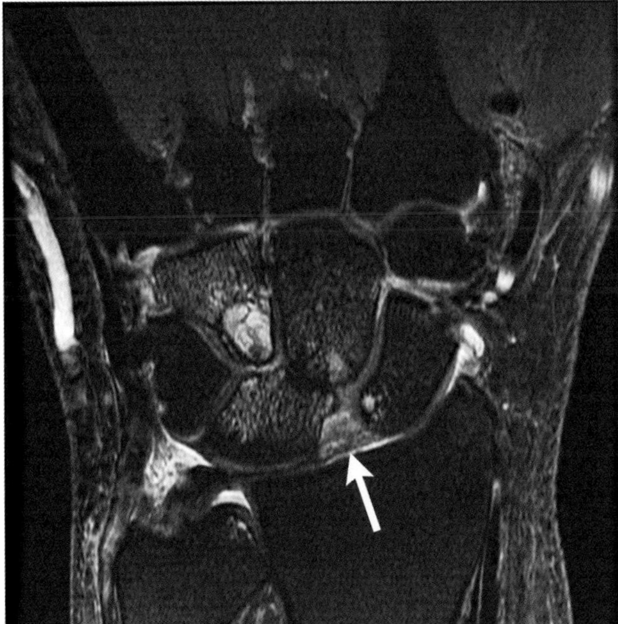

Fig. 4.32 Coronal fat-suppressed T2-weighted imaging from a second patient shows narrowed intercarpal joint spaces with subcortical geodes and reactive degenerative marrow edema. There is also a large scapholunate tear (arrow).

Table 4.6 (Cont.) Arthritis of the wrist

Abnormalities	MRI findings	Comments
Rheumatoid arthritis (RA) (▶ Fig. 4.33)	On FS T2WI a variety of different high signal abnormalities can be found, including bone erosions, synovial proliferation often associated with complex mixed signal joint effusion, bursal collections, and tenosynovitis. On postcontrast FS T1WI there is usually obvious enhancement corresponding to these zones of abnormal increased signal on FS T2WI. MRI may be most useful in follow-up evaluation of patients with known RA. MRI readily identifies zones of active inflammation as areas of abnormal increased enhancement on postcontrast FS T1WI. Serial follow-up radiographs may not demonstrate any interval changes.	RA is a systemic inflammatory disease of synovium that often results in radiographically obvious bony destruction. The small hand and feet joints are most commonly affected. RA occurs more frequently in women (3:1). Patients complain of symmetric joint pain and swelling, usually in the hands and feet. RA is associated with several laboratory abnormalities, including positive serum rheumatoid factor (RF), positive antinuclear antibody (ANA), and positive cyclic citrullinated peptide (CCP) antibody. There are a variety of new drugs used to treat RA, broadly known as biologics, which include Enbril and Remicade. These drugs have had a dramatic impact on the treatment of RA, although they do have side effects, particularly related to immune compromise.

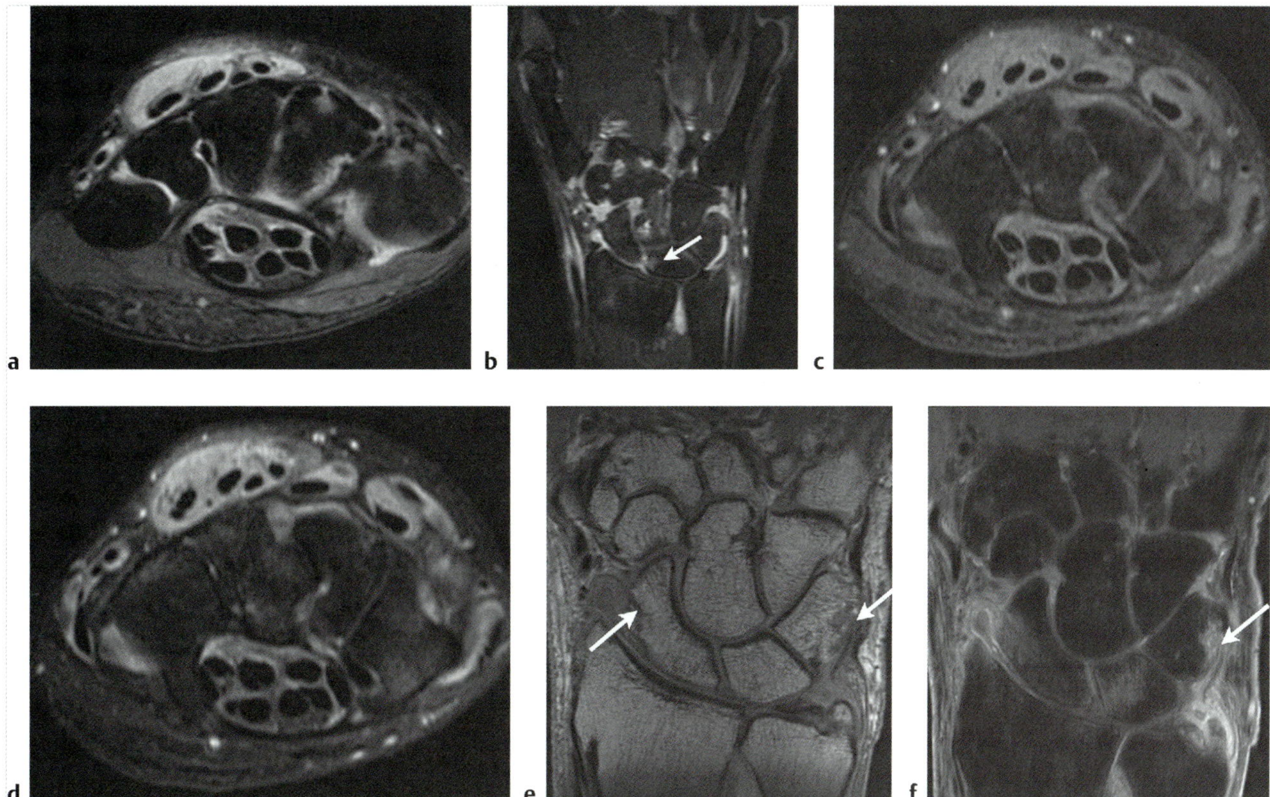

Fig. 4.33 (a) Axial fat-suppressed T2-weighted imaging (FS T2WI) shows diffuse flexor and extensor tenosynovitis. (b) Coronal FS T1-weighted imaging (T1WI) postcontrast shows diffuse enhancing synovitis and enhancing erosion in the radial aspect of the lunate (arrow). (c) Axial FS T1WI shows diffuse synovial thickening. (d) Axial FS T1WI postcontrast shows diffuse synovial enhancement. (e) Coronal proton density-weighted imaging from a second patient shows erosions of the scaphoid and triquetrum (arrows). (f) Coronal FS T1WI postcontrast from the same patient shows enhancing erosion in the triquetrum (arrow) and diffuse heterogeneous synovial enhancement.

4.6.1 Arthritis of the Wrist
Suggested Reading

[1] McGonagle D, Tan AL. What magnetic resonance imaging has told us about the pathogenesis of rheumatoid arthritis—the first 50 years. Arthritis Res Ther 2008; 10: 222

[2] Navalho M, Resende C, Rodrigues AM, et al. Bilateral MR imaging of the hand and wrist in early and very early inflammatory arthritis: tenosynovitis is associated with progression to rheumatoid arthritis. Radiology 2012; 264: 823–833

[3] Weber MA, von Stillfried F, Kloth JK, Rehnitz C. Cartilage imaging of the hand and wrist using 3-T MRI. Semin Musculoskelet Radiol 2012; 16: 71–87

Chapter 5

The Hand

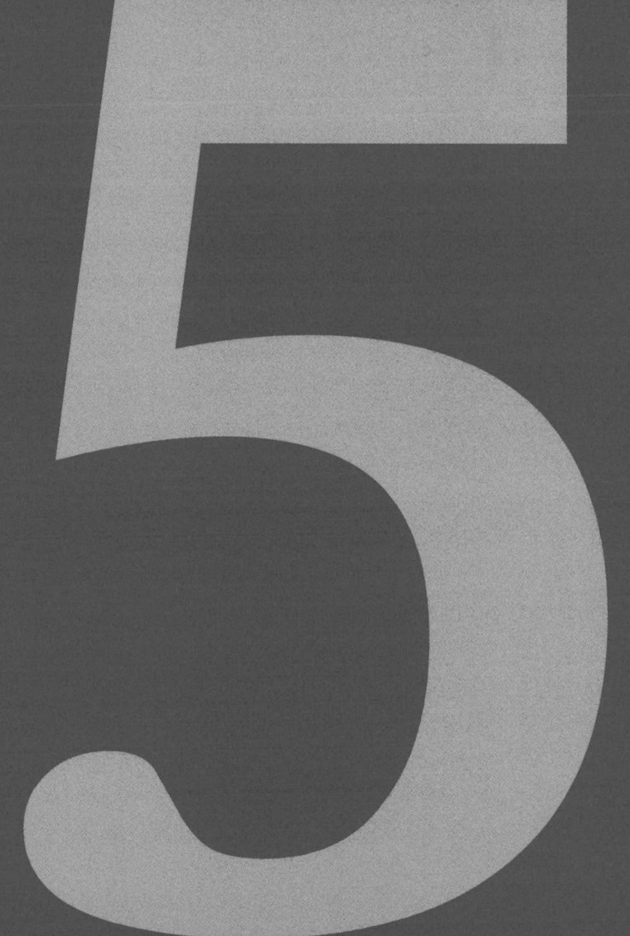

5 The Hand

Eric P. Weinberg

5.1 Ligament Injuries of the Hand

- Normal collateral ligaments and tears
- Ulnar collateral ligament tear of the thumb (gamekeeper's thumb)

Table 5.1 Ligament injuries of the hand

Abnormalities	MRI findings	Comments
Normal collateral ligaments and tears (▶ Fig. 5.1)	On both proton density–weighted imaging (PDWI) and fat-suppressed T2-weighted imaging (FS T2WI) all ligaments of the hand are low signal linear bands, which normally traverse both the ulnar and radial side of each joint. When there is a ligament tear it may be partial or complete. On FS T2WI a partial tear is seen as thickening and increased signal in a portion of the ligament, usually at its proximal or distal attachment. A complete ligament tear is seen as discontinuity or complete detachment of the ligament from its bony connection. This is often associated with high signal in the adjacent soft tissues on FS T2WI. There may also be fluid collection/hemorrhage at the site of ligament tear. Adjacent marrow edema or even small avulsion fractures are possible. The coronal plane is best for identifying collateral ligament injuries of the fingers.	Proximal interphalangeal (PIP) joint ligaments are more commonly injured than other locations in the fingers. The radial collateral ligaments are also more commonly injured. Athletes involved in contact sports such as basketball and football are more commonly affected. Distinction between partial and complete tears of the collateral ligaments is important in determining treatment. Surgery is often not needed even in complete tears. Joint stiffness is a major potential complication of these injuries.

(continued on page 124)

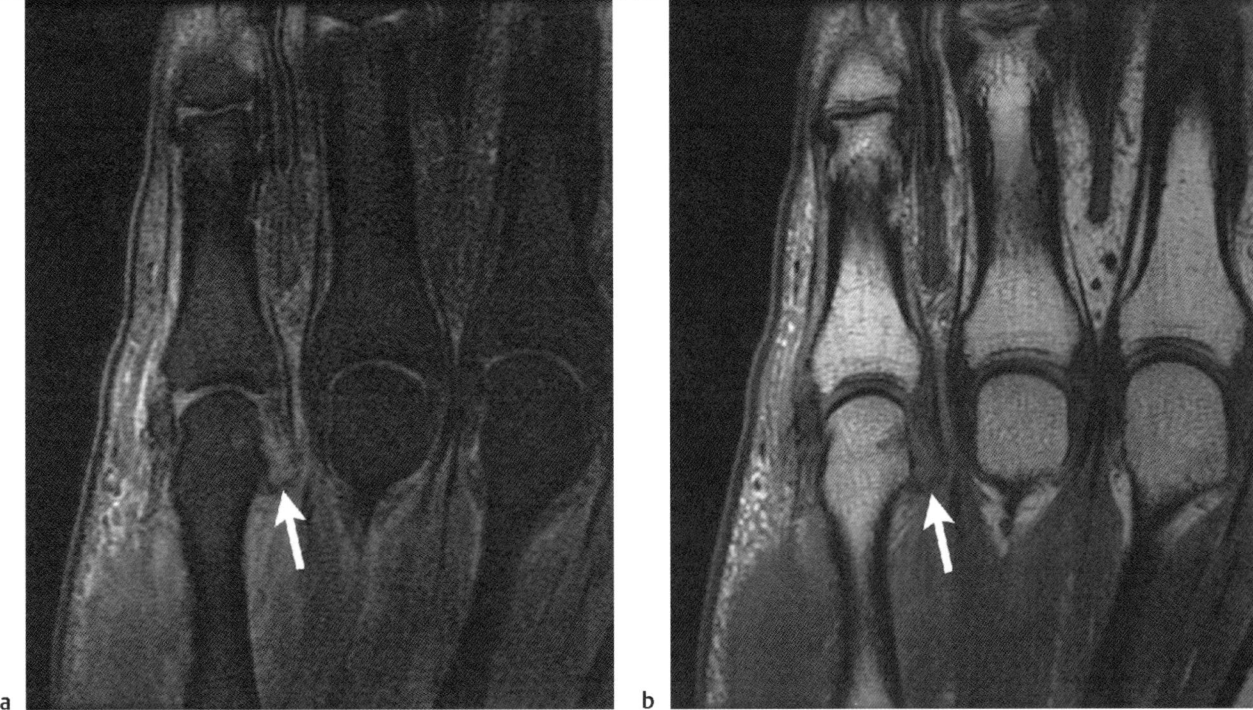

Fig. 5.1 (a) Coronal fast spin-echo (FSE) T2 imaging shows fifth proximal interphalangeal (PIP) joint proximal radial collateral ligament tear (arrow) and partial tear of the fifth ulnar collateral ligament at the fifth PIP. (b) Coronal proton density–weighted imaging shows a fifth radial collateral ligament tear at the fifth PIP joint proximally (arrow) and partial tear of the fifth ulnar collateral ligament at the fifth PIP joint.

Table 5.1 (Cont.) Ligament injuries of the hand

Abnormalities	MRI findings	Comments
Ulnar collateral ligament tear of the thumb (gamekeeper's thumb) (▶ Fig. 5.2; ▶ Fig. 5.3; ▶ Fig. 5.4; ▶ Fig. 5.5)	The normal first metacarpophalangeal (MCP) joint ulnar collateral ligament (UCL) has the same appearance on magnetic resonance imaging (MRI) as any other finger collateral ligament, a well-defined low signal band seen on both PDWI and FS T2WI. UCL tears at the first MCP joint may be partial or complete and in a minority of cases may be associated with a bony avulsion fracture fragment. Similar to the collateral ligaments at other joints in the fingers tears are seen as partial or complete disruption of the ligament and may be associated with surrounding edema or hemorrhage in the adjacent soft tissues as well as edema in adjacent bone marrow. An important special subset of first UCL tears is the Stener lesion. On MRI this is seen as retraction and displacement of the UCL such that there is interposition of the adductor aponeurosis between the torn ligament and the bone. The classic MRI appearance is referred to as the yo-yo on a string. The "string" is the adductor aponeurosis and the "yo-yo" is the balled-up torn and retracted collateral ligament. The coronal plane is best for identifying UCL injuries of the thumb. However, special care is needed to properly obtain this plane because it is coronal to the thumb and not coronal to the other four digits.	UCL tears of the thumb are easily identified on high-field MRI scanners. Determining if the patient has a Stener lesion is not always easy. This is the key distinction that the referring clinician is looking for. In the subset of first UCL tears, which are in fact Stener lesions, prompt diagnosis and surgical treatment are needed. In the Stener lesion the adductor aponeurosis is deep to the torn UCL ligament preventing nonsurgical healing because the aponeurosis is now between the ligament and the bone. The UCL tear of the thumb is usually secondary to abduction injury. This is now most commonly seen in skiers who fall while holding ski poles.

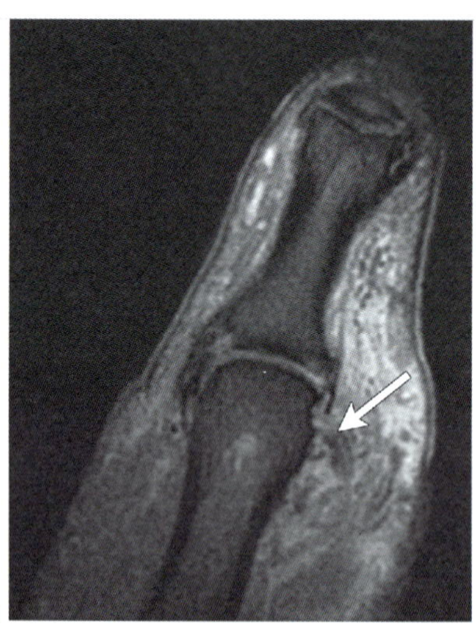

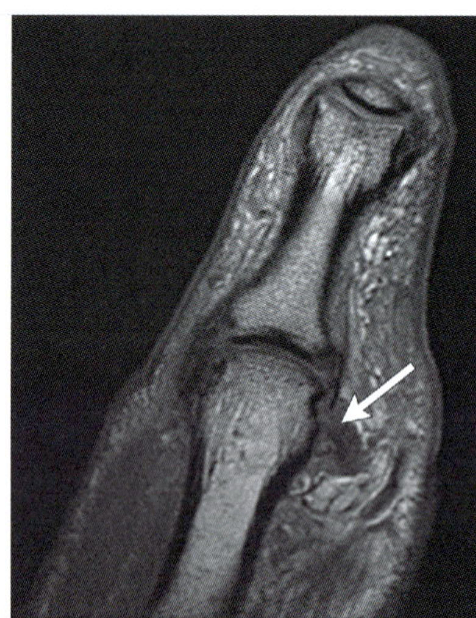

Fig. 5.2 (a) Coronal fat-suppressed T2-weighted imaging (FS T2WI) shows a proximal ulnar collateral ligament (UCL) tear with interposition of the palmar aponeurosis between the UCL and its bony attachment site (arrow). (b) Coronal proton density–weighted imaging shows a proximal UCL tear with interposition of the palmar aponeurosis between the UCL and its bony attachment site (arrow).

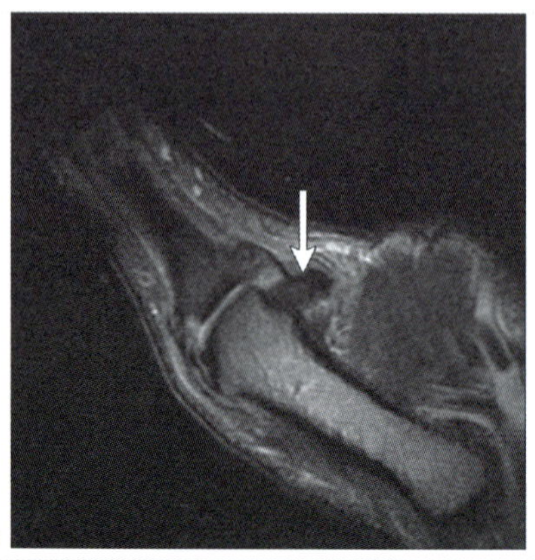

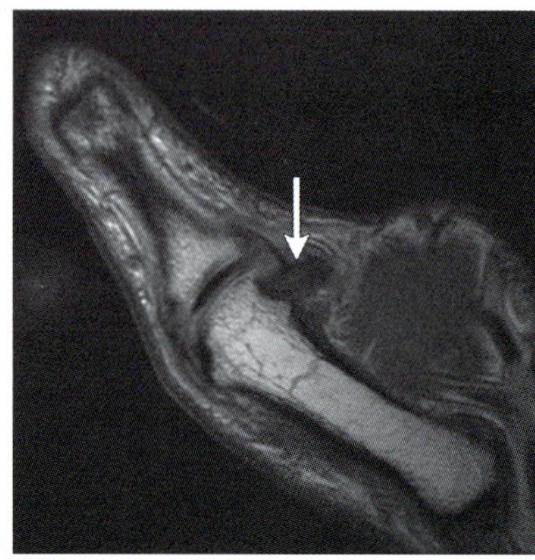

Fig. 5.3 (a) Coronal fat-suppressed T2-weighted imaging (FS T2WI) shows a proximal ulnar collateral ligament (UCL) tear with interposition of the palmar aponeurosis between the UCL and its bony attachment site (arrow). (b) Coronal proton density–weighted imaging shows a proximal UCL tear with interposition of the palmar aponeurosis between the UCL and its bony attachment site (arrow).

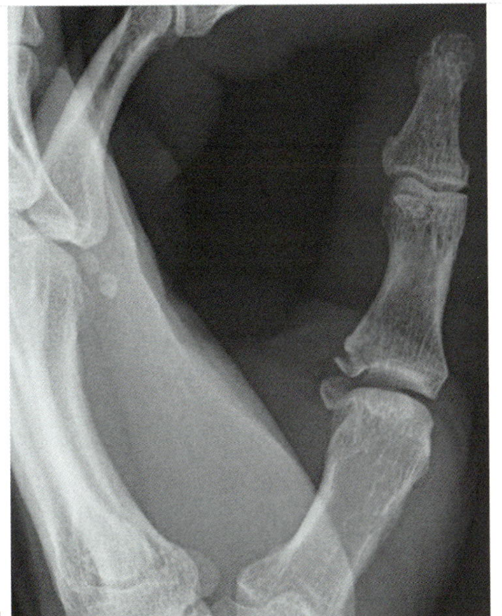
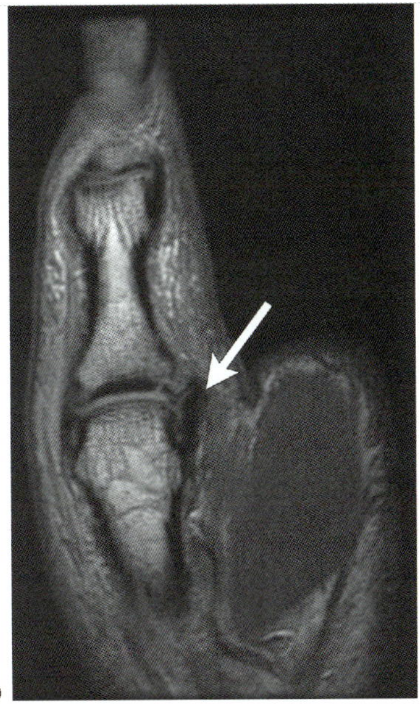
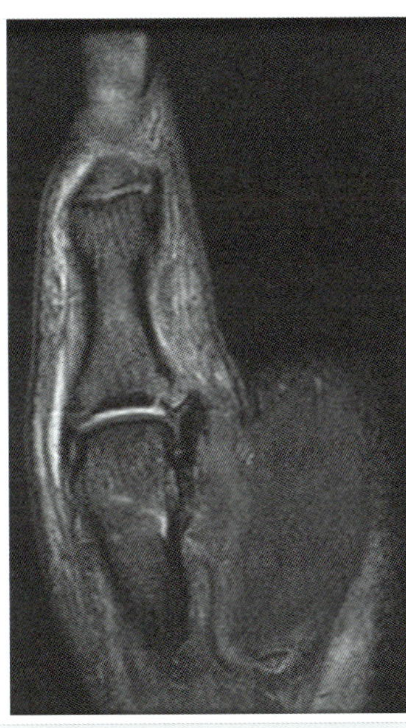

Fig. 5.4 (a) Anteroposterior radiograph of the thumb shows a small avulsion fracture at the base of the first proximal phalanx. (b) Coronal proton density-weighted imaging shows a thickened ulnar collateral ligament (UCL) still attached to the avulsed bony fragment arising from the ulnar aspect of the first proximal phalanx (arrow). (c) Coronal fat-suppressed T2-weighted imaging (FS T2WI) shows a thickened UCL still attached to the avulsed bony fragment arising from the ulnar aspect of the first proximal phalanx.

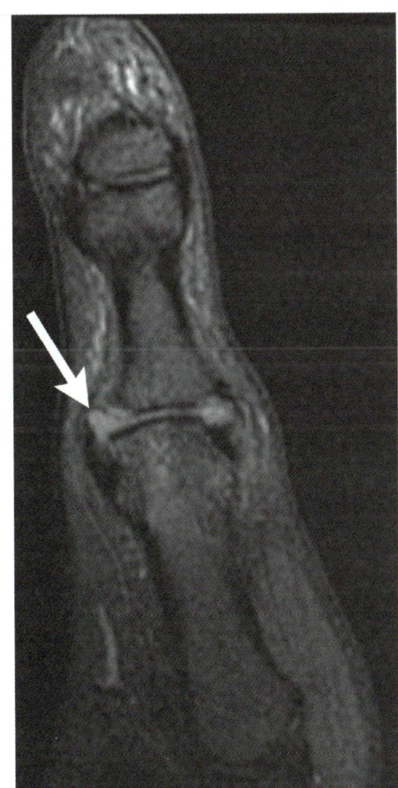
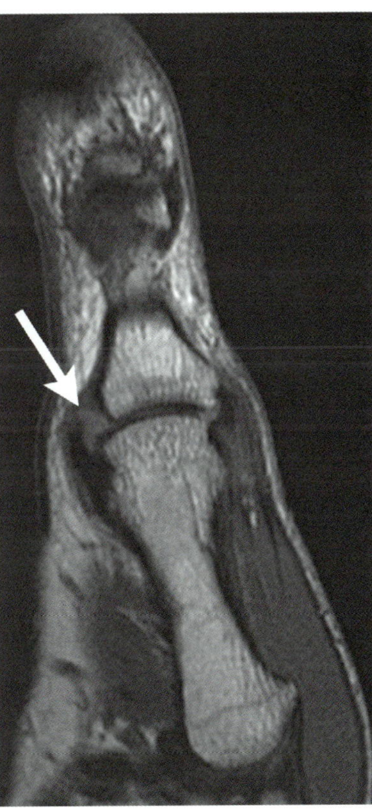

Fig. 5.5 (a) Coronal fat saturation T2-weighted imaging shows a tear of the ulnar collateral ligament (UCL) distally (arrow). There is also a bone bruise in the distal first metacarpal. (b) Coronal proton density-weighted imaging shows a distal UCL tear (arrow).

5.1.1 Ligament Injuries of the Hand Suggested Reading

[1] Clavero JA, Alomar X, Monill JM, et al. MR imaging of ligament and tendon injuries of the fingers. Radiographics 2002; 22: 237–256

[2] Deady LH, Salonen D. Skiing and snowboarding injuries: a review with a focus on mechanism of injury. Radiol Clin North Am 2010; 48: 1113–1124

[3] Lohman M, Vasenius J, Kivisaari A, Kivisaari L. MR imaging in chronic rupture of the ulnar collateral ligament of the thumb. Acta Radiol 2001; 42: 10–14

5.2 Tendon Lesions of the Hand

- Tenosynovitis
- Tendon tears
- Flexor annular pulley tears
- Volar plate injuries

Table 5.2 Tendon lesions of the hand

Abnormalities	MRI findings	Comments
Tenosynovitis (▶ Fig. 5.6)	On fat-suppressed T2-weighted imaging (FS T2WI) tenosynovitis is seen as circumferential bright signal fluid around the affected tendon. There is often increased signal seen within the substance of the tendon. There may also be thickening of the tendon. On post-contrast images there is often enhancement around and within the affected tendon(s). This is best seen on axial images. Normal tendons may have small amounts of fluid in the tendon sheath as well as internal foci of increased signal on FS T2WI.	Inflammation of tendons may commonly be secondary to chronic overuse and inflammatory arthritis. Infection is also possible.

(continued on page 128)

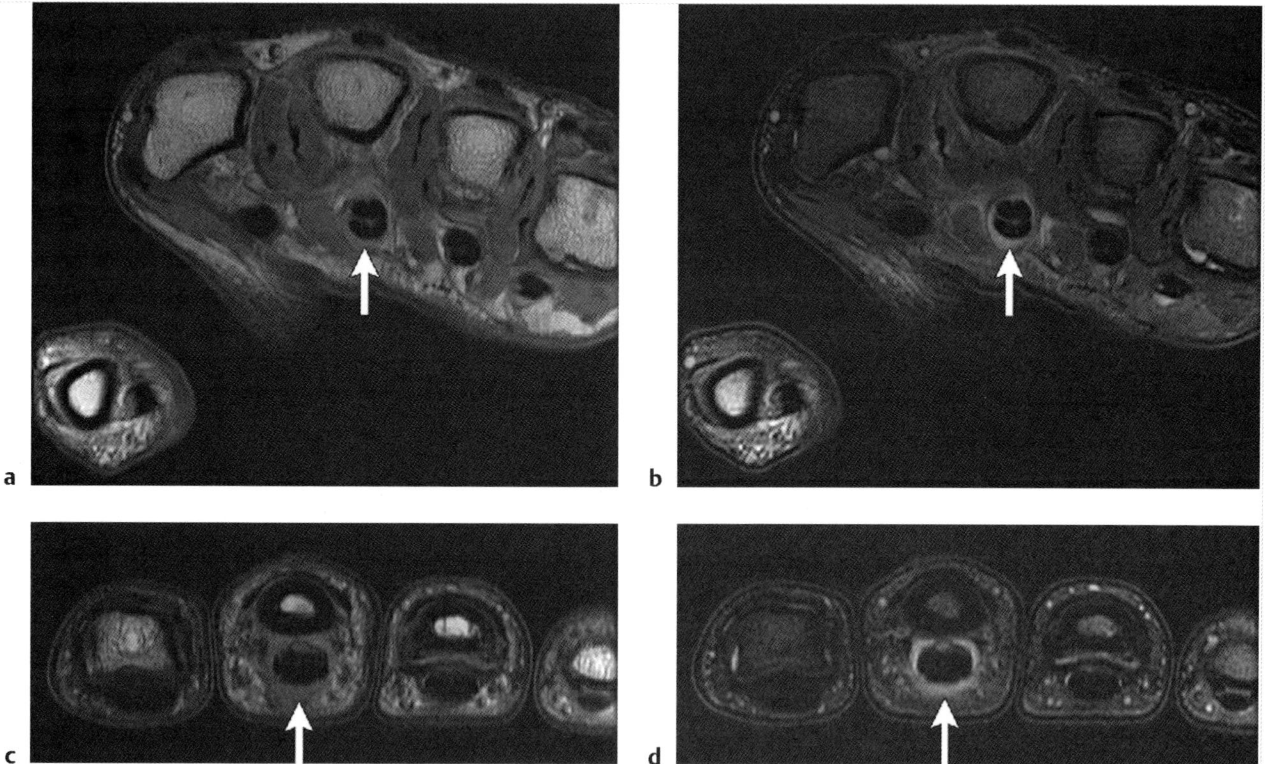

Fig. 5.6 (a) Axial proton density–weighted imaging (PDWI) shows increased signal surrounding the proximal third flexor tendons (arrow). (b) Axial fat-suppressed T2-weighted imaging (FS T2WI) shows increased signal fluid surrounding the proximal third flexor tendons (arrow). (c) Axial PDWI shows increased signal in the mid/distal third flexor tendon sheath (arrow). (d) Axial FS T2WI shows increased signal fluid surrounding the mid/distal third flexor tendon sheath (arrow).

Table 5.2 (Cont.) Tendon lesions of the hand

Abnormalities	MRI findings	Comments
Tendon tears (▶ Fig. 5.7; ▶ Fig. 5.8; ▶ Fig. 5.9)	Tears of the tendons may be partial or complete. This distinction can be made with MRI. Partial tears are seen as partial discontinuity of dark (low signal) linear tendon on both FS T2WI and proton density–weighted imaging (PDWI). There may or may not be increased fluid within the tendon sheath, seen as bright signal surrounding the remnant of injured tendon. Complete tendon tears are seen as a gap of variable length between the torn tendon ends. Complete tears can be seen best on axial and sagittal planes. In the gap between the torn ends there is loss of uniform low signal on both PDWI and FS T2WI with either intermediate signal material (granulation tissue) or bright signal fluid seen at the tear site on FS T2WI.	Most tendon tears in the fingers involve the extensors. The extensor tendons are more susceptible to lacerations. When a tendon tear is complete determining the size of the gap between the torn and retracted tendon ends provides an important piece of information for the referring clinician. When the gap is large approximating the torn tendon ends will not be possible, and a tendon graft interposed between the torn ends will be needed.

(continued on page 130)

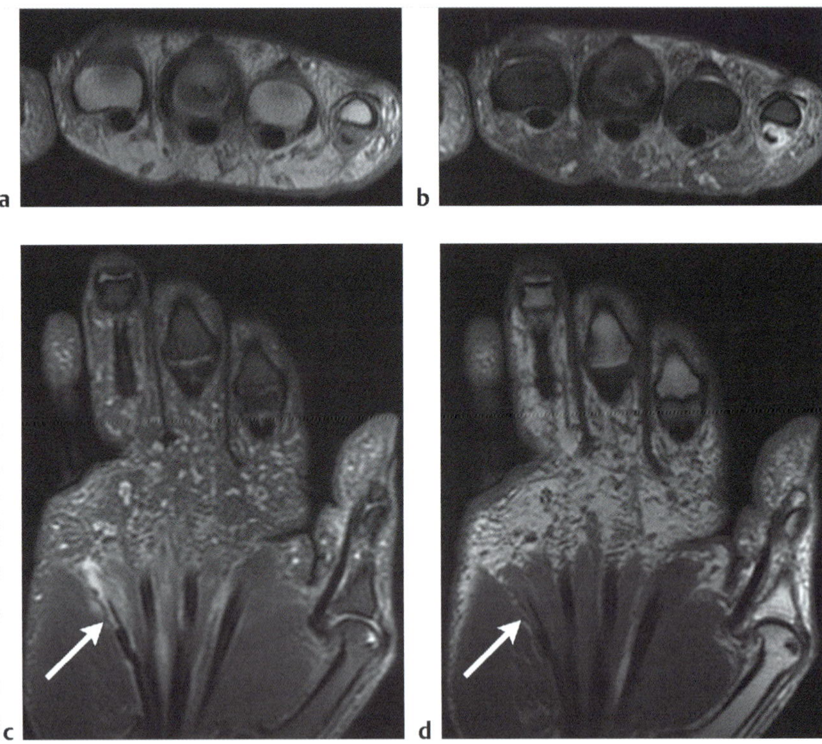

Fig. 5.7 (a) Axial proton density–weighted imaging (PDWI) shows a high-grade partial tear of the fifth superficial flexor and rupture of the fifth deep flexor. (b) Axial fat-suppressed T2-weighted imaging (FS T2WI) shows a high-grade partial tear of the fifth superficial flexor and rupture of the fifth deep flexor. (c) Coronal FS T2WI shows a few remnant fibers of the fifth flexor tendon (arrow). (d) Coronal PDWI shows a few remnant fibers of the fifth flexor tendon (arrow).

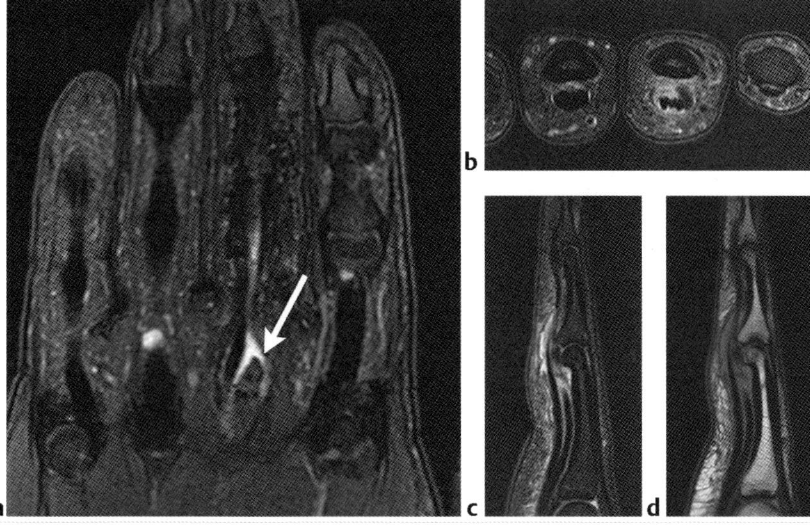

Fig. 5.8 (a) Coronal fat-suppressed T2-weighted imaging (FS T2WI) shows rupture of the third superficial flexor tendon (arrow). (b) Axial FS T2WI from a second patient shows absent superficial fourth flexor tendon with edema in the flexor tendon sheath. (c) Sagittal FS T2WI from the same patient shows a ruptured fourth superficial flexor tendon. (d) Corresponding sagittal proton density–weighted imaging shows a ruptured fourth superficial flexor tendon.

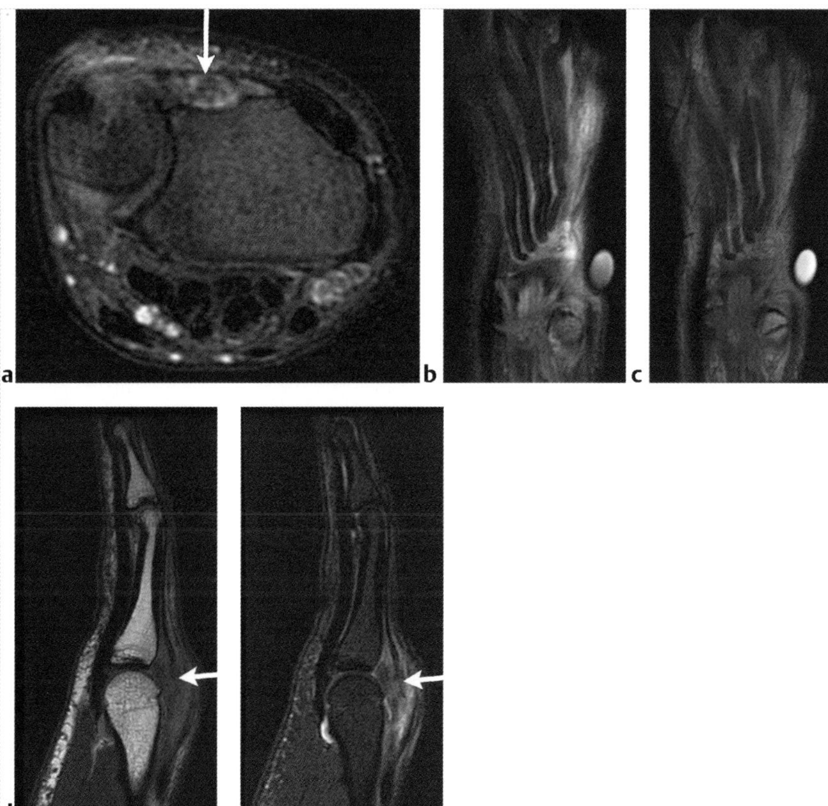

Fig. 5.9 (a) Axial fat-suppressed T2-weighted imaging (FS T2WI) shows absent extensor tendons (arrow). (b) Coronal FS T2WI shows transected second through fifth extensor tendons. (c) Coronal FS T2WI shows a large gap between torn ends of the second through fifth extensor tendons. (d) Sagittal proton density–weighted imaging from a second patient shows rupture of the fifth extensor tendon (arrow). (e) Corresponding FS T2WI shows rupture of the fifth extensor tendon (arrow).

Table 5.2 (Cont.) Tendon lesions of the hand

Abnormalities	MRI findings	Comments
Flexor annular pulley tears (▶ Fig. 5.10)	On both axial PDWI and FS T2WI the normal flexor pulley ligament system is visualized as an angled black band on each side of the flexor tendon, which connects the tendon with the adjacent bone. Normally there is very little space between the flexor tendons of the digits and the bones of the fingers. Direct visualization of pulley rupture is seen on axial images as disruption of the angled dark band connecting the bone to the tendon. This may occur on the radial or ulnar side of the tendon or may involve both sides. The classic indirect sign of pulley rupture is bowstringing. This is best seen on sagittal images and is caused by separation of the flexor tendon from the bone such that the appearance is that of a bow. This occurs when both ulnar and radial sides of the pulley are disrupted. When one side of the pulley is torn the tendon will often sublux toward the intact pulley. Additional associated findings include marrow edema in adjacent bone and joint effusion. These injuries can be subtle, and careful comparison to adjacent normal digits is often helpful.	The pulley system of the finger flexor tendons is a focal tendon sheath thickening. The pulley system is referred sequentially as A1 to A4 with the A2 segment the most commonly injured. Early diagnosis is important to prevent complications such as flexion contracture. These injuries are often associated with significant pain and swelling at the site of injury, which can limit accurate physical exam. Treatment may be conservative or may require surgical repair.

(continued on page 132)

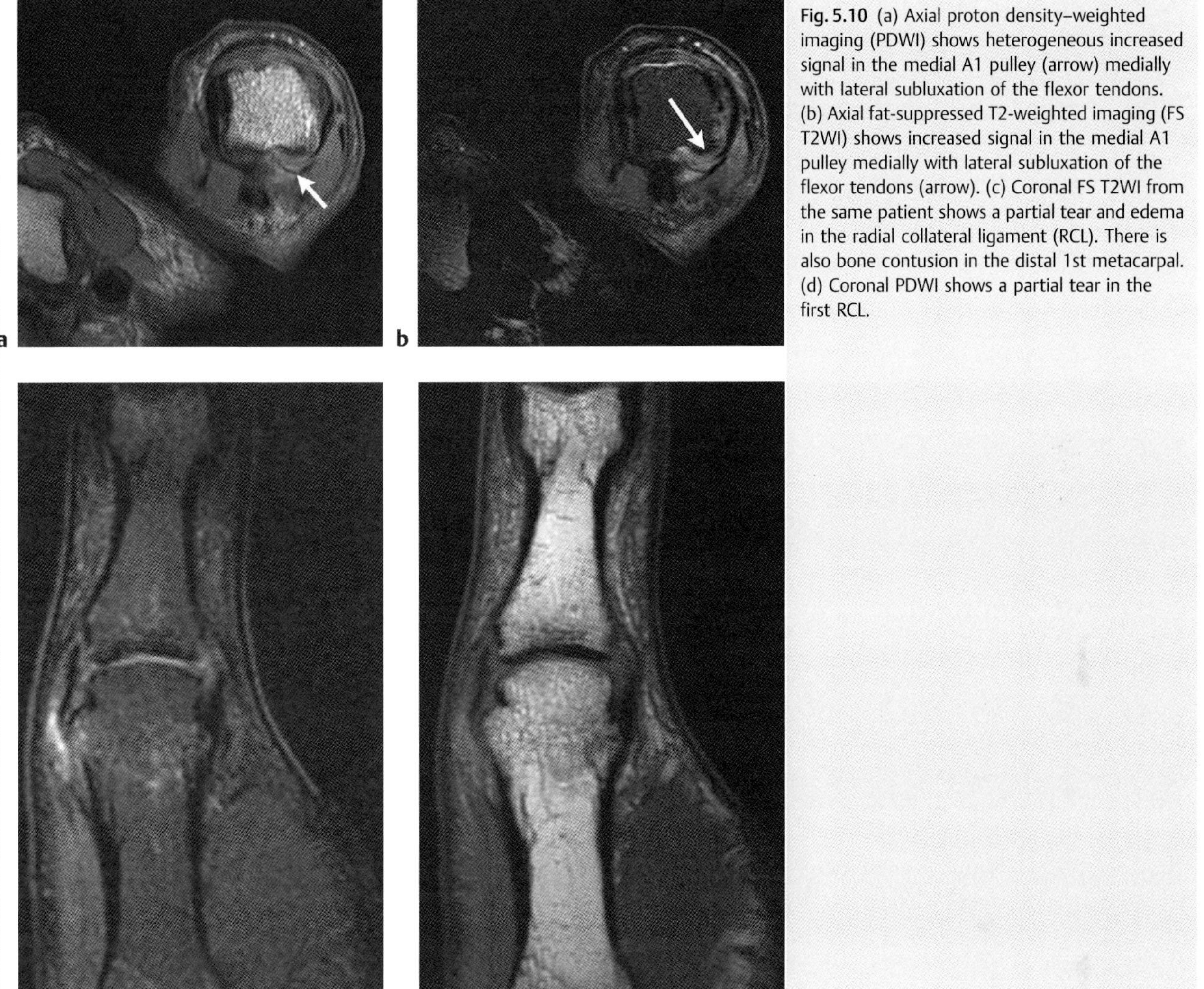

Fig. 5.10 (a) Axial proton density–weighted imaging (PDWI) shows heterogeneous increased signal in the medial A1 pulley (arrow) medially with lateral subluxation of the flexor tendons. (b) Axial fat-suppressed T2-weighted imaging (FS T2WI) shows increased signal in the medial A1 pulley medially with lateral subluxation of the flexor tendons (arrow). (c) Coronal FS T2WI from the same patient shows a partial tear and edema in the radial collateral ligament (RCL). There is also bone contusion in the distal 1st metacarpal. (d) Coronal PDWI shows a partial tear in the first RCL.

Table 5.2 (Cont.) Tendon lesions of the hand

Abnormalities	MRI findings	Comments
Volar plate injuries (▶ Fig. 5.11)	On both PDWI and FS T2WI the injured volar plate will have heterogeneous signal, abnormal contour, and thickening. When there is avulsion of the volar plate a gap is seen at the bony attachment. When there is volar plate avulsion high signal fluid is often seen at the site of detachment along with marrow edema in the adjacent bone. Volar plate injuries can occur at the proximal or distal attachment.	Volar plate injuries most commonly occur at the proximal interphalangeal (PIP) joints. There is often pain and swelling at the PIP joint. Some volar plate injuries are associated with small bony avulsion fractures. Injuries to the adjacent flexor tendon and collateral ligaments can also be seen. Hyperextension injury is the usual cause.

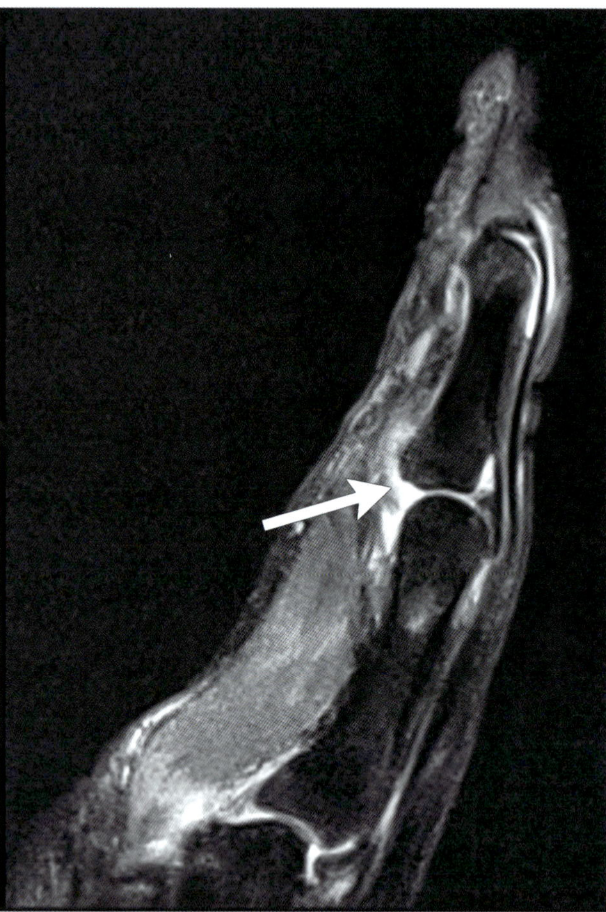

Fig. 5.11 Sagittal fat-suppressed T2-weighted imaging shows an avulsed torn volar plate at the first proximal phalanx (arrow). Note high signal fluid between the torn avulsed volar plate and the adjacent proximal phalanx. There is also mild marrow edema in the volar proximal portion of the first proximal phalanx.

5.2.1 Tendon Lesions of the Hand Suggested Reading

[1] Clavero JA, Alomar X, Monill JM, et al. MR imaging of ligament and tendon injuries of the fingers. Radiographics 2002; 22: 237–256

[2] Parellada JA, Balkissoon ARA, Hayes CW, Conway WF. Bowstring injury of the flexor tendon pulley system: MR imaging. AJR Am J Roentgenol 1996; 167: 347–349

[3] Tehranzadeh J, Ashikyan O, Anavim A, Tramma S. Enhanced MR imaging of tenosynovitis of hand and wrist in inflammatory arthritis. Skeletal Radiol 2006; 35: 814–822

5.3 Foreign Body, Infection, and Stress Fractures

- Foreign body
- Cellulitis
- Osteomyelitis
- Stress fracture (hand miscellaneous)

Table 5.3 Foreign body, infection, and stress fractures

Abnormalities	MRI findings	Comments
Foreign body (▶ Fig. 5.12, ▶ Fig. 5.13)	Foreign bodies have a variable appearance on MRI depending on their composition. Most foreign bodies are uniformly low signal on all sequences obtained. Metallic foreign bodies are associated with magnetic susceptibility artifacts, which can be highlighted with gradient echo sequences. Wood, plastic, and glass are common foreign bodies in the hand and will be seen as low signal on all pulse sequences. Fluid collections or granulation tissue or both are often associated with foreign bodies; when there is predominantly fluid this will be seen as high signal on fat-suppressed T2-weighted imaging (FS T2WI). Granulation tissue is often heterogeneous intermediate signal on both proton density–weighted imaging (PDWI) and FS T2WI and will usually enhance to some degree on postcontrast images. Postcontrast FS T1WI is often helpful in identifying associated soft tissue infection.	The hand is a common location for a variety of foreign bodies. MRI can be a valuable tool for identifying radiographically occult foreign bodies. MRI is also useful in identifying associated infection and injuries, including fractures and tendon tears. After imaging identification of foreign bodies, surgical removal is usually straightforward.
Cellulitis (▶ Fig. 5.14)	On FS T2WI there is ill-defined increased signal in the soft tissues, which has a corresponding low signal on PDWI and enhancement after intravenous contrast on FS T1-weighted imaging (T1WI). Soft tissue abscess is usually a defined fluid signal collection, high on FS T2WI, low on PDWI, and without evidence for internal enhancement on postcontrast FS T1WI. Abscesses often have increased enhancement peripherally.	Soft tissue infection in the hand can occur as cellulitis, abscess, and septic arthritis. There can also be infection of tendon sheaths. Sterile and infected tenosynovitis cannot be distinguished by MRI. Soft tissue infection of the hand can spread rapidly between compartments and along tendon sheaths. Soft tissue infection of the hand requires rapid diagnosis and treatment.

(continued on page 136)

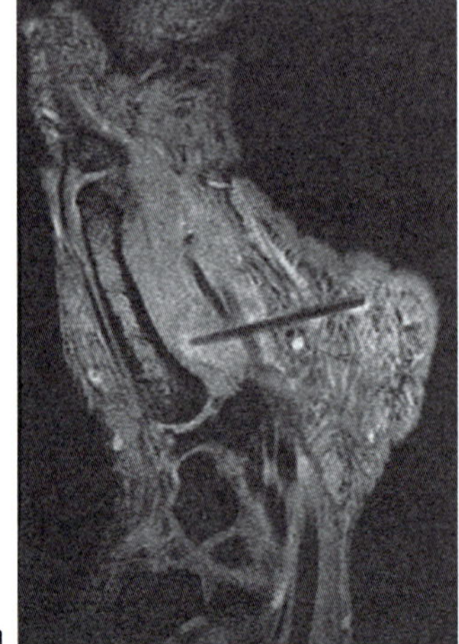

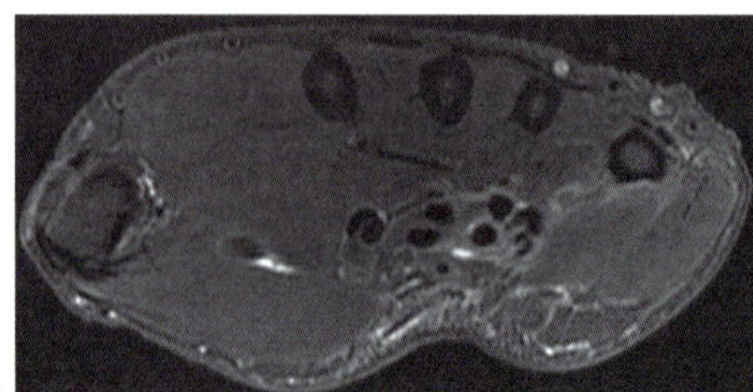

Fig. 5.12 (a) Sagittal gradient recall echo image shows a low signal linear sliver of wood traversing the hypothenar soft tissues and nearly reaching the fifth metacarpal. (b) Axial fat-suppressed T2-weighted imaging shows edema in the volar soft tissues deep to the fifth metacarpal. The foreign body is not well seen.

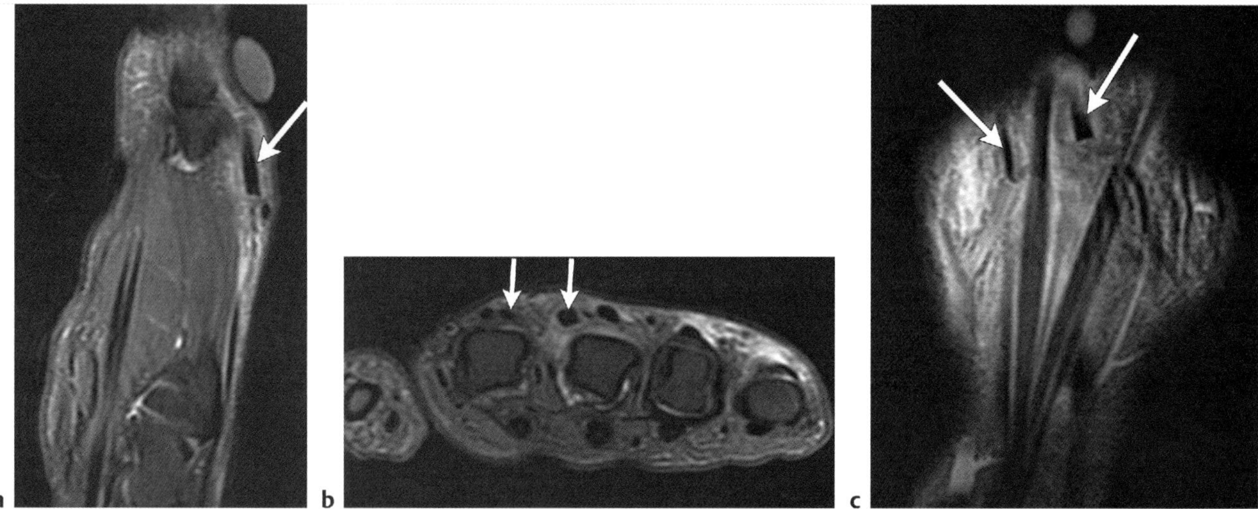

Fig. 5.13 (a) Sagittal fat-suppressed T2-weighted imaging (FS T2WI) shows a vitamin E capsule along the dorsum of the hand marking the area of concern. Just proximal to the skin marker is a subcutaneous low signal plastic foreign body from a plastic fork (arrow). (b) Axial FS T2WI image shows a round, low signal foreign body adjacent to the radial aspect of the third extensor tendon (arrow). An additional foreign body is seen adjacent to the second extensor tendon (arrow). (c) Coronal FS T2WI shows low signal foreign bodies adjacent to the extensor tendons (arrows).

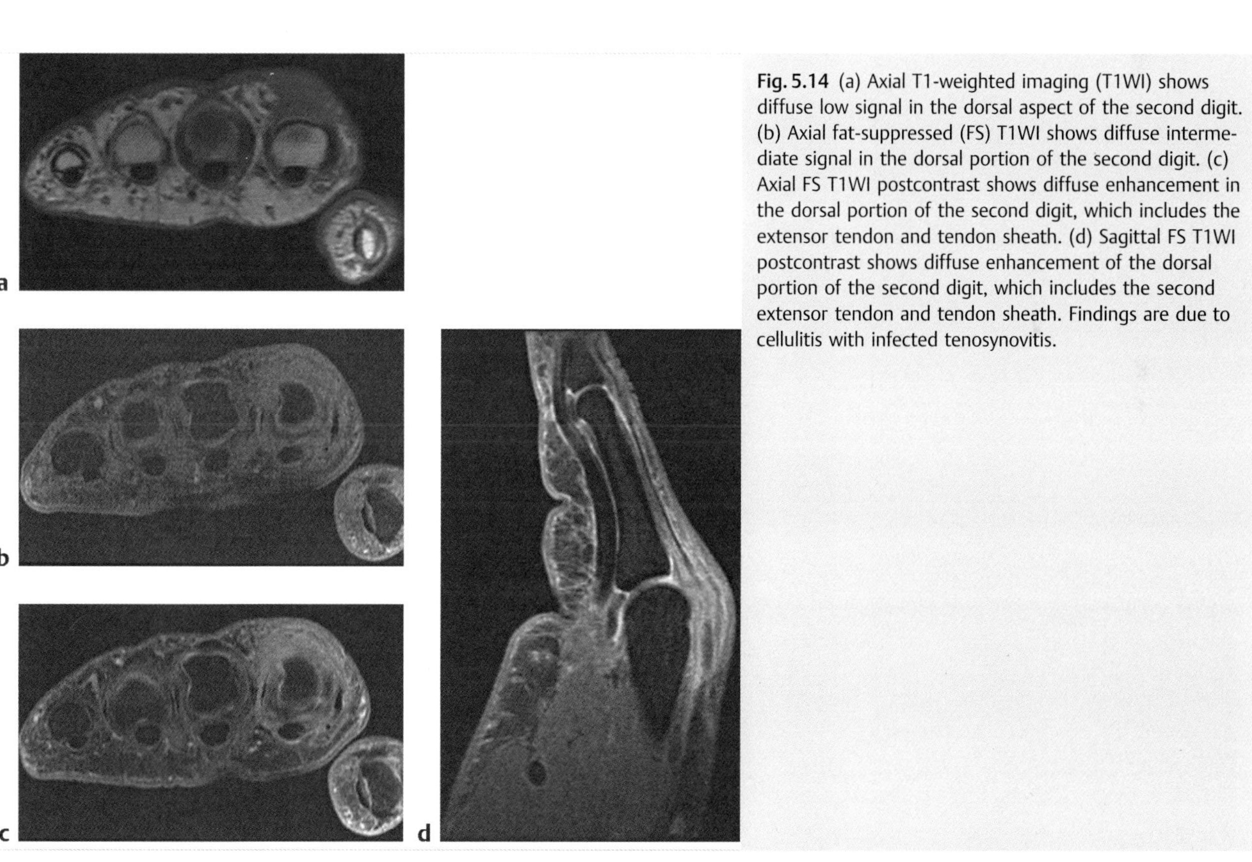

Fig. 5.14 (a) Axial T1-weighted imaging (T1WI) shows diffuse low signal in the dorsal aspect of the second digit. (b) Axial fat-suppressed (FS) T1WI shows diffuse intermediate signal in the dorsal portion of the second digit. (c) Axial FS T1WI postcontrast shows diffuse enhancement in the dorsal portion of the second digit, which includes the extensor tendon and tendon sheath. (d) Sagittal FS T1WI postcontrast shows diffuse enhancement of the dorsal portion of the second digit, which includes the second extensor tendon and tendon sheath. Findings are due to cellulitis with infected tenosynovitis.

Table 5.3 (Cont.) Foreign body, infection, and stress fractures

Abnormalities	MRI findings	Comments
Osteomyelitis (▸ Fig. 5.15)	MRI of osteomyelitis has a range of appearances. Often the initial finding on MRI consists of bone marrow edema with low signal seen on T1WI and high signal on FS T2WI, with enhancement on FS T1WI with contrast. There may also be evidence of cortical destruction and periosteal reaction. If there is an intraosseous abscess there is low signal on T1WI and high signal on FS T2WI with peripheral enhancement on FS T1WI. In some cases a sinus tract will be seen, with communication of the marrow space through a cortical defect to the skin surface. The appearance is usually low signal on T1WI and high signal on FS T2WI with enhancement of the sinus tract periphery.	Osteomyelitis may be acute, subacute, or chronic. Typically, osteomyelitis will develop via three possible routes; hematogenous seeding, direct implantation, and contiguous spread from adjacent soft tissues. The MRI appearance of osteomyelitis is affected by both the route of infection and chronicity. In hematogenous seeding the appearance and location of infection is also dependent on patient age. In children there is a predilection for involvement of the metaphysis of long bones and apophysis of flat bones. This is due to the nature of the blood supply to the metaphysis in children. Extension into the epiphysis is not uncommon. In certain joints, such as the hip and shoulder, septic arthritis is also more likely. *Staphylococcus aureas* is the most common organism affecting children. In the skeletally mature patient hematogenous seeding is typically found in the subchondral portion of long bones; as a result septic arthritis is not uncommon. In contiguous spread there is soft tissue infection, which spreads to adjacent periosteum and eventually to bone. Debilitated, diabetic, and patients on steroids are most commonly affected. In direct implantation a puncture wound is usually the cause of infection. Examples include human and animal bites, surgery, and open fracture. Most patients with infection secondary to direct implantation have both soft tissue and adjacent bony infection.
Stress fracture (hand miscellaneous) (▸ Fig. 5.16)	Stress fractures of the hand have a similar appearance on MRI to stress fractures in other parts of the body. On FS T2WI high signal is seen within the marrow space of the affected bone. Corresponding low signal is seen on PDWI. Periosteal reaction may or may not be present. Low signal fracture lines may also be seen in more advanced cases. These may or may not extend to involve the cortical bone. Long-axis sagittal plane images are often helpful to quickly determine the overall extent of the abnormality.	Upper extremity stress fractures are uncommon. There are several typical activities in which these injuries do occur, including high level gymnastics, tennis, and jackhammer operation. In the absence of accurate clinical information the interpreting radiologist may confuse the findings of stress fracture with more ominous entities such as Ewing sarcoma. After appropriate rest from the inciting activity, follow-up MRI will show interval improvement with decreased bone marrow edema.

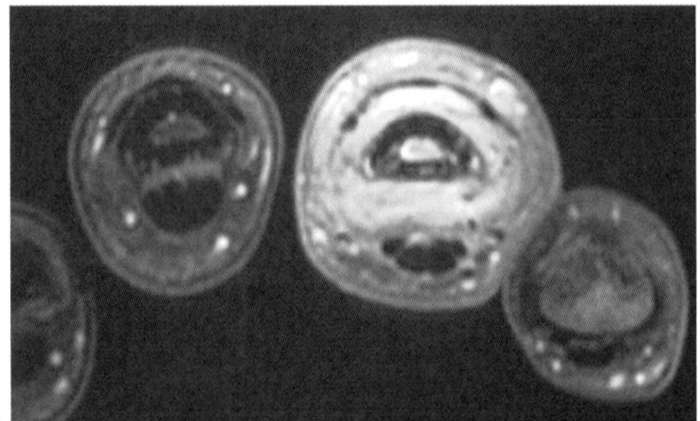
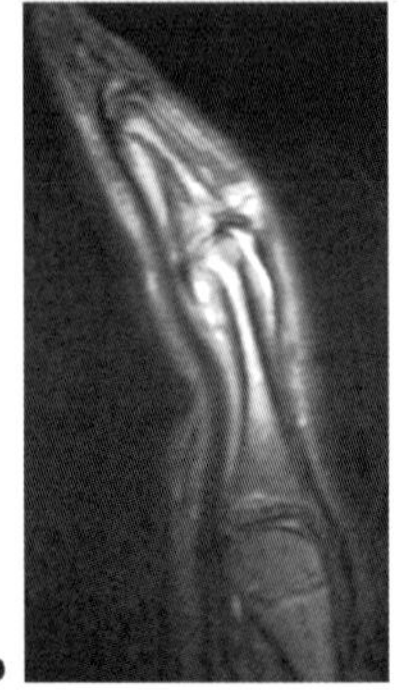
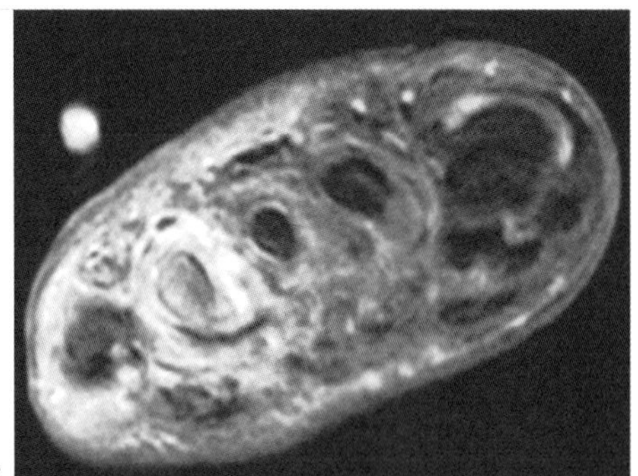

Fig. 5.15 (a) Axial fat-suppressed T2-weighted imaging (FS T2WI) shows high signal in the fourth middle phalanx with surrounding high signal periosteal reaction. (b) Sagittal FS T2WI shows high signal in the middle and distal fourth proximal phalanx and fourth middle phalanx. (c) Axial FS T2WI shows high signal in the fourth proximal phalanx with surrounding high signal periosteal reaction and extension into the subcutaneous soft tissue.

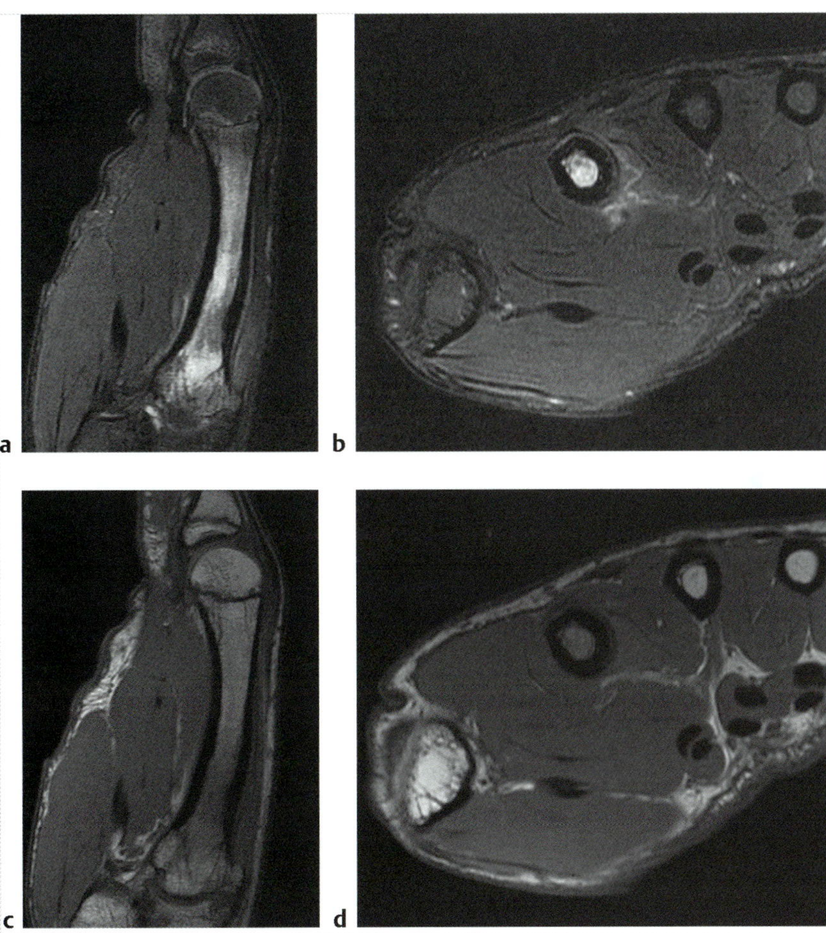

Fig. 5.16 (a) Sagittal fat-suppressed T2-weighted imaging (FS T2WI) shows a diffusely increased signal in the second metacarpal. (b) Axial FS T2WI shows increased signal in the medullary portion of the second metacarpal. There is also increased signal in the periosteum and surrounding soft tissues. (c) Sagittal proton density–weighted imaging (PDWI) shows diffuse low signal in the second metacarpal. (d) Axial PDWI reveals low signal in the medullary portion of the second metacarpal with no evidence of cortical fracture.

5.3.1 Foreign Body, Infection, and Stress Fractures Suggested Reading

[1] Balius R, Pedret C, Estruch A, Hernández G, Ruiz-Cotorro A, Mota J. Stress fractures of the metacarpal bones in adolescent tennis players: a case series. Am J Sports Med 2010; 38: 1215–1220

[2] Kornreich L, Katz K, Horev G, Zeharia A, Mukamel M. Preoperative localization of a foreign body by magnetic resonance imaging. Eur J Radiol 1998; 26: 309–311

[3] Helms CA, Major NM, Anderson MW, Kaplan PA, Dussault R. Musculoskeletal infections. In: Helms CA, Major NM, Anderson MW, Kaplan PA, Dussault R. Musculoskeletal MRI. 2nd ed. Philadelphia, PA; Saunders Elsevier; 2009:92–102

[4] Nelson EW, DeHart MM, Christensen AW, Smith DK. Magnetic resonance imaging characteristics of a lead pencil foreign body in the hand. J Hand Surg Am 1996; 21: 100–103

5.4 Soft Tissue Lesions of the Hand

- Giant cell tumor of tendon sheath (nodular type)
- Soft tissue lipoma
- Soft tissue hemangioma
- Hypothenar hammer syndrome

Table 5.4 Soft tissue lesions of the hand

Abnormalities	MRI findings	Comments
Giant cell tumor of tendon sheath (nodular type) (▶ Fig. 5.17)	These lesions are ovoid with well-defined margins. On proton density–weighted imaging (PDWI) these lesions are low to intermediate signal and on fat-suppressed T2-weighted imaging (FS T2WI) they are intermediate to high signal. There may be small zones of low signal on FS T2WI representing foci of hemosiderin. On postcontrast images there is enhancement, which may be uniform or heterogeneous. Erosion of adjacent bone may occur in some cases.	The hand and wrist are the most common locations for these tumors. Most lesions are painless, slowly growing, firm masses attached to the tendon sheath. In some cases patients will have mild pain with activity. Diffuse type giant cell tumor is uncommon in the hand. Nodular lesions are benign and commonly treated with surgery. Postsurgical recurrence is more common when there is invasion of adjacent bone. Malignant giant cell tumors of the tendon sheath are rare.
Soft tissue lipoma (▶ Fig. 5.18)	Soft tissue lipomas may or may not be intramuscular and are usually well defined. These tumors follow normal fat signal on all MRI pulse sequences. On occasion there may be a few thin, low signal septations. On postcontrast images there is often no enhancement with the exception of mild enhancement of thin internal septations.	Lipoma is the most common tumor of soft tissue. The hand and wrist are the least common locations. Most lipomas are painless and easily palpated on physical exam. Most lipomas are treated conservatively, with surgery reserved for tumors with decreased range of motion or disfigurement. Lipomas with more aggressive atypical features may also be removed.
Soft tissue hemangioma (▶ Fig. 5.19)	Soft tissue hemangiomas of the cavernous type have a variable appearance on MRI. On PDWI these lesions are usually low to intermediate signal with some linear zones of increased signal, which may be due to fat incorporated within the lesion or slow flow within veins. On FS T2WI there is heterogeneous increased signal. In the arteriovenous type dilated veins with flow voids may be present. Hemorrhage and phleboliths may be present. On postcontrast images there is usually prominent enhancement. On time-resolved magnetic resonance angiography (MRA) there is often early arterial phase flow seen within these lesions.	Soft tissue hemangiomas are benign lesions considered to represent a vascular hamartoma. These lesions may be found in subcutaneous soft tissue or in an intramuscular location. Most hemangiomas are lobulated, well circumscribed lesions. Hemangiomas are the fourth most common soft tissue tumor. These lesions are most common in the hand. If the lesion is close enough to the skin surface there may be a blue discoloration visible on physical exam. Most hemangiomas are asymptomatic, although intramuscular lesions may be associated with pain after exercise. Very large cavernous hemangiomas may be associated with platelet deficiency and congestive heart failure (Kasabach-Merritt syndrome). Multiple soft tissue hemangiomas combined with enchondromas of the digits is referred to as Maffucci syndrome.

(continued on page 140)

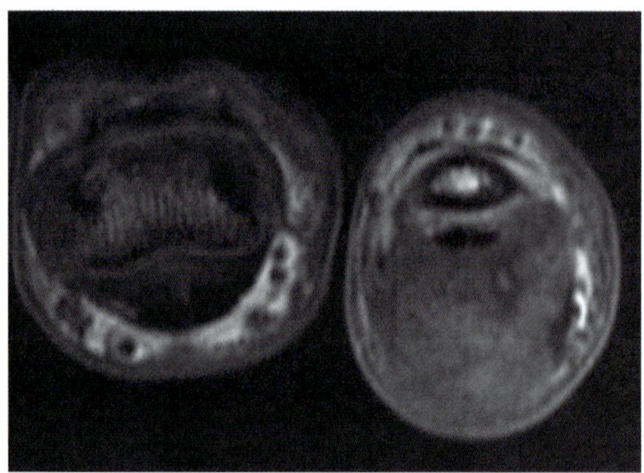

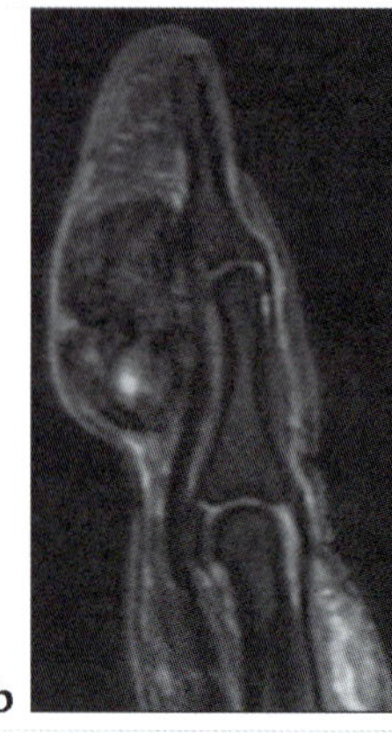

Fig. 5.17 (a) Axial fat-suppressed (FS) T1-weighted imaging shows a mixed contrast signal mass in the flexor compartment. (b) Sagittal FS T2-weighted imaging shows a low mixed low signal mass superficial to the flexor tendon.

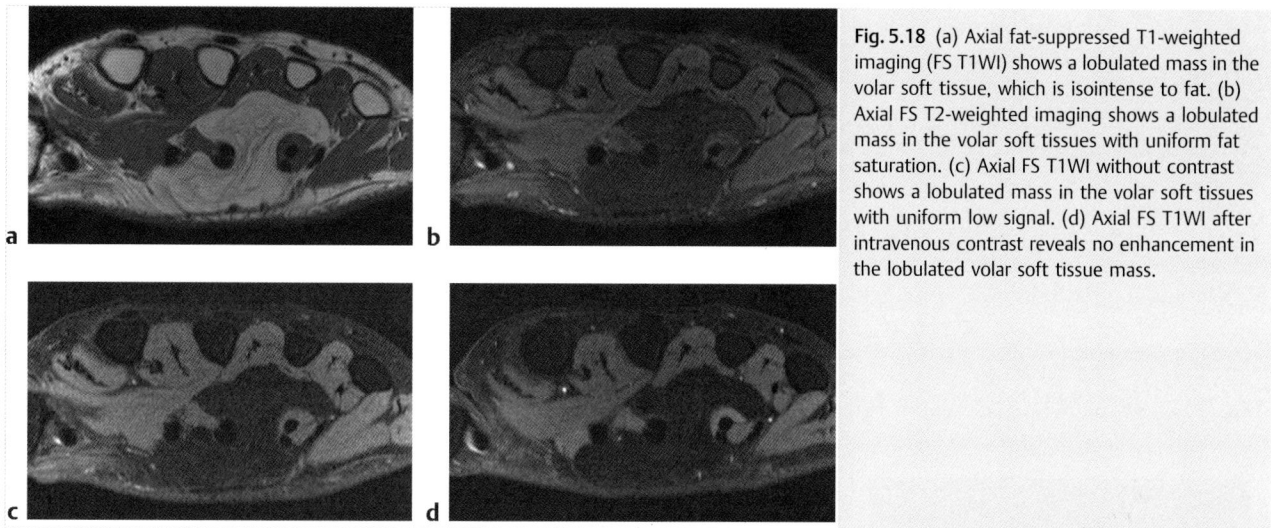

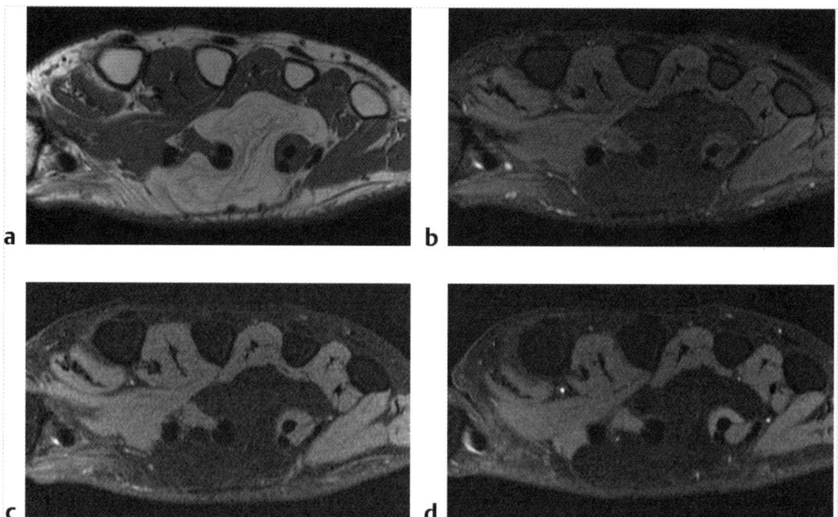

Fig. 5.18 (a) Axial fat-suppressed T1-weighted imaging (FS T1WI) shows a lobulated mass in the volar soft tissue, which is isointense to fat. (b) Axial FS T2-weighted imaging shows a lobulated mass in the volar soft tissues with uniform fat saturation. (c) Axial FS T1WI without contrast shows a lobulated mass in the volar soft tissues with uniform low signal. (d) Axial FS T1WI after intravenous contrast reveals no enhancement in the lobulated volar soft tissue mass.

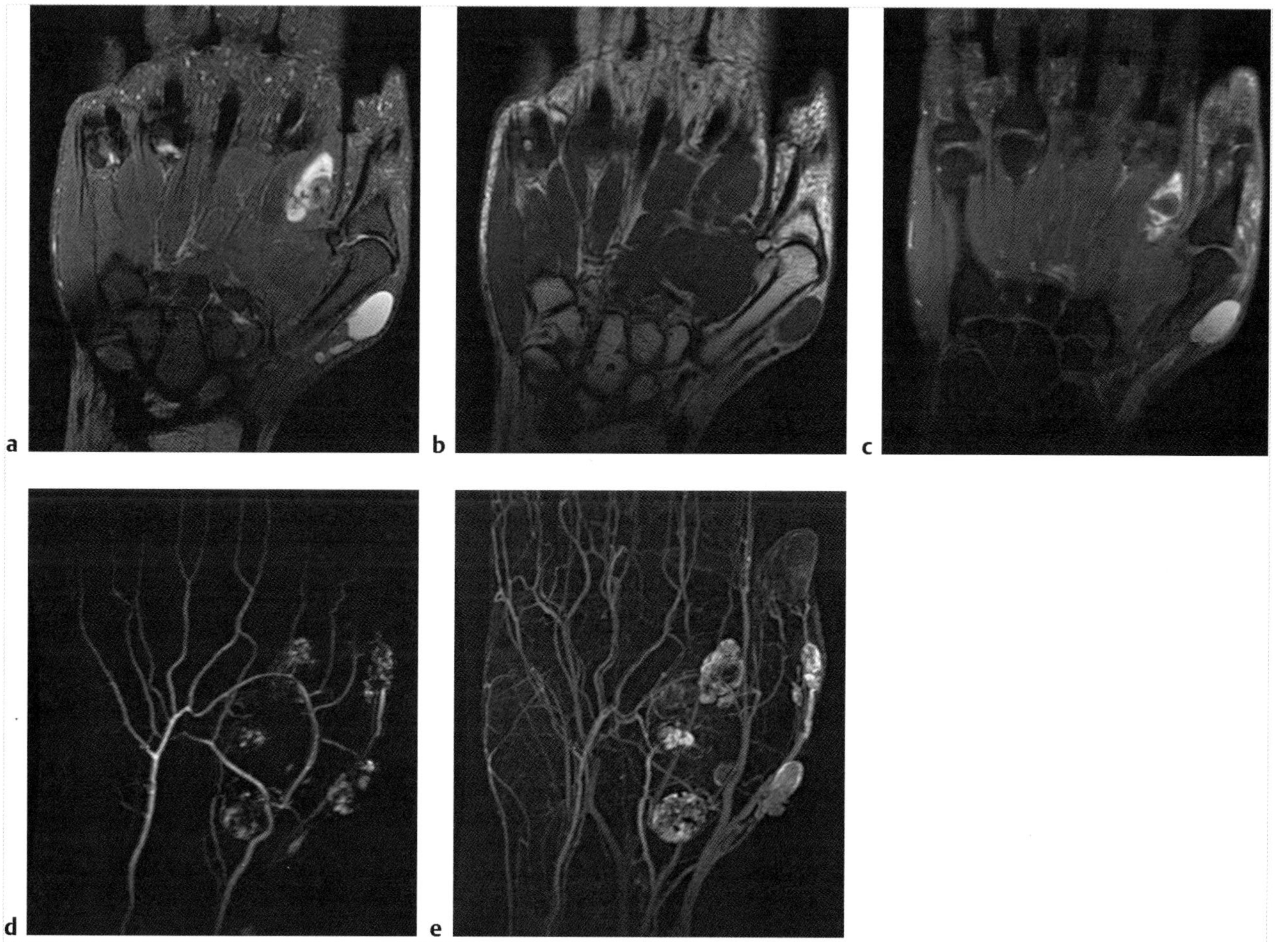

Fig. 5.19 (a) Coronal fat-suppressed T2-weighted imaging (FS T2WI) shows lobulated soft tissue masses with heterogeneous increased signal. (b) Coronal T1-weighted imaging (T1WI) shows lobulated intermediate signal masses. (c) Coronal FS T1WI postcontrast shows heterogeneously enhancing masses. (d) Time-resolved imaging of contrast kinetics (TRICKS) magnetic resonance angiography (MRA) shows multiple arterial phase, lobulated, heterogeneously enhancing masses. (e) TRICKS MRA in late arterial phase/early venous phase shows increased enhancement of multiple lobulated masses.

Table 5.4 (Cont.) Soft tissue lesions of the hand

Abnormalities	MRI findings	Comments
Hypothenar hammer syndrome (▸ Fig. 5.20)	On PDWI there is heterogeneous increased signal seen in a thickened ulnar artery, at the level of the Guyon canal. On FS T2WI there is a heterogeneous-signal nodular lesion seen in the expected location of the palmar ulnar artery. On postcontrast images there is low signal seen centrally within the thrombosed ulnar artery and enhancement of the arterial wall and adjacent connective tissue. Time-resolved contrast-enhanced MRA is also useful in delineating the location of thrombosis and evaluating for the possibility of emboli to downstream digital arteries.	This is an uncommon syndrome in which there is thrombosis of the palmar ulnar artery and possibly emboli to digital arteries resulting in symptomatic ischemia. Most cases are unilateral and occur in individuals with particular occupations, such as jackhammer operators.

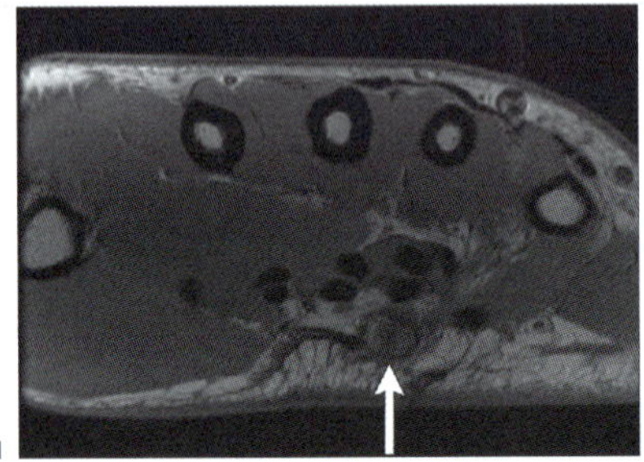

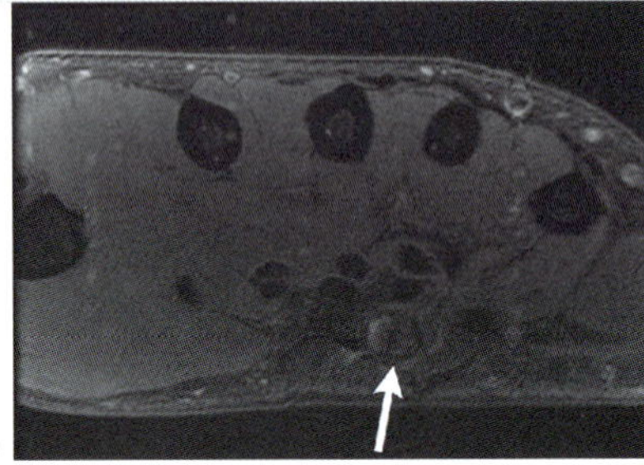

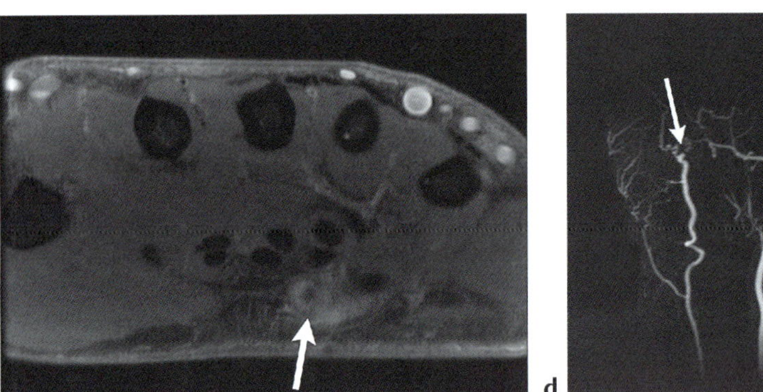

Fig. 5.20 (a) Axial proton density–weighted imaging shows a thickened palmar ulnar artery with heterogeneous signal (arrow). (b) Axial fat-suppressed (FS) T2-weighted imaging shows a thickened palmar ulnar artery with edema (arrow). (c) Axial FS T1-weighted imaging post-contrast shows a thickened palmar ulnar artery with peripheral arterial wall enhancement and central thrombosis (arrow). (d) Time-resolved imaging of contrast kinetics magnetic resonance angiography reveals thrombosis of the distal ulnar artery at the level of the palmar arch (arrow).

5.4.1 Soft Tissue Lesions of the Hand Suggested Reading

[1] Blum AG, Zabel JP, Kohlmann R, et al. Pathologic conditions of the hypothenar eminence: evaluation with multidetector CT and MR imaging. Radiographics 2006; 26: 1021–1044

[2] Connell DA, Koulouris G, Thorn DA, Potter HG. Contrast-enhanced MR angiography of the hand. Radiographics 2002; 22: 583–599

[3] Giant cell tumor of the tendon sheath and/or soft tissue (also referred to as nodular tenosynovitis, fibrous xanthoma, tenosynovial giant cell tumor, and benign synovioma) (A30). In: Meyers SP, ed. MRI of Bone and Soft Tissue Tumors and Tumorlike Lesions, Differential Diagnosis and Atlas. 1st ed. Stuttgart, Germany: Thieme; 2007:469–475

[4] Hemangiomas (also referred to as Vascular Hamartomas) (A34). In: Meyers SP. MRI of Bone and Soft Tissue Tumors and Tumorlike Lesions, Differential Diagnosis and Atlas. 1st ed. Stuttgart, Germany: Thieme; 2007: 491–492, 496–499

[5] Lipoma, atypical lipoma, and hibernoma (A43). In: Meyers, SP, ed. MRI of Bone and Soft Tissue Tumors and Tumorlike Lesions, Differential Diagnosis and Atlas. 1st ed. Stuttgart, Germany: Thieme; 2007: 543–549

Chapter 6

The Hip

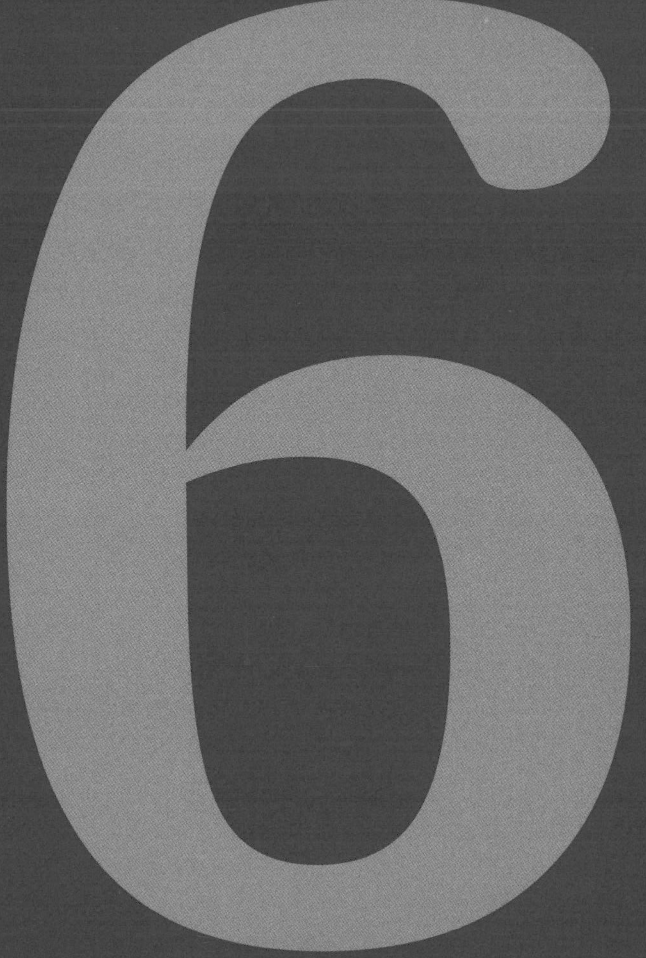

6 The Hip

Eric P. Weinberg

6.1 Bone Lesions of the Hip

- Avascular necrosis (AVN)
- Transient osteoporosis
- Subcortical insufficiency fractures
- Femoral stress (fatigue) fractures
- Femoral neck fractures
- Intertrochanteric fractures
- Acetabular fractures
- Pubic rami fractures
- Avulsion fractures of the ischial tuberosity
- Legg-Calvé-Perthes (LCP) disease
- Slipped capital femoral epiphysis (SCFE)
- Developmental dysplasia of the hip (DDH)
- Rapid osteolysis

Table 6.1 Bone lesions of the hip

Abnormalities	MRI findings	Comments
Avascular necrosis (AVN) (▶ Fig. 6.1)	The appearance of AVN on magnetic resonance imaging (MRI) depends on when the patient is imaged. Most cases of AVN are seen as diffuse high signal on fat-suppressed T2-weighted imaging (FS T2WI), and on T1-weighted imaging (T1WI) there is usually a sharply defined curvilinear serpiginous band of low signal surrounding variable signal marrow. Over time high signal seen on FS T2WI is more localized to the anterior superior femoral head. Eventually there may be flattening and subchondral collapse of the femoral head. Coronal images depict these findings to better advantage. The amount of weight-bearing surface of the femoral head that is abnormal has important prognostic significance, with greater involvement indicating worsened prognosis.	AVN of the hip is reported to occur bilaterally in up to 40% of patients. Therefore, both hips should be imaged when there is a question of AVN. Patients usually present with intermittent groin pain that will typically worsen over time. Weight bearing generally results in increased pain. There are many reported possible causes of AVN, with more common etiologies being idiopathic or resulting from trauma, use of steroids, or alcoholism. Trauma is the most common cause of AVN. Early diagnosis and treatment of AVN is important. Some of these treatments include core decompression, rotational osteotomy, and vascularized bone graft. Late diagnosis can result in significant complications, including femoral head flattening and fragmentation, which ultimately may require hip replacement surgery. Differential diagnostic considerations include transient osteoporosis and subchondral insufficiency fracture of the femoral head.
Transient osteoporosis (▶ Fig. 6.2)	On FS T2WI there is diffuse high signal edema involving the femoral head and neck with corresponding diffuse low signal on T1WI. Signal abnormalities often extend into the intertrochanteric region of the femur. On postcontrast FS T1WI there is abnormal enhancement, which corresponds to the signal abnormality seen on FS T2WI. Variable-size joint effusion is also often noted. Findings are unilateral with no involvement of the opposite hip. There are no serpiginous low signal lines on any imaging sequence, and there is no evidence for low signal line of a subcortical fracture.	Transient osteoporosis is a self-limited abnormality that spontaneously resolves, usually within 9 months. Patients present with rapid worsening pain in the inguinal region, buttock, or anterior thigh. Transient osteoporosis is an idiopathic disorder that occurs in patients without risk factors for AVN. Most patients are either pregnant women in the third trimester or middle-aged men. Treatment is nonsurgical with protected weight bearing and nonsteroidal anti-inflammatory drugs.

(continued on page 146)

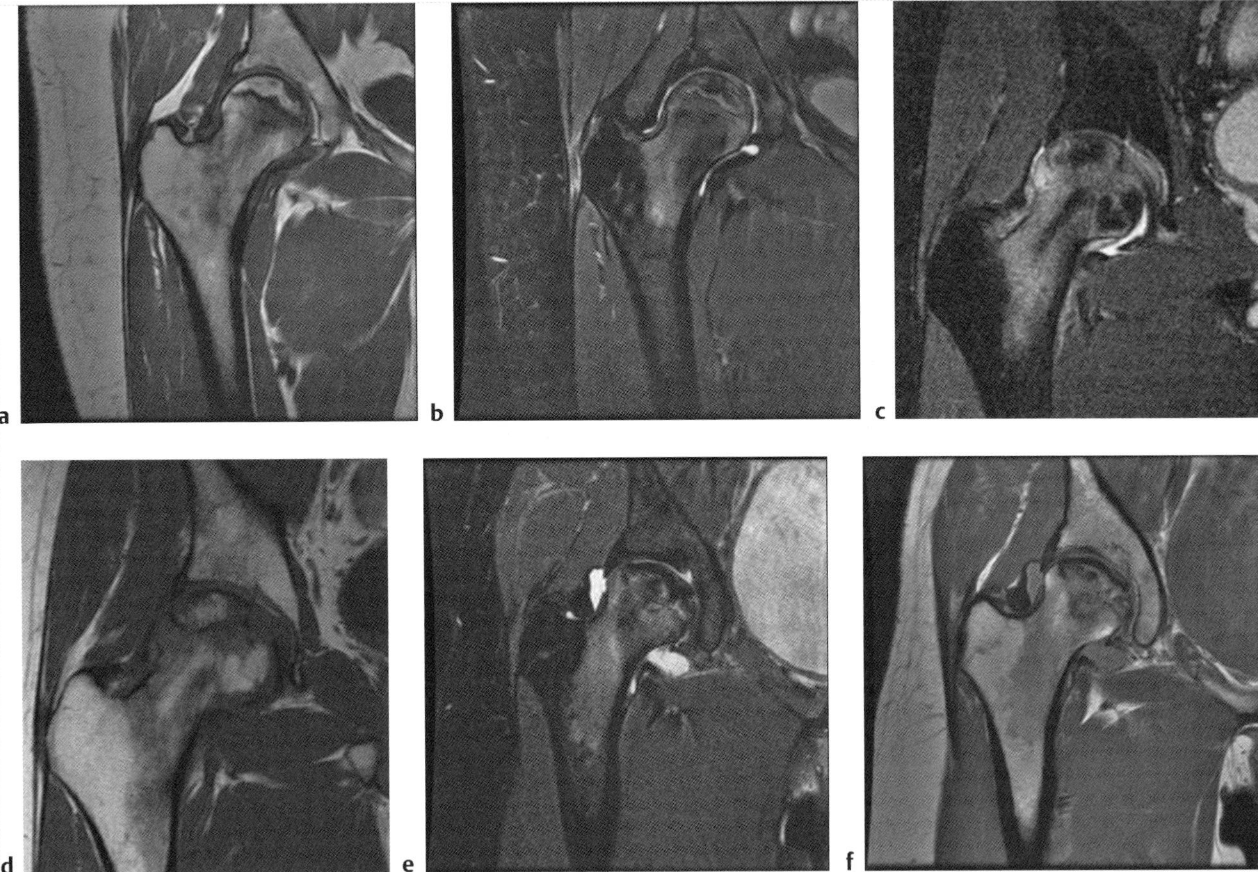

Fig. 6.1 (a) Coronal T1-weighted imaging (T1WI) shows a sharply defined curvilinear band of low signal in the femoral head with adjacent heterogeneous low signal. Note the femoral head contour remains normal. (b) Coronal fat-suppressed T2-weighted imaging (FS T2WI) shows a curvilinear band of low signal in the femoral head with adjacent patchy high signal marrow edema, which extends into the intertrochanteric region of the proximal femur. (c) Coronal FS T2WI from a second patient shows more extensive edema with extension into the intertrochanteric region. (d) Coronal proton density–weighted imaging (PDWI) from the same patient shows corresponding heterogeneous zones of low signal in the femoral head, neck, and intertrochanteric regions. The femoral head contour is still grossly maintained. (e) Coronal FS T2WI from a third patient shows more advanced changes of avascular necrosis, including early collapse of the femoral head with some flattening of the femoral head contour. Large joint effusion is also present. (f) Coronal PDWI from the same patient shows some collapse of the femoral head with flattening of the superior femoral head contour.

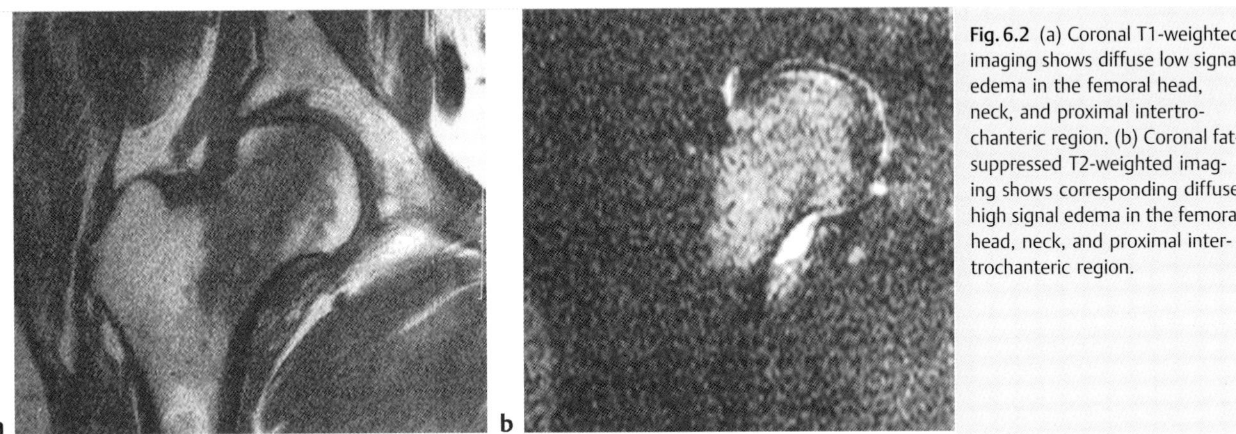

Fig. 6.2 (a) Coronal T1-weighted imaging shows diffuse low signal edema in the femoral head, neck, and proximal intertrochanteric region. (b) Coronal fat-suppressed T2-weighted imaging shows corresponding diffuse high signal edema in the femoral head, neck, and proximal intertrochanteric region.

Table 6.1 (Cont.) Bone lesions of the hip

Abnormalities	MRI findings	Comments
Subcortical insufficiency fractures (▶ Fig. 6.3)	On T1WI there is linear low signal seen in a subcortical location, which may closely parallel the articular surface. There is surrounding marrow edema extending beyond the margins of the fracture, which may be extensive.This is low signal on T1WI and high signal on FS T2WI.	Insufficiency fractures occur in abnormal osteopenic bone that has been subjected to normal stress. Most patients are female, older than 65, and overweight. Patients present with hip pain and some difficulty in weight bearing. Imaging of the entire pelvis is recommended because insufficiency fractures may also involve the sacrum and pubic rami.
Femoral stress (fatigue) fractures (▶ Fig. 6.4)	The MRI appearance of a proximal femur stress fracture depends on the stage at which the abnormality is imaged. In early stress injuries there may only be mild subcortical high signal edema in marrow on FS T2WI. This is usually seen in the femoral neck and intertrochanteric region and is often in the medial portion of the femur. As the injury progresses there is periosteal reaction followed by linear subcortical low signal fracture seen on both FS T2WI and proton density–weighted imaging (PDWI). Ultimately there can be cortical fracture, which may or may not be displaced.	MRI is the most accurate imaging method for detecting all types of stress fractures of the proximal femur. Stress fractures are injuries that occur when normal bone is subjected to abnormal stresses. The classic example is the long-distance runner. Patients typically present with groin or hip pain and pain that worsens with weight bearing. Early diagnosis of proximal femur stress fractures is needed to return the athlete to sport as soon as possible and to prevent the injury from progressing to a cortical fracture.
Femoral neck fractures (▶ Fig. 6.5)	MRI is the most sensitive, accurate method for detecting fractures of the femoral neck. Femoral neck fractures are sometimes radiographically occult. On FS T2WI there is high signal marrow edema centered on the femoral neck and corresponding low signal on PDWI. On both FS T2WI and PDWI there is often a low signal line surrounded by marrow edema indicating the presence of fracture. The adjacent cortex may or may not be involved, and the presence or absence of any bony displacement is variable. MRI is particularly useful when there is an incomplete fracture with no cortical involvement.	Femoral neck fractures typically occur in elderly patients after sustaining minor trauma. Symptoms include hip and groin pain with difficulty in weight bearing. In the setting of negative hip radiographs and clinical history of injury in an older patient, MRI examination of the hip should be performed. This can be of a limited nature such that coronal images are obtained. The goal of early accurate diagnosis is to prevent an incomplete fracture from progressing to a completed and displaced cortical fracture requiring hip-pinning surgery. Early diagnosis and treatment also decrease the incidence of femoral head AVN.
Intertrochanteric fractures	Intertrochanteric fractures may be radiographically occult. This is particularly true for incomplete intertrochanteric fractures, which involve the greater trochanter and intertrochanteric bone but do not involve the medial cortex. On FS T2WI there is high signal marrow edema in the intertrochanteric portion of the proximal femur, which surrounds linear low signal. On PDWI there is corresponding low signal marrow edema, which surrounds the lower signal fracture line. There may or may not be associated cortical fracture, and fracture displacement is variable.	Intertrochanteric fractures of the femur are most commonly seen in older osteoporotic patients. Most patients have a history of recent minor injury such as slipping or falling. Patients complain of severe hip pain and are unable to bear weight or move the affected limb without extreme pain. Treatment for most patients consists of open reduction internal fixation. In some patients with incomplete fractures surgery may not be indicated.

(continued on page 148)

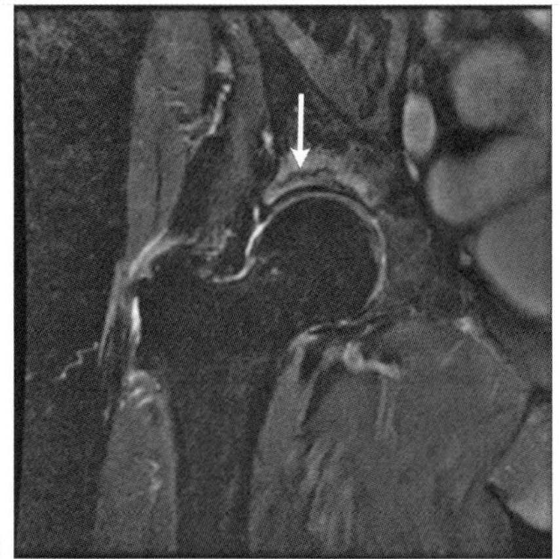

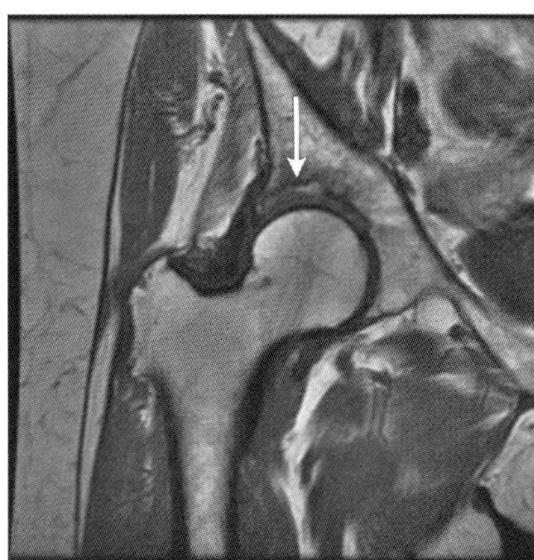

Fig. 6.3 (a) Coronal fat-suppressed T2-weighted imaging shows a low signal band near to and roughly parallel to the acetabular cortex with adjacent high signal marrow edema. (b) Coronal T1-weighted imaging shows a low signal band near to and roughly parallel to the acetabualar cortex with adjacent low signal marrow edema.

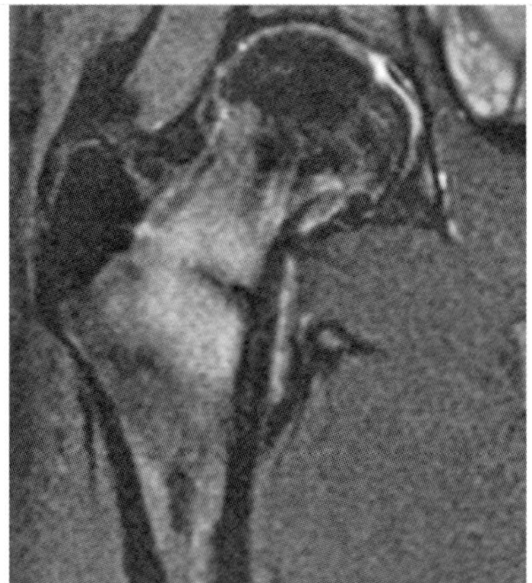

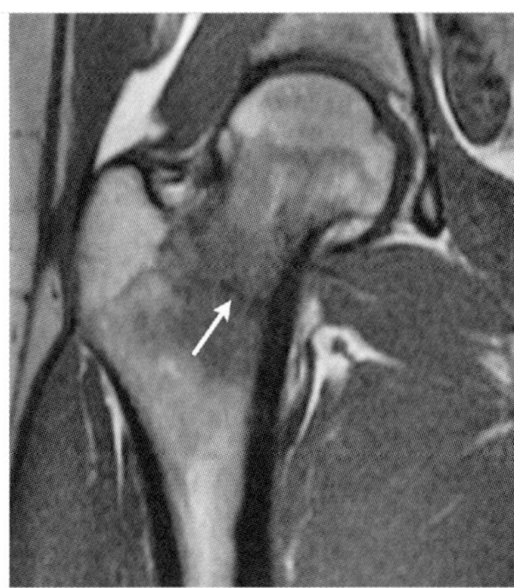

Fig. 6.4 (a) Coronal fat-suppressed T2-weighted imaging shows a linear low signal in the medial aspect of the intertrochanteric portion of the femur with adjacent extensive high signal marrow edema. There is no cortical fracture. (b) Coronal proton density–weighted imaging shows subtle linear low signal in the medial intertrochanteric portion of the femur (arrow) with adjacent low signal marrow edema.

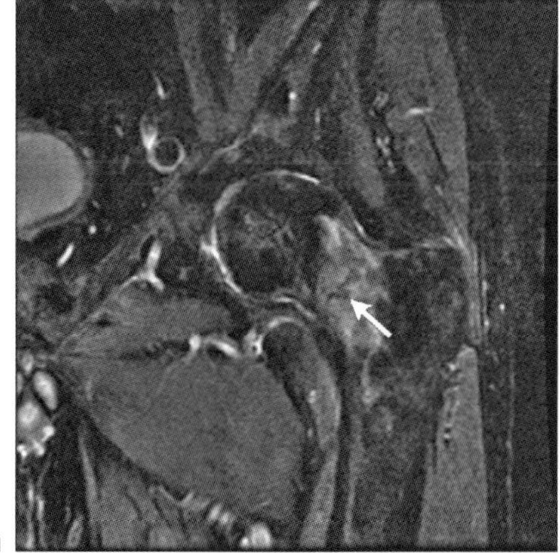

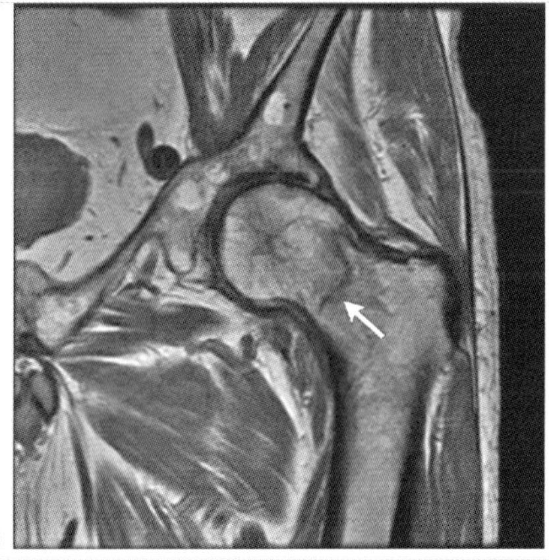

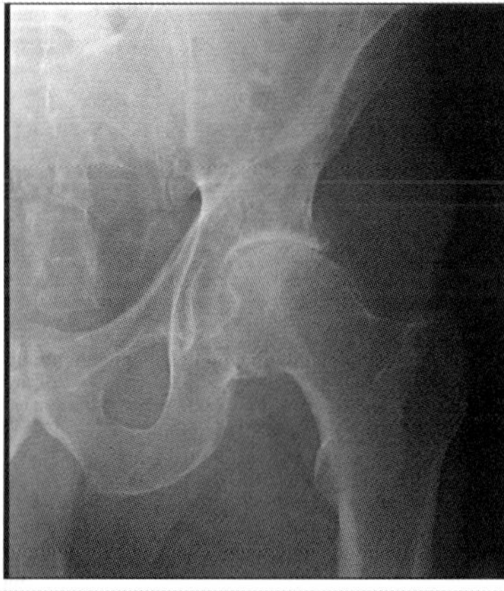

Fig. 6.5 (a) Coronal fat-suppressed T2-weighted imaging shows a curvilinear low signal traversing the femoral neck with adjacent high signal marrow edema. No cortical fracture is seen. (b) Coronal proton density–weighted imaging (PDWI) shows a curvilinear low signal traversing the femoral neck without evidence for cortical fracture. (c) Anteroposterior radiograph of the left hip from the same patient is without evidence of fracture. This is therefore a radiographically occult hip fracture, which is not uncommon in older patients.

Table 6.1 (Cont.) Bone lesions of the hip

Abnormalities	MRI findings	Comments
Acetabular fractures (▶ Fig. 6.6)	In most patients MRI is not needed to identify an acetabular fracture. Multislice computed tomography (CT) is the imaging modality of choice for evaluating the acetabulum. However, on occasion there may be an acetabualar fracture that is occult on both radiographs and CT scans. These fractures may be incomplete or nondisplaced. On FS T2WI there is high signal marrow edema surrounding a low signal line seen within the acetabulum. On PDWI there is low signal marrow edema surrounding the lower signal fracture line. The cortex is usually fractured though not in all cases.	Most acetabualar fractures result from severe trauma such as motor vehicle injuries. There are many possible acetabular fracture types, and a full discussion is beyond the scope of this book. The most common type of acetabular fracture involves the posterior wall. Most fractures of the acetabulum result in hip instability and require surgical fixation. Some posterior wall fractures can be treated conservatively.
Pubic rami fractures (▶ Fig. 6.7)	On FS T2WI there is high signal seen focally within the affected pubic rami. Low signal fracture line is often seen surrounded by high signal edema. Extensive callus formation is often seen if the injury is subacute. High signal edema may also be seen in adjacent muscles. On PDWI there is corresponding low signal edema surrounding lower signal linear fracture.	Most pubic rami fractures are due to stress injuries. In athletes, often long-distance runners, these injuries are due to increased repetitive stress in normal bone (fatigue fracture). In older patients, often with osteoporosis, these injuries are due to normal stress in abnormal bone (insufficiency fracture). Other causes of pubic rami fractures include prior pelvic radiation and trauma. In the case of trauma, particularly in older patients, these fractures may be associated with femoral neck fractures and sacral fractures. In acute trauma the concept of the bony ring applies to rami fractures such that often both the superior and inferior rami on the same side will be fractured. Patients with pubic rami fractures often present with hip and groin pain, which cannot be clinically distinguished from hip fractures.
Avulsion fractures of the ischial tuberosity	On FS T2WI there is a gap between the ischial tuberosity and inferior pubic ramus. In this gap there is high signal edema or hematoma or both. There is also likely some high signal marrow edema in the displaced bony fragment and the adjacent portion of the inferior pubic ramus. On PDWI there is corresponding low signal seen in the involved portions of bone and in the gap formed between the inferior pubic ramus and displaced ischial tuberosity. In some cases there may be a variable amount of bony fragmentation of the ischial tuberosity, which is seen to better advantage on PDWI. The axial plane is best for identifying this type of injury. In chronic cases there is often callous formation.	The ischial tuberosity is an apophysis and is most commonly avulsed in skeletally immature athletes. In particular this injury is seen in soccer players. In adults bony avulsion is less common, and there is often more severe injury of the conjoint tendon of the hamstrings, which attaches to the ischial tuberosity. Patients with acute avulsion fractures typically present with sudden onset of pain, which occurs during the causative sport or activity. Treatment is usually nonsurgical unless the gap between the bones is greater than 2 cm.

(continued on page 150)

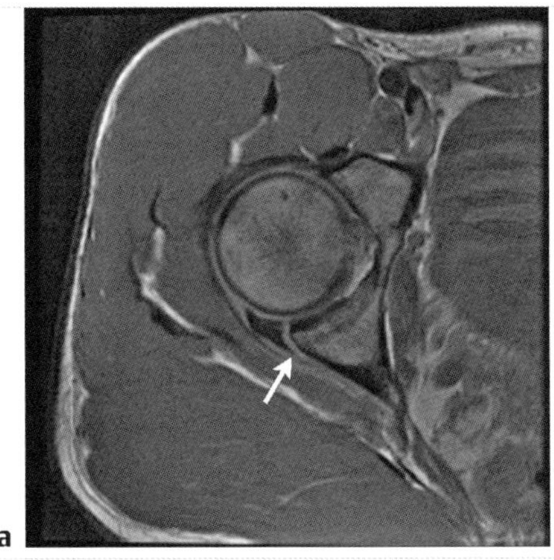

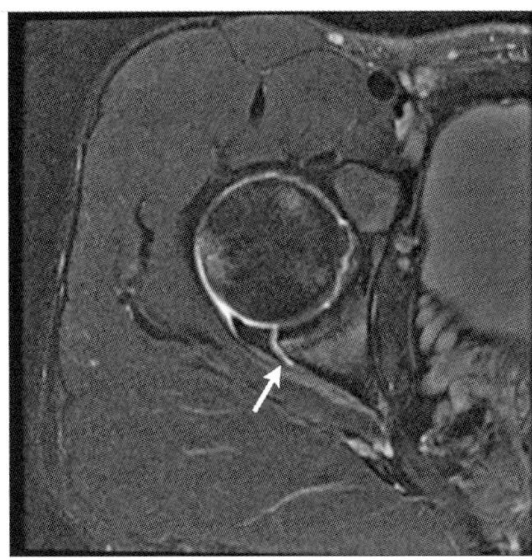

Fig. 6.6 (a) Axial proton density–weighted imaging shows a well-defined fracture through the posterior acetabulum. (b) Axial fat-suppressed T2-weighted imaging shows a well-defined high signal fracture line through the posterior acetabulum. Note several high signal bone contusions within the femoral head.

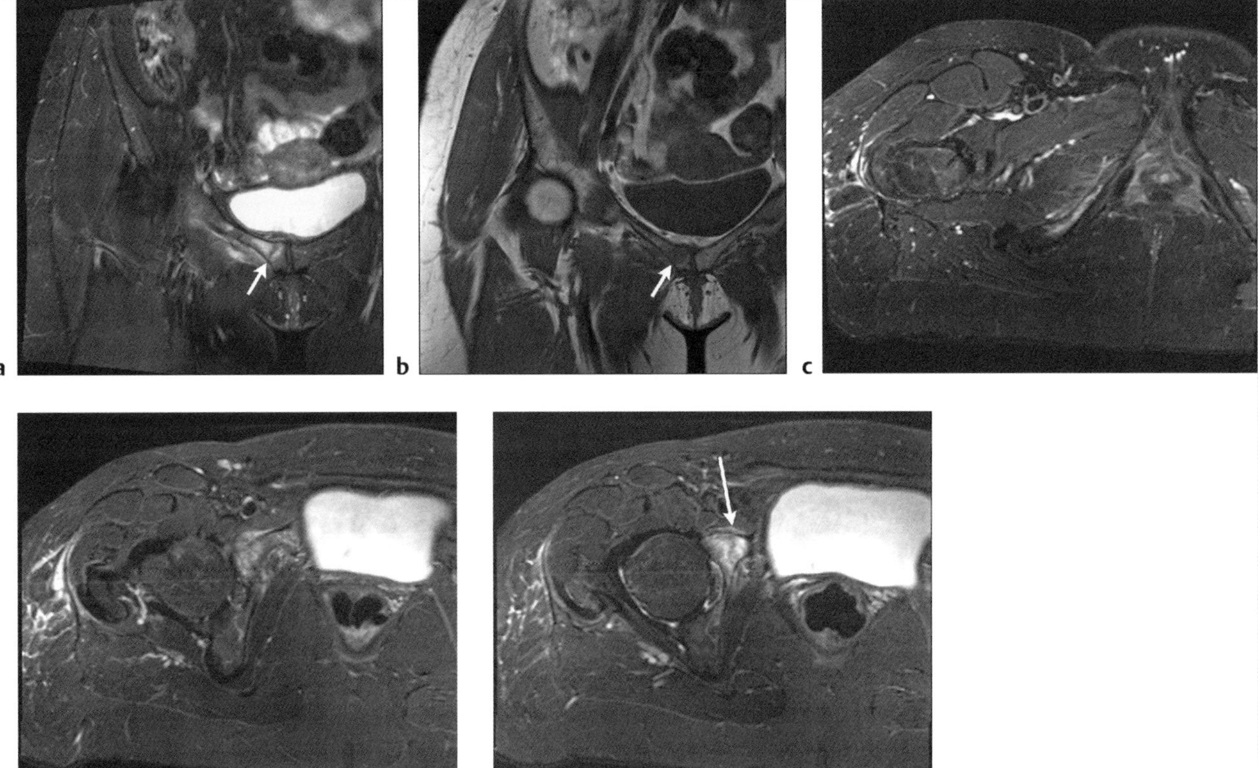

Fig. 6.7 (a) Coronal fat-suppressed T2-weighted imaging (FS T2WI) shows a vertical linear low signal fracture (arrow) in the right pubic ramus with surrounding marrow edema. (b) Corresponding coronal proton density–weighted imaging shows a low signal fracture line (arrow). (c) Axial FS T2WI shows diffuse marrow edema in the right inferior pubic ramus. (d) Axial FS T2WI shows diffuse marrow edema in the right superior pubic ramus. (e) Axial FS T2WI shows an anterior acetabular fracture to better advantage (arrow).

Table 6.1 (Cont.) Bone lesions of the hip

Abnormalities	MRI findings	Comments
Legg-Calvé-Perthes (LCP) disease (▶ Fig. 6.8)	The MRI findings in LCP disease are variable and depend on which phase of the disease is imaged. In the necrotic phase of the disease on both T1WI and PDWI there is low to intermediate signal in the proximal femoral epiphysis, which can be focal or diffuse. On FS T2WI there is heterogeneous increased signal seen focally or diffusely within the proximal femoral epiphysis. In some patients a curvilinear subchondral hyperintensity may be seen in the anterior superior portion of the femoral head indicating a subchondral fracture. On postcontrast FS T1WI there is variable enhancement of the proximal femoral epiphysis, which can range from no enhancement to focal zones of no enhancement. Other findings may include thickened articular cartilage with abnormal signal and flattening of the articular surface of the femoral head. Joint effusion and synovitis may also be present. In the revascularization and reparative phases of LCP disease the appearance of the proximal femoral epiphysis is variable. On FS T2WI revascularized portions of the femoral head are high signal intensity, and on postcontrast FS T1WI demonstrate high signal enhancement, which can persist if delayed images are obtained. In some patients there can be fragmentation of the epiphysis, and each fragment may demonstrate different signal characteristics indicating varying phases of the disease. In some patients there may also be abnormal signal and configuration of the proximal femoral physis. The physis may demonstrate increased undulation, cysts, and transphyseal bony bridging (bars).	LCP disease is a type of idiopathic osteonecrosis of the proximal femoral epiphysis that typically occurs in children ages 2 to 14. The peak age of onset is 5 to 6 years, with boys affected up to five times more frequently than girls. Most cases are unilateral, with approximately 15% of patients having bilateral disease. Patients complain of hip pain and may have a limp. Younger patients with LCP have a better prognosis than patients diagnosed at an older age. Early diagnosis is important so that prompt treatment may begin. MRI is often helpful in establishing an early diagnosis because radiography may be normal in early-stage LCP disease. MRI is also helpful in rejecting other possible diagnoses, including sickle cell disease, complications of corticosteroids, Gaucher disease, juvenile chronic arthritis, and epiphyseal dysplasia. MRI findings are also important in establishing an accurate disease prognosis. MRI accurately identifies the extent and location of femoral head necrosis, which is closely related to patient outcome. Fortunately, 60 to 70% of patients with LCP disease will spontaneously resolve without long-term complications. In the minority of patients who do not make a full recovery the major complication is early-onset osteoarthritis related to abnormal shape of the femoral head.
Slipped capital femoral epiphysis (SCFE) (▶ Fig. 6.9)	On FS T2WI high signal marrow edema is often present on both sides of the physis. There is disruption of the physis with variable to minimal displacement of the femoral epiphysis. There is disruption of the periosteum laterally and buckling of the periosteum medially. Joint effusion and synovitis are also often present. In more chronic cases there may be remodeling of bone. In some patients follow-up imaging may reveal spontaneous reduction of the slipped epiphysis.	Most patients with SCFE present with hip pain. The ability or inability to bear weight on the affected hip is a key clinical finding, and those patients that are unable to bear weight are considered to have instability. These patients often go on to surgical intervention. SCFE often results from a fall and is considered a Salter-Harris type I fracture. MRI is often needed to determine the severity of the SCFE so that proper treatment may be given.
Developmental dysplasia of the hip (DDH) (▶ Fig. 6.10)	The MRI findings in DDH depend on the age of the patient at the time of imaging and vary widely with the degree of severity. For the purposes of this discussion findings in patients with late presentation will be addressed. On all imaging sequences an elongated acetabular labrum is a typical finding along with a shallow acetabulum. On FS T2WI there is increased intrasubstance signal, often with irregularity and fissuring of the margins of the labrum. Abnormal signal and morphology are also seen at the labral chondral transition zone. On FS T2WI there are often high signal fissures and clefts. There may also be chondral thinning and subchondral cyst formation. These findings are often more accurately defined with postarthrographic FS T1WI. On these images high signal contrast may be seen entering into cartilage defects and clefts. Full-thickness cartilage defects may also be seen.	DDH represents a broad spectrum of disease. The severity of this disease ranges from hip instability, anatomical dysplasia, to hip dislocation. The most severe form, hip dislocation, presents in the early neonatal period. Less severe forms of DDH may be occult and present in young adults as hip pain with early changes of osteoarthritis. In the occult form of DDH there is a shallow acetabulum, which may be unstable. Patients with mild DDH that are not diagnosed may progress to early osteoarthritis and subsequent early hip replacement.

(continued on page 152)

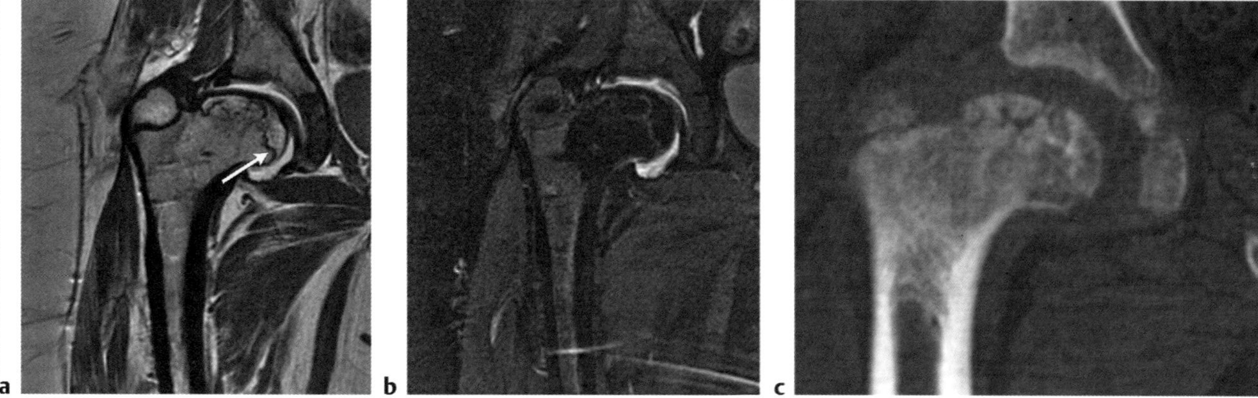

Fig. 6.8 (a) Coronal proton density–weighted imaging from a magnetic resonance imaging (MRI) arthrogram shows a flattened femoral capital epiphysis. There is also undulation of the physis. (b) Coronal fat-suppressed T2-weighted imaging from an MRI arthrogram shows a flattened femoral articular surface and irregular acetabular cartilage. (c) Coronal two-dimensional reformat from a hip computed tomographic scan shows a flattened femoral articular surface.

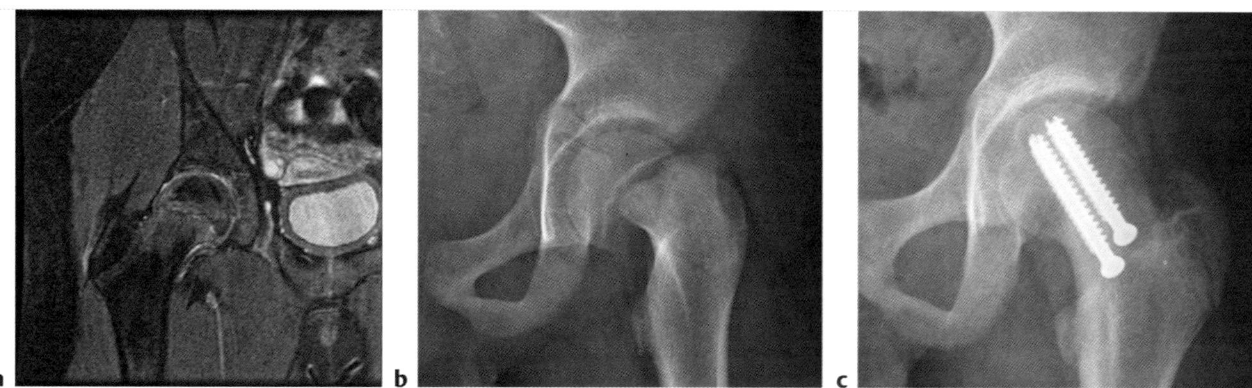

Fig. 6.9 (a) Coronal fat-suppressed T2-weighted imaging shows a mild marrow edema on both sides of the proximal femoral physis. (b) Anteroposterior (AP) radiograph from a second patient showing disruption of the physis with extensive slipping of the femoral capital epiphysis. (c) AP radiograph shows the postoperative appearance of a treated slipped capital femoral epiphysis.

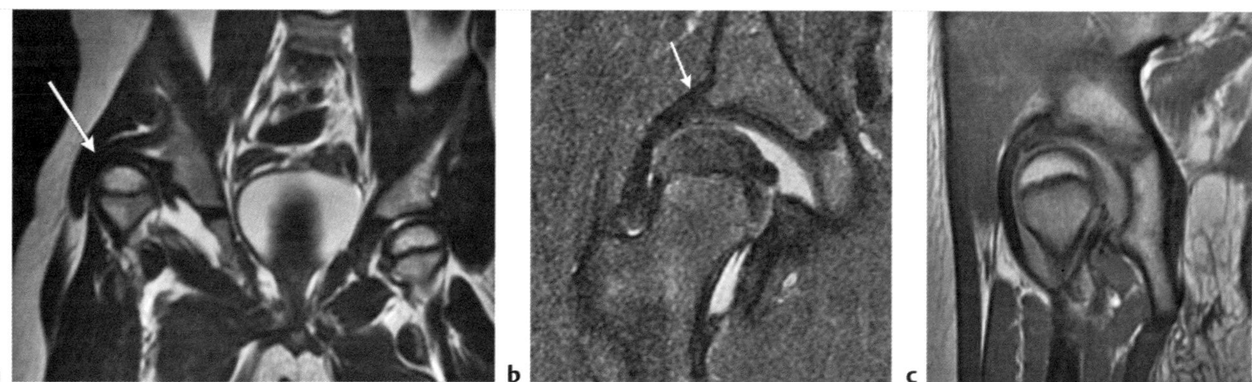

Fig. 6.10 (a) Coronal proton density–weighted imaging (PDWI) shows a shallow right acetabulum with an elongated acetabular labrum (arrow). (b) Coronal fat-suppressed T2-weighted imaging from a second patient shows a shallow acetabulum and an elongated labrum (arrow). (c) Coronal PDWI shows a shallow acetabulum and an elongated acetabular labrum.

Table 6.1 (Cont.) Bone lesions of the hip

Abnormalities	MRI findings	Comments
Rapid osteolysis (▶ Fig. 6.11)	MRI findings in rapid osteolysis are variable and depend on the stage of the disease. In general there is heterogeneous low signal on T1WI and heterogeneous high signal on FS T2WI in the femoral head and adjacent soft tissues. The signal changes are likely related to varying degrees of neovascularity in the affected bone and soft tissue. On postcontrast FS T1WI there is often strong enhancement.	Rapid osteolysis, also known as Gorham-Stout disease, is an idiopathic disorder that results in progressive massive spontaneous resorption of bone. Patients are usually young and often asymptomatic. The most commonly involved sites are the shoulder, pelvic girdle, and skull. Patients may not present until there has been a pathological fracture. The disease is characterized by increased benign vascular proliferation in bone with associated fibrous stroma and often fatty changes in the bone. The disease course is unpredictable and in some patients may spontaneously stop, whereas in others there is progression.

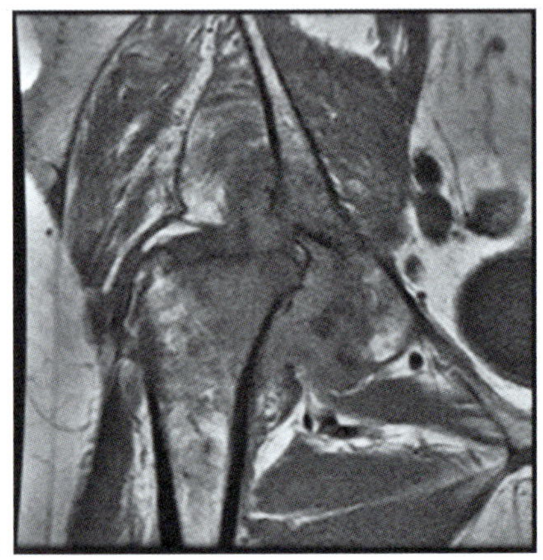
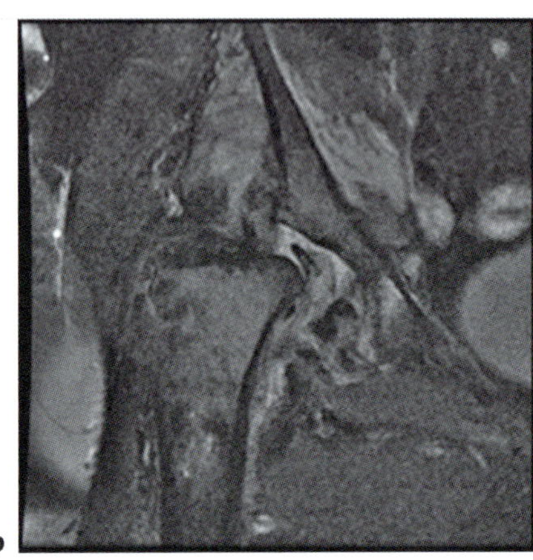
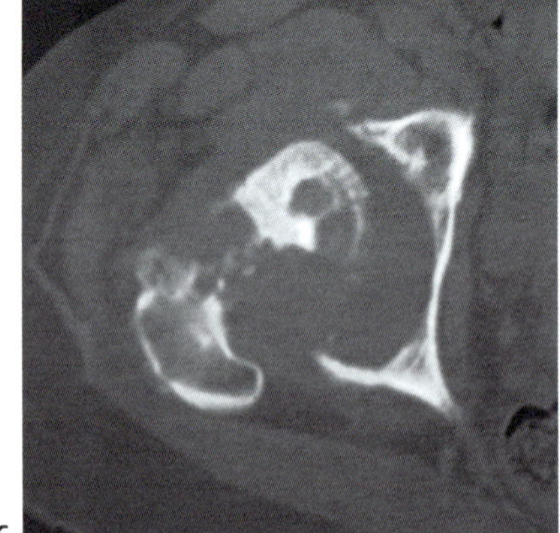
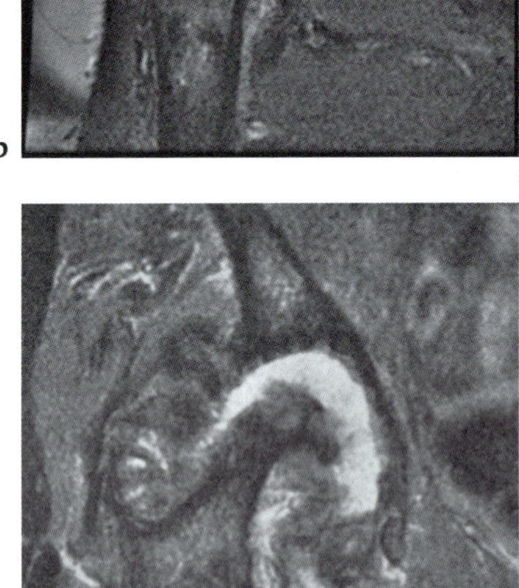

Fig. 6.11 (a) Coronal T1-weighted imaging shows advanced changes of osteolysis with destruction of the femoral head and low signal in the femoral neck, which extends into the intertrochanteric region. (b) Corresponding coronal fat-suppressed T2-weighted imaging (FS T2WI) shows destruction of the femoral head and high signal in the femoral neck and intertrochanteric regions. (c) Axial computed tomographic scan from a second patient with rapidly destructive osteoarthritis shows extensive destruction of the femoral head and neck with bony erosions, which are not featured in rapid osteolysis. (d) Coronal FS T2WI from the same patient shows erosions of the femoral head and neck with mixed zones of high signal edema and complex joint effusion with synovial proliferation.

6.1.1 Bone Lesions of the Hip Suggested Reading

[1] Dillman JR, Hernandez RJ. MRI of Legg-Calve-Perthes disease. AJR Am J Roentgenol 2009; 193: 1394–1407

[2] Hakkarinen DK, Banh KV, Hendey GW. Magnetic resonance imaging identifies occult hip fractures missed by 64-slice computed tomography. J Emerg Med 2012; 43: 303–307

[3] James S, Miocevic M, Malara F, Pike J, Young D, Connell D. MR imaging findings of acetabular dysplasia in adults. Skeletal Radiol 2006; 35: 378–384

[4] Malizos KN, Zibis AH, Dailiana Z, Hantes M, Karachalios T, Karantanas AH. MR imaging findings in transient osteoporosis of the hip. Eur J Radiol 2004; 50: 238–244

[5] Miese FR, Zilkens C, Holstein A, et al. MRI morphometry, cartilage damage and impaired function in the follow-up after slipped capital femoral epiphysis. Skeletal Radiol 2010; 39: 533–541

[6] Nguyen JT, Peterson JS, Biswal S, Beaulieu CF, Fredericson M. Stress-related injuries around the lesser trochanter in long-distance runners. AJR Am J Roentgenol 2008; 190: 1616–1620

[7] Roposch A, Wright JG. Increased diagnostic information and understanding disease: uncertainty in the diagnosis of developmental hip dysplasia. Radiology 2007; 242: 355–359

[8] Ruggieri P, Montalti M, Angelini A, Alberghini M, Mercuri M. Gorham-Stout disease: the experience of the Rizzoli Institute and review of the literature. Skeletal Radiol 2011; 40: 1391–1397

[9] Szewczyk-Bieda M, Thomas N, Oliver TB. Radiographically occult femoral and pelvic fractures are not mutually exclusive: a review of fractures detected by MRI following low-energy trauma. Skeletal Radiol 2012; 41: 1127–1132

[10] Tins B, Cassar-Pullicino V, McCall I. The role of pre-treatment MRI in established cases of slipped capital femoral epiphysis. Eur J Radiol 2009; 70: 570–578

[11] Watson RM, Roach NA, Dalinka MK. Avascular necrosis and bone marrow edema syndrome. Radiol Clin North Am 2004; 42: 207–219

6.2 Lesions of the Hip Joint

- Lesions of cartilage
- Lesions of the ligamentum teres
- Femoroacetabular impingement
- Osteoarthritis (OA)
- Rheumatoid arthritis (RA)

Table 6.2 Lesions of the hip joint

Abnormalities	MRI findings	Comments
Lesions of cartilage (▶ Fig. 6.12)	The normal hip has cartilage covering the femoral head with the exception of the fovea capitis. The normal acetabulum also has cartilage covering it with the exception of the supra-acetabular fossa, which is located near the 12 o'clock position. Normal cartilage is of intermediate signal on fat-suppressed T2-weighted imaging (FS T2WI). The cartilage is normally thin (up to 3 mm). Abnormal cartilage can have a variety of different appearances. Findings may include focal thinning, ulcerations, linear fissures, cartilaginous flaps, and focal defects. Many of these abnormalities are well seen on small field of view thin section (3 mm) FS T2WI. Cartilage fissure flaps and defects are seen as high signal defects in the otherwise intermediate signal cartilage. On conventional MRI exams it is helpful if there is a small amount of joint fluid present in the hip joint. Cartilage defects are seen to better advantage on MRI arthrograms with FS T1-weighted imaging (T1WI). The defect is well seen as high signal contrast–laden fluid extending into the normal cartilage and, in cases, with full-thickness defects, contacting the articular surface of the bone.	Patients with abnormal cartilage may have no symptoms or hip pain, sometimes with decreased range of motion. Cartilage defects are often seen with labral tears and in the setting of femoral acetabular impingement. As cartilage loss progresses there is joint space narrowing and subchondral sclerotic change seen in the bones of the hip joint.
Lesions of the ligamentum teres (▶ Fig. 6.13)	The normal ligamentum teres is variable in size and thickness with smooth margins and in general low signal on all pulse sequences. In some patients subtle striations may be seen within the substance of the ligament. The normal ligament extends from the transverse acetabular ligament to the fovea capitis of the femoral head. Complete tears are seen as discontinuity of the ligament and are most often located near the attachment on the fovea capitis. On FS T2WI there may be a high signal mass in the region of the tear. MRI arthrography is preferred in the evaluation of the ligmantum teres to more accurately define the contours of the tear and to separate normal structures form each other. Partial tears of the ligamentum teres are more difficult to identify. On FS T1WI with intra-articular contrast, high signal contrast–laden fluid can be seen to enter into the substance of the ligament. In partial tears there may be thinning of the ligament with fewer remaining intact fibers. On FS T2WI there may be increased signal within the ligamentum teres fibers. In both full-thickness and partial tears there are often associated injuries, including both labral tears and cartilage abnormalities. Synovitis and joint effusion may also be present.	Patients with injuries of the ligamentum teres often present with hip and groin pain and may complain of locking and catching. Traumatic tears of the ligamentum teres often occur in the setting of sports, including football and hockey. Martial arts and ballet are also associated with ligamentum teres injuries, due to the requirement for a large range of motion at the hip. The ligamentum teres is an important stabilizer of the hip and can be thought of as similar in function to the ACL in the knee. In patients with torn ligamentum teres a type of microinstability may occur, which in some patients may progress to early osteoarthritis. Treatment often consists of simple surgical debridement of remaining ligament fibers. In the future surgical ligament reconstruction may be both possible and desirable to preserve the hip joint.

(continued on page 156)

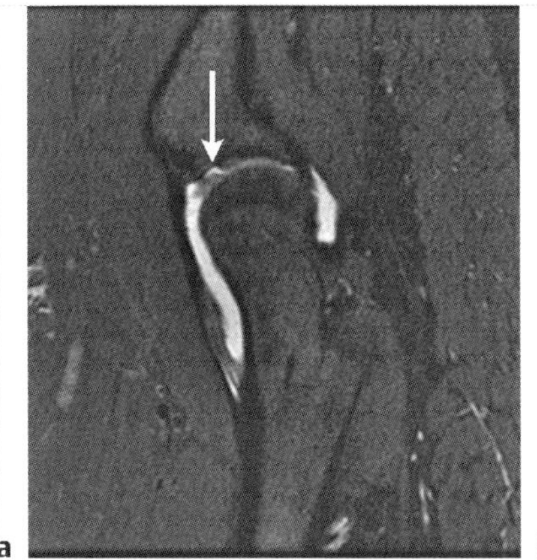

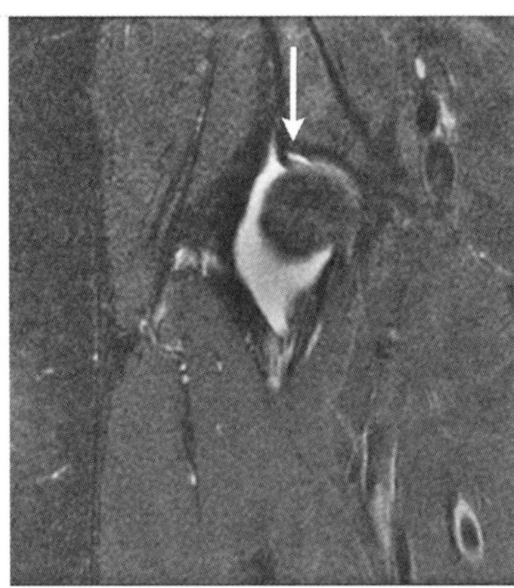

Fig. 6.12 (a) Sagittal fat-suppressed T2-weighted imaging (FS T2WI) from a magnetic resonance imaging arthrogram shows high signal fluid entering into a large delamination tear of the acetabular cartilage (arrow). (b) Coronal FS T2WI from the same patient also showing a large cartilage delamination tear (arrow).

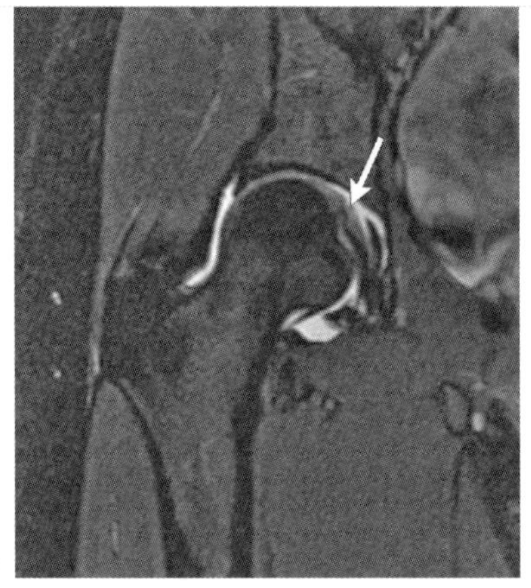

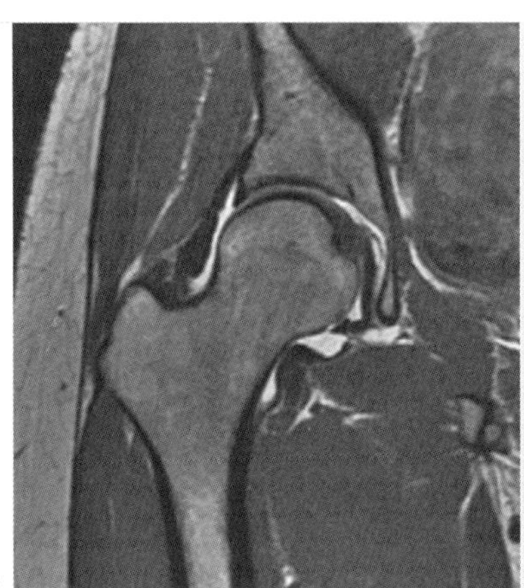

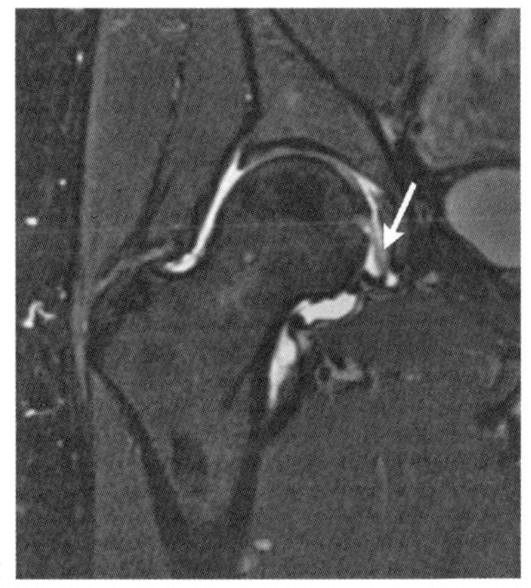

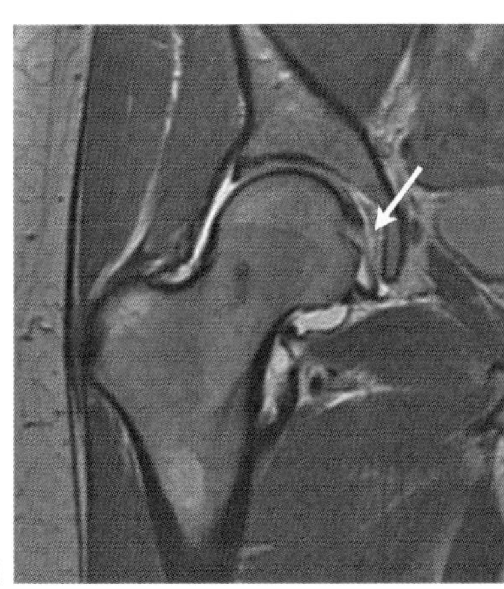

Fig. 6.13 (a) Coronal fat-suppressed T2-weighted imaging (FS T2WI) from an MRI arthrogram shows mildly increased signal and mild thickening in the ligamentum teres near its attachment to the fovea capitus (arrow). (b) Coronal proton density–weighted imaging (PDWI) from an MRI arthrogram shows a thickened ligamentum teres at its attachment on the fovea capitus. (c) Coronal FS T2WI from an MRI arthrogram in a second patient shows a high-grade partial tear of the ligamentum teres with only a few remnant fibers remaining (arrow). (d) Coronal PDWI from an MRI arthrogram shows a high-grade partial tear of the ligamentum teres with a few remaining fibers.

Table 6.2 (Cont.) Lesions of the hip joint

Abnormalities	MRI findings	Comments
Femoroacetabular impingement (FAI) (▸ Fig. 6.14)	There are two types of FAI: cam and pincer. Both types are associated with early-onset osteoarthritis, labral tears, and cartilage abnormalities. In cam type FAI there is decreased offset of the femoral head neck junction with an osseous bump at the anterior aspect of the femoral head and neck junction. This is best seen in the oblique axial plane known as the Swiss plane, which extends along the long axis of the trochanteric portion of the proximal femur. On proton density-weighted imaging (PDWI) this is seen as an osseous bump along the anterior portion of the femoral head and neck junction with an abnormal alpha angle of greater than 55 degrees. On coronal and sagittal FS T2WI there is often joint space narrowing and cartilage abnormalities, including thinning and cartilage delamination. This is best seen on MRI arthrography with FS T1WI. In cam type FAI the anterosuperior cartilage and labrum are often abnormal. In pincer type FAI there is overcoverage of the femoral head by the acetabulum. This is well seen on coronal FS T2WI. The cartilage and labrum in pincer type FAI are most often abnormal in the posteroinferior position. An os acetabuli or other separate bony fragment is often seen in pincer type FAI. Some patients may have a mixed type FAI, which is a combination of cam and pincer types.	FAI is increasingly recognized as a major cause of early-onset osteoarthritis. The critical issue in FAI is early diagnosis so that appropriate surgical treatment can be performed before there has been significant cartilage and labral damage. Patients with FAI may present as early as the second decade with hip pain; this is more common in athletes with FAI. In cam type FAI surgical treatment consists of recontouring the anterior portion of the femoral head–neck junction so that the bony impingement is relieved. Cam type FAI is more common in younger male athletes. In pincer type FAI the acetabulum is trimmed back so that the femoral head is no longer overcovered. Pincer type FAI is more common in middle-aged women. The etiology of some cases of FAI and in particular the CAM type is likely related to prior undiagnosed subclinical slipped capital femoral epiphysis.

(continued on page 158)

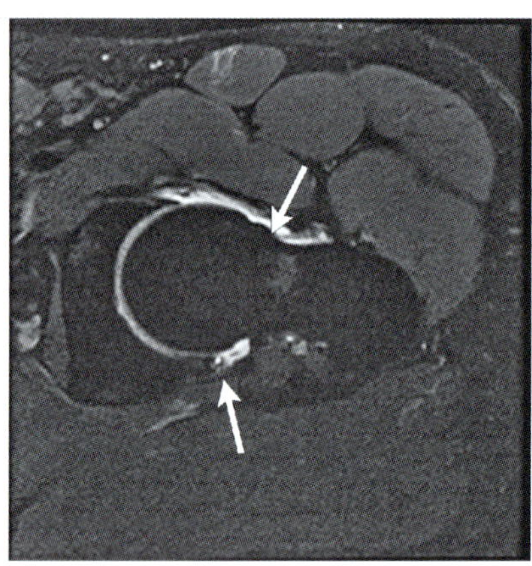

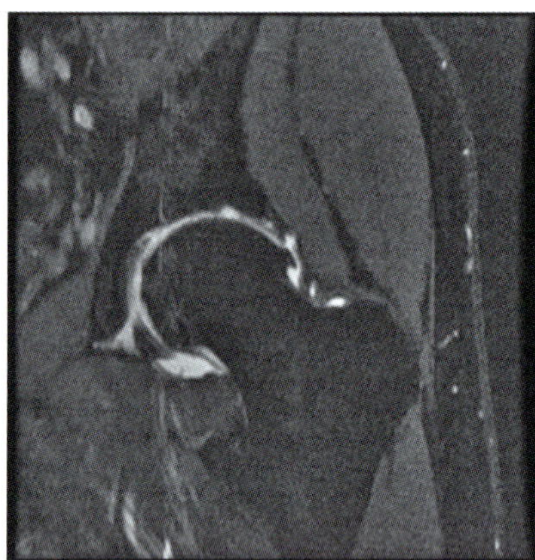

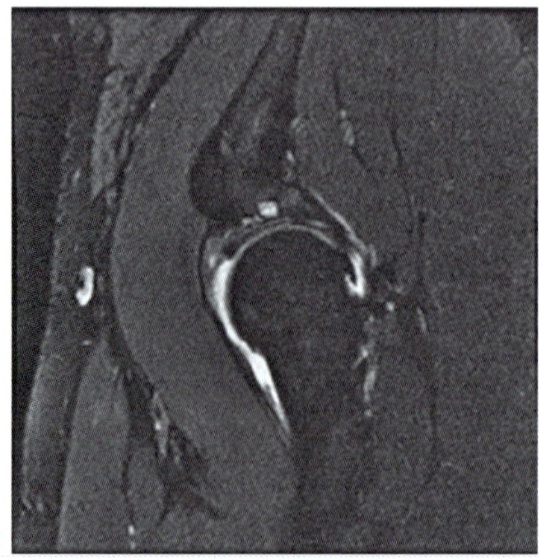

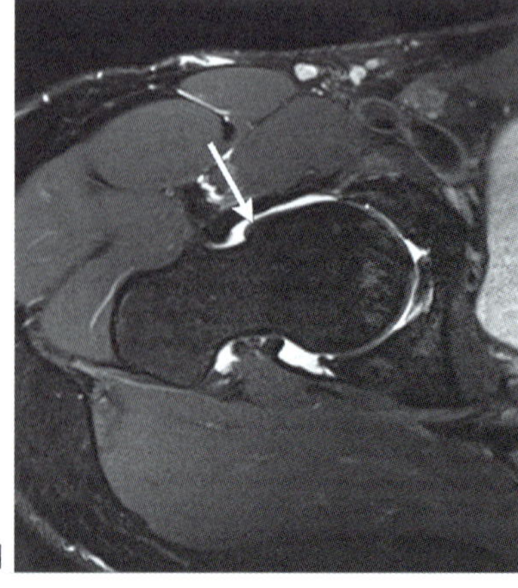

Fig. 6.14 (a) Oblique axial (Swiss) fat-suppressed T2-weighted imaging (FS T2WI) from an MRI arthrogram shows a decreased femoral head–neck junction offset with a small cam bump (arrow). Note abnormal posterior labrum (arrow). (b) Coronal FS T2WI from the same patient shows superior joint space narrowing, irregular acetabular articular cartilage, and large femoral-collar osteophytes. (c) Sagittal FS T2WI from the same patient shows joint space narrowing with several acetabular subcortical geodes and femoral osteophyte. (d) Oblique axial (Swiss) FS T2WI from an MRI arthrogram in a second patient shows a large cam bump at the femoral head–neck junction anteriorly. (*continued*)

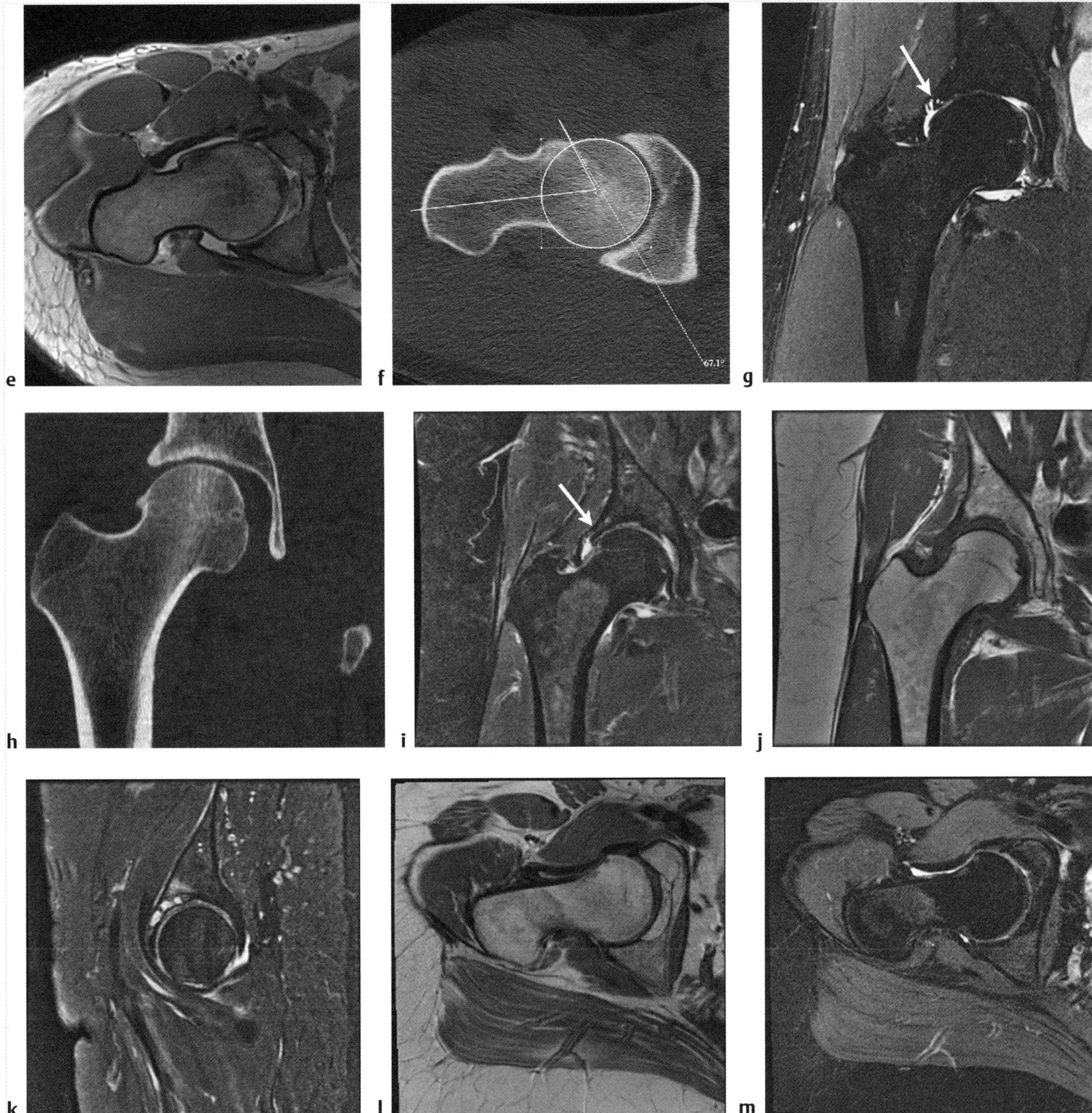

Fig. 6.14 (*continued*) (e) Oblique axial (Swiss) PDWI from the same patient also shows a large cam bump at the femoral head–neck junction. (f) Oblique axial two-dimensional reformat (Swiss) from a computed tomographic (CT) scan of the hip in the same patient shows a large alpha angle of 67 degrees, which is abnormal and indicates cam type femoroacetabular impingement (FAI). (g) Coronal FS T2WI from the same patient shows severe superior joint space narrowing and abnormal superior acetabular labrum. (h) Coronal 2-D reformat from a hip CT scan in the same patient shows superior joint space narrowing and femoral osteophyte. (i) Coronal FS T2WI from an MRI arthrogram in a third patient shows pincer type FAI with overcoverage of the femoral head by the acetabulum (arrow). (j) Corresponding proton density–weighted imaging (PDWI) from the same patient shows acetabular overcoverage. (k) Sagittal FS T2WI from the same patient shows several subcortical geodes with adjacent marrow edema in the acetabulum. (l) Axial oblique (Swiss) PDWI from a fourth patient shows postoperative appearance of the femoral head–neck junction in a patient previously diagnosed with cam type FAI. (m) Axial oblique (Swiss) FS T2WI from the same patient shows the postoperative appearance of the femoral head–neck junction in a patient treated for cam type FAI.

Table 6.2 (Cont.) Lesions of the hip joint

Abnormalities	MRI findings	Comments
Osteoarthritis (OA) (▶ Fig. 6.15)	On both PDWI and FS T2WI there is superolateral joint space narrowing and osteophyte formation. On FS T2WI there are often subchondral cysts seen in both the femoral head and the acetabulum. There may also be high signal subchondral marrow edema on both sides of the hip joint. Cartilage thinning and defects are best seen on MRI arthrography with FS T1WI and FS T2WI. Joint effusions, often with associated synovitis, may also be present and are best seen on FS T2WI as high signal fluid with ill-defined zones of lower signal corresponding to areas of thickened synovium. If intravenous gadolinium-contrast is given there is often thickened proliferating synovium with high signal enhancing zones and adjacent low signal joint fluid on FS T1WI. Other findings seen on MRI may include tears of the acetabular labrum, intra-articular loose bodies, synovial herniation pits, tendonitis, and bursitis.	OA of the hip is a progressive multifactorial condition in which there is continued loss of articular cartilage over time. Hip OA is in general age related with prevalence and severity increasing with increasing patient age. However, there is a group of younger patients presenting with hip OA sooner and with greater severity than would be expected. These patients often have some form of FAI or hip dysplasia. Patients with OA of the hip present with chronic hip pain, which progresses over time to the point where it can become incapacitating and require a hip joint replacement. Hip OA is a major U.S. public health problem. Other causes of hip pain that can be clinically confused with OA include insufficiency or stress fractures, tendonitis, and greater trochanteric bursitis. Many of these conditions can also be seen in the setting of hip OA. MRI is often needed to identify which of these abnormalities is present in any given patient with chronic hip pain.

(continued on page 160)

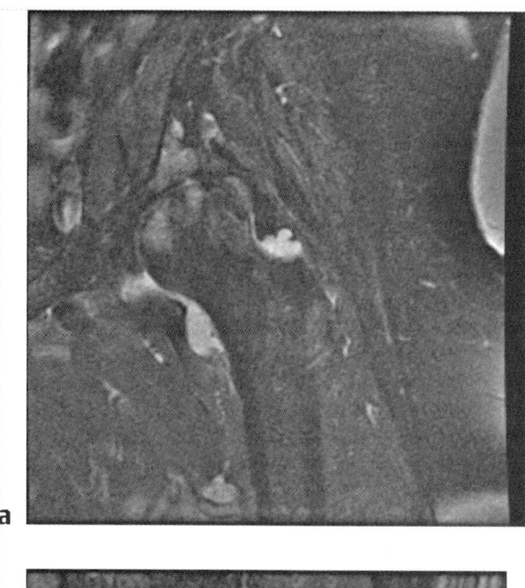

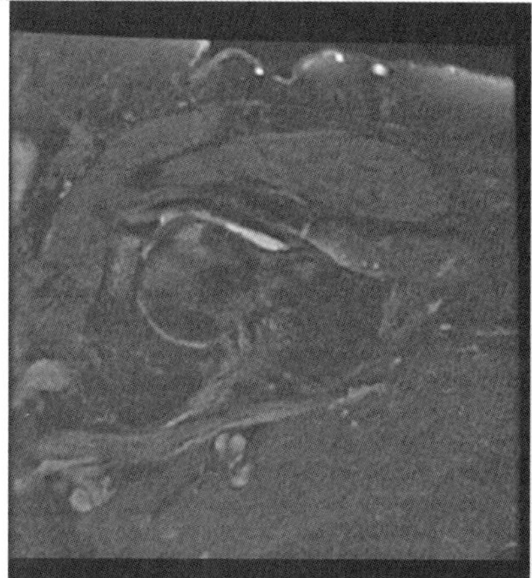

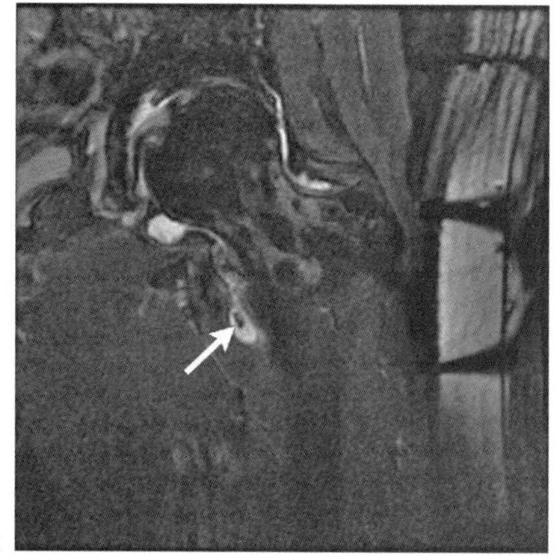

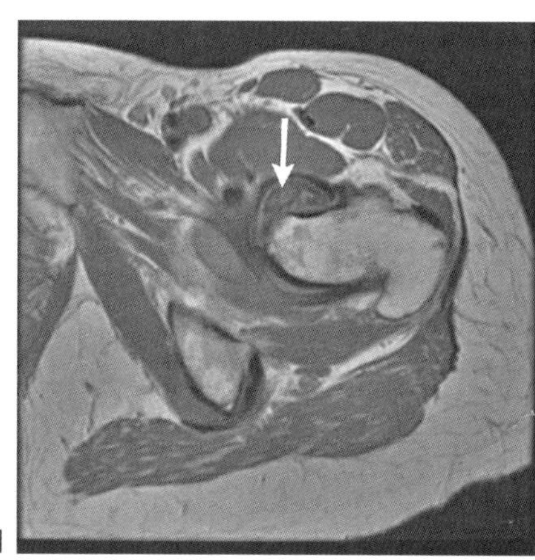

Fig. 6.15 (a) Coronal fat-suppressed T2-weighted imaging (FS T2WI) shows severe joint space narrowing with loss of articular cartilage and subcortical degenerative reactive marrow edema in the femoral head and opposite acetabulum. A large joint effusion is also present. (b) Axial FS T2WI shows joint space narrowing and degenerative reactive subcortical marrow edema. (c) Coronal FS T2WI from a second patient shows superior joint space narrowing with cartilage loss and joint effusion containing loose bodies (arrow). (d) Axial proton density–weighted imaging shows intra-articular loose bodies (arrow) as can be seen in secondary synovial osteochondromatosis.

Table 6.2 (Cont.) Lesions of the hip joint

Abnormalities	MRI findings	Comments
Rheumatoid arthritis (RA) (▶ Fig. 6.16)	On FS T2WI and postcontrast FS T1WI the earliest finding of RA is synovial proliferation. This is seen as heterogeneous increased signal fluid in the hip joint on FS T2WI and as ill-defined enhancement and thickening of synovium on FS T1WI. On FS T2WI there is often high signal subchondral marrow edema seen in one or both sides of the joint. As the disease progresses there are sharply marginated juxta-articular bony erosions. On FS T2WI there is high signal inflammatory material seen in the cortical defect. On FS T1WI postcontrast injection this inflammatory tissue will demonstrate high signal enhancement. When the hip joint is affected in RA the process is usually bilateral and symmetric with axial joint space narrowing. On FS T2WI there are also high signal subchondral cysts seen. In addition tenosynovitis in and around the affected joint is commonly seen.	RA is a chronic autoimmune disease. It causes synovial proliferation that can often lead to joint destruction. Patients present with joint pain and stiffness, which is usually though not always symmetric. Women are more commonly affected than men. When hip involvement is unilateral it is difficult to distinguish RA from septic arthritis. With introduction of new drug therapies for RA the importance of MRI in the follow-up evaluation of patients has increased because plain radiography is not adequate for evaluating response to treatment.

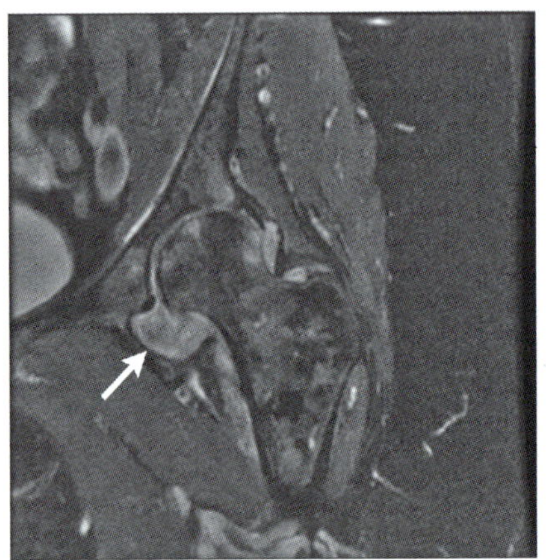

a

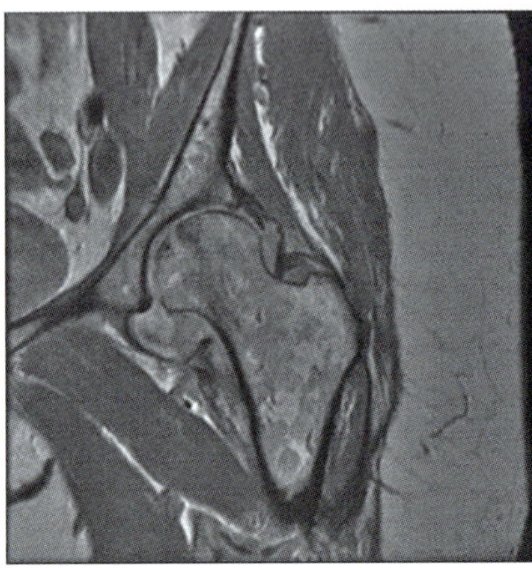

b

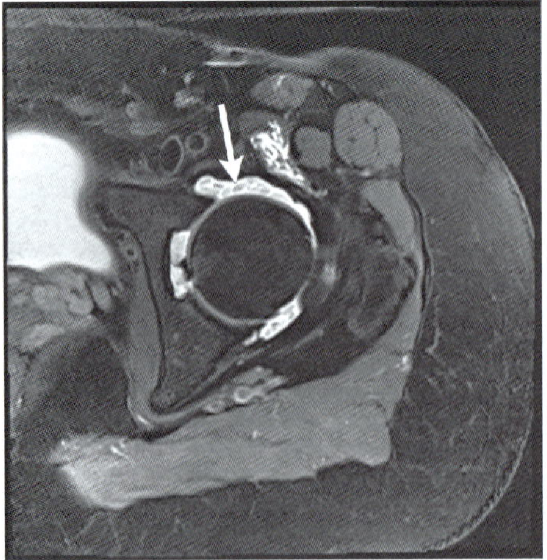

c

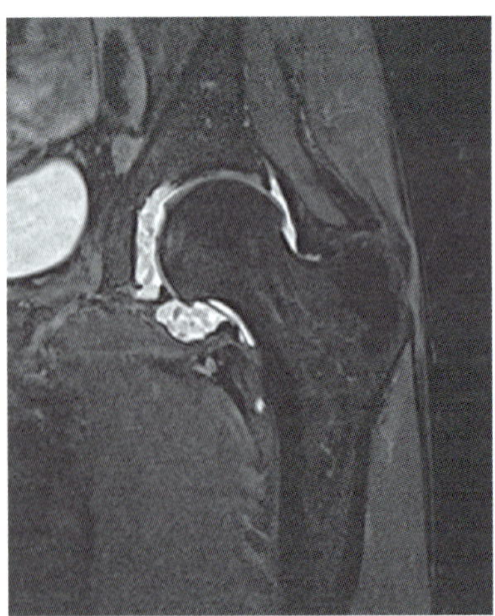

d

Fig. 6.16 (a) Coronal fat-suppressed T2-weighted imaging (FS T2WI) shows joint space narrowing, reactive subcortical marrow edema, and complex effusion with synovial hypertrophy (arrow). (b) Corresponding proton density–weighted imaging also shows joint space narrowing complex effusion with synovial hypertrophy. (c) Axial FS T2WI from an MRI arthrogram in a second patient shows low signal rice bodies (arrow). (d) Coronal FS T2WI from an MRI arthrogram shows multiple low signal rice bodies.

6.2.1 Lesions of the Hip Joint Suggested Reading

[1] Cerezal L, Kassarjian A, Canga A, et al. Anatomy, biomechanics, imaging, and management of ligamentum teres injuries. Radiographics 2010; 30: 1637–1651

[2] Dietrich TJ, Suter A, Pfirrmann CWA, Dora C, Fucentese SF, Zanetti M. Supra-acetabular fossa (pseudodefect of acetabular cartilage): frequency at MR arthrography and comparison of findings at MR arthrography and arthroscopy. Radiology 2012; 263: 484–491

[3] Pfirrmann CWA, Mengiardi B, Dora C, Kalberer F, Zanetti M, Hodler J. Cam and pincer femoroacetabular impingement: characteristic MR arthrographic findings in 50 patients. Radiology 2006; 240: 778–785

[4] Leydet-Quilici H, Le Corroller T, Bouvier C, et al. Advanced hip osteoarthritis: magnetic resonance imaging aspects and histopathology correlations. Osteoarthritis Cartilage 2010; 18: 1429–1435

[5] Roemer FW, Hunter DJ, Winterstein A, et al. Hip Osteoarthritis MRI Scoring System (HOAMS): reliability and associations with radiographic and clinical findings. Osteoarthritis Cartilage 2011; 19: 946–962

[6] Rowbotham EL, Grainger AJ. Rheumatoid arthritis: ultrasound versus MRI. AJR Am J Roentgenol 2011; 197: 541–546

6.3 Lesions of the Acetabular Labrum

- Tears of the acetabular labrum
- Lesions of the postoperative acetabular labrum
- Paralabral cysts of the hip

Table 6.3 Lesions of the acetabular labrum

Abnormalities	MRI findings	Comments
Tears of the acetabular labrum (▶ Fig. 6.17)	The normal acetabular labrum is uniformly low signal on all imaging sequences. The normal labrum has a smooth, well-defined contour with a triangular shape such that the base of the labrum is in contact with the bony acetabulum. Labral tears are most effectively identified with MRI arthrography. On fat-suppressed T1-weighted imaging (FS T1WI) high signal contrast is seen to enter the substance of the labrum. This may be a partial- or full-thickness defect. In some cases there may be detachment of the labrum with a displaced fragment. Other configurations are also possible, including fraying of the labral margins and flap tears. On FS T2-weighted imaging (T2WI) a labral tear may be seen as a linear high signal extending through or into the labrum. Most labral tears occur in the anterior superior portion. A normal anatomical variant known as a sublabral recess is also known to occur. These are most commonly located in the anterior inferior portion of the labrum, a location in which tears are less common. On FS T1WI postarthrography a linear high signal is seen to extend only partially into the base of the labrum. On FS T2WI no signal abnormality is seen in the substance of the labrum.	Acetabular labral tears are an important cause of hip pain, which can significantly limit a patient's ability to participate in athletic activity. Many tears of the acetabular labrum are now believed to be related to femoracetabular impingement. Early diagnosis and treatment of labral tears result in relief of symptoms and may reduce the incidence of early-onset osteoarthritis. Tears of the acetabular labrum may be seen in association with cartilage injuries. Labral tears are typically treated with arthroscopic debridement or repair.
Lesions of the postoperative acetabular labrum (▶ Fig. 6.18)	Re-tear of the acetabular labrum after prior labral surgery is best evaluated with MRI arthrography using dilute intra-articular gadolinium-based contrast material. If possible comparison to a previous preoperative MRI examination is suggested because differentiating between re-tear and postsurgical change can be difficult. On FS T1WI and FS T2WI the presence of a new high signal line extending to the labral surface is evidence of a new labral tear and is analogous to the criteria used in evaluating the postoperative meniscus. A new labral fragment or significant distortion or irregular contour of the labrum may also indicate a labral tear. A new paralabral cyst is also evidence for labral re-tear.	Patients with clinically suspected acetabular labral re-tear present with new-onset hip pain. After initially successful labral surgery many patients are able to return to their normal activities, which often include sports. In some cases the mechanism of labral reinjury may be similar to the original cause of labral tear. The incidence of acetabular labral re-tear is likely to increase over time because more patients are being treated successfully for labral tears and are able to return to high-level activity with the potential for labral reinjury. The ability to accurately diagnose labral re-tear is of similar importance to accurate diagnosis of the initial tear so that early treatment can be initiated and thereby reduce the likelihood of early-onset osteoarthritis.

(continued on page 164)

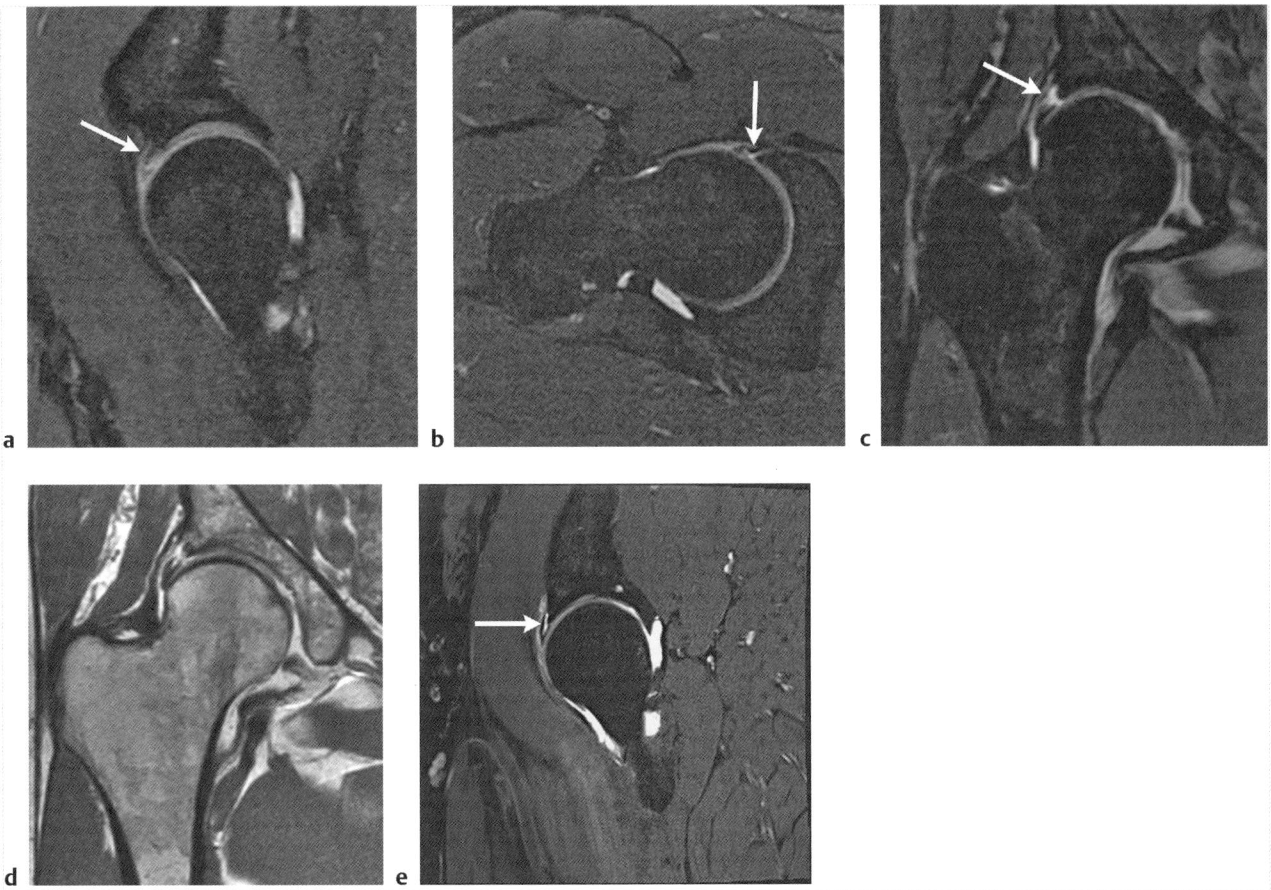

Fig. 6.17 (a) Sagittal fat-suppressed T2-weighted imaging (FS T2WI) from an MRI arthrogram shows a tear of the anterior acetabualar labrum (arrow). (b) Oblique axial (Swiss) FS T2WI shows an anterior labral tear (arrow). (c) Coronal FS T2WI from an MRI arthrogram in a second patient shows a large tear of the superior labrum (arrow). There is also joint space narrowing and cartilage irregularity. (d) Coronal proton density–weighted imaging (PDWI) from the same patient shows a large superior labral tear. (e) Sagittal FS T2WI from an MRI arthrogram in a third patient shows a large high signal tear in the anterior labrum (arrow).

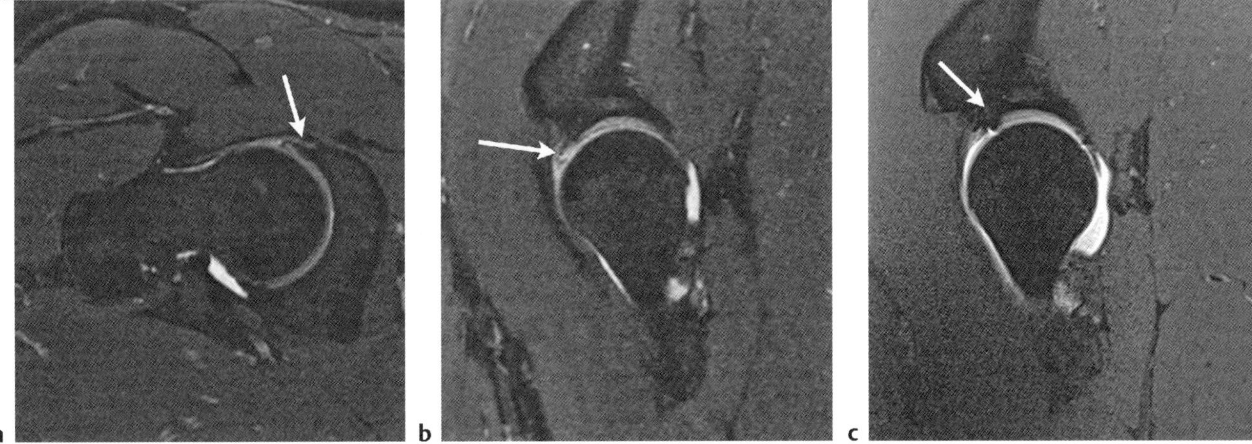

Fig. 6.18 (a) Axial oblique (Swiss) fat-suppressed T2-weighted imaging (FS T2WI) from a preoperative MRI arthrogram shows a linear high signal tear in the anterior superior labrum (arrow). (b) Sagittal FS T2WI from a preoperative MRI arthrogram shows the same anterior superior labral tear (arrow). (c) Sagittal FS T2WI from a postoperative MRI arthrogram in the same patient shows mild irregularity of the anterior superior labrum (arrow) and adjacent postoperative susceptibility artifact. There is no evidence for labral re-tear.

Table 6.3 (Cont.) Lesions of the acetabular labrum

Abnormalities	MRI findings	Comments
Paralabral cysts of the hip (▶ Fig. 6.19)	On FS T2WI a paralabral cyst is a rounded high signal lesion of variable size and may contain internal septation. On PDWI the paralabral cyst is low signal. The paralabral cyst is usually located in continuity with the adjacent labrum, and there is often though not always an identifiable labral tear. The most common location for paralabral cysts of the hip is anterior superior, which is the most common location of acetabular labral tears. Other locations for paralabral cysts are also possible though less common.	Paralabral cysts are strongly associated with tears of the acetabular labrum. These patients often complain of hip pain related to the presence of a labral tear and not due to the presence of the paralabral cyst. Paralabral cysts are likely caused by increased intra-articular pressure caused by altered joint mechanics when a labral tear is present. When intra-articular pressure is increased synovial fluid is forced through the labral tear, resulting in a paralabral cyst.

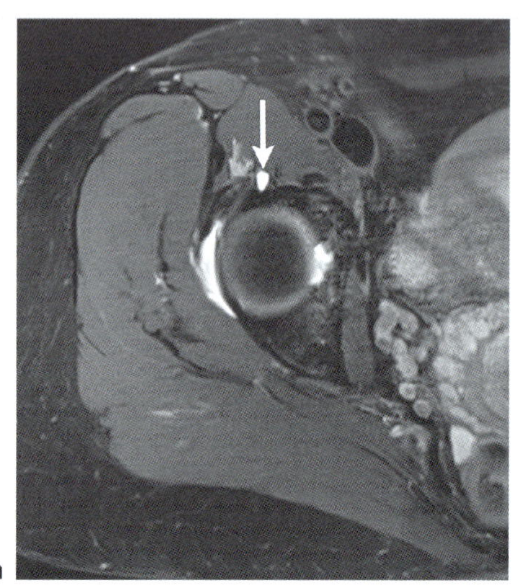
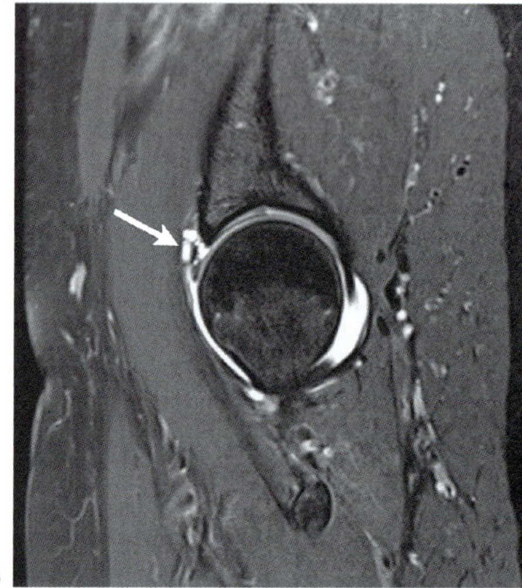
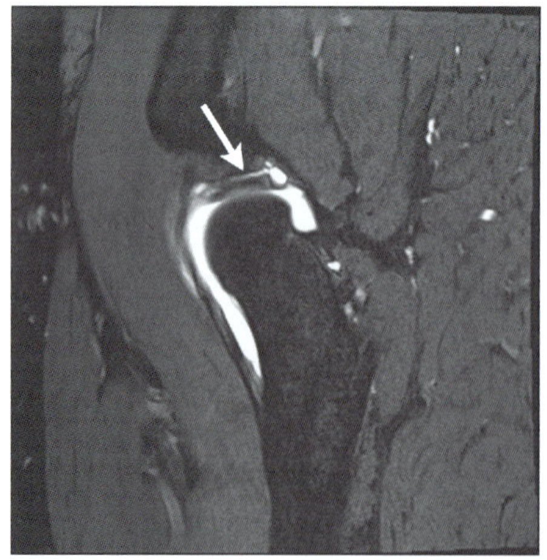
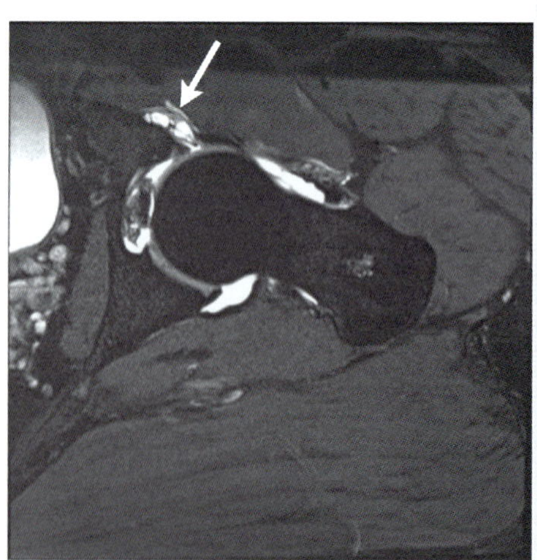

Fig. 6.19 (a) Axial fat-suppressed T2-weighted imaging (FS T2WI) from an MRI arthrogram shows an anterior paralabral cyst (arrow). (b) Sagittal FS T2WI from an MRI arthrogram shows a multiseptated anterior paralabral cyst from the same patient. (c) Sagittal FS T2WI from an MRI arthrogram in a second patient shows a large delaminating tear of the superior labrum (arrow) with a posterior paralabral cyst. (d) Axial oblique (Swiss) FS T2WI from an MRI arthrogram in the same patient shows a multiseptated anterior paralabral cyst (arrow).

6.3.1 Lesions of the Acetabular Labrum Suggested Reading

[1] Blankenbaker DG, De Smet AA, Keene JS. MR arthrographic appearance of the postoperative acetabular labrum in patients with suspected recurrent labral tears. AJR Am J Roentgenol 2011; 197: W1118–22

[2] Blankenbaker DG, De Smet AA, Keene JS, Fine JP. Classification and localization of acetabular labral tears. Skeletal Radiol 2007; 36: 391–397

[3] Mervak BM, Morag Y, Marcantonio D, Jacobson J, Brandon C, Fessell D. Paralabral cysts of the hip: sonographic evaluation with magnetic resonance arthrographic correlation. J Ultrasound Med 2012; 31: 495–500

[4] Perdikakis E, Karachalios T, Katonis P, Karantanas A. Comparison of MR-arthrography and MDCT-arthrography for detection of labral and articular cartilage hip pathology. Skeletal Radiol 2011; 40: 1441–1447

[5] Studler U, Kalberer F, Leunig M, et al. MR arthrography of the hip: differentiation between an anterior sublabral recess as a normal variant and a labral tear. Radiology 2008; 249: 947–954

6.4 Juxta-articular Lesions of the Hip

- Lesions of the gluteal tendons
- Hamstring tendon injuries
- Athletic pubalgia (sports hernia)
- Morel-Lavallée lesions

Table 6.4 Juxta-articular lesions of the hip

Abnormalities	MRI findings	Comments
Lesions of the gluteal tendons (▶ Fig. 6.20)	Abnormalities of the gluteal tendons, the gluteus medius and minimus, range in severity from mild peritendinitis to tendinosis, partial tear, and, most severe, a complete tendon rupture. On coronal and axial fat-suppressed T2-weighted imaging (FS T2WI) peritendinitis of the gluteus medius and minimus tendons is seen as high signal surrounding a tendon of normal thickness and with normal internal signal. On FS T2WI gluteal tendinitis is seen as a thickened tendon with some internal high signal. There may also be a small amount of trochanteric bursal fluid present. These findings are similar to what is seen on magnetic resonance imaging in shoulder rotator cuff tendinitis. Partial tear of the gluteus medius or minimus is seen on FS T2WI as loss of distal fibers at their attachment on the greater trochanter of the proximal femur. Often high signal edema is seen in and adjacent to the remaining tendon fibers. Complete tears of the gluteal tendons are seen on FS T2WI as discontinuity of fibers, often with some retraction away from their expected insertion on the greater trochanter. On FS T2WI there is often high signal fluid seen in the gap between the torn tendon and the greater trochanter.	Tendinopathy of the gluteus medius and minimus are common causes of lateral hip pain and weakness of hip abduction. This clinical entity has been referred to as the greater trochanteric pain syndrome (GTPS) and is more common in women than in men. GTPS is an extra-articular cause of hip pain and can be confused with other causes of extra-articular hip pain, including femoral neck stress fractures and referred pain from abnormalities of the lumbar spine. Trochanteric bursitis is now recognized as much less common than gluteal tendon pathology, and if present is often secondary to abnormalities of the gluteal tendons.

(continued on page 168)

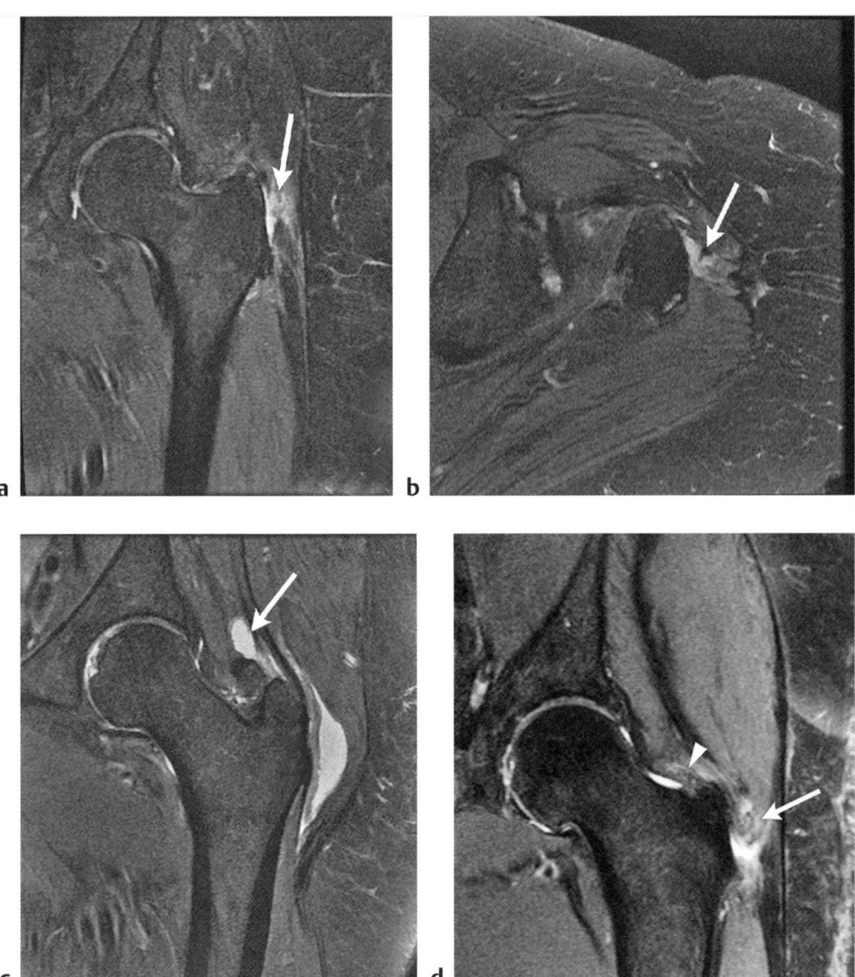

Fig. 6.20 (a) Coronal fat-suppressed T2-weighted imaging (FS T2WI) shows high signal at the site of a tear of the gluteus medius tendon (arrow). (b) Axial FS T2WI shows high signal at the site of a gluteus medius tendon tear. (c) Coronal FS T2WI from a second patient shows torn gluteus minimus tendon (arrow) with fluid in the trochanteric bursa. (d) Coronal FS T2WI from a third patient shows a tear of the gluteus medius (arrow) and tendinopathy of the distal gluteus minimus (arrowhead).

Table 6.4 (Cont.) Juxta-articular lesions of the hip

Abnormalities	MRI findings	Comments
Hamstring tendon injuries (▶ Fig. 6.21)	The hamstrings consist of the semimembranosus, semitendinosus, and biceps femoris. The long head of the biceps femoris and the semitendinosus have a common origin from the ischial tuberosity. A variety of different hamstring tendon injuries can occur. Tendinopathy at the origin of the conjoint tendon is seen as increased signal on FS T2WI, often with thickening of the proximal portion of the tendon. There may also be mild marrow edema seen as high signal in the adjacent ischial tuberosity on FS T2WI. Partial tears often occur near the origin of the conjoint tendon and are seen as high signal fluid within the thickened tendon on FS T2WI. Complete tears of the conjoint tendon usually occur at the ischial tuberosity and are seen as focal discontinuity of the tendon. In some cases there may be a variable degree of tendon retraction. In younger patients there is more often avulsion injury of the ischial tuberosity with high signal edema on FS T2WI.	The major function of the hamstring muscle group is hip extension and knee flexion. Hamstring injuries commonly occur in athletes participating in sports such as hurdling, long jumping, gymnastics, and cheerleading. The usual mechanism of injury is simultaneous hip flexion and knee extension. Some hamstring injuries can heal spontaneously, including muscle strain and tears along the musculotendinous junction. Tears at the tendon origin on the ischial tuberosity may require surgery.

(continued on page 170)

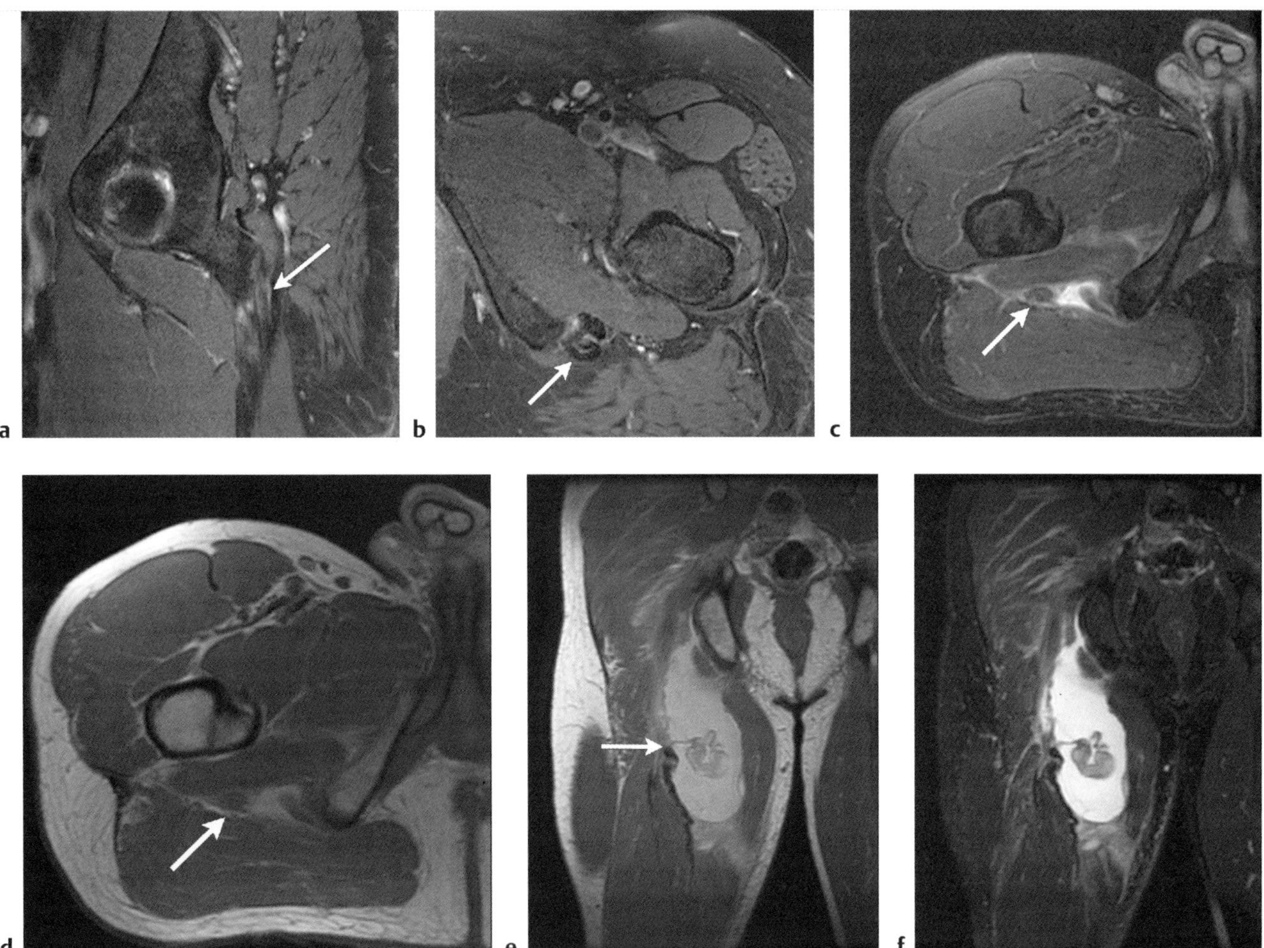

Fig. 6.21 (a) Sagittal fat-suppressed T2-weighted imaging (FS T2WI) shows high signal tendinopathy of the conjoint tendon of the hamstrings (arrow). (b) Axial FS T2WI from the same patient shows high signal tendinopathy in the conjoint tendon on the left at its attachment on the left ischial tuberosity. (c) Axial FS T2WI shows complete retracted tear of the conjoint tendon with high signal fluid between the torn tendon end (arrow) and the ischial tuberosity. (d) Axial proton density–weighted imaging (PDWI) also shows a gap between the torn end of the conjoint tendon and the ischial tuberosity with intervening fluid. (e) Coronal PDWI shows a retracted torn hamstring tendon (arrow) with adjacent large organizing hematoma. (f) Coronal FS T2WI shows a retracted torn tendon end with adjacent organizing hematoma.

Table 6.4 (Cont.) Juxta-articular lesions of the hip

Abnormalities	MRI findings	Comments
Athletic pubalgia (sports hernia) (▶ Fig. 6.22)	Athletic pubalgia encompasses a range of different possible abnormalities resulting in different patterns of injury. MRI evaluation of this condition should begin with large field of view FS T2WI centered on the pubic symphysis and continue with smaller field of view detailed images when the site of pathology is identified. On FS T2WI some patients will have findings of high signal edema along both sides of the pubic symphysis, which may be asymmetrically greater on the more symptomatic side. In some cases a secondary cleft with curvilinear high signal fluid is seen inferior and directly adjacent to the pubic bone. This finding is indicative of disruption of the rectus abdominis aponeurotic plate. The distal attachment of the rectus abdominis to the anterior pubic symphysis may be abnormal with high signal edema on one side indicating muscle strain, or there may be more severe injury with partial- or even full-thickness tear of the muscle attachment. Often the ipsilateral adductor longus origin is also partially or completely torn from the anterior portion of the pubic symphysis.	Patients with athletic pubalgia typically are athletes presenting with groin pain. In particular athletes involved in sports with twisting at the waist, sideways motion, and abrupt directional changes are considered to be most at risk for these injuries. Sports such as soccer, ice hockey, and football are often associated with groin injuries. Some patients will present with acute injury and resultant pain, whereas others have a more chronic course with groin pain that gradually increases over time. Other causes of groin pain in athletes must also be considered, including inguinal hernia, testicular torsion, acetabular labral tear, avascular necrosis of the femoral head, stress fracture, and others. Most patients can be treated with conservative therapy typically including rest and nonsteroidal anti-inflammatory drugs. In some patients surgery is required. This may consist of repairing the specific site of injury. Unfortunately, in some patients with recurrent injury there may be significant loss of playing time and even termination of an athlete's career.

(continued on page 172)

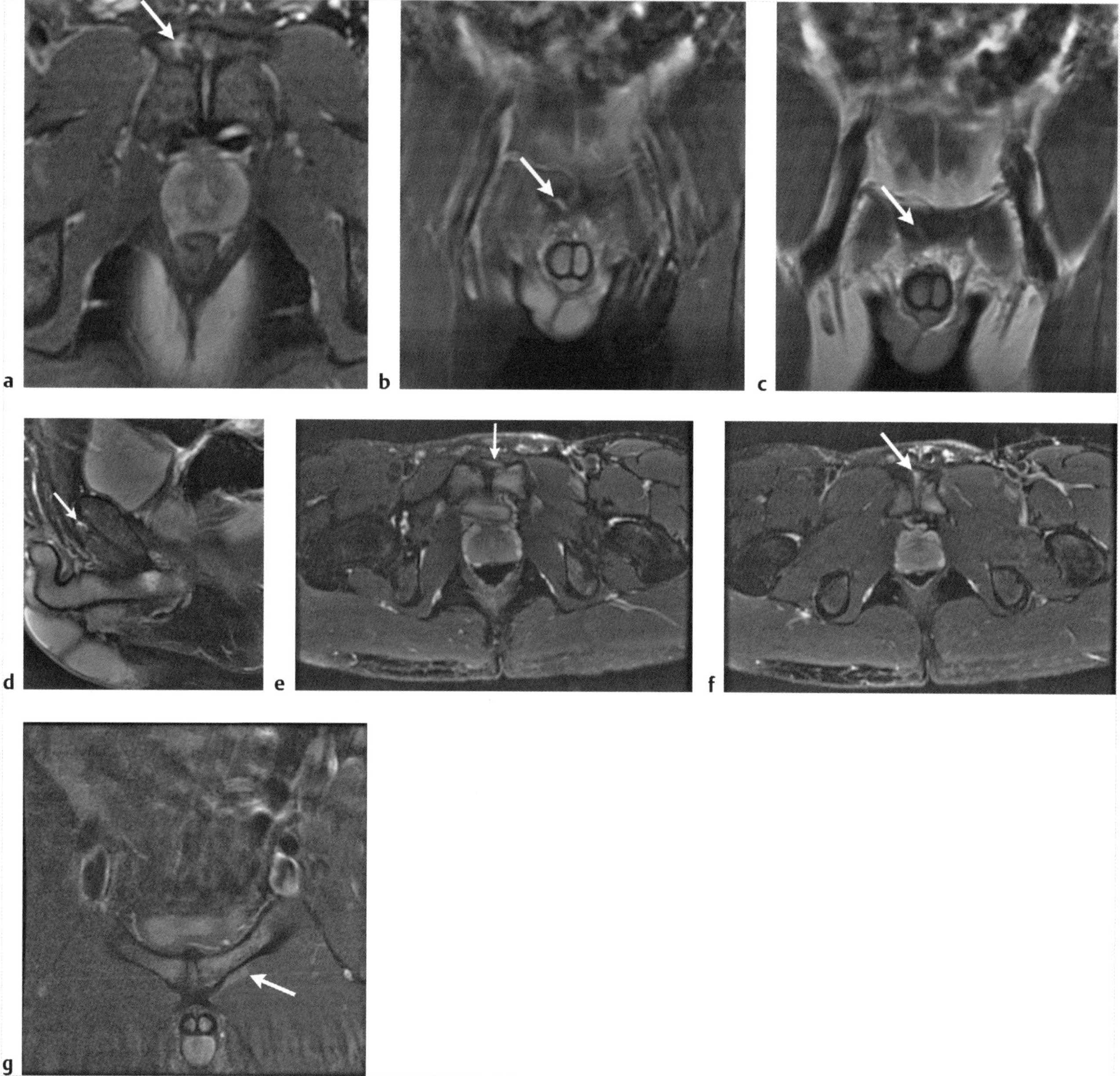

Fig. 6.22 (a) Axial fat-suppressed T2-weighted imaging (FS T2WI) shows an irregular high signal partial tear (arrow) of the right rectus abdominis tendon insertion. (b) Coronal FS T2WI shows an irregular high signal partial tear of the right rectus abdominis tendon insertion (arrow). (c) Corresponding proton density–weighted imaging (PDWI) shows an irregular intermediate signal partial tear of the right rectus abdominis tendon insertion (arrow). (d) Sagittal FS T2WI shows an irregular high signal partial tear of the right rectus abdominis tendon insertion (arrow). (e) Axial FS T2WI from a second patient shows a linear high signal tear of the rectus abdominis aponeurosis (arrow) and high signal marrow edema in the right and left pubic bones. (f) Axial FS T2WI from the same patient shows high signal edema in the pubic symphysis (arrow) with edema in the adjacent right and left pubic bones. (g) Coronal FS T2WI from the same patient shows a tear of the left adductor magnus (arrow) and edema in the right and left pubic rami.

Table 6.4 (Cont.) Juxta-articular lesions of the hip

Abnormalities	MRI findings	Comments
Morel-Lavallée lesions (▶ Fig. 6.23)	The Morel-Lavallée lesion is a type of post-traumatic hematoma that often occurs near the greater trochanter of the femur. The lesion is usually well circumscribed and will have a variable appearance on MRI depending on how old it is. On proton density–weighted imaging (PDWI) and T1-weighted imaging (T1WI) there is often mildly heterogeneous low signal. On FS T2WI there is heterogeneous high signal, often with foci of low signal indicating the presence of hemosiderin. On postcontrast FS T1WI there is mild peripheral enhancement without internal enhancement. In some cases there may be a fluid-fluid level.	The Morel-Lavallée lesion is a post-traumatic hematoma that results from acute traumatic separation of the skin and subcutaneous fatty tissue from the adjacent fascia. Small perforating arteries are often torn in this injury and a hematoma forms in the potential space that has been created. The overall pattern of injury is referred to as a closed degloving injury. Patients with this lesion often complain of pain, and over time this lesion will often grow, raising concern for a soft tissue neoplasm. Treatment often consists of surgery or percutaneous drainage.

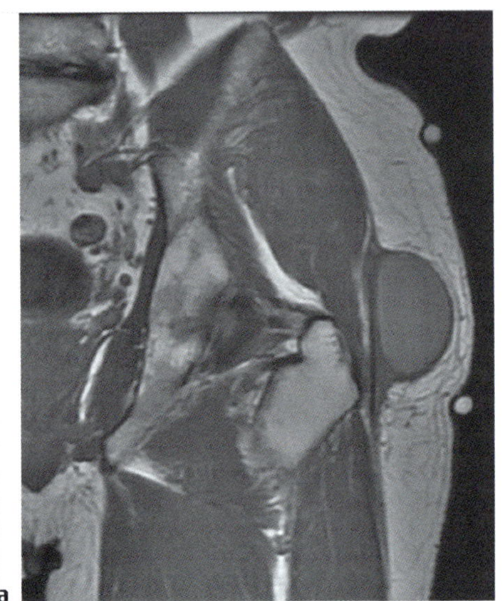

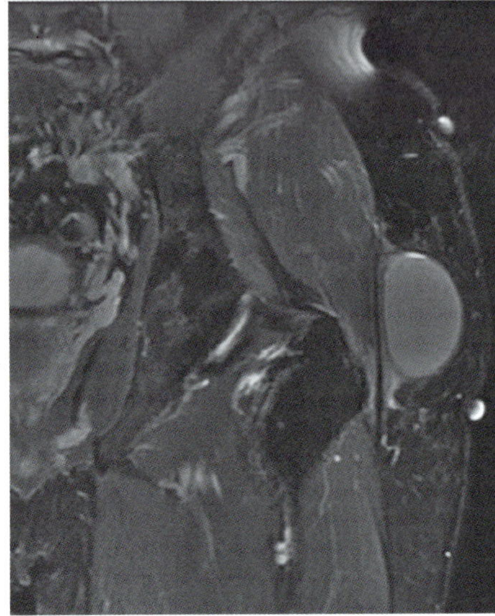

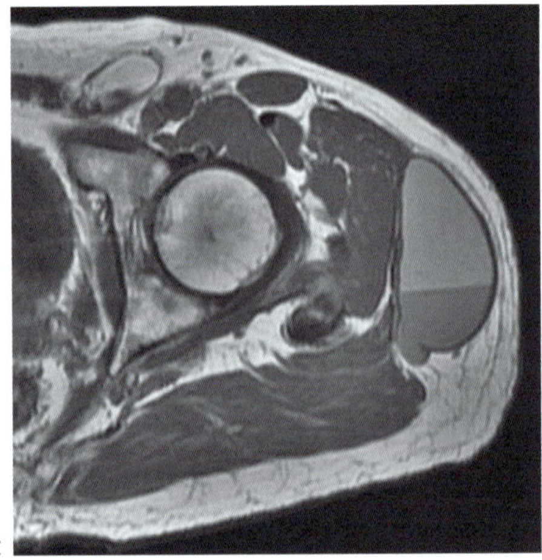

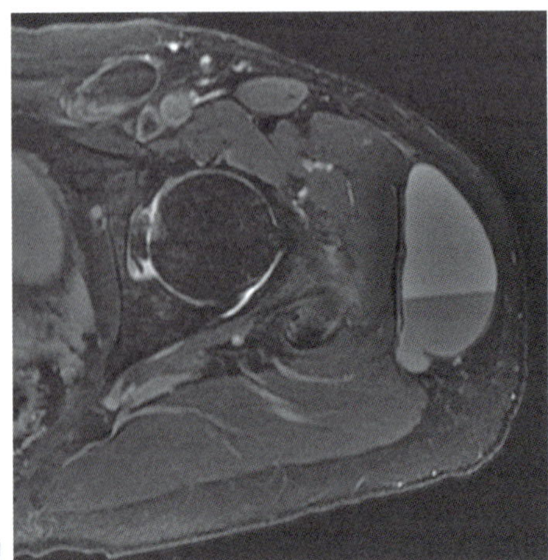

Fig. 6.23 (a) Coronal proton density–weighted imaging (PDWI) shows intermediate signal evolving hematoma in the subcutaneous fatty tissue adjacent to the fascia. (b) Coronal fat-suppressed T2-weighted imaging (FS T2WI) shows predominantly low signal evolving hematoma in the subcutaneous fatty tissue adjacent to the fascia. (c) Axial PDWI shows the fluid level in an evolving hematoma in the subcutaneous fatty tissue adjacent to the fascia. (d) Axial FS T2WI shows the fluid level in an evolving hematoma in the subcutaneous fatty tissue adjacent to the fascia.

6.4.1 Juxta-articular Lesions of the Hip Suggested Reading

[1] Kalaci A, Karazincir S, Yanat AN. Long-standing Morel-Lavallée lesion of the thigh simulating a neoplasm. Clin Imaging 2007; 31: 287–291

[2] Kingzett-Taylor A, Tirman PFJ, Feller J, et al. Tendinosis and tears of gluteus medius and minimus muscles as a cause of hip pain: MR imaging findings. AJR Am J Roentgenol 1999; 173: 1123–1126

[3] Kong A, Van der Vliet A, Zadow S. MRI and US of gluteal tendinopathy in greater trochanteric pain syndrome. Eur Radiol 2007; 17: 1772–1783

[4] Mullens FE, Zoga AC, Morrison WB, Meyers WC. Review of MRI technique and imaging findings in athletic pubalgia and the "sports hernia." Eur J Radiol 2012; 81: 3780–3792

[5] Omar IM, Zoga AC, Kavanagh EC, et al. Athletic pubalgia and "sports hernia": optimal MR imaging technique and findings. Radiographics 2008; 28: 1415–1438

Chapter 7

The Knee

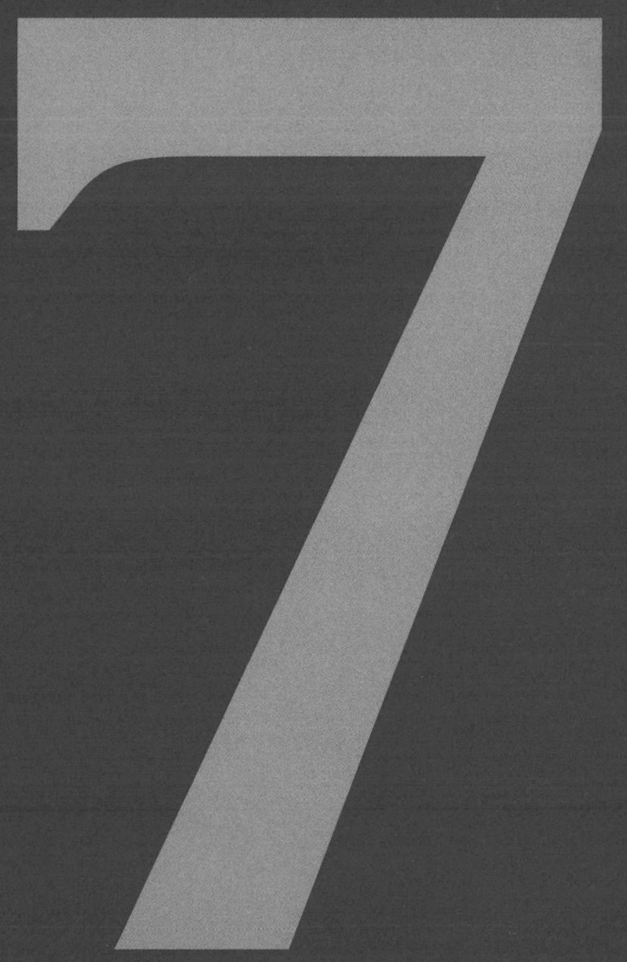

7 The Knee

Eric P. Weinberg

7.1 Lesions of the Menisci

- Normal meniscus
- Discoid meniscus
- Mucoid degeneration and intrasubstance tears
- Horizontal or oblique tears
- Bucket handle tears
- Radial tears
- Meniscal root tears
- Meniscocapsualar separation
- Meniscal cysts
- Postoperative meniscus

Table 7.1 Lesions of the menisci

Abnormalities	MRI findings	Comments
Normal meniscus (▶ Fig. 7.1)	The normal meniscus is composed of fibrocartilage and has a C-shaped configuration with uniform low signal proton density–weighted imaging (PDWI) and fat-suppressed T2-weighted imaging (FS T2WI). On images obtained in the Sagittal plane the normal meniscus has a bow tie configuration. The posterior horns of the menisci may have some intermediate increased signal in younger patients related to normal vascularity. The posterior horns of both menisci are larger than the anterior horns of both menisci. The medial meniscus is larger than the lateral meniscus.	The normal meniscus has several functions and is a critically important structure in the knee. The menisci act as cushions that help to evenly transmit weight-bearing forces along the femoral tibial articulation. The menisci are also important in maintaining knee joint stability during normal weight- bearing activities. In addition the menisci aid in joint lubrication. Given this increased understanding of the importance of the menisci orthopedic surgeons now approach the surgical treatment of the torn meniscus with the goal of preserving as much meniscal material as possible.

(continued on page 178)

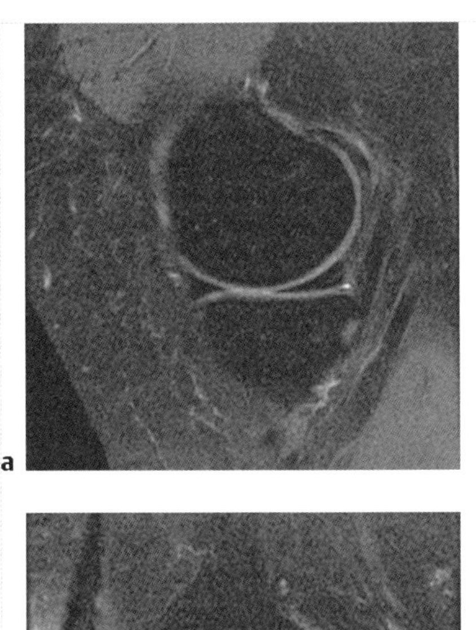
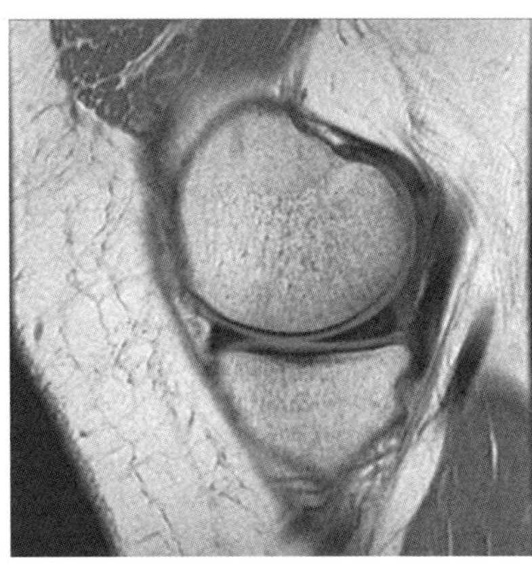
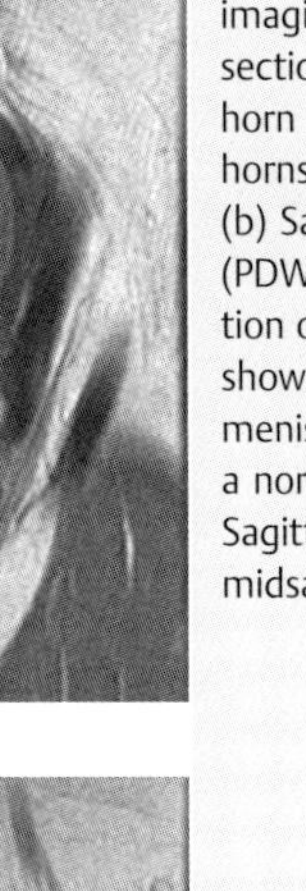
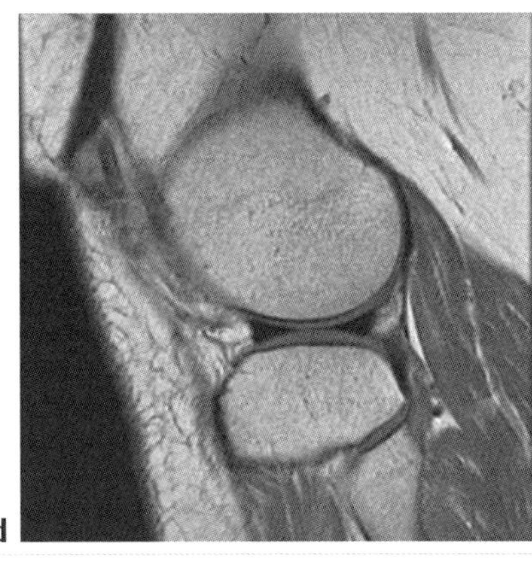

Fig. 7.1 (a) Sagittal fat-suppressed T2-weighted imaging (FS T2WI) shows a normal midsagittal section of the medial meniscus. The posterior horn is larger than the anterior horn, and both horns have a low signal triangular configuration. (b) Sagittal proton density–weighted imaging (PDWI) shows a corresponding midsagittal section of the medial meniscus. (c) Sagittal FS T2WI shows a normal midsagittal section of the lateral meniscus. The anterior and posterior horns have a normal low signal triangular configuration. (d) Sagittal PDWI shows a corresponding normal midsagittal section of the lateral meniscus.

Table 7.1 (Cont.) Lesions of the menisci

Abnormalities	MRI findings	Comments
Discoid meniscus (▶ Fig. 7.2)	Discoid menisci are enlarged with loss of the normal C shape. Discoid lateral meniscus is more common than discoid medial meniscus. The incidence of discoid lateral meniscus is reported as from 3 to 15%. Medial discoid meniscus is less common, from 0.1 to 0.3%. The magnetic resonance imaging (MRI) findings of discoid meniscus are described as more than two bow ties on consecutive sagittal images. This is a problematic definition because it assumes a slice thickness of 4 to 5 mm and an average-sized patient. Neither assumption may be true. Many MRI centers now routinely obtain thinner (3 to 3.5 mm) sagittal slices and some patients are of course larger than average. Additional findings are a lateral meniscus that is larger than the medial meniscus and distinct asymmetry in the size of the anterior and posterior meniscal horns. Also meniscal material extending into the intercondylar notch is indicative of a discoid meniscus. An important variant of discoid meniscus is the Wrisberg variant in which there is only one attachment of the posterior horn of lateral meniscus to the capsule, the ligament of Wrisberg.	The discoid lateral meniscus is a clinically significant finding due to a high associated incidence of meniscal tear and/or cystic degeneration of the meniscus. The discoid meniscus can be symptomatic without evidence of tear as seen in the case of the Wrisberg variant, which does not have the normal capsular attachments.

(continued on page 180)

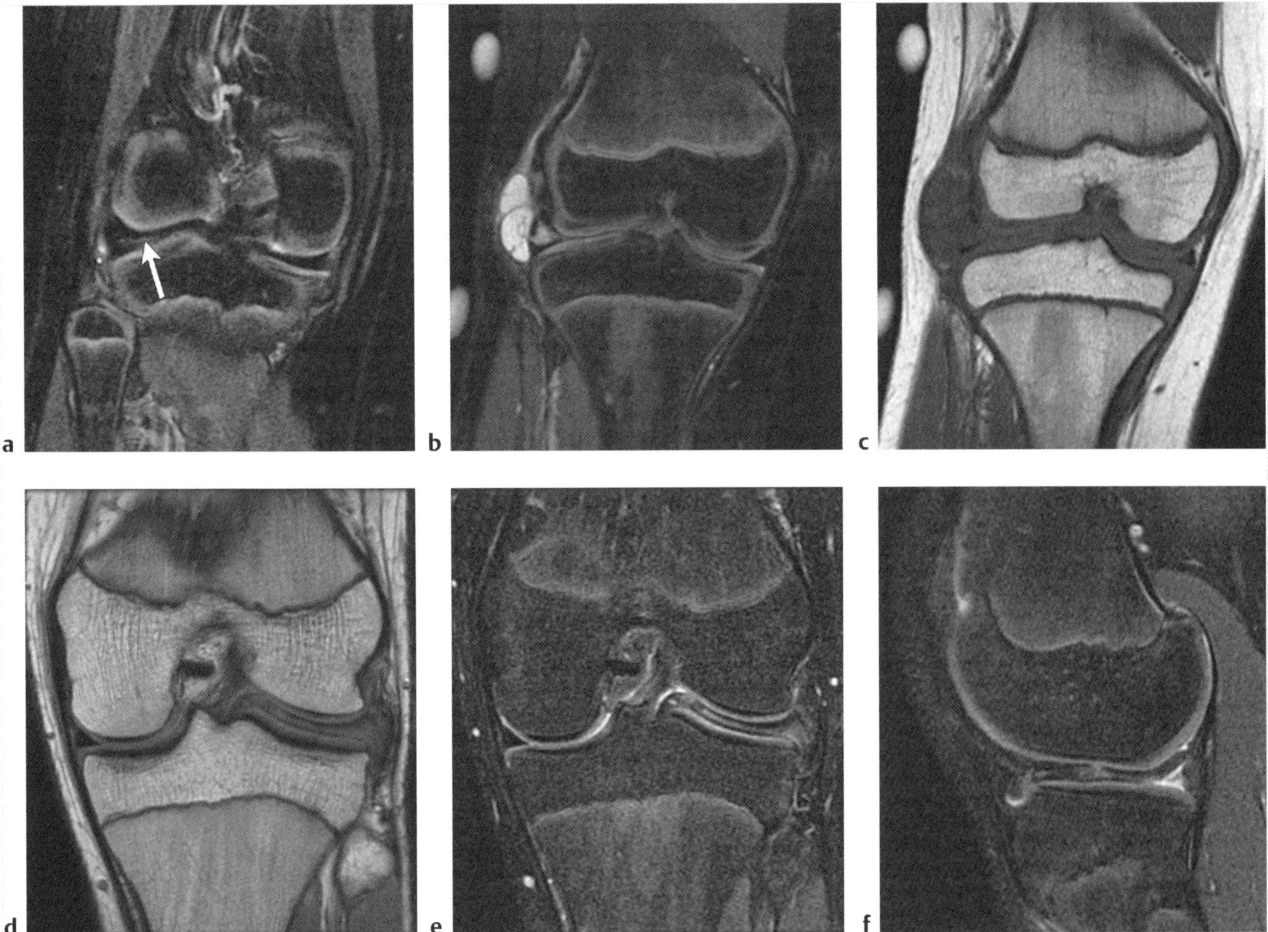

Fig. 7.2 (a) Coronal fat-suppressed T2-weighted imaging (FS T2WI) shows a discoid lateral meniscus with a tear (arrow) in a skeletally immature patient. (b) Coronal FS T2WI shows a large, high signal, multiseptated parameniscal cyst adjacent to the torn discoid lateral meniscus. (c) Coronal proton density–weighted imaging (PDWI) shows a low signal parameniscal cyst adjacent to a discoid lateral meniscus. (d) Coronal PDWI from a second patient shows a large tear in a discoid lateral meniscus. (e) Coronal FS T2WI from a second patient shows a large high signal tear in a discoid lateral meniscus. (f) Sagittal FS T2WI from a second patient shows a large tear in a discoid lateral meniscus.

Table 7.1 (Cont.) Lesions of the menisci

Abnormalities	MRI findings	Comments
Mucoid degeneration and intrasubstance tears (▶ Fig. 7.3; ▶ Fig. 7.4)	In mucoid degeneration on both FS T2WI and PDWI there is globular increased signal seen in either or both the medial and the lateral meniscus. This abnormality may be seen in either or both the anterior and the posterior horn of the meniscus. The body of the meniscus may also be involved. The abnormality may extend to a meniscal surface. Intrasubstance tear is seen as linear high signal on both FS T2WI and PDWI and may be present in the medial or lateral meniscus or both. The abnormality may involve the posterior horn, body, anterior horn, or any combination. Intrasubstance tears do not extend to a meniscal surface.	Mucoid degeneration and intrasubstance tear are not readily identified on arthroscopy because they do not contact the meniscal surface. Neither entity is considered a true tear. Both abnormalities are due to mucinous degeneration of the fibrocartilagenous meniscus. Both abnormalities are likely asymptomatic incidental findings on MRI exams. Neither abnormality is treated surgically.
Horizontal or oblique tears (▶ Fig. 7.5)	These tears are seen as linear increased signal on PDWI and FS T2WI in the sagittal and coronal planes. These signal changes often reach the inferior surface of the meniscus.	These tears are the most common type of meniscal tear and typically occur in the posterior horn of the medial meniscus. These tears are usually degenerative and not secondary to trauma.

(continued on page 182)

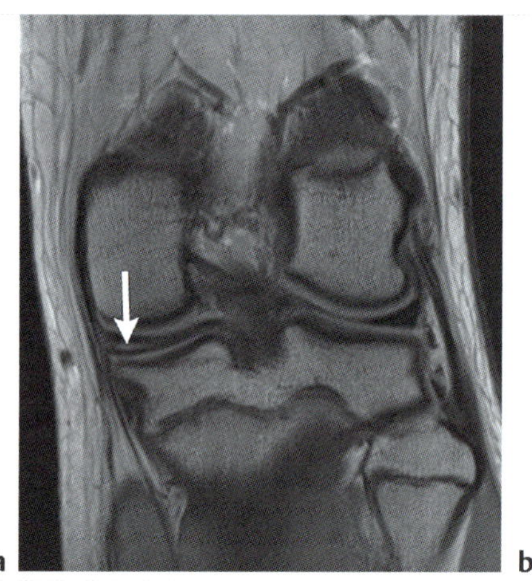
a

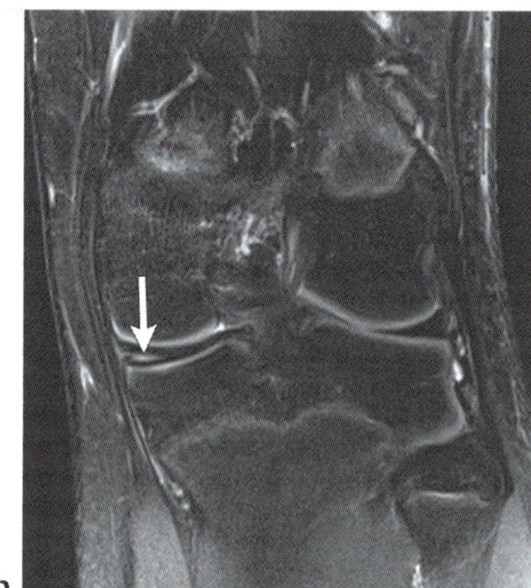
b

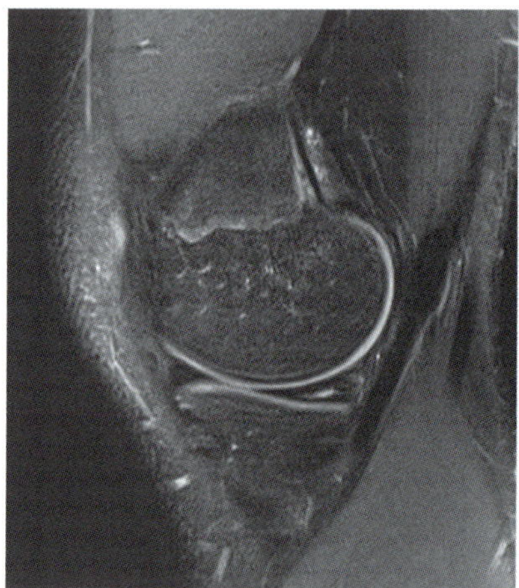
c

Fig. 7.3 (a) Coronal proton density–weighted imaging shows a linear high signal in the posterior horn of the medial meniscus that does not reach a meniscal surface (arrow). (b) Coronal fat-suppressed T2-weighted imaging (FS T2WI) shows a linear high signal in the posterior horn of the medial meniscus that does not reach a meniscal surface (arrow). (c) A sagittal FS T2WI shows linear high signal in the posterior horn of medial meniscus that does not extend to a meniscal surface.

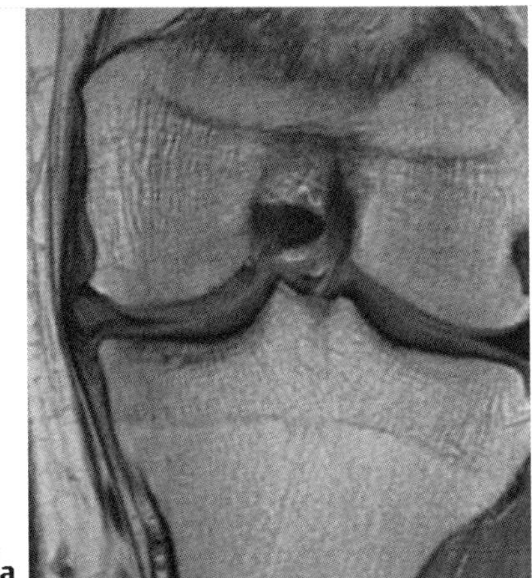

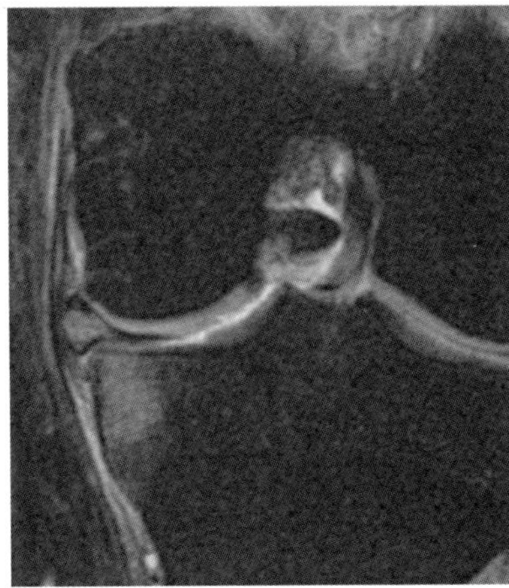

Fig. 7.4 (a) Coronal proton density–weighted imaging shows a globular high signal in the posterior horn of the medial meniscus. (b) Coronal fat-suppressed T2-weighted imaging shows a globular high signal in the posterior horn of the medial meniscus.

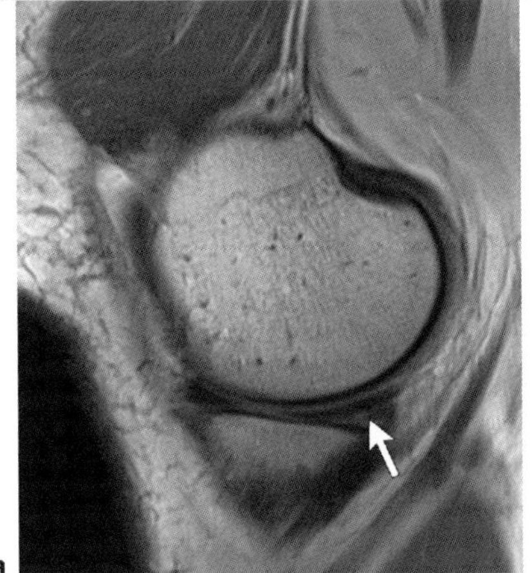

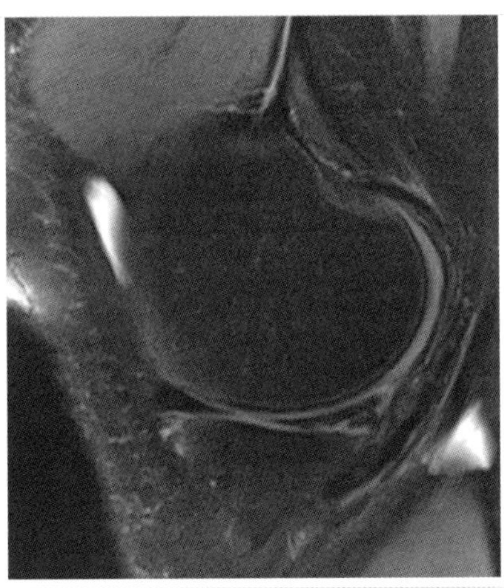

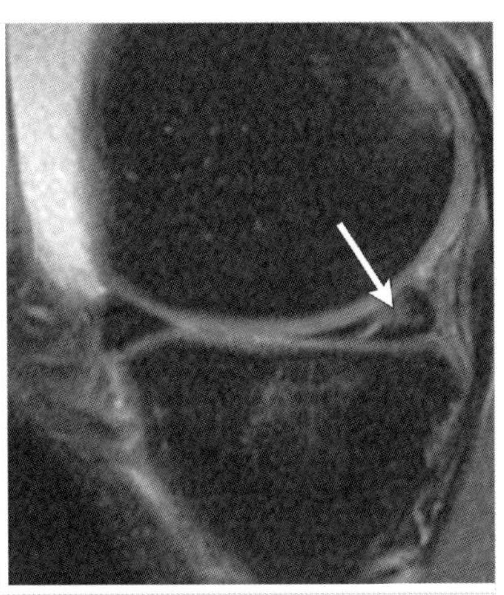

Fig. 7.5 (a) Sagittal proton density–weighted imaging shows an oblique tear of the posterior horn of the medial meniscus extending to the inferior meniscal surface. A smaller component of the tear extends to the superior surface (arrow). (b) Sagittal fat-suppressed T2-weighted imaging (FS T2WI) shows an oblique tear of the posterior horn of the medial meniscus extending to the inferior meniscal surface. A smaller component of the tear extends to the superior surface. (c) Sagittal FS T2WI from a second patient shows a linear, oblique high signal in the posterior horn of medial meniscus extending to the inferior meniscal surface. There is also superimposed adjacent mucoid degenerative change (arrow).

Table 7.1 (Cont.) Lesions of the menisci

Abnormalities	MRI findings	Comments
Bucket handle tears (▶ Fig. 7.6; ▶ Fig. 7.7)	The classic appearance of a bucket handle tear is the absent bow tie seen on sagittal images as fewer than two bow ties on 4-mm-thick sagittal images. There will often be the associated double posterior cruciate ligament (PCL) sign in which there is displaced meniscal material in the intercondylar region of the knee such that there appears to be a second low signal band paralleling the native PCL. The displaced meniscal material is located anterior to the PCL. This tear configuration occurs when the torn fragment maintains a connection with the anterior and posterior horns of the residual meniscus. Alternatively the displaced meniscal fragment may be seen to have flipped to the anterior knee such that it is now adjacent to the anterior horn. This posterior horn is then diminutive or absent. Sagittal, coronal, and sometimes axial planes are used to diagnose these tears.	Bucket handle tears are commonly seen in athletes involved in football and basketball. The classic presenting sign is knee locking. Although this typical finding may not be observed because these patients can be difficult to examine soon after injury due to guarding and overall decreased range of motion. Surgery is typically required in these patients.

(continued on page 184)

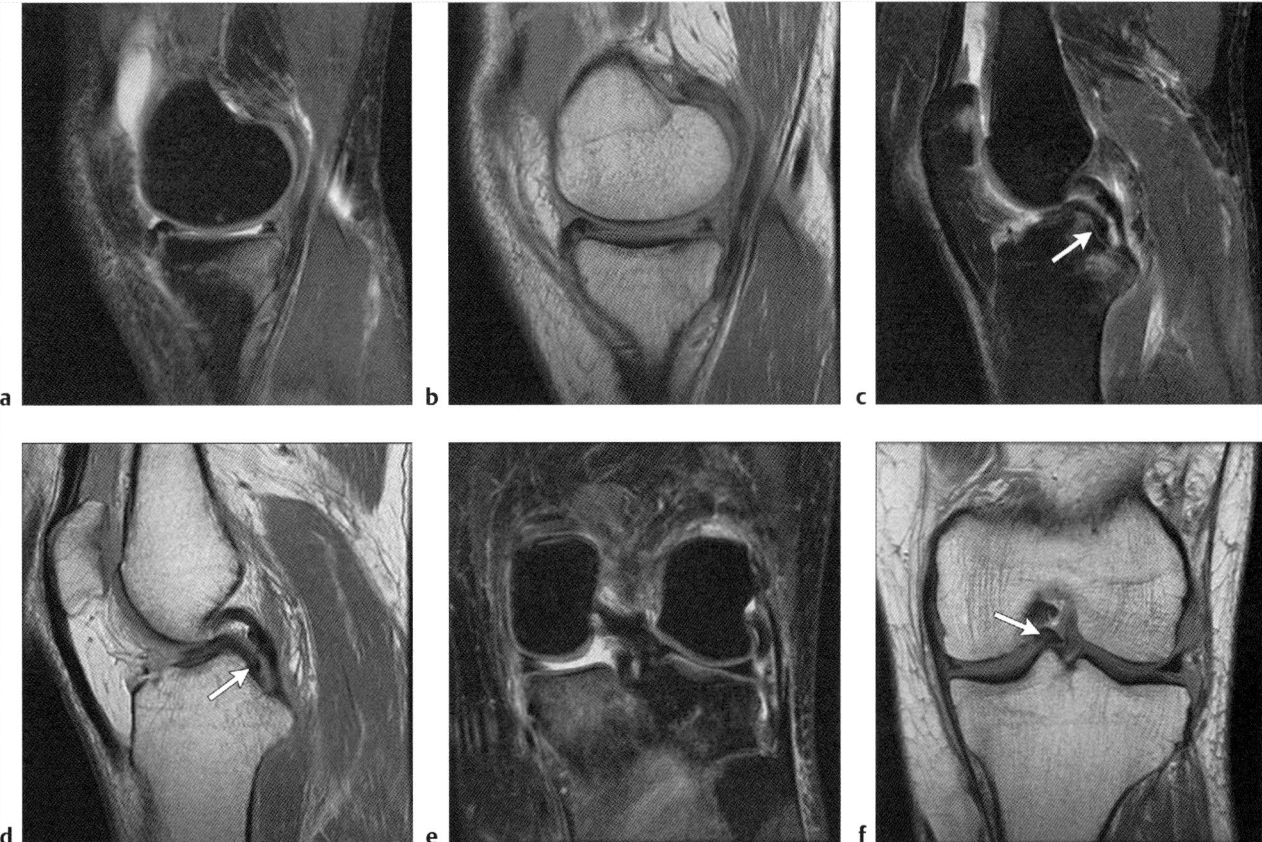

Fig. 7.6 (a) Sagittal fat-suppressed T2-weighted imaging (FS T2WI) shows a diminutive irregular posterior horn and body of the medial meniscus with bone contusion in the proximal posterior medial tibia. (b) Sagittal proton density–weighted imaging (PDWI) shows a diminutive irregular posterior horn and body of the medial meniscus. (c) Sagittal FS T2WI shows meniscal material anterior to the posterior cruciate ligament (PCL) in the central portion of the knee such that there is a double PCL sign (arrow). (d) Sagittal PDWI shows meniscal material anterior to the PCL in the central portion of the knee such that there is a double PCL sign (arrow). (e) Coronal FS T2WI shows a diminutive irregular posterior horn with bone contusion in the proximal medial tibia. (f) Coronal PDWI shows meniscal material displaced to the central portion of the knee (arrow).

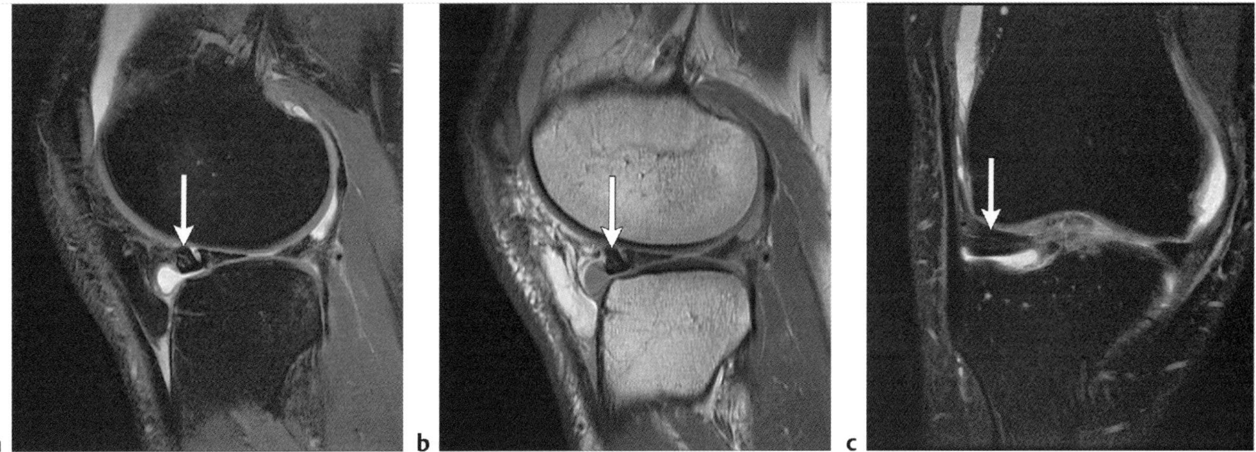

Fig. 7.7 (a) Sagittal fat-suppressed T2-weighted imaging (FS T2WI) shows a meniscal fragment adjacent to the anterior horn of the lateral meniscus (arrow). (b) Sagittal proton density–weighted imaging (PDWI) shows a meniscal fragment adjacent to the anterior horn of the lateral meniscus (arrow). (c) Coronal FS T2WI from the anterior portion of the knee shows a meniscal fragment adjacent to the anterior horn of the lateral meniscus (arrow).

Table 7.1 (Cont.) Lesions of the menisci

Abnormalities	MRI findings	Comments
Radial tears (▶ Fig. 7.8)	Radial tears are vertically oriented tears. On sagittal images there is loss of the normal bow tie configuration of the meniscus with a much smaller defect than is seen with bucket handle tears. Truncation of the normal triangular appearance of the meniscus and a small cleft are also signs of radial tears. On occasion axial plain images may also show these tears because they occur along the free edge of the meniscus.	Small radial tears may be asymptomatic, and larger tears are often painful. Large tears will prevent the meniscus from performing its normal cushioning function. Over time untreated larger radial tears will result in early-onset osteoarthritis with loss of adjacent articular cartilage and subcortical reactive marrow edema. Larger radial tears are often treated surgically.
Meniscal root tears (▶ Fig. 7.9)	Meniscal root tears are a special type of radial tear. These tears are most frequently seen in the medial meniscus posterior root. These tears are vertically oriented and can be seen on sagittal images as irregularity of the inner margin of the meniscus, or in larger tears there is absence of the inner margin. The coronal plane may directly reveal the tear as a discontinuity of meniscal material at or adjacent to the meniscal root. There may also be a fluid-filled gap between the torn ends of the meniscus, which is best seen on the coronal plane. This is often the case when there is extrusion of the meniscus. Meniscal extrusion is an important, often associated finding in the case of meniscal root tears. Extrusion of meniscal material is seen when the meniscus extends beyond the margins of the distal femur and proximal tibia. Care must be taken in the presence of large marginal osteophytes because an intact meniscus may be seen to extend parallel to the osteophytes. In some respects this appearance is not unlike a disk bulge osteophyte complex seen in lumbar spine MRI exams.	Meniscal root tears are often symptomatic. There is severe loss of meniscal hoop strength associated with these tears. Early-onset osteoarthritis is typically the result of these tears. There are the expected findings of extensive articular cartilage loss and degenerative reactive marrow edema in the adjacent subcortical bone.
Meniscocapsular separation (▶ Fig. 7.10)	Increased fluid seen between the meniscus and the joint capsule occurs when there is tearing of the meniscal attachment to the joint capsule. This type of injury usually occurs in the posterior horn of the medial meniscus. On coronal images fluid separating the medial meniscus and the medial collateral ligament (MCL) is indicative of meniscocapsular separation. On sagittal images uncovering of the posterior peripheral portion of the tibia is a suggestive though not definitive sign of meniscocapsular separation. There can be confusion when there is fluid seen in the superior and inferior capsular recesses. This finding does not indicate a meniscocapsular tear.	These are often symptomatic and result in hypermobility of the normally less mobile posterior horn of the medial meniscus. Small tears may heal without surgical treatment. Larger tears will usually respond well to surgical treatment because there is a rich blood supply in the periphery of the meniscus.

(continued on page 186)

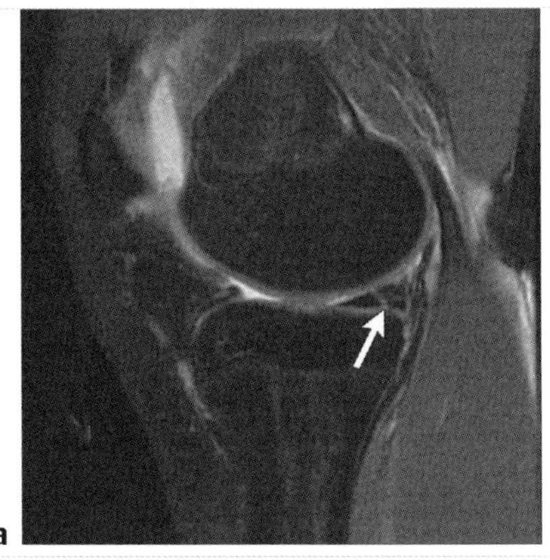

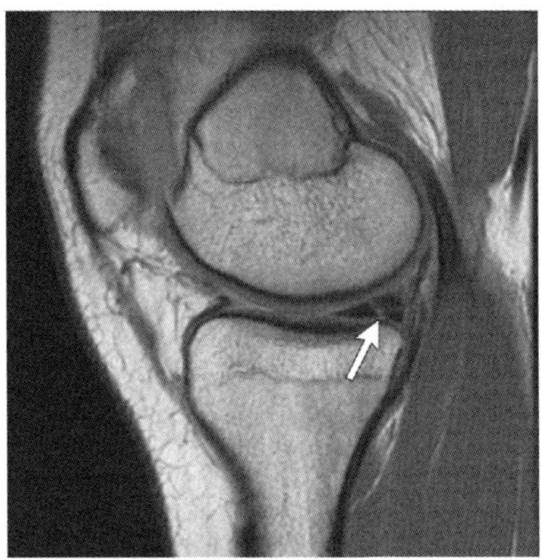

Fig. 7.8 (a) Sagittal fat-suppressed T2-weighted imaging (FS T2WI) shows a vertically oriented high signal tear that extends to the superior and inferior meniscal surfaces (arrow). (b) Sagittal proton density–weighted imaging (PDWI) shows a vertically oriented high signal linear tear contacting both meniscal surfaces (arrow).

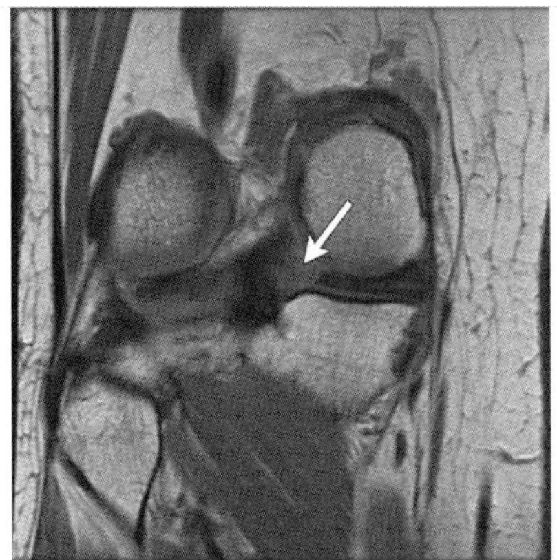

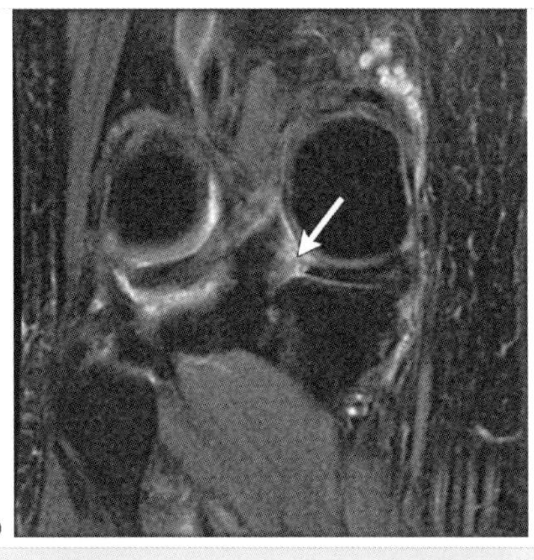

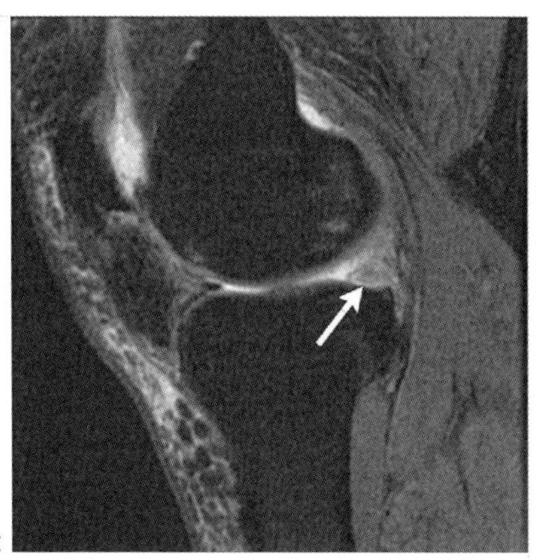

Fig. 7.9 (a) Coronal proton density–weighted imaging (PDWI) shows disruption of the medial meniscal posterior root (arrow). (b) Coronal fat-suppressed T2-weighted imaging (FS T2WI) shows disruption of the medial meniscal posterior root (arrow). (c) Sagittal FS T2WI shows a torn high signal remnant of the posterior root of the medial meniscus (arrow).

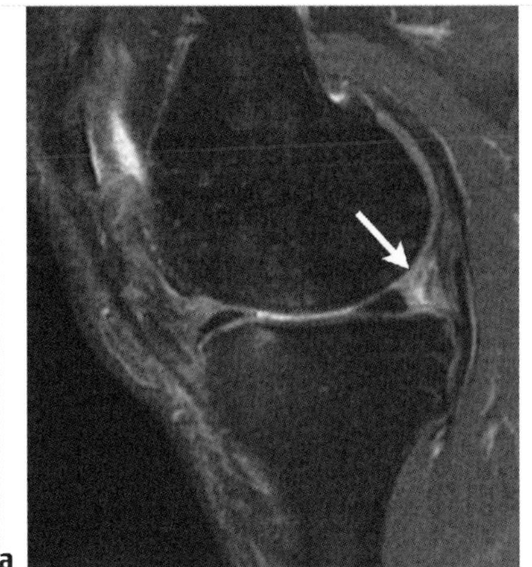

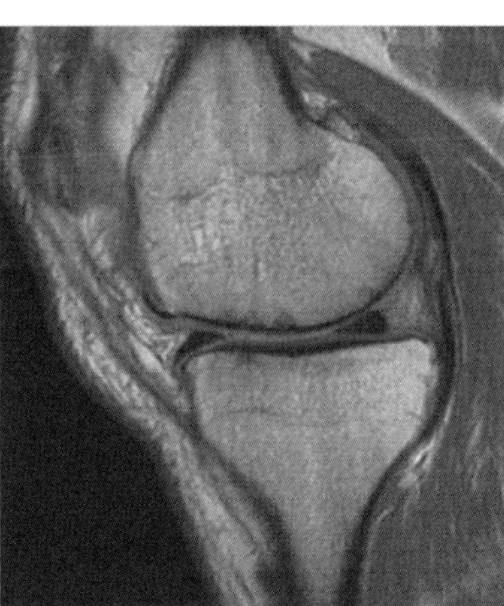

Fig. 7.10 (a) Sagittal fat-suppressed T2-weighted imaging shows high signal fluid between the medial meniscus posterior horn and the joint capsule (arrow) and uncovering of the posterior peripheral portion of the tibia. (b) Sagittal proton density–weighted imaging shows intermediate signal between the medial meniscus posterior horn and the joint capsule.

Table 7.1 (Cont.) Lesions of the menisci

Abnormalities	MRI findings	Comments
Meniscal cysts (▶ Fig. 7.11; ▶ Fig. 7.12)	Meniscal cysts are seen as high signal on FS T2WI and low signal on PDWI. These cysts are often septated and are highly variable in size, ranging from a few millimeters to several centimeters. Meniscal cysts are usually seen along the periphery of the meniscus and often can be seen to communicate with a meniscal tear. Not all meniscal cysts are associated with a meniscal tear. Some meniscal cysts are entirely located within the meniscus, an intrameniscal cyst. Intrameniscal cysts can also extend beyond the margins of the meniscus into the adjacent soft tissues.	Most meniscal cysts occur on the medial side. Most of these cysts are associated with the posterior horn. Meniscal cysts are thought to occur as a result of synovial fluid extending through a meniscal tear. Meniscal cysts may be symptomatic and may require surgical treatment.

(continued on page 188)

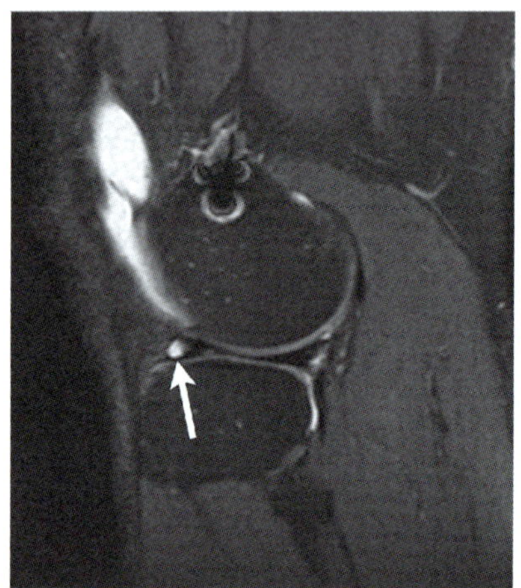
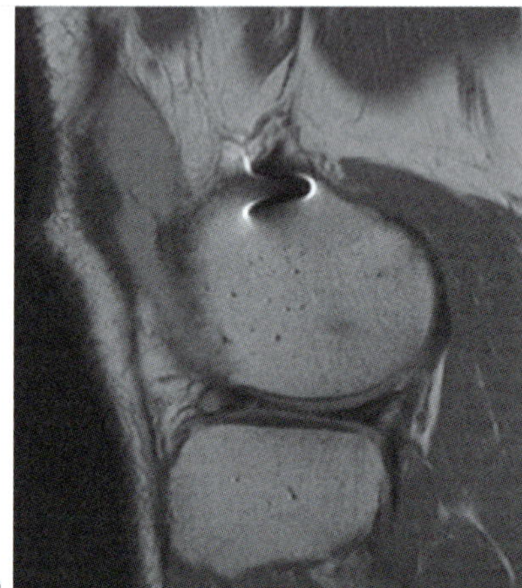
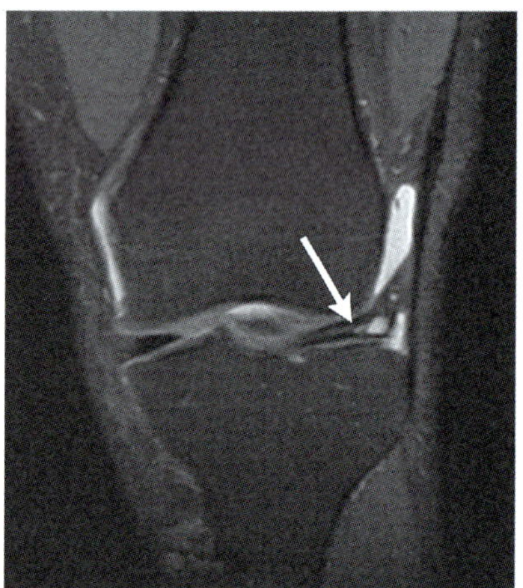

Fig. 7.11 (a) Sagittal fat-suppressed T2-weighted imaging (FS T2WI) shows a high signal intrameniscal cyst within the anterior horn of the lateral meniscus (arrow). (b) Sagittal image shows an intermediate signal intrameniscal cyst within the anterior horn of lateral meniscus. (c) Coronal FS T2WI shows a high signal intrameniscal cyst within the anterior horn of the lateral meniscus with an adjacent tear of the meniscus (arrow).

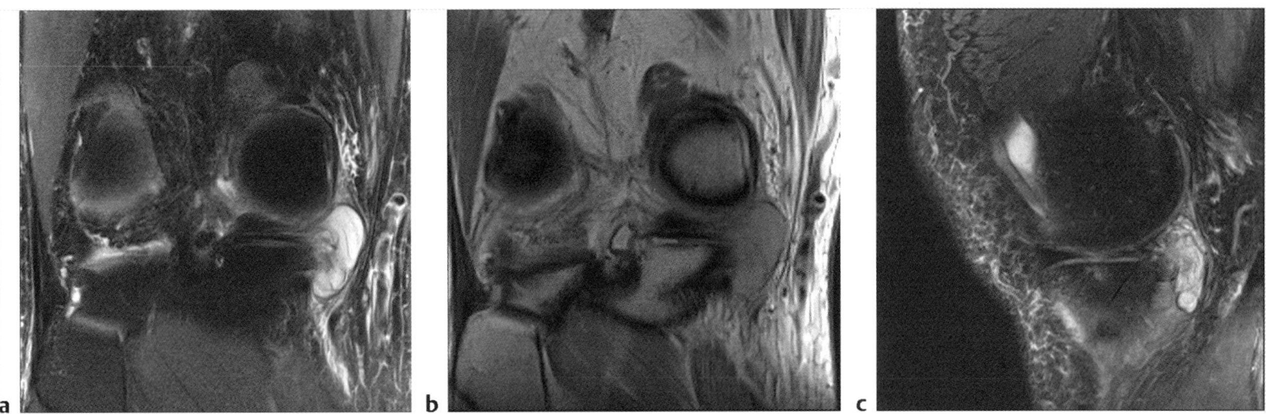

Fig. 7.12 (a) Coronal fat-suppressed T2-weighted imaging (FS T2WI) shows a large high signal multiseptated medial parameniscal cyst adjacent to a torn medial meniscus. (b) Coronal proton density–weighted imaging shows a septated intermediate signal medial parameniscal cyst. (c) Sagittal FS T2WI shows a large high signal medial parameniscal cyst.

Table 7.1 (Cont.) Lesions of the menisci

Abnormalities	MRI findings	Comments
Postoperative meniscus (▶ Fig. 7.13; ▶ Fig. 7.14)	Recurrent and residual meniscal tears are difficult to accurately diagnose with conventional MRI. On conventional MRI a recurrent or residual tear will be seen as a linear zone of high signal on FS T2WI that reaches an articular surface. Unfortunately the postsurgical appearance of the residual meniscus can have a similar appearance with no new or residual tear present. A free fragment is a more convincing sign of meniscal re-tear. If a prior postoperative MRI is available for comparison this could be helpful in finding a re-tear if there is an interval change in the appearance of the residual meniscus. MRI arthrography of the knee is very helpful in distinguishing postoperative meniscal changes from recurrent or residual meniscal tear. On FS T1-weighted imaging (T1WI) injected saline with dilute gadolinium chelate can be seen as linear high signal extending into a residual or recurrent tear. A postsurgical change without recurrent or residual meniscal tear will have linear high signal on FS T2WI and no evidence of corresponding high signal on FS T1WI.	The question of residual and recurrent tear versus postoperative change is a common indication for MRI of the knee. Unfortunately this is usually a difficult diagnostic challenge on conventional MRI. MRI arthrography seems to be superior to conventional MRI for this indication. Recurrent meniscal tears are a common occurrence and may require additional surgery.

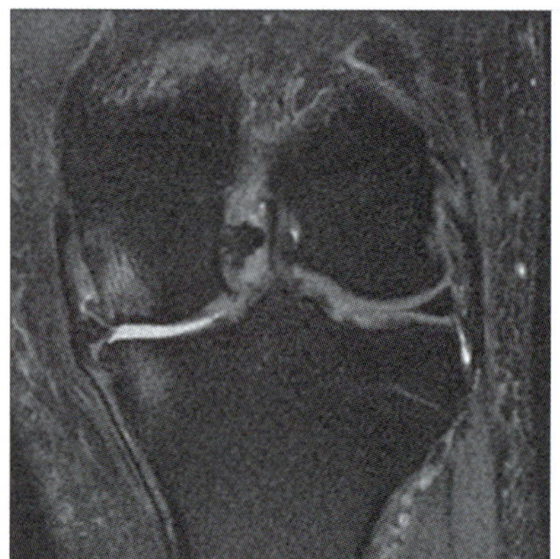
a

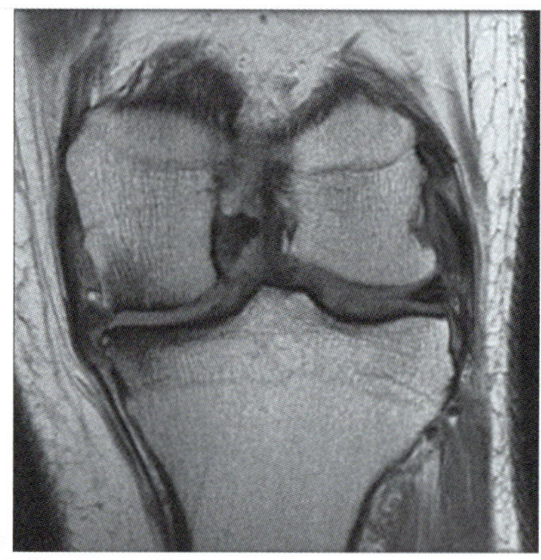
b

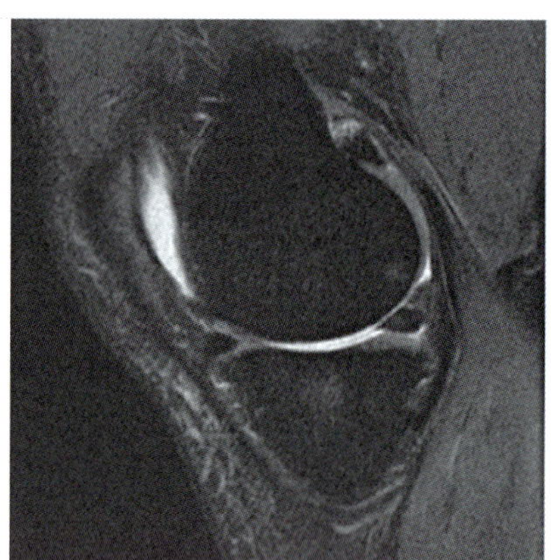
c

Fig. 7.13 (a) Coronal fat-suppressed T2-weighted imaging (FS T2WI) shows a diminutive residual medial meniscus with medial compartment cartilage loss, degenerative reactive marrow edema in the medial femoral condyle and opposite proximal tibia (bright signal), and marginal osteophytes. (b) Coronal proton density–weighted imaging shows a small residual medial meniscus with degenerative changes in the medial compartment. (c) Sagittal FS T2WI shows postoperative residual medial meniscus with some internal high signal in the residual posterior horn.

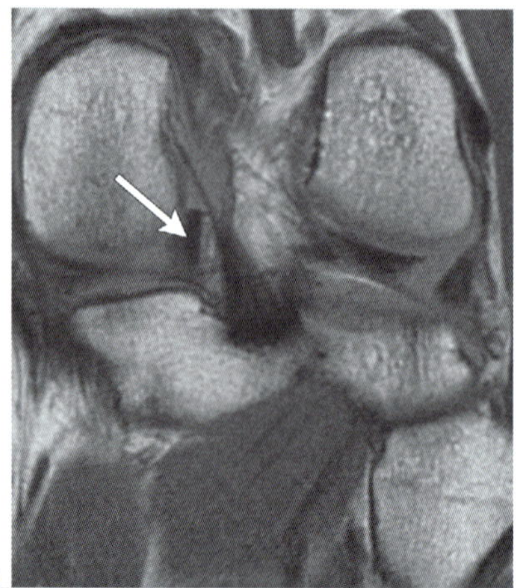
a

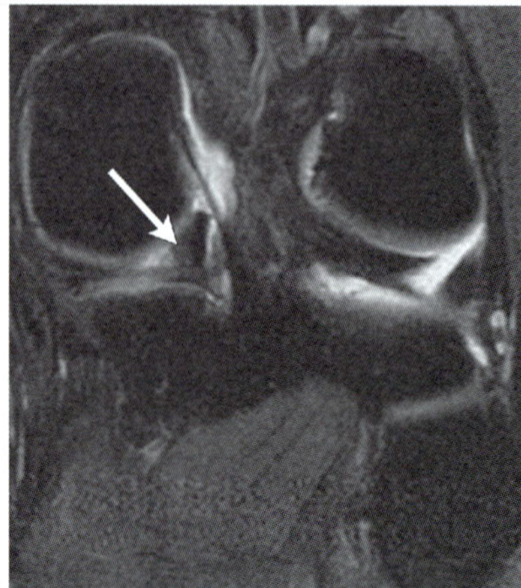
b

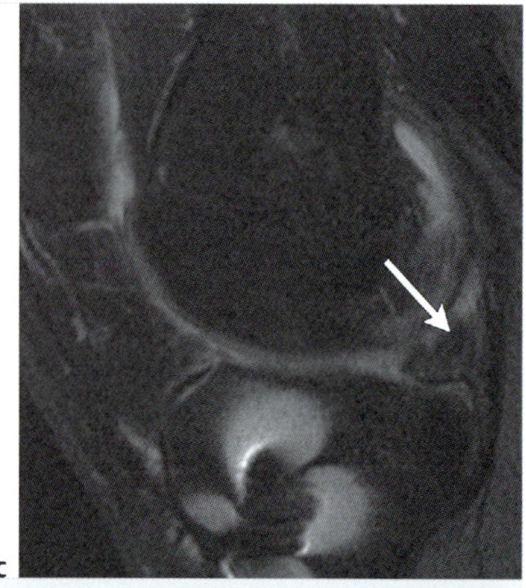
c

Fig. 7.14 (a) Coronal proton density–weighted imaging (PDWI) shows a medial meniscal fragment adjacent to the inner margin of the posterior horn of the medial meniscus (arrow) in a patient with prior partial meniscectomy. (b) Coronal fat-suppressed T2-weighted imaging (FS T2WI) shows a medial meniscal fragment adjacent to the inner margin of the posterior horn of the medial meniscus (arrow). (c) Sagittal FS T2WI of the inner medial meniscus shows a diminutive anterior horn with extra meniscal material in the posterior horn that includes a displaced meniscal fragment (arrow). *(continued)*

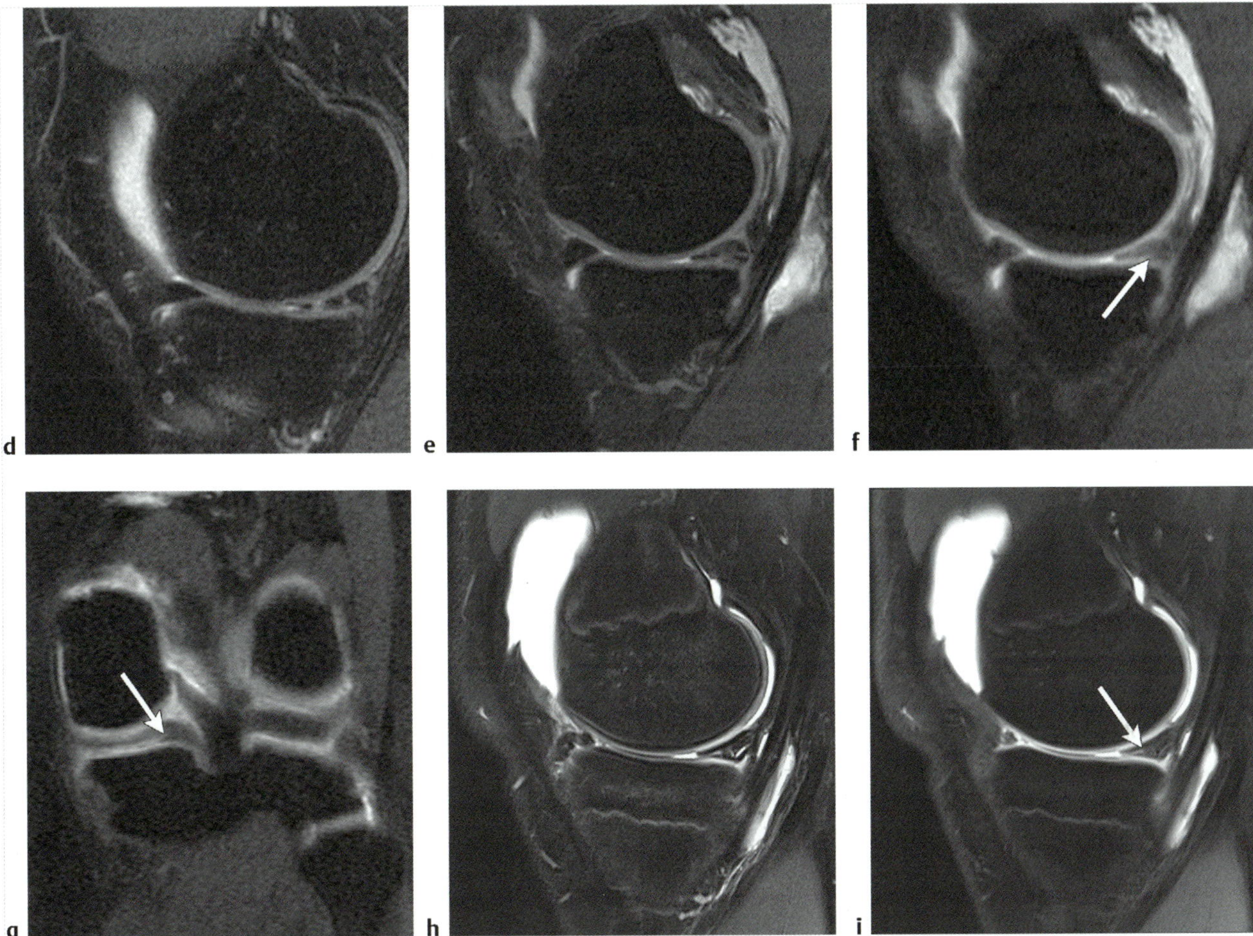

Fig. 7.14 *(continued)* (d) Sagittal FS T2WI shows postoperative changes of prior partial medial meniscectomy in the posterior horn of the medial meniscus. (e) MRI arthrographic sagittal FS T2WI from a second patient shows irregular linear high signal in the posterior horn of the medial meniscus, which has had prior partial meniscectomy. (f) MRI arthrographic sagittal FS T1WI from a second patient shows high signal contrast-laden fluid entering into the substance of the posterior horn of the residual medial meniscus (arrow) indicating a re-tear. (g) MRI arthrographic coronal FS T2WI from a second patient shows high signal contrast-laden fluid extending into the substance of the posterior horn medial meniscus (arrow). (h) MRI arthrographic sagittal FS T2WI from a third patient who had prior partial meniscectomy shows linear high signal in the posterior horn of the residual medial meniscus. (i) MRI arthrographic sagittal FS T1WI from a third patient shows high signal contrast-laden fluid extending into the posterior horn of the medial meniscus indicating re-tear (arrow).

7.1.1 Lesions of the Menisci Suggested Reading

[1] Alatakis S, Naidoo P. MR imaging of meniscal and cartilage injuries of the knee. Magn Reson Imaging Clin N Am 2009; 17: 741–756, vii

[2] De Maeseneer M, Shahabpour M, Vanderdood K, Van Roy F, Osteaux M. Medial meniscocapsular separation: MR imaging criteria and diagnostic pitfalls. Eur J Radiol 2002; 41: 242–252

[3] De Smet AA, Graf BK, del Rio AM. Association of parameniscal cysts with underlying meniscal tears as identified on MRI and arthroscopy. AJR Am J Roentgenol 2011; 196: W180-W186

[4] De Smet AA. MR imaging and MR arthrography for diagnosis of recurrent tears in the postoperative meniscus. Semin Musculoskelet Radiol 2005; 9: 116–124

[5] Engstrom BI, Vinson EN, Taylor DC, Garrett WE, Helms CA. Hemi-bucket-handle tears of the meniscus: appearance on MRI and potential surgical implications. Skeletal Radiol 2012; 41: 933–938

[6] Grossman JW, De Smet AA, Shinki K. Comparison of the accuracy rates of 3-T and 1.5-T MRI of the knee in the diagnosis of meniscal tear. AJR Am J Roentgenol 2009; 193: 509–514

[7] Jung JY, Jee WH, Park MY, Lee SY, Kim JM. Meniscal tear configurations: categorization with 3D isotropic turbo spin-echo MRI compared with conventional MRI at 3 T. AJR Am J Roentgenol 2012; 198: W173-W180

[8] Kijowski R, Woods MA, McGuine TA, Wilson JJ, Graf BK, De Smet AA. Arthroscopic partial meniscectomy: MR imaging for prediction of outcome in middle-aged and elderly patients. Radiology 2011; 259: 203–212

[9] Rubin DA. MR imaging of the knee menisci. Radiol Clin North Am 1997; 35: 21–44

[10] Venkatanarasimha N, Kamath A, Mukherjee K, Kamath S. Potential pitfalls of a double PCL sign. Skeletal Radiol 2009; 38: 735–739

[11] White LM, Kramer J, Recht MP. MR imaging evaluation of the postoperative knee: ligaments, menisci, and articular cartilage. Skeletal Radiol 2005; 34: 431–452

7.2 Lesions of the Knee Ligaments

- Anterior cruciate ligament (ACL) tears
- Partial ACL tears
- Mucoid cystic degeneration of the ACL and posterior cruciate ligament (PCL)
- Postoperative ACL and Re-tear
- Arthrofibrosis
- PCL tears
- Medial collateral ligament (MCL) tears
- Lateral collateral ligament (LCL) complex tears
- Iliotibial band syndrome

Table 7.2 Lesions of the knee ligaments

Abnormalities	MRI findings	Comments
Anterior cruciate ligament (ACL) tears (▶ Fig. 7.15; ▶ Fig. 7.16)	The ACL is well seen in both sagittal and coronal planes. The normal ACL is nonuniform in signal on fat-suppressed T2-weighted imaging (FS T2WI). The distal tibial attachment is usually heterogeneously increased in signal with the proximal femoral attachment more uniformly low signal. When the ACL is torn it is often completely disrupted such that there may be no remaining identifiable fibers in its expected location in the intercondylar notch. On occasion there may be a few residual fibers remaining. In acute ACL tears there are often associated findings that vary depending on the nature of the injury. The most common associated findings include bone bruises in the lateral femoral condyle and proximal posterior tibia. In some cases there may be significant impaction of the lateral femoral condyle, which can be seen on radiographs of the knee. Other associated injuries can include meniscal tears and tears of the collateral ligaments. Posterolateral corner injuries can also occur when the ACL is torn.	The most common causes of acute ACL tears are athletic injuries sustained in sports such as football, basketball, soccer, and alpine skiing. ACL tears result in knee instability, which can result in the inability of patients to return to their sport unless repaired surgically. Surgical treatment of acute ACL tears is becoming more common as patients are leading more active life styles at ever increasing older ages. MRI is very sensitive and specific in identifying tears of the ACL. However, even in the setting of a clinically obvious ACL tear MRI is often used to evaluate for the range of associated injuries that can be seen. The presence or absence of these associated injures will often determine what treatment options will be recommended.

(continued on page 192)

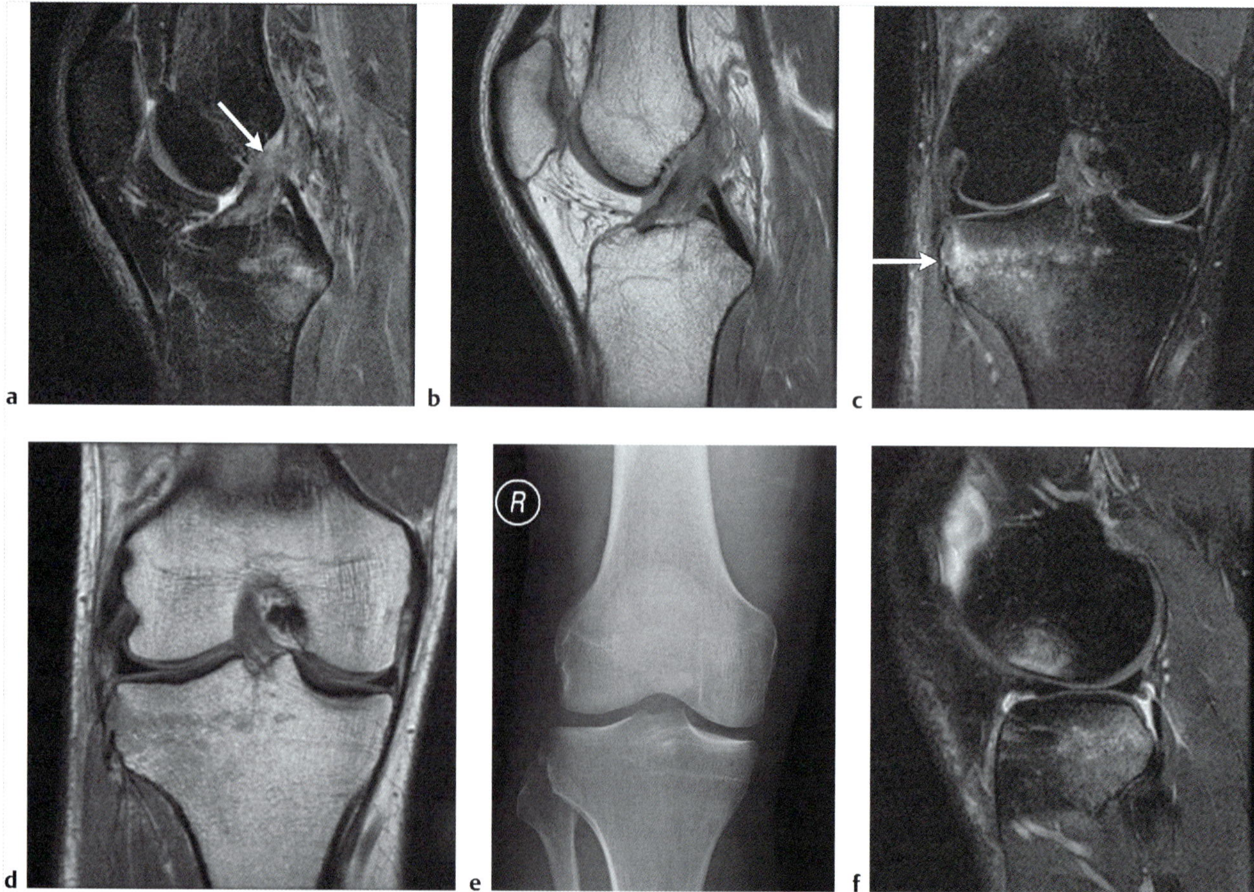

Fig. 7.15 (a) Sagittal fat-suppressed T2-weighted imaging (FS T2WI) shows a thickened edematous anterior cruciate ligament (ACL), which is torn at the femoral attachment (arrow). Marrow edema from contusion is also seen in the posterior proximal tibia. (b) Sagittal proton density–weighted imaging (PDWI) shows a thickened ACL, which is torn from its femoral attachment. (c) Coronal FS T2WI shows a contusion of the proximal lateral tibia with avulsion fracture of the proximal lateral tibia (the Gerdy tubercle) (arrow). (d) Coronal PDWI shows a proximal lateral tibia avulsion fracture with adjacent low signal edema. (e) Anteroposterior radiograph shows avulsion fracture at the Gerdy tubercle. (f) Sagittal FS T2WI shows a typical pattern of bone bruises in an ACL tear that includes the lateral femoral condyle and the posterior proximal tibia.

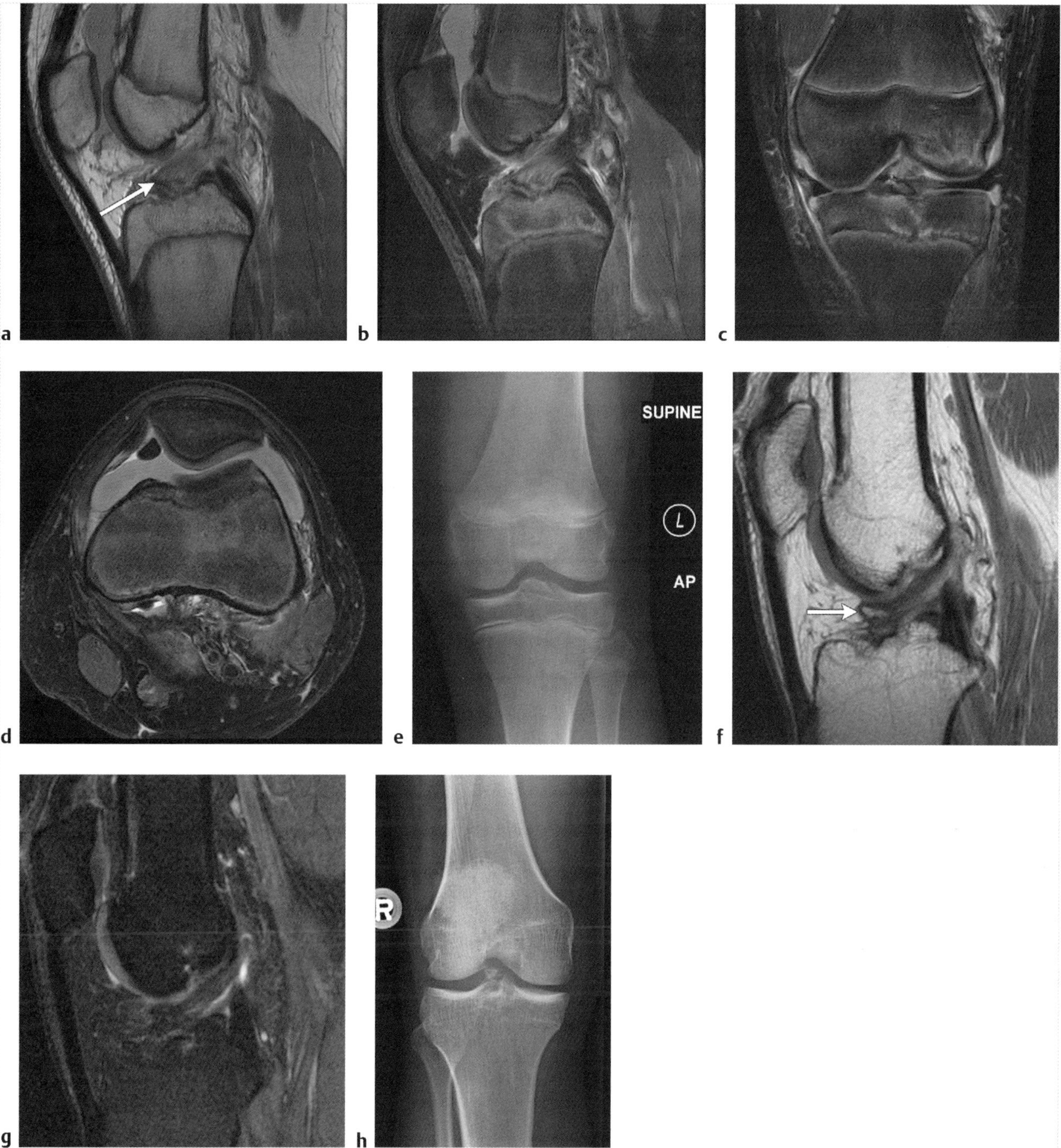

Fig. 7.16 (a) Sagittal proton density–weighted imaging (PDWI) shows a tibial spine avulsion fracture (arrow) and thickened edematous anterior cruciate ligament (ACL). (b) Sagittal fat-suppressed T2-weighted imaging (FS T2WI) shows a tibial spine avulsion fracture with an adjacent bone contusion and thickened edematous ACL. (c) Coronal FS T2WI shows bone contusion in the lateral femoral condyle with a tibial spine avulsion fracture and adjacent bone contusion. (d) Axial FS T2WI shows a large lipohemarthrosis. (e) Anteroposterior (AP) radiograph of the knee shows a fracture of the tibial spines in a skeletally immature patient. (f) Sagittal PDWI from a different patient shows a tibial spine avulsion fracture (arrow) with an intact ACL. (g) Sagittal FS T2WI shows an old tibial spine avulsion fracture with an intact ACL. (h) AP radiograph shows a tibial spine avulsion fracture in a skeletally mature patient.

Table 7.2 (Cont.) Lesions of the knee ligaments

Abnormalities	MRI findings	Comments
Partial ACL tears (▶ Fig. 7.17)	Partial tears of the ACL are often more difficult to accurately diagnose with MRI than complete ACL tears. On FS T2WI there is often thickening of the ACL with heterogeneously increased signal either focally or diffusely throughout the ACL. Other findings of partial ACL tear may include bowing or buckling of ACL fibers and thinning of the ACL with overall fewer fibers than would normally be expected. There may also be associated findings of the typical pattern of bone marrow edema that is seen with complete ACL tears. Evidence of ACL laxity may also be observed. This could include anterior subluxation of the tibia with respect to the femur.	Partial tears of the ACL may or may not be clinically significant. If there is evidence of knee instability in addition to MRI findings of partial ACL tear this would be clinically significant. Conversely, the MRI finding of partial ACL tear in the absence of knee instability is less likely to be clinically significant. In general more severe partial ACL tears are associated with greater knee instability on physical exam.

(continued on page 194)

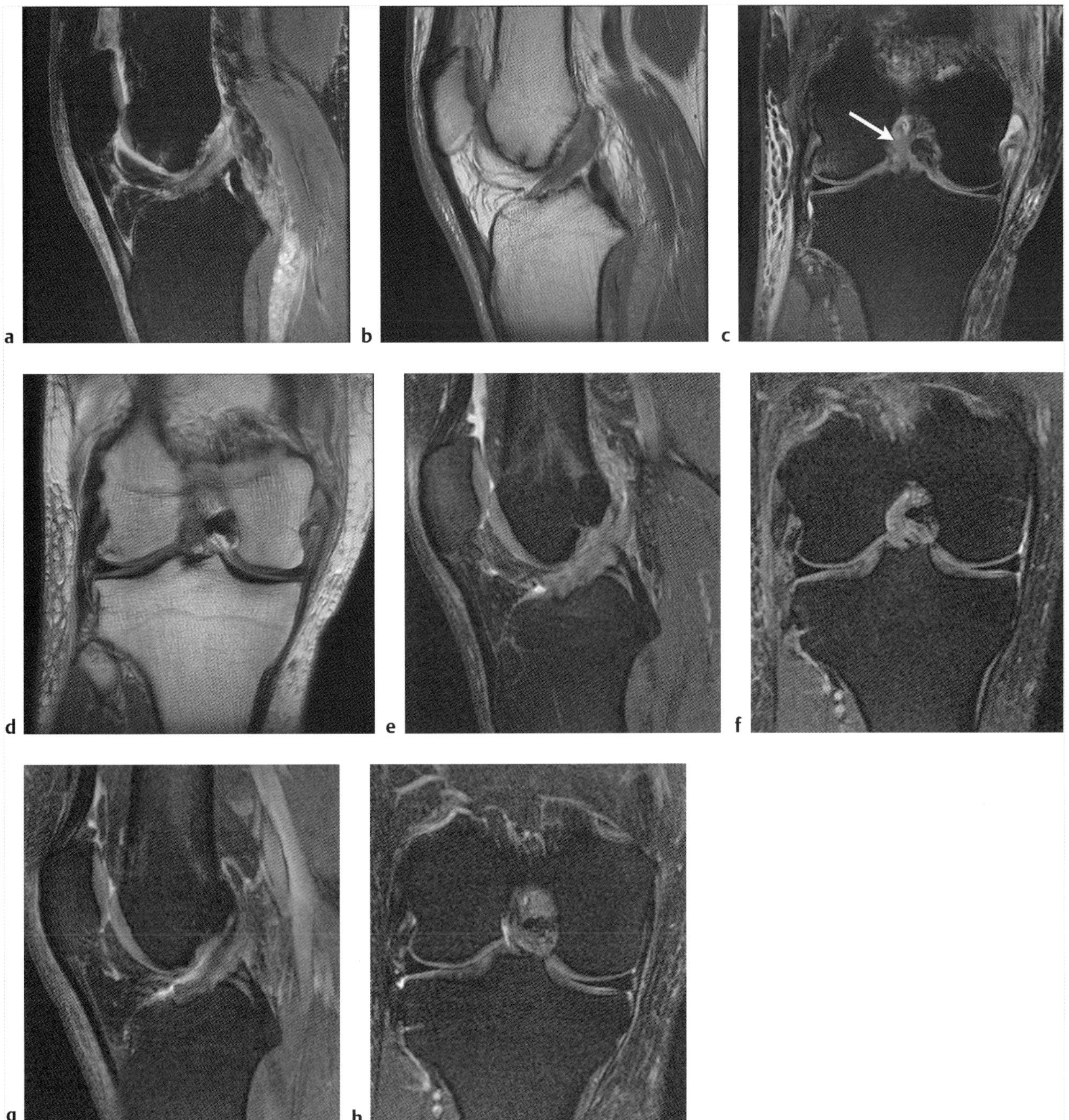

Fig. 7.17 (a) Sagittal fat-suppressed T2-weighted imaging (FS T2WI) shows a thickened partially torn anterior cruciate ligament (ACL) with internal high signal. (b) Sagittal proton density–weighted imaging (PDWI) shows a thickened partially torn ACL with internal high signal. (c) Coronal FS T2WI shows a thickened high signal partially torn ACL (arrow). (d) Coronal PDWI shows a thickened partially torn ACL. (e) Sagittal FS T2WI from a second patient shows high signal in an apparent severe partial ACL tear. (f) Coronal FS T2WI from the same patient shows diffuse high signal in a severe partial ACL tear. (g) Sagittal FS T2WI from the same patient 1 year later shows a marked decrease in signal in the ACL with substantial remaining fibers. (h) Corresponding coronal FS T2WI from the same patient shows evidence for interval healing of the previously partially torn ACL.

Table 7.2 (Cont.) Lesions of the knee ligaments

Abnormalities	MRI findings	Comments
Mucoid cystic degeneration of the ACL and PCL (▶ Fig. 7.18; ▶ Fig. 7.19)	On FS T2WI a rounded high signal structure is seen within the ACL or PCL. These cysts can be seen to be located in between the ACL or PCL fibers such that they are splayed apart. On sagittal images these intraligamentous cysts may have a "drumstick" appearance. These cysts are of variable size and can be seen to occupy a portion of or the majority of the ACL or PCL.	The cysts found in mucoid cystic degeneration of the ACL and PCL are intraligamentous ganglion cysts. These cysts are of unclear clinical significance and etiology. These cysts may be associated with knee pain that in some patients is worsened with activity. In some patients mucoid cystic degeneration may be due to remote prior trauma. However, this is not proven. Some patients may benefit from surgical debridement.

(continued on page 196)

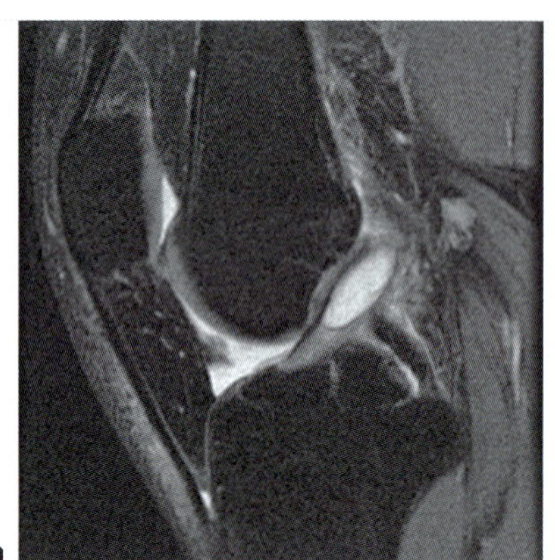
a

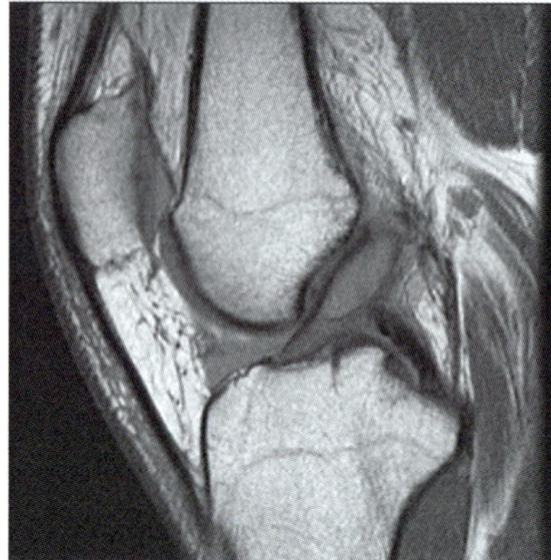
b

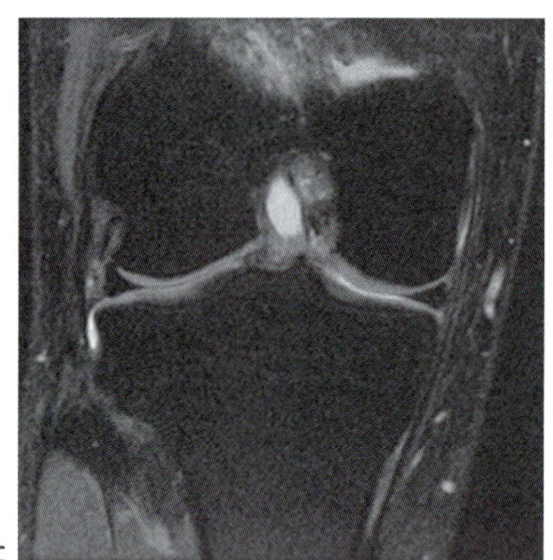
c

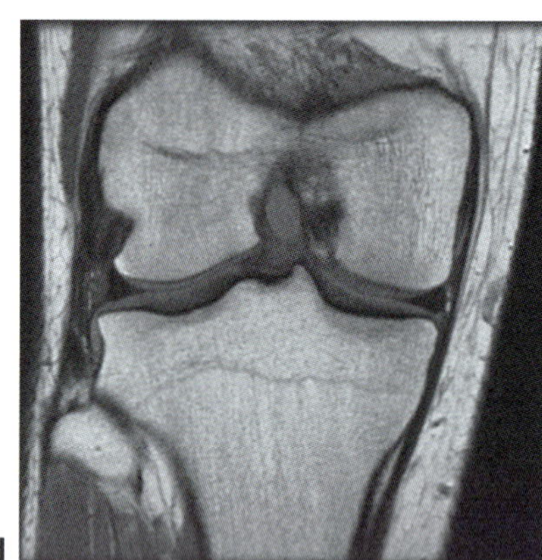
d

Fig. 7.18 (a) Sagittal fat-suppressed T2-weighted imaging (FS T2WI) shows a high signal cystic lesion within the proximal portion of the anterior cruciate ligament (ACL) with a typical "drumstick appearance of the ACL." (b) Sagittal proton density–weighted imaging (PDWI) shows an intermediate signal lesion in the proximal ACL. (c) Coronal FS T2WI shows a high signal cystic lesion in the proximal ACL. (d) Coronal PDWI shows an intermediate signal lesion in the proximal ACL.

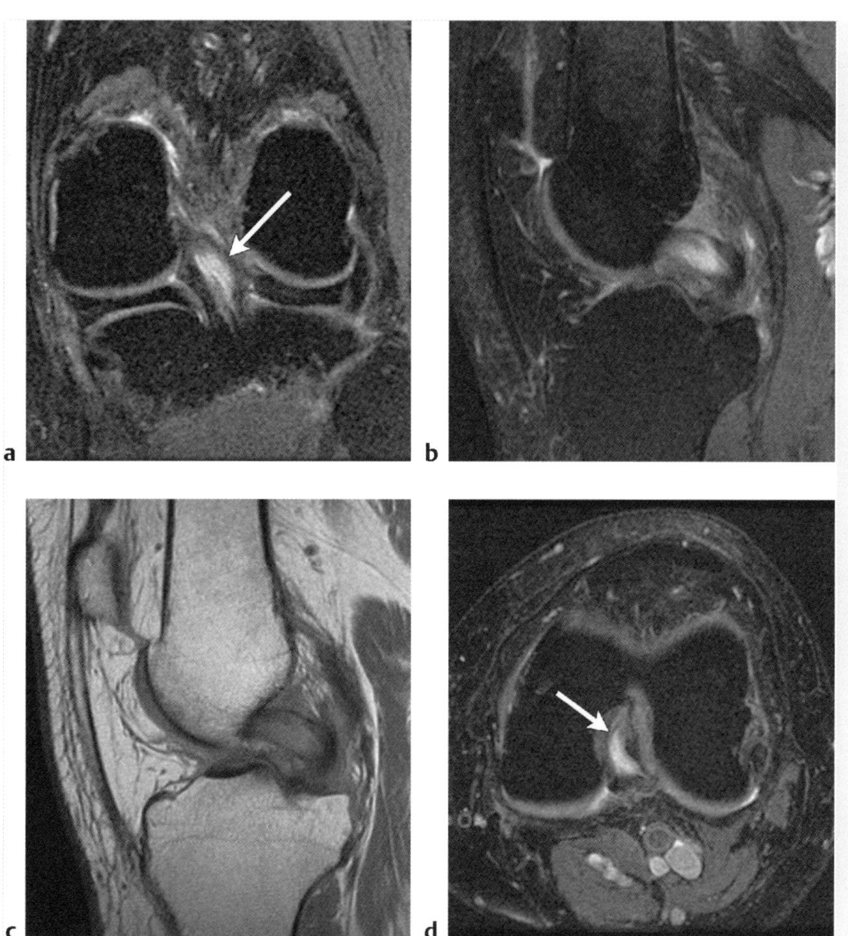

Fig. 7.19 (a) Coronal fat-suppressed T2-weighted imaging (FS T2WI) shows an expanded posterior cruciate ligament (PCL) with high signal separating the ligament fibers (arrow). (b) Sagittal FS T2WI shows a globular high signal in an expanded PCL. (c) Sagittal proton density–weighted imaging (PDWI) shows an intermediate globular signal in an expanded PCL. (d) Axial FS T2WI shows a globular increased signal in an expanded PCL (arrow).

Table 7.2 (Cont.) Lesions of the knee ligaments

Abnormalities	MRI findings	Comments
Postoperative ACL and re-tear (▶ Fig. 7.20; ▶ Fig. 7.21)	The MRI appearance of the repaired ACL is variable depending on the type of repair performed. The major types of ACL repair include ACL allograft, split native patellar tendon, and native semitendinosus/gracilis. The normal ACL repair is uniformly low signal on all MRI sequences. The repaired ACL may be poorly seen on standard MRI sequences such as FS T2WI. This is often the case when ACL allograft repair is performed because there are metallic interference screws placed in the distal femur and proximal tibia. These screws may produce a variable amount of magnetic susceptibility artifact depending on the exact composition and location of the screw. FS T2WI scans are very sensitive to the presence of metal, which will cause localized failure of fat suppression. Short TI inversion recovery (STIR) images are less affected by metal. A new sequence known as IDEAL on GE magnets is the least affected by the presence of metal. This new sequence results in excellent visualization of the ACL graft as well as other structures of the knee that would otherwise be obscured.	In ACL graft re-tears the graft will be disrupted in similar fashion to the native ACL. In addition there are often identical associated findings of typical bone bruise pattern and possibly meniscal and collateral ligament tears. These findings can also be obscured by metal susceptibility artifacts, and metal suppressive sequences such as IDEAL are very helpful in defining the true extent of knee injury. ACL repairs are becoming increasingly common in a wide variety of patient ages. This is likely due to a variety of factors, including older patients engaged in higher levels of athletic activity than in the past and increased overall success of ACL repairs. Unfortunately, ACL re-tears are quite common and are often caused by the same activity and mechanism of injury that resulted in the original ACL tear. In many patients the re-tear will be surgically repaired with similar need to identify any commonly associated injuries, including meniscal tears, cartilaginous injuries, and collateral ligament injuries.

(continued on page 198)

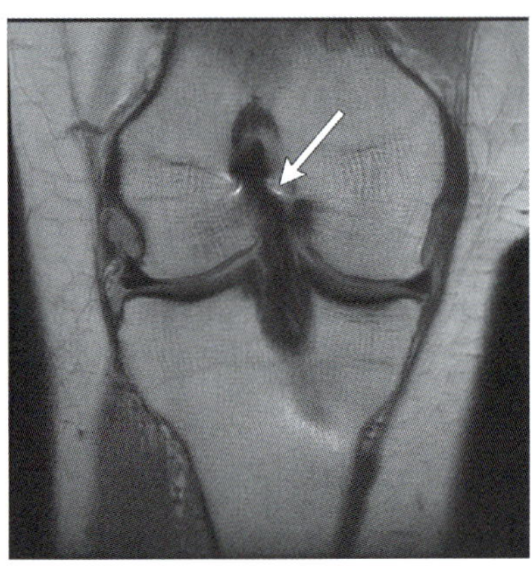

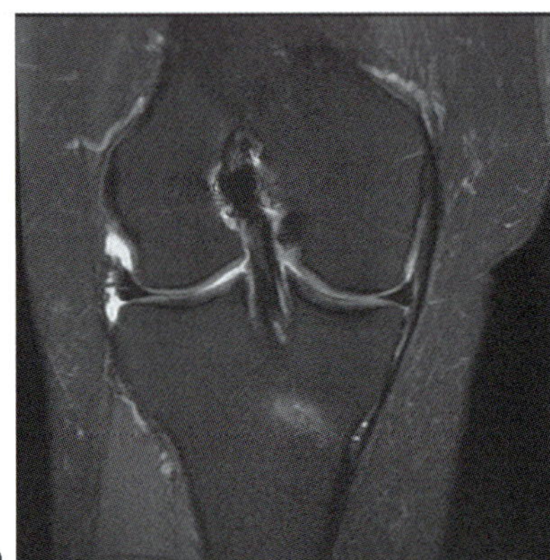

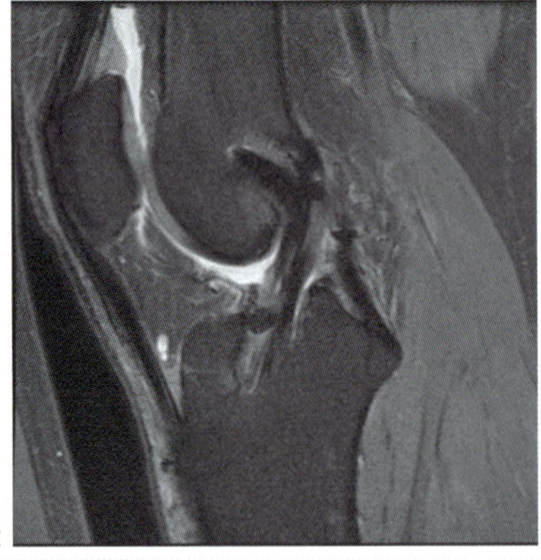

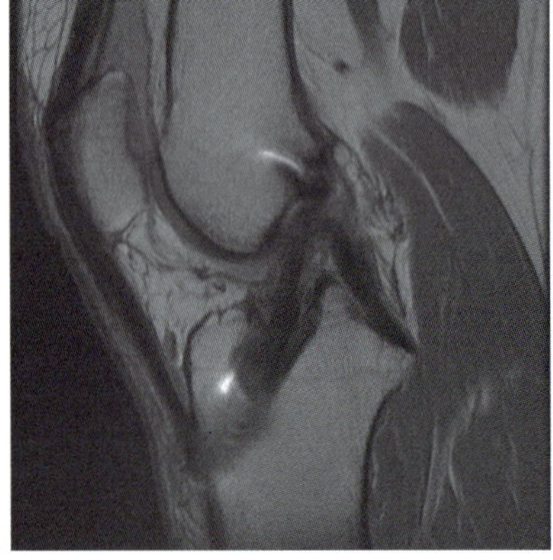

Fig. 7.20 (a) Coronal proton density–weighted imaging (PDWI) shows an intact anterior cruciate ligament (ACL) graft with partial visualization of the femoral and tibial tunnels. Note some expected magnetic susceptibility from interference screws (arrow). (b) Coronal iterative decomposition of water and fat with echo asymmetry and least squares estimation (IDEAL) water image shows an intact low signal ACL graft with markedly reduced magnetic susceptibility artifact compared with conventional FS T2WI. (c) Sagittal IDEAL water image shows an intact low signal ACL graft and a portion of the femoral and tibial tunnels. (d) Sagittal PDWI shows an intact low signal ACL graft.

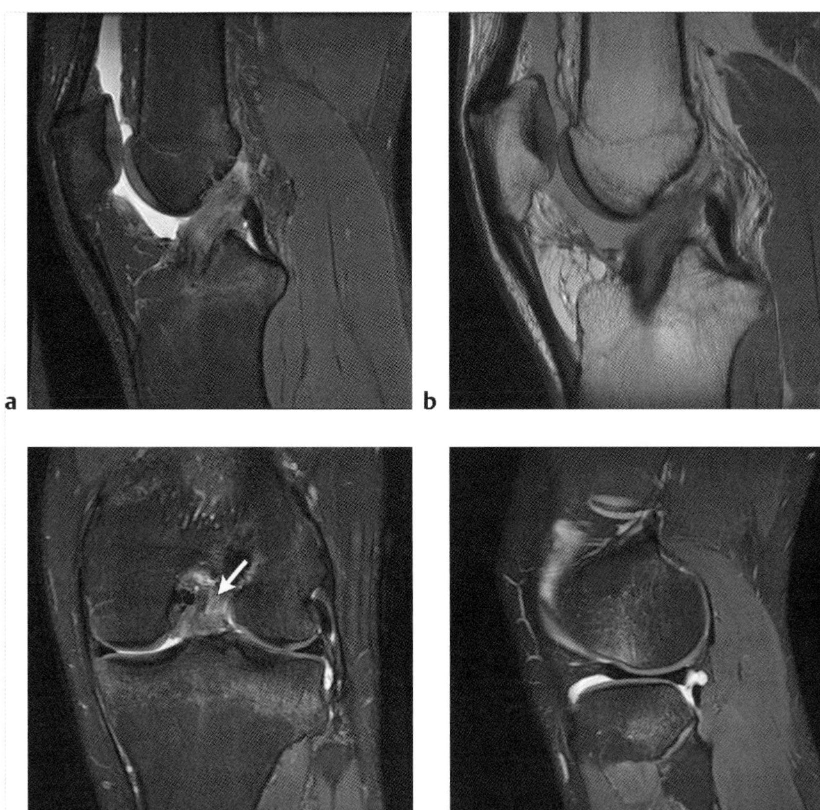

Fig. 7.21 (a) Sagittal iterative decomposition of water and fat with echo asymmetry and least squares estimation (IDEAL) water image shows a thickened high signal torn anterior cruciate ligament (ACL) graft. (b) Sagittal proton density–weighted imaging shows a thickened torn ACL graft. (c) Coronal IDEAL water image shows amorphous high signal material in the expected location of the ACL graft (arrow). (d) Sagittal IDEAL water image shows high signal bone bruises in the lateral femoral condyle and proximal posterior tibia. This is the same pattern of bone bruising seen in acute tears of the native ACL.

Table 7.2 (Cont.) Lesions of the knee ligaments

Abnormalities	MRI findings	Comments
Arthrofibrosis (▶ Fig. 7.22)	The MRI appearance is variable. Most commonly there is a rounded area of mixed heterogeneous signal on FS T2WI located anterior to the ACL graft and in or adjacent to Hoffa fat. On PDWI the abnormality is often heterogeneous low signal. This abnormality is best seen in the sagittal plane. The zone of abnormal signal is caused by postoperative scar formation and when viewed arthroscopically is referred to as a cyclops lesion.	Arthrofibrosis may cause a combination of pain and decreased range of motion in patients who have had prior ACL reconstruction. In some cases surgery is required.

(continued on page 200)

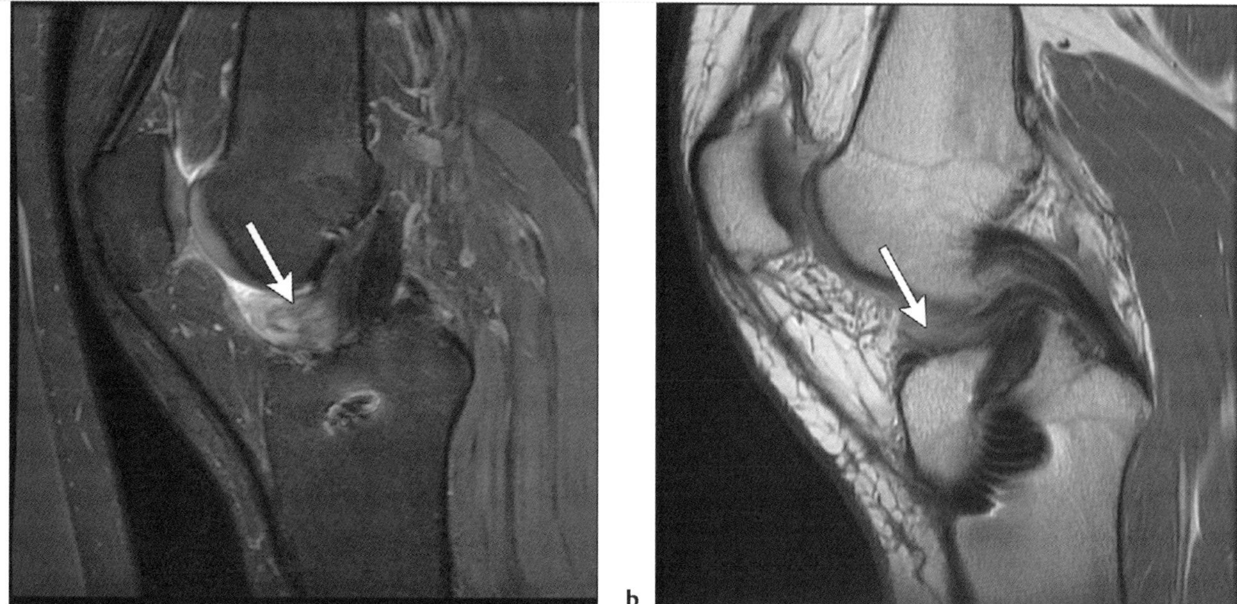

Fig. 7.22 (a) Sagittal fat-suppressed T2-weighted imaging shows a mixed high signal rounded structure anterior to the anterior cruciate ligament graft consistent with a cyclops lesion (arrow). (b) Sagittal proton density–weighted imaging shows a mixed signal structure anterior to the cruciate ligaments consistent with a cyclops lesion (arrow).

Table 7.2 (Cont.) Lesions of the knee ligaments

Abnormalities	MRI findings	Comments
PCL tears (▶ Fig. 7.23; ▶ Fig. 7.24; ▶ Fig. 7.25)	The normal PCL is low signal throughout its course on all pulse sequences. In some patients there may be subtle variation in signal in the proximal third of the PCL, possibly related to magic angle phenomenon. The PCL is best evaluated on sagittal images. The normal PCL may appear thickened in its middle third on sagittal plane images. This is due to adjacent meniscofemoral ligaments of Humphrey (anterior to the PCL) and Wrisberg (posterior to the PCL). Most tears of the PCL are complete and appear as discontinuity of the ligament. In some cases the PCL is not visualized at all. Partial tears of the PCL can occur and have variable appearance. A common appearance of partial PCL tear is heterogeneous increased signal within the substance of the PCL on FS T2WI and proton density–weighted imaging (PDWI) with intact borders along the anterior and posterior margins. Mucoid cystic change can also occur in the PCL and has a similar appearance to mucoid cystic degeneration of the ACL.	PCL tears are less common than ACL tears. Most PCL tears occur in high-level athletes such as college and professional football players or as a result of car accidents with the flexed knee striking the dashboard. The PCL is a stronger ligament than the ACL, and injuries require more force than is seen in the ACL. PCL injuries are also commonly associated with other injuries including fracture and injury of the posterolateral corner. PCL tears occur in true knee dislocations (femoral tibial dislocation). If this is suspected the popliteal artery should be carefully evaluated, with absence of the normal popliteal signal void raising suspicion for a possible posttraumatic dissection. The frequency of PCL reconstruction is much lower than that of ACL reconstruction. PCL reconstruction is usually reserved for high-level athletes. Some patients with PCL tears may be asymptomatic and unaware that the ligament is torn. PCL tears do predispose to early-onset osteoarthritis.

(continued on page 202)

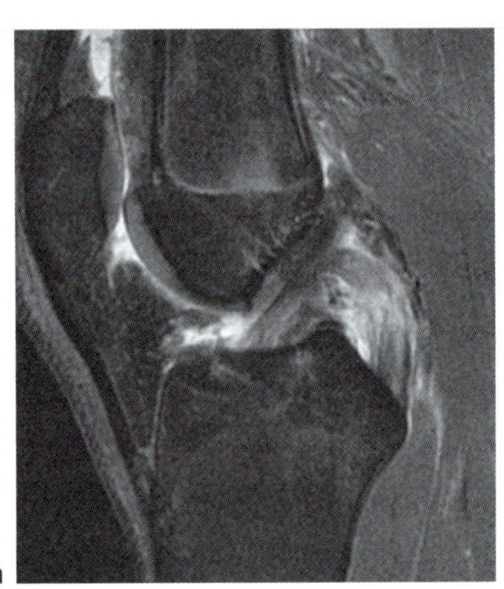
a

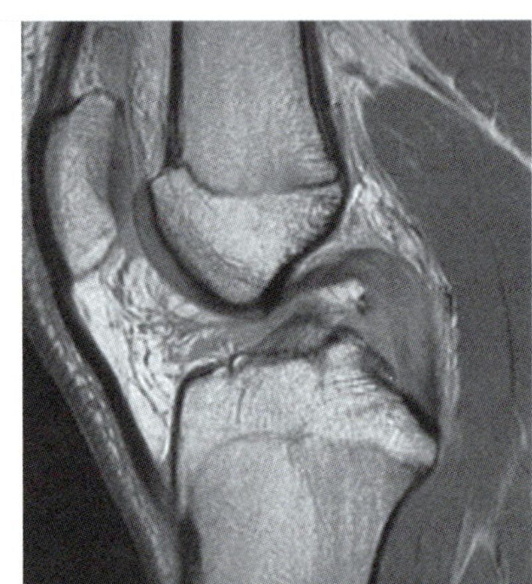
b

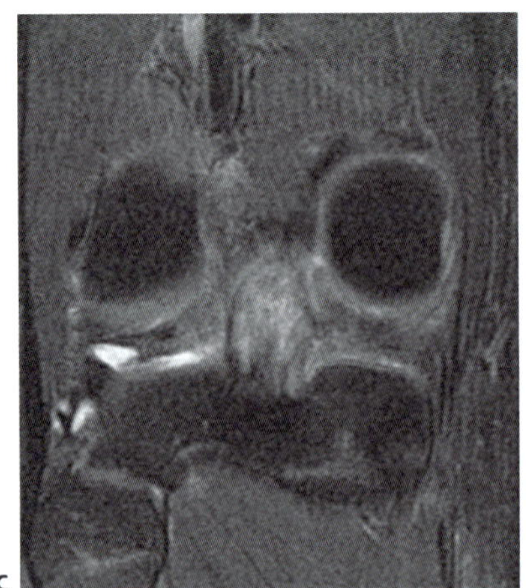
c

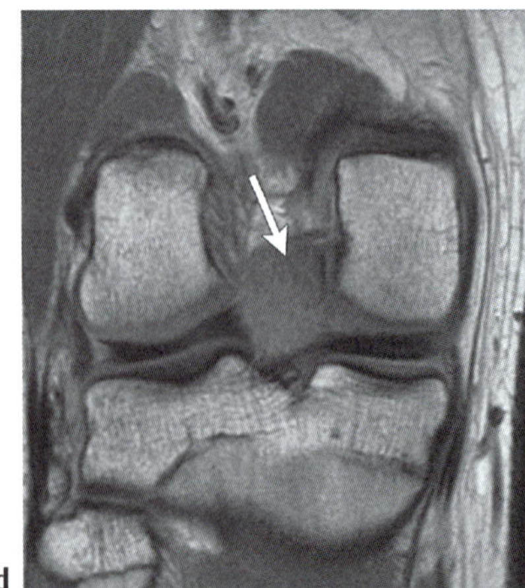
d

Fig. 7.23 (a) Sagittal fat-suppressed T2-weighted imaging (FS T2WI) shows a thickened high signal posterior cruciate ligament (PCL) with disruption of fibers. (b) Sagittal proton density–weighted imaging (PDWI) shows a thickened heterogeneous PCL with disruption of fibers. (c) Coronal FS T2WI shows a high signal PCL with disrupted fibers. (d) Coronal PDWI shows amorphous remnants of a disrupted PCL (arrow).

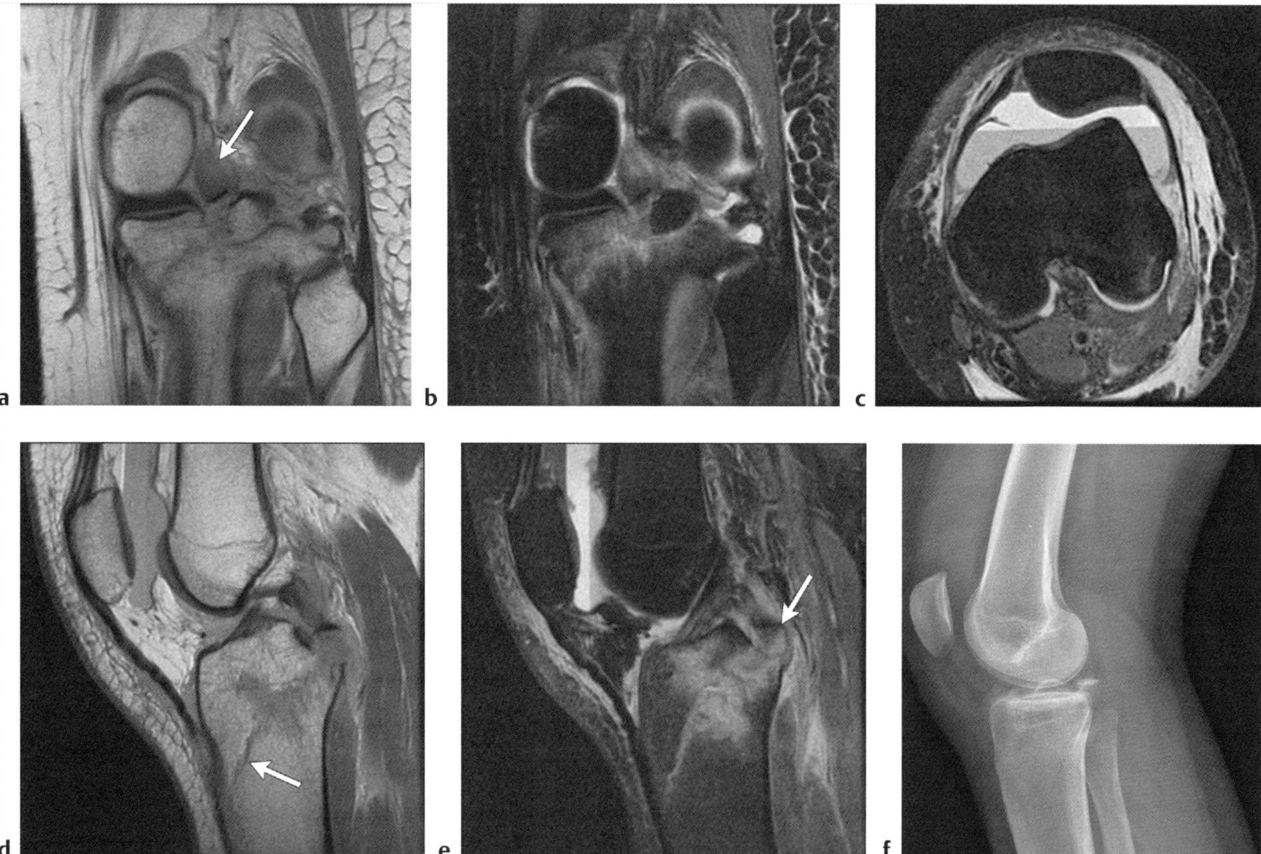

Fig. 7.24 (a) Coronal proton density–weighted imaging (PDWI) shows a torn posterior cruciate ligament (PCL) with an attached avulsion fracture of the tibial spine (arrow). (b) Coronal fat-suppressed T2-weighted imaging (FS T2WI) shows a torn, ill-defined PCL attached to an avulsed fracture of the tibial spine. Note extensive marrow edema of the adjacent proximal tibia. (c) Axial FS T2WI shows a large lipohemarthrosis. (d) Sagittal PDWI shows a PCL tear with an attached avulsion fracture fragment. There is also an intramedullary fracture of the proximal tibia (low signal line extending obliquely and inferiorly toward the anterior tibial cortex (arrow). (e) Sagittal FS T2WI shows a PCL tear with an attached avulsed fracture fragment (arrow) and adjacent marrow edema with an oblique high signal intramedullary fracture of the proximal tibia. Note the lipohemarthrosis. (f) Lateral radiograph shows a displaced avulsion fracture of the proximal posterior tibia. There is also a large joint effusion.

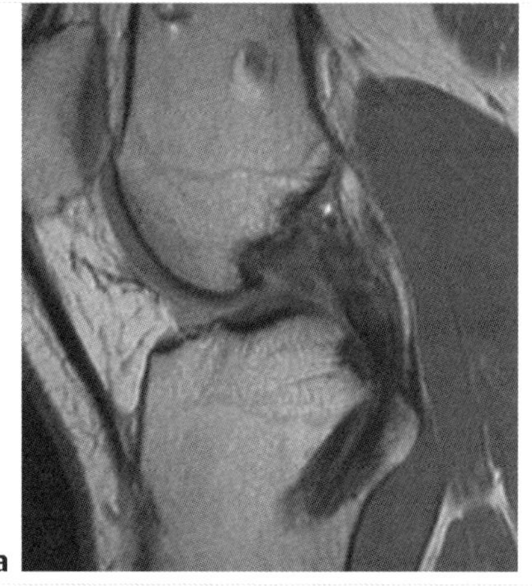

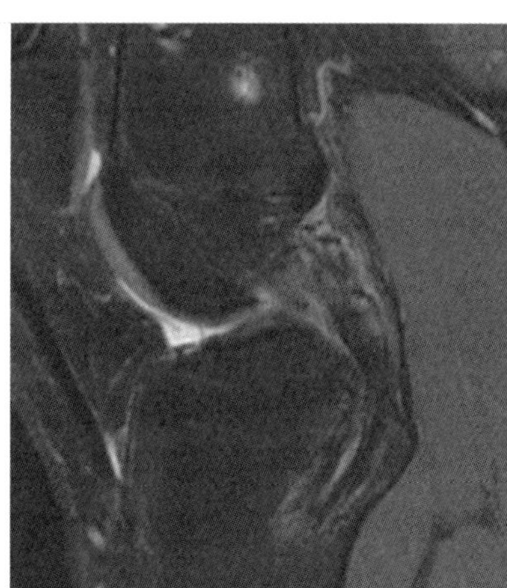

Fig. 7.25 (a) Sagittal proton density–weighted imaging shows an intact posterior cruciate ligament (PCL) graft with foci of magnetic susceptibility artifact related to the presence of metal. (b) Sagittal fat-suppressed T2-weighted imaging shows an intact PCL graft with some adjacent magnetic susceptibility artifact.

Table 7.2 (Cont.) Lesions of the knee ligaments

Abnormalities	MRI findings	Comments
Medial collateral ligament (MCL) tears (▶ Fig. 7.26; ▶ Fig. 7.27; ▶ Fig. 7.28)	The normal anatomy of the MCL is complicated, with both deep and superficial components. The MCL is well seen on coronal plane images and is low signal on both PDWI and FS T2WI. Tears of the deep fibers are common and of lesser significance than tears of the superficial fibers. Tears of the MCL may be partial or complete. Partial tears usually have increased edema signal surrounding the ligament on coronal FS T2WI with intact low signal ligament fibers. A more severe partial tear has surrounding edema and increased signal within the substance of the ligament as seen on FS T2WI. Complete tears of the MCL reveal disruption of the ligament fibers with surrounding edema. Most tears occur near the proximal femoral attachment of the MCL with tears of the midsubstance and distal tibial attachment of the MCL occurring less frequently. Chronic injuries of the MCL are also commonly seen on MRI exams of the knee. Old partial tears are seen as low signal thickened ligaments on coronal plane PDWI and FS T2WI. In some cases old injuries of the MCL may be seen on radiographs as calcification in the expected location of the MCL (Pellegrini-Stieda disease).	Injuries of the MCL are common and typically occur in athletes participating in football or skiing. Patients often complain of medial knee pain and may demonstrate instability with valgus stress. MCL injuries are often associated with other injuries including meniscal tears and ACL tears. Most patients with MCL injuries do not require surgery. The severity of the injury will often correlate with the length of time required before the patient can resume full activity and return to sport.

(continued on page 204)

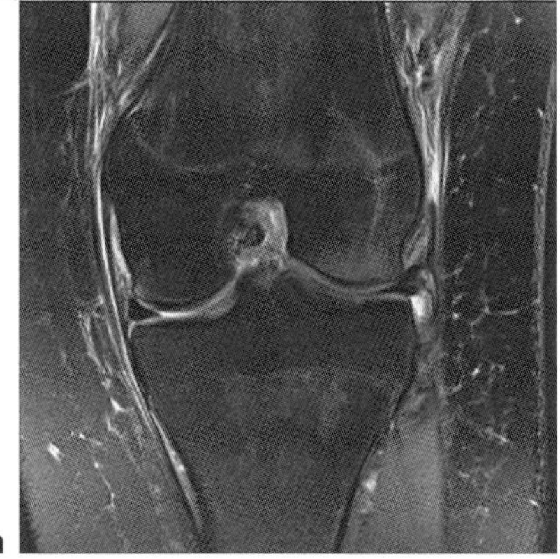
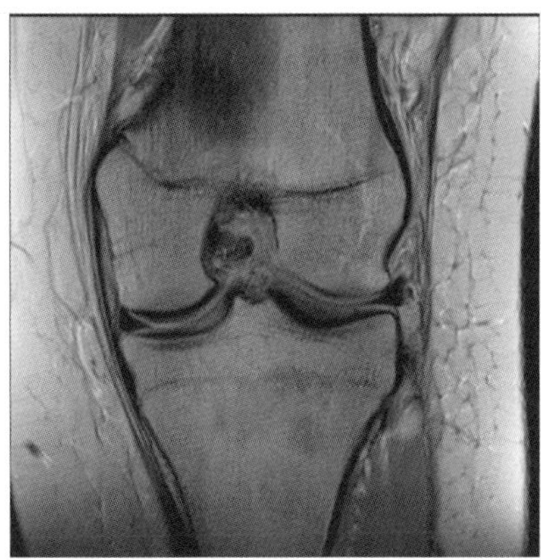

Fig. 7.26 (a) Coronal fat-suppressed T2-weighted imaging shows high signal fluid on both sides of an intact medial collateral ligament (MCL). This is a sprain of the MCL. (b) Coronal proton density–weighted imaging shows intermediate signal fluid on both sides of an intact MCL.

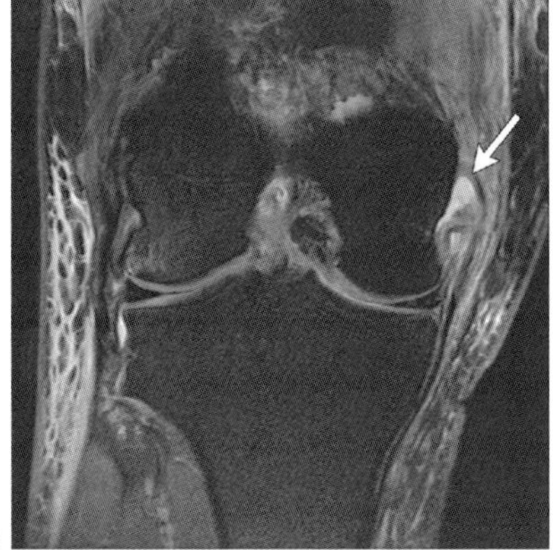
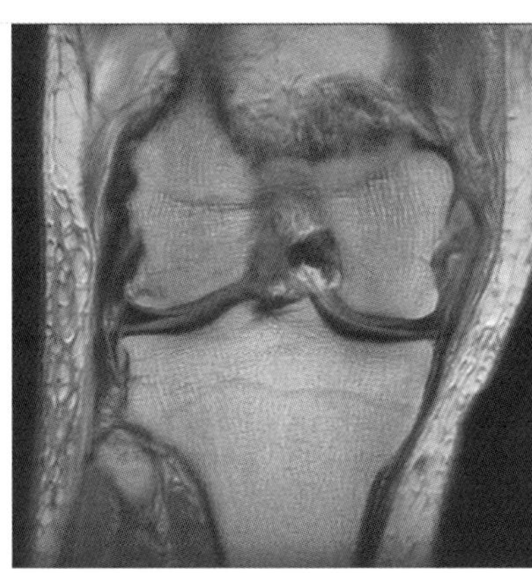

Fig. 7.27 (a) Coronal fat-suppressed T2-weighted imaging shows a high signal thickened partially torn proximal medial collateral ligament (MCL) (arrow). (b) Coronal proton density–weighted imaging shows a thickened partially torn proximal MCL.

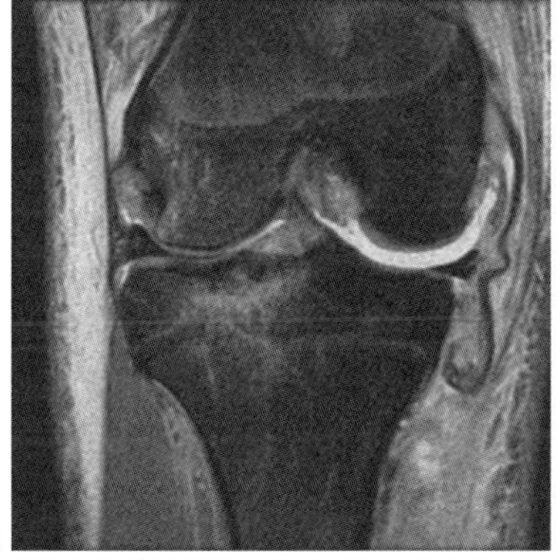
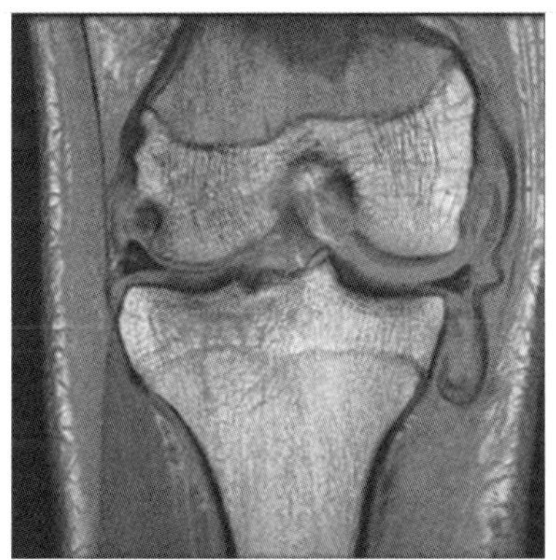
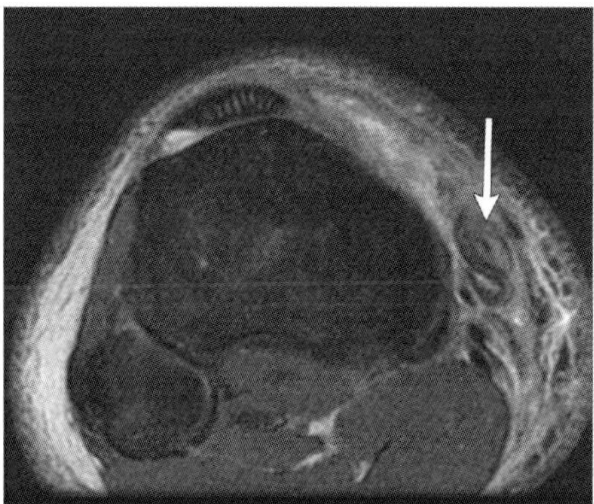

Fig. 7.28 (a) Coronal fat-suppressed T2-weighted imaging (FS T2WI) shows a redundant ruptured medial collateral ligament (MCL) with bone bruises in the lateral femoral condyle and proximal lateral tibia. (b) Coronal proton density–weighted imaging (PDWI) shows a redundant ruptured MCL. (c) Axial FS T2WI shows a high signal thickened torn MCL (arrow).

Table 7.2 (Cont.) Lesions of the knee ligaments

Abnormalities	MRI findings	Comments
Lateral collateral ligament (LCL) complex tears (▶ Fig. 7.29; ▶ Fig. 7.30)	The LCL complex is composed of several structures with the most important consisting of the fibular collateral ligament (the true LCL), the biceps femoris tendon, and the iliotibial band. In addition there are two other structures that are not normally always seen; the arcuate ligament and the popliteofibular ligament. In general the coronal plane is best for evaluating the LCL complex. The fibular collateral ligament, iliotibial band, biceps femoris, and popliteofibular ligament are well seen as dark signal linear bands on PDWI and FS T2WI. The axial plane is best for evaluating the arcuate ligament if it can be seen at all. The normal arcuate ligament is a dark signal band on PDWI and FS T2WI in the expected location of the posterior capsule. FS T2WI is best for identifying abnormalities of the LCL complex. Minor injuries including sprains will appear as high signal on both sides of the abnormal structure. Tears are seen as discontinuity of the ligament. The posterolateral corner is a subset of the LCL complex with the most important components consisting of the fibular collateral ligament, biceps femoris tendon, arcuate ligament, and popliteofibular ligament.	LCL complex injuries are less common than MCL injuries. Injuries of the more posterior structures, including the fibular collateral ligament, biceps femoris tendon, and arcuate ligament are more likely to cause clinically significant loss of knee stability and increased knee pain. Posterior LCL ligament complex injuries (also known as posterolateral corner injuries) often occur in association with cruciate ligament injuries. The combination of cruciate tear and postererolateral corner injury often requires surgery, and the surgeon needs to know this information because ACL grafts are thought to fail more often if the there is an untreated simultaneous posterolateral corner tear. Typical causes of LCL complex injuries include sports and motor vehicle accidents.
Iliotibial (IT) band syndrome (▶ Fig. 7.31)	The IT band is the anterior portion of the LCL complex and is normally well seen on coronal images as a well-defined low signal band attaching to the anterior portion of the distal tibia. The normal IT band passes close to the anterior portion of the lateral femoral condyle (LFC). In IT band syndrome there is increased fluid seen between the IT band and the anterior portion of the lateral femoral condyle. On coronal FS T2WI high signal fluid is seen replacing the low signal normal fat between the IT band and the anterior LFC.	IT band syndrome often presents as anterolateral knee pain in a patient with a history of running. There is increased incidence in runners with recent significant increase in running distance. The cause of this syndrome is friction between the IT band and the LFC.

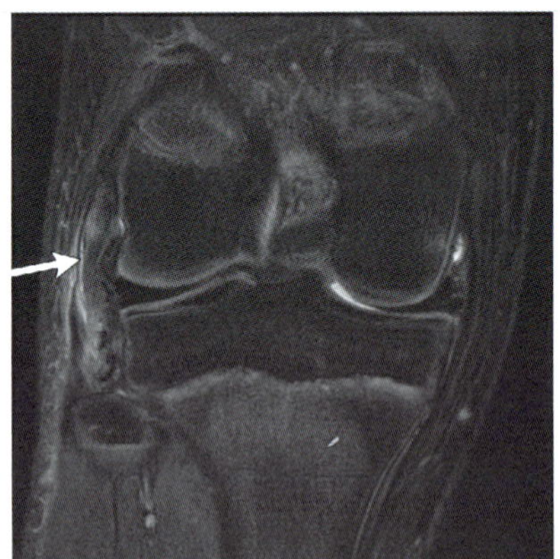

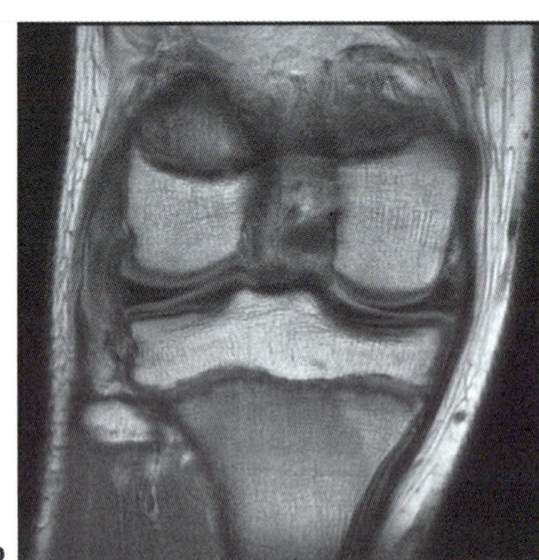

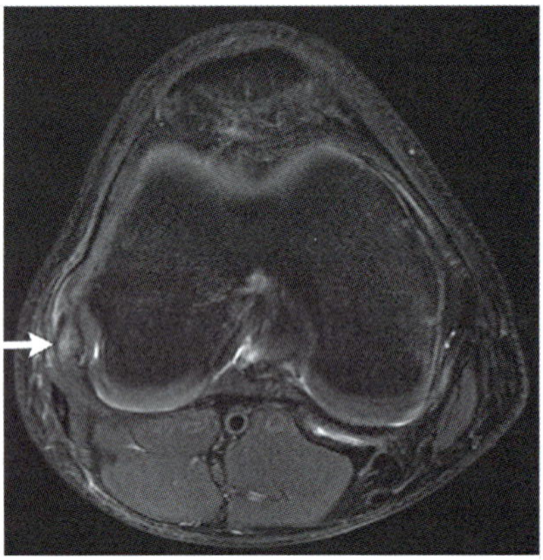

Fig. 7.29 (a) Coronal fat-suppressed T2-weighted imaging (FS T2WI) shows a thickened high signal fibular collateral ligament that is torn distally (arrow). (b) Coronal proton density–weighted imaging shows a thickened torn fibular collateral ligament. (c) Axial FS T2WI shows a thickened high signal torn fibular collateral ligament (arrow).

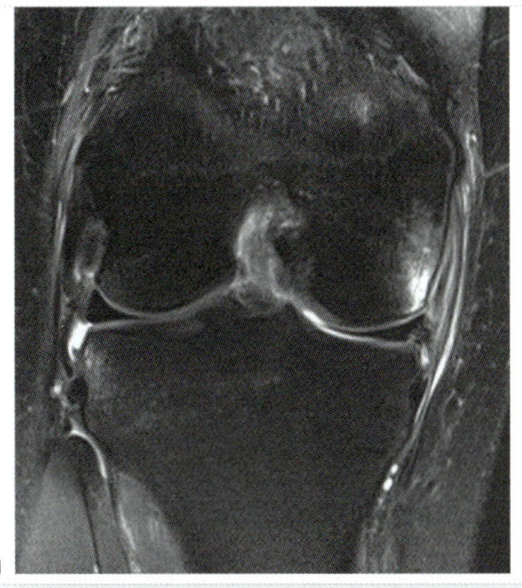

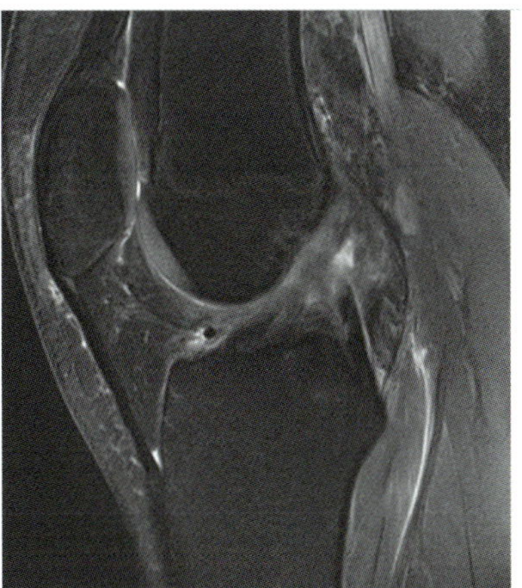

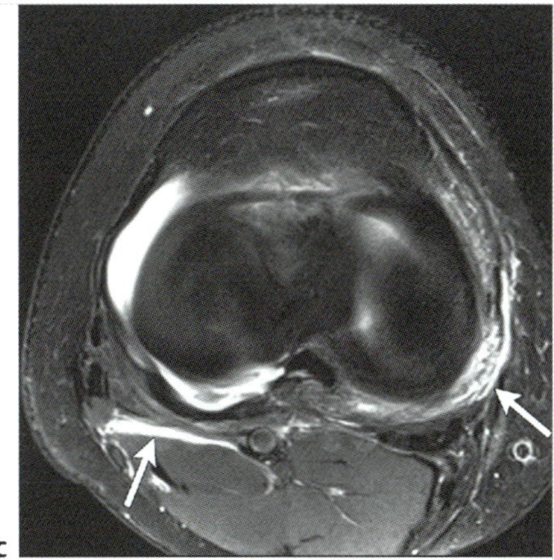

Fig. 7.30 (a) Coronal fat-suppressed T2-weighted imaging (FS T2WI) shows a torn anterior cruciate ligament (ACL) with remnant fibers in the intercondylar notch. There is also a high grade medial collateral ligament (MCL) tear and bone contusions in the medial femoral condyle and proximal tibia. (b) Sagittal FS T2WI shows a torn ACL with some remnant fibers in the intercondylar notch. (c) Axial FS T2WI shows fluid posterolaterally beyond the margins of the joint capsule (arrow) indicating a tear of the arcuate ligament, which is a component of the posterolateral corner. There is also fluid posteromedially (arrow), which is seen in posteromedial corner injuries.

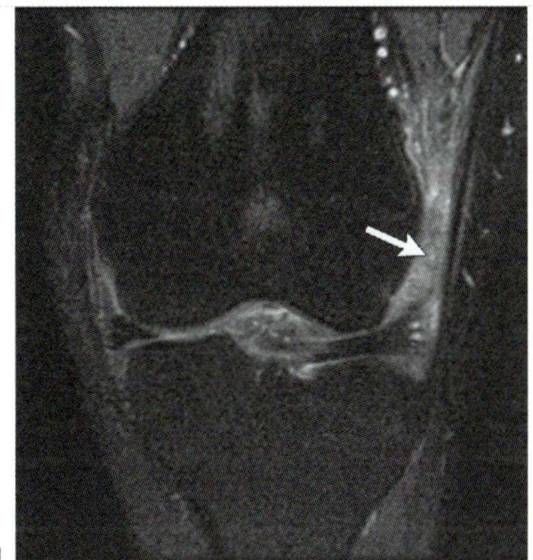

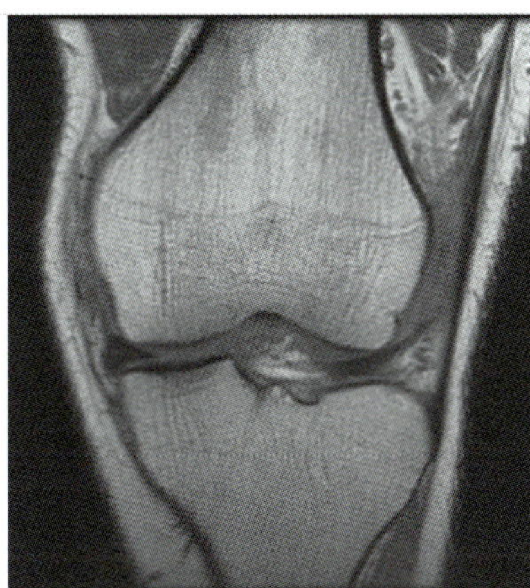

Fig. 7.31 (a) Coronal fat-suppressed T2-weighted imaging (FS T2WI) shows heterogeneous high signal fluid between the anterior lateral femur and iliotibial band (arrow). (b) Coronal proton density–weighted imaging shows intermediate signal fluid between the anterior lateral femoral condyle and the iliotibial band.

7.2.1 Lesions of the Knee Ligaments Suggested Reading

[1] Casagranda BU, Maxwell NJ, Kavanagh EC, Towers JD, Shen W, Fu FH. Normal appearance and complications of double-bundle and selective-bundle anterior cruciate ligament reconstructions using optimal MRI techniques [published correction in AJR Am J Roentgenol 2009;192(6):1454. Casagranda, Bethany C corrected to Casagranda, Bethany U]. AJR Am J Roentgenol 2009; 192: 1407–1415

[2] Davis KW. Imaging pediatric sports injuries: lower extremity. Radiol Clin North Am 2010; 48: 1213–1235

[3] Lintz F, Pujol N, Boisrenoult P, Bargoin K, Beaufils P, Dejour D. Anterior cruciate ligament mucoid degeneration: a review of the literature and management guidelines. Knee Surg Sports Traumatol Arthrosc 2011; 19: 1326–1333

[4] Pacheco RJ, Ayre CA, Bollen SR. Posterolateral corner injuries of the knee: a serious injury commonly missed. J Bone Joint Surg Br 2011; 93: 194–197

[5] Rodriguez W, Vinson EN, Helms CA, Toth AP. MRI appearance of posterior cruciate ligament tears. AJR Am J Roentgenol 2008; 191: 1031

[6] Van Dyck P, Vanhoenacker FM, Gielen JL, et al. Three tesla magnetic resonance imaging of the anterior cruciate ligament of the knee: can we differentiate complete from partial tears? Skeletal Radiol 2011; 40: 701–707

7.3 Cartilage Lesions of the Knee

- Cartilage defects
- Osteochondral injuries
- Osteochondritis dissecans

Table 7.3 Cartilage lesions of the knee

Abnormalities	MRI findings	Comments
Cartilage defects (▸ Fig. 7.32)	The appearance of normal cartilage on MRI is dependent on which type of MRI sequence is used. Currently fat-suppressed T2-weighted imaging (FS T2WI) is widely used to examine cartilage. The cartilage is easily identified as the structure of intermediate signal between dark cortical bone and bright fluid. Proton density–weighted imaging (PDWI) is also useful, with cartilage well seen as higher signal than the adjacent cortical bone. Cartilage defects are of several types and well seen on FS T2WI. Cartilage defects may be acute or chronic. Cartilage fissures are linear high signal defects extending from the articular surface partially or fully to the cortical bone. When there are many cartilage fissures this is referred to as cartilage fibrillation. An ulcer of cartilage is a contour defect arising from the cartilage articular surface and extending to a variable depth though not to the cortical bone. A full-thickness defect is a focal or diffuse complete loss of articular cartilage. Cartilage defects are often associated with adjacent subcortical marrow edema and subcortical geodes. The axial, coronal and sagittal planes are needed to fully evaluate the cartilage of the patellofemoral, medial, and lateral knee compartments.	Cartilage may be injured acutely or chronically over many years. Acute injuries of cartilage often result in focal partial- or full-thickness defects and are often associated with injury to other components of the knee. Often the adjacent subchondral bone may be injured acutely as well. Transient patellar dislocation is a typical example of a mechanism of possible acute cartilage injury of the patella. In this case the cartilage may be normal, or damaged with partial- or full-thickness defect or even an osteochondral fracture. Chronic cartilage injuries may also be partial or full thickness. Typical patterns of chronic injury are fibrillation and surface ulceration. Over time the joint compartment may progressively narrow with increasing loss of cartilage. Other typical findings include subchondral sclerosis, subcortical geodes, and subcortical degenerative reactive marrow edema, often on both sides of the affected joint compartment. The overall appearance is typical of osteoarthritis. One common cause of this type of gradual joint degeneration is a meniscal tear in which there is loss of the normal hoop strength. This results in loss of the normal cushioning with increased abnormal stresses on the articular cartilage. Over time the cartilage may suffer a gradual degeneration progressing from minor partial-thickness loss to severe full-thickness loss. Not all patients with cartilage injury go on to progressive worsening. Options for patients needing surgery for cartilage defects include microfracture of the underlying bone, which results in formation of a blood clot. Within this clot there are some stem cells that differentiate into chondroblasts. Ultimately, there is some restoration of the overlying cartilage, although this new cartilage is usually inferior to the original cartilage. Another type of repair is cartilage implantation, which may be performed with an autogenic or allogenic graft.

(continued on page 208)

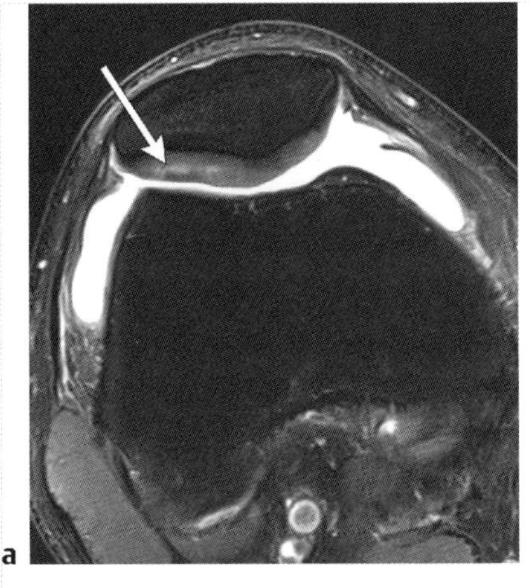

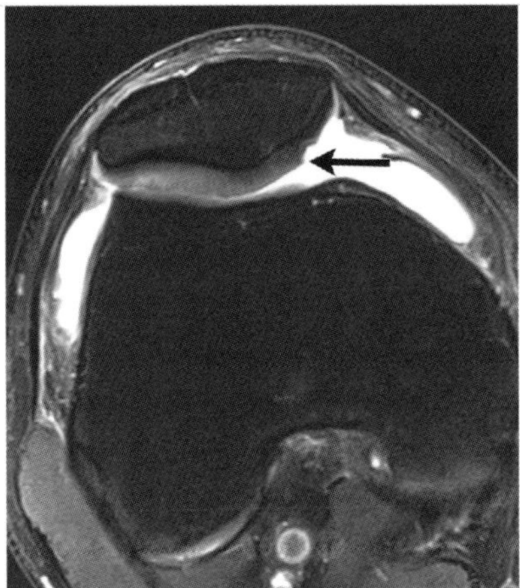

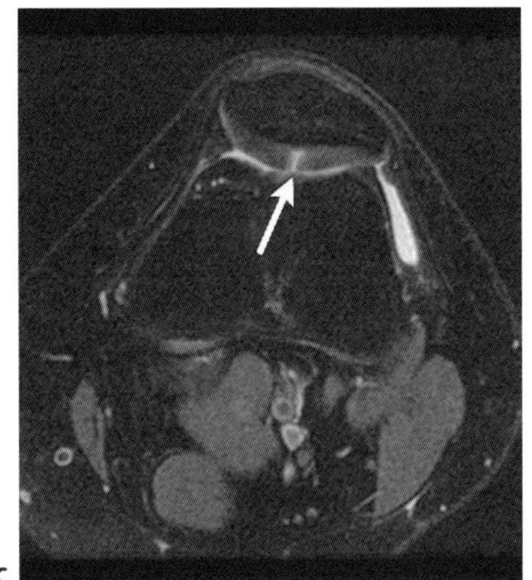

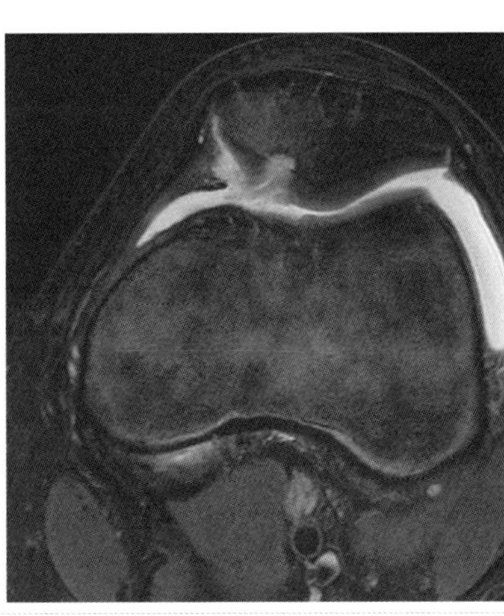

Fig. 7.32 (a) Axial fat-suppressed T2-weighted imaging (FS T2WI) shows increased signal in the substance of the lateral patellar facet cartilage (arrow). The articular surface remains intact. This is the earliest identifiable abnormality of cartilage with magnetic resonance imaging. (b) Axial FS T2WI from a second patient shows a surface ulcer of the medial patellar facet cartilage (arrow). (c) Axial FS T2WI from a third patient shows a high signal fissure of cartilage at the patellar vertex (arrow). (d) Axial FS T2WI from a fourth patient shows a full-thickness defect of the medial facet patellar articular cartilage.

Table 7.3 (Cont.) Cartilage lesions of the knee

Abnormalities	MRI findings	Comments
Osteochondral injuries (▶ Fig. 7.33)	An osteochondral injury is any injury in which both articular cartilage and the adjacent underlying bone are injured. Examples include osteochondral fractures in which a fragment of both bone and cartilage forms a loose body with a readily identifiable donor site defect. This type of injury is common and may occur in transient patellar dislocation. In this situation a fragment containing both bone and cartilage may be fractured off the medial patellar facet resulting in a loose osteochondral fragment, which on fat-suppressed T2-weighted imaging (FS T2WI) has typical low signal cortical bone with overlying intermediate signal cartilage. The donor site is easily identified by the presence of a contour defect in the medial patellar facet and adjacent high signal marrow edema. Because there is cortical fracture a lipohemarthrosis is often identified. A less severe example of osteochondral injury is a cortical impaction with injury of the overlying cartilage. This pattern of injury is often seen in the lateral femoral condyle in patients with acute anterior cruciate ligament (ACL) tears. On FS T2WI there is contour deformity of the impacted lateral femoral condyle articular surface with adjacent high signal subcortical marrow edema.	Osteochondral injuries can be acute or chronic. Osteochondral injuries are often associated with knee pain or decreased range of motion or both. Some patients with osteochondral injury may go on to develop progressive osteoarthritis of the affected joint compartment(s). In some patients a loose osteochondral fracture fragment can be reattached surgically.

(continued on page 210)

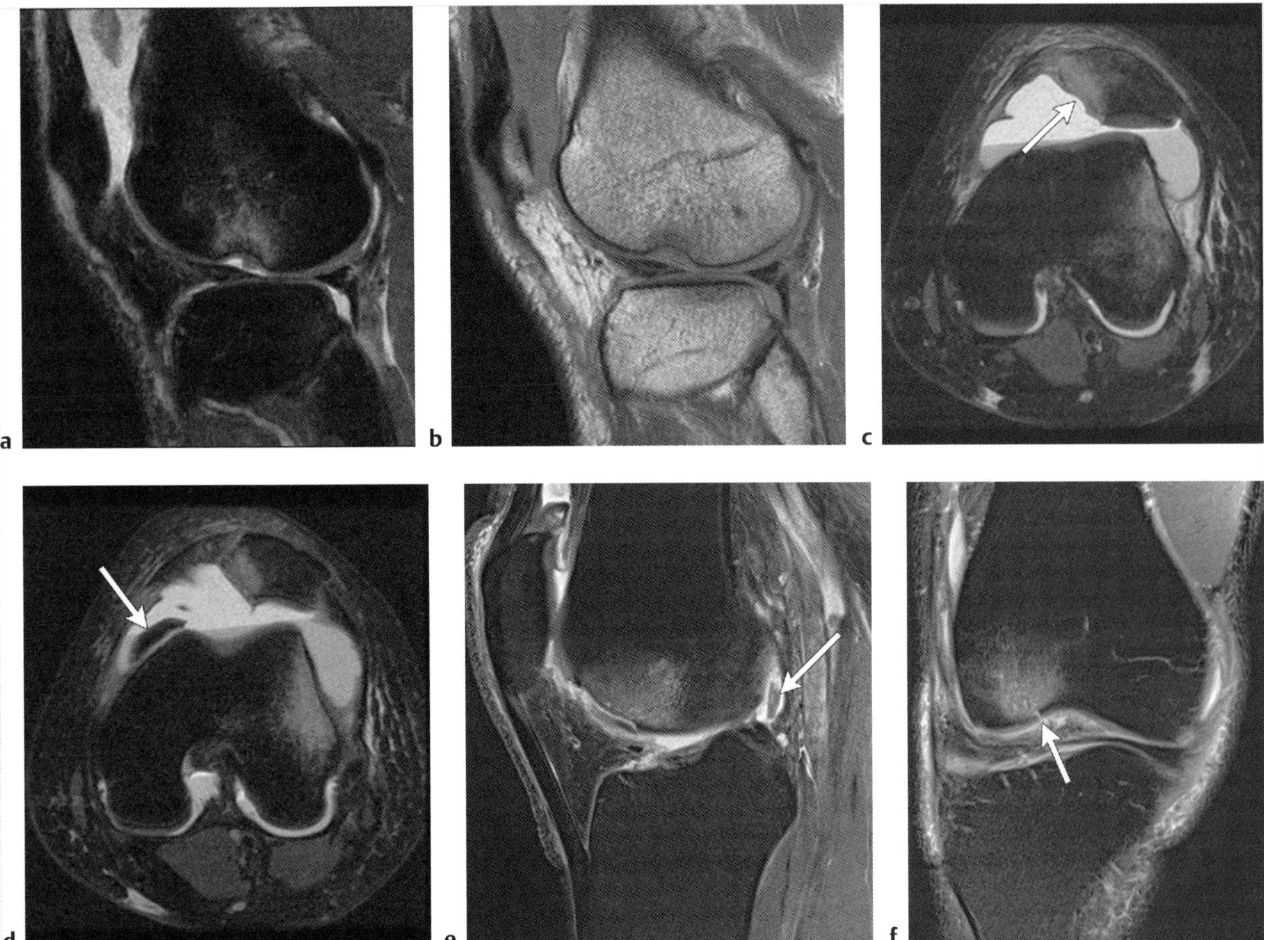

Fig. 7.33 (a) Sagittal fat-suppressed T2-weighted imaging (FS T2WI) shows osteochondral injury of the lateral femoral condyle with a large subcortical impaction, adjacent marrow edema, and irregular overlying cartilage with some fragmentation. (b) Corresponding proton density–weighted imaging (PDWI) shows deep cortical impaction of the lateral femoral condyle (LFC). (c) Axial FS T2WI from a second patient shows an osteochondral fracture of the medial patellar facet with osteocartilagenous defect (arrow) and lipohemarthrosis in a patient with patellar dislocation. (d) Axial FS T2WI from the same patient shows a displaced osteocartilagenous fragment adjacent to the anterior aspect of the medial femoral condyle (MFC) (arrow). Note the typical bone contusion pattern of patellar dislocation, which includes the medial patella and anterior LFC. (e) Sagittal FS T2WI from a third patient shows fluid undermining a mildly displaced osteochondral fracture of the LFC anteriorly. There is extensive high signal marrow contusion in the adjacent LFC. Note a small cartilage loose body posteriorly (arrow). (f) Coronal FS T2WI from the same patient shows the same osteochondral fracture (arrow) of the anterior LFC with adjacent high signal marrow contusion.

Table 7.3 (Cont.) Cartilage lesions of the knee

Abnormalities	MRI findings	Comments
Osteochondritis dissecans (▶ Fig. 7.34)	The appearance of osteochondritis dissecans on MRI depends on the stage in which it is observed. In stage 1 there is focal subchondral marrow edema, which is seen as high signal on FS T2WI. The overlying cartilage is abnormal but intact. In stage 2 there is high signal edema with a central subchondral cyst seen on FS T2WI. In stage 3 there is a high signal line on FS T2WI seen surrounding the osteochondral fragment, which remains in place. There can be some fragmentation of the bony portion of the osteochondral lesion. In stage 4 the osteochondral fragment(s) are displaced from their donor site. The stage 3 and 4 lesions are unstable, whereas stages 1 and 2 are considered stable. The goal of MRI is primarily to distinguish stable from unstable lesions.	The cause of osteochondritis dissecans is unknown, though repetitive trauma is suspected as a cause. The most common location in the knee for this lesion is the lateral aspect of the medial femoral condyle. In the skeletally immature patient the preferred treatment is often conservative and consists of several months of non-weight bearing to allow for healing and ultimately remodeling of the lesion. In the skeletally mature patient surgical fixation of an unstable lesion may be needed.

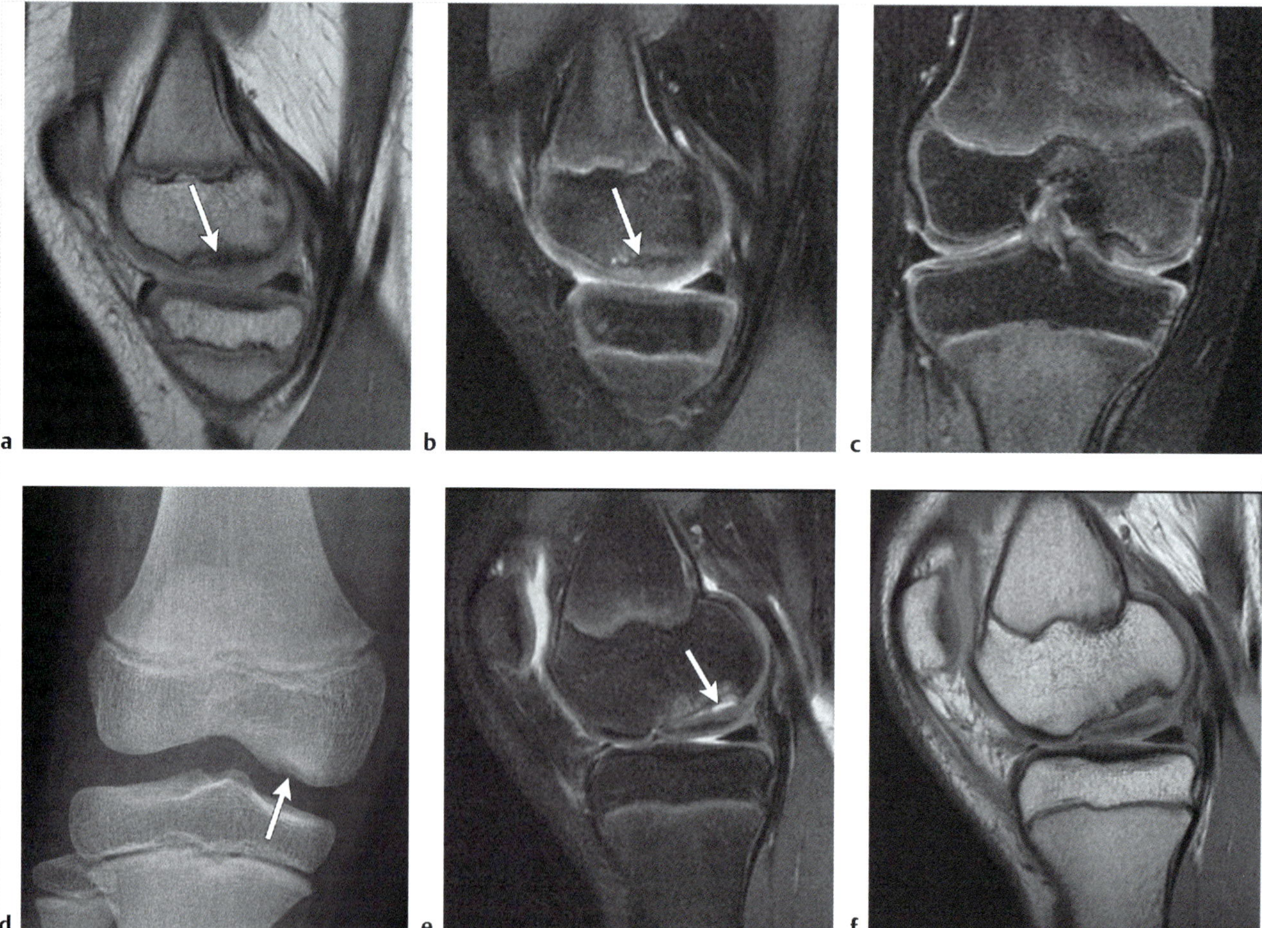

Fig. 7.34 (a) Sagittal proton density–weighted imaging (PDWI) shows osteochondral defect (OCD) of the medial femoral condyle with intact overlying cartilage (arrow). (b) Sagittal fat-suppressed T2-weighted imaging (FS T2WI) shows OCD of the medial femoral condyle with intact overlying cartilage (arrow). (c) Coronal FS T2WI shows OCD of the medial femoral condyle with intact overlying cartilage. (d) Anteroposterior radiograph shows OCD of the medial femoral condyle (arrow). (e) Sagittal FS T2WI from a second patient shows OCD of the medial femoral condyle with high signal fluid (arrow) undermining the osteochondral fragment, which is not yet displaced. (f) Corresponding sagittal PDWI. (*continued*)

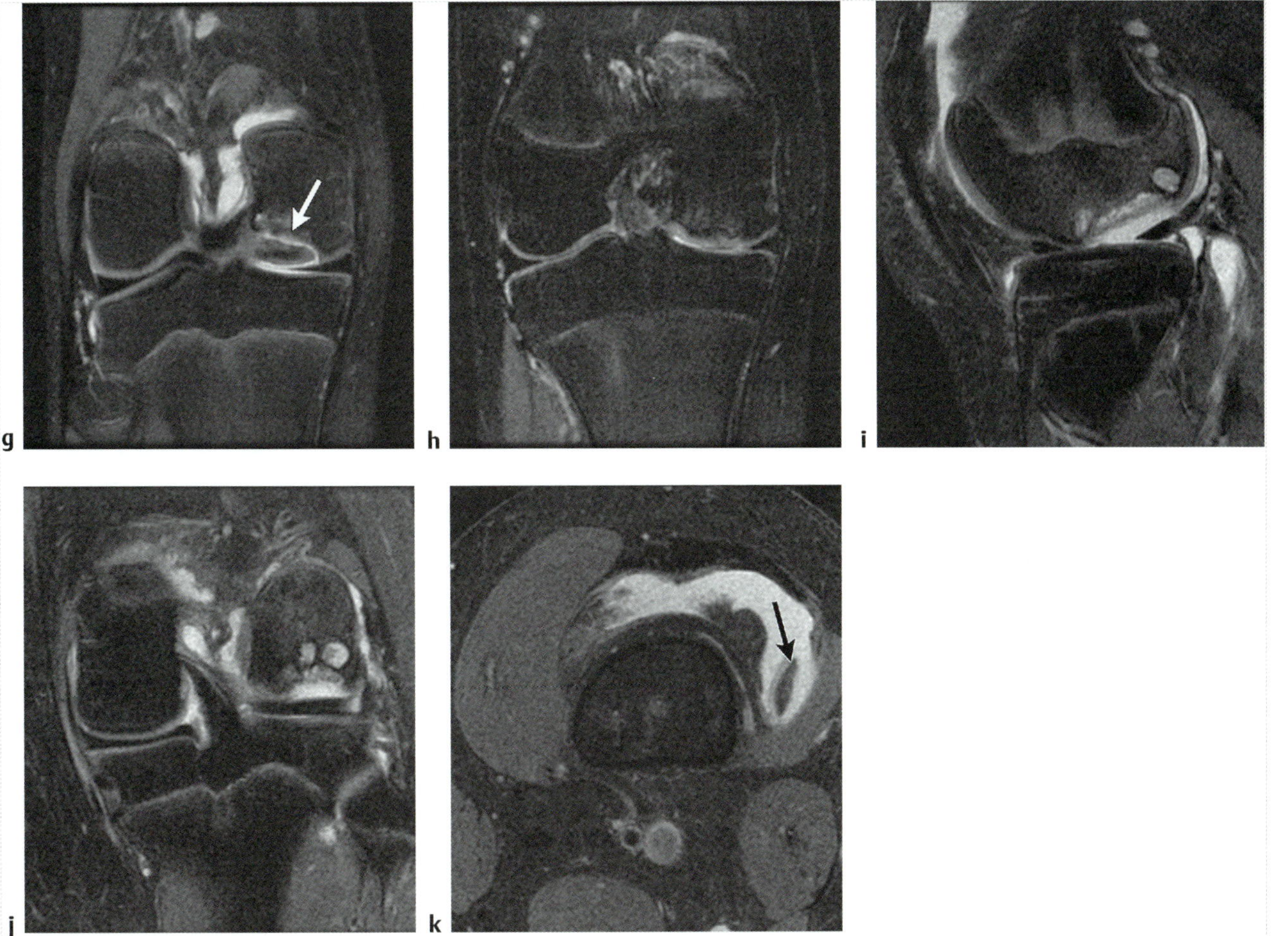

Fig. 7.34 *(continued)* (g) Corresponding coronal FS T2WI again shows high signal fluid (arrow) undermining the osteochondral fragment. (h) Same patient, coronal FS T2WI shows marked improvement in OCD after treatment. (i) Sagittal FS T2WI from a third patient shows a large lateral femoral condyle OCD with subcortical geodes. (j) Corresponding coronal FS T2WI from the same patient shows a large lateral femoral condyle defect with subcortical geodes. (k) Axial FS T2WI from the same patient shows displaced osteochondral fragment (arrow).

7.3.1 Cartilage Lesions of the Knee Suggested Reading

[1] Crema MD, Roemer FW, Marra MD, et al. Articular cartilage in the knee: current MR imaging techniques and applications in clinical practice and research. Radiographics 2011; 31: 37–61

[2] Heywood CS, Benke MT, Brindle K, Fine KM. Correlation of magnetic resonance imaging to arthroscopic findings of stability in juvenile osteochondritis dissecans. Arthroscopy 2011; 27: 194–199

[3] Kijowski R. Clinical cartilage imaging of the knee and hip joints. AJR Am J Roentgenol 2010; 195: 618–628

[4] Kijowski R, Blankenbaker DG, Shinki K, Fine JP, Graf BK, De Smet AA. Juvenile versus adult osteochondritis dissecans of the knee: appropriate MR imaging criteria for instability. Radiology 2008; 248: 571–578

7.4 Bone Lesions of the Knee

- Fractures
- Stress fracture (fatigue fracture)
- Stress fracture (insufficiency fracture)
- Bone infarct (osteonecrosis)
- Blount disease
- Dysplasia epiphysealis hemimelica (DEH) (Trevor disease)

Table 7.4 Bone lesions of the knee

Abnormalities	MRI findings	Comments
Fractures (▶ Fig. 7.35; ▶ Fig. 7.36; ▶ Fig. 7.37; ▶ Fig. 7.38)	The MRI appearance of fracture is variable depending on the severity of the injury. The mildest form of bony injury is contusion or bone bruise, which is in fact a micofracturing of the medullary bone trabecula. On fat-suppressed T2-weighted imaging (FS T2WI) this pattern of injury is seen as increased signal, which is usually in a subarticular location and not associated with a cortical break. On proton density–weighted imaging (PDWI) there is corresponding low signal. An incomplete fracture is a fracture confined to the medullary portion of bone and is seen as a linear focus of low signal surrounded by high signal edema on FS T2WI. A complete fracture occurs when there is a cortical discontinuity. These fractures may be nondisplaced or displaced. On FS T2WI the low signal fracture line is seen to extend to include the cortex, which is disrupted. There is adjacent high signal marrow edema which over time decreases in intensity. Often there is an associated lipohemarthrosis. This has a distinctive appearance on MRI. On FS T2WI the fat fluid level is seen as two separate signal components. The fat portion is low signal and located antidependent compared with the heavier fluid/blood component. A sharply defined linear separation is seen between both components.	In general radiography is often sufficient to diagnose bony fractures. However, there are some situations in which MRI plays a critical role in accurate diagnosis. Bone bruises and incomplete fractures are radiographically occult and can result in severe pain, which is explained by the MRI findings. Untreated these injuries can worsen over time. The radiographic finding of joint effusion without obvious fracture may also be an indication for MRI because a radiographically occult fracture may be present. Additional indications for MRI occur when there is a need to assess the articular surface for cartilage injury and when there is suspicion for associated soft tissue injuries such as anterior cruciate ligament (ACL) and meniscal tears.

(continued on page 216)

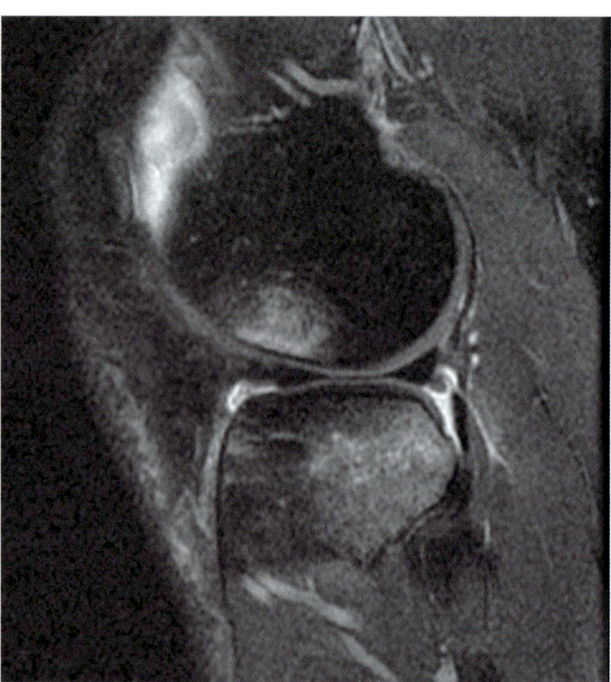

Fig. 7.35 Sagittal fat-suppressed T2-weighted imaging shows high signal bone contusion in the lateral femoral condyle and proximal lateral tibia.

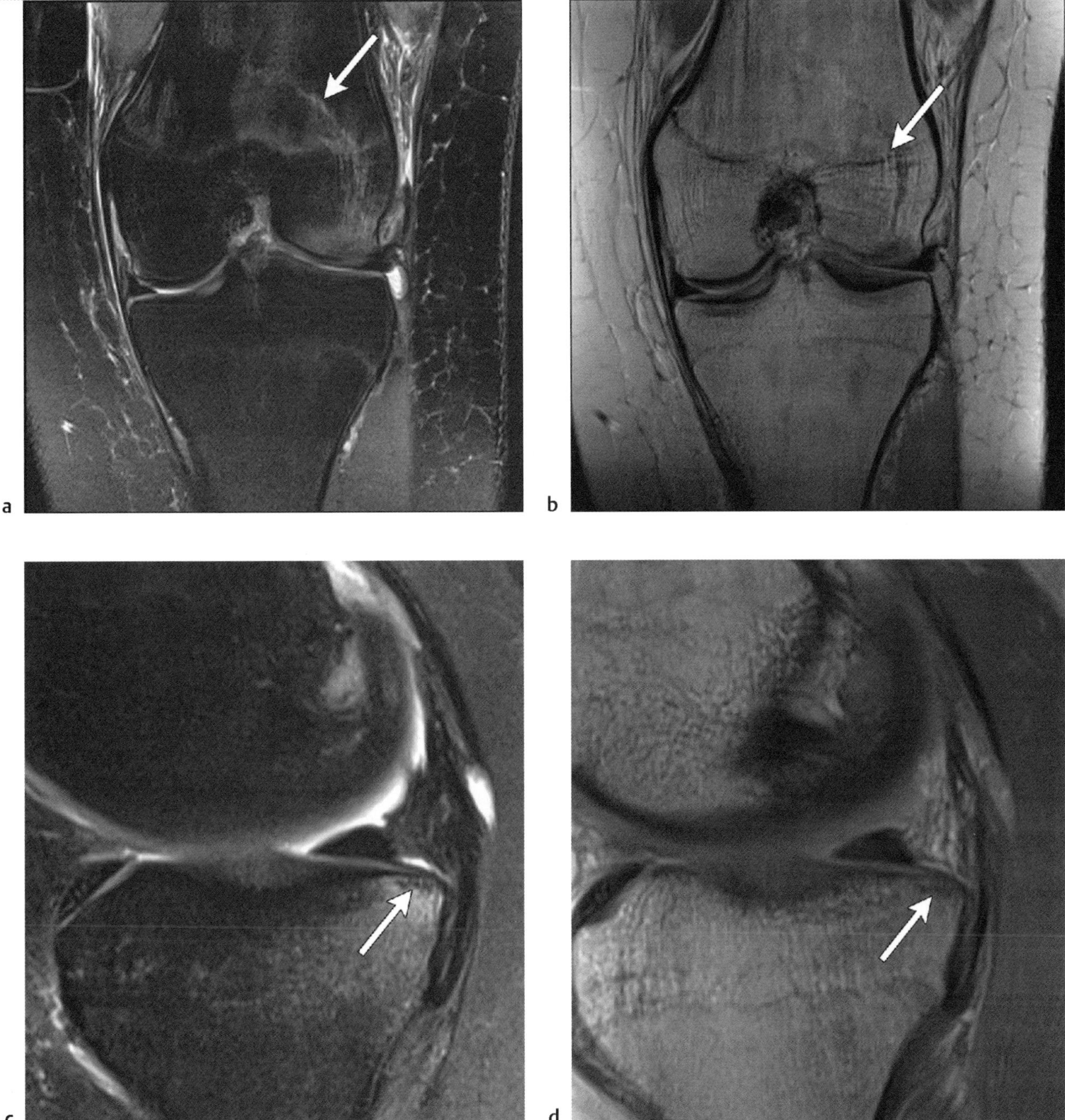

Fig. 7.36 (a) Coronal fat-suppressed T2-weighted imaging (FS T2WI) shows a linear high signal incomplete fracture extending from the lateral femoral condyle across the physeal scar and into the distal femoral metaphysis (arrow). There is adjacent bone contusion without a cortical fracture. (b) Coronal proton density–weighted imaging (PDWI) shows a corresponding linear low signal incomplete fracture in the distal lateral femur (arrow). (c) Sagittal FS T2WI from a second patient shows a small linear subcortical low signal fracture (arrow) in the proximal medial posterior tibia, which is surrounded by high signal bone contusion. There is no cortical fracture. (d) Sagittal PDWI from the same patient shows a small linear low signal subcortical incomplete fracture in the proximal posterior medial tibia (arrow).

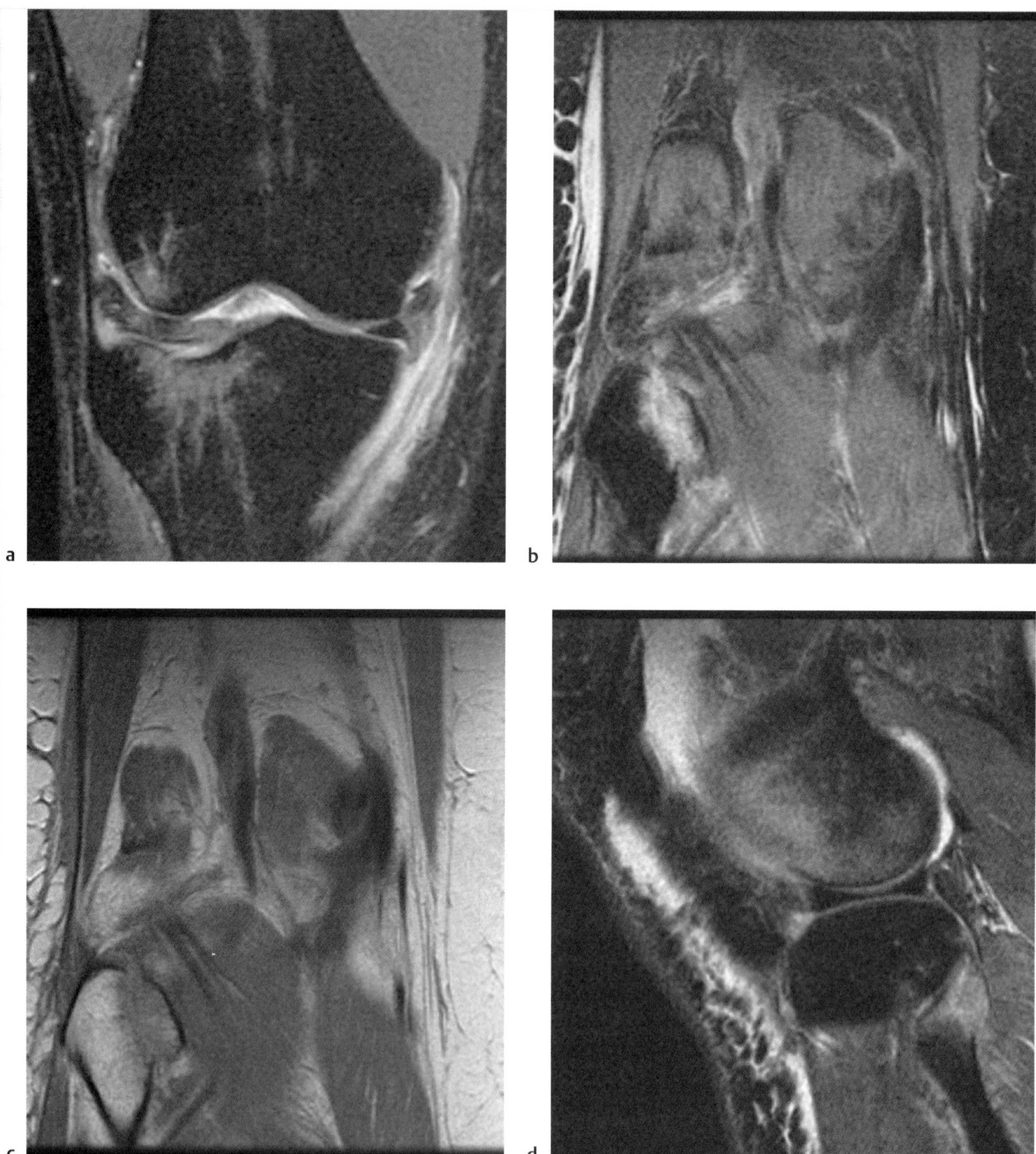

Fig. 7.37 (a) Coronal fat-suppressed T2-weighted imaging (FS T2WI) shows a depressed cortical fracture of the lateral tibial plateau with adjacent bone marrow edema. (b) Coronal FS T2WI from a second patient shows a displaced intra-articular fracture of the fibular head. (c) Coronal PDWI from a second patient shows a displaced intra-articular fracture of the fibular head. (d) Sagittal FS T2WI from a second patient shows a displaced fracture of the fibular head.

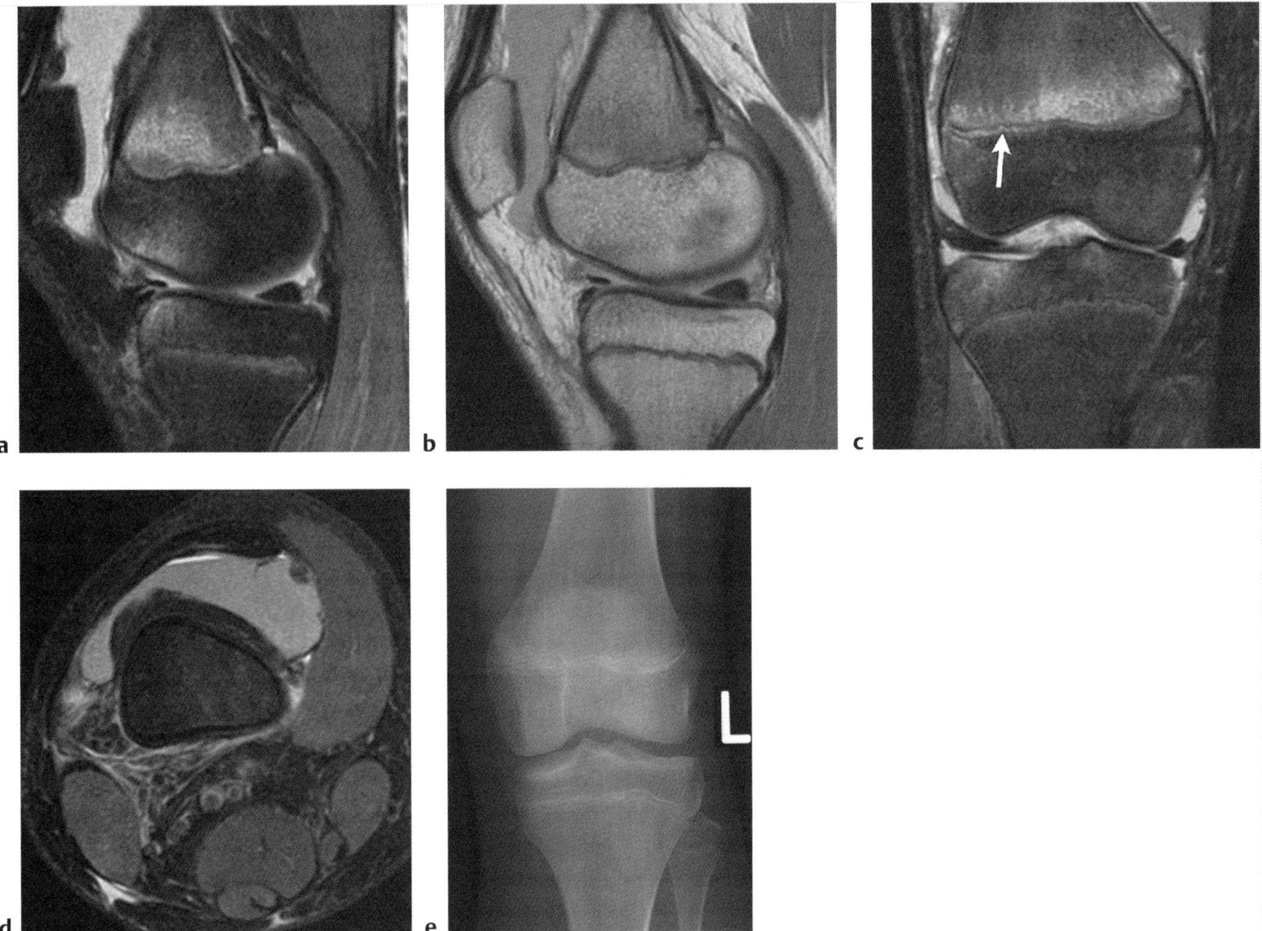

Fig. 7.38 (a) Sagittal fat-suppressed T2-weighted imaging (FS T2WI) shows high signal edema in the metaphysis extending to the distal femoral physis. This is a Salter-Harris I fracture. (b) Sagittal proton density–weighted imaging (PDWI) shows a corresponding low signal in the distal femoral metaphysis. (c) Coronal FS T2WI from the same patient shows high signal edema in the distal femoral metaphysis extending to the physis, which is slightly widened medially (arrow). (d) Axial FS T2WI from the same patient shows a large effusion with fluid level indicating the presence of a fracture. (e) Anteroposterior radiograph with no evidence of a Salter-Harris I fracture, which is typical.

Table 7.4 (Cont.) Bone lesions of the knee

Abnormalities	MRI findings	Comments
Stress fracture (fatigue fracture) (▶ Fig. 7.39)	The MRI findings of stress fracture depend on the severity of the injury. In the early phase of injury there is often mild focal subcortical marrow edema seen as focal high signal on FS T2WI and focal low signal on PDWI and T1-weighted imaging (T1WI). As the injury progresses in severity there is a mild high signal periosteal reaction seen on FS T2WI. Eventually there may be cortical edema, which is high signal on FS T2WI, and finally there is outright cortical fracture seen as linear low signal surrounded by high signal in the cortex with confluent subcortical marrow edema (high signal and high signal periosteal reaction on FS T2WI).	Fatigue fractures are abnormal stress applied to normal bone. These are potentially significant injuries that can progress to cortical fracture if left untreated. Early diagnosis and treatment result in optimal outcome for the patient. These injuries typically occur in athletes such as long-distance runners and individuals participating in jumping sports. In the early stage of stress-related injury there are often no radiographic findings. If there is clinical suspicion for stress injury further evaluation with MRI is indicated. This is particularly true in high-performance athletes. In these patients early diagnosis with MRI not only helps to prevent a more serious cortical fracture but can result in earlier appropriate treatment thereby allowing earlier return to sport. In general MRI is considered superior to nuclear medicine in the diagnosis of stress fractures. MRI is more sensitive than nuclear medicine bone scan in the identification of the earliest findings of stress injury, and there is also inherently more information on the MRI scan, including the precise location of the injury within the bone (i.e., cortical or medullary or both). This degree of precision affects both patient prognosis and treatment. In addition, MRI is not associated with ionizing radiation, which is an advantage because these patients are often young.
Stress fracture (insufficiency fracture) (▶ Fig. 7.40)	On FS T2WI there is a zone of high signal indicating marrow edema, and there is often a linear zone of low signal in a subcortical location. Often the cortex is not disrupted, and the MRI findings are radiographically occult. On PDWI or T1WI there is low signal corresponding to the high signal zone of edema.	Insufficiency fractures occur when normal stress is applied to abnormal bone. Most commonly this occurs in older osteoporotic patients. Other causes include prior irradiation to the affected site, steroids, hyperparathyroidism, and rheumatoid arthritis. Spontaneous osteonecrosis (SONC) in the knee is likely; in fact subcortical insufficiency fracture often occurs in the femoral condyles in older osteoporotic patients with recent minor trauma.

(continued on page 218)

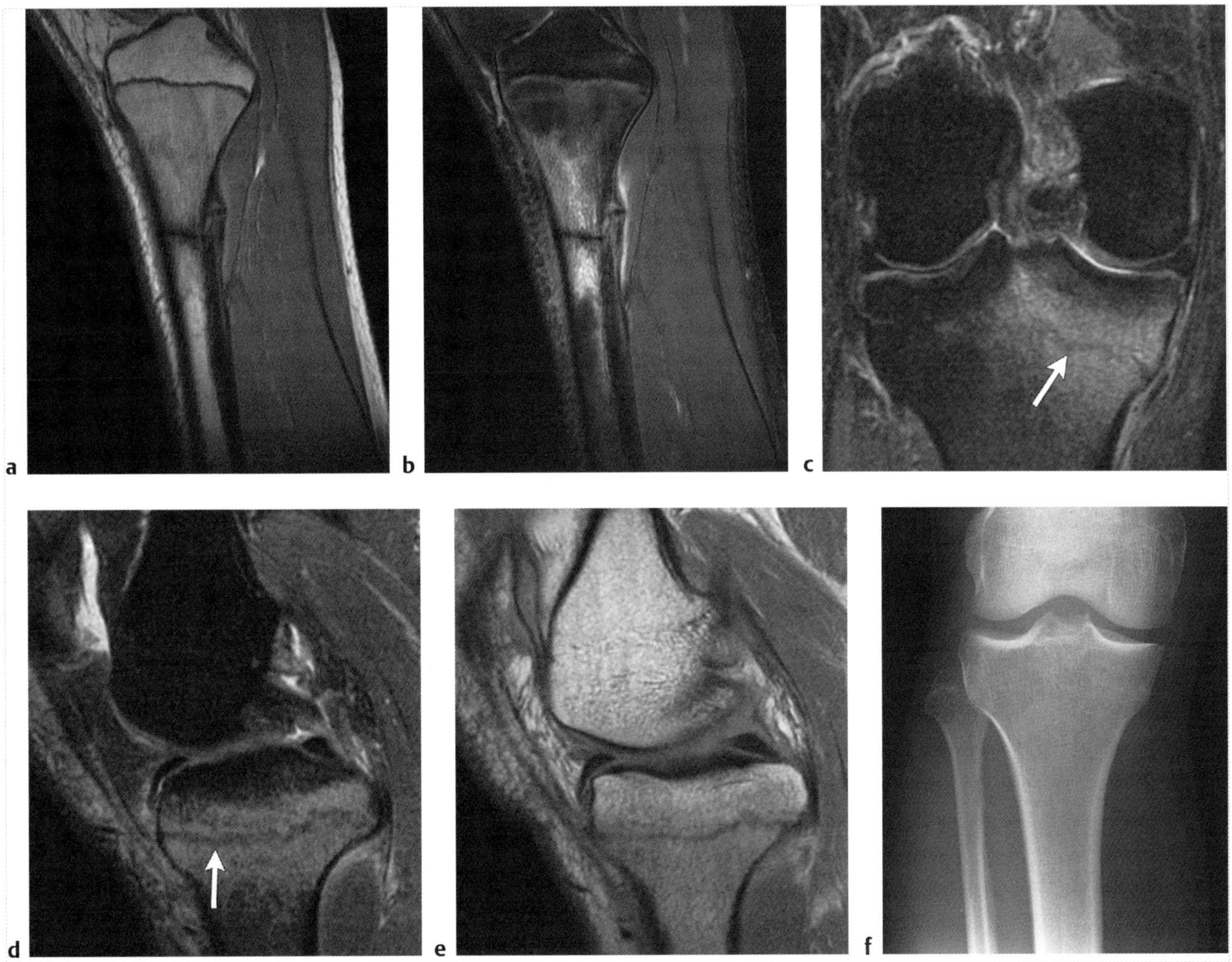

Fig. 7.39 (a) Sagittal proton density–weighted imaging (PDWI) shows a low signal linear defect traversing the proximal tibia diaphysis with extension to the posterior cortex and adjacent periosteal reaction. (b) Sagittal fat-suppressed T2-weighted imaging (FS T2WI) shows extensive marrow edema in the proximal tibial diaphysis with a low signal linear fracture extending to the posterior cortex and adjacent periosteal reaction. (c) Coronal FS T2WI from a second patient shows linear low signal in the proximal medial tibia (arrow) with surrounding marrow edema. The patient had recently completed a marathon. (d) Sagittal FS T2WI from the same patient shows a band of low signal in the proximal tibia (arrow) surrounded by high signal marrow edema. (e) Sagittal PDWI from the same patient shows linear low signal in the proximal tibia with no evidence of cortical fracture. (f) Anteroposterior radiograph is normal demonstrating the greater sensitivity of MRI in detecting stress fractures.

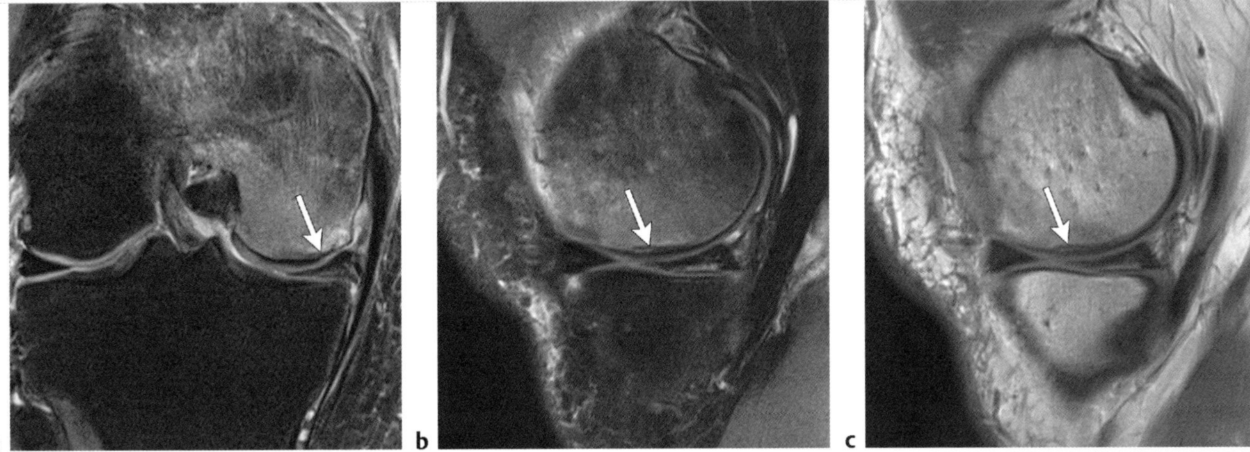

Fig. 7.40 (a) Coronal fat-suppressed T2-weighted imaging (FS T2WI) in a 57-year-old female shows diffuse marrow edema in the medial femoral condyle with a subtle linear low signal subcortical insufficiency fracture (arrow). (b) Sagittal FS T2WI shows a linear low signal subcortical insufficiency fracture in the medial femoral condyle (arrow) with adjacent extensive marrow edema. Note that there is a posterior horn medial meniscal tear. (c) Sagittal proton density–weighted imaging shows a linear low signal subcortical fracture in the medial femoral condyle (arrow).

Table 7.4 (Cont.) Bone lesions of the knee

Abnormalities	MRI findings	Comments
Bone infarct (osteonecrosis) (▶ Fig. 7.41)	The appearance of osteonecrosis is variable. In the earliest phase the only finding may be nonspecific marrow edema seen as high signal on FS T2WI and low signal on PDWI and T1WI. There is often rapid progression to the characteristic double line sign. This sign refers to the often serpentine line that separates viable from necrotic bone. On FS T2WI there is a low signal line marking the periphery of the infarcted bone, often with an adjacent high signal line just deep to the low signal line. The bone within the zone of infarction is often low signal (isointense to fat) on FS T2WI and high signal on T1WI. In some cases there may be a mixed pattern of low and/or high signal within the zone of infarction on FS T2WI.	There are many causes of osteonecrosis, including steroids, systemic lupus erythematosus (SLE), sickle cell disease, caisson disease, and idiopathic causes. The epiphyses and diaphysis of long bones are most commonly affected. MRI is the most sensitive and specific imaging modality for diagnosing suspected osteonecrosis. Untreated osteonecrosis can progress to the point where there is collapse of affected bone. If an articular surface is involved this can result in early-onset osteoarthritis.
Blount disease (▶ Fig. 7.42)	The key features of Blount disease are best seen on sagittal and coronal planes. These include widening and depression of the medial tibial growth plate and both small and deep extensions of the cartilage into the proximal tibial metaphysis, which is seen as abnormal linear high signal on FS T2WI. Additional findings often include varus deformity of the lower leg; widening of the lateral proximal tibial growth plate; hypertrophy of the medial meniscus, which may also have abnormal signal best seen on FS T2WI that is often in the posterior horn; osteochondral injury of the medial femoral condyle; bony bars across the proximal tibial physis; and thicker unossified proximal tibial epiphysis.	Blount disease is a developmental disorder of abnormal growth of the medial proximal tibial epiphysis. Patients are often overweight and have varus deformity of the lower extremity. The cause of this abnormality may be related to excessive force on the medial aspect of the proximal tibial physis. This is then thought to cause abnormal function and structure of the affected physeal chondrocytes with delay in ossification. Surgical treatment is typically required.

(continued on page 220)

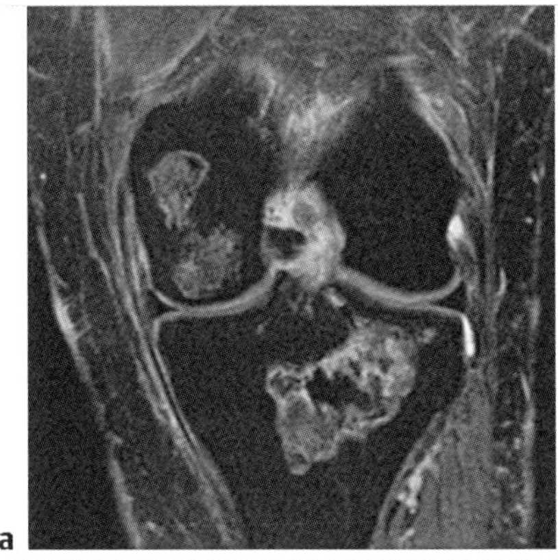

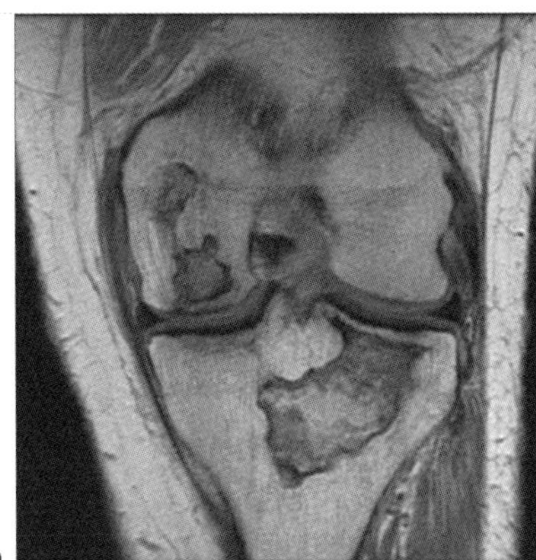

Fig. 7.41 (a) Coronal fat-suppressed T2-weighted imaging (FS T2WI) shows serpiginous zones of mixed predominantly high signal with low signal sharply demarcated borders in the medial femoral condyle and proximal tibia. (b) Coronal proton density–weighted imaging shows corresponding zones of mixed predominantly low signal with sharply demarcated low signal borders in the medial femoral condyle and proximal tibia.

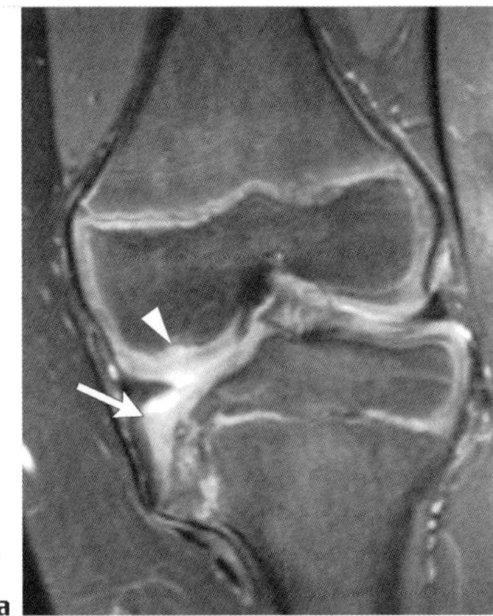

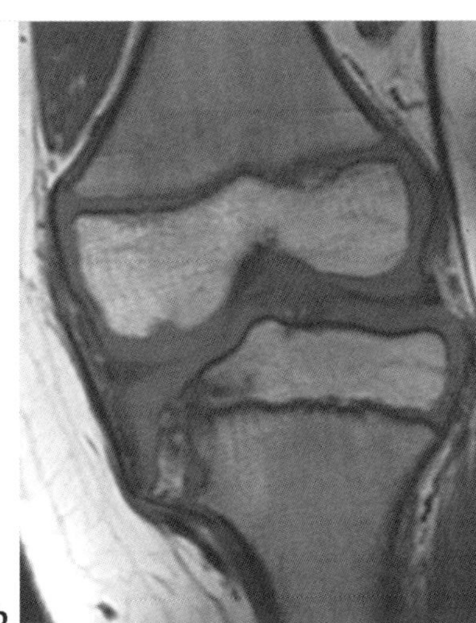

Fig. 7.42 (a) Coronal fat-suppressed T2-weighted imaging (FS T2WI) shows widening and depression of the medial tibial growth plate, thicker unossified tibial epiphysis (arrow), and medial femoral condyle osteochondral injury (arrowhead). (b) Coronal proton density–weighted imaging also shows depression of the medial tibial growth plate, thick unossified medial tibial epiphysis, and medial femoral condyle osteochondral injury.

Table 7.4 (Cont.) Bone lesions of the knee

Abnormalities	MRI findings	Comments
Dysplasia epiphysealis hemimelica (DEH) (Trevor disease) (▶ Fig. 7.43)	On PDWI there is an irregular lobulated mass, of intermediate signal with low signal foci of calcification, arising from the medial or lateral aspect of the epiphysis. This can be in the femur or tibia. On FS T2WI the lesion is heterogeneously increased in signal with a variable degree of low signal foci depending on the amount of calcification. Lesions may be connected to or separate from the parent bone and can mimic a loose body.	DEH is a rare disorder of the epiphysis or equivalent occurring on one side of the body in children. The classic feature of the disorder is an osteocartilagenous mass involving the epiphysis. The majority of cases occur in the lower extremity, most commonly the knee or ankle or both. Three forms have been described: localized (affects one location), classical (affects more than one location on the same side of the body), and generalized (affects the entire limb on one side). Patients usually present with a painless asymmetric mass. Varus or valgus deformity may also be present. Boys are reported to be three times more commonly affected as girls. Treatment for DEH is surgery.

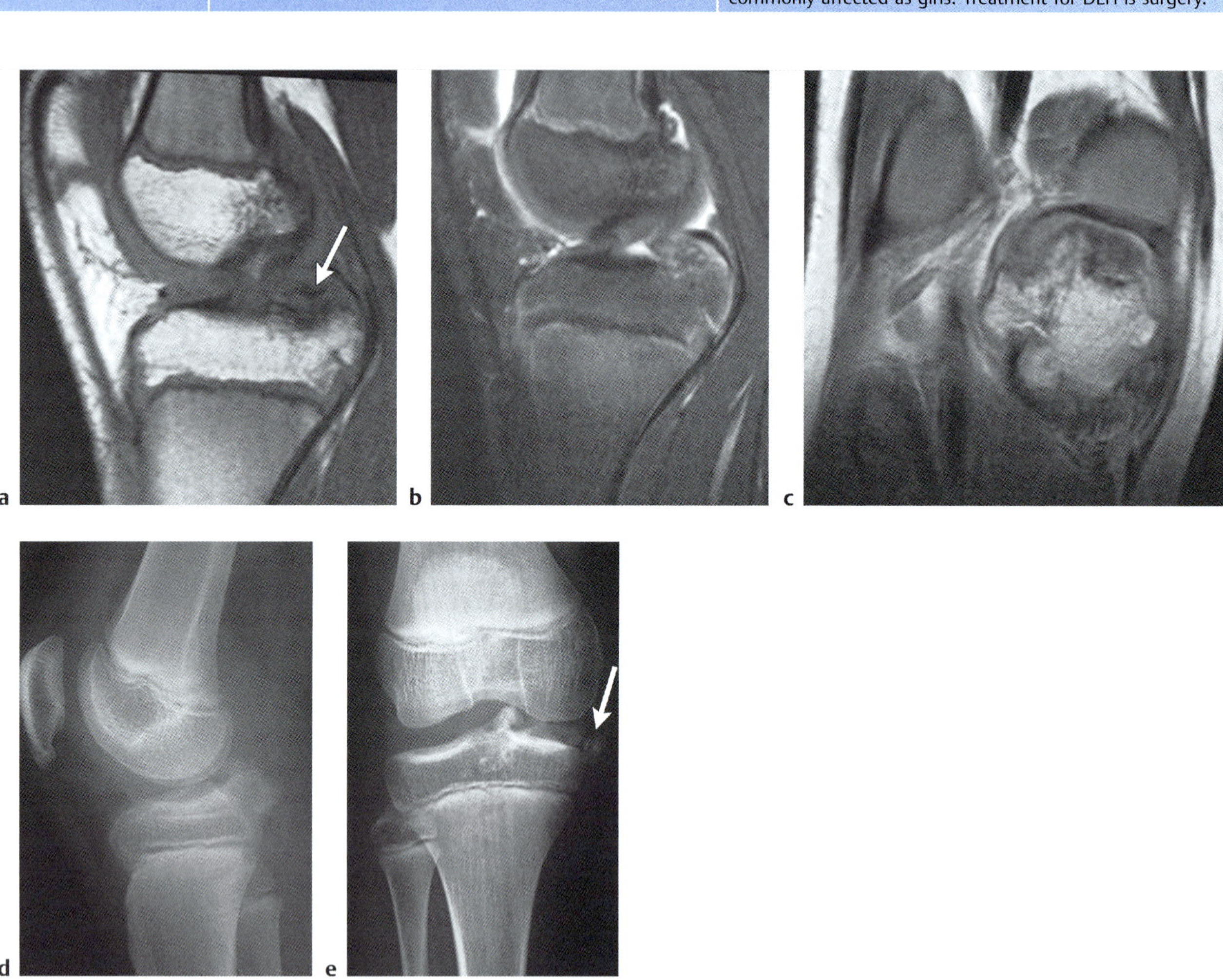

Fig. 7.43 (a) Sagittal proton density–weighted imaging (PDWI) shows a lobulated mass arising from the proximal medial tibial epiphysis (arrow), which is heterogeneously low signal indicating the presence of calcification. (b) Corresponding sagittal fat-suppressed T2-weighted imaging (FS T2WI) shows a lobulated mass arising from the proximal medial tibial epiphysis, which has heterogeneous signal with foci of both high and low signal. (c) Corresponding coronal PDWI shows a lobulated mass with a zone of heterogeneous low signal arising from the medial proximal tibial epiphysis. (d) The corresponding lateral radiograph shows a lobulated osseous mass arising from the proximal medial tibial epiphysis. (e) The corresponding anteroposterior radiograph shows a lobulated osseous mass arising from the proximal medial tibial epiphysis with some components mimicking loose bodies (arrow).

7.4.1 Bone Lesions of the Knee Suggested Reading

[1] Bahk WJ, Lee HY, Kang YK, Park JM, Chun KA, Chung YG. Dysplasia epiphysealis hemimelica: radiographic and magnetic resonance imaging features and clinical outcome of complete and incomplete resection. Skeletal Radiol 2010; 39: 85–90

[2] Craig JG, van Holsbeeck M, Zaltz I. The utility of MR in assessing Blount disease. Skeletal Radiol 2002; 31: 208–213

[3] Deangelis JP, Spindler KP. Traumatic bone bruises in the athlete's knee. Sports Health 2010; 2: 398–402

[4] Kidwai AS, Hemphill SD, Griffiths HJ. Radiologic case study. Spontaneous osteonecrosis of the knee reclassified as insufficiency fracture. Orthopedics 2005; 28: 236–, 333–336

[5] Kritsaneepaiboon S, Shah R, Murray MM, Kleinman PK. Posterior periosteal disruption in Salter-Harris Type II fractures of the distal femur: evidence for a hyperextension mechanism. AJR Am J Roentgenol 2009; 193: W540-W545

[6] Lang IM, Azouz EM. MRI appearances of dysplasia epiphysealis hemimelica of the knee. Skeletal Radiol 1997; 26: 226–229

[7] Niva MH, Kiuru MJ, Haataja R, Pihlajamäki HK. Bone stress injuries causing exercise-induced knee pain. Am J Sports Med 2006; 34: 78–83

[8] Sabharwal S, Wenokor C, Mehta A, Zhao C. Intra-articular morphology of the knee joint in children with Blount disease: a case-control study using MRI. J Bone Joint Surg Am 2012; 94: 883–890

7.5 Lesions of the Extensor Mechanism

- Patellar tendinosis
- Patellar tendon tears
- Osgood-Schlatter disease
- Sinding-Larsen-Johansson syndrome
- Quadriceps tendon tears
- Transient patellar dislocation
- Hoffa disease

Table 7.5 Lesions of the extensor mechanism

Abnormalities	MRI findings	Comments
Patellar tendinosis (▶ Fig. 7.44)	On sagittal fat-suppressed T2-weighted imaging (FS T2WI) there is a focal zone of increased signal intensity most commonly seen in the proximal posterior portion of the tendon. This focus of abnormal signal is of variable size and signal intensity. Larger lesions of higher signal intensity are often more symptomatic. Adjacent structures may also become inflamed and demonstrate patchy increased signal on FS T2WI. Typically the lower pole of the patella and the adjacent portion of Hoffa fat may be involved. On proton density-weighted imaging(PDWI) the zone of increased signal corresponds to a zone of decreased signal. The findings of patellar tendinopathy are best seen on sagittal plane images. The axial plane can also be helpful.	Patellar tendinosis (tendinopathy) is most often seen in young, high-level athletes engaged in jumping sports such as basketball and volleyball. Patients present with infrapatellar knee pain. Ultrasonography is an alternative imaging modality for the diagnosis of this entity. However, if there is a different cause of infrapatellar region pain such as a chondral injury of the lower pole of the patella then ultrasound will not identify the abnormality. The high signal region seen in the proximal posterior portion of the patellar tendon corresponds to granulation tissue with increased neovascularity. Treatment of most patients with patellar tendinosis is conservative with eventual return to sport. In a small percentage of patients the condition becomes chronic, and surgery to excise the abnormal portion of the tendon can be performed. In many patients patellar tendinosis is bilateral, although often asymmetric in severity.
Patellar tendon tears (▶ Fig. 7.45)	The most common site of patellar tendon rupture is the proximal attachment to the lower pole of the patella. On sagittal images there is obvious discontinuity and often redundancy of the torn end such that the torn end has an appearance of being rolled up into a ball. In an acute tear there is often high signal edema or some hemorrhage or both at the site of rupture.	Patellar tendon tears most often occur in young adults. Most tears occur at the site of underlying patellar tendinopathy. Patients with patellar tendon rupture are unable to extend the knee and often complain of infrapatellar pain.
Osgood-Schlatter disease (▶ Fig. 7.46)	On sagittal FS T2WI there is fragmentation of the anterior tibial tubercle with thickening of the distal portion of the patellar tendon and variable high signal edema in the distal portion of the tendon with variable edema in the fragmented tibial tubercle. In addition there is often fluid in the infrapatellar bursa.	This type of injury is most often secondary to overuse related to certain sports such as football, soccer, and basketball. Patients complain of pain over the anterior aspect of the tibia. Adolescents are most commonly seen with this disorder. It should be noted that the radiographic finding of fragmentation of the anterior tibial tubercle without any symptoms is possible and is therefore not diagnostic of the disease.

(continued on page 224)

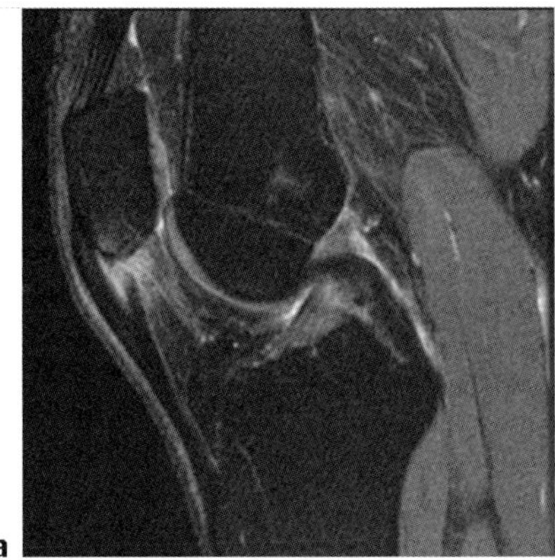

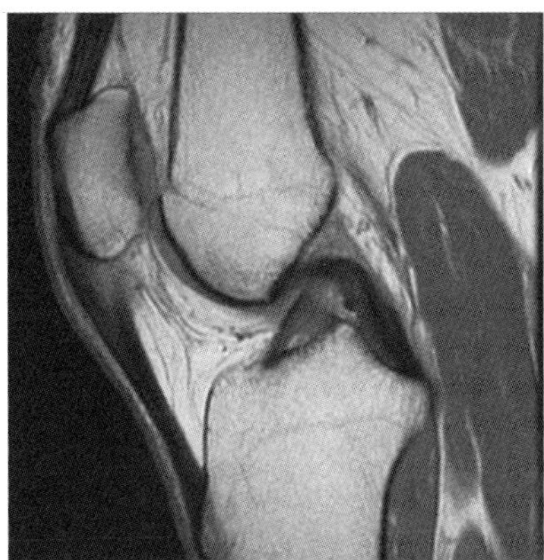

Fig. 7.44 (a) Sagittal fat-suppressed T2-weighted imaging (FS T2WI) shows high signal edema and granulation tissue in the proximal posterior portion of a thickened patellar tendon. Note adjacent reactive edema in the lower pole of the patella and the adjacent Hoffa fat. (b) Sagittal proton density–weighted imaging shows a thickened proximal patellar tendon with intermediate signal in the proximal posterior portion of the tendon.

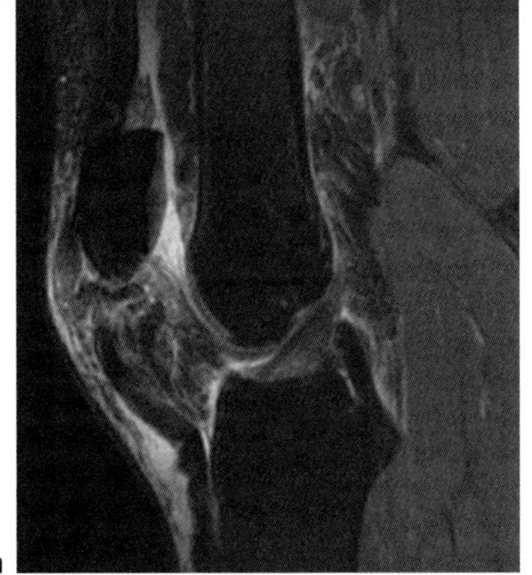

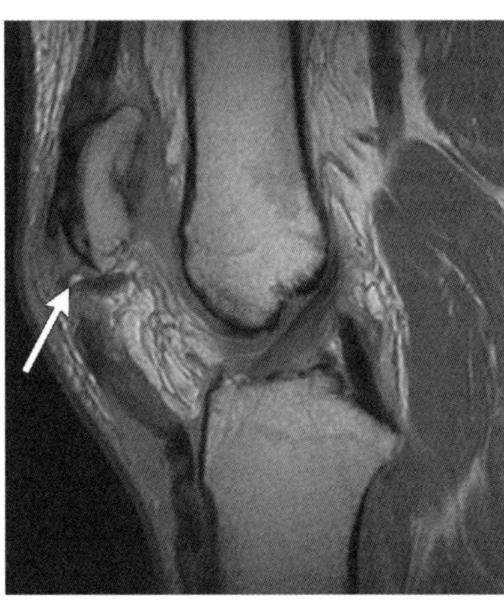

Fig. 7.45 (a) Sagittal fat-suppressed T2-weighted imaging (FS T2WI) shows the patellar tendon torn, thickened, and retracted from the lower pole of the patella. (b) Sagittal proton density–weighted imaging shows a thickened, torn, and retracted patellar tendon with a small avulsed fragment of bone from the patella (arrow).

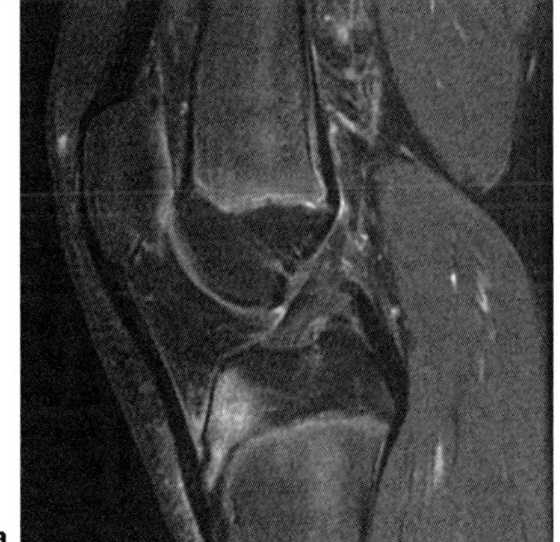

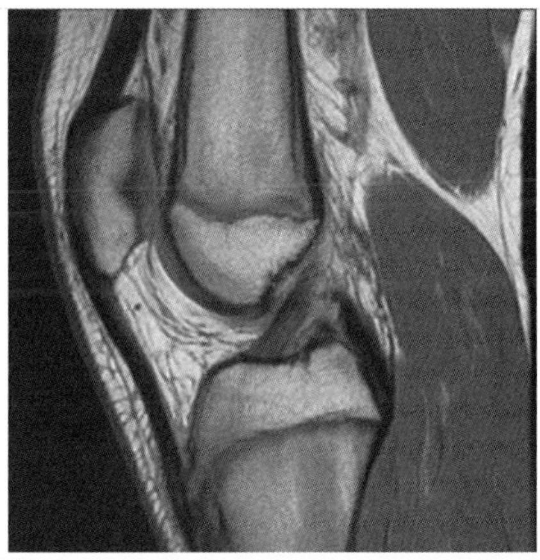

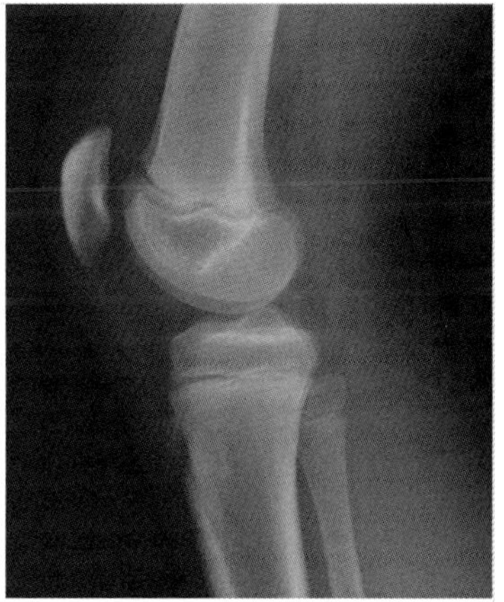

Fig. 7.46 (a) Sagittal fat-suppressed T2-weighted imaging (FS T2WI) shows high signal marrow edema in the anterior tibial tubercle. (b) Sagittal proton density–weighted imaging shows some fragmentation of the anterior tibial tubercle. (c) Lateral radiograph shows a fragmented anterior tibial tubercle in a skeletally immature patient.

Table 7.5 (Cont.) Lesions of the extensor mechanism

Abnormalities	MRI findings	Comments
Sinding-Larsen-Johansson syndrome (▶ Fig. 7.47)	On sagittal images there is thickening of the proximal patellar tendon with high signal seen in the region of tendon thickening on FS T2WI and low signal on PDWI. There is also some fragmentation of the lower pole of the patella, often with high signal edema on FS T2WI.	This abnormality is mostly seen in teenage patients. This injury is most commonly associated with overuse and is often seen in athletes playing soccer, basketball, and football. It should be noted that the radiographic finding of fragmentation of the lower pole of the patella without associated symptoms is possible and is therefore not diagnostic of the syndrome.
Quadriceps tendon tears (▶ Fig. 7.48; ▶ Fig. 7.49)	On sagittal FS T2WI and PDWI acute tendon rupture is seen as separation of the torn distal tendon end from the normal attachment on the upper portion of the patella. The amount of tendon retraction from the patella is variable, and there is often high signal edema seen on FS T2WI in the distal torn tendon end as well as in the gap between the bone and tendon.	This injury is more common in adults and in particular patients with underlying tendinopathy. Some chronic diseases are associated with this injury, including diabetes and rheumatoid arthritis. Surgery is usually required in retracted ruptures. In general partial tears and nonretracted tears can be treated nonsurgically.

(continued on page 226)

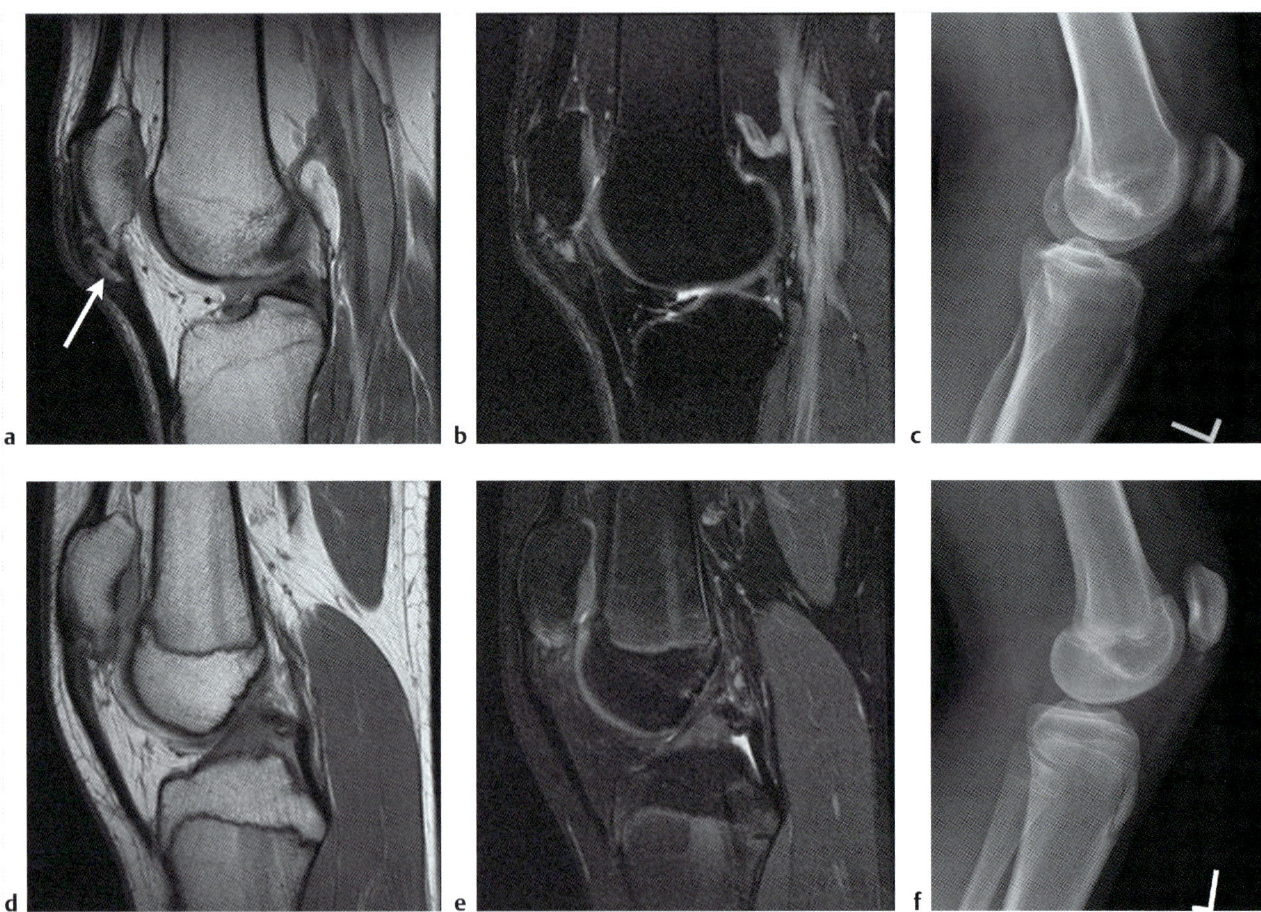

Fig. 7.47 (a) Sagittal proton density–weighted imaging (PDWI) shows a fragmented lower pole of the patella (arrow). (b) Sagittal fat-suppressed T2-weighted imaging (FS T2WI) shows high signal edema in the thickened proximal patellar tendon. (c) Lateral radiograph of the knee shows an osseous fragment of the lower pole patella. (d) Sagittal PDWI from a second patient shows a fragmented lower pole of the patella. (e) Sagittal FS T2WI from the same patient shows high signal edema in the lower pole of the patella and mild edema in the proximal patellar tendon. (f) Lateral radiograph from the same patient shows osseous fragment adjacent to the lower pole of the patella.

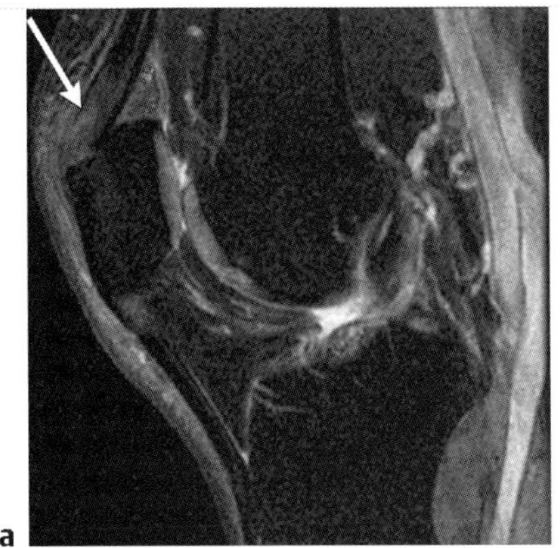

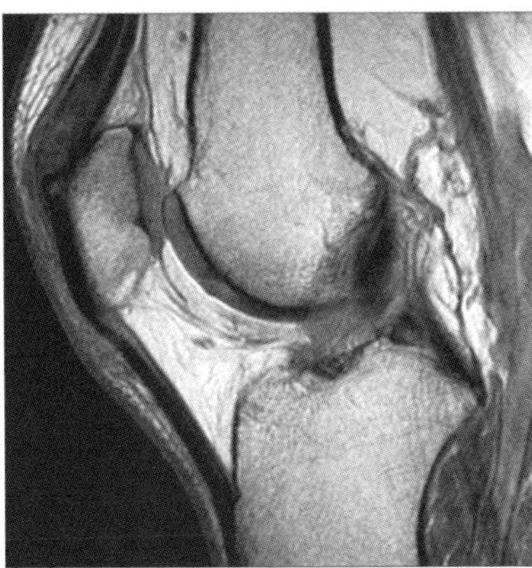

Fig. 7.48 (a) Sagittal fat-suppressed T2-weighted imaging (FS T2WI) shows high signal edema in a thickened distal quadriceps tendon with tendonopathy and partial thickness tear (arrow). (b) Sagittal proton density–weighted imaging (PDWI) shows a thickened distal quadriceps tendon with intermediate signal.

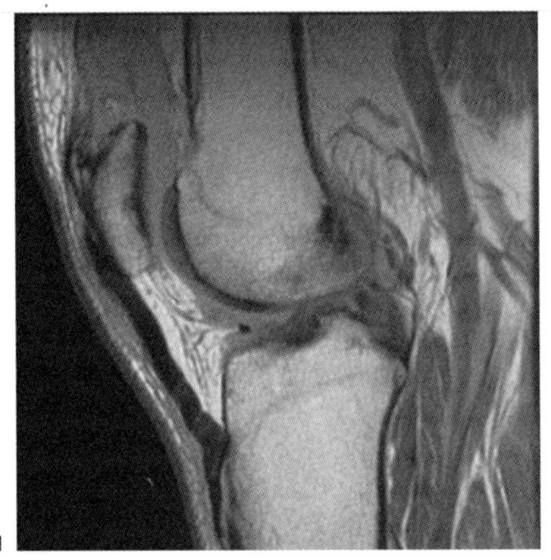

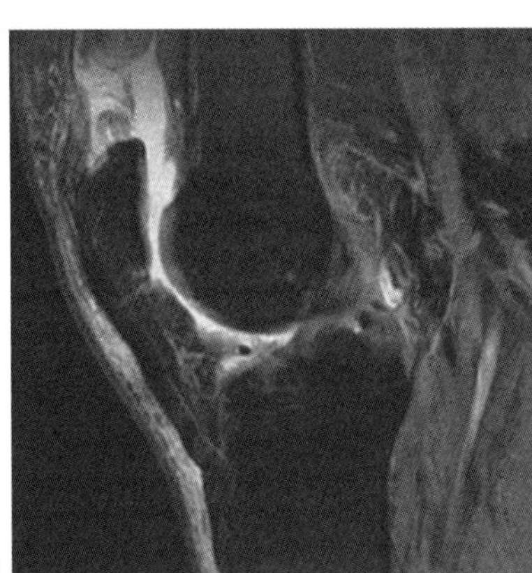

Fig. 7.49 (a) Sagittal proton density–weighted imaging shows a ruptured retracted quadriceps tendon. (b) Sagittal fat-suppressed T2-weighted imaging shows a ruptured retracted quadriceps tendon.

Table 7.5 (Cont.) Lesions of the extensor mechanism

Abnormalities	MRI findings	Comments
Transient patellar dislocation (▶ Fig. 7.50)	On axial FS T2WI there are often high signal bone bruises seen in the inferior medial patella and the anterior aspect of the lateral femoral condyle. In some cases there may be a chondral or osteochondral fracture of the inferior medial patellar facet. In this situation the location and size of the fragment should be described as well as the donor site. If there is an osteochondral fracture there will also likely be a lipohemarthrosis with obvious fat fluid level on axial images. Additional findings may include partial or complete tear of the medial patellar retinaculum. There may also be edema in the infrapatellar fat. The position of the patella is variable with some cases demonstrating a return to normal position with respect to the femoral trochlea. In other patients there may be abnormal persistent lateral patellar subluxation with a variable degree of abnormal patellar tilt.	In patellar dislocation the patella dislocates laterally with respect to the distal femur. This may occur in athletes involved in sports such as football, basketball, and soccer or in situations where the patient landed abnormally after jumping. It is likely that some patients are prone to patellar dislocation, particularly those with high-riding patella and lateral patellar subluxation.
Hoffa disease (▶ Fig. 7.51)	The typical appearance on FS T2WI is variable though is usually seen as diffuse high signal within normally low signal fat. There may also be heterogeneous mixed signal seen, sometimes with low signal foci of hemosiderin. On PDWI intermediate signal is often seen in place of normally high signal fat.	Inflammation of the Hoffa fat (also referred to as the infrapatellar fat pad) can occur due to acute or chronic trauma. Hyperextension injuries can result in hemorrhage and swelling within the fat pad. Patients typically complain of anterior knee pain. This can be difficult to differentiate from other causes of anterior knee pain.

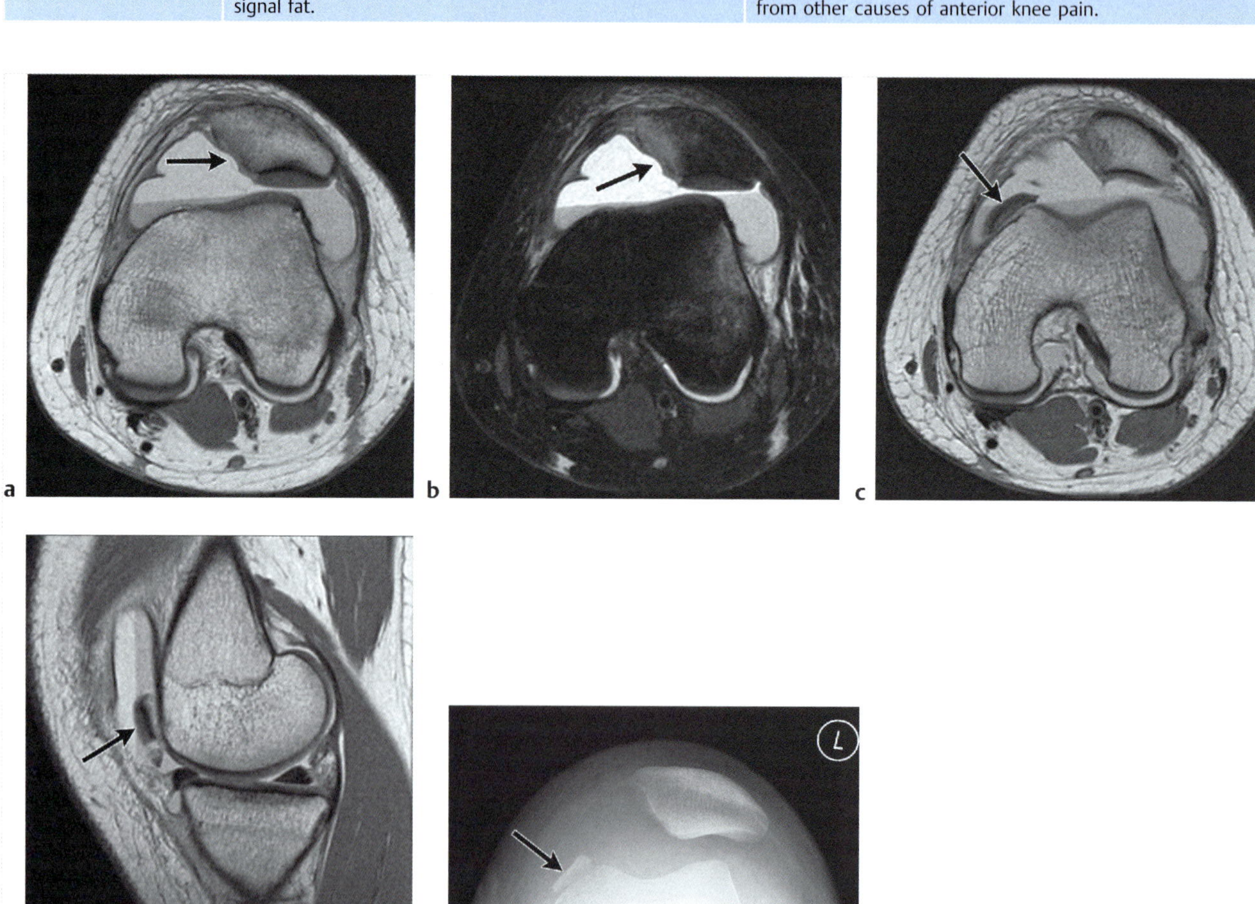

Fig. 7.50 (a) Axial proton density–weighted imaging (PDWI) shows an osteocartilaginous defect involving the medial patellar facet (arrow) with lipohemarthrosis and lateral subluxation of the patella. (b) Axial fat-suppressed T2-weighted imaging shows an osteocartilaginous defect involving the medial patellar facet (arrow) with lipohemarthrosis and lateral subluxation of the patella. Note the high signal bone contusion in the anterior lateral femoral condyle and medial patellar facet. (c) Axial PDWI shows an osteocartilaginous fracture fragment floating in the medial portion of the lipohemarthrosis (arrow). (d) Sagittal PDWI shows osteocartilaginous fragments anterior to the medial femoral condyle (arrow). (e) Sunrise view shows fracture fragment adjacent to the anterior medial distal femur.

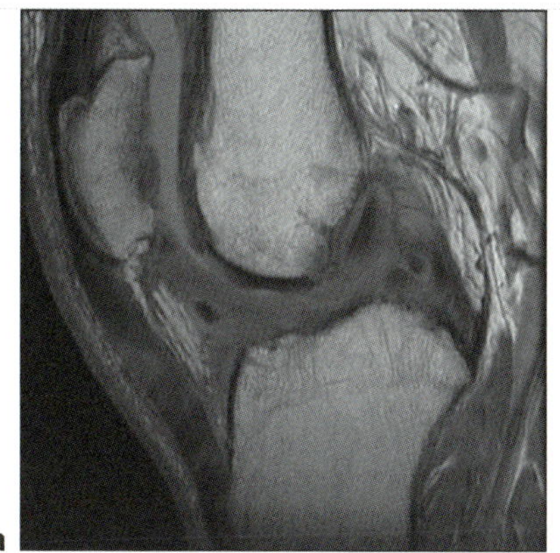

a

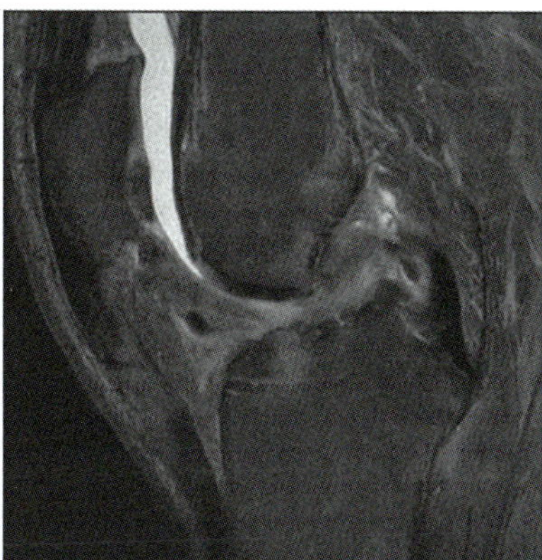

b

Fig. 7.51 (a) Sagittal proton density–weighted imaging shows extensive intermediate signal obliterating the Hoffa fat. (b) Sagittal fat-suppressed T2-weighted imaging shows intermediate signal in the Hoffa fat.

7.5.1 Lesions of the Extensor Mechanism Suggested Reading

[1] Boublik M, Schlegel T, Koonce R, Genuario J, Lind C, Hamming D. Patellar tendon ruptures in National Football League players. Am J Sports Med 2011; 39: 2436–2440

[2] Diederichs G, Issever AS, Scheffler S. MR imaging of patellar instability: injury patterns and assessment of risk factors. Radiographics 2010; 30: 961–981

[3] Gottsegen CJ, Eyer BA, White EA, Learch TJ, Forrester D. Avulsion fractures of the knee: imaging findings and clinical significance. Radiographics 2008; 28: 1755–1770

[4] Hirano A, Fukubayashi T, Ishii T, Ochiai N. Magnetic resonance imaging of Osgood-Schlatter disease: the course of the disease. Skeletal Radiol 2002; 31: 334–342

[5] Saddik D, McNally EG, Richardson M. MRI of Hoffa's fat pad. Skeletal Radiol 2004; 33: 433–444

[6] Sonin AH, Fitzgerald SW, Bresler ME, Kirsch MD, Hoff FL, Friedman H. MR imaging appearance of the extensor mechanism of the knee: functional anatomy and injury patterns. Radiographics 1995; 15: 367–382

7.6 Lesions of the Synovium and Bursae and Arthropathy

- Baker cyst
- Prepatellar bursitis
- Pes anserinus bursitis
- Plicae
- Pigmented villonodular synovitis (PVNS)
- Synovitis
- Synovial chondromatosis
- Osteoarthritis (OA)

Table 7.6 Lesions of the synovium and bursae and arthropathy

Abnormalities	MRI findings	Comments
Baker cyst (▶ Fig. 7.52)	Fluid-filled, well-defined mass, often bilobed, located between the semimembranosus tendon and the medial gastrocnemius tendon. These lesions are low signal on proton density–weighted imaging (PDWI) and high signal on fat-suppressed T2-weighted imaging (FS T2WI) with axial plane imaging being the best. There may be debris or evidence of hemorrhage and synovial thickening in some cases. This can result in heterogeneous mixed signal appearance on FS T2WI. On post contrast images no enhancement is seen. In some cases the cyst will be large and may extend cranially or caudally toward the ankle or in both directions. Baker cysts often leak or rupture; both situations are seen on MRI as poorly defined high signal fluid on axial FS T2WI extending beyond the margins of the cyst.	Baker cysts are common in adults and uncommon in children. These cysts are often associated with other knee pathology such as meniscal tears, joint effusions and rheumatoid arthritis. Baker cysts are often painful and when they rupture can be difficult to differentiate from deep venous thrombosis. Treatment of patients with symptomatic Baker cyst is often conservative consisting of rest and NSAIDs. In some case aspiration or steroid injection may be needed.
Prepatellar bursitis (housemaid's knee) (▶ Fig. 7.53)	On sagittal FS T2WI there is a well-defined high signal fluid collection located between the subcutaneous skin and the anterior aspect of the patella. There are often some mixed foci of low signal seen within this fluid indicating the presence of internal debris. On PDWI there is low signal fluid seen.	Patients often have obvious swelling over the knee, which can be painful. The cause of the fluid collection can be secondary to acute trauma with a fall or direct blow to the anterior knee at the level of the patella resulting initially in a hematoma, which can then evolve into a simple fluid collection. Chronic repetitive injury such as in floor cleaning on the knees can also result in fluid collections occurring in this bursa.
Pes anserinus bursitis	This bursa is located between the distal portion of the medial collateral ligament and the pes anserine tendons (sartorius, gracilis, and semitendinosus). On axial and sagittal FS T2WI a high signal fluid collection is seen in this location. The collection is often locultated.	These bursal collections may be painful and can result in medial knee swelling. Treatment is similar to that of other symptomatic bursal collections.
Plicae (▶ Fig. 7.54)	Plicae are intra-articular linear bands of persistent fetal tissue. Symptomatic plicae are seen as thickened low signal bands on FS T2WI and are best identified when a joint effusion is present, which helps to define the low signal band with high signal fluid on either side.	There are several commonly occurring plicae that are synovial bands. The most commonly symptomatic is the medial plicae. Most patients with symptomatic plicae complain of anterior knee pain, sometimes with clicking. Other causes of anterior knee pain can have a similar clinical presentation, including patellar tendinosis and meniscal tears involving the anterior horns. MRI is often needed to distinguish among these abnormalities. Most patients respond well to conservative therapy. If there are continued symptoms surgical resection of the plica can be performed.

(continued on page 230)

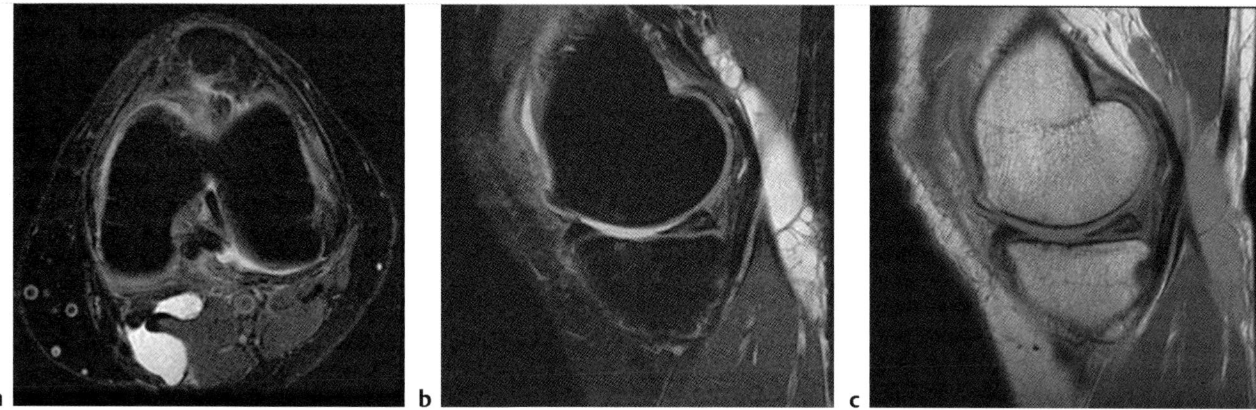

Fig. 7.52 (a) Axial fat-suppressed T2-weighted imaging (FS T2WI) shows a bilobed high signal cyst in the posterior medial knee between the semimembranosus tendon and the medial gastrocnemius. (b) Sagittal FS T2WI shows the same high signal Baker cyst to be multiseptated and to extend significantly in length. Note there is also a posterior horn medial meniscal tear. (c) Sagittal proton density–weighted imaging shows a large multiseptated intermediate signal Baker cyst.

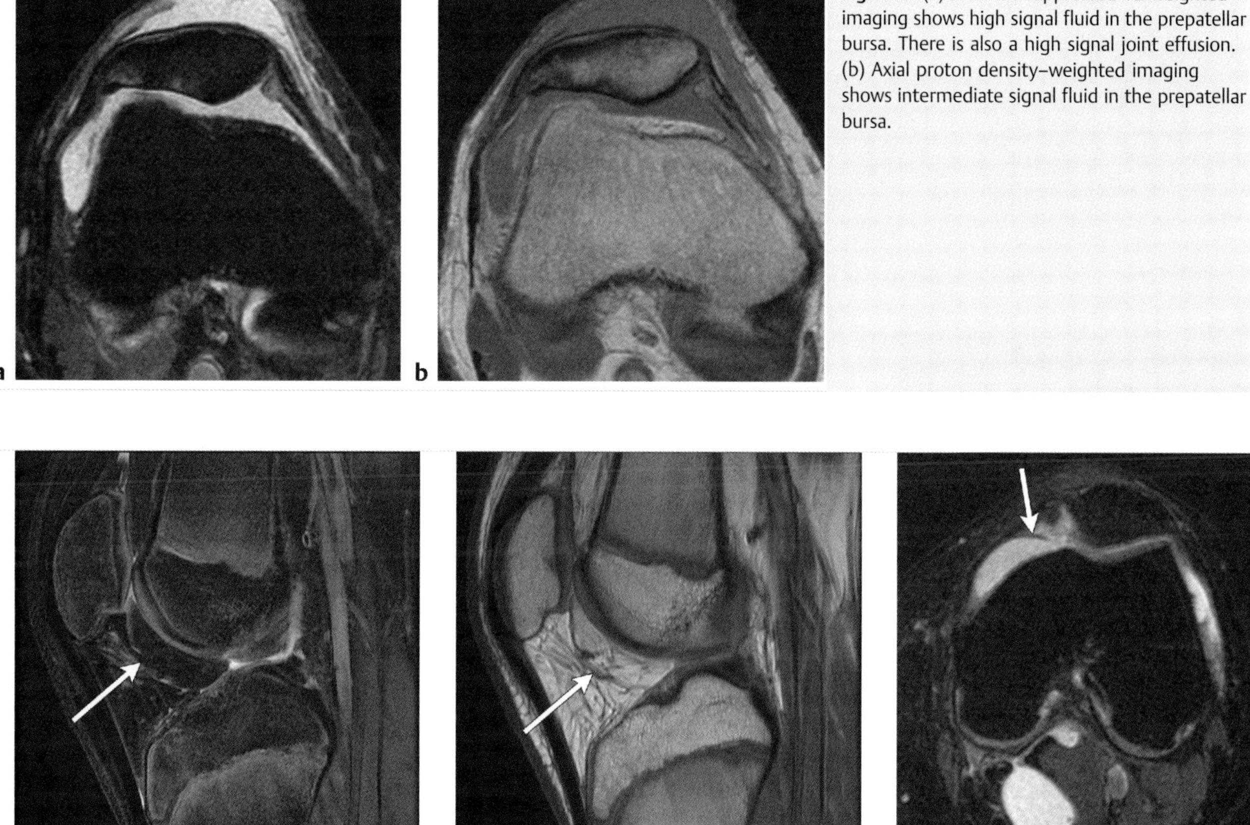

Fig. 7.53 (a) Axial fat-suppressed T2-weighted imaging shows high signal fluid in the prepatellar bursa. There is also a high signal joint effusion. (b) Axial proton density–weighted imaging shows intermediate signal fluid in the prepatellar bursa.

Fig. 7.54 (a) Sagittal fat-suppressed T2-weighted imaging (FS T2WI) shows a thickened low signal band running obliquely through the Hoffa fat (arrow) with adjacent high signal. (b) Sagittal proton density–weighted imaging (PDWI) shows a low signal band in the Hoffa fat (arrow). (c) Axial FS T2WI from a second patient shows a thickened medial patellar low signal plica (arrow) with adjacent high signal fluid from joint effusion.

Table 7.6 (Cont.) Lesions of the synovium and bursae and arthropathy

Abnormalities	MRI findings	Comments
Pigmented villonodular synovitis (PVNS) (▶ Fig. 7.55; ▶ Fig. 7.56)	PVNS may be of diffuse or nodular type. Both types have similar signal characteristics with low signal on fat-suppressed T2-weighted imaging (FS T2WI) and low signal on both proton density–weighted imaging (PDWI) and T1-weighted imaging (T1WI). Enhancement with gadolinium chelate is variable, often moderate in degree. One characteristic that is helpful in identifying this lesion on MRI is the pronounced blooming effect on gradient echo sequences due to the presence of hemosiderin within the lesion. This is easily seen on high field strength MRI where the effect is stronger. Erosion of adjacent bone may also be seen. Joint effusion is often present.	Most cases are seen in the knee in an intra-articular location. Many patients with PVNS complain of pain that is slowly progressive. Other symptoms may include stiffness and locking. Most patients are treated surgically with synovectomy. If the lesion is small then radiation may be sufficient. Up to 50% of patients treated for PVNS may have recurrence.

(continued on page 232)

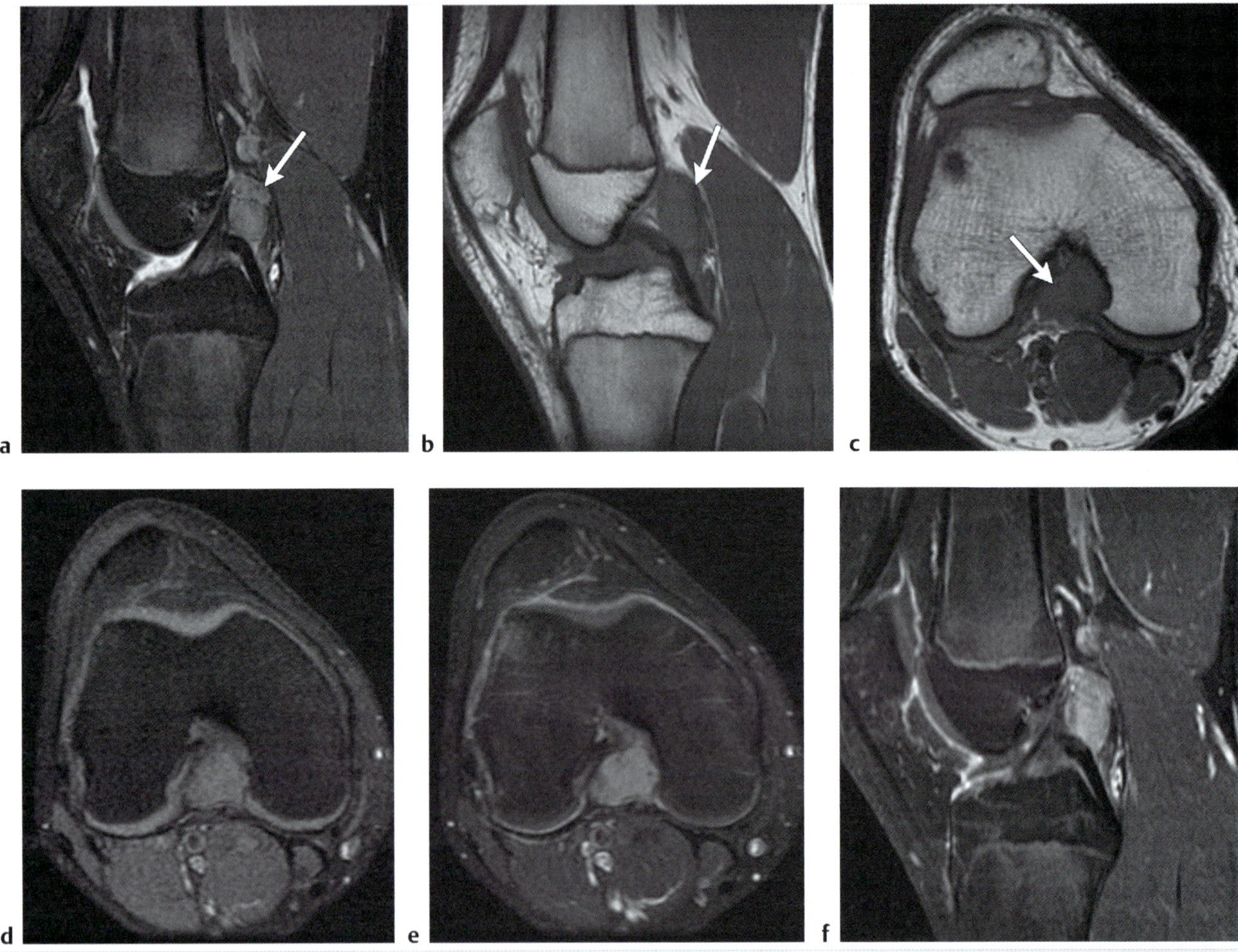

Fig. 7.55 (a) Sagittal fat-suppressed T2-weighted imaging (FS T2WI) shows a mildly increased signal mass posterior to the cruciate ligaments (arrow). This is nodular type pigmented villonodular synovitis (PVNS). (b) Sagittal proton density–weighted imaging (PDWI) shows an intermediate signal mass posterior to the cruciate ligaments (arrow). (c) Axial T1-weighted imaging (T1WI) shows a low to intermediate signal mass posterior to the cruciate ligaments (arrow). (d) Axial FS T1WI shows a mass that is nearly isointense to muscle and posterior to the cruciate ligaments. (e) Axial FS T1WI postcontrast shows a mild to moderately enhancing mass posterior to the cruciate ligaments. (f) Sagittal FS T1WI postcontrast shows a moderately enhancing mass posterior to the cruciate ligaments.

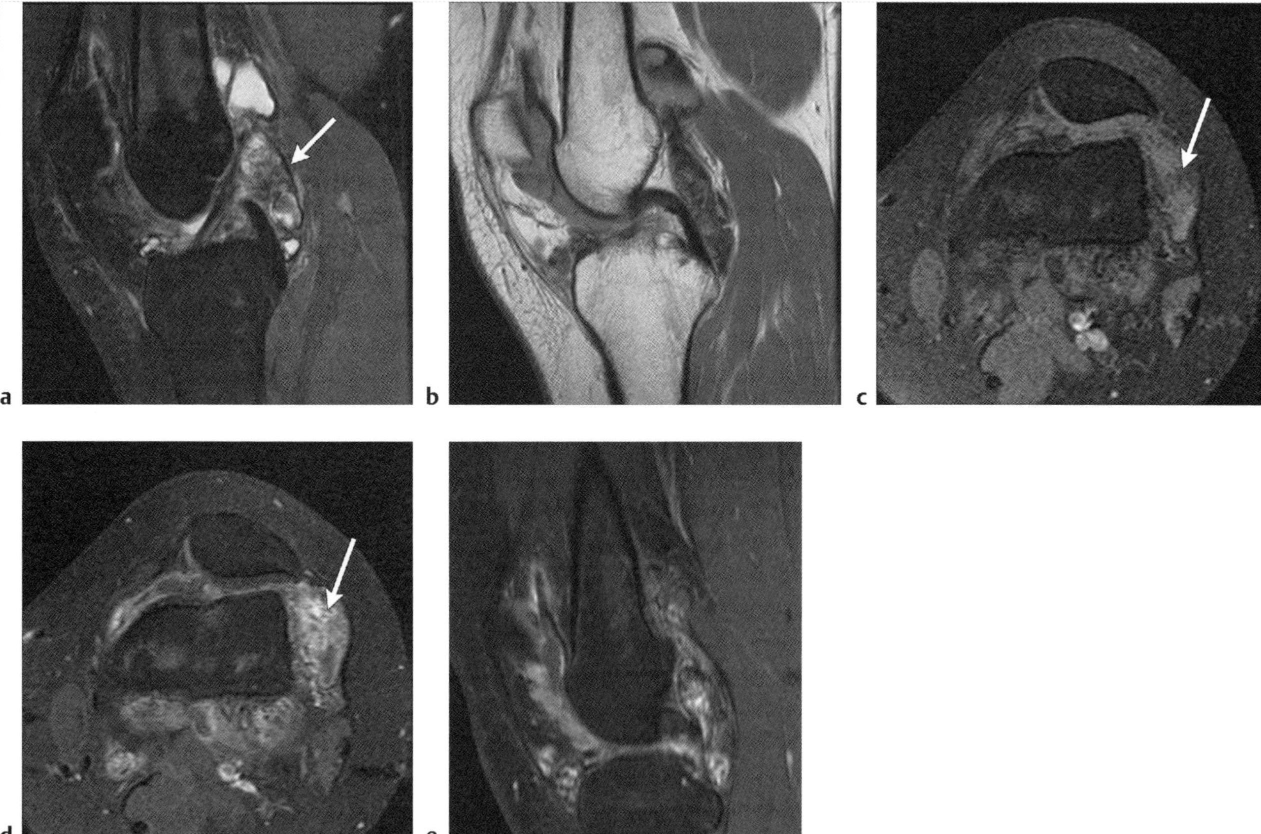

Fig. 7.56 (a) Sagittal fat-suppressed T2-weighted imaging (FS T2WI) shows ill-defined zones of mixed high and low signal, predominantly in the posterior portion of the knee (arrow). This is diffuse type pigmented villonodular synovitis. (b) Sagittal proton density–weighted imaging (PDWI) shows ill-defined zones of heterogeneous signal in the anterior and posterior portions of the knee. (c) Axial FS T1-weighted imaging (T1WI) shows ill-defined zones of mixed signal in the anterior and posterior portions of the knee with small foci of low signal (arrow) likely representing deposits of hemosiderin. (d) Corresponding axial FS T1WI postcontrast shows moderate heterogeneous zones of ill-defined enhancement (arrow). (e) Corresponding sagittal FS T1WI postcontrast shows heterogeneous zones of ill-defined enhancement.

Table 7.6 (Cont.) Lesions of the synovium and bursae and arthropathy

Abnormalities	MRI findings	Comments
Synovitis (▸ Fig. 7.57)	On FS T2WI there are often heterogeneous, somewhat nodular zones of mixed low signal seen within a high signal joint effusion. On FS T1WI after intravenous contrast administration there is enhancement of these zones of proliferating synovium, which is adjacent to nonenhancing low signal joint effusion.	In normal joints there is a thin, smooth synovial lining that demonstrates minimal thin linear enhancement with intravenous contrast. When the synovium becomes inflamed it will become thickened and often have zones of nodularity that demonstrate strong enhancement. This represents synovial proliferation, which can have several causes, including many different arthropathies.
Synovial chondromatosis (▸ Fig. 7.58)	Primary and secondary synovial chondromatosis has a variable MRI appearance dependent on the amount of ossification relative to cartilage. In cases where there is extensive calcification the lesion will appear as multiple intra-articular rounded signal voids on all MRI sequences. On postcontrast images there may be minimal enhancement of the periphery of these lesions. In cases with a higher proportion of cartilage content there is intermediate signal on PDWI and slightly to moderately high signal on FS T2WI. In late stages of this disease there are often associated changes of secondary osteoarthritis, including subchondral sclerosis, loss of articular cartilage, subcortical reactive marrow edema, and joint effusion.	Synovial chondromatosis is divided into two types, primary and secondary, with secondary being much more common. Primary type is a benign disorder in which there is nodular cartilaginous metaplasia of intra-articular synovium. This can progress to form small loose bodies, which can ultimately ossify. This disorder can also occur in the synovium of bursae and tendon sheaths. Secondary osteochondromatosis occurs in the setting of other joint diseases such as osteoarthritis, avascular necrosis (AVN), prior joint trauma, and others. The underlying cause is disruption of articular cartilage with the formation of loose bodies, which go on to osseous metaplasia. These loose bodies receive nutrients from the synovial fluid that surrounds them. Most patients complain of joint pain and decreased range of motion. The knee is the most common location. Surgical treatment consisting of removal of the loose bodies with synovectomy is often effective, although recurrence is possible if there has been incomplete synovectomy.

(continued on page 234)

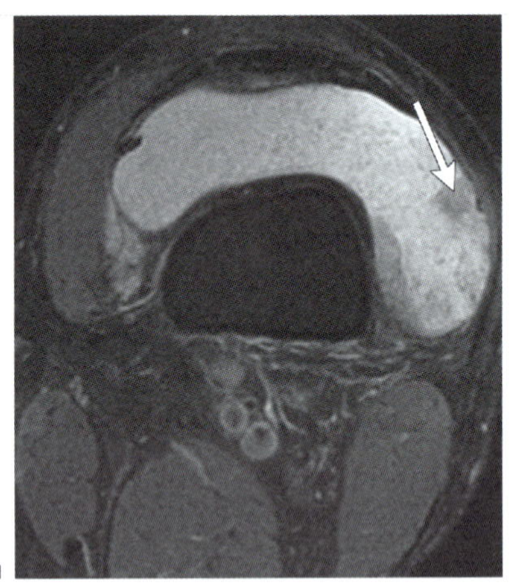

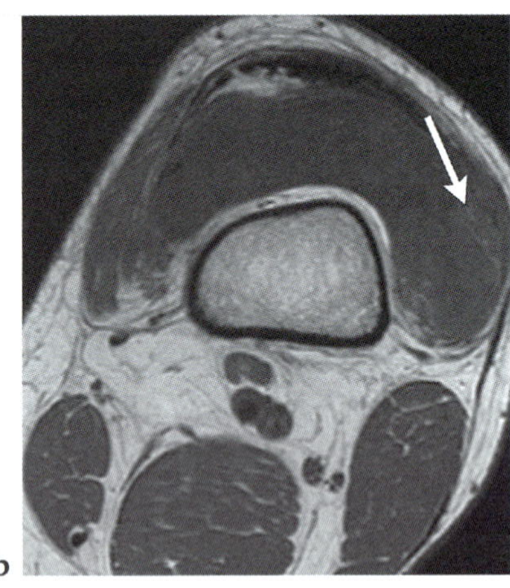

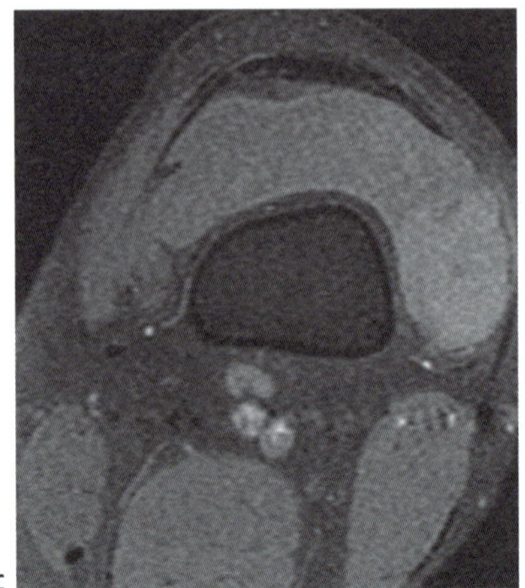

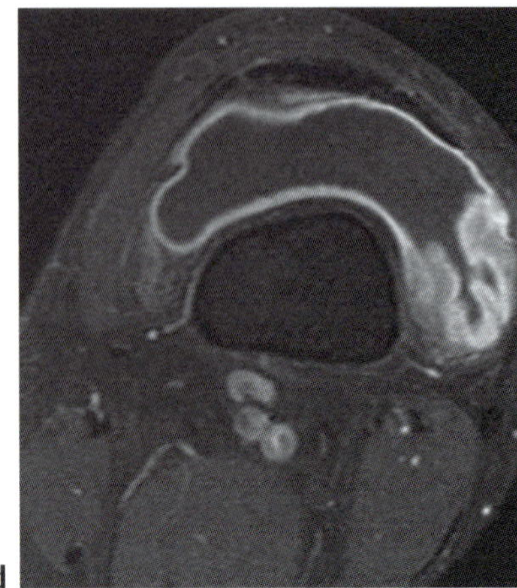

Fig. 7.57 (a) Axial fat-suppressed T2-weighted imaging (FS T2WI) shows a large joint effusion with some zones of lower signal nodularity (arrow). (b) Axial T1-weighted imaging (T1WI) shows a low signal effusion with a zone intermediate signal (arrow). (c) Corresponding axial FS T1WI shows a large effusion. (d) Axial FS T1WI post–intravenous contrast shows a thick, inflamed, enhancing synovium.

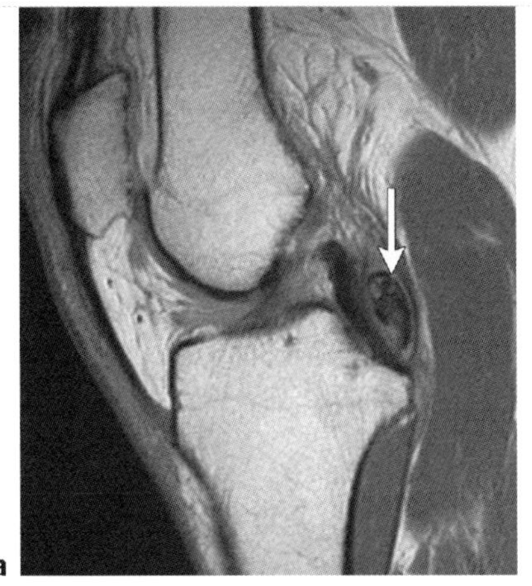

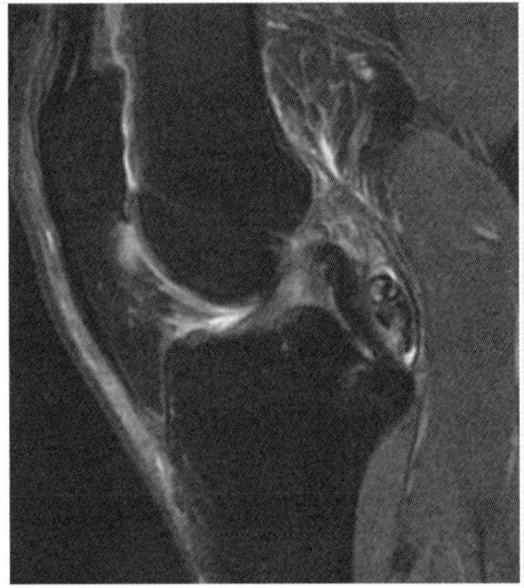

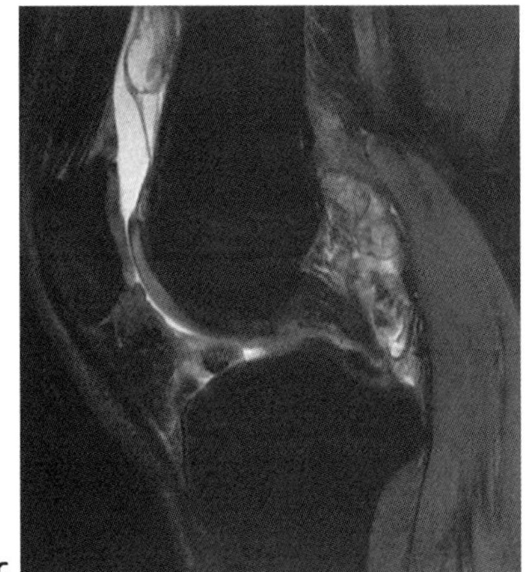

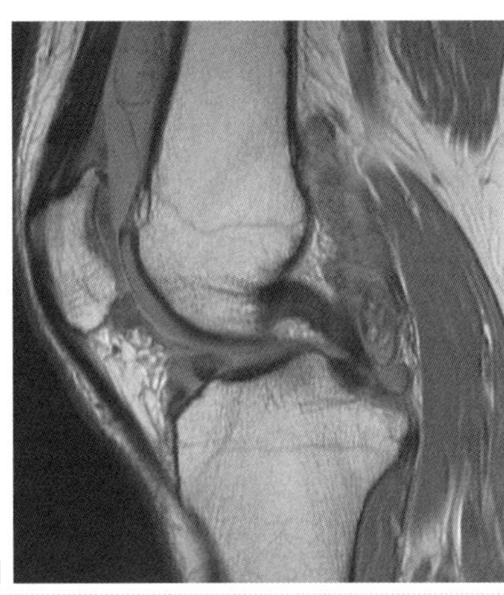

Fig. 7.58 (a) Sagittal proton density–weighted imaging (PDWI) shows a cluster of adjacent low signal loose bodies posterior to the posterior cruciate ligament (PCL) (arrow). (b) Sagittal fat-suppressed T2-weighted imaging (FS T2WI) shows a cluster of predominantly low signal loose bodies with foci of high signal posterior to the PCL. (c) Sagittal FS T2WI from a second patient shows multiple large mixed signal loose bodies posterior to the PCL. (d) Sagittal PDWI from the same patient shows multiple mixed signal loose bodies posterior to the PCL. In both patients this is secondary osteochondromatosis.

Table 7.6 (Cont.) Lesions of the synovium and bursae and arthropathy

Abnormalities	MRI findings	Comments
Osteoarthritis (OA) (▶ Fig. 7.59)	The goal of MRI in evaluation of OA of the knee is assessment of articular cartilage and adjacent subchondral bone. On fat-suppressed T2-weighted imaging (FS T2WI) a range of cartilage abnormalities can be seen, including minor surface irregularities with progression to more severe abnormalities, including surface ulcers, fissures, fibrillation, partial-thickness defects, and ultimately full-thickness defects, which may be small or large. Commonly associated with cartilage abnormalities are signal changes in the adjacent subcortical bone. These may be mild or severe and usually correspond to the degree of cartilage damage. On FS T2WI there is often patchy high signal seen in the adjacent subcortical bone. This is degenerative reactive marrow edema and is often on both sides of a joint in a fairly symmetric pattern unlike a posttraumatic bone contusion, which often affects a bone on only one side of the joint. Other typical findings on FS T2WI are round high signal subcortical cysts (geodes), which are variable in size and number. Marginal osteophytes and subcortical sclerosis, low signal in the subcortical region on PDWI and T1WI, are also commonly seen. In advanced cases there may also be flattening of bony articular contours.	OA is the most common arthropathy. Cartilage destruction and resultant changes in the underlying bone are the distinctive features of OA. There are many causes of OA, all of which ultimately lead to cartilage destruction. Typical causes include acute traumatic injuries and repetitive injuries, sometimes related to work. Other predisposing factors include obesity, older age, and anatomical variation, including bony alignment. Patients often present with joint pain, which will increase in severity with increasing levels of activity. Eventually, patients may complain of knee joint instability. OA can be treated both medically and surgically. Medical treatment typically consists of nonsteroidal anti-inflammatory drugs for pain and in some patients with supplements such as glucosamine and chondroitin sulfate. Surgery often consists of total joint replacement. In selected patients new cartilage transplantation techniques are being performed. This is an evolving technique.

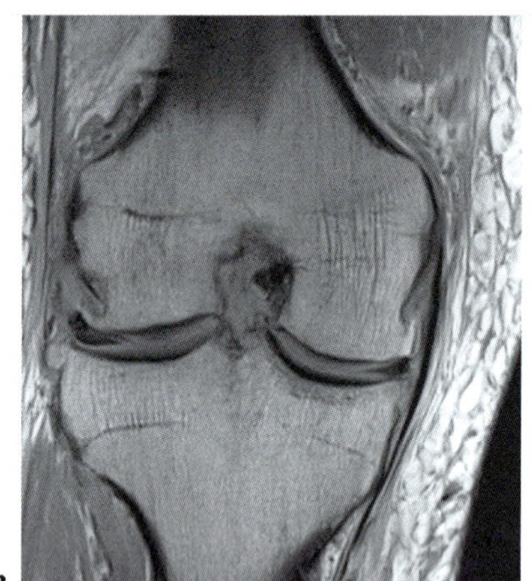

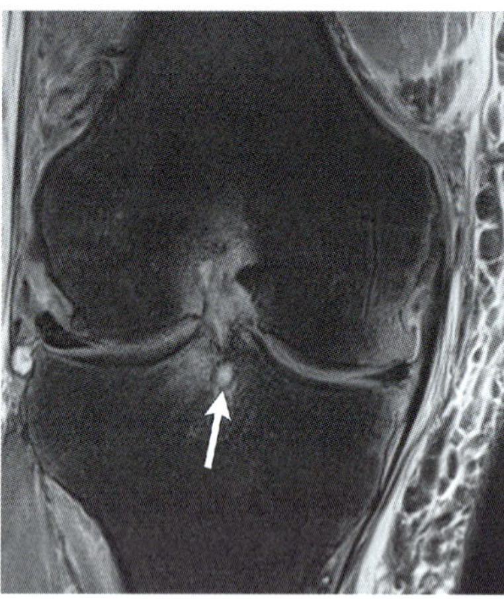

Fig. 7.59 (a) Coronal proton density–weighted imaging shows large marginal osteophytes arising from the distal femur and smaller proximal tibial osteophytes. (b) Coronal fat-suppressed T2-weighted imaging shows subcortical degenerative reactive marrow edema in the medial femoral condyle and opposite medial tibia with additional degenerative reactive marrow edema in the central proximal tibia extending into the tibial spines. A small geode is also present between the tibial spines (arrow). There is also some thinning and irregularity of the femoral articular cartilage.

7.6.1 Lesions of the Synovium and Bursae and Arthropathy

[1] Boles CA, Butler J, Lee JA, Reedy ML, Martin DF. Magnetic resonance characteristics of medial plica of the knee: correlation with arthroscopic resection. J Comput Assist Tomogr 2004; 28: 397–401

[2] Huétink K, Nelissen RGHH, Watt I, van Erkel AR, Bloem JL. Localized development of knee osteoarthritis can be predicted from MR imaging findings a decade earlier. Radiology 2010; 256: 536–546

[3] Marra MD, Crema MD, Chung M, et al. MRI features of cystic lesions around the knee. Knee 2008; 15: 423–438

[4] Murphey MD, Rhee JH, Lewis RB, Fanburg-Smith JC, Flemming DJ, Walker EA. Pigmented villonodular synovitis: radiologic-pathologic correlation. Radiographics 2008; 28: 1493–1518

[5] Roemer FW, Crema MD, Trattnig S, Guermazi A. Advances in imaging of osteoarthritis and cartilage. Radiology 2011; 260: 332–354

Chapter 8

The Ankle and Foot

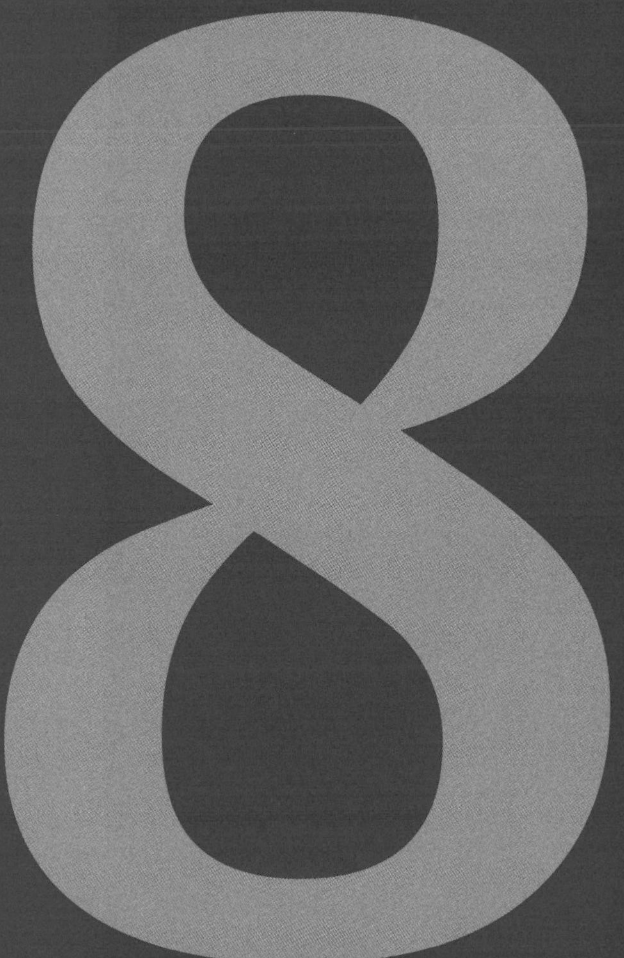

8 The Ankle and Foot

Gary M. Hollenberg

8.1 Lesions of the Ankle and Foot Tendons

- Noninsertional Achilles tendinosis
- Insertional Achilles tendinosis
- Achilles tendon tears
- Posterior tibial tendon (PTT) abnormalities
- Flexor hallucis longus (FHL) tendon abnormalities
- Peroneus brevis (PB) tendon abnormalities
- Peroneus longus (PL) tendon abnormalities
- Tibialis anterior (TA) tendon abnormalities

Table 8.1 Lesions of the ankle and foot tendons

Abnormalities	MRI findings	Comments
Noninsertional Achilles tendinosis (▶ Fig. 8.1)	Look for tendon enlargement (normally 7 mm in short axis), anterior convex bowing of the tendon, and increased intratendinous signal on proton density–weighted imaging (PDWI) and fat-suppressed T2-weighted imaging (FS T2WI). This is commonly seen 4 to 6 cm proximal to the calcaneal insertion. To distinguish tendinopathy from a partial tear, check for fluid signal on FS T2WI seen with tears. Assess the paratenon for abnormal signal. Inflammation adjacent to the tendon reflects paratendonitis.	Noninsertional tendinosis occurs in the hypovascular/watershed area of the tendon 4 to 6 cm proximal to the insertion. A paratenon surrounds the tendon on all but its anterior margin. Tendinosis is associated with partial tears. Other differential considerations for an enlarged Achilles tendon or abnormal tendon signal include xanthomas in patients with familial hyperlipidemia types II and III and gouty deposits.

(continued on page 240)

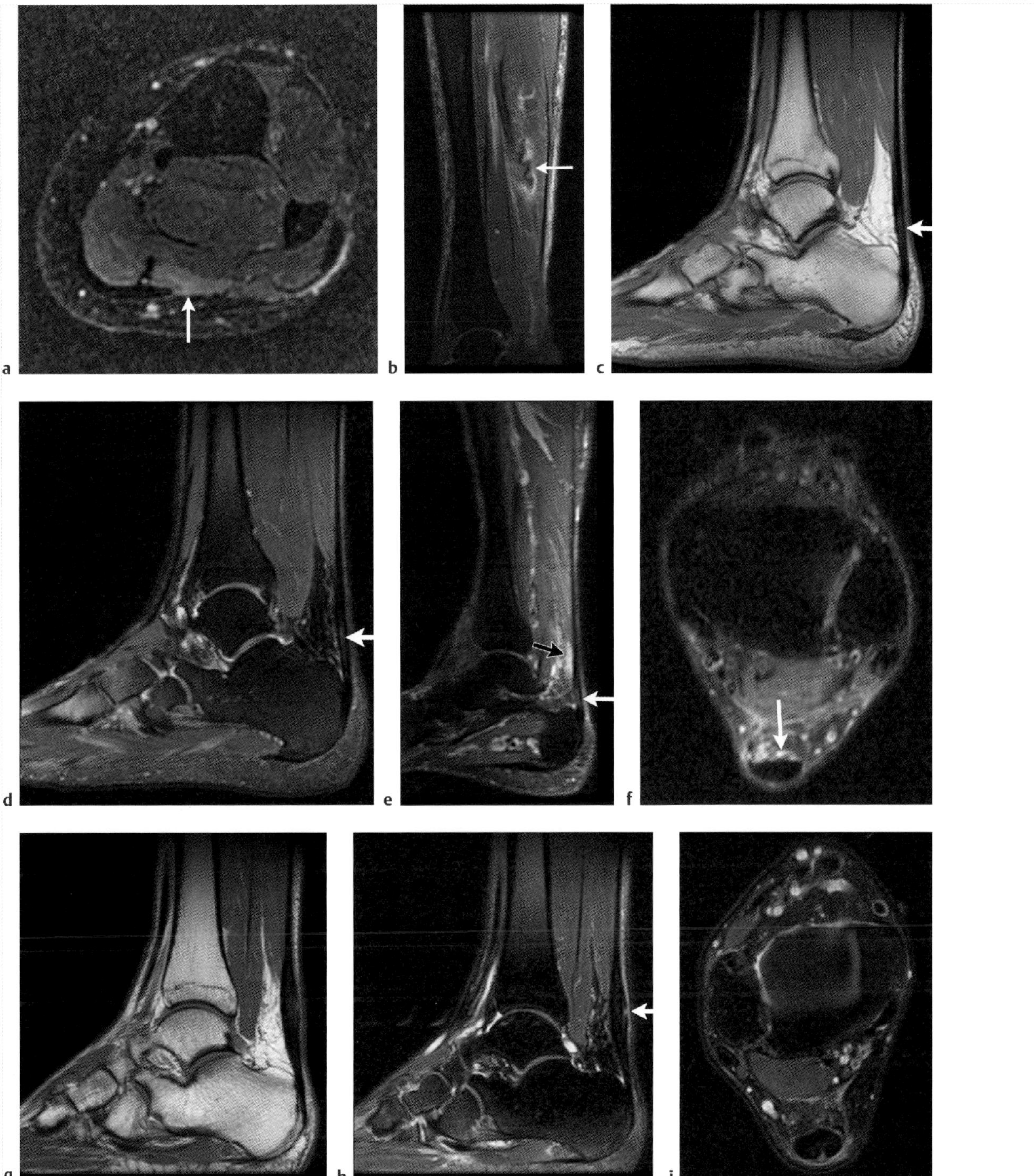

Fig. 8.1 (a) Mild soleus muscle strain may mimic a musculotendinous junction injury of the Achilles tendon. Note mild soleus muscle edema posteriorly on axial fat-suppressed T2-weighted imaging (FS T2WI). (b) A different patient with a partial soleus tendon tear with wavy torn tendon fibers surrounded by mild edema posteriorly on sagittal FS T2WI. (c) Minimal distal Achilles tendinopathy with abnormal increased signal in the distal tendon (arrow) and mild anterior tendon bowing on sagittal proton density–weighted imaging (PDWI) and (d) on sagittal FS T2WI. (e) In a different patient, note paratendonitis with abnormal high T2 signal anterior to the Achilles tendon (black arrow) and more subtle increased signal within the distal tendon (white arrow) on sagittal FS T2WI and (f) on axial FS T2WI. (g) In a more severe case of tendinosis, note focal thickening and anterior bowing of the tendon on sagittal PDWI. (h) There is a superimposed tiny partial tear along the posterior tendon (arrow) on sagittal FS T2WI. (i) Note increased signal of paratendonitis posterior to the Achilles tendon partial tear on axial FS T2WI. An intact plantaris tendon is seen anteromedial to the Achilles tendon.

Table 8.1 (Cont.) Lesions of the ankle and foot tendons

Abnormalities	MRI findings	Comments
Insertional Achilles tendinosis (▶ Fig. 8.2)	Abnormal tendon enlargement and increased signal on PDWI and FS T2WI (as with noninsertional tendinosis) seen distally at the calcaneal insertion.	Insertional Achilles tendinosis is often associated with retrocalcaneal and retro-Achilles bursitis. Look for increased signal fluid on FS T2WI in the retrocalcaneal bursa posterior to the calcaneus and in the retro-Achilles bursa posterior to the Achilles tendon. Haglund syndrome consists of insertional Achilles tendinosis, bursitis, and Haglund deformity (a prominent calcaneal tuberosity). Note that the retro-Achilles bursa is an adventitial bursa, discussed later.

(continued on page 242)

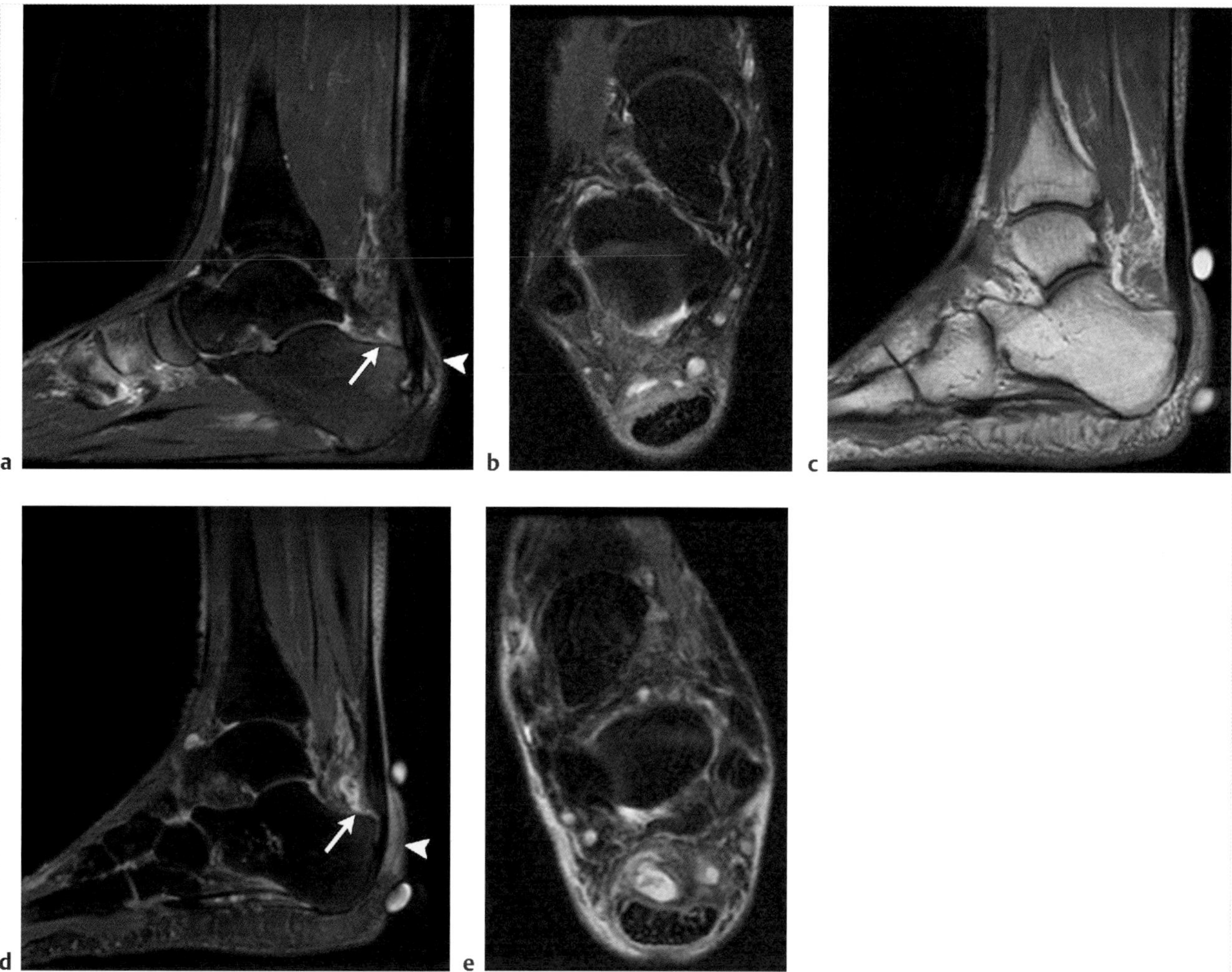

Fig. 8.2 (a) Distal Achilles tendinopathy with degenerative geode formation and reactive marrow edema of the posterior calcaneus. Note distal tendon thickening and adjacent increased signal edema and fluid in the retrocalcaneal (arrow) and retro-Achilles (arrowhead) bursae on sagittal fat-suppressed T2-weighted imaging (FS T2WI). (b) Corresponding axial FS T2WI demonstrates slight anterior bowing of the thickened portion of the distal Achilles tendon with surrounding edema/fluid. (c) In a similar patient with Achilles tendinopathy note the thickened distal Achilles tendon on sagittal proton density–weighted imaging. (d) There is fluid in the retrocalcaneal bursa (white arrow) and edema in the retro-Achilles bursa (arrowhead) on sagittal FS T2WI. (e) Correlative axial FS T2WI also demonstrates fluid in the retrocalcaneal bursa.

Table 8.1 (Cont.) Lesions of the ankle and foot tendons

Abnormalities	MRI findings	Comments
Achilles tendon tears (▸ Fig. 8.3)	Rupture commonly occurs 2 to 6 cm proximal to the insertion of the tendon on the calcaneus, or more proximally at the musculotendinous junction. Look for disrupted tendon architecture with abnormal tendon morphology including bulging of the anterior tendon margin, tendon enlargement, and wavy retracted tendon ends in complete tears. Abnormal increased signal on PDWI and fluid signal on FS T2WI will be seen at the tear site, versus intermediate signal abnormalities on FS T2WI seen with tendinosis. The sagittal plane is the most helpful in initial evaluation. Assess the size of the gap between torn tendon ends in complete tears. This gap will vary depending on degree of plantar flexion.	The presence and size of the gap at the tear site is important in determining the choice of conservative or surgical management. Complete tears may present with apposed or overlapping torn ends, particularly if the patient is casted in plantar flexion. Partial tears may be diagnosed by assessing for contour abnormality at the suspected tear site. Proximal tendon imaging is essential to exclude a musculotendinous junction injury. Do not mistake an intact plantaris tendon (seen medially) for the Achilles tendon. Tendon enlargement due to infiltration by a xanthoma may occur in familial hyperlipidemia, and mimics tendinosis, but tends to be bilateral. Re-tear of postoperative Achilles tendons may be identified by the presence of susceptibility artifact from suture material.

(continued on page 244)

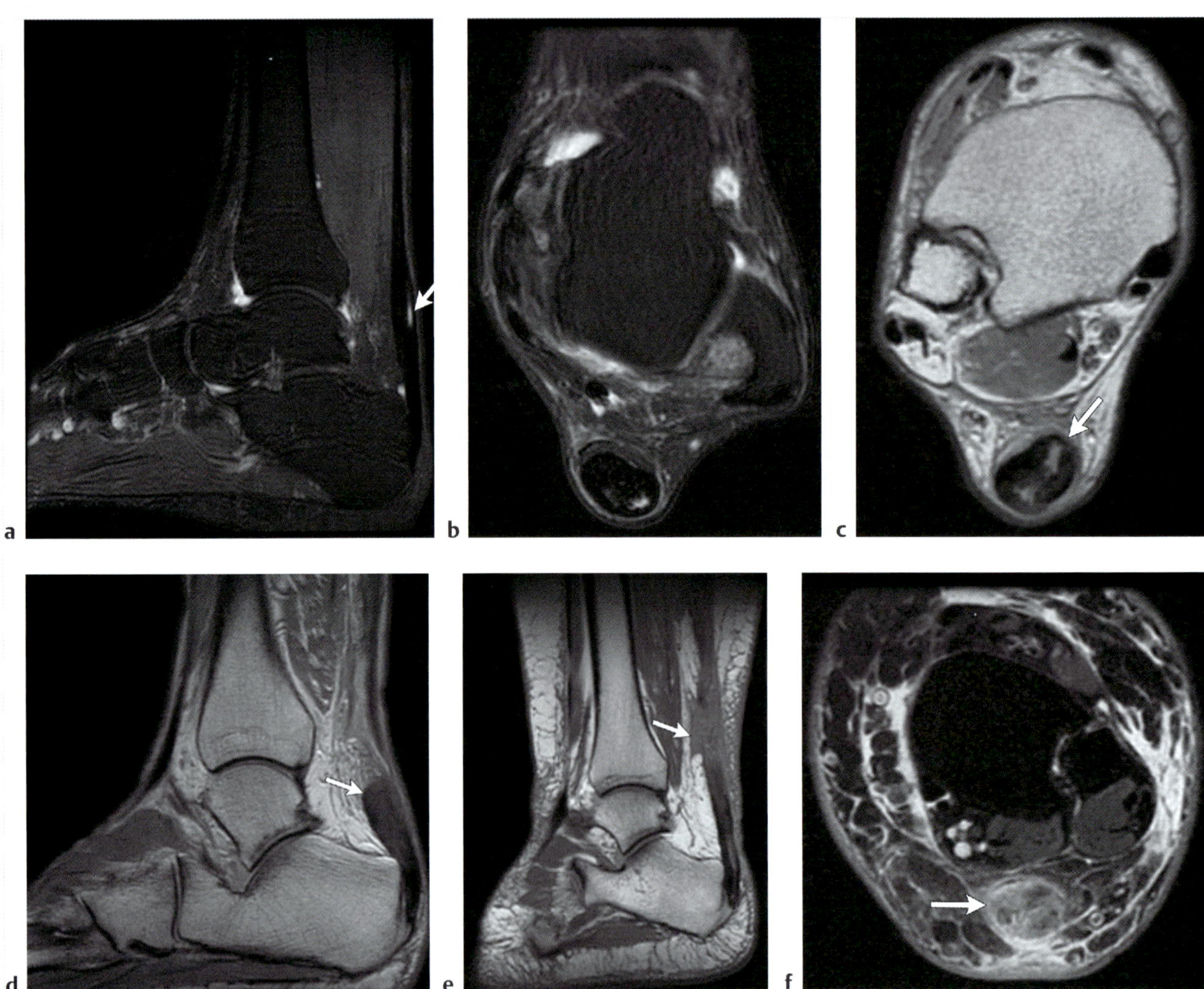

Fig. 8.3 (a) Small partial tear of the Achilles tendon demonstrating fluid signal at the tear site posteriorly (arrow) on sagittal fat-suppressed T2-weighted imaging (FS T2WI) and (b) on axial FS T2WI. Note abnormal tendon thickening and anterior bowing. (c) Larger partial Achilles tendon tear on axial proton density–weighted imaging (PDWI). Note irregular separation of the torn ends along an oblique plane (arrow) and intermediate signal fluid within the tear site. Note asymmetric ovoid configuration of the torn ends, which remain apposed. (d) Complete Achilles tendon tear with abnormal signal and thickening of the distal torn end (arrow) and irregular thinning and poor definition of the proximal end on sagittal PDWI. Patient is in a neutral position with separation of the torn ends in this subacute case of a torn Achilles tendon. (e) A more proximal Achilles tear with intermediate signal fluid within the tear site (arrow) and fluid extending anteriorly. Note linear increased signal more distally representing tendinosis on sagittal PDWI. (f) Corresponding axial FS T2WI through the tear site (arrow) demonstrates ill-defined fluid, hemorrhage, and torn tendon ends. *(continued)*

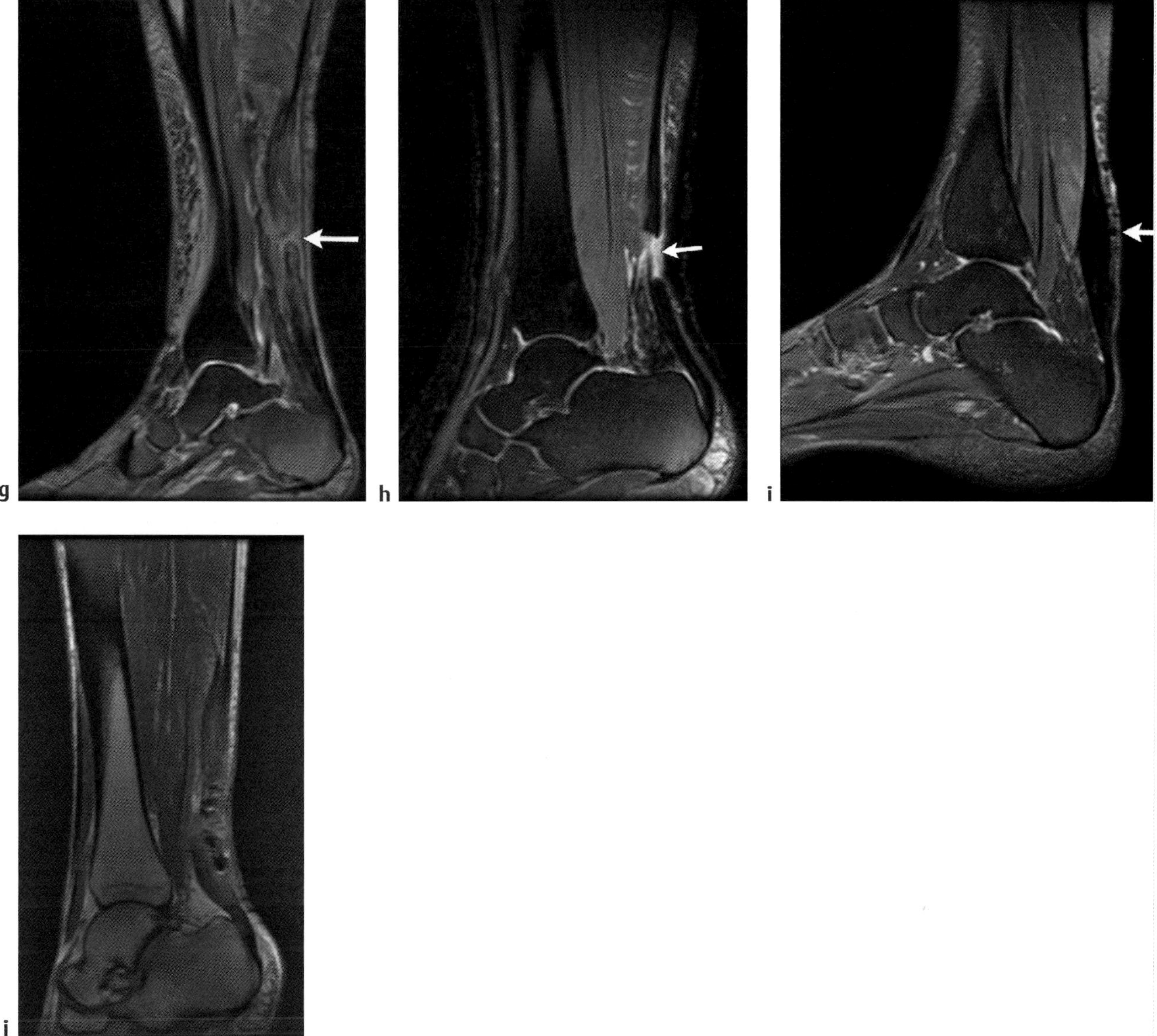

Fig. 8.3 *(continued)* (g) A different case of a proximal Achilles tendon tear with nearly opposed torn ends (arrow) on sagittal FS T2WI. Note severe tendinosis of the proximal and distal torn ends. (h) Laceration of an Achilles tendon following injury. Note the fluid-filled gap (arrow) between the tendon ends and a lack of adjacent tendinosis on sagittal FS T2WI. (i) Postoperative appearance of a repaired tendon with residual thickening and magnetic susceptibility artifact (arrow) on sagittal FS T2WI. (j) Re-rupture of a previously repaired tendon. Note the ill-defined tear site and low signal foci of magnetic susceptibility artifact on sagittal PDWI.

Table 8.1 (Cont.) Lesions of the ankle and foot tendons

Abnormalities	MRI findings	Comments
Posterior tibial tendon (PTT) abnormalities (► Fig. 8.4)	A spectrum of signal and morphological abnormalities ranging from tenosynovitis to complete tendon tear. Tenosynovitis presents with abnormal fluid signal on FS T2WI surrounding an otherwise intact tendon. Tendon enlargement and increased signal within the tendon on PDWI and FS T2WI are indicative of tendinosis, often seen at and distal to the medial malleolus. The presence of fluid within the tendon substance on FS T2WI differentiates tendinosis from a tear. Note that the normal tendon can be up to twice the size of the adjacent flexor digitorum longus tendon. Vertical split tears present with tendon thickening and variable increased linear signal on PDWI and FS T2WI. The tendon may appear attenuated due to subtendons along a split tear. Marrow edema may be seen in the adjacent medial malleolus. Complete tears are indicated by absence of the tendon along its expected course.	Typically affects middle-aged women and is associated with flatfoot deformity. The posterior tibial tendon normally increases in size and signal as it inserts on the navicular tubercle and divides to insert on the cuneiforms, the second to fourth metatarsals, and the cuboid. Patients with a type II accessory navicular demonstrate a synchondrosis between the ossicle and the navicular. The tendon inserts on the ossicle resulting in abnormal stress and an increased incidence of tendon pathology. Angled axial magnetic resonance (MR) images are useful to maximize short axis image orientation to tendons as they cross the malleoli. This also helps minimize magic angle effect on short TE sequences. PTT dysfunction is usually degenerative. Pannus of rheumatoid arthritis will appear more complex and nodular than routine tenosynovitis.

(continued on page 246)

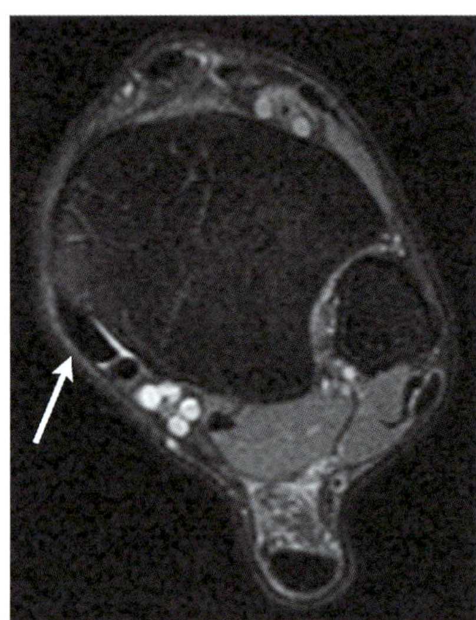

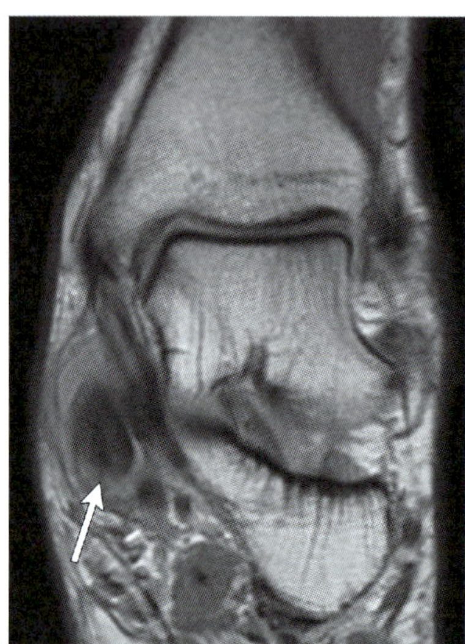

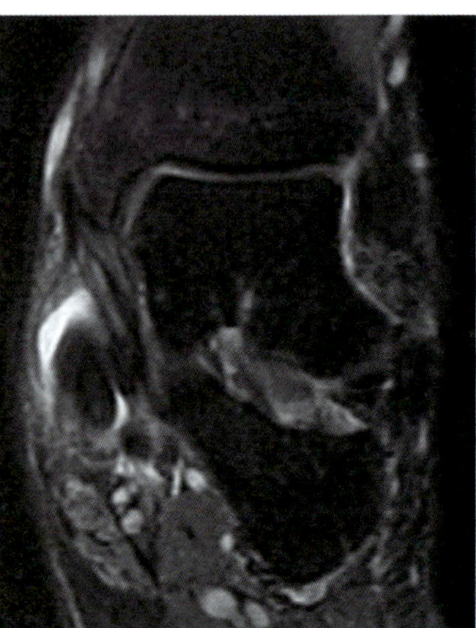

Fig. 8.4 (a) Normally low signal but mildly thickened posterior tibial tendon (PTT) (arrow) on axial fat-suppressed T2-weighted imaging (FS T2WI). (b) Severe posterior tibial tendinopathy with tendon enlargement (arrow) on coronal proton density–weighted imaging (PDWI). (c) High signal fluid surrounding the enlarged and thickened PTT represents tenosynovitis and tendinopathy on coronal FS T2WI. (*continued*)

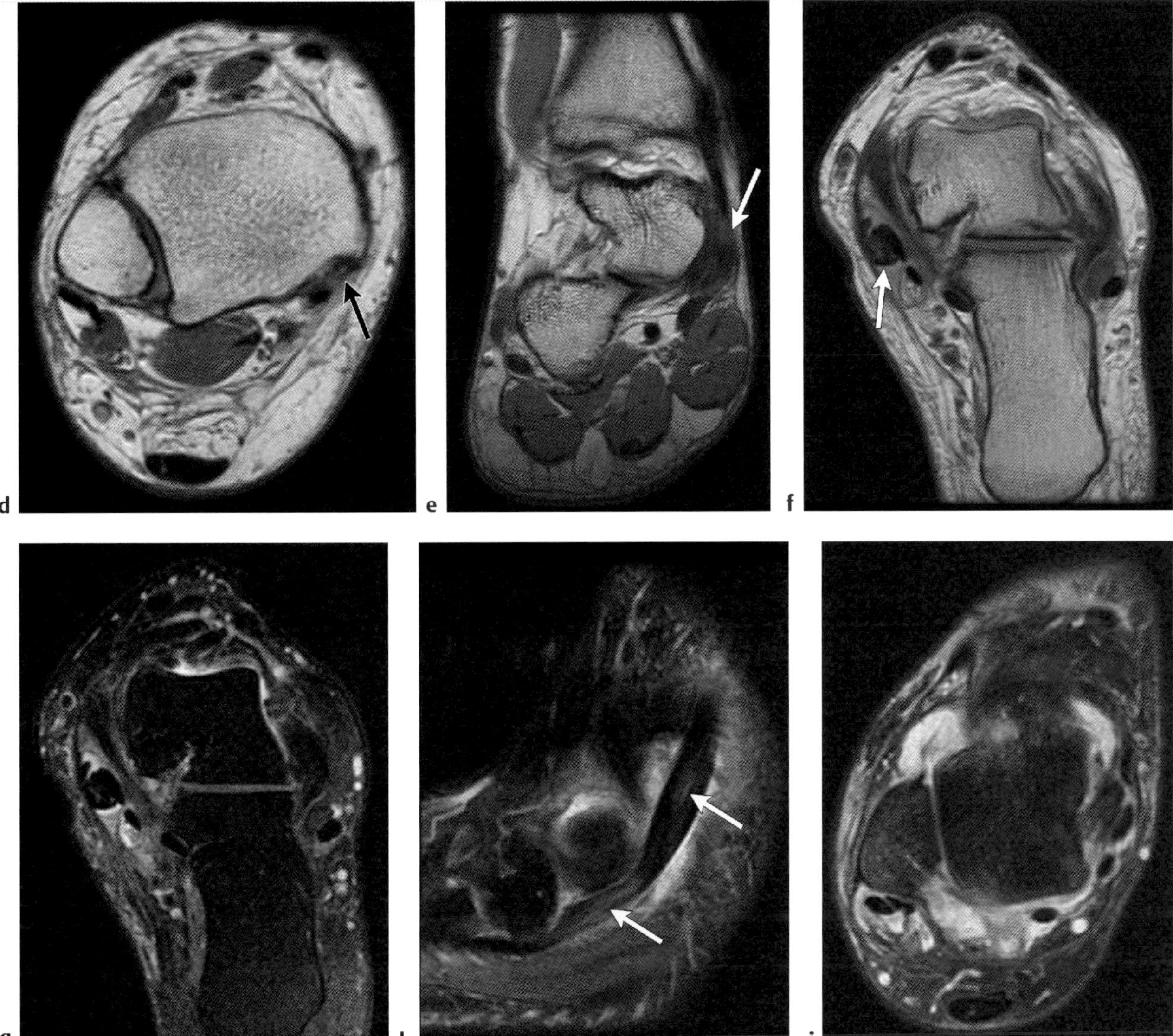

Fig. 8.4 (*continued*) (d) Small PTT with a split tear (arrow) on axial PDWI. Note linear increased signal through the substance of the tendon. (e) In a different patient, an ill-defined tear of the PTT (arrow) with abnormally increased signal on coronal PDWI. (f) Complex split tear of the PTT with subtendons (arrow) on angled axial PDWI. (g) Note surrounding high signal tenosynovitis on angled axial FS T2WI. Tenosynovitis also extends to surround the flexor digitorum tendon more posteriorly. (h) Both tenosynovitis and tendinopathy with tendon thickening and linear split tears (arrows) involve the PTT on sagittal FS T2WI. (i) Note extensive heterogeneous high signal pannus surrounding the medial and lateral tendon groups in a patient with rheumatoid arthritis on axial FS T2WI. The pannus should not be confused with simple fluid.

Table 8.1 (Cont.) Lesions of the ankle and foot tendons

Abnormalities	MRI findings	Comments
Flexor hallucis longus (FHL) tendon abnormalities (▶ Fig. 8.5)	The key to diagnosis of tenosynovitis is a disproportionate amount of high T2 signal fluid along the tendon sheath when compared to the amount of fluid in the tibiotalar joint. Finding is usually well seen on sagittal images. FHL tendinopathy appears similar to that seen involving other ankle tendons. Stenosing tenosynovitis occurs as a result of inflammation and fibrosis, interrupting the flow of synovial fluid with resultant pooling or lobulation of fluid along the tendon sheath.	The flexor hallucis longus tendon commonly communicates with the ankle joint, allowing fluid to enter the tendon sheath. Stenosing tenosynovitis is often associated with os trigonum syndrome. With repeated plantar flexion (e.g. dancers) the os trigonum and flexor hallucis longus tendon become pinched between the calcaneus and posterior malleolus. Complete tendon tears are uncommon.

(continued on page 248)

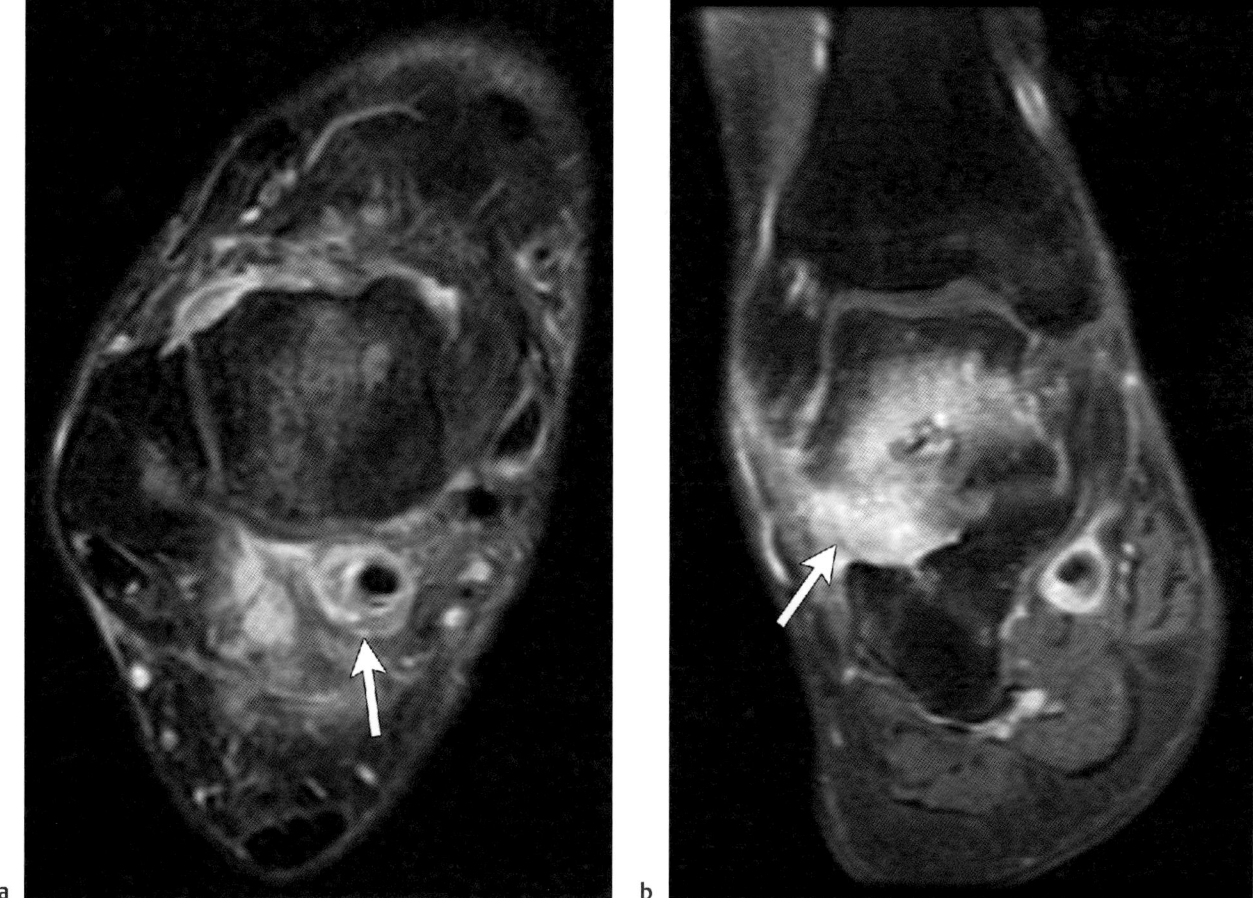

Fig. 8.5 (a) Extensive high signal heterogeneous pannus surrounding the flexor hallucis longus (FHL) tendon (arrow) on axial fat-suppressed T2-weighted imaging (FS T2WI) in a patient with known rheumatoid arthritis. (b) Note the pannus within the sinus tarsi (arrow), and adjacent reactive marrow edema of the talus, on coronal FS T2WI.

Table 8.1 (Cont.) Lesions of the ankle and foot tendons

Abnormalities	MRI findings	Comments
Peroneus brevis (PB) tendon abnormalities (▶ Fig. 8.6)	Spectrum of abnormalities including tenosynovitis that demonstrates high signal fluid surrounding the tendon on FS T2WI. Tendinopathy or partial tendon tears will usually show attenuation of the tendon and abnormally increased tendon signal on PDWI and FS T2WI. A peroneus brevis tendon split tear is typically centered at the tip of the lateral malleolus with a C- or chevron-shaped tendon with variably increased signal on PDWI and FS T2WI. A split tear may also present as two separate subtendons. Check for interposition of the larger peroneus longus tendon within a split tear of the peroneus brevis. Assess the insertion of the PB on the fifth metatarsal base.	Peroneus brevis split tear may be associated with antero-lateral tendon subluxation due to a tear of the overlying superior peroneal retinaculum. Look for associated lateral ankle ligament injuries in cases of peroneal tendon abnormalities. Beware of a normal variant, the peroneus quartus muscle, which can result in erroneous diagnosis of a split tear. Visualization of a separate muscle belly more proximally confirms this variant.

(continued on page 250)

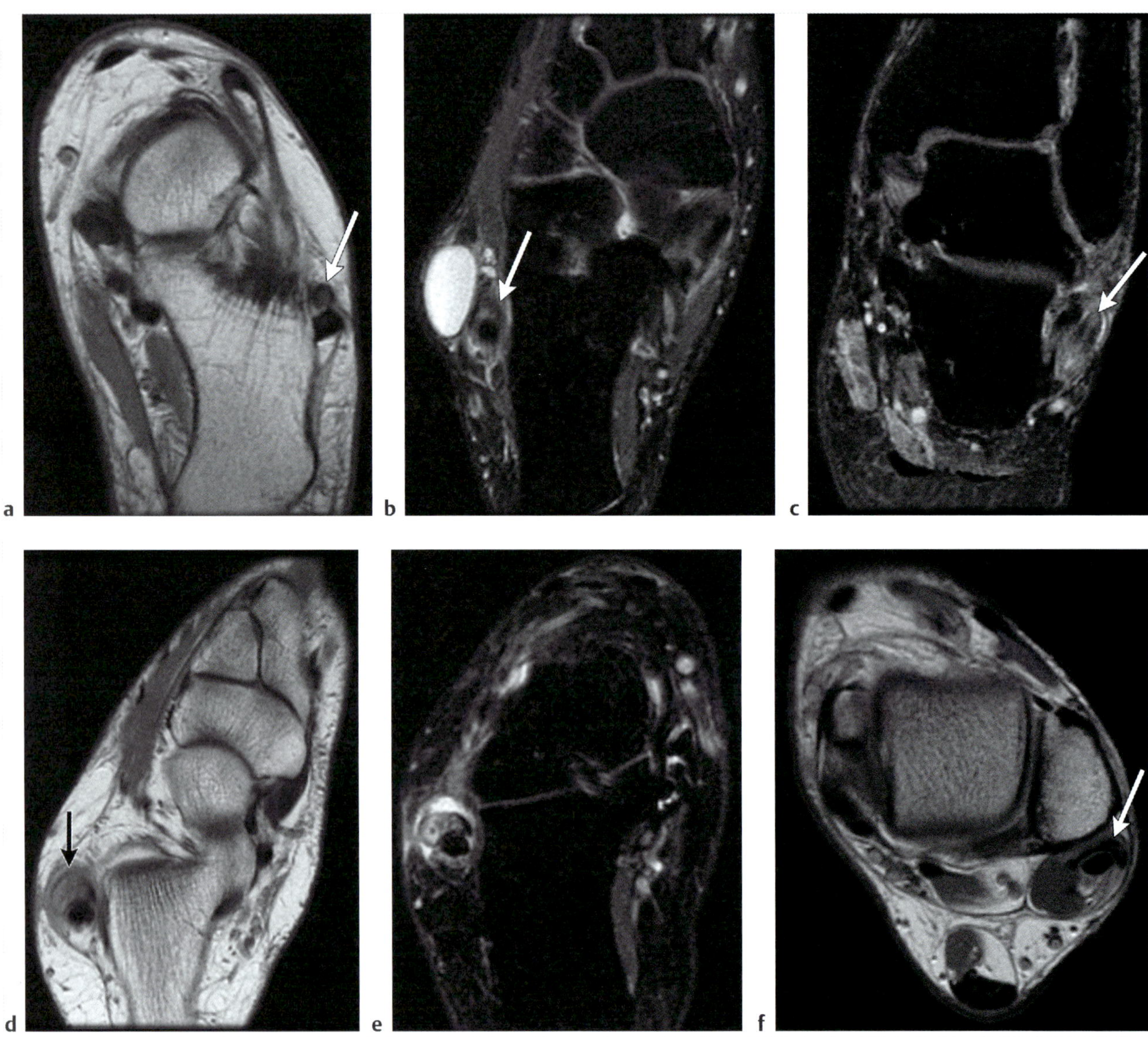

Fig. 8.6 (a) Mild tendinopathy of the peroneus brevis (PB) tendon with increased signal within the tendon (arrow) on axial proton density–weighted imaging (PDWI). (b) Typical chevron- or C-shaped (arrow) appearance of a split tear of the PB tendon. Tendon is irregular and of increased signal. Note the adjacent ganglion cyst in the subcutaneous tissues on axial fat-suppressed T2-weighted imaging (FS T2WI). (c) Well-defined PB split tear (arrow) with surrounding high signal tenosynovitis, on coronal FS T2WI. (d) Marked tendon enlargement and abnormal signal are noted in this example of tendinopathy and partial tear of the PB tendon (arrow) on axial PDWI and (e) on axial FS T2WI. Note surrounding high signal tenosynovitis. (f) A different patient with PB tendinopathy and partial tears on axial PDWI. Note tendon thinning and lobulated contour (arrow). (*continued*)

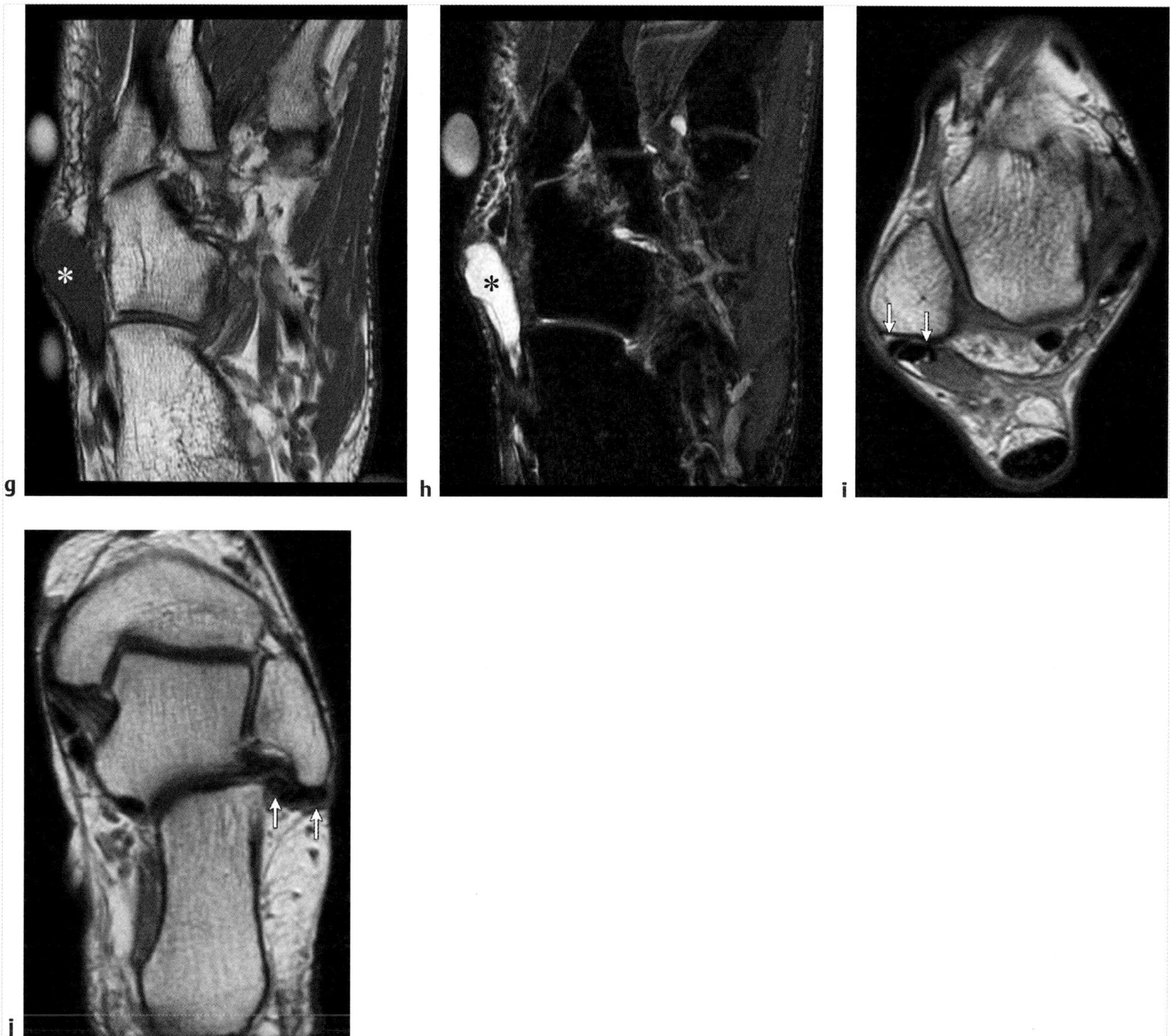

Fig. 8.6 (*continued*) (g) Intermediate signal fluid (asterisk) separating a PB split tear on axial PDWI and (h) corresponding high signal fluid (asterisk) within the PB split tear on axial FS T2WI. (i) Two cases of well-defined PB split subtendons (arrows) on either side of an intact PL tendon on axial PDWI and (j) oblique axial PDWI. Note tendons are not subluxed, which may accompany peroneal tears.

Table 8.1 (Cont.) Lesions of the ankle and foot tendons

Abnormalities	MRI findings	Comments
Peroneus longus (PL) tendon abnormalities (▶ Fig. 8.7)	The tendon may demonstrate tendinosis or split tears with MR findings of increased signal on PDWI and FS T2WI. Fluid signal replacing the expected tendon location on FS T2WI or other fluid-sensitive sequence is indicative of a tear, rather than tendinopathy. Check for an os peroneum of the PL tendon proximal to the cuboid tunnel. Marrow edema or fracture of the ossicle is seen with peroneal tendon dysfunction. Displacement of the ossicle proximally is a subtle plain film finding of a tendon tear.	The peroneus brevis and longus tendons have a shared tendon sheath proximally, making visual separation difficult. Tendons normally pass below the fibula through the retromalleolar groove, held in place by the superior peroneal retinaculum. Check for the flat peroneus brevis tendon anterior to a larger and more rounded PL tendon. The peroneus brevis tendon can be followed to the fifth metatarsal base and the PL tendon will pass beneath the cuboid to insert on the first metatarsal and medial cuneiform.

(continued on page 252)

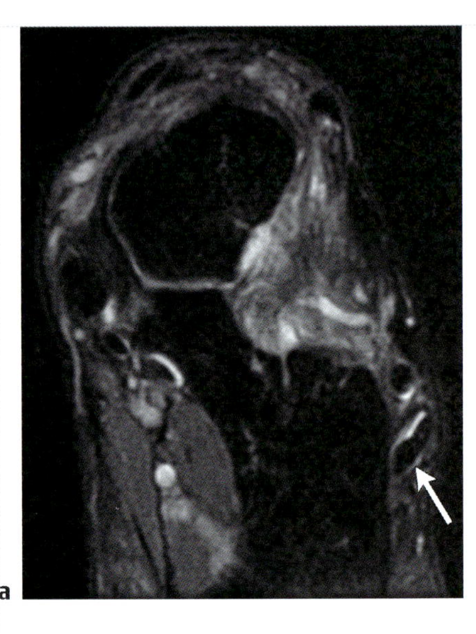

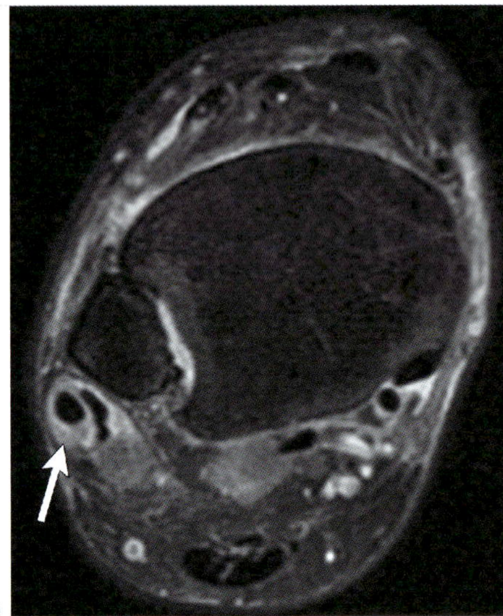

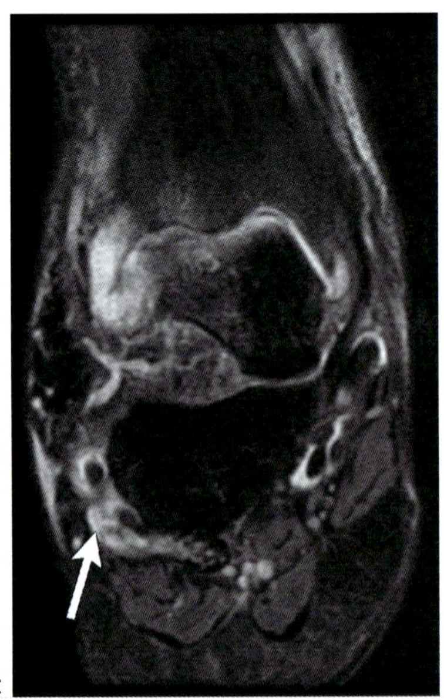

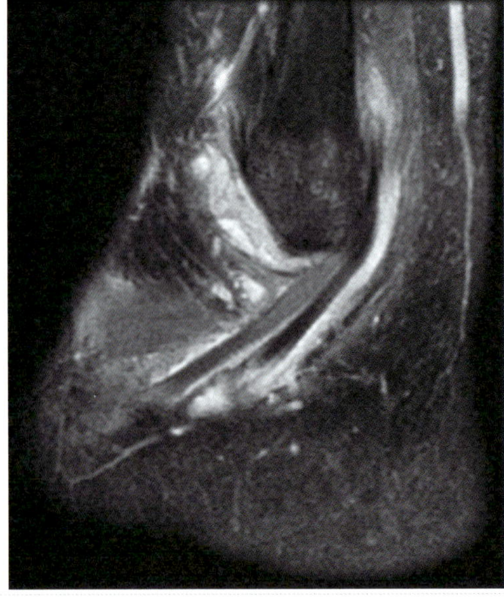

Fig. 8.7 (a) A thin rim of high signal fluid (arrow) surrounds the peroneus longus (PL) tendon in an example of mild tenosynovitis with only subtle signal changes of tendinopathy on axial fat-suppressed T2-weighted imaging (FS T2WI). (b) Tenosynovitis with increased signal pannus (arrow) in the tendon sheath of the PL and peroneus brevis (PB) tendons in a patient with rheumatoid arthritis on axial FS T2WI. (c) Note slightly increased signal in the peroneal tendons reflecting tendinopathy with surrounding tenosynovitis (arrow) on coronal FS T2WI and (d) sagittal FS T2WI. *(continued)*

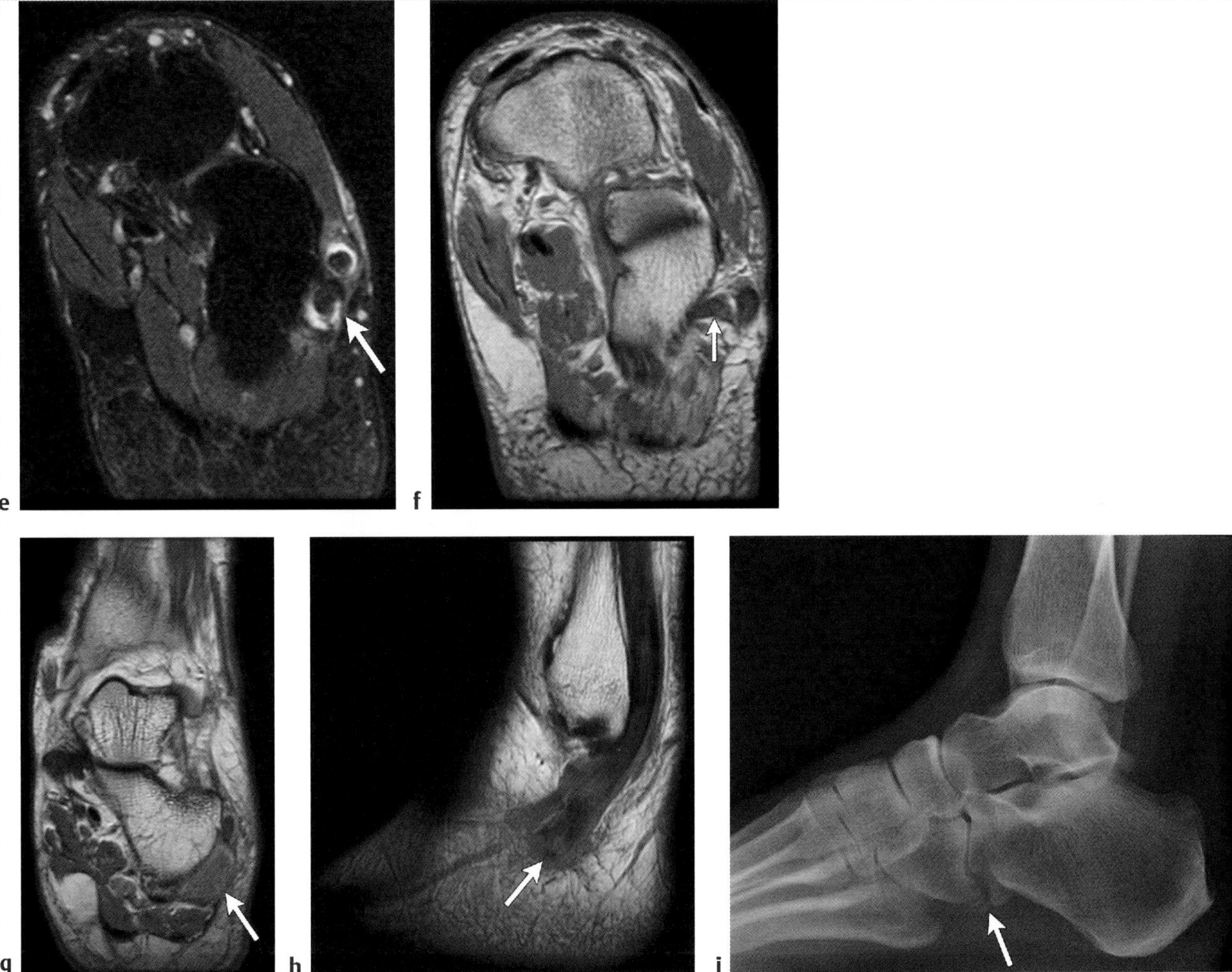

Fig. 8.7 (*continued*) (e) More severe cases of PL tendinosis with abnormal tendon shape and partial tears (arrows) on axial FS T2WI and (f) proton density–weighted imaging (PDWI). (g) Complete tear of the PL tendon with an empty sheath (arrow) on coronal PDWI and (h) retracted tendon end (arrow) on sagittal PDWI. (i) Corresponding lateral ankle X-ray demonstrates fragmented os perineum, a finding associated with PL tendon abnormalities.

Table 8.1 (Cont.) Lesions of the ankle and foot tendons

Abnormalities	MRI findings	Comments
Tibialis anterior (TA) tendon abnormalities (▶ Fig. 8.8)	With suspected TA tears look for high signal fluid on fluid-sensitive sequences. PDWI demonstrates a thinned tendon in cases of partial tears. Oblique axial images oriented perpendicular to the tendon at the level of the ankle may best profile tendon pathology. Imaging in the oblique axial and sagittal planes is useful to assess the degree of tendon retraction in complete tears.	Patients often present with decreased ability to dorsiflex the ankle. The tendon tear may present as an anterior ankle mass with intermediate signal on PDWI and FS T2WI. Differential considerations include tenosynovitis, talar dome lesions, and osteoarthritis of the tibiotalar joint.

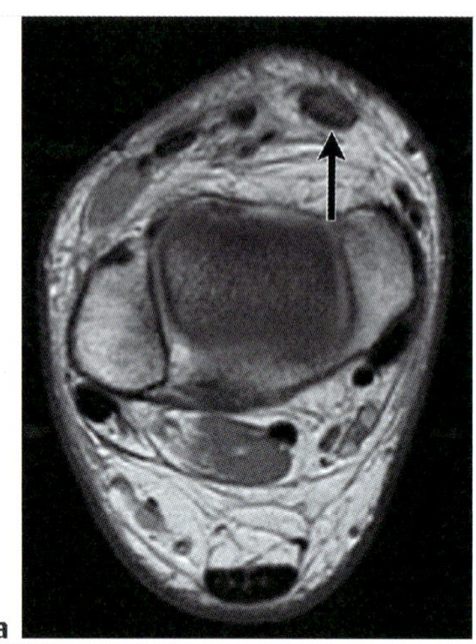

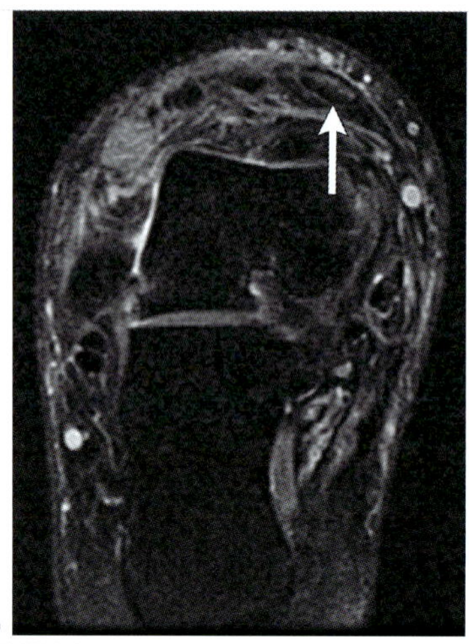

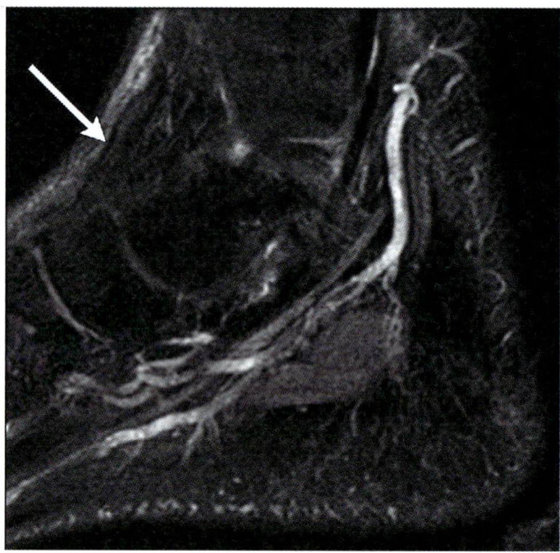

Fig. 8.8 (a) Note abnormal signal and enlargement of the tibialis anterior tendon (arrows) on axial proton density–weighted imaging and (b) coronal fat-suppressed T2-weighted imaging (FS T2WI). (c) On sagittal FS T2WI, the tendon is noted to be wavy in contour and is partly torn (arrow). Evaluation of tendon abnormalities often requires evaluation in multiple planes.

8.1.1 Lesions of the Ankle and Foot Tendons Suggested Reading

[1] Arnold G, Vohra S, Marcantonio D, Doshi S. Normal magnetic resonance imaging anatomy of the ankle & foot. Magn Reson Imaging Clin N Am 2011; 19: 655–679

[2] Kijowski R, De Smet A, Mukharjee R. Magnetic resonance imaging findings in patients with peroneal tendinopathy and peroneal tenosynovitis. Skeletal Radiol 2007; 36: 105–114

[3] Rodriguez CP, Goyal M, Wasdahl DA. Best cases from the AFIP: atypical imaging features of bilateral Achilles tendon xanthomatosis. Radiographics 2008; 28: 2064–2068

[4] Wang XT, Rosenberg ZS, Mechlin MB, Schweitzer ME. Normal variants and diseases of the peroneal tendons and superior peroneal retinaculum: MR imaging features. Radiographics 2005; 25: 587–602

8.2 Lesions of the Ankle and Foot Ligaments

- Lateral ligaments: anterior talofibular ligament (ATFL) sprain
- Lateral ligaments: calcaneofibular (CF) ligament sprain
- Lateral ligaments: syndesmotic ligament injuries/high ankle sprain
- Lateral ligaments: anterolateral impingement
- Medial ligaments: deltoid ligament–deep tibiotalar and superficial tibiocalcaneal ligaments
- Medial ligaments: calcaneonavicular ligament (CNL) spring ligament complex
- Sinus tarsi syndrome

Table 8.2 Lesions of the ankle and foot ligaments

Abnormalities	MRI findings	Comments
Lateral ligaments: anterior talofibular ligament (ATFL) sprain (▶ Fig. 8.9)	Normally a low signal structure coursing obliquely between the lateral malleolus and anterior talus. Best evaluated on axial images at the level of the malleolar fossa. The ligament is easily identified by beginning at the tip of the lateral malleolus and scrolling proximally until a triangle formed by the ATFL, posterior talofibular ligament, and tibia is identified. ATFL injuries span a spectrum of appearances. Acute tears present with increased signal on fat-suppressed T2-weighted imaging (FS T2WI) with blurring and intermediate signal of remaining intact ligament fibers on T1-weighted imaging (T1WI) and proton density–weighted imaging (PDWI). High signal fluid may be identified around the torn ligament with marrow edema in the adjacent fibula and tibia. Loss of surrounding fat signal is a useful finding for identifying ligament injury. Look for an avulsion fragment from the distal fibula. In chronic injuries, the ligament may appear wavy or irregular. Abnormal thinning or thickening of a healed ligament sprain may be seen. Complete tears are distinguished by identification of discontinuity of fibers and an appreciable gap on PDWI and FS T2WI.	The ATFL is the weakest and most commonly injured ankle ligament. The severity of lateral ankle ligament sprains increases from ATFL sprain, to partial ATFL tear with sprain of the calcaneofibular (CF) ligament, and finally to complete tears of both ligaments. The posterior talofibular ligament is rarely injured. ATFL sprains are often associated with injury to other ligaments, including the deltoid, syndesmotic, and sinus tarsi ligaments. Injury to the lateral ligaments is also associated with peroneal tendon abnormalities and sinus tarsi syndrome.

(continued on page 256)

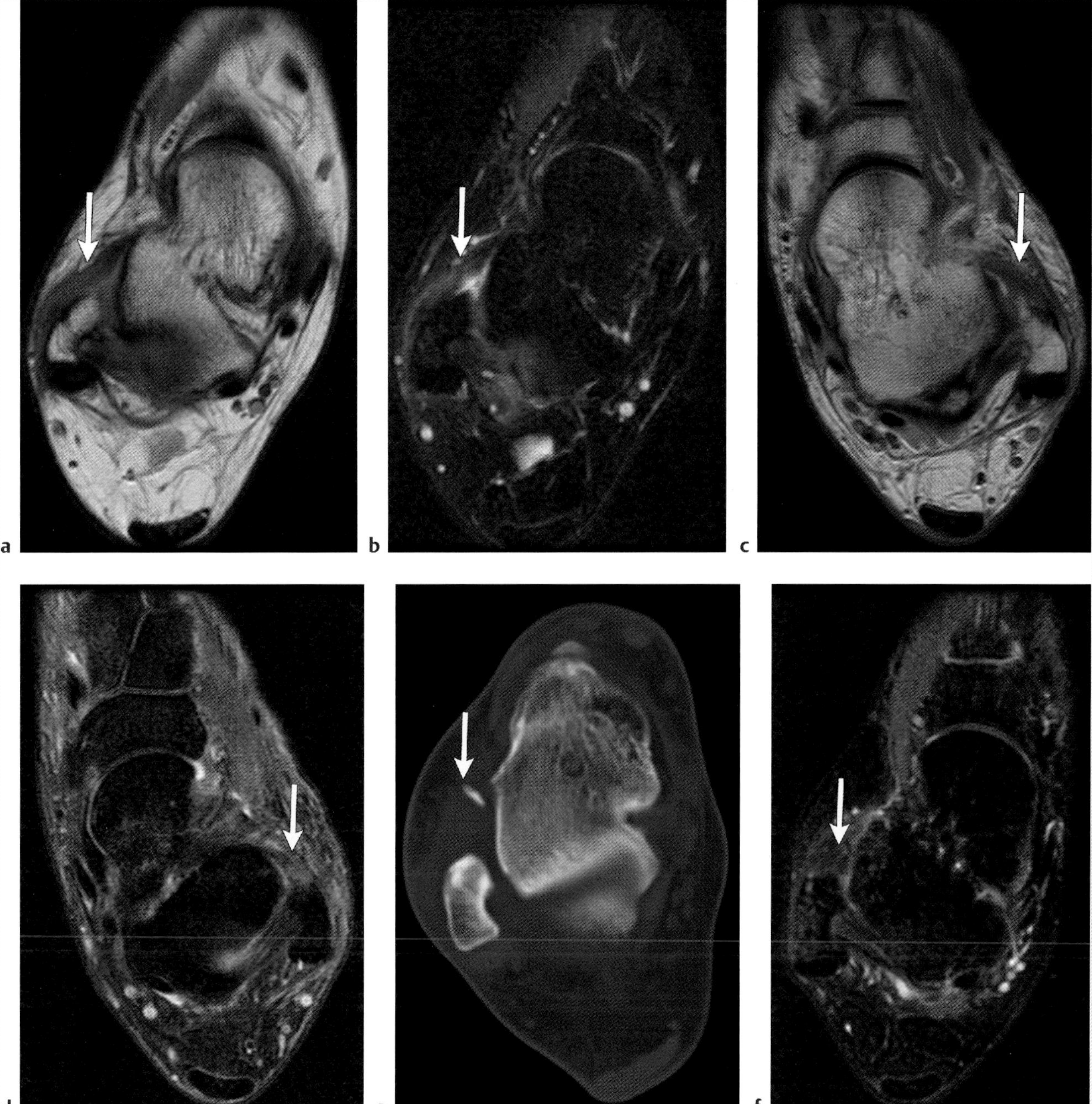

Fig. 8.9 (a) In a patient with a history of ankle sprains, note an anterior talofibular ligament (ATFL) sprain with a thickened and wavy ATFL (arrow) coursing from the anterior aspect of the lateral malleolus to the talus. Although the ligament is intact, it demonstrates increased signal and blurred margins near the fibula on axial proton density–weighted imaging (PDWI). (b) Corresponding mild increased signal edema in the ATFL (arrow) is seen on axial fat-suppressed T2-weighted imaging (FS T2WI). Note the different scan location than that shown in (a). (c) Different patient with a more severe ATFL sprain (arrows). Note blurred irregular ATFL fibers on axial PDWI and (d) corresponding increased signal on axial FS T2WI. The irregularity is related to tearing and subsequent scar tissue formation. (e) On axial computed tomography from another patient, note the avulsed fragment (arrow) related to an ATFL tear. (f) Corresponding axial FS T2WI demonstrates a torn ATFL (arrow).

Table 8.2 (Cont.) Lesions of the ankle and foot ligaments

Abnormalities	MRI findings	Comments
Lateral ligaments: calcaneofibular ligament (CF) sprain (▶ Fig. 8.10)	The CF ligament is normally identified on coronal images of the ankle posterior to the ATFL coursing deep to the peroneal tendons between the lateral fibular tip and lateral calcaneus. This ligament is often difficult to identify. As with ATFL injuries, look for low to intermediate signal on PDWI and increased signal on FS T2WI within and surrounding the CF ligament. In cases of sprain, the CF ligament may appear attenuated with altered morphology. The normally sharp ligament margins may be ill defined in cases of chronic injury.	CF ligament tears are typically seen in association with ATFL tears. The CF ligament is the most commonly injured ligament after the ATFL. Look for associated peroneal tendon injury. The posterior talofibular ligament is the thickest of the three lateral ankle ligaments and is rarely injured. Do not mistake the normally striated appearance of the posterior talofibular ligament for a sprain.

(continued on page 258)

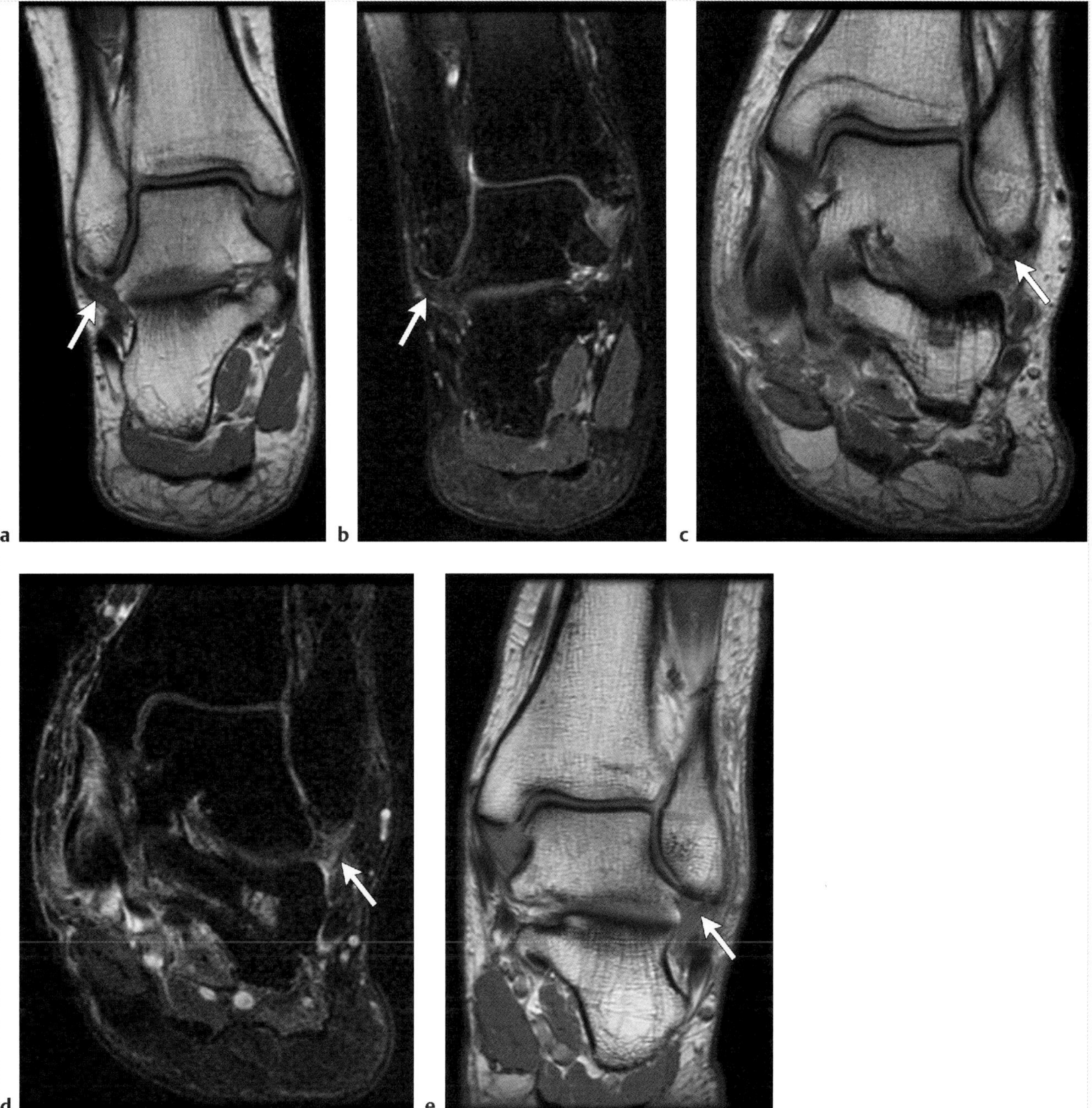

Fig. 8.10 (a) Mild sprain of the calcaneofibular (CF) ligament (arrows) with increased signal along its course on coronal proton density–weighted imaging (PDWI) and (b) coronal fat-suppressed T2-weighted imaging (FS T2WI). (c) A more severe case of a CF ligament sprain (arrow) with proximal torn fibers visualized on coronal PDWI. (d) Note abnormal increased signal surrounding the torn ligament on corresponding coronal FS T2WI. (e) In a different patient, tear of the CF ligament (arrow) with nonvisualization of the CF ligament and intermediate signal replacing the expected location of the ligament on coronal PDWI.

Table 8.2 (Cont.) Lesions of the ankle and foot ligaments

Abnormalities	MRI findings	Comments
Lateral ligaments: syndesmotic ligament injuries/high ankle sprain (▶ Fig. 8.11)	The syndesmotic ligament complex of the distal tibiofibular joint consists of the anteroinferior tibiofibular (AITF) ligament, the posteroinferior tibiofibular (PITF) ligament, the inferior transverse ligament, and the inferior interosseus ligament. These ligaments are best identified at the level of the talar dome where the fibula has an oval configuration. The AITF ligament is the most commonly injured and demonstrates abnormal increased signal, wavy contour, or discontinuity following injury. Surrounding fluid and ligamentous edema is well seen on axial FS T2WI at the level of the tibial plafond. Discontinuity or visualization of the avulsed ligament may be seen. Helpful secondary findings include edema or fluid extending proximally into the tibiofibular recess, lateral subluxation of the fibula, and calcifications of the interosseus membrane in chronic injury seen as low signal foci on routine sequences.	Injury is often seen with high-contact athletic activities. Syndesmotic sprains associated with diastasis of the syndesmosis usually require surgical fixation. Note the AITF ligament may demonstrate an inferior fascicle known as the Bassett ligament, which parallels the AITF ligament. Injury to the thicker PITF ligament is unusual, but may present with magnetic resonance (MR) findings of thickening and increased signal indicative of edema.

(continued on page 260)

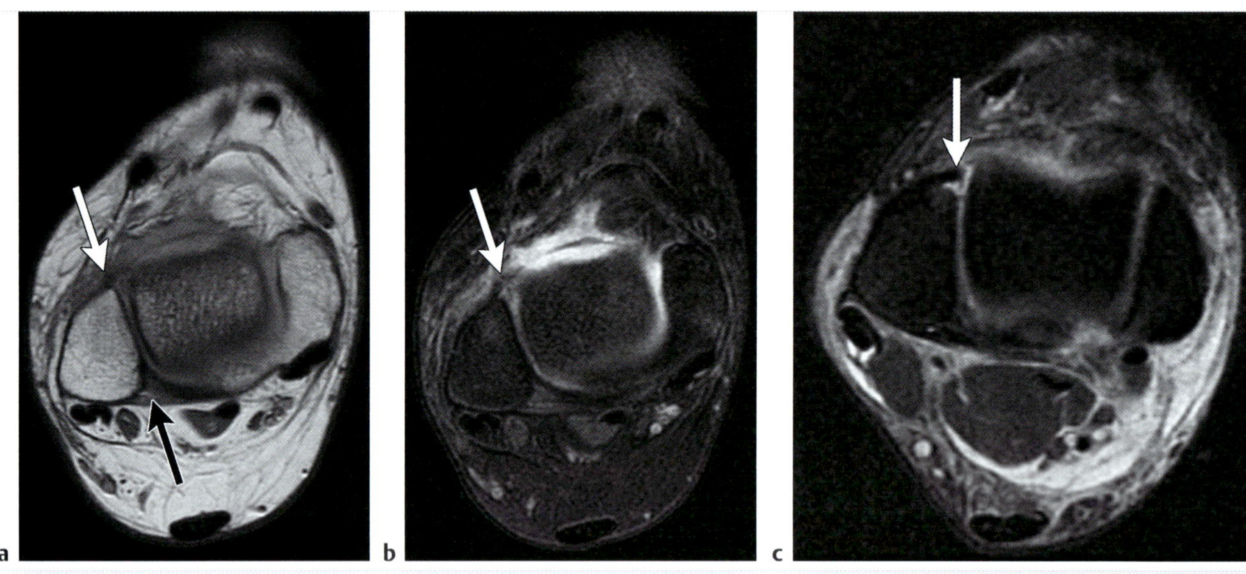

Fig. 8.11 (a) Tear of the normally low signal anteroinferior tibiofibular (AITF) ligament (white arrow) on axial proton density–weighted imaging (PDWI). The thick, normally striated posteroinferior tibiofibular (PITF) ligament is intact (black arrow). (b) Note an ankle joint effusion and discontinuity of the ligament (white arrow) as it courses from the anterior fibula to the anterior tibial attachment on axial fat-suppressed T2-weighted imaging (FS T2WI). (c) In a different patient note a well-defined tear of the AITF ligament (white arrow) from the anterior tibia on axial FS T2WI. *(continued)*

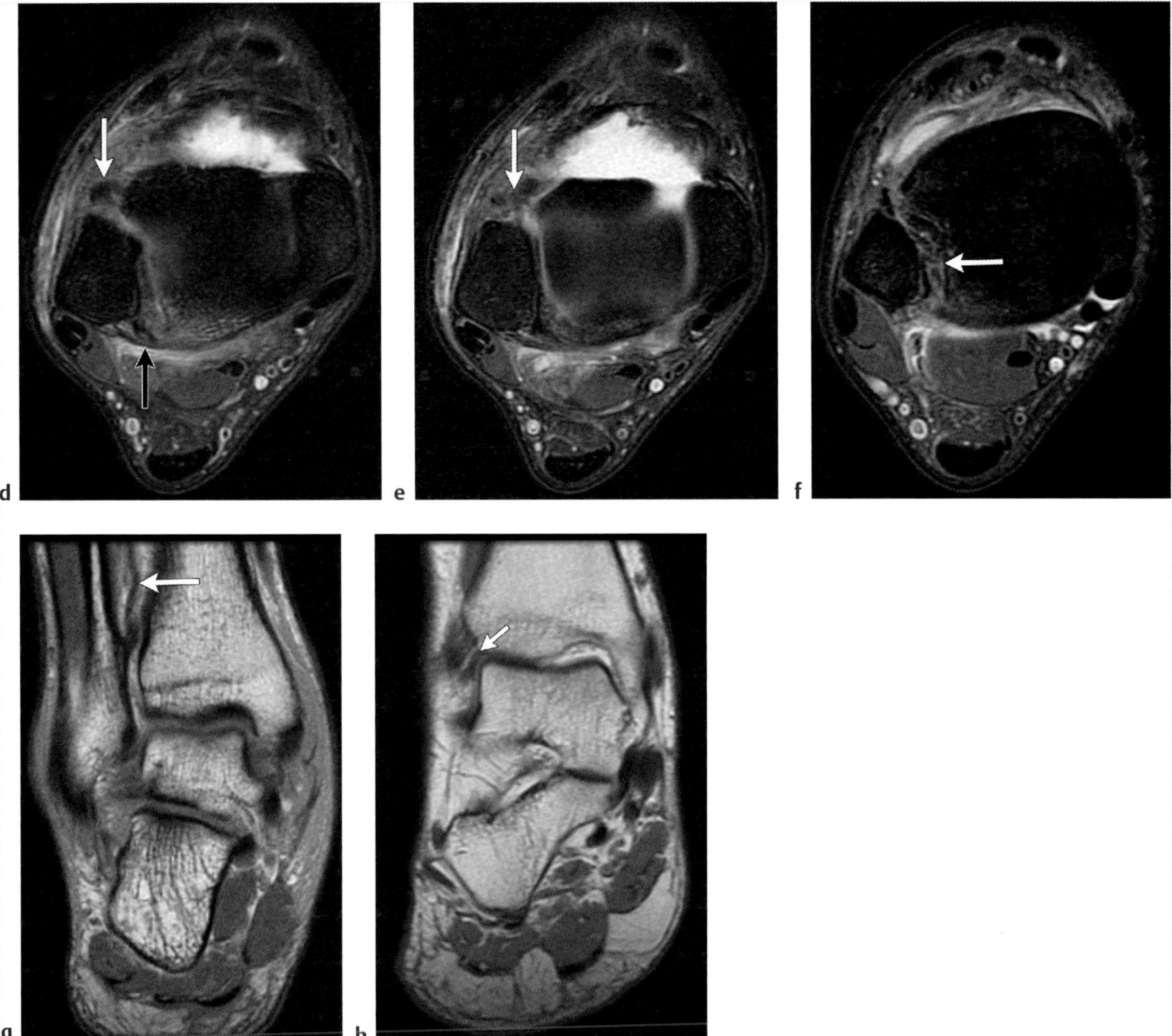

Fig. 8.11 *(continued)* (d) Tear of the AITF (white arrow) with abnormal lobulated morphology of the torn ligament. Also note a sprain of the PITF ligament (black arrow) on axial FS T2WI. (e) Contiguous axial FS T2WI demonstrates a complex appearance of the torn AITF ligament more inferiorly. (f) Example of interosseus ligament injury (arrow) with irregular wavy fibers proximal to the level of the talar dome on axial FS T2WI. (g) Note wavy fibers of the torn interosseus membrane more proximally (arrow) in a different patient on coronal PDWI. (h) Example of the Bassett ligament–a normal separate fascicle of the AITF on coronal PDWI.

Table 8.2 (Cont.) Lesions of the ankle and foot ligaments

Abnormalities	MRI findings	Comments
Lateral ligaments: anterolateral impingement (▶ Fig. 8.12)	In anterolateral impingement an intermediate to low signal soft tissue mass or "meniscoid lesion" consisting of scar or synovium entrapped in the anterolateral gutter anteriorly is often seen in association with tears of the ATFL and AITF ligaments. Abnormal tissue is of intermediate to low signal on axial T1WI and PDWI and intermediate signal on FS T2WI, replacing the normal fat in this location.	This condition is seen in younger patients following inversion injury, with tenderness along the syndesmosis and anterolateral ankle. Look for spurs and ossicles at the fibular tip and cartilage abnormalities of the talus. Check for loose bodies in the anterolateral gutter.
Medial ligaments: deltoid ligament–deep tibiotalar and superficial tibiocalcaneal ligaments (▶ Fig. 8.13)	The largest and easiest medial ankle ligament to consistently identify is the deep tibiotalar component of the deltoid ligament. With an acute sprain look for loss of the normal striated ligament appearance and increased signal on coronal PDWI and FS T2WI images. More chronic injury may result in abnormal ligament contour or thickening, embedded ossific fragments, and cystic change at the attachment sites at the tip of the medial malleolus and adjacent medial talus.	Deltoid ligament sprains as an isolated injury are uncommon. The four main components are injured in the following order: tibiocalcaneal and tibionavicular followed by the stronger tibiospring ligament and posterior tibiotalar ligaments.

(continued on page 262)

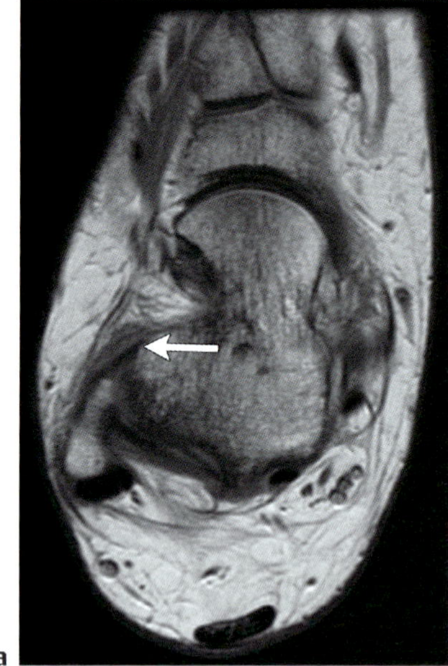

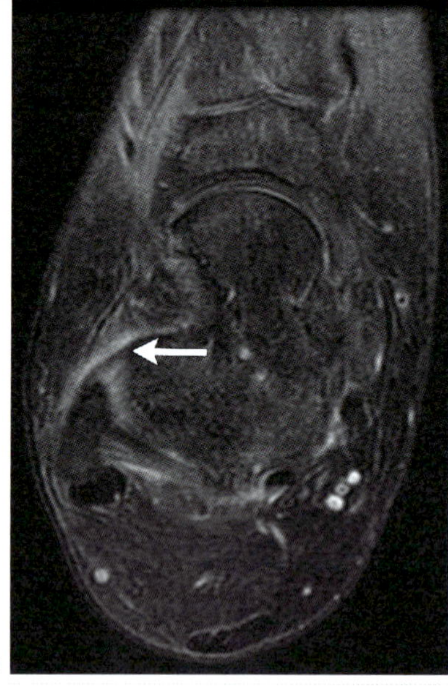

Fig. 8.12 (a) A patient with pain along the anterolateral ankle. Note abnormal low signal both anterior and posterior to the anterior talofibular ligament (ATFL) (arrow) on axial proton density–weighted imaging (PDWI). (b) On fat-suppressed T2-weighted imaging (FS T2WI), the ATFL (arrow) is of mildly abnormal signal with surrounding increased signal synovitis/scar replacing normal fat in the anterolateral gutter.

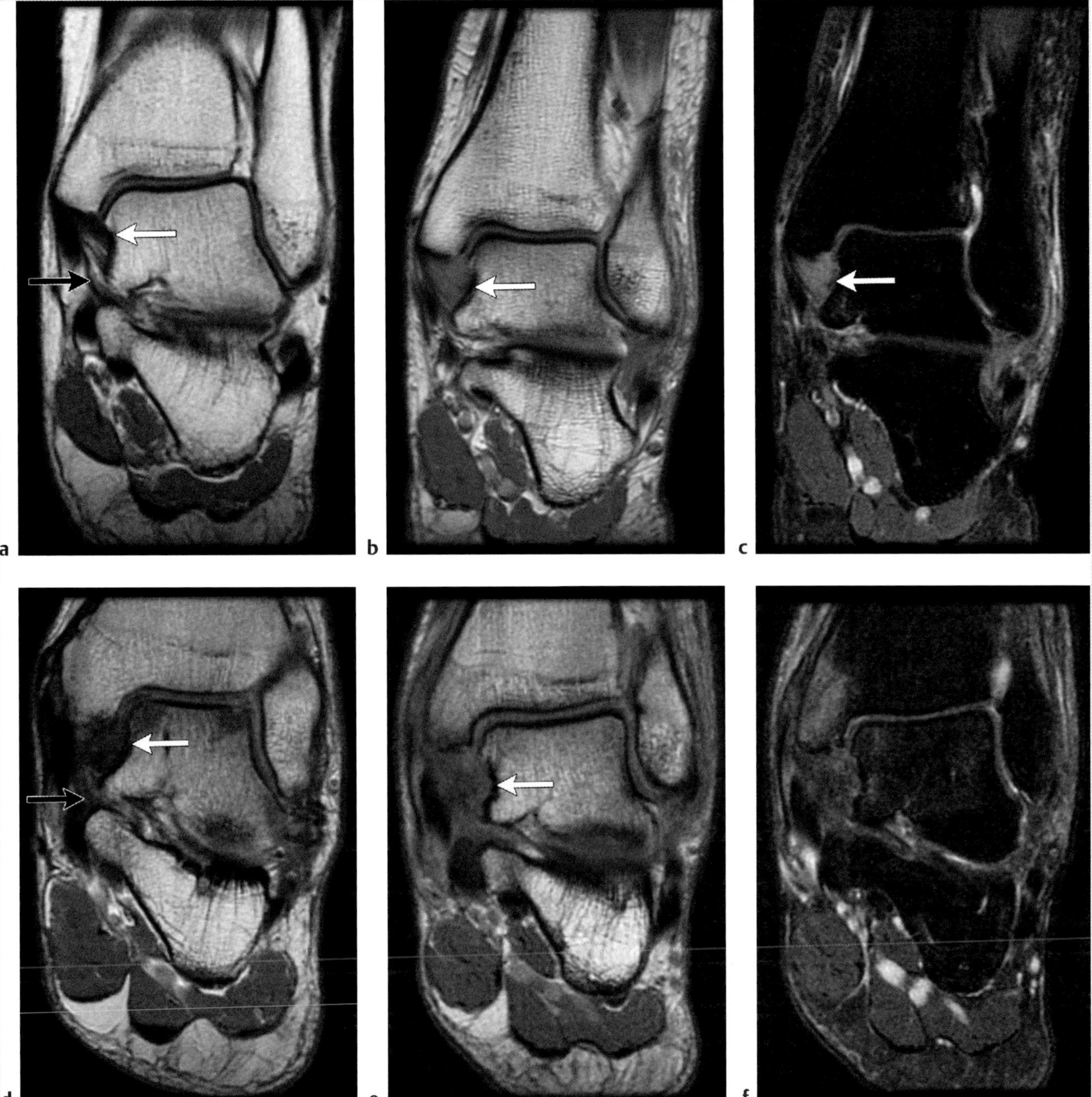

Fig. 8.13 (a) Normal striated appearance of the deep tibiotalar portion of the deltoid ligament (white arrow). The thinner superficial tibiocalcaneal portion of the deltoid ligament (black arrow) is also seen without striations on coronal proton density–weighted imaging (PDWI). (b) In this case of deltoid ligament sprain (arrow), note the loss of the normal tibiotalar ligament striation and the loss of definition of fibers on coronal PDWI. (c) Corresponding coronal fat-suppressed T2-weighted imaging (FS T2WI) demonstrates diffuse abnormally increased signal (arrow) in the normally low signal tibiotalar deltoid ligament. (d) Note heterogeneous disorganized appearance of the ligament in this case of chronic tibiotalar deltoid ligament sprain (white arrow). Also note thickening and increased signal in the sprained tibiocalcaneal portion of the deltoid ligament (black arrow) on coronal PDWI. (e) In a different patient, tibiotalar and tibiocalcaneal deltoid ligament sprains with bone irregularity at the medial malleolus and medial talar attachment sites (arrow) on coronal PDWI. (f) Corresponding reactive/posttraumatic marrow edema is seen in the medial malleolus on coronal FS T2WI.

Table 8.2 (Cont.) Lesions of the ankle and foot ligaments

Abnormalities	MRI findings	Comments
Medial ligaments: calcaneonavicular ligament (CNL) spring ligament complex (▶ Fig. 8.14)	Although three components of the calcaneonavicular spring ligament complex have been described, the superomedial calcaneonavicular ligament is most commonly torn. The two other components are the medial plantar oblique ligament and the short inferoplantar oblique ligament. With suspected injury, look for thickening or thinning of the superomedial CNL deep to an abnormal posterior tibial tendon. Abnormalities of this ligament are commonly associated with flatfoot deformity.	The spring ligament complex supports the head of the talus and is covered by fibrocartilage at its site of contact with the talus. The posterior tibial tendon crosses over the superomedial calcaneonavicular spring ligament at the "gliding zone." This relationship is best profiled on axial oblique and coronal images. The tibiospring component of the deltoid ligament attaches to the superomedial CNL anterior to the sustentaculum talus.

(continued on page 264)

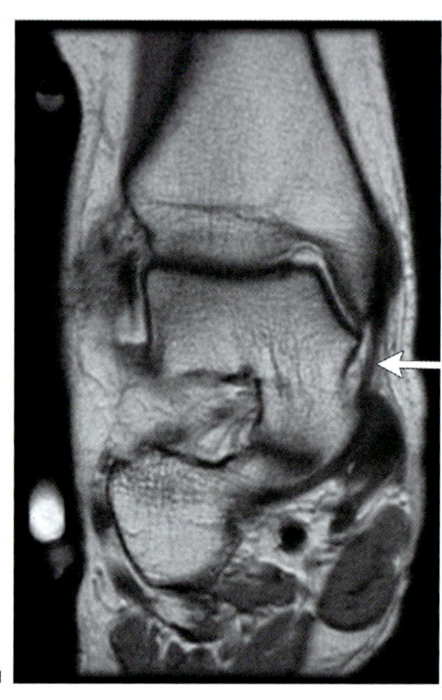
a

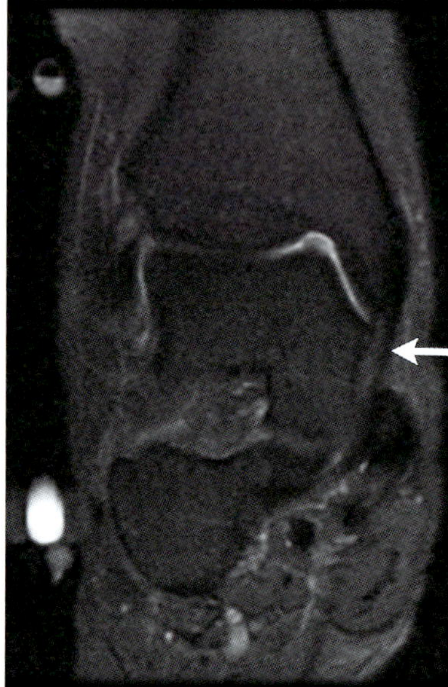
b

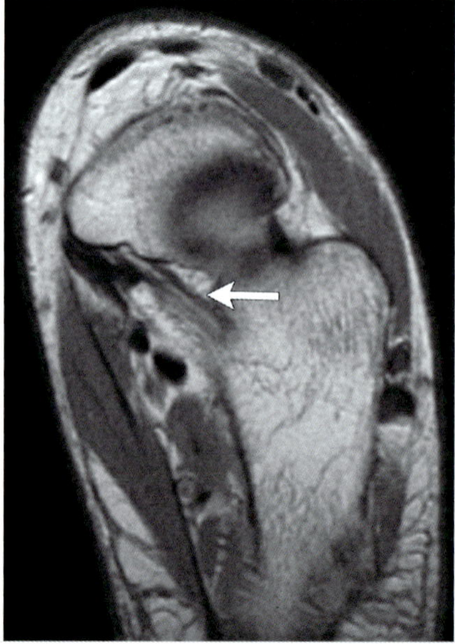
c

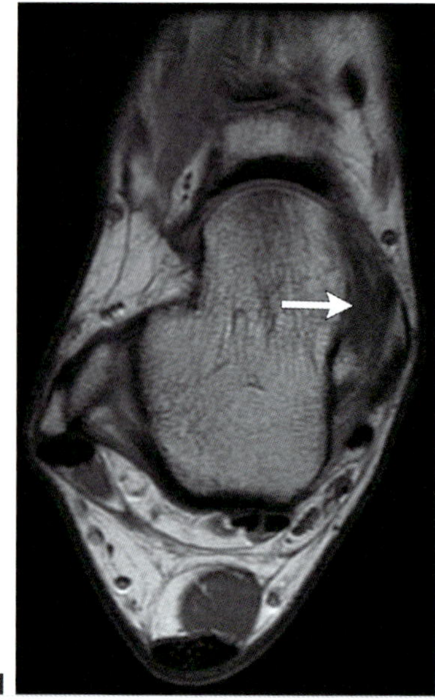
d

Fig. 8.14 (a) Normal spring ligament components. Superomedial calcaneonavicular ligament (CNL) (arrows) coursing deep to the posterior tibial tendon on coronal proton density–weighted imaging (PDWI) and (b) on coronal fat-suppressed T2-weighted imaging (FS T2WI). (c) The medioplantar oblique CNL (arrow) runs between the coronoid fossa of the calcaneus and the navicular on axial PDWI. (d) Moderate thickening and abnormal signal of the superomedial CNL (arrows) on axial PDWI (*continued*)

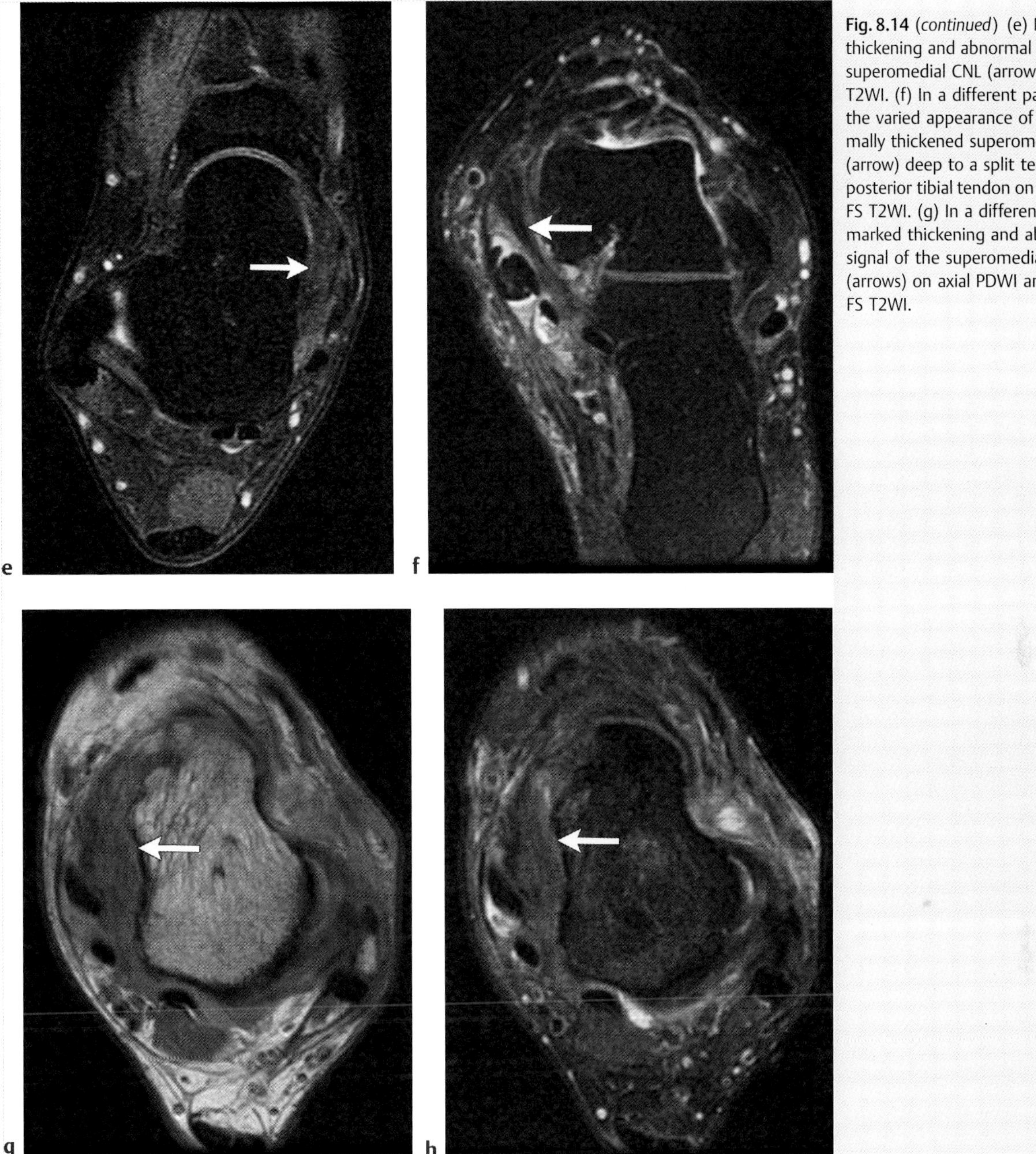

Fig. 8.14 (*continued*) (e) Moderate thickening and abnormal signal of the superomedial CNL (arrow) on axial FS T2WI. (f) In a different patient, note the varied appearance of an abnormally thickened superomedial CNL (arrow) deep to a split tear of the posterior tibial tendon on oblique axial FS T2WI. (g) In a different patient, marked thickening and abnormal signal of the superomedial CNL (arrows) on axial PDWI and (h) axial FS T2WI.

Table 8.2 (Cont.) Lesions of the ankle and foot ligaments

Abnormalities	MRI findings	Comments
Sinus tarsi syndrome (▶ Fig. 8.15)	On sagittal T1WI and PDWI, look for replacement of the normally high signal sinus tarsi fat by lower signal material representing fluid, synovitis, or fibrosis. On sagittal FS T2WI the normally low signal fat is replaced by relatively increased signal fluid, synovitis, or fibrosis. Interruption of the sinus tarsi cervical and interosseus ligaments may also be visible. Also check for associated lateral ligament tears and posterior tibial tendon pathology.	The sinus tarsi is a conical channel with a larger lateral opening that lies between the anterior and posterior portions of the subtalar joint. Patients often present with lateral pain near the sinus tarsi and a history of prior ankle sprain. A minority of patients have a history of inflammatory arthropathy. Displacement of a portion of the sinus tarsi fat by joint fluid does not indicate the presence of sinus tarsi syndrome.

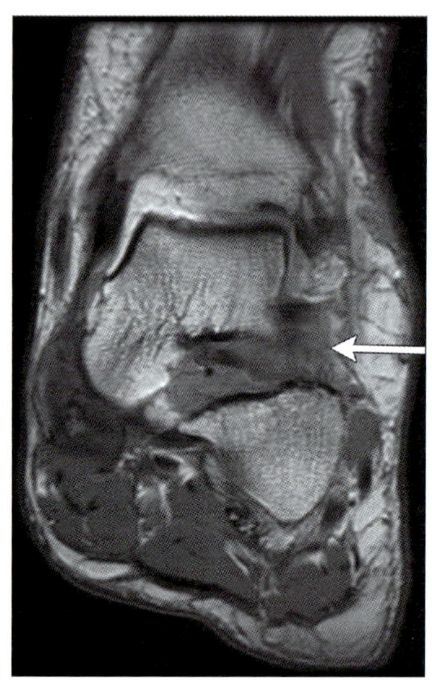

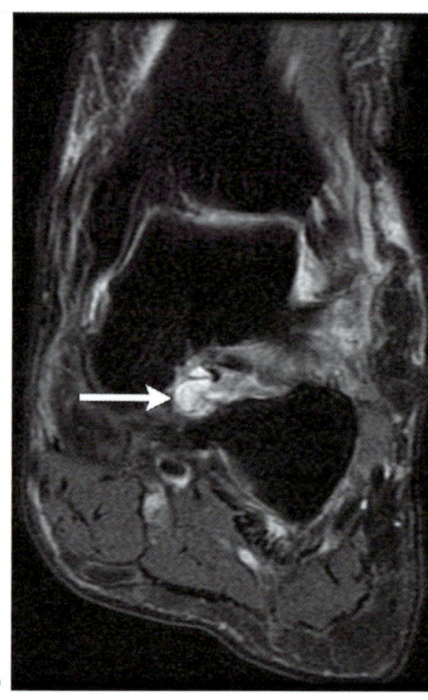

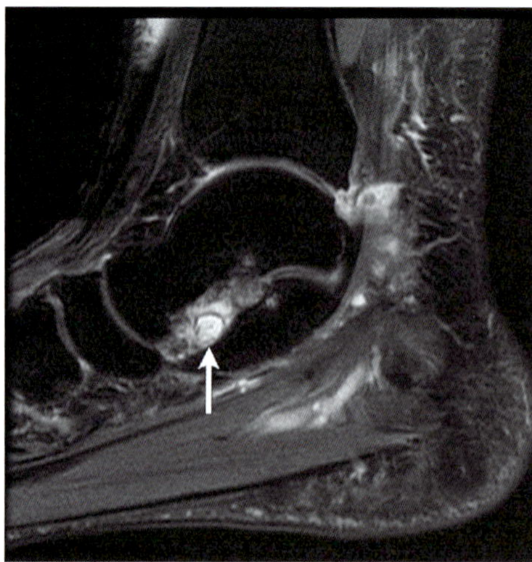

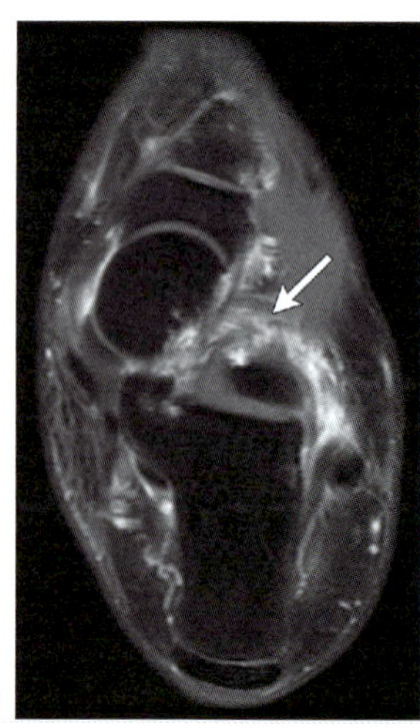

Fig. 8.15 (a) Replacement of the normal fat in the sinus tarsi (arrows) by intermediated signal fluid or synovitis on coronal proton density–weighted imaging (PDWI) and (b) corresponding increased signal on coronal fat-suppressed T2-weighted imaging (FS T2WI) and (c) sagittal FS T2WI. (d) Note corresponding extensive gadolinium-contrast enhancement (arrow) on axial FS T1-weighted imaging (T1WI). (*continued*)

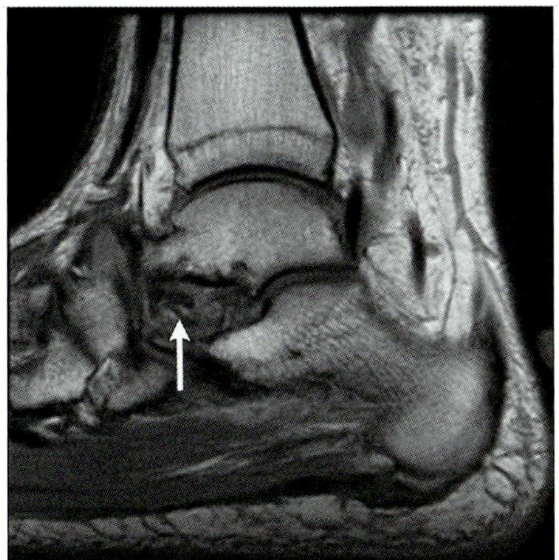

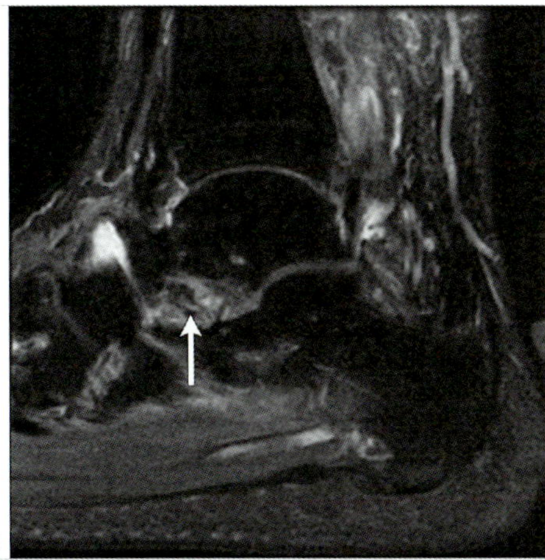

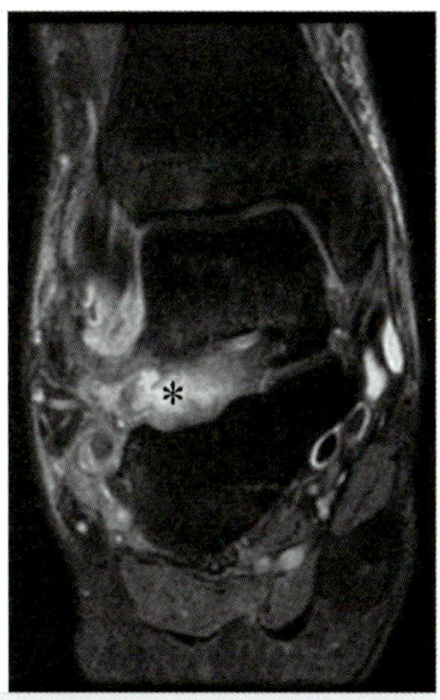

Fig. 8.15 *(continued)* (e) In another patient note low signal bodies and abnormal signal (arrows) replacing the sinus tarsi fat on sagittal PDWI and (f) on sagittal FS T2WI. (g) In a different patient with known rheumatoid arthritis, note high signal pannus and fluid (asterisk) replacing the sinus tarsi fat and surrounding the peroneal tendons on coronal FS T2WI.

8.2.1 Lesions of the Ankle and Foot Ligaments Suggested Reading

[1] Campbell SE, Warner M. MR imaging of ankle inversion injuries. Magn Reson Imaging Clin N Am 2008; 16: 1–18

[2] Datir A, Connell D. Imaging of impingement lesions in the ankle. Top Magn Reson Imaging 2010; 21: 15–23

[3] Desai KR, Beltran LS, Bencardino JT, Rosenberg ZS, Petchprapa C, Steiner G. The spring ligament recess of the talocalcaneonavicular joint: depiction on MR images with cadaveric and histologic correlation. AJR Am J Roentgenol 2011; 196: 1145–1150

[4] Perrich KD, Goodwin DW, Hecht PJ, Cheung Y. Ankle ligaments on MRI: appearance of normal and injured ligaments. AJR Am J Roentgenol 2009; 193: 687–695

[5] Toye LR, Helms CA, Hoffman BD, Easley M, Nunley JA. MRI of spring ligament tears. AJR Am J Roentgenol 2005; 184: 1475–1480

8.3 Abnormalities/Injuries of Soft Tissues and Ossicles in the Ankle and Foot

- Plantar fasciitis
- Os trigonum (posterior impingement) syndrome
- Accessory navicular (type II)
- Painful os peroneum syndrome (POPS)
- Diabetic foot: osteomyelitis
- Diabetic foot: neuropathic changes/Charcot neuroarthropathy
- Pressure lesion/adventitial bursa
- Morton neuroma/interdigital neuroma
- Sesamoid abnormalities
- Turf toe

Table 8.3 Abnormalities/injuries of soft tissues and ossicles in the ankle and foot

Abnormalities	MRI findings	Comments
Plantar fasciitis (▶ Fig. 8.16)	The plantar fascia is normally of low signal on sagittal T1-weighted imaging (T1WI) and proton density–weighted imaging (PDWI). With plantar fasciitis look for thickening (> 4 mm) of the proximal attachment of the plantar fascia/plantar aponeurosis on the calcaneus and abnormal intermediate signal on T1 and PDWI. On fat-suppressed T2-weighted imaging (FS T2WI), variable amounts of edema involve the abnormal portion of the aponeurosis. This condition may be associated with edema/inflammation of adjacent subcutaneous tissues. Assess calcaneus for a heel spur/enthesophyte, erosion, and marrow edema. Discontinuity of the plantar fascia on any sequence is indicative of a tear.	Most common site of involvement is at the medial calcaneal tuberosity where the thicker central cord of the plantar fascia arises. This condition is usually caused by microtrauma to the fascia. Patients present with focal pain medially at the calcaneal tuberosity that is worse upon rising in the morning. Whereas focal degenerative tears or detachment is seen at the calcaneal attachment, acute rupture typically occurs more distally.

(continued on page 268)

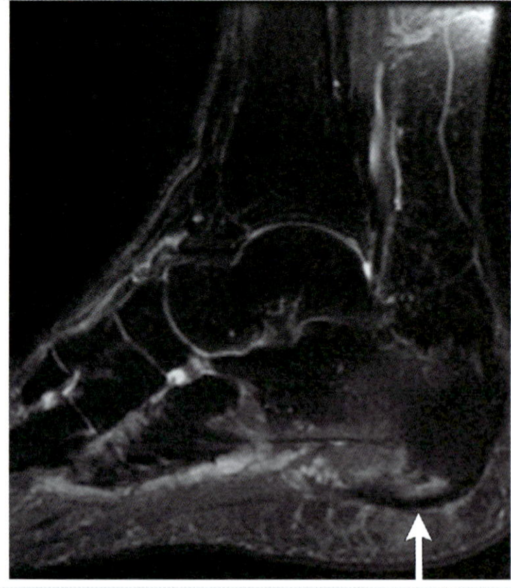

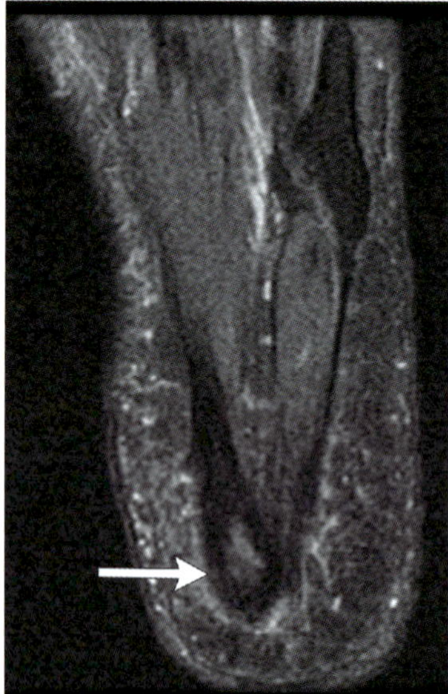

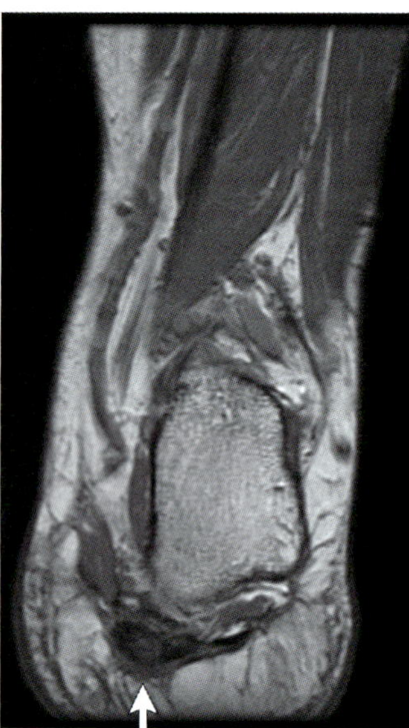

Fig. 8.16 (a) Note the abnormally thickened proximal plantar fascia (arrow) with abnormal signal within and adjacent to the tendon on sagittal fat-suppressed T2-weighted imaging (FS T2WI). (b) Axial FS T2WI demonstrates involvement of the medial cord (arrow) of the plantar fascia. (c) Asymmetric tendon thickening and increased abnormal signal within and surrounding the medial cord of the plantar fascia (arrows) in another case of plantar fasciitis on coronal proton density–weighted imaging (PDWI) and (*continued*)

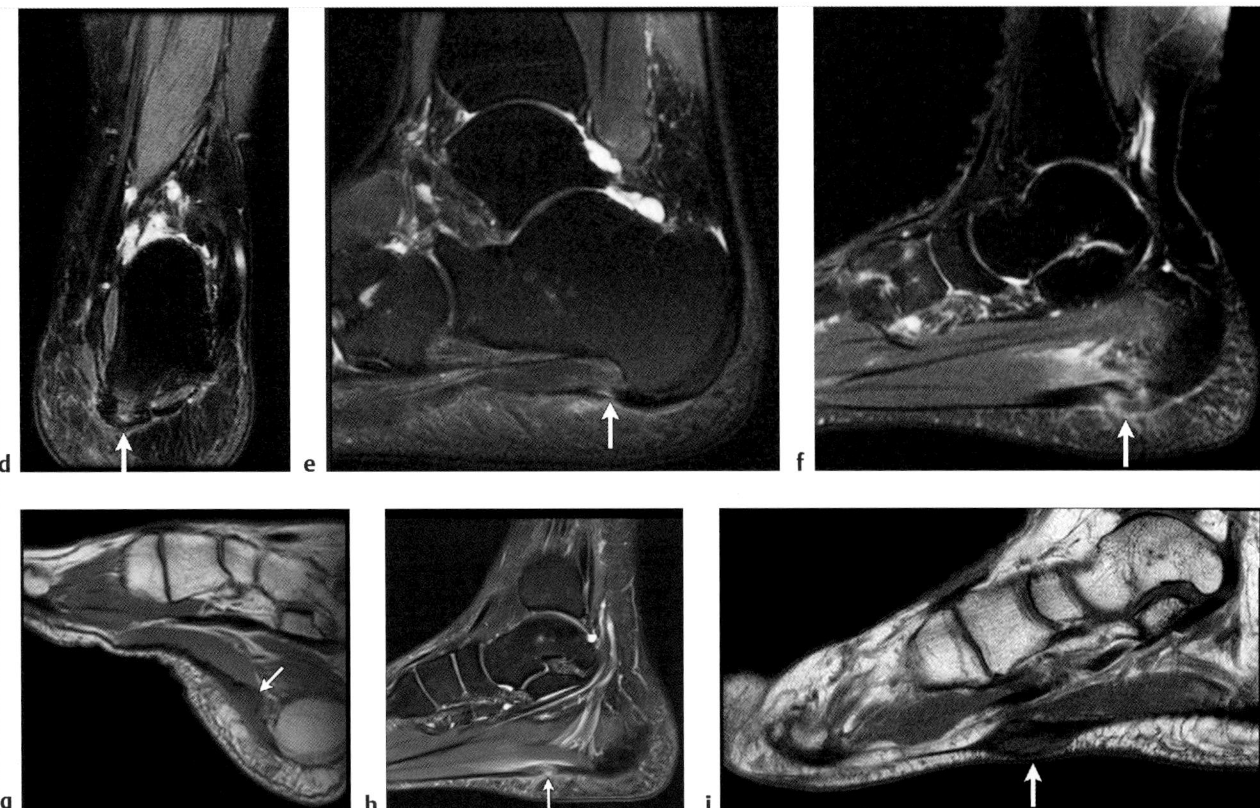

Fig. 8.16 (*continued*) (d) coronal FS T2WI. Central signal changes reflect partial tearing/detachment of the medial cord from the calcaneus. (e) Example of a partial tear of the proximal medial cord of the plantar fascia (arrow) with edema superficial to the tendon on sagittal FS T2WI. (f) A more pronounced example of a medial cord plantar fascia tear in a different patient with partial retraction of the torn thickened end on sagittal FS T2WI. (g) Near complete tear of the plantar fascia with retraction and a wavy aponeurosis with a calcaneal enthesophyte on sagittal PDWI. (h) More distal focal tear of the plantar fascia on sagittal FS T2WI, demonstrates abnormal signal at the site of tear. (i) Consider other causes of plantar pain such as a plantar fibroma (white arrow) on sagittal PDWI.

Table 8.3 (Cont.) Abnormalities/injuries of soft tissues and ossicles in the ankle and foot

Abnormalities	MRI findings	Comments
Os trigonum (posterior impingement) syndrome (▶ Fig. 8.17)	Abnormally increased T2 signal across the synchondrosis between the os trigonum and posterior talus is seen. T1WI and PDWI may also demonstrate degenerative cyst formation or sclerosis at the synchondrosis. Alternatively, one may see marrow edema of an intact lateral tubercle of the posterior process of the talus (Stieda process). Look for associated increased signal fluid/ganglia on FS T2WI about the posterior ankle ligaments on sagittal and axial images.	With pronounced recurrent plantar flexion seen, for example, in ballet dancers, there is compression of the posterior talus, resulting in microtrauma and subsequent rupture of the synchondrosis or fracture of the lateral tubercule. This condition may also result in compression of the medially adjacent flexor hallucis longus (FHL) tendon with resultant tendinosis, tenosynovitis, and/or stenosing tenosynovitis. Soft tissue posterior impingement is related to inflammation involving/surrounding the posterior ankle ligaments.
Accessory navicular (type II) (▶ Fig. 8.18)	A type II accessory navicular may demonstrate edema on either side of the synchondrosis seen on sagittal or axial FS T2WI. Low signal and cystic change may be seen on T1WI and PDWI. Look for associated posterior tibial tendon pathology. Distinguish the larger triangular type II accessory navicular from the smaller type I, which is not associated with posterior tibial tendon pathology.	Adventitial bursitis may be seen medial to a type II navicular. Assess the distal posterior tibial tendon for tendinosis or for enlargement more than seen normally at the insertion of this tendon on the navicular. The presence of a type III or cornuate navicular (prominent medial navicular tubercle) is also associated with posterior tibial tendon dysfunction.

(continued on page 270)

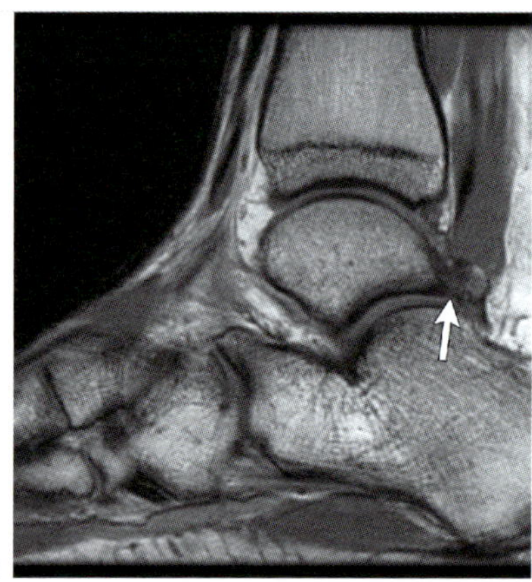

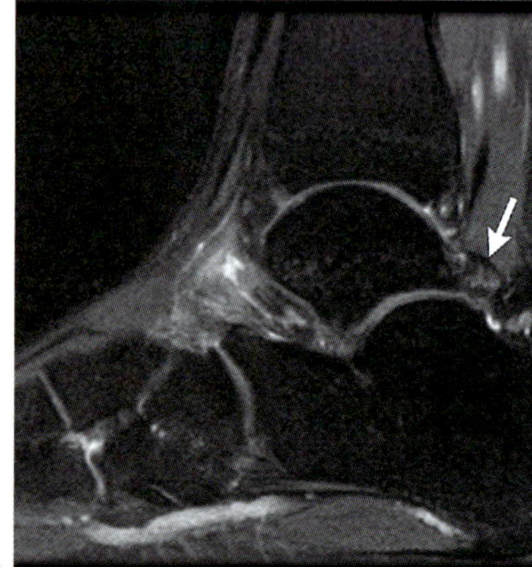

Fig. 8.17 (a) Note degenerative low signal and irregularity at the articulation (arrow) between the os trigonum and lateral tubercle of the posterior process of the talus on sagittal proton density–weighted imaging (PDWI). (b) Note irregular increased signal involving the synchondrosis between the talus and os trigonum (arrow) and marrow edema of the os trigonum on sagittal fat-suppressed T2-weighted imaging.

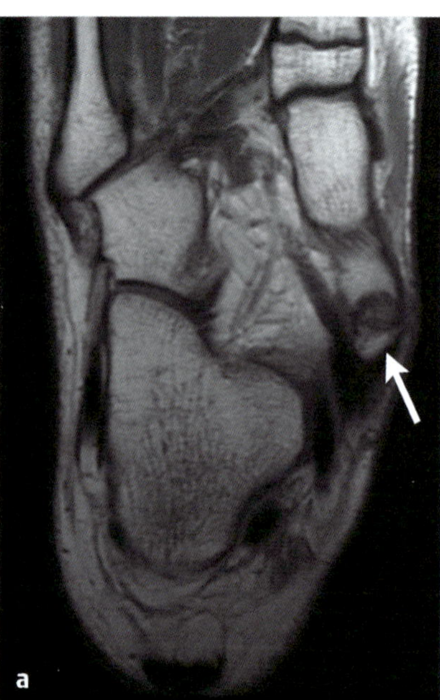

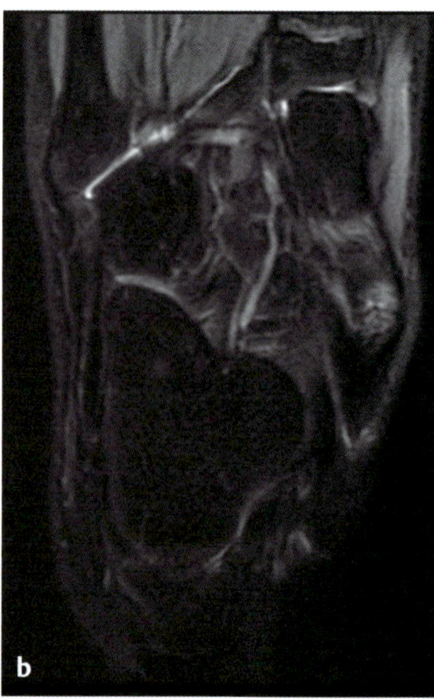

Fig. 8.18 (a) Type II accessory navicular (arrow) with subtle reactive low signal on either side of the synchondrosis on axial proton density–weighted imaging (PDWI). (b) Corresponding marrow edema is well seen across the synchondrosis on axial fat-suppressed T2-weighted imaging (FS T2WI). *(continued)*

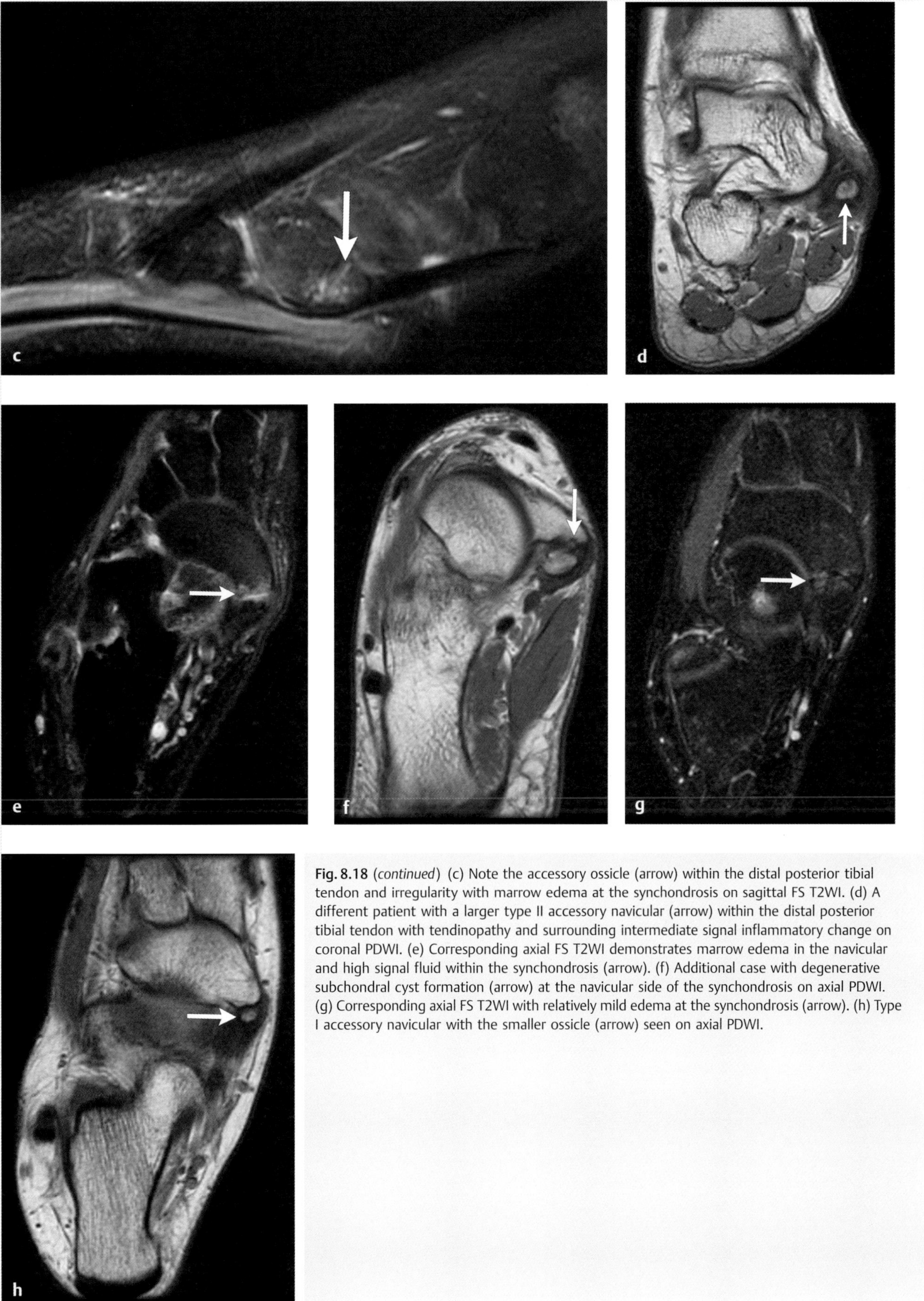

Fig. 8.18 (*continued*) (c) Note the accessory ossicle (arrow) within the distal posterior tibial tendon and irregularity with marrow edema at the synchondrosis on sagittal FS T2WI. (d) A different patient with a larger type II accessory navicular (arrow) within the distal posterior tibial tendon with tendinopathy and surrounding intermediate signal inflammatory change on coronal PDWI. (e) Corresponding axial FS T2WI demonstrates marrow edema in the navicular and high signal fluid within the synchondrosis (arrow). (f) Additional case with degenerative subchondral cyst formation (arrow) at the navicular side of the synchondrosis on axial PDWI. (g) Corresponding axial FS T2WI with relatively mild edema at the synchondrosis (arrow). (h) Type I accessory navicular with the smaller ossicle (arrow) seen on axial PDWI.

Table 8.3 (Cont.) Abnormalities/injuries of soft tissues and ossicles in the ankle and foot

Abnormalities	MRI findings	Comments
Painful os peroneum syndrome (POPS) (▶ Fig. 8.19)	An os peroneum is a sesamoid that is ossified in a minority of patients and found within the distal peroneus longus tendon near the cuboid. Fragmentation and proximal migration of the ossicle seen on PDWI and associated edema seen on FS T2WI can be seen with peroneus longus tendon pathology.	Proximal displacement of the os peroneum is a subtle radiographic sign of complete tear of the peroneus longus tendon. Similar finding may be assessed on sagittal magnetic resonance (MR) images.
Diabetic foot: osteo-myelitis (▶ Fig. 8.20)	Osteomyelitis is seen with an associated soft tissue ulcer or sinus tract adjacent to an area of abnormal marrow. Abnormal marrow will demonstrate low T1 signal and increased signal on FS T2WI. Periosteal reaction may be seen along with cortical destruction and soft tissue abscess. Abnormal marrow edema on FS T2WI without T1 signal changes often indicates reactive marrow edema secondary to the adjacent soft tissue inflammatory process.	Soft tissue ulcers are common at pressure points, including the first and fifth metatarsal heads, malleoli, and calcaneus. Marrow signal changes seen on MR not within the proximity of a soft tissue ulcer are unlikely to be related to osteomyelitis.

(continued on page 272)

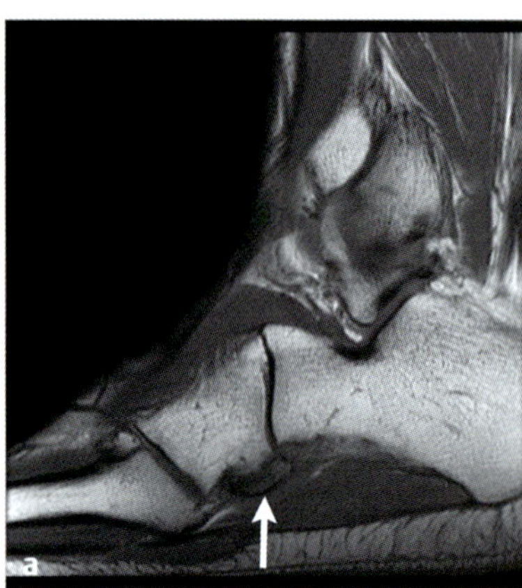

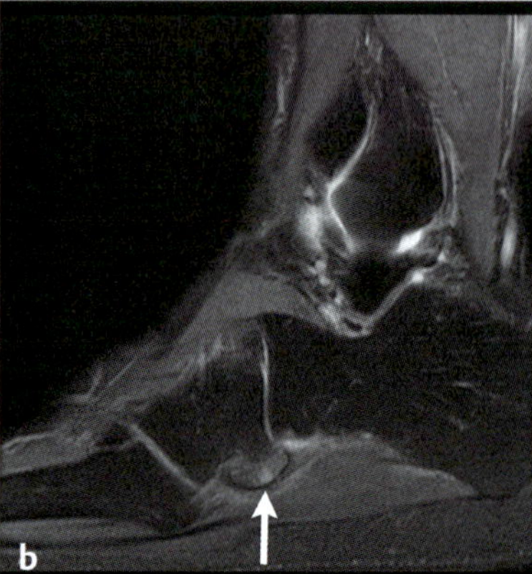

Fig. 8.19 (a) Note loss of normal fat signal and cortical irregularity in this abnormal os peroneum (arrow) on sagittal proton density–weighted imaging (PDWI). (b) Extensive marrow edema within the os (arrow), and mild surrounding soft tissue edema on sagittal fat-suppressed T2-weighted imaging. The peroneus longus tendon is partly seen proximal to the ossicle.

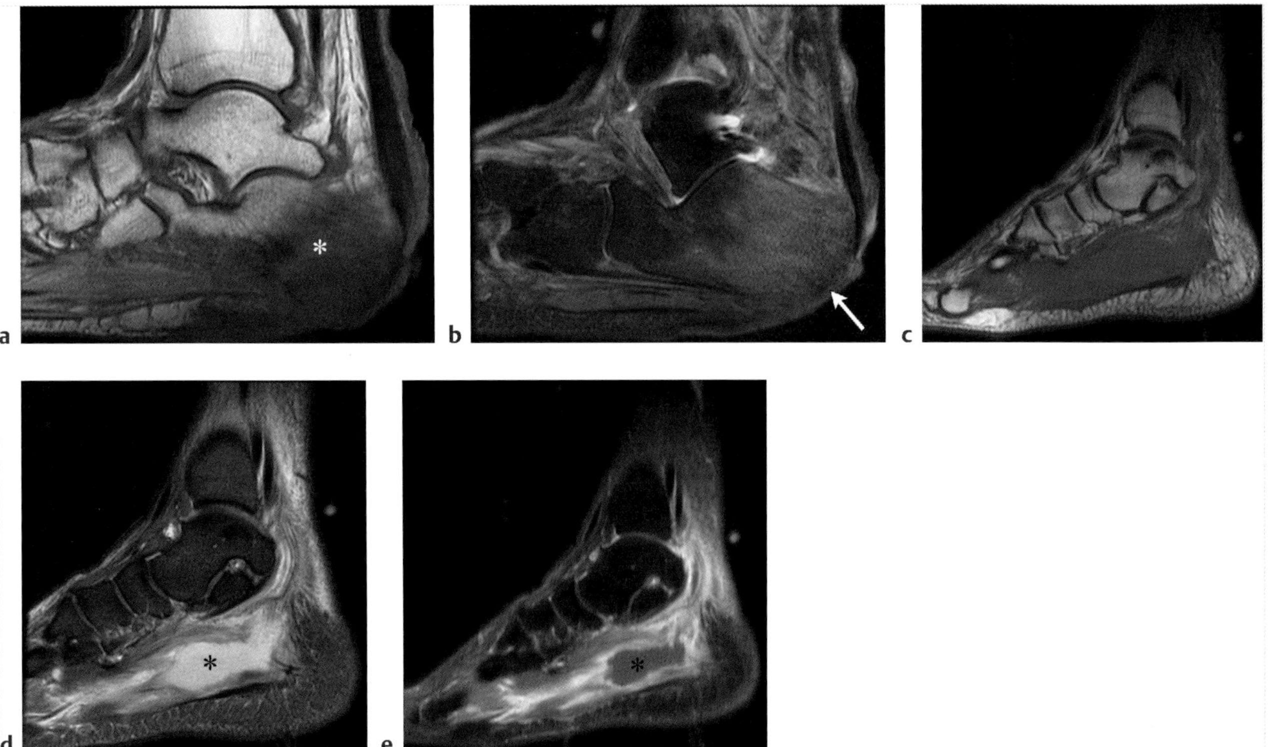

Fig. 8.20 Diabetic patient with long-standing heel ulcer and osteomyelitis. (a) Sagittal T1-weighted imaging (T1WI) demonstrates loss of overlying plantar soft tissues and low signal in the adjacent calcaneus (asterisk) representing osteomyelitis. Fatty infiltration of the plantar foot musculature is seen as well. (b) Note diffuse high signal marrow edema and erosion of the cortex (arrow) on the plantar aspect of the calcaneus on corresponding sagittal fat-suppressed T2-weighted imaging (FS T2WI). (c) In the differential for osteomyelitis is a soft tissue abscess. Note a fluid-filled abscess cavity within the plantar foot musculature demonstrating low signal on T1WI, and (d) high signal on FS T2WI (asterisk) with surrounding soft tissue edema. (e) Soft tissues surrounding the low signal abscess cavity (asterisk) demonstrate gadolinium-contrast enhancement on sagittal FS T1WI.

Table 8.3 (Cont.) Abnormalities/injuries of soft tissues and ossicles in the ankle and foot

Abnormalities	MRI findings	Comments
Diabetic foot: neuropathic changes/ Charcot neuroarthropathy (▶ Fig. 8.21)	Marrow signal changes in Charcot neuroarthropathy are seen without or distant from a soft tissue ulcer. This helps distinguish this entity from osteomyelitis. Bone destruction and fragmentation with neuropathic changes typically involve the midfoot–tarsometatarsal, intertarsal, and metatarsophalangeal joints. Fragmentation of bone with joint involvement demonstrates low signal on T1WI and either low or high signal on FS T2WI or short TI inversion recovery (STIR) images.	In later stages, infection may be superimposed on neuropathic changes as foot deformity leads to soft tissue ulceration. Diabetic foot changes present with nonhealing ulcers, whereas Charcot arthropathy often presents with swelling without pain. The etiology of Charcot arthropathy is believed to be due to a combination of repetitive trauma, loss of sensation, and autonomic dysfunction with decreased blood flow to involved bones. Look for associated tendon pathology, muscle edema, and fatty replacement due to neuropathic changes.
Pressure lesion/ adventitial bursa (▶ Fig. 8.22)	MR features include soft tissue regions of low signal on T1 and PDWI at the site of pain. Look for mixed signal on FS T2WI depending on fluid content. Lesion may be ill defined but may be mistaken for a true mass. Gadolinium-contrast (Gd-contrast) enhancement may be seen due to the presence of fibrous and fatty tissue and superimposed inflammation. With the presence of a superimposed adventitial bursa, look for fluid signal centrally within these lesions, well seen on Gd-contrast enhanced images.	Pressure lesions are seen in the subcutaneous tissues at sites of weight bearing or physical pressure such as the plantar subcutaneous tissues at the first and fifth metatarsal heads, retro-Achilles region, or points of malleolar prominence. They often demonstrate ill-defined signal change, which along with location helps distinguish this finding from a true mass lesion. They are composed of fat and fibrous tissue with intermixed central fluid when a bursa is present.

(continued on page 274)

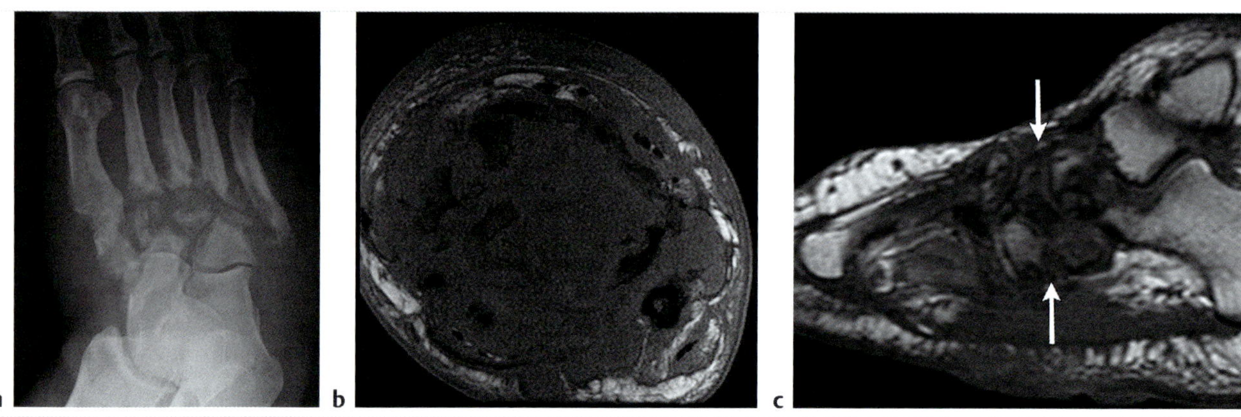

Fig. 8.21 (a) Diabetic patient with painless midfoot swelling and no overlying skin ulcer. Note bone fragmentation and destruction at the tarsometatarsal joints on an oblique radiograph of the foot. (b) Extensive abnormal low signal, bone fragmentation, and soft tissue swelling are seen on axial T1-weighted imaging (T1WI) corresponding to the X-ray findings. (c) Additional example of neuropathic change with low signal in the midfoot bone marrow, areas of bone destruction, and bone fragmentation (arrows) on sagittal T1WI. Although there is plantar soft tissue thickening, no ulcer was present.

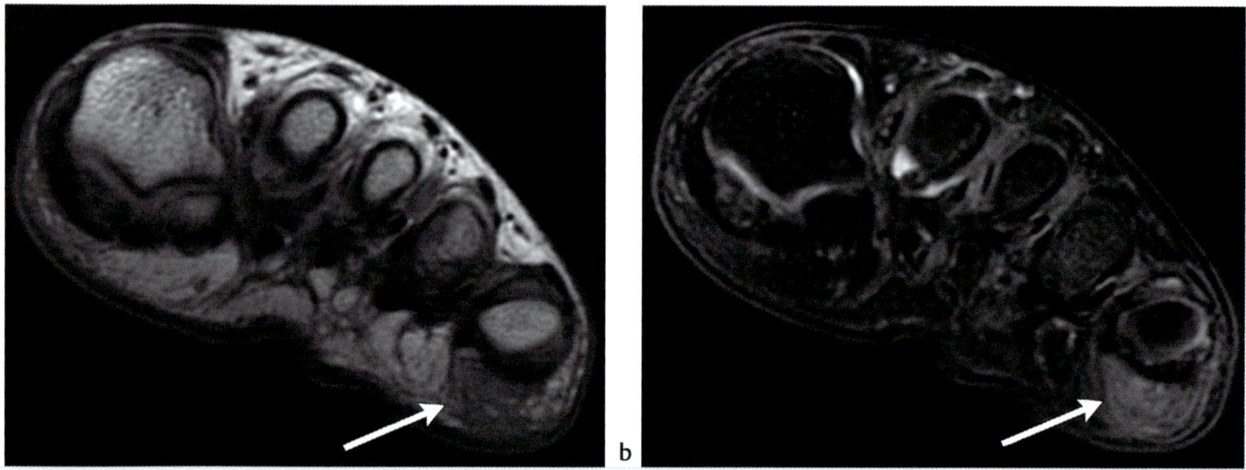

Fig. 8.22 (a) Patient with plantar pain at the fifth metatarsal head. Note intermediate signal infiltrative change of a pressure lesion (arrow) in the plantar subcutaneous fatty tissues on axial proton density–weighted imaging (PDWI). (b) Corresponding edematous changes (arrow) with soft tissue swelling are seen on axial fat-suppressed T2-weighted imaging (FS T2WI). *(continued)*

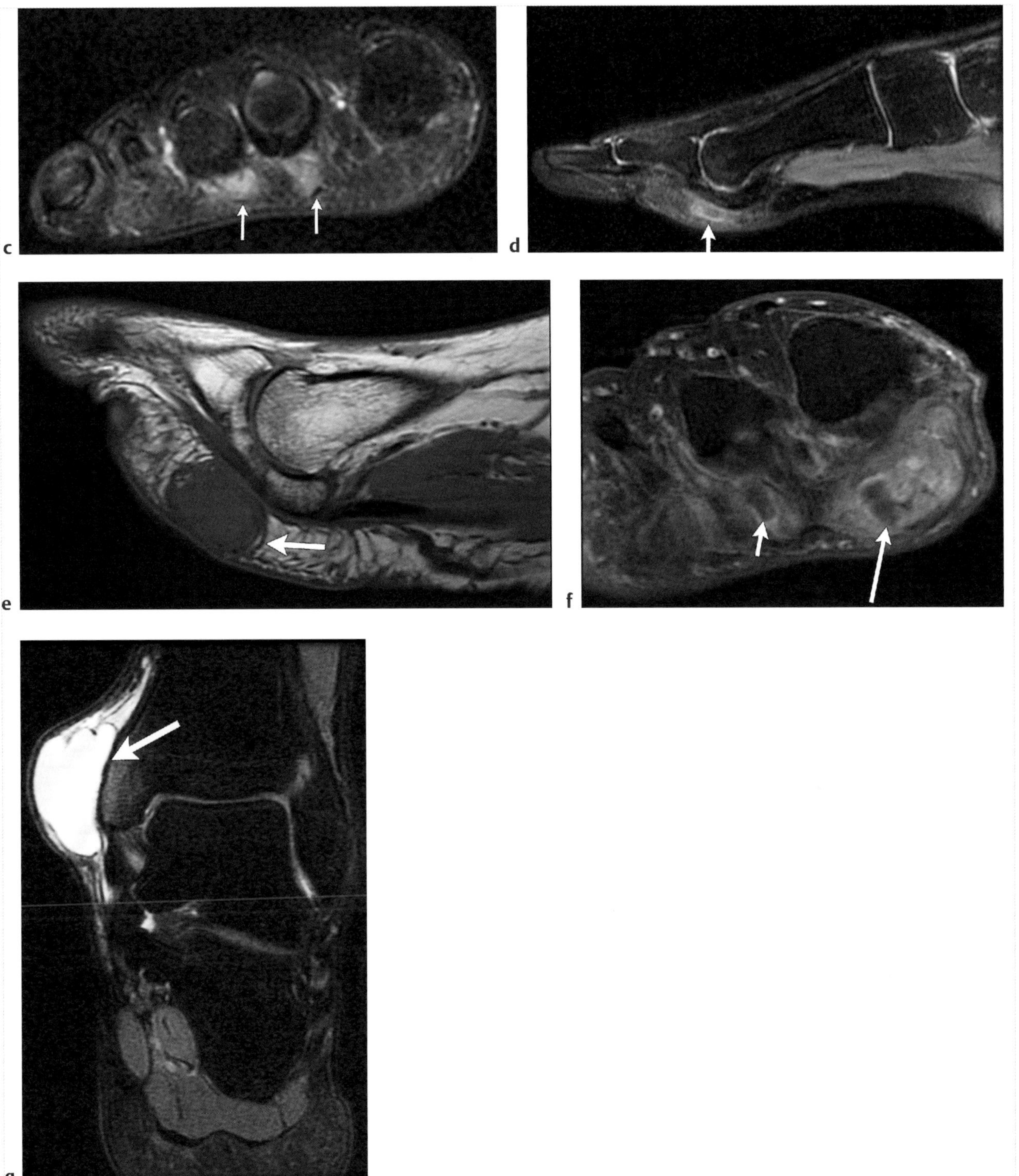

Fig. 8.22 *(continued)* (c) Two adjacent pressure lesions (arrows) in a different patient at the second and third metatarsal heads on axial FS T2WI. (d) In a more advanced case of a pressure lesion (arrow), note the plantar soft tissue enhancement surrounding a central area of low signal fluid representing development of an adventitial bursa on sagittal gadolinium-contrast (Gd-contrast) enhanced FS T1-weighted imaging (T1WI). (e) Large pressure lesion (arrow) along the plantar aspect of the first metatarsophalangeal joint demonstrating uniform low to intermediate signal on sagittal PDWI. (f) Note corresponding Gd-contrast enhancement on axial FS T1WI, with a low signal nonenhancing fluid portion (long arrow) indicative of an adventitial bursa. A similar lesion is seen at the second metatarsal (short arrow). (g) A large adventitial bursa/medial malleolar bursa (white arrow) adjacent to the medial malleolus may be caused by friction from tight boots. High signal fluid fills the bursa on coronal FS T2WI. Adjacent mild medial malleolus marrow edema and surrounding soft tissue edema are typical of this entity.

Table 8.3 (Cont.) Abnormalities/injuries of soft tissues and ossicles in the ankle and foot

Abnormalities	MRI findings	Comments
Morton neuroma/inter-digital neuroma (▸ Fig. 8.23)	Soft tissue signal mass consisting of perineural fibrosis typically seen at the metatarsal head level of the third intermetatarsal space. Lesions are typically teardrop shaped extending between the metatarsals into the plantar fat best seen on short axis images of the foot. Lesions are low to intermediate signal on T1WI and variable signal on T2WI. Morton neuroma can be distinguished from the more dorsal intermetatarsal bursitis, which will be fluid signal on FS T2WI.	Morton neuroma is not a true neuroma but rather the result of chronic plantar digital nerve entrapment and resultant perineural fibrosis. It may be seen in association with intermetatarsal bursitis. Differential considerations for pain in this region include a true nerve sheath tumor or foreign body reaction. This entity may be seen as an incidental MR finding in asymptomatic patients.

(continued on page 276)

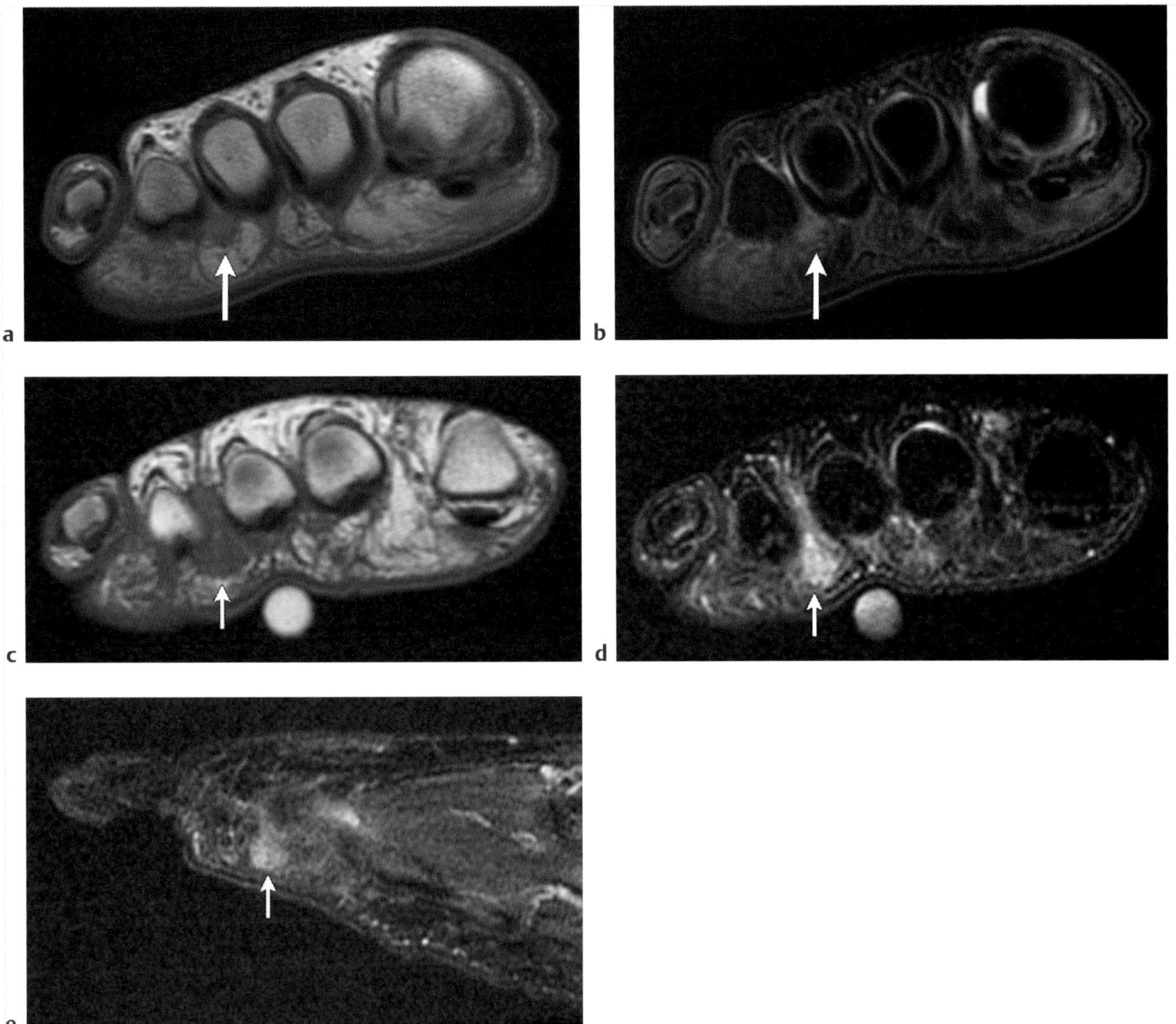

Fig. 8.23 (a) Teardrop-shaped mass (arrow) plantar to the third and fourth metatarsal heads in the interspace on axial T1-weighted imaging (T1WI). (b) Corresponding axial fat-suppressed T2-weighted imaging (FS T2WI) demonstrates increased signal of this lesion. (c) A larger example of a Morton neuroma (arrow), with a teardrop low signal lesion in the third interspace at the level of the third and fourth metatarsal heads on axial T1WI. (d) Note increased signal of this symptomatic Morton neuroma (arrows) on axial FS T2WI and (e) sagittal FS T2WI.

Table 8.3 (Cont.) Abnormalities/injuries of soft tissues and ossicles in the ankle and foot

Abnormalities	MRI findings	Comments
Sesamoid abnormalities (▶ Fig. 8.24)	Normally, a bipartite medial sesamoid at the first metatarsophalangeal (MTP) joint demonstrates irregular margins of the adjacent fragments with normal marrow signal on T1WI, PDWI, and FS T2WI. Sesamoid fracture, more common medially, results in a well-defined fracture line and marrow edema on FS T2WI. Displacement of the fragments may be seen. Osteochondritis followed by osteonecrosis more typically involves the lateral sesamoid and may demonstrate fragmentation and low signal on T1WI and intermediate signal (acute or subacute phase) to low signal (chronic phase) on FS T2WI. In osteoarthritis involving the sesamoids there is subchondral sclerosis and/or geode formation at the articulation between the dorsal margin of the sesamoid and adjacent plantar articular surface of the first metatarsal head.	Sesamoid abnormalities include a spectrum of abnormalities: sesamoiditis, osteochondritis/osteonecrosis, acute fracture, stress fracture, and osteoarthritis. Symptoms of pain about the plantar sesamoids are often described as a result of overuse. The term "sesamoiditis" typically refers to general symptoms of pain about the first MTP joint sesamoids. However, it has also been more narrowly defined as posttraumatic sesamoid chondromalacia associated with swelling of the MTP joint. Imaging findings often demonstrate overlap, regardless of etiology.

(continued on page 278)

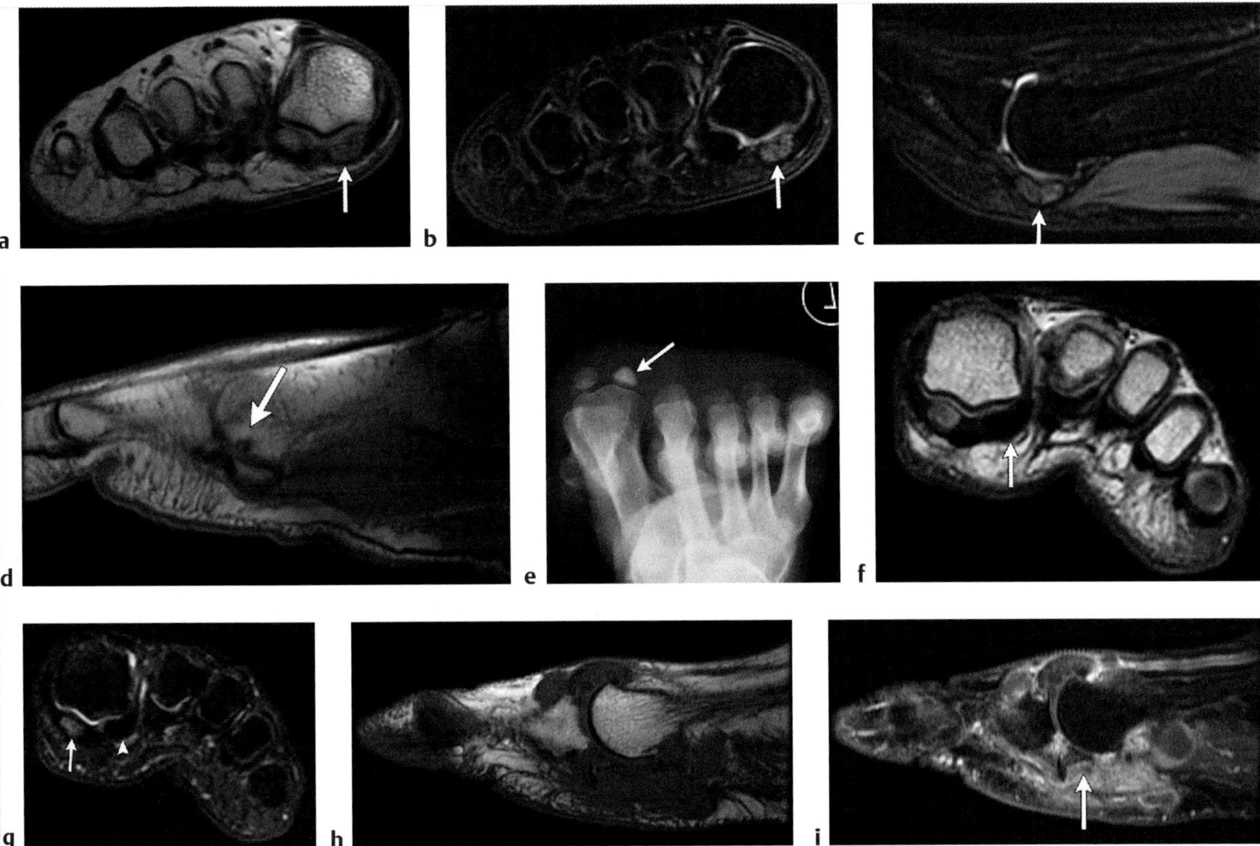

Fig. 8.24 (a) Note an abnormal medial sesamoid (arrow) with slightly decreased marrow signal on axial proton density–weighted imaging (PDWI). (b) There is corresponding increased signal (arrow) representing marrow edema on axial fat-suppressed T2-weighted imaging (FS T2WI). Changes were consistent with prior trauma based on history. (c) In a different patient with a history of acute pain after trauma, a well-defined low signal line (arrow) separates the medial sesamoid fragments on sagittal FS T2WI. Differential therefore favored sesamoid fracture rather than sesamoiditis involving a bipartite sesamoid. (d) Differential for pain at the first metatarsophalangeal joint also includes osteoarthritis as seen in this case with a low signal geode in the plantar aspect of the first metatarsal head (arrow). Note normal marrow signal in the sesamoid on sagittal PDWI. (e) Osteonecrosis more commonly involves the lateral sesamoid. Note sclerosis of the lateral sesamoid (arrow) on this sesamoid-view radiograph. (f) There is corresponding markedly low signal involving the lateral sesamoid (arrow) on axial PDWI and (g) on axial FS T2WI (arrowhead). Also note marrow edema of the medial sesamoid (white arrow) thought to be posttraumatic. (h) In a patient with known gout, note extensive intermediate signal tophus and synovitis on sagittal PDWI. (i) Note increased signal of an eroded sesamoid (arrow), and Gd-contrast enhancement of the surrounding synovial pannus on sagittal FS T1-weighted imaging.

Table 8.3 (Cont.) Abnormalities/injuries of soft tissues and ossicles in the ankle and foot

Abnormalities	MRI findings	Comments
Turf toe (▶ Fig. 8.25)	This injury results in a plantar capsular ligament sprain at the level of the first metatarsal secondary to forced dorsiflexion. Capsuloligamentous tears are seen as a defect in the normally low signal capsule on sagittal PDWI and FS T2WI. Look for edema/fluid within the gap, potential sesamoid subluxation, and surrounding soft tissue injury.	This injury to the first MTP joint was first described associated with artificial turf. The plantar plate serves to stabilize the joint and includes the tendon sheath of the flexor digitorum longus and brevis tendons. Tears of the plantar plate may also be seen at the lesser MTP joints. Note the lack of stabilizing sesamoids at the lesser MTP joints.

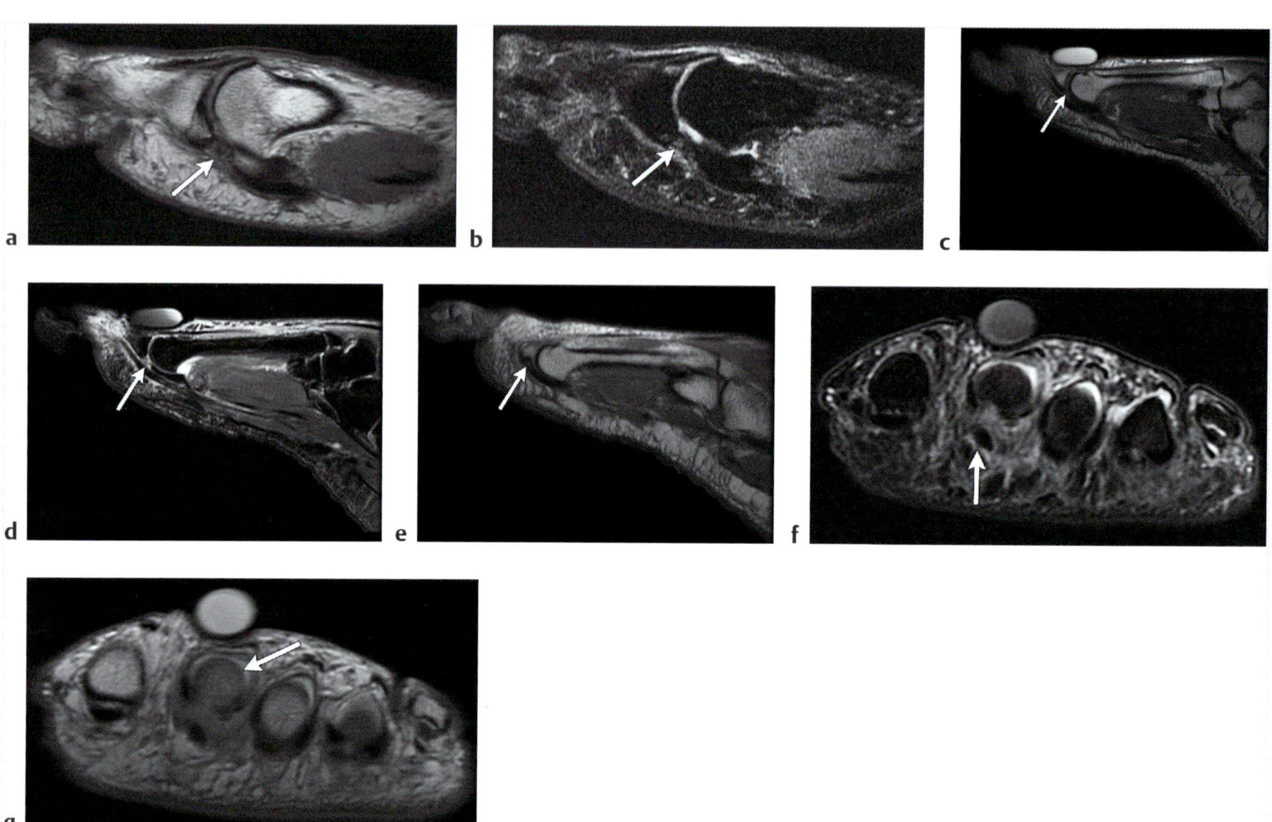

Fig. 8.25 (a) Note indistinct and heterogeneous capsuloligamentous attachment between the sesamoid and base of the proximal first phalanx (arrow) consistent with a history of prior injury on sagittal proton density-weighted imaging (PDWI). (b) Corresponding fat-suppressed T2-weighted imaging (FS T2WI) demonstrates mild edema distal to the sesamoid at the capsuloligamentous attachment (arrow). (c) In this case of plantar plate rupture at the second metatarsophalangeal joint, there is widening of the distance between the plantar plate and the adjacent proximal phalanx on sagittal proton density-weighted imaging (PDWI). (d) Corresponding increased signal edema (arrow) is seen in the gap on sagittal FS T2WI. (e) A normal plantar plate for comparison–note the close approximation between the plantar plate and the second proximal phalangeal base (arrow) on sagittal PDWI. (f) A more severe case of complete plantar plate rupture with extensive edema about the torn capsule and mild medial displacement of the flexor tendons (arrow) seen on axial FS T2WI. (g) Corresponding axial PDWI demonstrates slight dorsal subluxation of the phalanx (arrow) due to capsular injury.

8.3.1 Abnormalities/Injuries of Soft Tissues and Ossicles in the Ankle and Foot Suggested Reading

[1] Ahmadi ME, Morrison WB, Carrino JA, Schweitzer ME, Raikin SM, Ledermann HP. Neuropathic arthropathy of the foot with and without superimposed osteomyelitis: MR imaging characteristics. Radiology 2006; 238: 622–631

[2] Brown RR, Sadka Rosenberg Z, Schweitzer ME, Sheskier S, Astion D, Minkoff J. MRI of medial malleolar bursa. AJR Am J Roentgenol 2005; 184: 979–983

[3] Crain JM, Phancao JP, Stidham K. MR imaging of turf toe. Magn Reson Imaging Clin N Am 2008; 16: 93–103

[4] Donovan A, Schweitzer ME. Use of MR imaging in diagnosing diabetes-related pedal osteomyelitis. Radiographics 2010; 30: 723–736

[5] Jeswani T, Morlese J, McNally EG. Getting to the heel of the problem: plantar fascia lesions. Clin Radiol 2009; 64: 931–939

[6] Linklater JM. Imaging of sports injuries in the foot. AJR Am J Roentgenol 2012; 199: 500–508

[7] Murphey MD, Ruble CM, Tyszko SM, Zbojniewicz AM, Potter BK, Miettinen M. From the archives of the AFIP: musculoskeletal fibromatoses: radiologic-pathologic correlation. Radiographics 2009; 29: 2143–2173

[8] Shortt CP. Magnetic resonance imaging of the midfoot and forefoot: normal variants and pitfalls. Magn Reson Imaging Clin N Am 2010; 18: 707–715

[9] Toledano TR, Fatone EA, Weis A, Cotten A, Beltran J. MRI evaluation of bone marrow changes in the diabetic foot: a practical approach. Semin Musculoskelet Radiol 2011; 15: 257–268

8.4 Osseous Lesions and Trauma of the Ankle and Foot

- Tarsal coalition
- Osteochondral lesions of the talar dome
- Avascular necrosis (AVN)/osteonecrosis
- Freiberg infraction
- Metatarsal stress fracture
- Lisfranc ligament injury
- Navicular fracture
- Calcaneal stress fracture
- Tibial stress reaction

Table 8.4 Osseous lesions and trauma of the ankle and foot

Abnormalities	MRI findings	Comments
Tarsal coalition (▶ Fig. 8.26)	In cases of suspected osseous talocalcaneal coalition look for bony continuation/synostosis at the level of the middle facet/sustentaculum on coronal images. Calcaneonavicular bony coalition will be seen along the anterior facet on sagittal images. Fibrous or cartilaginous coalitions are identified by articular irregularity and sclerosis on T1-weighted imaging (T1WI) and proton density–weighted imaging (PDWI). On fat-suppressed T2-weighted imaging (FS T2WI) subchondral reactive marrow edema is often identified and associated with degenerative irregularity. Radiographic findings such as a talar beak may be associated with a coalition.	Calcaneonavicular and talocalcaneal coalition are most common. Talonavicular coalition is uncommon. Coalition types include bony, fibrous, cartilaginous, or fibrocartilaginous. Coalitions may be developmental or secondary due to prior trauma or arthritis. Patients typically present with limited subtalar joint motion and pain. Check for flatfoot deformity.

(continued on page 282)

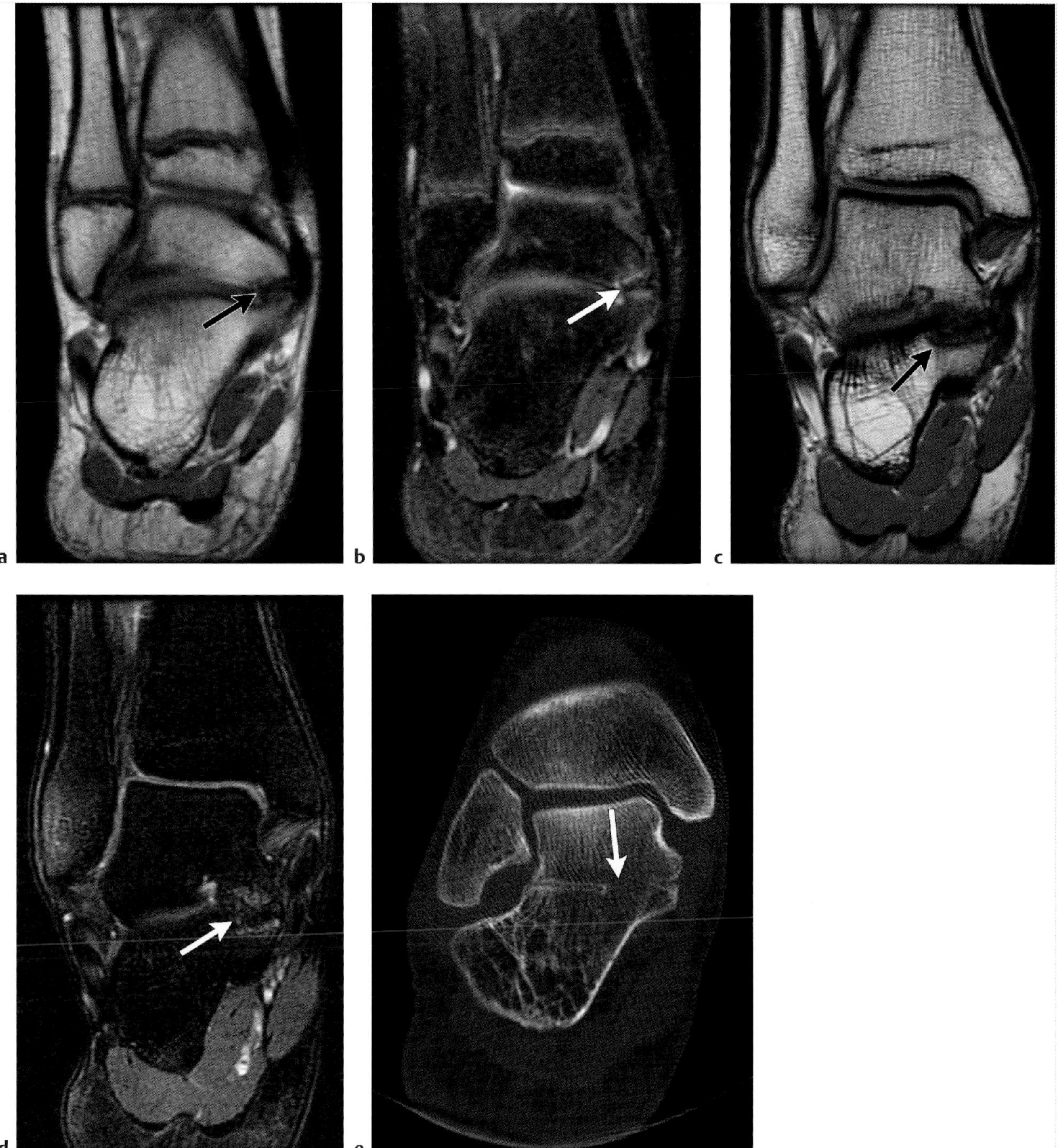

Fig. 8.26 (a) Talocalcaneal fibrocartilaginous coalition in a pediatric patient with narrowing of the middle facet of the subtalar joint. Note subchondral signal changes and articular irregularity on coronal proton density–weighted imaging (PDWI) (arrow). (b) Corresponding coronal fat-suppressed T2-weighted imaging (FS T2WI) demonstrates marrow edema of the sustentaculum tali and adjacent talus at the middle facet of the subtalar joint (arrow). (c) More advanced case of a fibrocartilaginous talocalcaneal coalition in a skeletally mature patient with low signal bordering the coalition at the subtalar joint on coronal PDWI (arrow). (d) Note corresponding marrow edema (arrow) on coronal FS T2WI. No bony coalition is seen. (e) Example of a bony talocalcaneal coalition (arrow) on coronal computed tomographic image.

Table 8.4 (Cont.) Osseous lesions and trauma of the ankle and foot

Abnormalities	MRI findings	Comments
Osteochondral lesions of the talar dome (▶ Fig. 8.27)	On coronal and sagittal T1WI and PDWI look for low signal along the talar dome with surrounding edema on FS T2WI. Intact cartilage, chondral fissures, or flaps may be seen overlying the lesion. Marrow edema is typically larger than the lesion. Look for fluid surrounding the lesion on FS T2WI as a sign of an unstable osteochondral fragment. In more severe cases, fragment displacement or loose bodies will be seen. The presence of joint fluid helps identify loose bodies.	Medial talar dome osteochondral lesions are often seen posteromedially, whereas lateral talar dome lesions are typically seen anterolaterally. There is typically a history of ankle inversion injury leading to impaction injury. Magnetic resonance (MR) is useful to determine the stability of osteochondral lesions and to detect early lesions not visible on radiographs. Lesion stability is presumed if no increased signal is seen deep to the lesion. Instability is presumed when fluid signal material or subchondral cyst formation is seen separating the osteochondral fragment from the adjacent talar dome. In more advanced cases, the fragment may be displaced or become necrotic.

(continued on page 284)

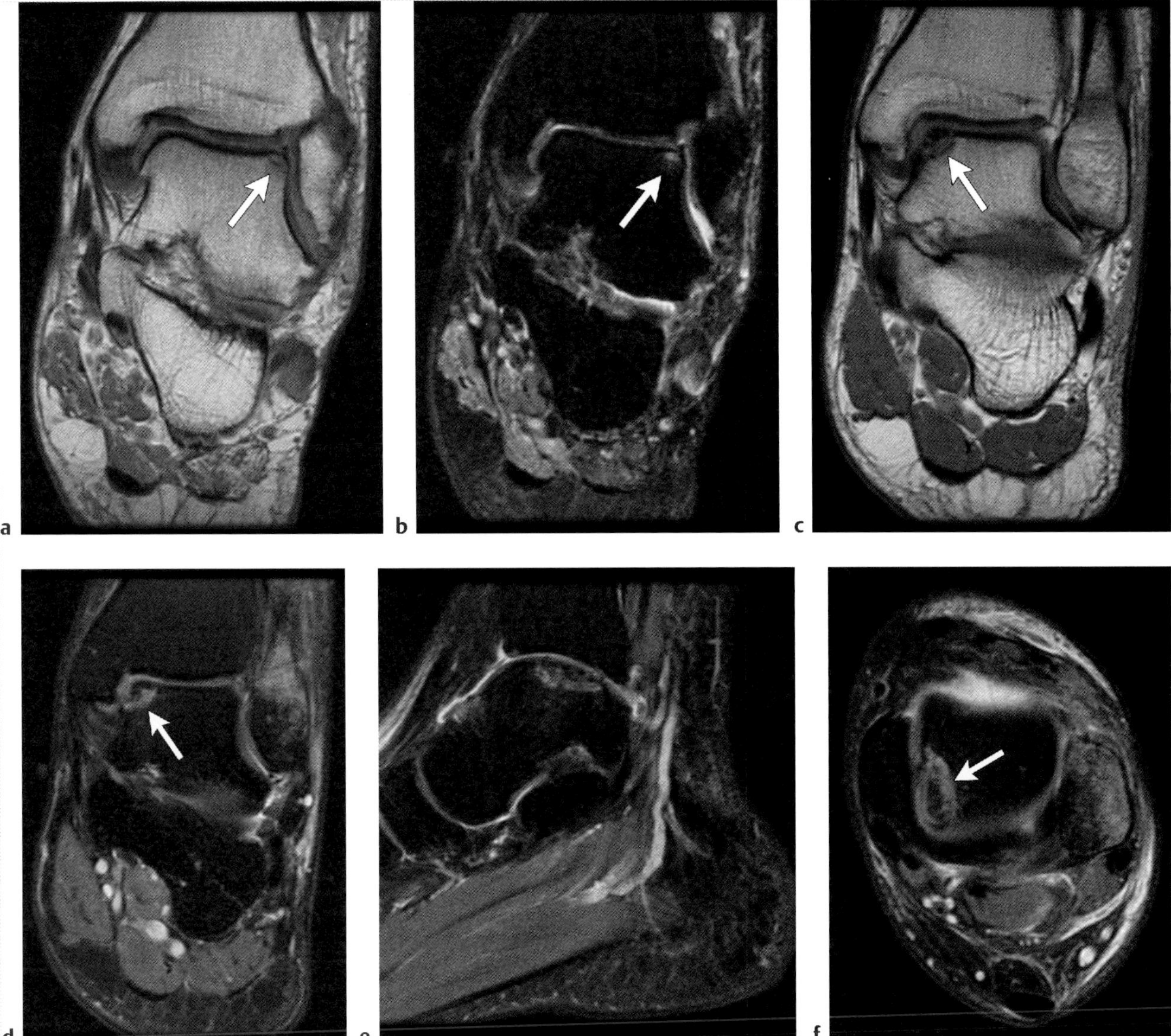

Fig. 8.27 (a) Small osteochondral lesion of the lateral talar dome (arrow) with abnormal curvilinear low signal in the subchondral bone and signal changes of the overlying cartilage on coronal proton density–weighted imaging (PDWI). (b) Corresponding coronal fat-suppressed T2-weighted imaging (FS T2WI), demonstrates increased signal in the subchondral bone with heterogeneous signal of the overlying cartilage (arrow). (c) A more pronounced example of an osteochondral lesion of the medial talar dome (arrow) with a low signal osteochondral fragment on coronal PDWI. (d) Note increased signal granulation tissue surrounding the osteochondral fragment (arrow) on coronal FS T2WI. A healing lateral malleolus fracture is noted. (e) The extent of the osteochondral lesion is often best appreciated on sagittal images as on sagittal FS T2WI. (f) Slight displacement of the fragment (arrow) is well seen on axial FS T2WI.

Table 8.4 (Cont.) Osseous lesions and trauma of the ankle and foot

Abnormalities	MRI findings	Comments
Avascular necrosis (AVN)/osteonecrosis (▶ Fig. 8.28)	On T1WI and PDWI a low signal serpiginous sclerotic line surrounding marrow fat is often seen in the subchondral bone in cases of AVN. Findings also include focal low signal zones of osteonecrosis. On FS T2WI look for diffuse marrow edema surrounding areas of low signal osteonecrosis. The double line sign on T2WI is an increased signal inner rim of granulation tissue surrounded by an outer rim of low signal.	AVN is commonly seen in the talus following talar neck fracture or dislocation but may also be seen with other causes including diabetes and steroid use. It is important to differentiate AVN from transient bone marrow edema where no area of low signal necrosis will be seen. Transient bone marrow edema will resolve spontaneously. Osteonecrosis of the talus will involve a larger area than the smaller osteochondral lesion of the dome described above.
Freiberg infraction (▶ Fig. 8.29)	On sagittal and coronal T1WI and PDWI low signal osteonecrosis is demonstrated by sclerosis typically at the second metatarsal head. This may be later accompanied by flattening, subchondral cystic change, and fragmentation. On FS T2WI marrow edema is appreciated. There may also be a curved subchondral line of osteonecrosis.	Freiberg infraction is a form of osteonecrosis most typically seen at the second, but also the third or fourth metatarsal head. It is usually isolated to the subchondral region. To distinguish this entity from osteoarthritis, look for arthritic changes in adjacent joints. Lack of erosion helps to rule out inflammatory arthropathy and gout.
Metatarsal stress fracture (▶ Fig. 8.30)	When assessing for radiographically occult metatarsal stress fractures, the key finding is marrow edema on FS T2WI. In more advanced cases, one may see surrounding soft tissue edema, periostitis, and an early low signal fracture line. Subacute cases will demonstrate periosteal reaction representing healing. On T1WI and PDWI look for variable decreased signal of the normal marrow fat and low signal periosteal thickening around the fracture site. The base of the fifth metatarsal is a common location for a stress fracture. Findings are best seen with a long axis view of the symptomatic metatarsal.	Stress fractures are seen involving normal bone undergoing abnormal stresses, such as march fractures, and in runners and dancers. Fractures are typically perpendicular to the involved metatarsal. The role of MR is to diagnose early stress reaction before cortical fracture occurs. Periosteal reaction may be exuberant and aggressive in appearance with heterogeneous marrow edema in more advanced cases. A similar aggressive appearance may be seen with recurrent injury and incomplete healing. The clinical history is helpful in excluding neoplastic disease or infection as a cause of periosteal reaction.

(continued on page 286)

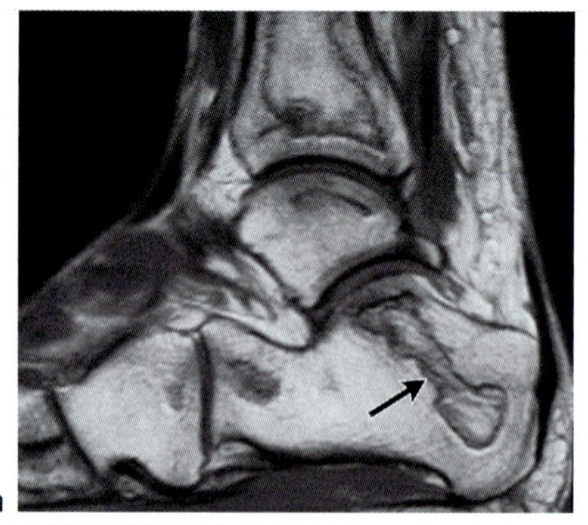

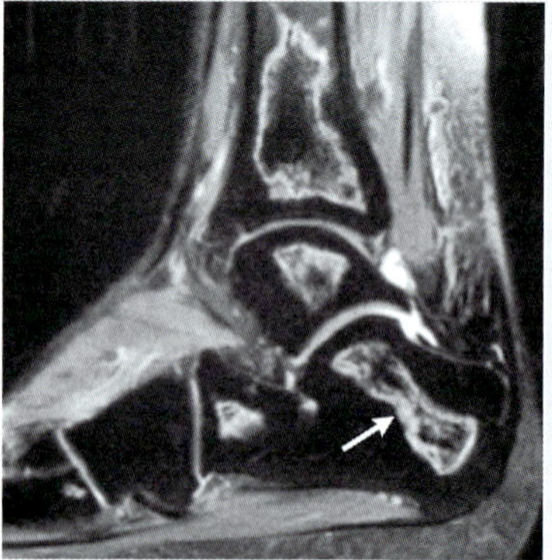

Fig. 8.28 (a) Bone infarcts about the included distal femur and hindfoot in a patient with sickle cell trait. Note serpiginous zones of low signal (arrow) on sagittal proton density–weighted imaging (PDWI) adjacent to zones of normal signal marrow. (b) The double-line sign is seen with curved adjacent zones of low and high signal on sagittal fat-suppressed T2-weighted imaging (FS T2WI) (arrow). This occurs at the border of bone resorption and healing.

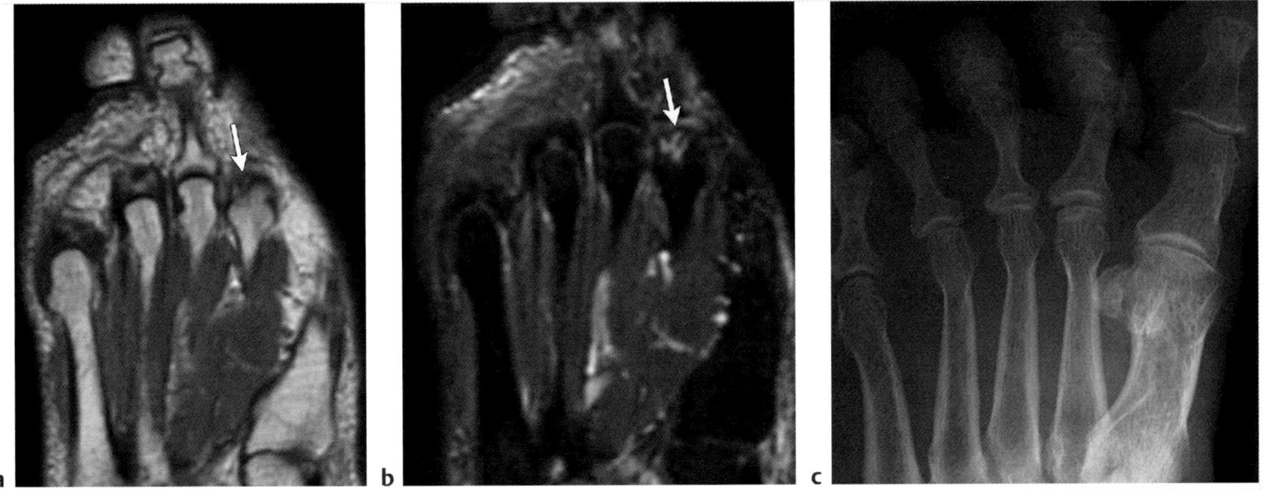

Fig. 8.29 (a) Subchondral low signal in the second metatarsal head (arrow) on coronal proton density–weighted imaging (PDWI). (b) Note the corresponding marrow edema and slight subchondral flattening of the second metatarsal head (arrow) on coronal fat-suppressed T2-weighted imaging. (c) Subchondral lucency and sclerosis of the metatarsal head are seen on the corresponding anteroposterior radiograph.

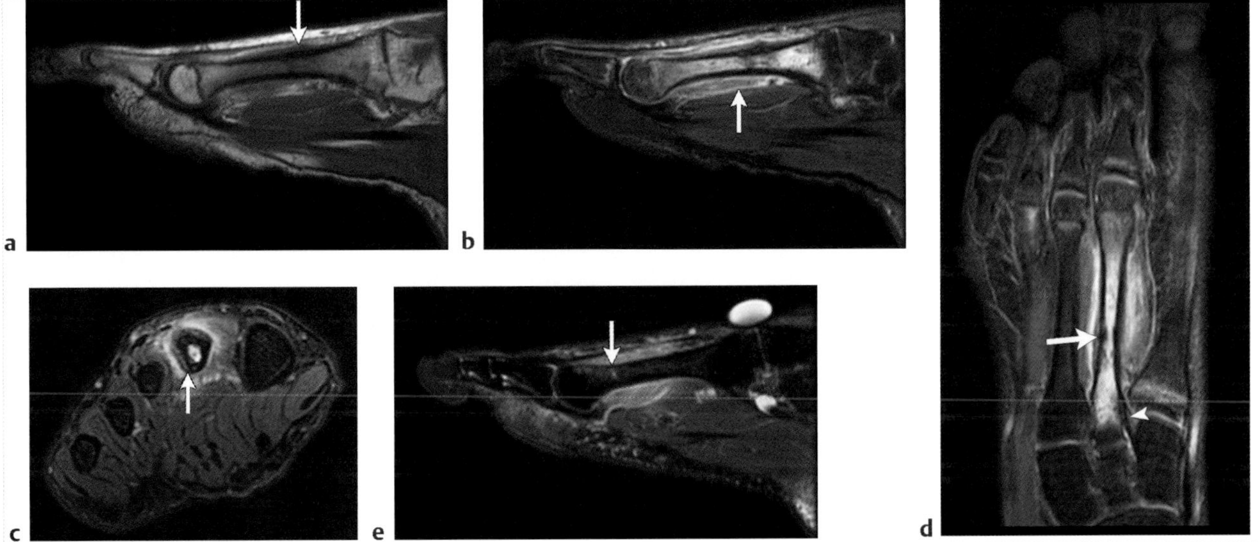

Fig. 8.30 (a) A nondisplaced second metatarsal stress fracture demonstrating low signal across the proximal shaft and low signal periostitis (arrow) on sagittal proton density–weighted imaging (PDWI). (b) Note extensive marrow edema and surrounding soft tissue edema (arrow) on corresponding sagittal fat-suppressed T2-weighted imaging (FS T2WI). (c) Short axis images through the fracture show a thickened cortex with periosteal reaction (arrow) and soft tissue edema on axial FS T2WI. (d) Extent of the periosteal reaction (arrow) and soft tissue edema is well seen on coronal FS T2WI. Note the intact Lisfranc ligament (arrowhead) coursing obliquely between the second metatarsal base and medial cuneiform. (e) In a different patient with a second metatarsal neck stress fracture note high signal fracture line perpendicular to the metatarsal (arrow) on sagittal FS T2WI. Note extensive surrounding edema.

Table 8.4 (Cont.) Osseous lesions and trauma of the ankle and foot

Abnormalities	MRI findings	Comments
Lisfranc ligament injury (▶ Fig. 8.31)	Normally the low signal Lisfranc ligament extends obliquely from the medial cuneiform to the second metatarsal base. With a sprain, look for increased signal within the ligament on coronal (long axis to metatarsals) PDWI of the foot, and surrounding high signal edema on coronal FS T2WI. Look for a flake/avulsion fracture from the lateral tip of the medial cuneiform on axial or coronal T1WI or PDWI. This indicates disruption of the Lisfranc ligament, which may be accompanied by widening of the first to second intermetatarsal distance. Assess the metatarsal bases and cuneiforms for associated bone bruises and fractures as a sign of Lisfranc fracture/dislocation.	A Lisfranc ligament sprain may occur without displacement of the tarsometatarsal joints. Check for alignment of the medial margins of the medial cuneiform and second metatarsal base. Note that the Lisfranc ligaments consist of a thinner dorsal component extending obliquely between the medial cuneiform and the second metatarsal, and a thicker plantar component extending from the medial cuneiform to the medial second metatarsal as well as in between the second and third metatarsal. These may be seen as separate ligaments on coronal images. Note that with a greater degree of injury, Lisfranc fracture dislocation may be seen. Injuries may be homolateral with all metatarsals displaced laterally, or divergent with medial displacement of the first metatarsal.

(continued on page 288)

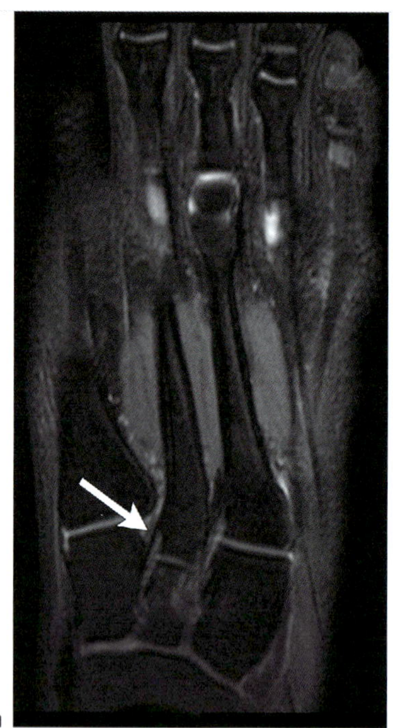
a

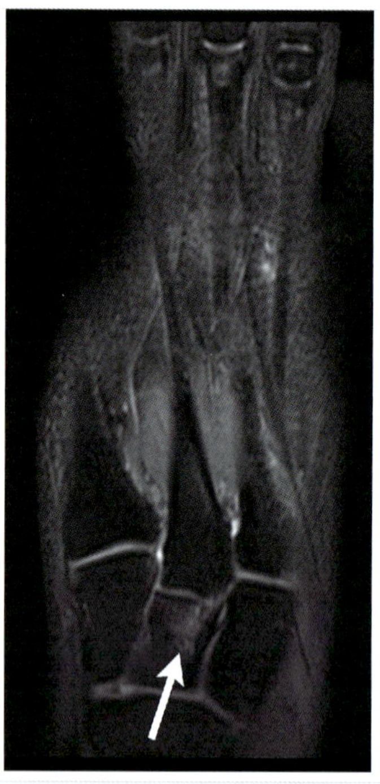
b

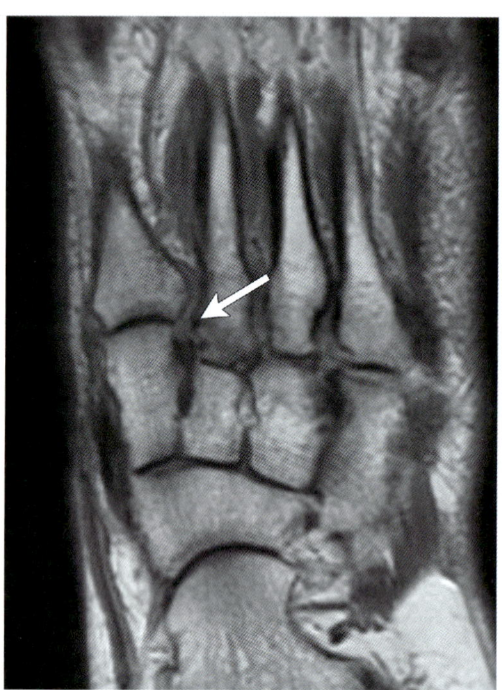
c

Fig. 8.31 (a) In a patient with recent trauma, an intact Lisfranc ligament (arrow) is seen between the medial cuneiform and second metatarsal base on coronal fat-suppressed T2-weighted imaging (FS T2WI). (b) On a contiguous image, posttraumatic marrow edema is seen involving the intermediate (arrow) and medial cuneiforms on coronal FS T2WI. (c) A torn Lisfranc ligament on coronal proton density–weighted imaging (PDWI) (arrow). Note lack of the normal ligament between the second metatarsal base and medial cuneiform. (*continued*)

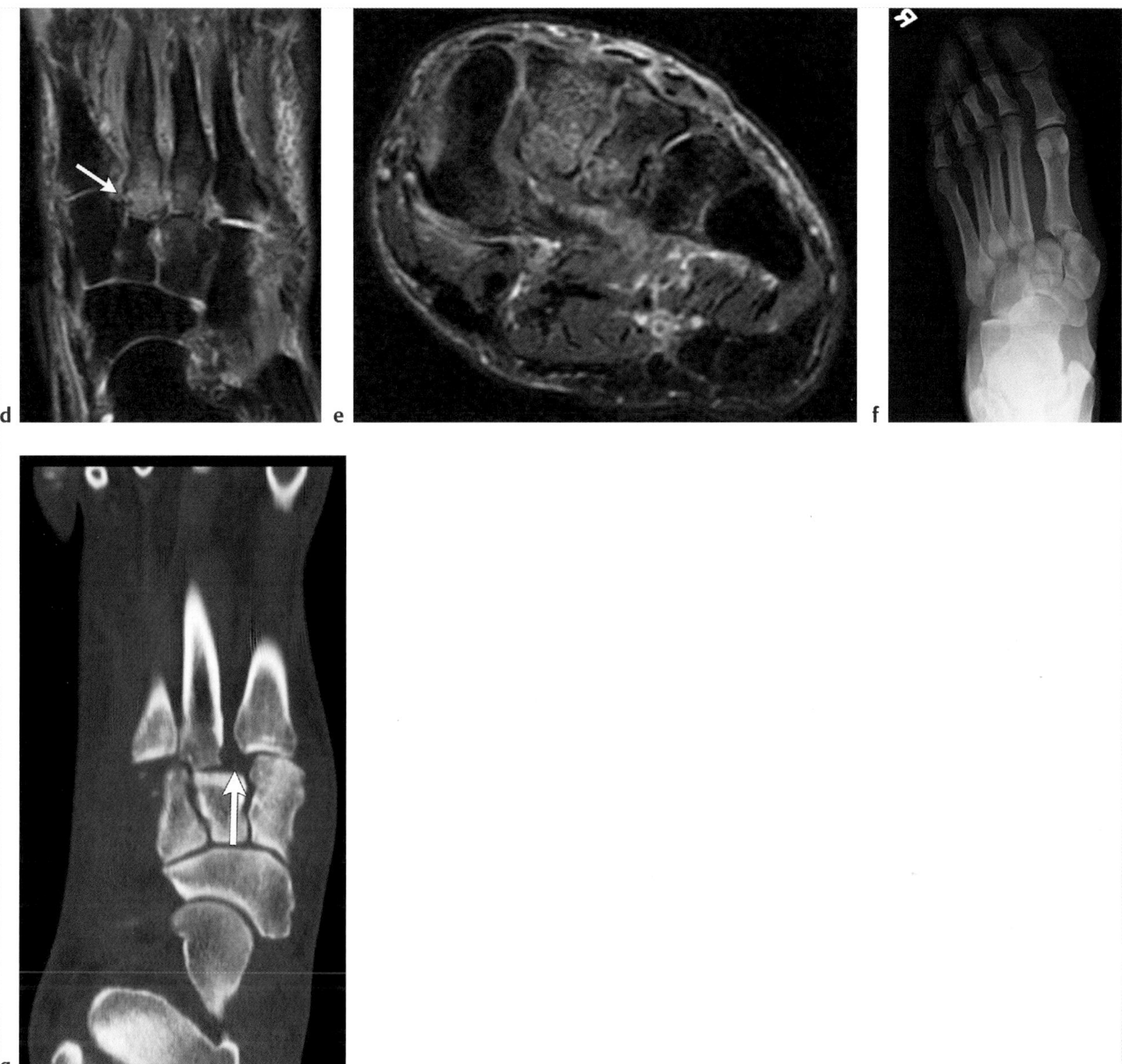

Fig. 8.31 (*continued*) (d) Corresponding coronal FS T2WI reveals the disrupted Lisfranc ligament (arrow) and extensive marrow edema due to fracture of the second and third metatarsal bases. Tarsal–metatarsal alignment is, however, maintained. (e) Subtle fractures of the metatarsal bases and the extent of soft tissue injury to the tarsalmetatarsal joints are also seen on corresponding axial FS T2WI. (f) Case of homolateral Lisfranc fracture-dislocation with lateral displacement of the first through fifth metatarsals on a posteroanterior foot radiograph. (g) Lateral offset of the first to third metatarsals relative to the cuneiforms and tiny avulsion fracture fragments including one related to the torn Lisfranc ligament (arrow) are seen on the coronal computed tomographic image.

Table 8.4 (Cont.) Osseous lesions and trauma of the ankle and foot

Abnormalities	MRI findings	Comments
Navicular fracture (▶ Fig. 8.32)	To image suspected fractures of the navicular and other tarsal bones use short- and long-axis FS T2WI images to identify marrow edema, and use T1WI or PDWI to assess for low signal fracture lines. Fracture lines may be obscured on sagittal images because the fracture line may parallel the plane of image acquisition. Distinguish the marrow edema of a simple bone bruise seen on fluid-sensitive sequences from that of a cortical fracture by identifying a low signal fracture line on T1WI or PDWI.	The tarsal navicular is susceptible to osteonecrosis following occult fracture. The central portion of the navicular has relatively decreased vascularity and is a common site of stress fracture. This may lead to delayed or nonunion if not diagnosed and treated. Navicular fractures are usually seen in jumping or running athletes with nonspecific midfoot and arch pain made worse with activity.

(continued on page 290)

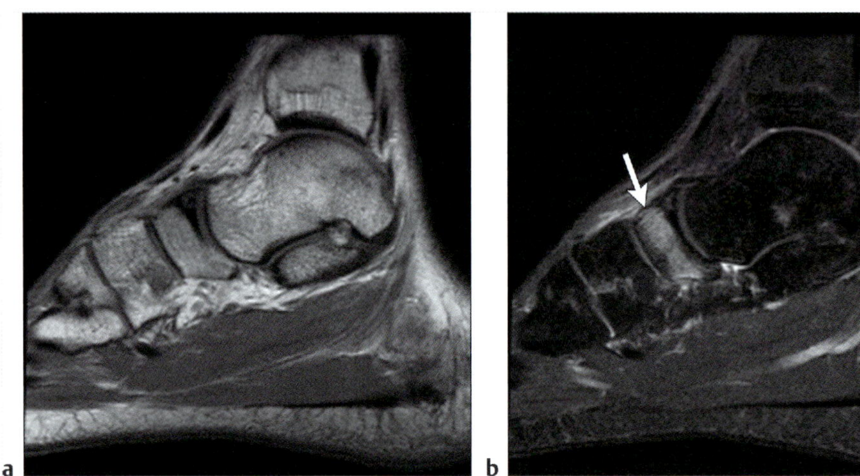

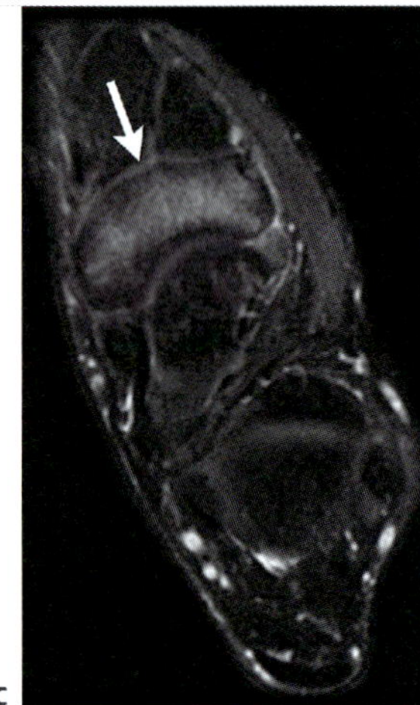

Fig. 8.32 (a) Early stress fractures are often difficult to detect on T1-weighted imaging or proton density–weighted imaging (PDWI) as demonstrated on this sagittal PDWI with only subtle decreased marrow signal in the navicular. (b) The corresponding sagittal FS T2WI and (c) coronal fat-suppressed T2-weighted imaging (FS T2WI) demonstrate extensive marrow edema of the navicular (arrows) with a suspected low signal cortical fracture on the sagittal image. (*continued*)

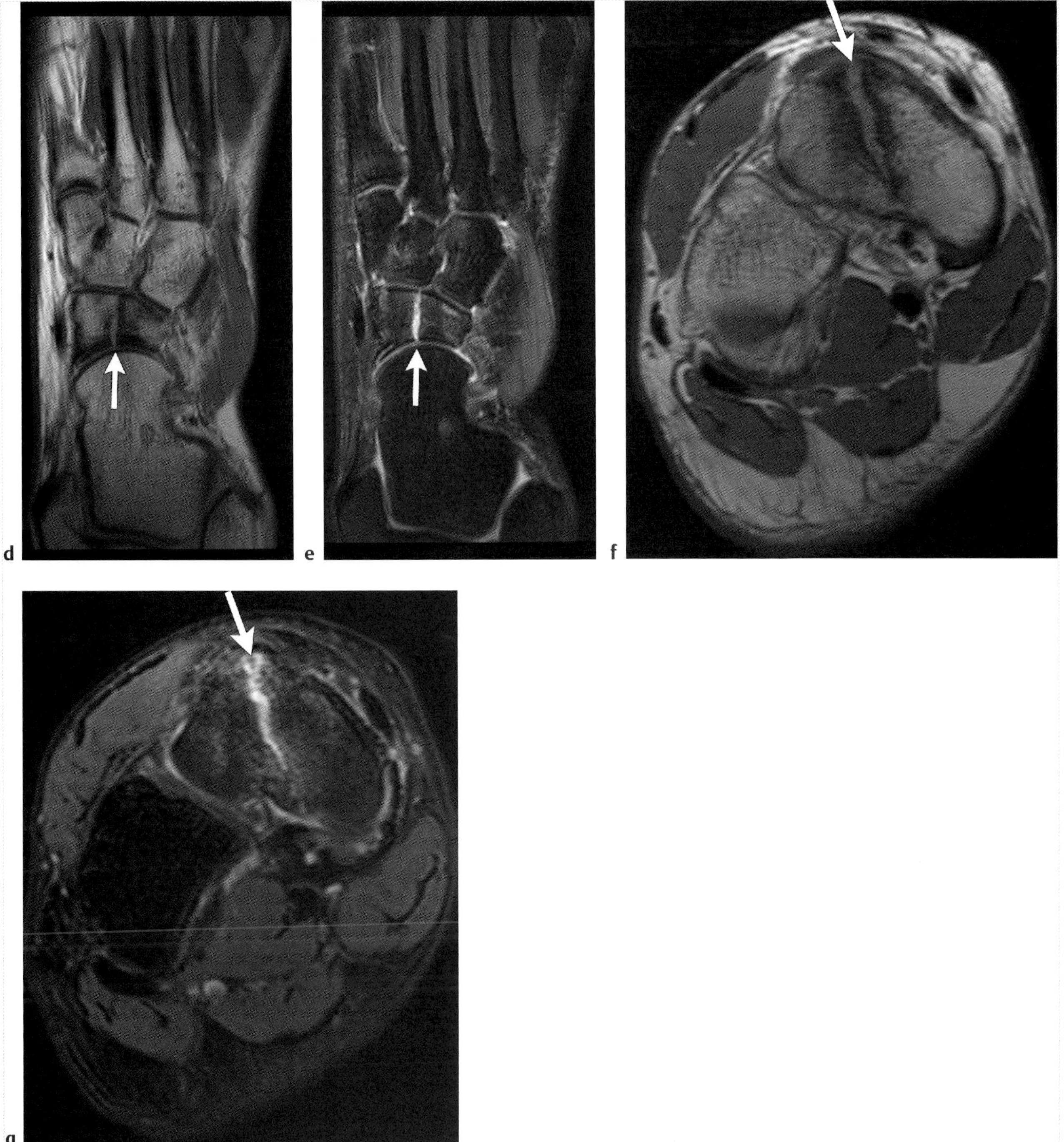

Fig. 8.32 (*continued*) (d) An example of a navicular fracture (arrow) with a well-defined fracture line on coronal PDWI. (e) The corresponding coronal FS T2WI demonstrates high signal fluid/granulation tissue at the fracture line (arrow) and surrounding marrow edema. (f) Comparison axial PDWI and (g) axial FS T2WI demonstrate dorsal separation of the fracture fragments (arrows) not appreciated on other planes.

Table 8.4 (Cont.) Osseous lesions and trauma of the ankle and foot

Abnormalities	MRI findings	Comments
Calcaneal stress fracture (▶ Fig. 8.33)	In patients with a calcaneal stress fracture a curvilinear band of low signal on sagittal PDWI will be surrounded by marrow edema on FS T2WI. Similar findings may also be seen in other planes. Distinguish a stress fracture from osteomyelitis by history, and the absence of an adjacent soft tissue ulcer.	Calcaneal stress fractures are seen in walkers and runners. Radiographs are often diagnostic, but magnetic resonance imaging (MRI) is of use with negative radiographs. Pain is noted posteriorly. Diabetic insufficiency fractures may be seen with involvement of the superior cortex.
Tibial stress reaction (▶ Fig. 8.34)	The earliest MR findings in stress reaction are mild marrow edema and subperiosteal edema/ periosteal reaction seen on FS T2WI or short TI inversion recovery (STIR). In our experience, marrow signal higher than that of surrounding muscle on FS T2WI is considered abnormal and is indicative of marrow edema. Higher grades of stress injury result in signal abnormalities on both T1 and fluid-sensitive sequences with subsequent visualization of a low signal fracture line perpendicular to the cortex. Shin splints, the earliest form of stress-related change, will demonstrate edema along the posteromedial tibial cortex on FS T2WI. This is well seen on axial or sagittal images.	Tibial stress fracture is the most commonly seen lower extremity stress fracture. Although stress fractures in athletes (abnormal stress on normal bone) commonly occur in the mid- to proximal shaft of the tibia, insufficiency fractures (normal stress on abnormal bone) are seen more distally. The role of imaging is to identify early stress-related changes prior to cortical fracture. This provides for faster recovery and return to activity.

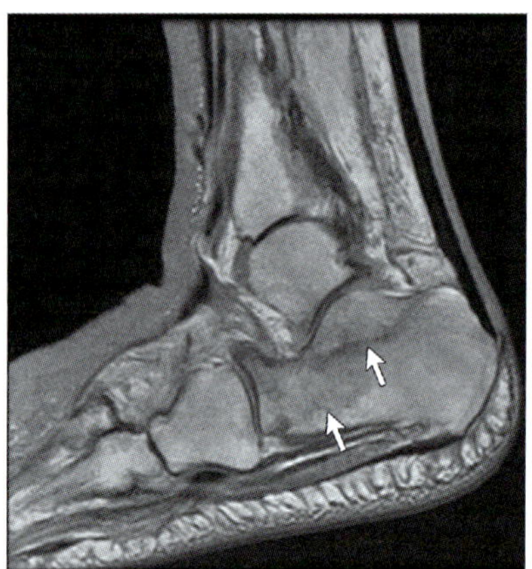
a

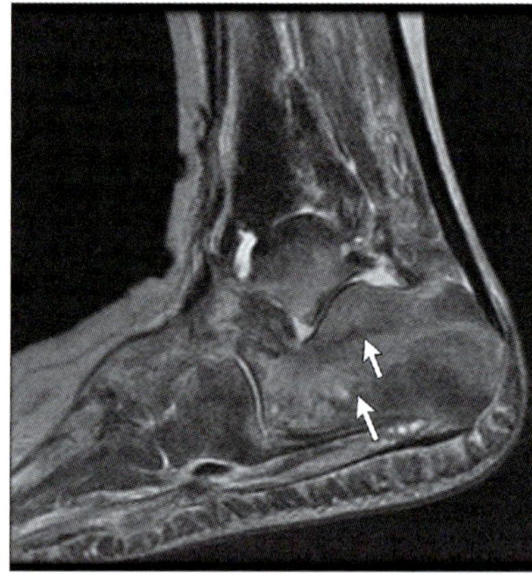
b

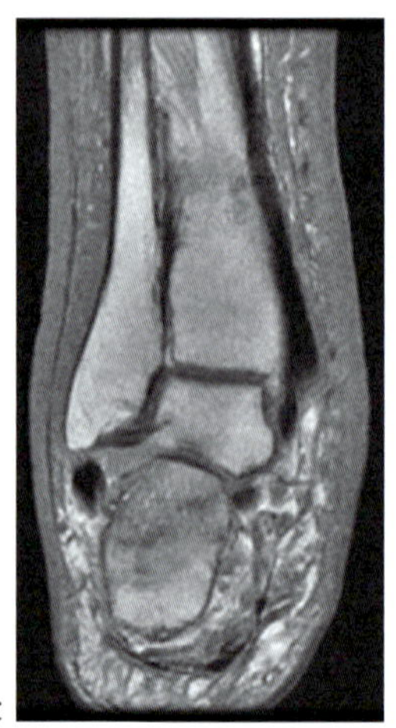
c

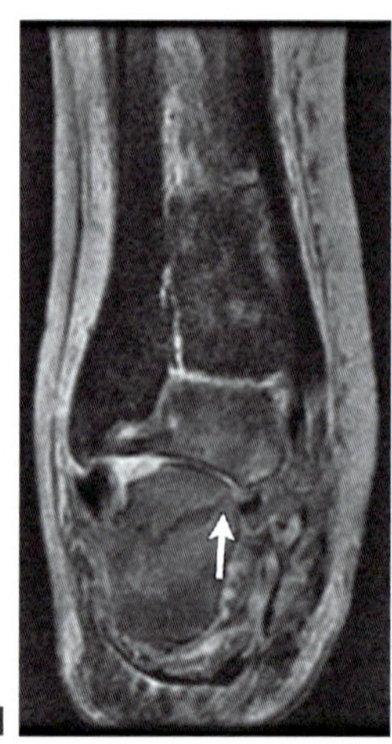
d

Fig. 8.33 (a) Calcaneal insufficiency fracture with several low signal fracture lines (arrows) within the calcaneus on sagittal proton density–weighted imaging (PDWI). (b) Note extensive high signal marrow edema with low signal fracture lines (arrows) demonstrated on sagittal fat-suppressed T2-weighted imaging (FS T2WI). (c) Comparison coronal PDWI better demonstrates the fracture lines. (d) Note extension of the fracture lines (arrow) into the subtalar joint on coronal FS T2WI.

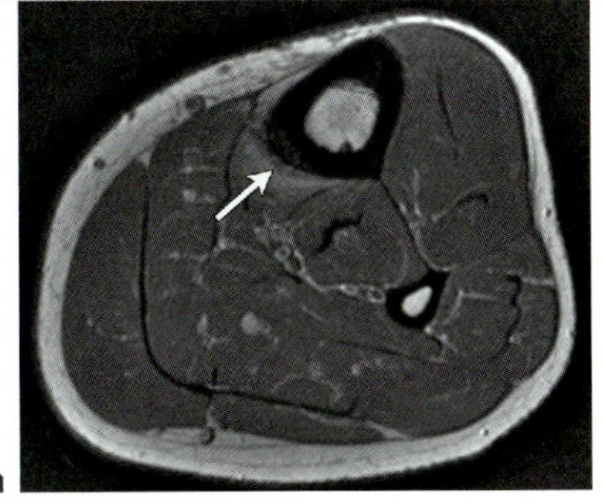

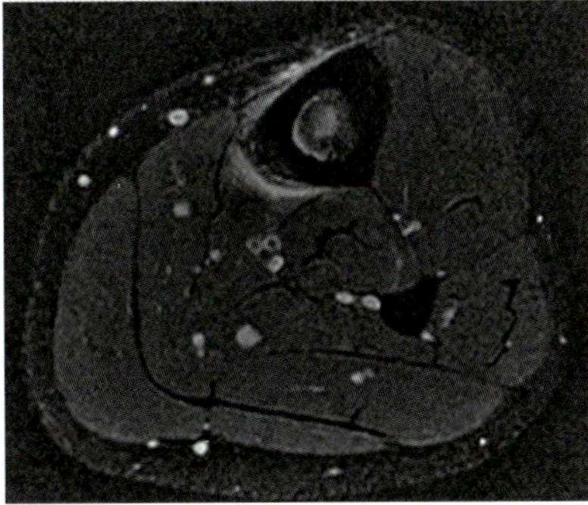

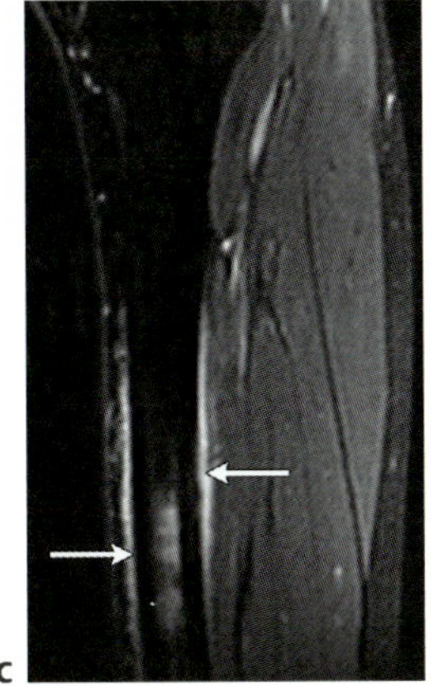

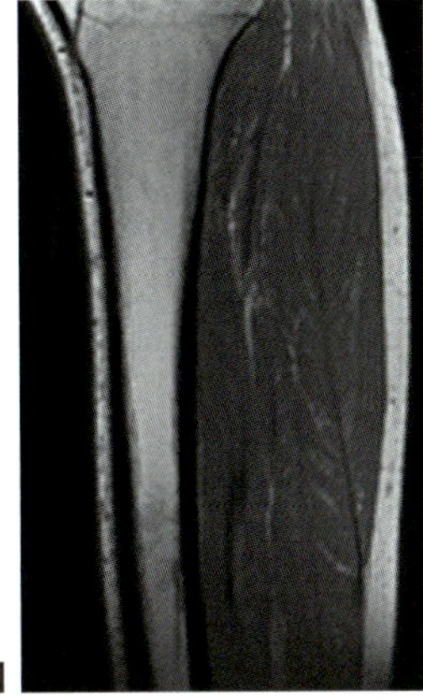

Fig. 8.34 (a) Early stress reaction of the mid tibia with periosteal reaction (arrow) on axial T1-weighted imaging. (b) Corresponding fat-suppressed T2-weighted imaging (FS T2WI) demonstrates marrow edema, periosteal reaction, and soft tissue edema along the anterior, medial, and posterior tibial shaft. (c) Sagittal FS T2WI demonstrates the extent of periosteal reaction and marrow edema (arrows). (d) Corresponding sagittal proton density–weighted imaging demonstrates the lack of a cortical fracture.

8.4.1 Osseous Lesions and Trauma of the Ankle and Foot Suggested Reading

[1] Davis KW. Imaging pediatric sports injuries: lower extremity. Radiol Clin North Am 2010; 48: 1213–1235

[2] Forney M, Subhas N, Donley B, Winalski CS. MR imaging of the articular cartilage of the knee and ankle. Magn Reson Imaging Clin N Am 2011; 19: 379–405

[3] Kalia V, Fishman EK, Carrino JA, Fayad LM. Epidemiology, imaging, and treatment of Lisfranc fracture-dislocations revisited. Skeletal Radiol 2012; 41: 129–136

[4] Linklater JM. Imaging of talar dome chondral and osteochondral lesions. Top Magn Reson Imaging 2010; 21: 3–13

[5] Patel CV. The foot and ankle: MR imaging of uniquely pediatric disorders. Magn Reson Imaging Clin N Am 2009; 17: 539–547

[6] Rios AM, Rosenberg ZS, Bencardino JT, Rodrigo SP, Theran SG. Bone marrow edema patterns in the ankle and hindfoot: distinguishing MRI features. AJR Am J Roentgenol 2011; 197: W720-W729

8.5 Suggested Reading: The Ankle and Foot

[1] Ballehr LO. Ankle/foot: technical aspects, normal anatomy, common variants, and basic biomechanics. In: Pope TL, Bloem HL, Beltran J, Morrison WB, Wilson DJ, eds. Imaging of the Musculoskeletal System. Philadelphia, PA: Saunders; 2008:690–712

[2] Cheung YY, Rosenberg ZS. Soft tissue injury to the ankle: ligaments. In: Pope TL, Bloem HL, Beltran J, Morrison WB, Wilson DJ, eds. Imaging of the Musculoskeletal System. Philadelphia, PA: Saunders; 2008:749–789

[3] Durand DJ, Carrino JA, Shatby MW, Moshirfar A, Campbell JT. The foot and ankle. In: Khanna AJ, ed. MRI for Orthopaedic Surgeons. New York, NY: Thieme; 2010;202–228

[4] Helms CA, Major NM, Anderson MW, Kaplan PA, Dussault R. Foot and ankle. In: Musculoskeletal MRI. 2nd ed. Philadelphia, PA: Saunders; 2009:384–430

[5] Spouge AR, Willits KR. Soft tissue injury to the ankle: tendons. In: Pope TL, Bloem HL, Beltran J, Morrison WB, Wilson DJ, eds. Imaging of the Musculoskeletal System. Philadelphia, PA: Saunders; 2008:790–810

[6] Stoller DW, Ferkel RD, Li AE, Mann RA, Lindauer KR. The ankle and foot. In: Stoller DW, ed. Magnetic Resonance Imaging in Orthopaedics and Sports Medicine. 3rd ed. Baltimore, MD: Lippincott Williams & Wilkins; 2007:733–1050

[7] Stoller DW, Tirman PFJ, Bredella MA, Beltran S, Branstetter RM, Blease SCP. Ankle and foot. In: Diagnostic Imaging Orthopaedics. Vol 6. Salt Lake City, UT: Amirsys; 2004:2–149

[8] Ulmans H. Imaging of the forefoot. In: Pope TL, Bloem HL, Beltran J, Morrison WB, Wilson DJ, eds. Imaging of the Musculoskeletal System. Philadelphia, PA: Saunders; 2008:864–878

Chapter 9

Magnetic Resonance Imaging of Bone and Soft Tissue Tumors and Tumor-Like Lesions: An Overview

9

9 Magnetic Resonance Imaging of Bone and Soft Tissue Tumors and Tumor-Like Lesions: An Overview

Steven P. Meyers

9.1 Classification of Bone Tumors and Tumors Involving Musculoskeletal Soft Tissues

The classification of bone and soft tissue neoplasms has evolved with the combined and coordinated use of clinical, imaging, macroscopic, histological, immunohistochemical cytogenetic, and molecular genetic information.[1–10] The classification scheme on which this book is based is from the World Health Organization (WHO), which itself was derived from an Editorial and Consensus Conference of the International Academy of Pathology in Lyon, France, in April 2002. The WHO Classification of bone tumors is listed in ▶ Table 9.1. The WHO Classification of soft tissue tumors is listed in ▶ Table 9.2. These classifications incorporate immunohistochemical reactivity profiles to distinguish between lesions that have overlapping morphological features or have uncertain histogenesis.[7,8,11] In addition, the new *WHO Classification of Tumours of Soft Tissue and Bone* also uses data from cytogenetic and molecular genetic analyses.[3–6,9,10,12,13]

Table 9.1 The World Health Organization Classification of bone tumors

Type of tumor	(ICD-O CODE)*
Cartilage tumors	
Osteochondroma	9210/0
Chondroma • Enchondroma • Periosteal chondroma • Multiple chondromatosis	• 9220/0 • 9220/0 • 9221/0 • 9220/1
Chondroblastoma	9230/0
Chondromyxoid fibroma	9241/0
Chondrosarcoma • Central, primary, and secondary • Peripheral • Dedifferentiated • Mesenchymal • Clear cell	9220/3 • 9220/3 • 9221/3 • 9243/3 • 9240/3 • 9242/3
Osteogenic tumors	
Osteoid osteoma	9191/0
Osteoblastoma	9200/0
Osteosarcoma	9180/3
• Conventional ◦ Chondroblastic ◦ Fibroblastic ◦ Osteoblastic Telangiectatic Small cell Low grade central Secondary Parosteal Periosteal High grade surface	• 9180/3 ◦ 9181/3 ◦ 9182/3 ◦ 9180/3 9183/3 9185/3 9187/3 9180/3 9192/3 9193/3 9194/3
Fibrogenic tumors	
Desmoplastic fibroma	8823/0
Fibrosarcoma	8810/3
Fibrohistiocytic Tumors	
Benign fibrous histiocytoma	8830/0
Malignant fibrous histiocytoma	8830/3
Ewing Sarcoma/Primitive Neuroectodermal Tumor	
Ewing sarcoma	9260/3
Hematopoietic Tumors	
Plasma cell myeloma	9732/3
Malignant lymphoma, NOS	9590/3
Giant cell tumor	
Giant cell tumor	9250/1
Malignancy in giant cell tumor	9250/3
Notochordal tumors	
Chordoma	9370/3
Vascular tumors	
Haemangioma	9120/0
Angiosarcoma	9120/3
Smooth muscle tumors	
Leiomyoma	8890/0
Leiomyosarcoma	8890/3
Lipogenic tumors	
Lipoma	8850/0
Liposarcoma	8850/3
Neural tumors	
Neurilemmoma	9560/0
Miscellaneous tumors	
Adamantinoma	9261/3
Metastatic malignancy	
Miscellaneous lesions	
Aneurysmal bone cyst	
Simple cyst	
Fibrous dysplasia	
Osteofibrous dysplasia	
Langerhans cell histiocytosis	9751/1
Erdheim-Chester disease	
Chest wall hamartoma	
Joint lesions	
Synovial chondromatosis	9220/0

*Morphology codes of the International Classification of Diseases for Oncology (ICD-O) and the Systematized Nomenclature of Medicine (http://snomed.org). Behavior is coded /0 for benign tumors; /1 for unspecified, borderline, or uncertain behavior; /2 for in situ carcinomas and grade III intraepithelial neoplasia; and /3 for malignant tumors.

Table 9.2 The World Health Organization Classification of soft tissue tumors

Type of tumor	(ICD-O CODE)
Adipocytic tumors	
Benign	
Lipoma	8850/0
Lipomatosis	8850/0
Lipomatosis of nerve	8850/0
Lipoblastoma/Lipoblastomatosis	8881/0
Angiolipoma	8861/0
Myolipoma	8890/0
Chondroid lipoma	8862/0
Extrarenal angiomyolipoma	8860/0
Extra-adrenal myelolipoma	8870/0
Spindle cell • Pleomorphic lipoma	8857/0 8854/0
Hibernoma	8880/0
Intermediate (locally aggressive)	
Atypical lipomatous tumor/well differentiated liposarcoma	8851/3
Malignant	
Dedifferentiated liposarcoma	8858/3
Myxoid liposarcoma	8852/3
Round cell liposarcoma	8853/3
Pleomorphic liposarcoma	8854/3
Mixed-type liposarcoma	8855/3
Liposarcoma, not otherwise specified	8850/3
Fibroblastic/myofibroblastic tumors	
Benign	
Nodular fasciitis	
Proliferative fasciitis	
Proliferative myositis	
Myositis ossificans • Fibro-osseous pseudotumor of digits	
Ischemic fasciitis	
Elastofibroma	8820/0
Fibrous hamartoma of infancy	
Myofibroma/myofibromatosis	8824/0
Fibromatosis colli	
Juvenile hyaline fibromatosis	
Inclusion body fibromatosis	
Fibroma of tendon sheath	8810/0
Desmoplastic fibroblastoma	8810/0
Mammary-type myofibroblastoma	8825/0
Calcifying aponeurotic fibroma	8810/0
Angiomyofibroblastoma	8826/0
Cellular angiofibroma	9160/0
Nuchal-type fibroma	8810/0
Gardner fibroma	8810/0
Calcifying fibrous tumor	
Giant cell angiofibroma	9160/0

Table 9.2 (Cont.) The World Health Organization Classification of soft tissue tumors

Type of tumor	(ICD-O CODE)
Intermediate (locally aggressive)	
Superficial fibromatoses (palmar/plantar)	
Desmoid-type fibromatoses	8821/1
Lipofibromatosis	
Intermediate (rarely metastasizing)	
Solitary fibrous tumor • and hemangiopericytoma (including lipomatous hemangiopericytoma)	8815/1 9150/1
Inflammatory myofibroblastic tumor	8825/1
Low grade myofibroblastic sarcoma	8825/3
Myxoinflammatory fibroblastic sarcoma	8811/3
Infantile fibrosarcoma	8814/3
Malignant	
Adult fibrosarcoma	8810/3
Myxofibrosarcoma	8811/3
Low grade fibromyxoid sarcoma	8811/3
Hyalinizing spindle cell tumor	
Sclerosing epithelioid fibrosarcoma	8810/3
So-called fibrohistiocytic tumors	
Benign	
Giant cell tumor of tendon sheath	9252/0
Diffuse-type giant cell tumor	9251/0
Deep benign fibrous histiocytoma	8830/0
Intermediate (rarely metastasizing)	
Plexiform fibrohistiocytic tumor	8835/1
Giant cell tumor of soft tissues	9251/1
Malignant	
Pleomorphic "MFH"/undifferentiated pleomorphic sarcoma	8830/3
Giant cell "MFH"/undifferentiated pleomorphic sarcoma with giant cells	8830/3
Inflammatory "MFH"/ undifferentiated pleomorphic sarcoma with prominent inflammation	8830/3
Smooth muscle tumors	
Angioleiomyoma	8894/0
Deep leiomyoma	8890/0
Genital leiomyoma	8890/0
Leiomyosarcoma (excluding skin)	8890/3
Pericytic (perivascular) tumors	
Glomus tumor (and variants) • Malignant glomus tumor	8711/0 8711/3
Myopericytoma	8713/1
Skeletal muscle tumors	
Benign	
Rhabdomyoma • Adult type	8900/0 8904/0

Table 9.2 (Cont.) The World Health Organization Classification of soft tissue tumors

Type of tumor	(ICD-O CODE)
• Fetal type • Genital type	8903/0 8905/0
Malignant	
Embryonal rhabdomyosarcoma (including spindle cell, botryoid, anaplastic)	8910/3 8912/3 8910/3
Alveolar rhabdomyosarcoma (including solid, anaplastic)	8920/3
Pleomorphic rhabdomyosarcoma	8901/3
Vascular tumors	
Benign	
Hemangiomas of	
• subcut/deep soft tissue • capillary • cavernous • arteriovenous • venous • intramuscular • synovial	9120/0 9131/0 9121/0 9123/0 9122/0 9132/0 9120/0
Epithelioid hemangioma	9125/0
Angiomatosis	
Lymphangioma	9170/0
Intermediate (locally aggressive)	
Kaposiform hemangioendothelioma	9130/1
Intermediate (rarely metastasizing)	
Retiform hemangioendothelioma	9135/1
Papillary intralymphatic angioendothelioma	9135/1
Composite hemangioendothelioma	9130/1
Kaposi sarcoma	9140/3
Malignant	
Epithelioid hemangioendothelioma	9133/3
Angiosarcoma of soft tissue	9120/3
Chondro-osseous tumors	
Soft tissue chondroma	9220/0
Mesenchymal chondrosarcoma	9240/3
Extraskeletal osteosarcoma	9180/3

Table 9.2 (Cont.) The World Health Organization Classification of soft tissue tumors

Type of tumor	(ICD-O CODE)
Tumors of uncertain differentiation	
Benign	
Intramuscular myxoma (including cellular variant)	8840/0
Juxta-articular myxoma	8840/0
Deep (aggressive) angiomyxoma	8841/0
Pleomorphic hyalinizing angiectatic tumor	
Ectopic hamartomatous thymoma	8587/0
Intermediate (rarely metastasizing)	
Angiomatoid fibrous histiocytoma	8836/1
Ossifying fibromyxoid tumor (including atypical/malignant)	8842/0
Mixed tumor • Myoepithelioma • Parachordoma	8940/1 8982/1 9373/1
Malignant	
Synovial sarcoma	9040/3
Epithelioid sarcoma	8804/3
Alveolar soft part sarcoma	9581/3
Clear cell sarcoma of soft tissue	9044/3
Extraskeletal myxoid chondrosarcoma (chordoid type)	9231/3
PNET/extraskeletal Ewing tumor	
• pPNET • Extraskeletal Ewing tumor	9364/3 9260/3
Desmoplastic small round cell tumor	8806/3
Extrarenal rhabdoid tumor	8963/3
Malignant mesenchymoma	8990/3
Neoplasms with perivascular epithelioid • Cell differentiation (PEComa) • Clear cell myomelanocytic tumor	
Intimal sarcoma	8800/3

9.2 Frequency of Occurrence of Bone Tumors

Bone neoplasms can be primary lesions arising from osseous structures or secondary to metastatic disease. Metastatic carcinoma is the most frequent malignant tumor involving bone.[14–16] In adults, metastatic lesions to bone occur most frequently from carcinomas of the lung, breast, prostate, kidney, and thyroid, as well as from sarcomas.[14–16] The exact incidence of metastatic skeletal disease is unknown.[16] Up to 50% of patients who die from disseminated carcinoma have evidence of skeletal metastases at autopsy.[16] Approximately 245,000 patients die in the United States each year from carcinoma of the lung, breast, prostate, kidney, and thyroid.[17] Using these data, up to 123,000 oncology patients who die each year may have metastatic skeletal disease. Metastatic skeletal disease has also been reported to occur in approximately 30% of all cancer cases.[14,15] Thirty percent of the 1,638,910 annual new cancer cases in the United States[17] is 491,673. In comparison, only 2,890 primary malignant bone tumors occur in the United States per year.[17] Metastatic lesions may therefore occur from 43 to 170 times more frequently than primary malignant bone tumors.

Primary bone sarcomas represent only 0.2% of all neoplasms.[4] The incidence of primary bone sarcomas has been reported to be approximately 8 per million.[4] Primary bone sarcomas occur 10 times less frequently than sarcomas in the soft tissues.[4] The most frequent type of primary bone sarcoma is osteosarcoma followed by chondrosarcoma and Ewing sarcoma.[4] Bone

Table 9.3 Primary malignant bone tumors

Tumors	Mayo Clinic % malignant (N = 7,086)	NCBT % malignant (N = 3,355)	Mayo % total (N = 9,973)	NCBT % total (N = 5,133)	Age range (years), median age
Myeloma	15	2	11	1	16–80, 60
Osteosarcoma	29	34	21	22	2–92, 16–39
Chondrosarcoma	20	21	15	14	7–91, 26–59
Lymphoma	13	3	9	2	18-69
Ewing sarcoma	9	11	6	7	6–30, 14
Chordoma	6	2	4	1	30–80, 58
Fibrosarcoma	4	5	3	4	10–75, 43
Malignant fibrous histiocytoma	1	5	< 1	3	11–80, 48
Giant cell tumor	< 1	2	< 1	1	10–55, 30
Angiosarcoma	2	1	1	< 1	10–80, 51
Hemangioendothelioma	< 1	< 1	< 1	< 1	15–60, 34
Adamantinoma	< 1	< 1	< 1	< 1	10–60, 25
Hemangiopericytoma	< 1	< 1	< 1	< 1	1–90, 40
Liposarcoma	< 1	< 1	< 1	< 1	Not reported
Synovial sarcoma		2		1	5–60, 25
Paget sarcoma		1		< 1	50–80, 66

Data from:
Mayo Clinic:
1. Unni KK, Inwards CY. Introduction and scope of study. In: Dahlin's Bone Tumors General Aspects and Data in 10,165 Cases. 6th ed. Wolters Kluwer/ Lippincott-Raven; 2010:1–8.
Netherlands Committee on Bone Tumors (NCBT):
2. Mulder JD, Schutte HE, Kroon HM, Taconis WK. Introduction. In: Radiologic Atlas of Bone Tumors. Elsevier; 1993:3–6.
3. Mulder JD, Schutte HE, Kroon HM, Taconis WK. The diagnosis of bone tumors. In: Radiologic Atlas of Bone Tumors. Elsevier; 1993:9–46.

sarcomas have a bimodal incidence rate with one peak occurring in the second decade (osteosarcoma, chondrosarcoma) and the other in patients over 60 years (chordoma, chondrosarcoma, osteosarcoma).[4] The relative frequencies of primary malignant bone tumors and primary nonmalignant bone tumors are listed in ▶ Table 9.3 and ▶ Table 9.4, respectively.[18,19] The relative frequencies of tumor-like bone lesions are listed in ▶ Table 9.5.[18,19] Other lesions or abnormalities involving bone are listed below. The imaging features of some of these abnormalities may overlap those of bone tumors.

Table 9.4 Primary nonmalignant bone tumors

Tumors	Mayo Clinic % benign tumors	NCBT % benign tumors	Mayo Clinic % total tumors	NCBT % total tumors	Age range (years), median age
Osteochondroma	31	14	9	5	1–50, 20
Giant cell tumor	24	22	7	8	10–55, 30
Enchondroma	15	17	4	6	3–83, 35
Osteoid osteoma	14	11	4	4	6–30, 17
Chondroblastoma	5	9	1	3	10–30, 17
Hemangioma	5	2	1	< 1	1–84, 33
Osteoblastoma	4	6	1	2	1–30, 15
Juxtacortical chondroma	2	5	< 1	2	4–77, 26
Chondromyxoid fibroma	2	4	< 1	1	1–40, 17
Neurilemoma	< 1	1	< 1	< 1	2–65, 30
Fibrous histiocytoma	< 1		< 1		
Lipoma	< 1	< 1	< 1	< 1	
Hamartoma	< 1		< 1		
Osteoma		< 1		< 1	
Lymphangioma		< 1		< 1	
Desmoplastic fibroma		< 1		< 1	1–71, 21

Data from:
Mayo Clinic:
1. Unni KK, Inwards CY. Introduction and scope of study. In: Dahlin's Bone Tumors General Aspects and Data in 10,165 Cases. 6th ed. Wolters Kluwer/ Lippincott-Raven; 2010:1–8.
Netherlands Committee on Bone Tumors (NCBT):
2. Mulder JD, Schutte HE, Kroon HM, Taconis WK. Introduction. In: Radiologic Atlas of Bone Tumors. Elsevier; 1993:3–6.
3. Mulder JD, Schutte HE, Kroon HM, Taconis WK. The diagnosis of bone tumors. In: Radiologic Atlas of Bone Tumors. Elsevier; 1993:9–46.

Table 9.5 Tumor-like bone lesions

Lesion	Relative frequency (%) (N = 2,287)	Age range (years), median age
Fibrous dysplasia	18	1–50, 20
Osteomyelitis	14	
Fibrous cortical defect/nonossifying fibroma	13	5–20, 14
Aneurysmal bone cyst	11	1–25, 14
Traumatic injury (fracture/callus)	10	
Solitary bone cyst	9	1–62, 11
Eosinophilic granuloma	8	1–35, 10
Heterotopic bone Formation/reaction	5	1–45, 22
Pigmented villonodular synovitis	3	15–60, 32
Geode	1	25–85, 52
Brown tumor	1	40–70, 52
Ganglion	< 1	20–70, 38
Epidermoid cyst	< 1	19–71, 38
Neuropathic arthropathy	< 1	
Melorheostosis	< 1	

Data from Netherlands Committee on Bone Tumors (NCBT):
1. Mulder JD, Schutte HE, Kroon HM, Taconis WK. Introduction. In: Radiologic Atlas of Bone Tumors. Elsevier; 1993:3–6.
2. Mulder JD, Schutte HE, Kroon HM, Taconis WK. The diagnosis of bone tumors. In: Radiologic Atlas of Bone Tumors. Elsevier; 1993:9–46.

- Malignant lesions
  - Metastatic disease
  - Leukemia
  - Desmoid tumors
- Benign lesions
  - Aneurysmal bone cyst
  - Unicameral bone cyst
  - Fibrous cortical defect
  - Nonossifying fibroma
  - Fibrous dysplasia
  - Eosinophilic granuloma
  - Osteofibrous dysplasia
  - Paget disease
  - Plexiform neurofibromas
  - Ganglion cysts
  - Geode
  - Bone Island
  - Melorrheostosis
- Metabolic disorders
  - Thalassemia
  - Sickle cell disease
  - Hemophilia
  - Osteopetrosis
  - Gaucher disease
  - Hyperparathyroidism
  - Vitamin deficiencies
- Radiation injury
  - Fat conversion
  - Bone infarcts
- Inflammatory diseases
  - Pyogenic osteomyelitis
  - TB osteomyelitis
  - Fungal osteomyelitis
- Langerhans cell histiocytosis/eosinophilic granuloma (EG)
  - Erdheim-Chester disease
  - Sarcoid
- Traumatic lesions
  - Fractures
  - Hematomas
  - Pseudarthrosis
  - Neuropathic joint
  - Bone infarct
  - Osteochondritis dissecans

9.3 Frequency of Occurrence of Soft Tissue Tumors

Benign tumors of the soft tissues are 100 times more frequent than sarcomas.[6,20,21] The annual incidence of benign tumors has been estimated to be approximately 3,000 per million, and 30 per million for sarcomas.[5] Sarcomas of the musculoskeletal system account for less than 1% of all malignant tumors.[5] The relative frequencies of primary malignant tumors and primary nonmalignant tumors of the soft tissues are listed in ▶ Table 9.6 and ▶ Table 9.7, respectively.[20,21]

Table 9.6 Malignant soft tissue tumors: 12,370 malignant tumors representing approximately 40% of total benign and malignant soft tissue lesions (31,047)

Tumor	Percent malignant	Percent total	Age range (years), mean age
Malignant fibrous histiocytoma	24	10	32–80, 59
Liposarcoma	14	6	18–78, 47
Sarcoma (not further classified)	12	5	
Leiomyosarcoma	8	3	35–79, 58
Malignant schwannoma	6	2	17–70, 42
Dermatofibrosarcoma protuberans	6	2	19–60, 38
Synovial sarcoma	5	2	14–58, 32
Fibrosarcoma	4	2	14–72, 41
Extraskeletal chondrosarcoma	2	< 1	22–71, 49
Angiosarcoma	2	< 1	17–77, 49
Rhabdomyosarcoma	2	< 1	2–40, 18
Epitheloid sarcoma	1	< 1	15–54, 31
Kaposi sarcoma	1	< 1	34–84, 64
Malignant hemangiopericytoma	1	< 1	22–73, 46
Extraskeletal Ewing	1	< 1	11–42, 25
Clear cell sarcoma	1	< 1	15–60, 37
Extraskeletal osteosarcoma	< 1	< 1	33–77, 57
Neuroblastoma	< 1	< 1	1–47, 19
Hemangioendothelioma	< 1	< 1	17–60, 40
Malignant granular cell tumor	< 1	< 1	14–70, 39

Data from:
Kransdorf MJ, Murphy MD. Soft tissue tumors in a large referral population: prevalence and distribution of diagnoses by age, sex, and location. In: Imaging of Soft Tissue Tumors. W.B. Saunders; 1997:3–35.
Kransdorf MJ. Malignant soft-tissue tumors in a large referral population: distribution of diagnoses by age, sex, and location. AJR 1995;164:129–134.

9.4 Grading and Staging of Bone Tumors

Two systems that are currently used for staging of primary malignant bone tumors include the American Joint Committee on Cancer (AJCC) system that was recently revised in 2002, and the Musculoskeletal Tumor Society (MSTS) system.[4,22]

For the revised AJCC system, four criteria are used for stages IA to IVB. T1 refers to tumors measuring less than 8 cm in greatest dimension and T2 for tumors greater than 8 cm. N0 refers to no regional lymph node metastasis, and N1 for the occurrence of regional lymph node metastasis. M0 refers to the absence of distant metastasis and M1 for the presence of distant metastasis. The last criterion is based on tumor grade with G1 assigned to low grade or well differentiated, G2 for moderately differentiated (also low grade), G3 for poorly differentiated (high grade), and G4 for undifferentiated (high grade) (▶ Table 9.8). The AJCC system is used for all primary malignant tumors of bone (osteosarcoma, Ewing sarcoma), except for primary malignant lymphoma or myeloma.[22]

For the MSTS system, three criteria are used for stages IA to III. T refers to whether the tumor is localized to a single compartment (T1) or involves more than one compartment (T2); M0 designation for absence of metastases and M1 for the presence of metastases; and G1 for low grade tumors and G2 for high grade tumors.[22]

9.5 Grading and Staging of Soft Tissue Tumors

The World Health Organization (WHO) has developed a classification system for soft tissue tumors with lesions assigned to four groups: benign, intermediate (locally aggressive), intermediate (rarely metastasizing), and malignant.[5] Two systems currently used for grading soft tissue sarcomas include the U.S. National Cancer Institute (NCI) system and the French Federation Nationale des Centres de Lutte Contre le Cancer (FNCLCC) system[5] (▶ Table 9.9).

The NCI grading system for tumors takes into account the histological type, cellularity, pleomorphism, mitotic rate, and presence of necrosis.[5] The FNCLCC system uses tumor differentiation, mitotic rate, and presence/extent of necrosis.[5] Two important histological features that have been associated with prognosis include high mitotic indices and presence of necrosis.[5] The FNCLCC system has been reported to result in a better correlation with overall and metastasis-free survival than the NCI system.[5] Staging of malignant soft tissue tumors is based on the extent of tumor from imaging, histological features of the tumors, and clinical data.[5] The main system used for staging for soft tissue sarcomas is the TNM system developed by the American Joint Committee on Cancer (AJCC) and the International Union against Cancer (see ▶ Fig. 9.1)[5] The TNM system has been shown to be clinically useful for prognostic purposes.

Table 9.7 Soft tissue tumors/lesions: 18,677 benign tumors representing approximately 60% of total benign and malignant soft tissue lesions (31,047)

Tumor/Lesion	Percent of benign	Percent total	Age range (years), mean age
Lipoma	16	10	26–68, 48
Fibrous histiocytoma	13	8	13–57, 33
Nodular fasciitis	11	7	11–51, 31
Hemangioma	8	5	1–65, 32
Fibromatosis	7	4	13–65, 36
Neurofibroma	5	3	16–66, 37
Schwannoma	5	3	22–72, 46
Giant cell tumor of tendon sheath	4	2	18–64, 39
Myxoma	3	2	24–74, 52
Granuloma annulare	2	1	2–58, 23
Hemangiopericytoma	2	1	23–70, 44
Granular cell tumor	2	1	15–56, 35
Leiomyoma	2	1	14–67, 40
Chondroma	1	< 1	16–70, 44
Fibroma of tendon sheath	1	< 1	15–75, 35
Fibroma	1	< 1	11–67, 40
Myofibromatosis	1	< 1	< 1–52, 14
Glomus tumor	< 1	< 1	19–71, 47
Pigmented villonodular synovitis (PVNS)	< 1	< 1	18–59, 38
Lymphangioma	< 1	< 1	1–50, 19
Ganglion	< 1	< 1	19–65, 40
Proliferative fasciitis	< 1	< 1	33–71, 54
Myositis ossificans	< 1	< 1	13–64, 35
Lipoblastoma	< 1	< 1	1–10, 4
Proliferative myositis	< 1	< 1	
Paraganglioma	< 1	< 1	24–70, 47
Synovial chondromatosis	< 1	< 1	
Ganglioneuroma	< 1	< 1	4–44, 22
Hibernoma	< 1	< 1	21–50, 32

Data from:
Kransdorf MJ, Murphy MD. Soft tissue tumors in a large referral population: prevalence and distribution of diagnoses by age, sex, and location. In: Imaging of Soft Tissue Tumors. W.B. Saunders; 1997:3–35.
Kransdorf MJ. Benign soft-tissue tumors in a large referral population: distribution of specific diagnoses by age, sex, and location. AJR 1995;164: 395–402.

Table 9.8 American Joint Committee on Cancer Staging System for Primary Malignant Tumors of Bone for Those Tumors Diagnosed on or After January 1, 2003[43]

Stage	Tumor	Lymph node	Metastases	Grade
IA	T1	N0	M0	G1 or G2
IB	T2	N0	M0	G1 or G2
IIA	T1	N0	M0	G3 or G4
IIB	T2	N0	M0	G3 or G4
III	T3	N0	M0	Any G
IVA	Any T	N0	M1a	Any G
IVB	Any T	N1	Any M	Any G
IVB	Any T	Any N	M1b	Any G

Tx = primary tumor cannot be assessed, T0 = no evidence of primary tumor, T1 = tumor 8 cm or less in greatest dimension; T2 = tumor more than 8 cm in greatest dimension, T3 = discontinuous tumors in the primary bone; Nx = regional lymph nodes not assessed, N0 = no regional lymph node metastases, N1 = regional lymph node metastasis; Mx = distant metastasis cannot be assessed, M0 = no distant metastasis, M1 = distant metastasis, M1a = lung, M1b = other distant sites; and Gx = grade cannot be assessed, G1 = well differentiated (low grade), G2 = moderately differentiated (low grade), G3 = poorly differentiated (high grade), G4 = undifferentiated (high grade).

Table 9.9 FNCLCC grading system: definition of parameters.[14] Modified from Trojani et al. Int J Cancer 1984;33:37–42

Tumor differentiation	
Score 1	Sarcomas closely resembling normal adult mesenchymal tissue (e.g., low grade leiomyosarcoma)
Score 2	Sarcomas for which histological typing is certain (e.g., myxoid liposarcoma)
Score 3	Embryonal and undifferentiated sarcomas, sarcomas of doubtful type, synovial sarcomas, osteosarcomas, PNET
Mitotic count	
Score 1	0–9 mitoses per 10 HPF*
Score 2	10–19 mitoses per 10 HPF
Score 3	≥ 20 mitoses per 10 HPF
Tumor necrosis	
Score 0	No necrosis
Score 1	< 50% tumor necrosis
Score 2	≥ 50% tumor necrosis
Histological grade	
Grade 1	Total score 2, 3
Grade 2	Total score 4, 5
Grade 3	Total score 6, 7, 8

PNET, primitive neuroectodermal tumor.
*A high power field (HPF) measures 0.1734 square millimeters.

Primary tumor (**T**)	TX:	primary tumor cannot be assessed
	T0:	no evidence of primary tumor
	T1:	tumor ≤ 5cm in greatest dimension
		T1a: superficial tumor*
		T1b: deep tumor
	T2:	tumor > 5cm in greatest dimension
		T2a: superficial tumor
		T2b: deep tumor
Regional lymph nodes (**N**)	NX:	regional lymph nodes cannot be assessed
	N0:	no regional lymph node metastasis
	N1:	regional lymph node metastasis

Note: Regional node involvement is rare and cases in which nodal status is not assessed either clinically or pathologically could be considered N0 instead of NX or pNX.

Distant metastasis (**M**)	M0:	no distant metastasis
	M1:	distant metastasis

G Histopathological Grading

Translation table for three and four grade to two grade (low vs. high grade) system

TNM two grade system	Three grade systems	Four grade systems
Low grade	Grade 1	Grade 1
		Grade 2
High grade	Grade 2	Grade 3
	Grade 3	Grade 4

Stage IA	T1a	N0,NX	M0	Low grade
	T1b	N0,NX	M0	Low grade
Stage IB	T2a	N0,NX	M0	Low grade
	T2b	N0,NX	M0	Low grade
Stage IIA	T1a	N0,NX	M0	High grade
	T1b	N0,NX	M0	High grade
Stage IIB	T2a	N0,NX	M0	High grade
Stage III	T2b	N0,NX	M0	High grade
Stage IV	Any T	N1	M0	Any grade
	Any T	Any N	M1	Any grade

*Superficial tumor is located exclusively above the superficial fascia without invasion of the fascia; deep tumor is located either exclusively beneath the superficial fascia, or superficial to the fascia with invasion of or through the fascia. Retroperitoneal, mediastinal and pelvic sarcomas are classified as deep tumors.

Fig. 9.1 TNM system developed by the American Joint Committee on Cancer

The TNM system uses data consisting of tumor size and depth, histological tumor grade, regional lymph node involvement, and presence of distant metastases.

9.6 Imaging Evaluation of Bone and Soft Tissue Tumors and Tumor-Like Lesions

The diagnosis of bone tumors is often made on conventional radiographs.[3] Osteolytic lesions from tumors, however, may not be visible on conventional radiographs until there is 30 to 50% loss of mineralization.[14,22,23] Because of superior soft tissue contrast, magnetic resonance imaging (MRI) can detect marrow-based tumors before they are evident on radiographs. In addition, MRI can be used to further characterize lesions with regard to extent and extraosseous extension. With progressive increased use of MRI for evaluation of musculoskeletal disorders, tumors and other bone lesions may also be found incidentally.

Features used to characterize bone tumors and other lesions on conventional radiographs include the following:

1. Lesion location (metaphyseal/diaphyseal/epiphyseal, cortical, intramedullary, eccentric, central)
2. Lesion size
3. Lesion density (radiolucent, sclerotic, presence of matrix mineralization)
4. Margins (well-defined geographic with or without sclerotic borders, poorly defined geographic, "moth-eaten" and/or "permeative" radiolucent patterns)
5. Presence of cortical destruction with or without extraosseous tumor extension
6. Presence of periosteal reaction (interrupted versus noninterrupted pattern, lamellated/onion-skin pattern, perpendicular pattern, sunburst pattern, Codman triangles)[3,4,24–26]

Many bone tumors and nonneoplastic osseous lesions arise within medullary bone. As these intraosseous lesions enlarge within marrow, they can distort, erode, remodel, and/or destroy bone trabeculae resulting in radiographic

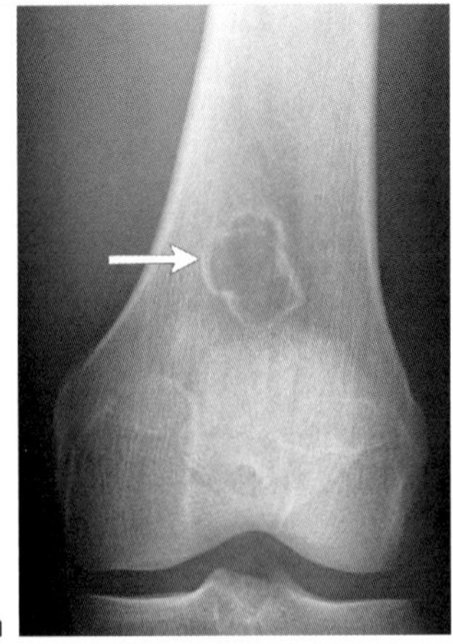

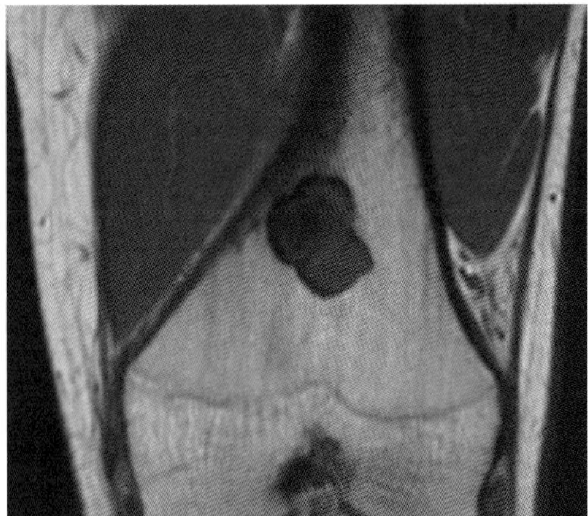

Fig. 9.2 Geographic lesion pattern type 1A in a 16-year-old boy with a nonossifying fibroma in the distal femur. (a) The geographic radiolucent lesion has a sharp zone of transition with normal bone, and has a thin peripheral sclerotic margin (arrow). (b) The lesion also has well-defined margins on coronal T1-weighted imaging.

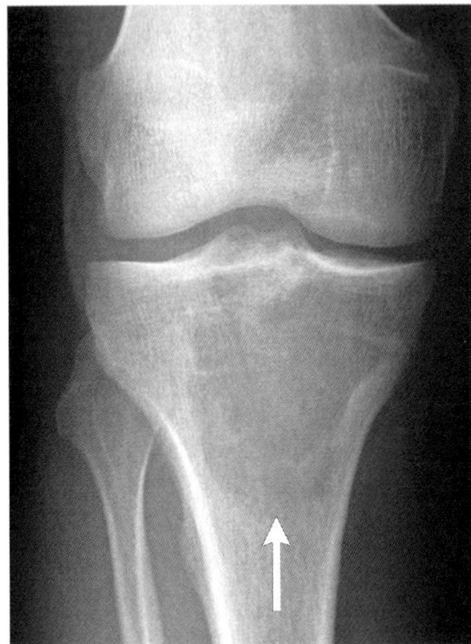

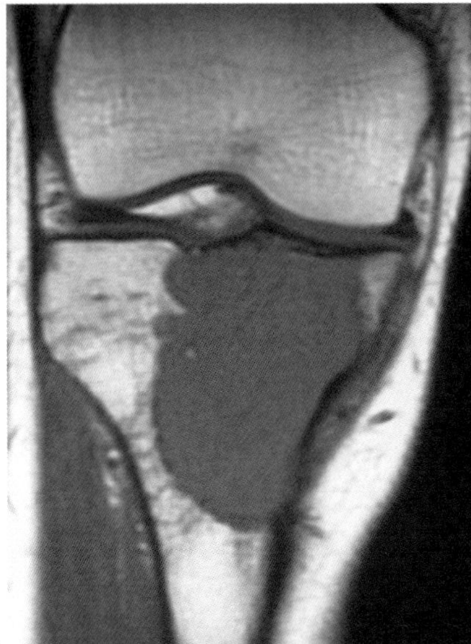

Fig. 9.3 Geographic lesion pattern type 1B in a 28-year-old man with a giant cell tumor involving the proximal tibia. (a) The geographic radiolucent lesion lacks a sclerotic margin on radiograph (arrow). (b) The lesion has intermediate signal on coronal T1-weighted imaging and has a sharp zone of transition with normal marrow.

findings. On conventional radiographs, most bone tumors are radiolucent.[3,4,14,23,25,26] The appearance of the bone tumor margins on conventional radiographs is often predictive of the aggressiveness of the neoplasms. Radiolucent lesions with margins that appear as abrupt zones of transition relative to normal-appearing bone are referred to as having a geographic pattern (type 1), usually indicating a slow-growing lesion (▶ Fig. 9.2; ▶ Fig. 9.3; ▶ Fig. 9.4).[4,14,19,25,27]

Geographic-pattern lesions can be subdivided into those with thin peripheral sclerotic margins (**type 1A**), those that lack peripheral sclerotic margins (**type 1B**), and those with slightly indistinct margins (**type 1C**). More aggressive patterns of bone destruction are classified as ***"moth-eaten"* radiolucent lesions (type II)** and ***"permeative"* radiolucent lesions (type III)**. The ***moth-eaten* radiolucent pattern (type II)** consists of multiple radiolucent round or oval foci of varying sizes (often between 2 and 5 mm), and wide zones of transition with adjacent normal-appearing bone (▶ Fig. 9.5).

The ***permeative* radiolucent pattern (type III)** consists of small (often 1 mm), poorly defined radiolucent zones with indistinct margins and wide zones of transition with adjacent normal-appearing bone (▶ Fig. 9.6). The ***moth-eaten*** and ***permeative*** radiolucent patterns are often associated with

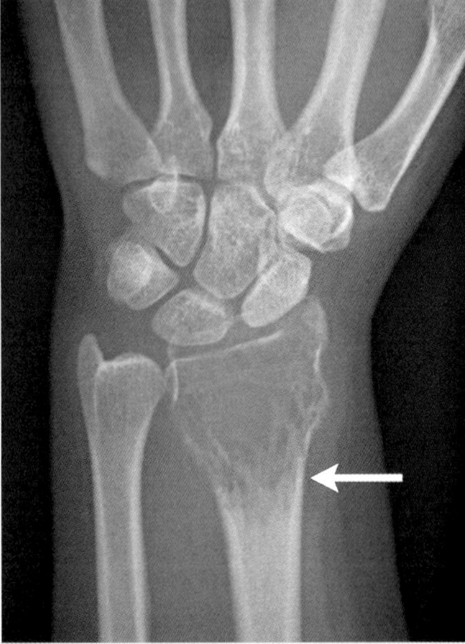

Fig. 9.4 Geographic lesion pattern type 1C in a 19-year-old woman involving the distal radius. The geographic radiolucent lesion has indistinct margins (arrow).

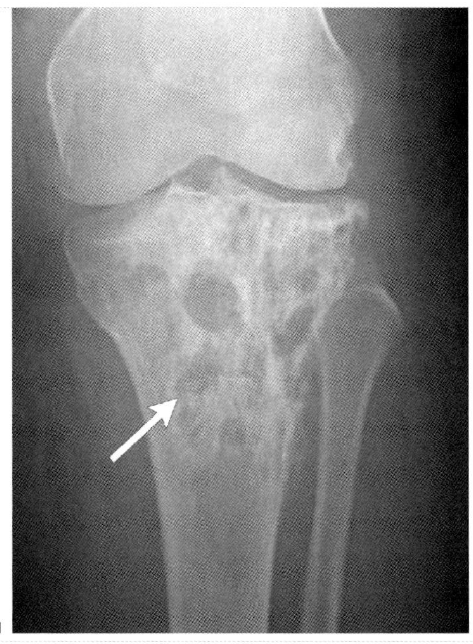
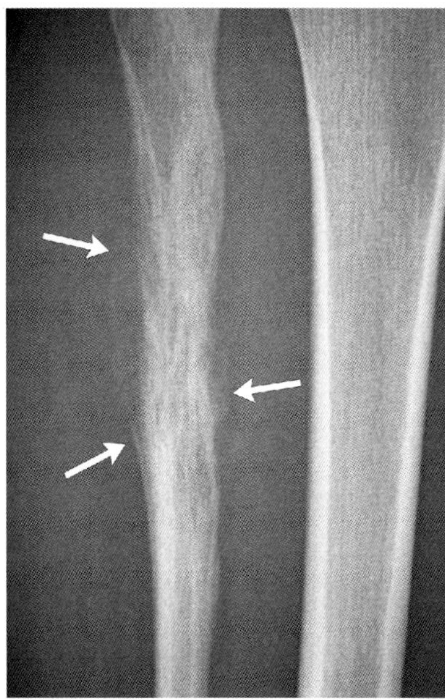

Fig. 9.5 "Moth-eaten" radiolucent destructive pattern (type II) in a patient with a plasmacytoma in the proximal tibia (a) and another with a Ewing sarcoma in the diaphysis of the fibula (b). Multiple round and oval intramedullary radiolucent foci of varying sizes are seen (arrow in a), as well as wide zones of transition with adjacent normal-appearing bone, and cortical bone destruction. Interrupted periosteal reaction is also seen (arrows in b).

aggressive lesions, including malignant neoplasms.[4,14,19,25,27] There can, however, be occasional overlapping patterns of bone destruction with benign and malignant neoplasms as well as with osteomyelitis.[4,14,19,25,27]

The presence of matrix mineralization (calcification, ossification) in tumors may allow a narrowing of the differential diagnosis. The presence of arc- or ring-shaped calcifications is highly suggestive of a cartilaginous tumor, whereas amorphous, cloudlike, ill-defined densities can be seen with osteosarcomas (▶ Fig. 9.7; ▶ Fig. 9.8).[4,14,19,25,27] Intraosseous lesions with a ground-glass radiographic appearance are typical for fibrous dysplasia (▶ Fig. 9.9).

The ***periosteum*** at the outer surface of bone is composed of an *outer hypocellular fibrous layer* and an *inner vascular cellular portion* (**cambium**).[27] The inner cellular (**cambium**) layer of periosteum is connected to bone cortex via perpendicularly oriented collagen fibers (Sharpey fibers).[27] The normal periosteum is radiolucent. In the settings of trauma, infection, inflammation, neoplasm, and tumor-like lesions that involve bone cortex and periosteum, the cellular layer of periosteum enlarges resulting in a greater separation of the outer fibrous periosteal layer from the bone cortex. Subsequent mineralization of the altered periosteum after 10 to 21 days results in radiographically observed *"periosteal reaction."*

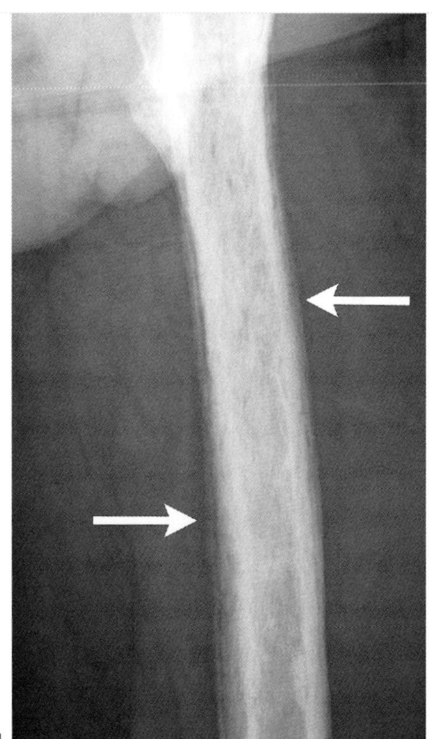
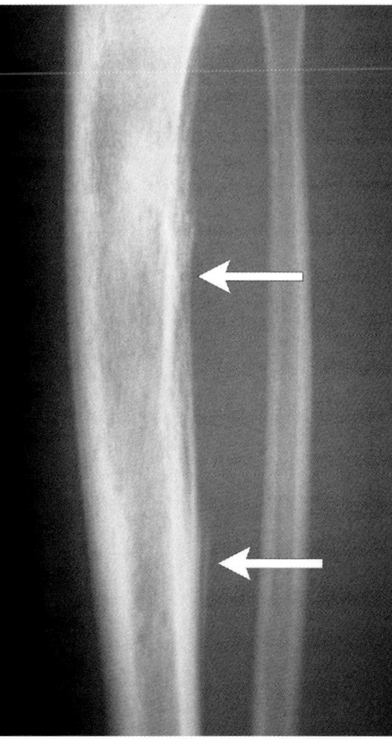

Fig. 9.6 "Permeative" radiolucent pattern (type III) in a patient with non-Hodgkin lymphoma in the diaphysis of the femur (a) and another with Ewing sarcoma involving the diaphysis of the tibia (b). Multiple small, poorly defined radiolucent intramedullary zones with indistinct margins are seen as well as wide zones of transitions with adjacent normal-appearing bone, and cortical bone destruction. Interrupted periosteal reaction is seen in both images (arrows).

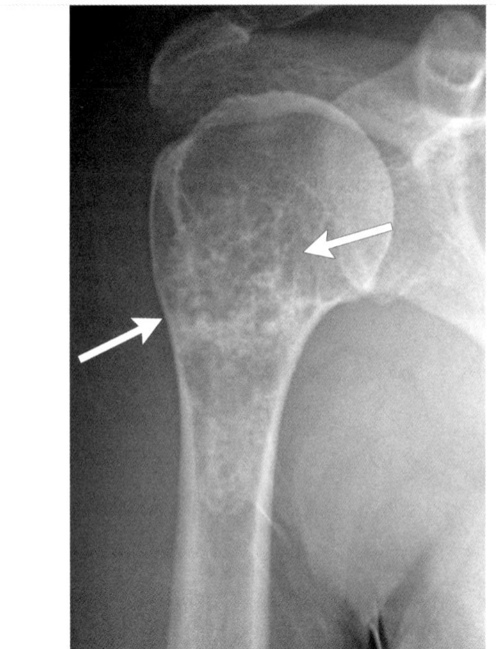

Fig. 9.7 Arc- and ring-shaped chondroid mineralization is seen within a chondrosarcoma involving the proximal humerus of a 46-year-old woman (arrows).

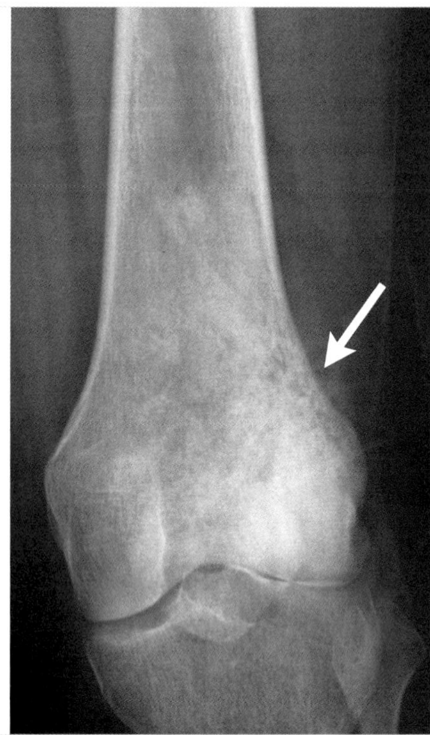

Fig. 9.8 Dense, amorphous, mineralized-tumor osteoid is seen with an osteoblastic osteosarcoma involving the distal femur of a 19-year-old woman (arrow).

As intraosseous lesions grow, they can erode or destroy adjacent bone cortex. Some intraosseous lesions erode bone cortex slightly faster than the overlying periosteum can produce periosteal new bone, resulting in expansile bone lesions with thin peripheral rims of bone[27] (▶ Fig. 9.10). This pattern is referred to as *negative perisosteal reaction.*[27] These expansile shell-type bone reactions can be seen with slow-growing benign lesions such as aneurysmal bone cysts, giant cell tumors, nonossifying fibromas, and fibrous dysplasia, as well as slow-growing malignant tumors such as low grade chondrosarcomas and some plasmacytomas (▶ Fig. 9.11). In contrast to *negative periosteal reaction, positive periosteal reaction* refers to when new

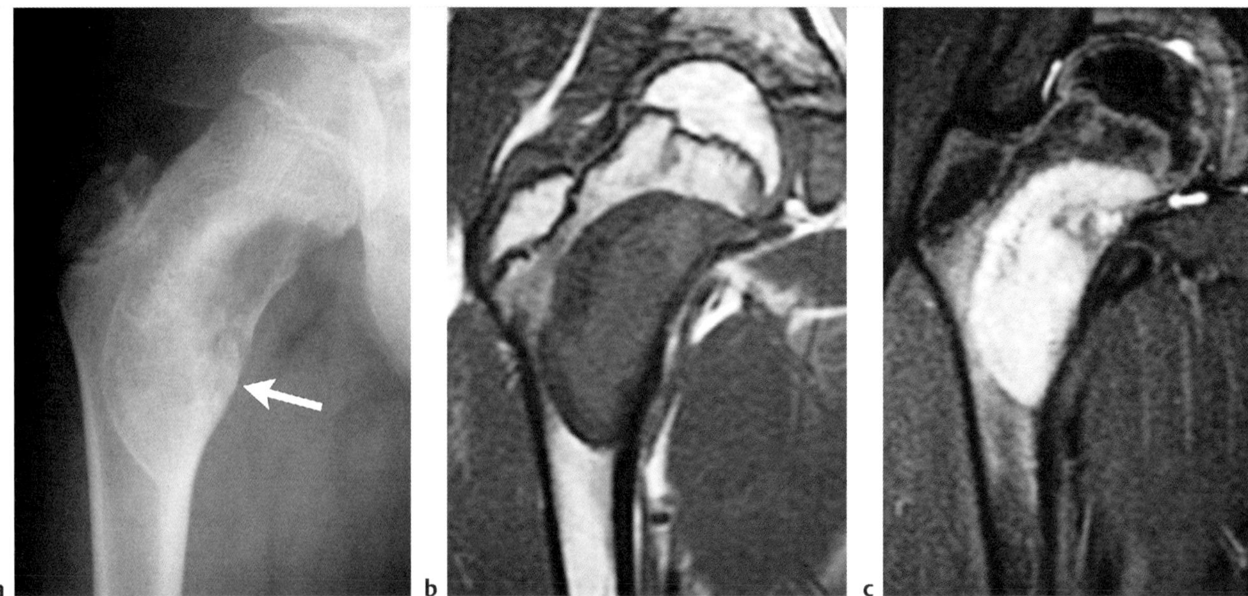

Fig. 9.9 A 10-year-old boy with fibrous dysplasia involving the metadiaphyseal portion of the proximal femur, which has a ground-glass radiographic appearance (arrow) (a). The circumscribed lesion has a margin of low signal surrounding a central zone with intermediate signal on coronal T1-weighted imaging (b). The lesion has high signal on coronal fat-suppressed T2-weighted imaging (c).

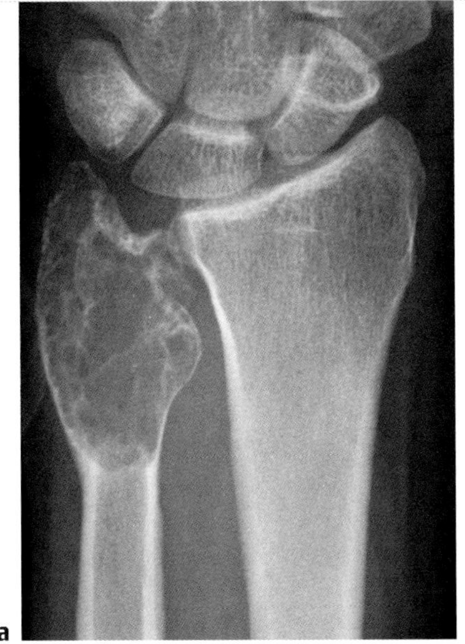
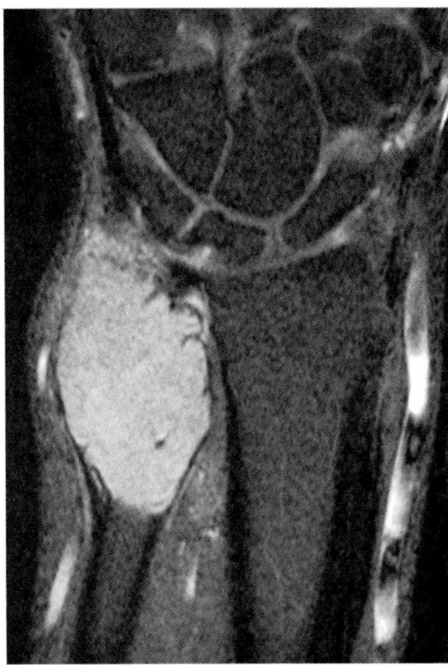
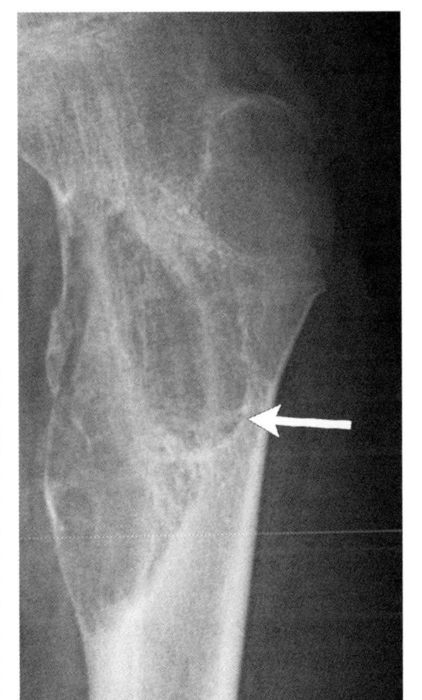
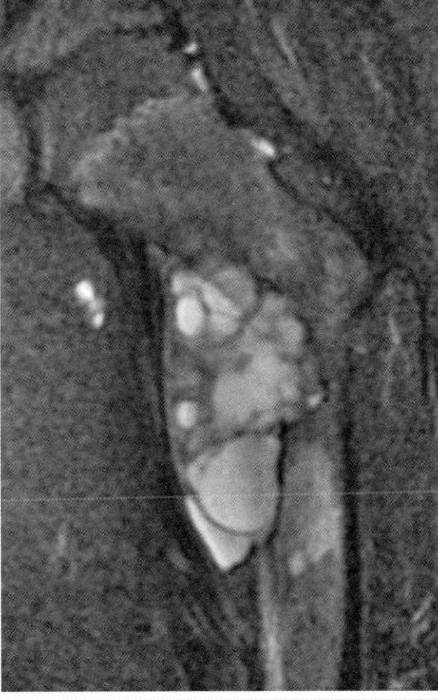

Fig. 9.10 Giant cell tumor involving the distal ulna in a 52-year-old man. Anteroposterior (AP) radiograph (a) shows an expansile radiolucent lesion with a thinned cortex and narrow zone of transition with adjacent normal medullary bone. The tumor has circumscribed margins and has high signal on coronal fat-suppressed T2-weighted imaging (FS T2WI). (b) An 11-year-old boy with an aneurysmal bone cyst involving the medial proximal shaft of the femur. AP radiograph (c) shows an expansile radiolucent lesion with thinned cortex (arrow). Coronal FS T2WI (d) shows a multiseptated lesion with fluid-fluid levels containing high and low-intermediate signal.

periosteal bone is added to the outer margin of bone cortex.[27] Patterns of periosteal reaction can vary related to growth of neoplasmas as well as with other bone lesions.[4,26–28] Slow-growing tumors (osteoma, osteoid osteoma, etc.) and inflammatory lesions (osteomyelitis, Langerhans cell histiocytosis) that involve bone cortex can elevate the periosteum, resulting in noninterrupted, single, mineralized layers of periosteal formation and cortical thickening (▶ Fig. 9.12; ▶ Fig. 9.13).[4,14,19,25–27]

Single-layered noninterrupted periosteal reaction can also occur with healing fractures, hypertrophic pulmonary osteoarthropathy, venous stasis, myositis ossificans, thyroid acropachy, and Gaucher disease. Zones of cortical destruction are commonly seen with malignant neoplasms as well as extraosseous tumor extension.[4,14,19,25–27] Aggressive and/or malignant tumors (osteosarcoma, Ewing sarcoma, chondrosarcoma, lymphoma) as well as inflammatory lesions (osteomyelitis, Langerhans cell histiocytosis) can elevate the periosteum as well as eventually destroy and interrupt portions of the elevated periosteum (▶ Fig. 9.5; ▶ Fig. 9.6; ▶ Fig. 9.13; ▶ Fig. 9.14).[4,14,19,25–27]

Triangular zones of periosteal reaction may be seen at the borders of cortical destruction and extraosseous tumor extension and are referred to as Codman triangles (▶ Fig. 9.14).[4,14,19,25–27] Codman triangles can be seen with malignant primary bone neoplasms, osteomyelitis, or trauma.[26,27] Various types of interrupted periosteal may be coexistent in malignant bone tumors.

Tumor-induced bone formation can occur within medullary bone as well as within extraosseous portions of neoplasms. Tumor-induced bone formation within extraosseous portions of

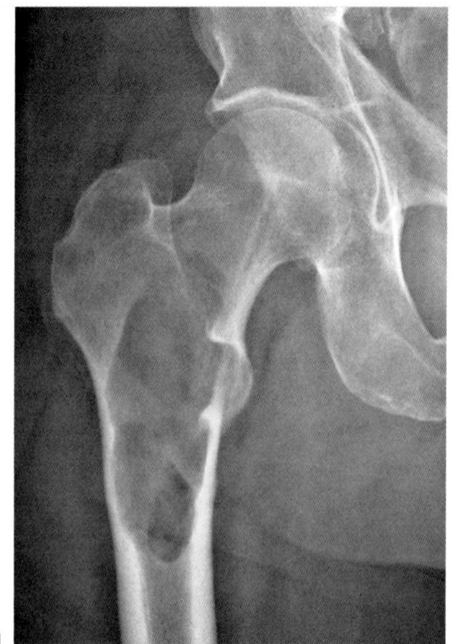

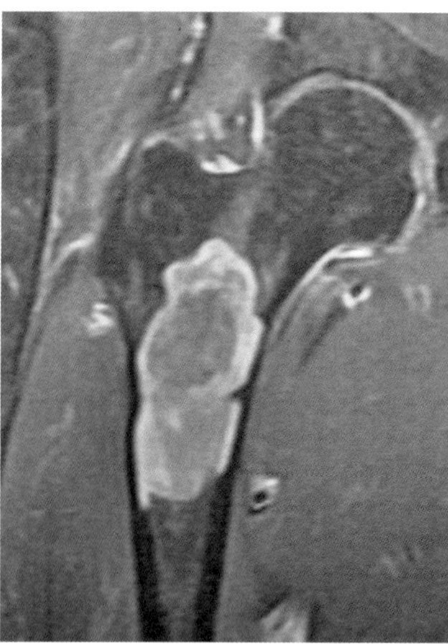

Fig. 9.11 A 56-year-old man with a plasmacytoma involving the proximal shaft of the femur. The radiolucent lesion has sharp intramedullary margins, and erodes, thins, and slightly expands the adjacent bone cortex (a). The tumor shows gadolinium-contrast enhancement on coronal fat-suppressed T1-weighted imaging (b).

the neoplasms, also referred to as periosteal reaction, can have various configurations. Tumor-induced bone formation from malignant neoplasms can be oriented perpendicular to the long axis of bone with "velvet," "hair on end," "sunburst," "cumulus cloud," or disorganized/complex configurations (▶ Fig. 9.15; ▶ Fig. 9.16).[4,14,19,25–27] Multilayered zones of periosteal reaction with an "onion-peel" or lamellated appearance can also be seen with aggressive tumors and inflammatory lesions (▶ Fig. 9.17).

With MRI, features used to evaluate and characterize bone and soft tissue tumors include the following:

1. Lesion location
2. Lesion size
3. Margins (well-defined geographic with or without low signal margins versus poorly defined margins)
4. Signal of the lesion on T1-weighted images, proton-density weighted images with and/or without fat suppression,

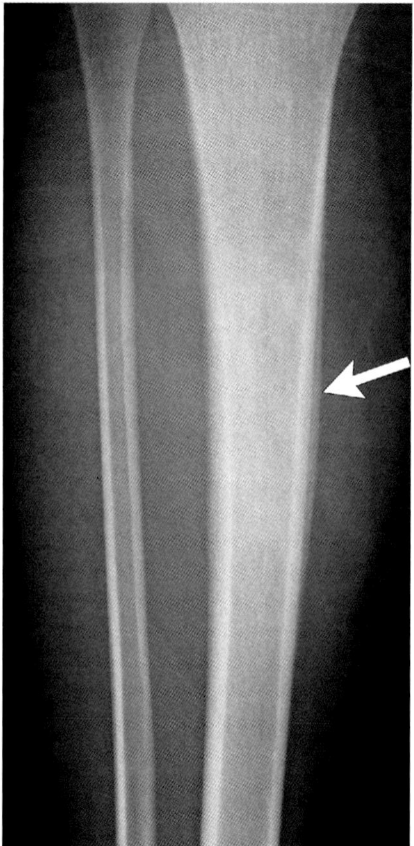

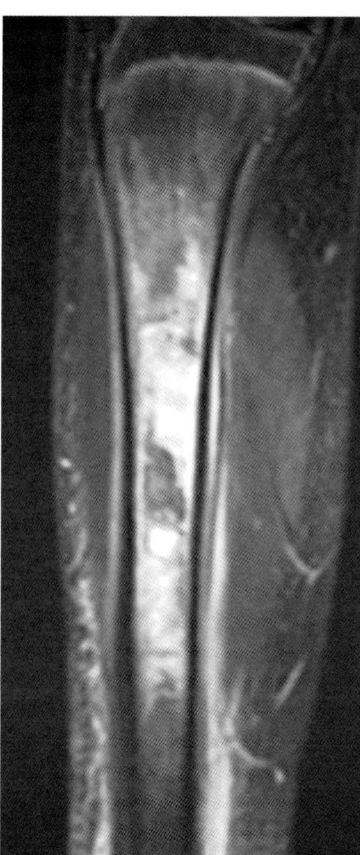

Fig. 9.12 A 13-year-old boy with pyogenic osteomyelitis involving the diaphysis of the tibia with noninterrupted single layer of periosteal reaction (arrow) on radiograph (a). A poorly defined zone of high signal on coronal fat-suppressed T2-weighted imaging (b) is seen in the marrow associated with periosteal elevation and poorly defined abnormal high T2 signal in the adjacent extraosseous soft tissues.

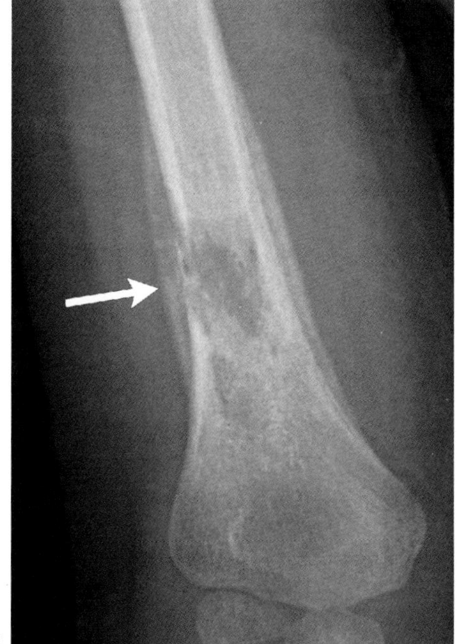
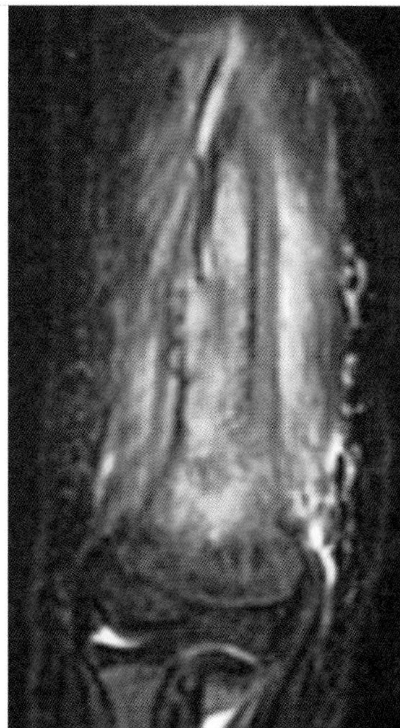

Fig. 9.13 Eosinophilic granuloma involving the distal humerus in a 5-year-old boy. Anteroposterior radiograph (a) shows a radiolucent intramedullary lesion with irregular margins, cortical disruption, and single layer of smooth perisoteal reaction at the medial (ulnar) aspect. A zone of disruption of the periosteum is seen laterally at the radial aspect (arrow). Magnetic resonance imaging shows an intramedullary poorly defined lesion with heterogeneous slightly high to high signal on coronal fat-suppressed T2-weighted imaging (FS T2WI) (b) with extension of the lesion from the marrow into adjacent soft tissues as seen through areas of cortical disruption. Zones of high signal on FS T2WI are seen superficial and deep to the elevated periosteum, which is seen as a linear zone of low signal.

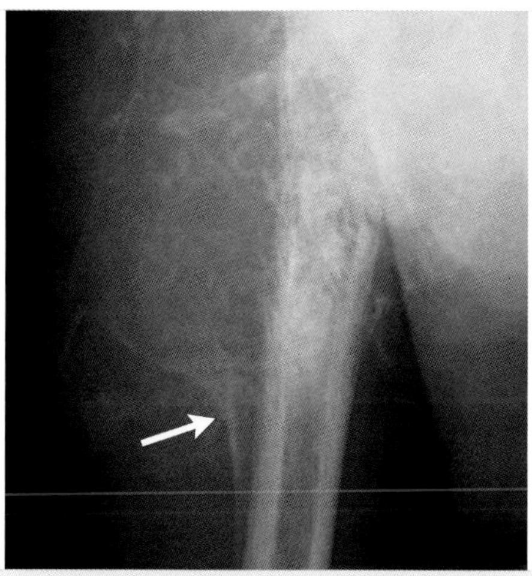

Fig. 9.14 A 12-year-old girl with an intramedullary osteogenic osteosarcoma involving the humerus with cortical destruction, extraosseous extension, and interrupted periosteal elevation. Anteroposterior radiograph shows a destructive intraosseous lesion with mineralized ossified matrix, cortical destruction, extraosseous tumor extension with disorganized tumoral bone formation, and a Codman triangle at the inferior lateral border (arrow).

T2-weighted images with and/or without fat suppression, short TI inversion recovery (STIR) images

5. Enhancement after intravenous administration of gadolinium-based contrast material
6. Presence of cortical destruction

For bone tumors, MRI can accurately demonstrate the size, configuration, and margins of extraosseous neoplastic extension from the medullary canal through sites of cortical destruction.

MRI findings may be useful for diagnosis and narrowing the list of differential possibilities of bone and soft tissue tumors. For example, extra- and intraosseous lipomas have signal similar to fat, and unicameral bone cysts usually have circumscribed margins and contain fluid signal. Nonossifying fibromas in bone often have circumscribed margins and have internal low signal on T2-weighted images reflecting their histological features. The locations of lesions combined with MRI features may also be highly suggestive of lesions such as with osteofibrous dysplasia, osteoid osteoma, juxtacortical chondroma, enchondroma, osteochondroma, chondroblastoma, fibrous dysplasia, chordoma, chondromyxoid fibroma, and Paget sarcoma. Features commonly associated with malignant bone tumors

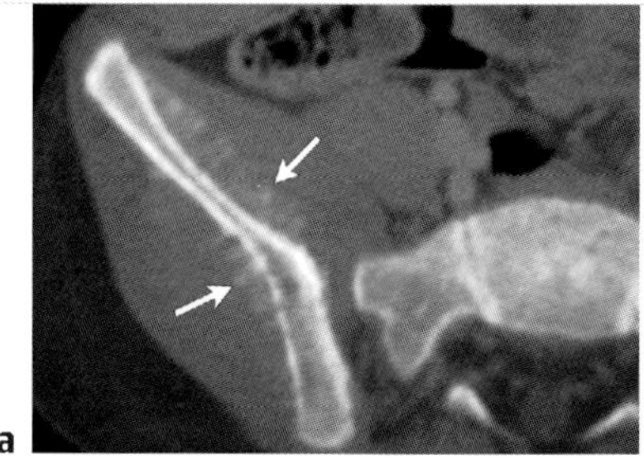
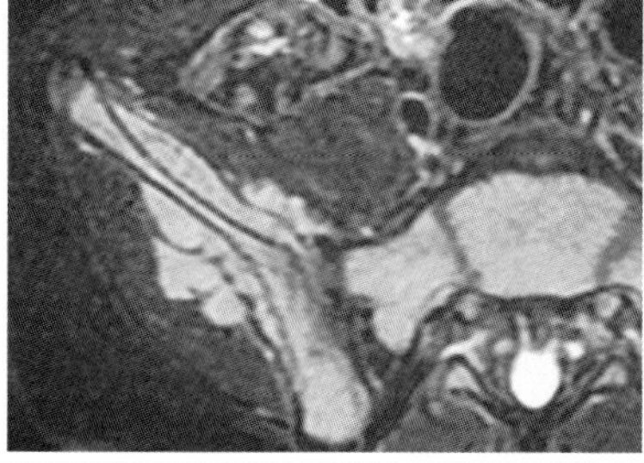
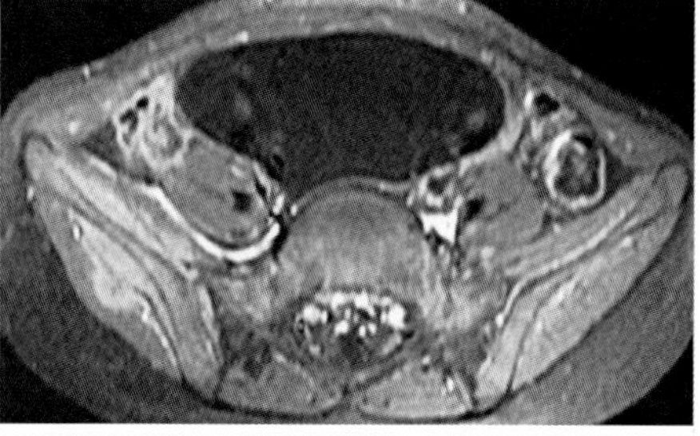

Fig. 9.15 A 3-year-old boy with metastatic neuroblastoma involving the right iliac bone. The tumor is associated with cortical destruction and extraosseous extension with "hair on end" as well as divergent striated/"sunburst-type" zones of periosteal reaction (arrows) (a). Intraosseous tumor has high signal on axial fat-suppressed (FS) T2-weighted imaging (T2WI) (b), and shows gadolinium-contrast enhancement on axial FS T1-weighted imaging (c). Tumor is seen extending through destroyed bone cortex both deep and superficial to the elevated low-signal band of interrupted periosteum.

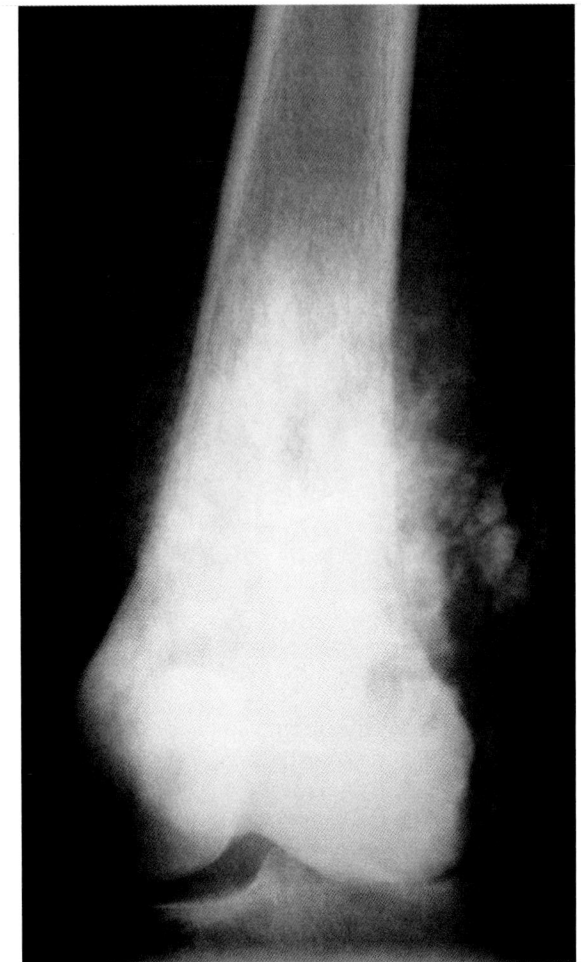

Fig. 9.16 A 19-year-old woman with an intramedullary osteogenic osteosarcoma involving the distal femur humerus with cortical destruction, extraosseous extension, and interrupted periosteal elevation. Anteroposterior radiograph shows the intraosseous and extraosseous portions of the lesion to have dense cloudlike and disorganized mineralized ossified matrix.

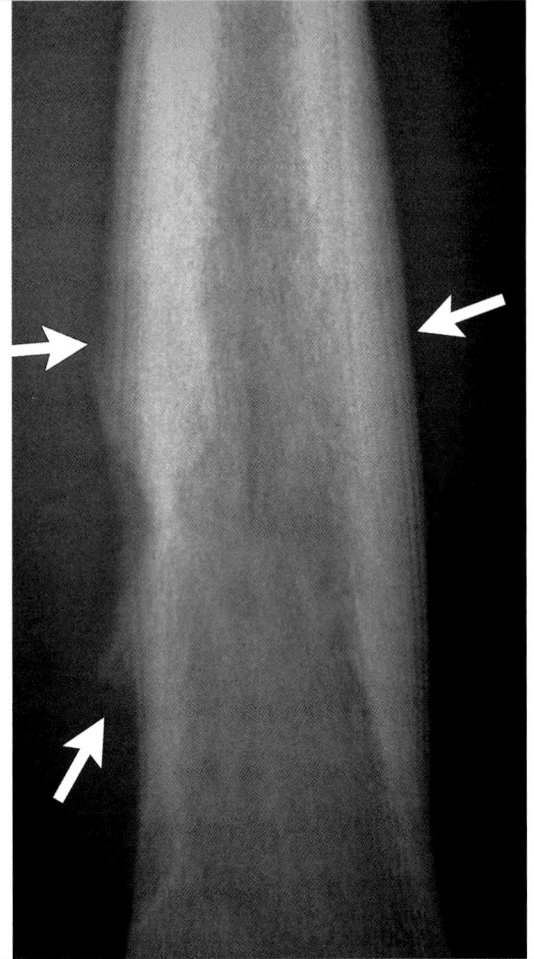

Fig. 9.17 Intramedullary telangiectatic osteosarcoma in the distal femur associated with cortical destruction with extraosseous tumor extension. Multiple layers of periosteal reaction oriented parallel to cortical bone ("onion skin" pattern) (white arrows) and a Codman triangle inferiorly (lower arrow) are seen on an anteroposterior radiograph.

include poorly defined margins, extension of tumor from marrow through sites of cortical destruction, irregular contrast enhancement with zones of necrosis, and skip lesions. Overlapping MRI features of many malignant tumors require biopsies for diagnosis and treatment planning. MRI is, however, recommended and routinely used for staging of bone and soft tissue tumors because of its superior contrast resolution and multiplanar imaging capabilities in determining tumor size and extent.[4,25,28–35] MRI provides a more accurate assessment of tumor volume compared with radiographs and computed tomography and is also useful in detecting fluid-fluid levels in tumors as well as nonenhancing necrotic and hemorrhagic zones.[4] MRI also provides detailed information regarding tumor margins, presence of tumor invasion of neurovascular structures, and bone.[5,36,37] MRI can also confirm the presence of hemorrhage, cystic, fibrotic, and myxoid changes within tumors.[5,38]

Contrast-enhanced MRI often provides useful information in the evaluation of musculoskeletal lesions.[27,28,31,33,39–50] For evaluation of musculoskeletal neoplasms, dynamic MRI after bolus intravenous administration of gadolinium-chelate contrast can sometimes be useful in distinguishing rapidly enhancing tumor from initially nonenhancing perineoplastic edema or necrosis.[39–41] Combining information from static and dynamic contrast-enhanced MRI with results from nonenhanced MRI may allow improved differentiation between benign and malignant soft tissue tumors.[47] The presence of liquefaction, large tumor size, and early patterns of dynamic contrast enhancement were features that were more commonly associated with malignant than with benign soft tissue tumors.[47] Responses of malignant tumors such as osteosarcomas and Ewing sarcomas to chemotherapy can also be assessed by detecting nonenhancing zones of necrosis or sites of persistent early enhancement that are typically associated with remaining viable tumor. Newer MRI techniques, such as diffusion-weighted imaging and MR spectroscopy, have been used in clinical research studies for the evaluation of musculoskeletal neoplasms, although their clinical relevance requires further study.[51,52]

The information provided by MRI is valuable for planning biopsies and surgical resection.[5] Knowledge of the MRI features and associated findings from conventional radiographs and computed tomographic scans can provide comprehensive and detailed evaluation of musculoskeletal tumors and tumor-like lesions.

This portion of the book is focused on the differential diagnosis, description, and categorization of the MRI features of both benign and malignant bone and soft tissue tumors and tumor-like lesions involving the musculoskeletal system. The actual definition of the English word "tumor" is derived from the Latin word "tumere," which is translated as "swelling." The lesions described in this book include both neoplasms and tumor-like masses involving the appendicular skeleton. This portion of the book groups musculoskeletal lesions into lists of differential diagnoses based on anatomical locations and/or MRI features illustrated with MR images.

For this book, MRI signal of the various entities will be described as low, intermediate, high, or mixed on T1-weighted imaging (T1WI), proton density–weighted imaging or intermediate-weighted imaging (PDWI), and T2-weighted imaging (T2WI), and whether there is gadolinium-contrast (Gd-contrast) enhancement or not. When available, comments and examples will be given regarding MRI features with fat-suppression techniques such as frequency-selective fat-presaturation (FS) applied on T1WI, PDWI, T2WI, or utilization of the short TI inversion recovery sequence (STIR). Both techniques enable distinction of pathological processes (e.g., neoplasm, infection, inflammation, edema) from normal anatomical structures with high signal from intrinsic fat, such as marrow and subcutaneous soft tissues.

9.7 References

[1] Arndt CA, Crist WM. Common musculoskeletal tumors of childhood and adolescence. N Engl J Med 1999; 341: 342–352

[2] Balach T, Stacy GS, Haydon RC. The clinical evaluation of soft tissue tumors. Radiol Clin North Am 2011; 49: 1185–1196, vi

[3] Bridge JA, Orndal C. Cytogenetic analysis of bone and joint neoplasms. In: Helliwell TR. ed. Pathology of Bone and Joint Neoplasms. Philadelphia, PA: Saunders; 1999:59–78

[4] Dorfman HD, Czerniak B, Kotz R, Vanel D, Park YK, Unni KK. WHO classification of tumors of bone: introduction. In: Fletcher CDM, Unni KK, Mertens F, eds. World Health Organization Classification of Tumors. Pathology and Genetics of Tumors of Soft Tissue and Bone. Lyon, France: IARC Press; 2002:227–232

[5] Fletcher CDM, Ryholm A, Singer S, Sundaram M Coindre. Soft tissue tumors: epidemiology, clinical features, histopathological typing and grading. In: Fletcher CDM, Unni KK, Mertens F, eds. World Health Organization Classification of Tumors. Pathology and Genetics of Tumors of Soft Tissue and Bone. Lyon, France: IARC Press; 2002:12–18

[6] Fletcher JA. Cytogenetic analysis of soft-tissue tumors. In: Weiss SW, Goldblum JR, eds. Enzinger and Weiss's Soft Tissue Tumors. 4th ed. St. Louis, MO: Mosby; 2001:125–146

[7] Folpe AL, Gown AM. Immunohistochemistry for analysis of soft tissue tumors. In: Weiss SW, Goldblum JR, eds. Enzinger and Weiss's Soft Tissue Tumors. 4th ed. St. Louis, MO: Mosby; 2001:199–245

[8] Gao Z, Kahn LB. The application of immunohistochemistry in the diagnosis of bone tumors and tumor-like lesions. Skeletal Radiol 2005; 34: 755–770

[9] Sandberg AA. Cytogenetics and molecular genetics of bone and soft-tissue tumors. Am J Med Genet 2002; 115: 189–193

[10] Scholz RB, Christiansen H, Kabisch H, Winkler K. Molecular markers in the evaluation of bone neoplasms. In: Helliwell TR, ed. Pathology of Bone and Joint Neoplasms. Philadelphia, PA: Saunders; 1999:79–105

[11] Kransdorf MJ, Meis JM. From the archives of the AFIP. Extraskeletal osseous and cartilaginous tumors of the extremities. Radiographics 1993; 13: 853–884

[12] Bridge JA, Sandberg AA. Cytogenetic and molecular genetic techniques as adjunctive approaches in the diagnosis of bone and soft tissue tumors. Skeletal Radiol 2000; 29: 249–258

[13] Slominski A, Wortsman J, Carlson A, Mihm M, Nickoloff B, McClatchey K. Molecular pathology of soft tissue and bone tumors. A review. Arch Pathol Lab Med 1999; 123: 1246–1259

[14] Balach T, Stacy GS, Peabody TD. The clinical evaluation of bone tumors. Radiol Clin North Am 2011; 49: 1079–1093, v

[15] Kim SH, Smith SE, Mulligan ME. Hematopoietic tumors and metastases involving bone. Radiol Clin North Am 2011; 49: 1163–1183, vi

[16] Salisbury JR. Bone neoplasms containing epithelial and epithelioid cells. In: Orthopedic Surgical Pathology: Diagnosis of Tumors and Pseudotumoral Lesions of Bone and Joints. New York: Churchill Livingstone; 1998:345–368

[17] Siegel R, Naishadham D, Jemal A. Cancer statistics, 2012. CA Cancer J Clin 2012; 62: 10–29

[18] Mulder JD, Schutte HE, Kroon HM, Taconis WK. Introduction. In: Radiologic Atlas of Bone Tumors. New York: Elsevier; 1993:3–6

[19] Mulder JD, Schutte HE, Kroon HM, Taconis WK. The diagnosis of bone tumors. In: Radiologic Atlas of Bone Tumors. New York: Elsevier; 1993:9–46

[20] Kransdorf MJ. Benign soft-tissue tumors in a large referral population: distribution of specific diagnoses by age, sex, and location. AJR Am J Roentgenol 1995; 164: 395–402

[21] Kransdorf MJ. Malignant soft-tissue tumors in a large referral population: distribution of diagnoses by age, sex, and location. AJR Am J Roentgenol 1995; 164: 129–134

[22] Stacy GS, Mahal RS, Peabody TD. Staging of bone tumors: a review with illustrative examples. AJR Am J Roentgenol 2006; 186: 967–976

[23] Murphey MD, Smith WS, Smith SE, Kransdorf MJ, Temple HT. From the archives of the AFIP. Imaging of musculoskeletal neurogenic tumors: radiologic-pathologic correlation. Radiographics 1999; 19: 1253–1280

[24] Miller SL, Hoffer FA. Malignant and benign bone tumors. Radiol Clin North Am 2001; 39: 673–699

[25] Ritchie DA, Davies AM. Imaging studies in bone neoplasia. In: Helliwell TR. ed. Pathology of Bone and Joint Neoplasms. Philadelphia, PA: Saunders; 1999:106–127

[26] Wenaden AET, Szyszko TA, Saifuddin A. Imaging of periosteal reactions associated with focal lesions of bone. Clin Radiol 2005; 60: 439–456

[27] Nichols RE, Dixon LB. Radiographic analysis of solitary bone lesions. Radiol Clin North Am 2011; 49: 1095–1114, v

[28] Stacy GS, Kapur A. Mimics of bone and soft tissue neoplasms. Radiol Clin North Am 2011; 49: 1261–1286, vii

[29] Choi H, Varma DG, Fornage BD, Kim EE, Johnston DA. Soft-tissue sarcoma: MR imaging vs sonography for detection of local recurrence after surgery. AJR Am J Roentgenol 1991; 157: 353–358

[30] Pettersson H, Gillespy T, Hamlin DJ, et al. Primary musculoskeletal tumors: examination with MR imaging compared with conventional modalities. Radiology 1987; 164: 237–241

[31] Rajiah P, Ilaslan H, Sundaram M. Imaging of primary malignant bone tumors (nonhematological). Radiol Clin North Am 2011; 49: 1135–1161, v

[32] Shuman WP, Patten RM, Baron RL, Liddell RM, Conrad EU, Richardson ML. Comparison of STIR and spin-echo MR imaging at 1.5 T in 45 suspected extremity tumors: lesion conspicuity and extent. Radiology 1991; 179: 247–252

[33] Stacy GS, Heck RK, Peabody TD, Dixon LB. Neoplastic and tumorlike lesions detected on MR imaging of the knee in patients with suspected internal derangement, I: Intraosseous entities. AJR 2002; 178: 589–594

[34] States LJ. Imaging of metabolic bone disease and marrow disorders in children. Radiol Clin North Am 2001; 39: 749–772

[35] Vade A, Eissenstadt R, Schaff HB. MRI of aggressive bone lesions of childhood. Magn Reson Imaging 1992; 10: 89–96

[36] Berquist TH, Ehman RL, King BF, Hodgman CG, Ilstrup DM. Value of MR imaging in differentiating benign from malignant soft-tissue masses: study of 95 lesions. AJR Am J Roentgenol 1990; 155: 1251–1255

[37] Biondetti PR, Ehman RL. Soft-tissue sarcomas: use of textural patterns in skeletal muscle as a diagnostic feature in postoperative MR imaging. Radiology 1992; 183: 845–848

[38] Bush CH. The magnetic resonance imaging of musculoskeletal hemorrhage. Skeletal Radiol 2000; 29: 1–9

[39] Dyke JP, Panicek DM, Healey JH, et al. Osteogenic and Ewing sarcomas: estimation of necrotic fraction during induction chemotherapy with dynamic contrast-enhanced MR imaging. Radiology 2003; 228: 271–278

[40] Erlemann R, Reiser MF, Peters PE, et al. Musculoskeletal neoplasms: static and dynamic Gd-DTPA–enhanced MR imaging. Radiology 1989; 171: 767–773

[41] Erlemann R. Dynamic, gadolinium-enhanced MR imaging to monitor tumor response to chemotherapy. Radiology 1993; 186: 904–905

[42] Garner HW, Kransdorf MJ, Peterson JJ. Posttherapy imaging of musculoskeletal neoplasms. Radiol Clin North Am 2011; 49: 1307–1323, vii

[43] Moore SG, Bisset GS, Siegel MJ, Donaldson JS. Pediatric musculoskeletal MR imaging. Radiology 1991; 179: 345–360

[44] Motamedi K, Seeger LL. Benign bone tumors. Radiol Clin North Am 2011; 49: 1115–1134, v

[45] Navarro OM. Soft tissue masses in children. Radiol Clin North Am 2011; 49: 1235–1259, vi–vii

[46] van der Woude HJ, Bloem JL, Pope TL. Magnetic resonance imaging of the musculoskeletal system. Part 9. Primary Tumors. Clin Orthop Relat Res 1998; 347: 272–286

[47] van Rijswijk CSP, Geirnaerdt MJA, Hogendoorn PCW, et al. Soft-tissue tumors: value of static and dynamic gadopentetate dimeglumine-enhanced MR imaging in prediction of malignancy. Radiology 2004; 233: 493–502

[48] Vanel D, Shapeero LG, De Baere T, et al. MR imaging in the follow-up of malignant and aggressive soft-tissue tumors: results of 511 examinations. Radiology 1994; 190: 263–268

[49] Walker EA, Fenton ME, Salesky JS, Murphey MD. Magnetic resonance imaging of benign soft tissue neoplasms in adults. Radiol Clin North Am 2011; 49: 1197–1217, vi

[50] Walker EA, Salesky JS, Fenton ME, Murphey MD. Magnetic resonance imaging of malignant soft tissue neoplasms in the adult. Radiol Clin North Am 2011; 49: 1219–1234, vi

[51] Sostman HD, Prescott DM, Dewhirst MW, et al. MR imaging and spectroscopy for prognostic evaluation in soft-tissue sarcomas. Radiology 1994; 190: 269–275

[52] Wang CK, Li CW, Hsieh TJ, Chien SH, Liu GC, Tsai KB. Characterization of bone and soft-tissue tumors with in vivo 1 H MR spectroscopy: initial results. Radiology 2004; 232: 599–605

Chapter 10

Lesions Involving Bones

10 Lesions Involving Bones

Steven P. Meyers

10.1 Lesions Involving the Outer Surface of Bone

- Nonmalignant lesions
  - Degenerative lesions
    - Osteophyte
    - Synovial cyst
    - Ganglion cyst
  - Benign tumors and tumor-like lesions
    - Osteochondroma
    - Juxtacortical chondroma
    - Bizarre parosteal osteocartilaginous proliferation
    - Chondromyxoid fibroma
    - Periosteal osteoid osteoma
    - Fibrous cortical defect (FCD) and nonossifying fibroma (NOF)
    - Cortical desmoid
    - Osteoma
    - Parosteal lipoma
    - Melorheostosis
    - Heterotopic ossification
    - Schwannoma
    - Neurofibroma
    - Giant cell tumor of tendon sheath
    - Glomus tumor
    - Nonmalignant giant cell tumor eroding through bone cortex
  - Inflammatory lesions
    - Myositis/cellulitis associated with infection of bone
    - Osteomyelitis
    - Chronic recurrent multifocal osteomyelitis
    - Syndromes of hyperostosis, osteitis, and skin lesions (SAPHO syndrome)
    - Eosinophilic granuloma eroding through bone cortex
    - Rheumatoid pannus adjacent to and eroding bone
    - Gout
    - Pigmented villonodular synovitis (PVNS)
    - Calcific tendinitis eroding into bone
  - Abnormalities involving the periosteum
    - Noninterrupted periosteal reaction from fracture
    - Subperiosteal hematoma
    - Hemophilic pseudotumor
    - Noninterrupted periosteal reaction from primary hypertrophic osteoarthropathy (pachydermoperiostosis)
    - Noninterrupted periosteal reaction from secondary hypertrophic osteoarthropathy
    - Noninterrupted periosteal reaction from venous stasis
    - Noninterrupted periosteal reaction from infantile cortical hyperostosis (Caffey disease)
    - Noninterrupted periosteal reaction from thyroid acropachy
    - Progressive diaphyseal dysplasia (Camurati-Engleman disease
    - Noninterrupted periosteal reaction from hypervitaminosis A
    - Periosteal reaction from hypovitaminosis C (scurvy)
    - Neurofibromatosis type 1
    - Periostitis associated with acute/subacute bone infarction
- Malignant lesions
  - Parosteal osteosarcoma
  - Periosteal osteosarcoma
  - Chondrosarcoma
  - Hemangioendothelioma
  - Sarcoma of soft tissue eroding into bone
  - Intramedullary primary sarcoma eroding through bone cortex
  - Metastatic lesions
  - Myeloma/plasmacytoma
  - Lymphoma
  - Leukemia
  - Malignant tumor with interrupted periosteal reaction: sunburst or divergent pattern
  - Malignant tumor with interrupted periosteal reaction: Codman triangle
  - Malignant tumor with interrupted periosteal reaction: disorganized pattern
  - Malignant tumor with interrupted periosteal reaction: "hair on end" or perpendicularly oriented spicules of periosteal reaction
  - Malignant tumor with interrupted periosteal reaction: "onion skin" multilayered, or multilamellated periosteal reaction oriented parallel to the long axis of bone

Table 10.1 Lesions involving the outer surface of bone

Abnormalities	MRI findings	Comments
Nonmalignant lesions		
Degenerative lesions		
Osteophyte (▶ Fig. 10.1)	Bone spurs (osteophytes) occur at the margins of synovial joints, and have low peripheral signal on T1-weighted imaging (T1WI) and T2-weighted imaging (T2WI) overlying fatty marrow with or without edematous reaction. In the axial skeleton, smooth undulating zones of ossification involving the anterior longitudinal ligament can be seen along the anterior margins of the vertebral bodies and extending across the disks.	Bony outgrowths usually related to degenerative athropathy at synovial joints, or degenerative disk disease adjacent to the anterior and posterior longitudinal ligaments. At synovial joints, these bony protrusions may be a response to increase the articular surface to reduce load. At the spine, osteophytes occur as a metaplastic bone response related to degenerative disk bulges displacing the longitudinal ligaments. Flowing or bridging osteophytes at four or more adjacent vertebral bodies have been referred to as diffuse idiopathic skeletal hyperostosis (DISH).

(continued on page 314)

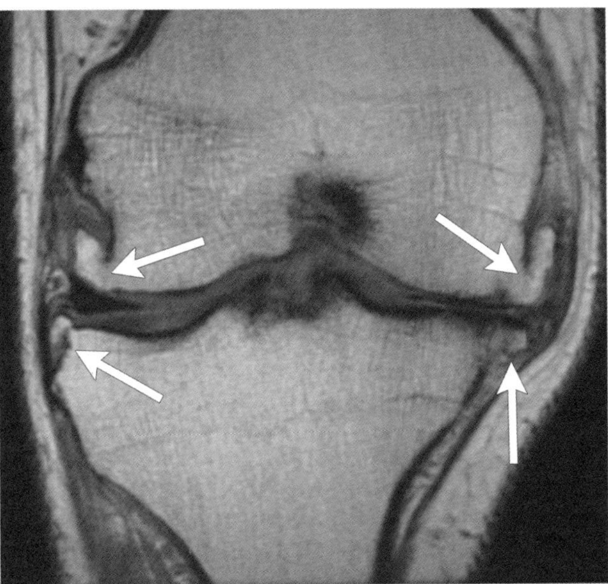

Fig. 10.1 A 54-year-old man with degenerative arthropathy at the knee with prominent osteophytes (arrows) at the distal femur and proximal tibia on coronal proton density–weighted imaging.

Table 10.1 (Cont.) Lesions involving the outer surface of bone

Abnormalities	MRI findings	Comments
Synovial cyst (▶ Fig. 10.2)	Spheroid or ovoid circumscribed collections, which often show a site of communication with the adjacent joint. The contents of the synovial cyst usually have low to intermediate signal on T1WI and proton density–weighted imaging (PDWI), and high signal on T2WI and fat-suppressed (FS) T2WI. A thin or slightly thick rim of low signal on T2WI and FS T2WI is typically seen at the periphery of the cysts. Some synovial cysts may have intermediate to high signal on T1WI, and/or intermediate or low signal on T2WI secondary to calcifications, cartilage formation, and/or hemorrhage. After gadolinium (Gd)-contrast administration, thin marginal enhancement may be seen.	Synovium-lined fluid collections that frequently occur at or near joints of the extremities, occasionally occur at facet joints of the spine, as well as bursae and tendon sheaths. In adults, synovial cysts are often associated with osteoarthritis, rheumatoid arthritis, and trauma.
Ganglion cyst (▶ Fig. 10.3)	Sharply defined lesions with low signal on T1WI, low-intermediate signal on PDWI, and homogeneous high signal on T2WI. Peripheral rimlike Gd-contrast enhancement can be seen as well as complete lack of enhancement. Lesions can erode and/or invade adjacent bone.	Ganglia are juxta-articular benign myxoid lesions that arise from degeneration of periarticular connective tissue, prior trauma, or prior inflammation. Ganglia may be derived from tendons, tendon sheaths, joint capsules, bursae, or ligaments.

(continued on page 316)

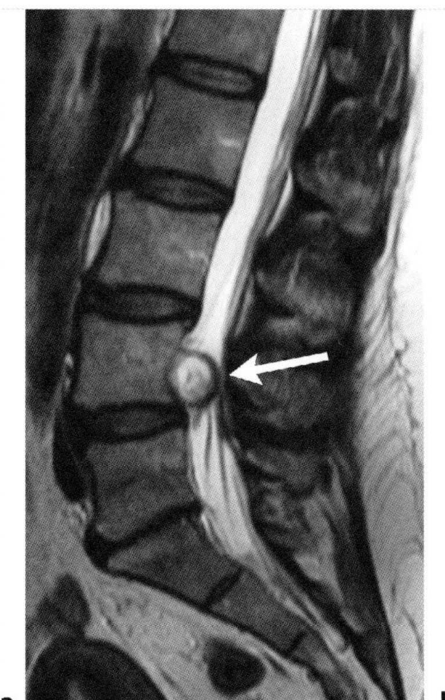

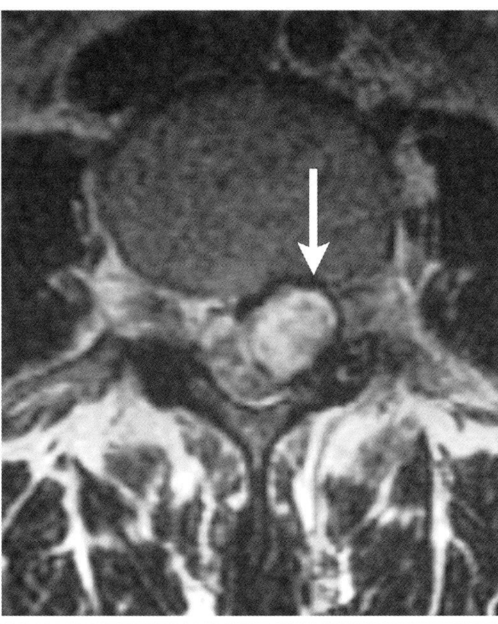

Fig. 10.2 Sagittal (a) and axial (b) T2-weighted imaging shows a synovial cyst (arrows) at the medial aspect of the left facet joint causing erosive changes at the vertebral body.

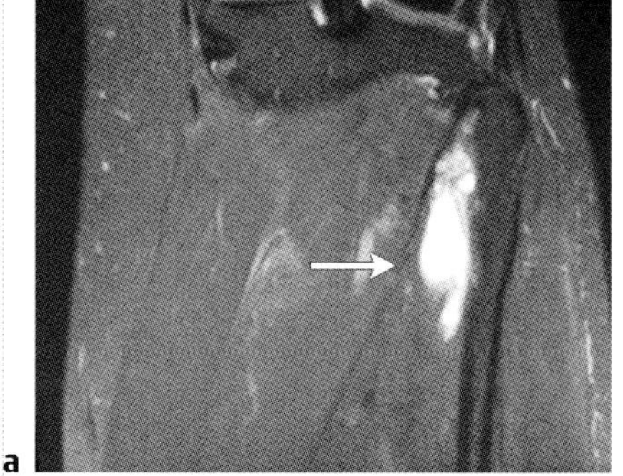

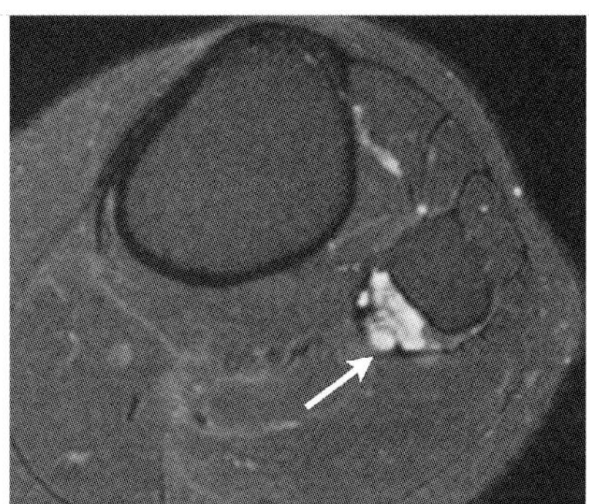

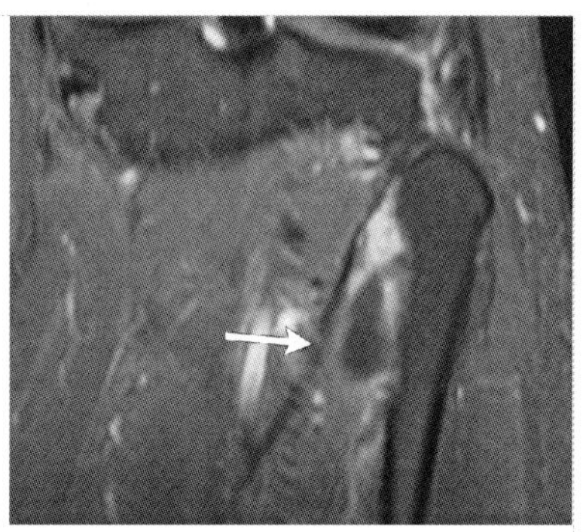

Fig. 10.3 Ganglion cyst along the outer surface of the fibula (arrows) which has high signal on coronal (a) and axial (b) fat-suppressed (FS) T2-weighted imaging. Thin peripheral gadolinium-contrast enhancement is seen at the lesion on coronal FS T1-weighted imaging (c).

Table 10.1 (Cont.) Lesions involving the outer surface of bone

Abnormalities	MRI findings	Comments
Benign tumors and tumor-like lesions		
Osteochondroma (▶ Fig. 10.4)	Circumscribed protruding lesion arising from outer cortex with a central zone with intermediate signal on T1WI and T2WI similar to marrow surrounded by a peripheral zone of low signal on T1 W and T2 W images.A cartilaginous cap with high signal on T2WI and FS T2WI is usually present in children and young adults. Increased malignant potential when cartilaginous cap is > 2 cm thick.	Benign cartilaginous tumors arising from defect at periphery of growth plate during bone formation with resultant bone outgrowth covered by a cartilaginous cap. Usually benign lesions unless associated with pain and increasing size of cartilaginous cap. Osteochondromas are common lesions, accounting for 14 to 35% of primary bone tumors. Occur with median age of 20 years, up to 75% of patients are less than 20 years.
Juxtacortical chondroma (▶ Fig. 10.5)	Lesions are located at the bone surface and can be sessile or slightly lobulated with low-intermediate signal on T1WI, which is hypo- or isointense relative to muscle. Lesions usually have heterogeneous predominantly high signal on T2WI. Lesions are surrounded by low signal borders on T2WI representing thin sclerotic reaction. Areas of low signal on T2WI are secondary to matrix mineralization. Edema is not typically seen in nearby medullary bone. Lesions often show a peripheral pattern of Gd-contrast enhancement.	Benign protuberant hyaline cartilaginous tumors that arise from the periosteum and are superficial to bone cortex. Juxtacortical chondromas account for < 1% of bone lesions. Occur with median age of 26 years.

(continued on page 318)

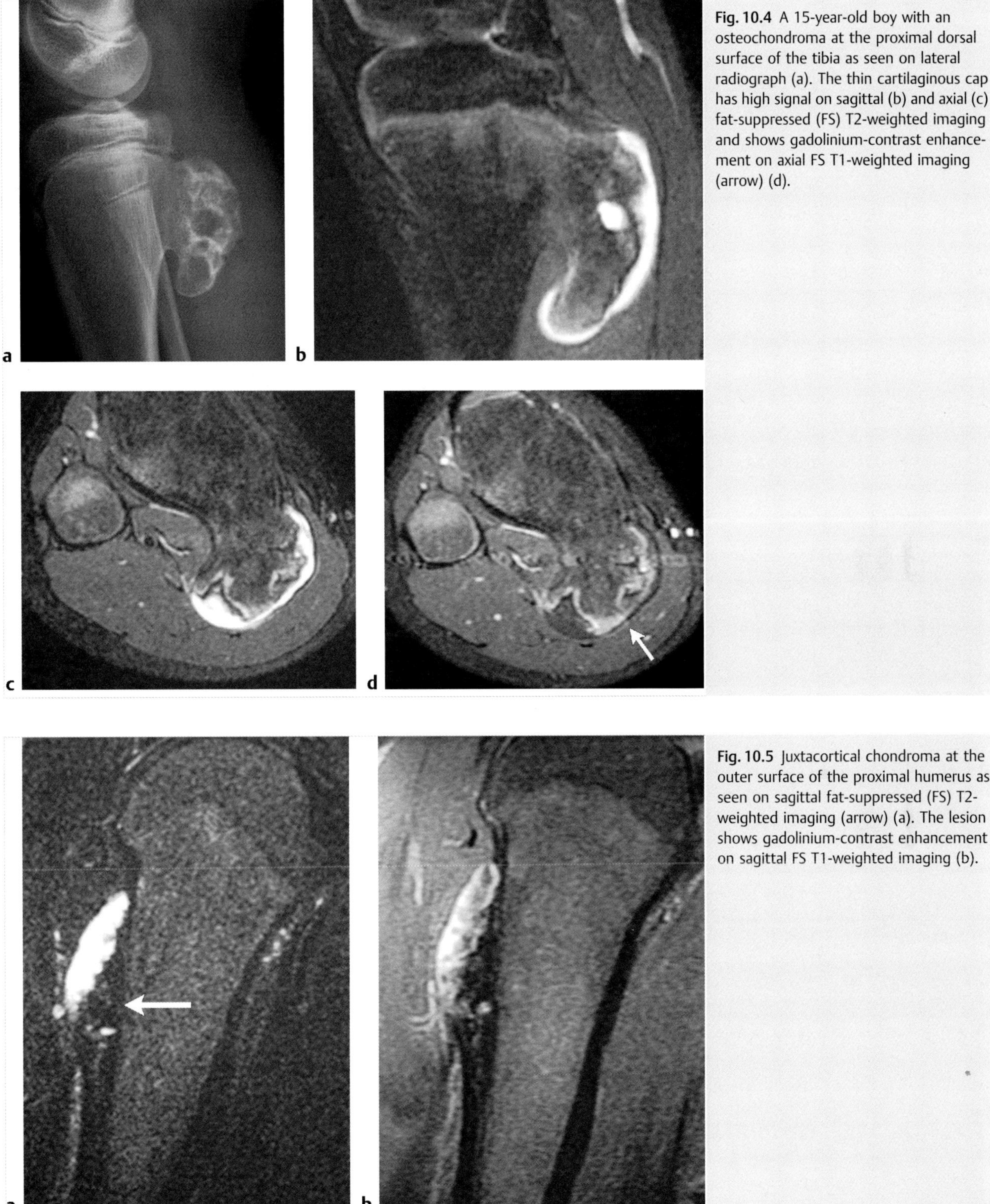

Fig. 10.4 A 15-year-old boy with an osteochondroma at the proximal dorsal surface of the tibia as seen on lateral radiograph (a). The thin cartilaginous cap has high signal on sagittal (b) and axial (c) fat-suppressed (FS) T2-weighted imaging and shows gadolinium-contrast enhancement on axial FS T1-weighted imaging (arrow) (d).

Fig. 10.5 Juxtacortical chondroma at the outer surface of the proximal humerus as seen on sagittal fat-suppressed (FS) T2-weighted imaging (arrow) (a). The lesion shows gadolinium-contrast enhancement on sagittal FS T1-weighted imaging (b).

Table 10.1 (Cont.) Lesions involving the outer surface of bone

Abnormalities	MRI findings	Comments
Bizarre parosteal osteocartilaginous proliferation (▶ Fig. 10.6)	Smooth and/or lobulated calcified and/or ossified lesions often with a broad base or stalk of attachment to an intact outer cortical surface of bone. Remodeling of adjacent bone cortex can occur. Typically displaces, but does not invade, adjacent extraosseous soft tissues.	Lesions adjacent to or attached to the outer periosteal surface of bone consisting of disorganized conglomerations of bone with short trabeculae, cartilage containing enlarged dysmorphic binucleate chondrocytes, spindle cells, fibrous tissue, and/or myxoid regions. Commonly occurs in the hands and feet (70%), less commonly in long bones. Peak age in fourth decade. May represent a type of heterotopic ossification versus benign tumor. Can be cured by surgical excision, although local recurrence is common.
Chondromyxoid fibroma (▶ Fig. 10.7)	Lesions are often slightly lobulated with low-intermediate signal on T1WI, intermediate signal on PDWI, and heterogeneous, predominantly high signal on T2WI secondary to myxoid and hyaline chondroid components with high water content. Magnetic resonance (MR) signal heterogeneity on T2WI is related to the proportions of myxoid, chondroid, and fibrous components within the lesions. Thin low signal septa within lesions on T2WI are secondary to fibrous strands. Lesions are surrounded by low signal borders representing thin sclerotic reaction. Edema is not typically seen in medullary bone. Lesions show prominent diffuse Gd-contrast enhancement.	Rare, benign, slow-growing bone lesions, which contain chondroid, myxoid, and fibrous components. Chondromyxoid fibromas represent 2 to 4% of primary benign bone lesions, and < 1% of primary bone lesions. Most chondromyxoid fibromas occur between the ages of 1 and 40 years, with a median of 17 years, and peak incidence in the second to third decades.

(continued on page 320)

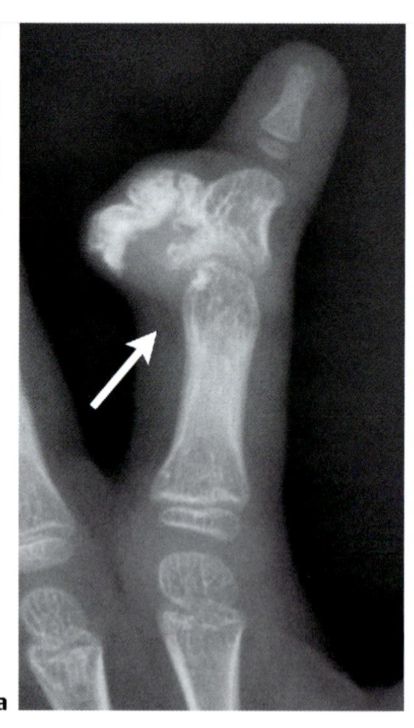
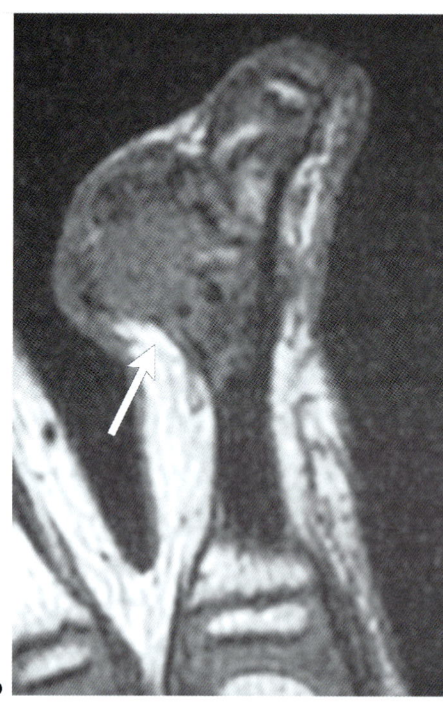
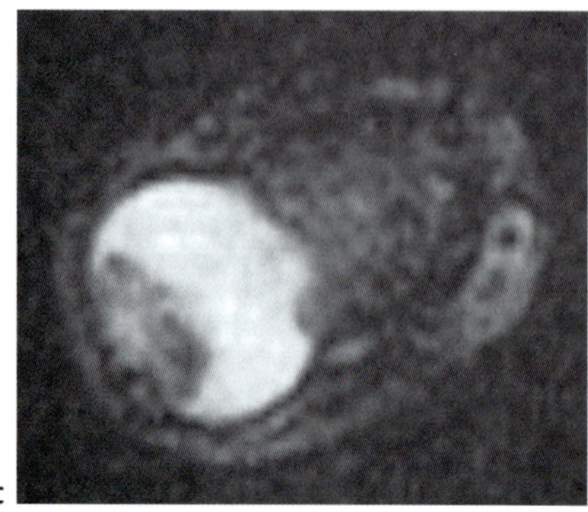
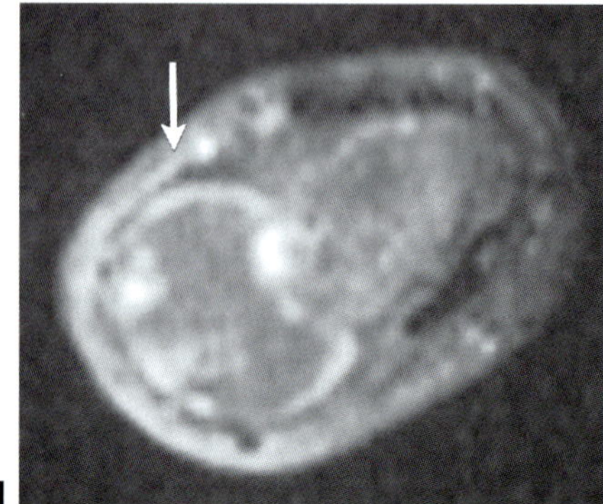

Fig. 10.6 Bizzare parosteal osteocartilaginous proliferation in a 5-year-old female. Calcified and ossified lesion (arrow) (a) with a broad base of attachment to an intact outer cortical surface of a middle phalange. The lesion has heterogeneous intermediate signal on coronal T1-weighted imaging (arrow) (b), mixed high and low signal on axial fat-suppressed T2-weighted imaging (FS T2WI) (c), and shows peripheral gadolinium-contrast enhancement (arrow) on axial FS T1WI (d). The lesion displaces but does not invade adjacent extraosseous soft tissues.

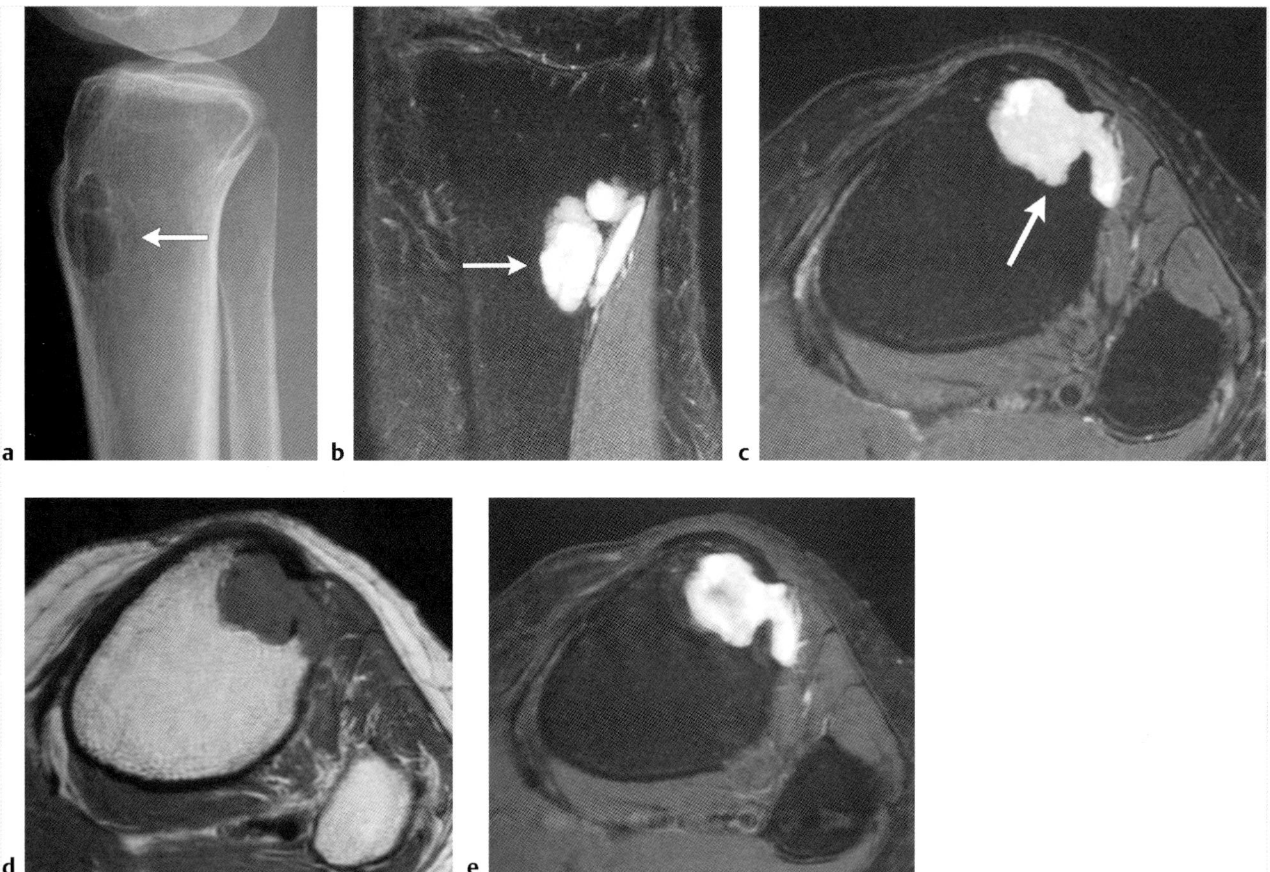

Fig. 10.7 Chondromyxoid fibroma in a 48-year-old woman involving the superifical portion of the proximal tibia. The radiolucent lesion has well-defined margins (arrow) on lateral radiograph (a). The lesion expands and thins the outer cortical margin, and has high signal (arrow) on coronal (b) and axial fat-suppressed (FS) T2-weighted imaging (arrow) (c), intermediate signal on axial T1-weighted imaging (T1WI), (d) and shows prominent gadolinium-contrast enhancement on axial FS T1WI (e).

Table 10.1 (Cont.) Lesions involving the outer surface of bone

Abnormalities	MRI findings	Comments
Periosteal osteoid osteoma (▶ Fig. 10.8)	Typically shows dense fusiform thickening of the cortex, which has low-intermediate signal on T1WI, PDWI, T2WI, and FS T2WI. Within the thickened cortex, a spheroid or ovoid zone (nidus) measuring less than 1.5 cm is seen in the region of the original external surface of bone cortex. The nidus can have irregular, distinct, or indistinct margins relative to the adjacent region of cortical thickening. The nidus can have low-intermediate signal on T1WI and PDWI, and low-intermediate or high signal on T2WI and FS T2WI. Calcifications in the nidus can be seen as low signal on T2WI. After Gd-contrast administration, variable degrees of enhancement are seen at the nidus, adjacent bone cortex, marrow, periosteum, and adjacent soft tissues.	Benign osteoblastic lesion composed of a circumscribed nidus less than 1.5 cm, and usually surrounded by reactive bone formation. These lesions are usually painful and have limited growth potential. Osteoid osteoma accounts for 11 to 13% of primary benign bone tumors. Occurs in patients age 6 to 30 years, median = 17 years. Approximately 75% occur in patients less than 25 years.
Fibrous cortical defect (FCD) and nonossifying fibroma (NOF) (▶ Fig. 10.9; ▶ Fig. 10.10)	FCDs: Circumscribed oval lesions involving bone cortex of long bones, which have low to intermediate signal on T1WI and PDWI, and low, intermediate, and/or high signal on FS T2WI surrounded by varying thickness of low signal from corresponding marginal sclerosis. FCDs with or without fracture can show variable degrees of Gd-contrast enhancement. NOFs have MRI features similar to FCDs, although they are larger and eccentrically involve the marrow in the dimetaphyseal regions of long bones. Cortical thinning or thickening, and bone expansion can be seen.	FCDs and NOFs are benign fibrohistiocytic lesions in the metaphyseal portions of long bones, which are composed of whorls of fibroblastic cells combined with smaller amounts of multinucleated giant cells and xanthomatous cells. Both lesions have similar pathologic findings, although they differ in size. FCDs are small lesions in bone cortex, whereas the larger NOFs are located eccentrically in the medullary cavity. Both lesions are considered in the spectrum of the same disorder of fibrohistiocytic origins. FCDs and NOFs are common benign lesions, which are usually asymptomatic and are often detected as incidental findings. Incidence may be up to 30 to 40% of children. Both lesions occur in patients age 1 to 45 years, median = 14 years, 95% occur between the ages of 5 and 20 years.

(continued on page 322)

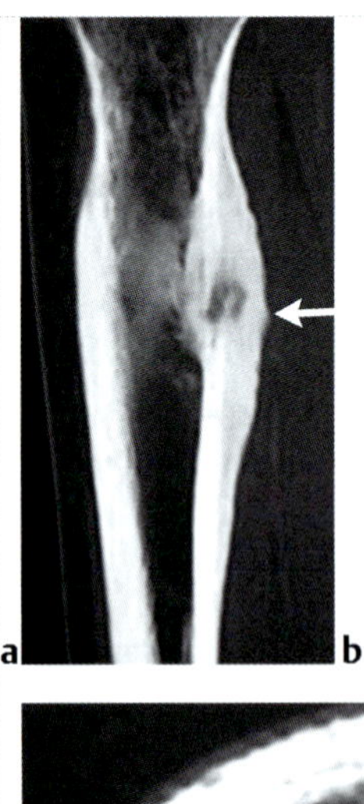
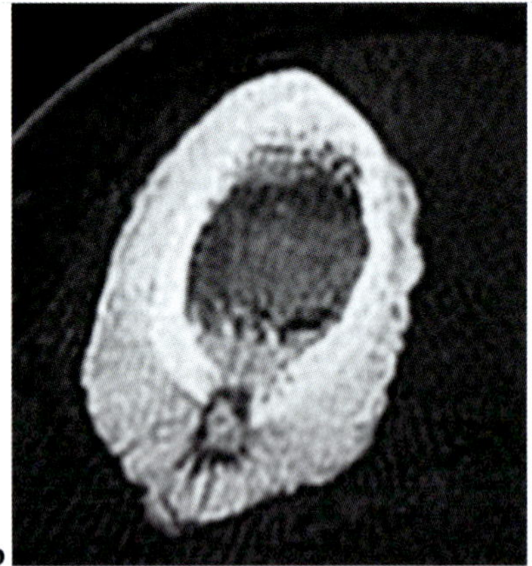
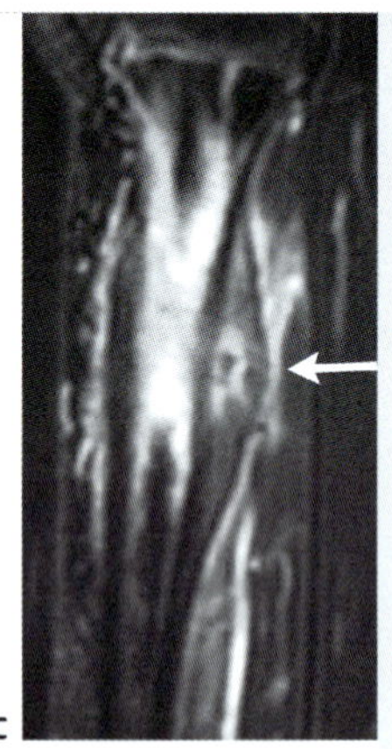
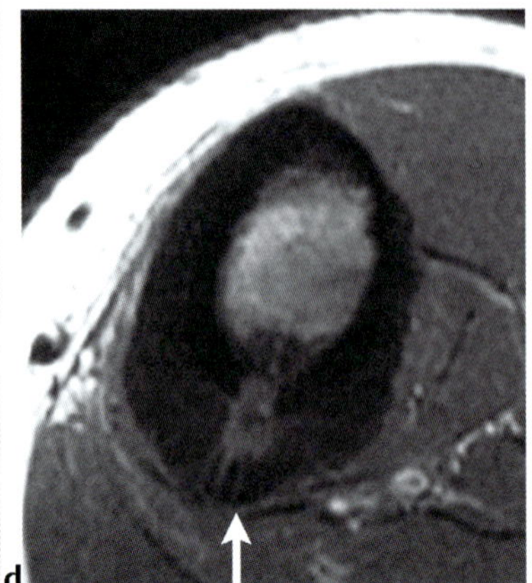
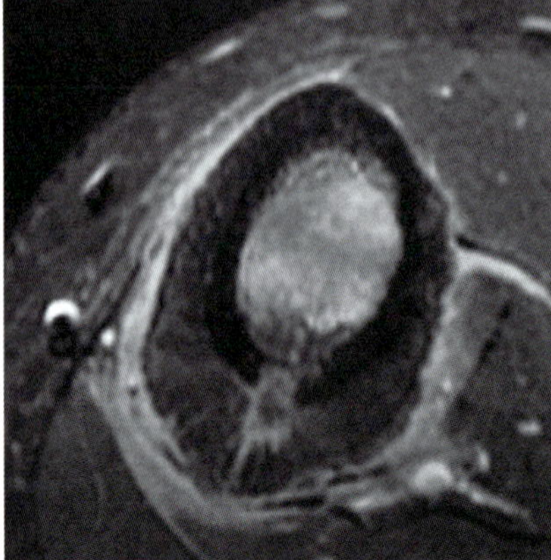

Fig. 10.8 Periosteal osteoid osteoma involving the tibia in a 15-year-old girl. Sagittal (a) and axial (b) computed tomographic images show a lucent nidus within thickened periosteal bone formation (arrow). The nidus has high signal (arrow) on sagittal fat-suppressed T2-weighted imaging (FS T2WI) (c), intermediate signal (arrow) on axial T1-weighted imaging (T1WI) (d), and shows gadolinium-contrast enhancement on axial FS T1WI (e). Prominent thickened periosteal bone formation is seen, which has heterogeneous intermediate and low signal on FS T2WI. Zones with high signal on FS T2WI with corresponding gadolinium-contrast enhancement are seen in the marrow and soft tissues superficial to the periosteal bone formation secondary to inflammatory and edematous changes from prostaglandin production by the lesion.

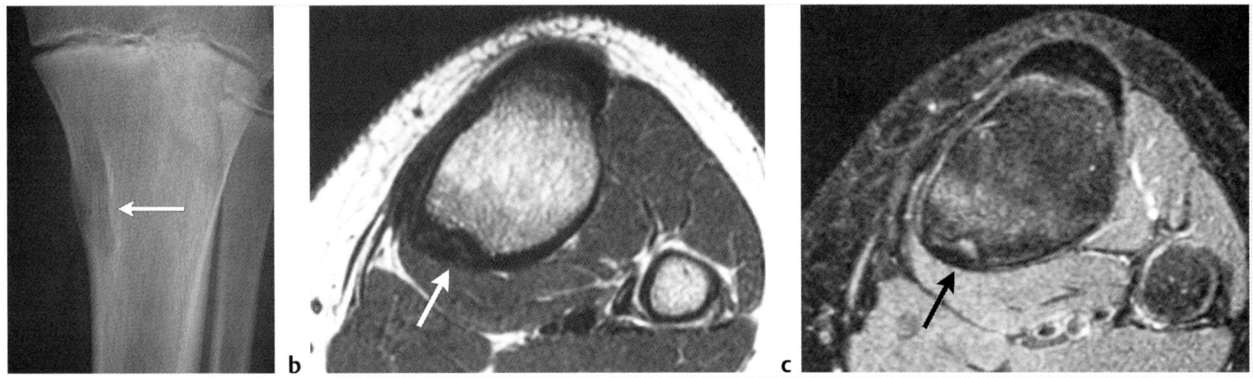

Fig. 10.9 A 13-year-old boy with a fibrous cortical defect involving the posterior medial tibia in the dimetaphyseal region. Anteroposterior radiograph (a) shows an oval sharply marginated radiolucent zone in the cortex surrounded by a thin rim of sclerotic bone (arrow). Centrally, the lesion has low-intermediate signal on axial T1-weighted imaging (arrow) (b) similar to muscle, and intermediate to slightly high signal on axial fat saturation T2-weighted imaging (arrow) (c). A thin zone of low signal is seen at the medullary border of the lesion.

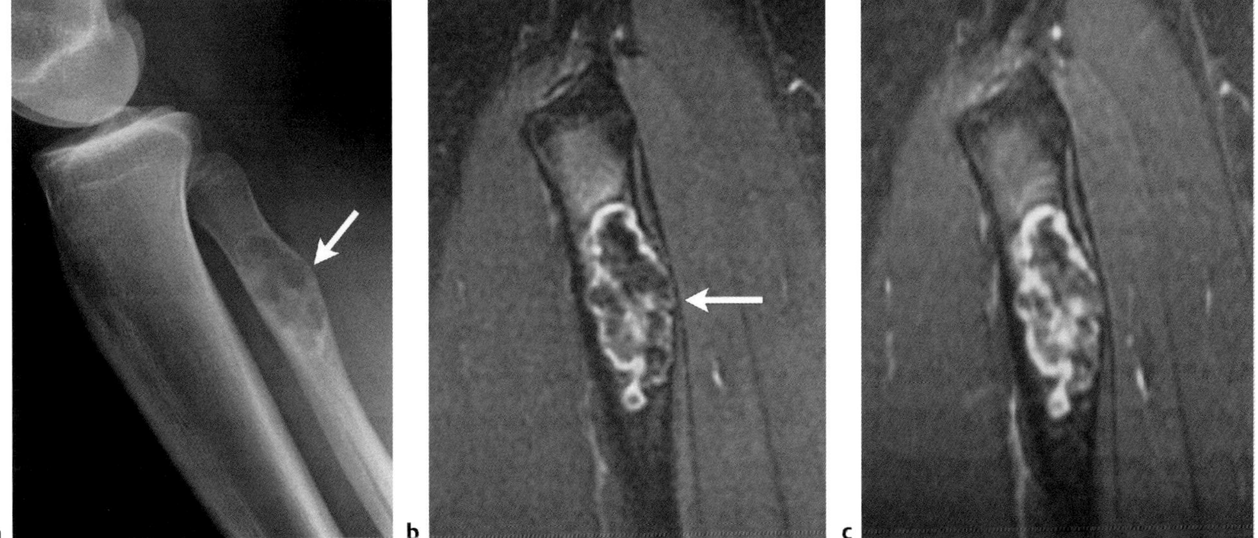

Fig. 10.10 Nonossifying fibroma in the marrow of the proximal fibula of a 15-year-old girl. Oblique radiograph (a) shows a circumscribed radiolucent intramedullary lesion associated with thinning and expansion of the outer cortical margins (arrow). The lesion has mostly low signal centrally surrounded by thin zones with high signal (arrow) on sagittal fat-suppressed (FS) T2-weighted imaging (b) and gadolinium-contrast enhancement on sagittal FS T1-weighted imaging (c). The lesion expands and thins the outer cortical margins.

Table 10.1 (Cont.) Lesions involving the outer surface of bone

Abnormalities	MRI findings	Comments
Cortical desmoid (▶ Fig. 10.11)	Cortical desmoids are located at the bone cortex at the distal posterior medial portions of the femur, and usually have low to intermediate signal on T1WI and PDWI, and intermediate to slightly high signal on T2WI, and slightly high to high signal on FS T2WI. A thin border of low signal on T1WI and T2WI is often seen at the inner margin of the lesion which corresponds to a thin zone of sclerosis seen on plain films and/or computed tomography (CT). Bone marrow deep and peripheral to the lesion may have slightly high signal on FS T2WI. After Gd-contrast administration, enhancement can be seen at the lesion and occasionally in the adjacent marrow.	Cortical desmoids (also referred to as periosteal desmoid or distal femoral cortical irregularity) are fibrous defects at the distal posteromedial femur, which may arise from an avulsive injury or stress reaction at the insertion site of the medial head of the gastrocnemius muscle or adductor magnus. Similar-appearing irregularities of bone cortex at sites where other tendons attach to bone are referred to as tug lesions.
Osteoma (▶ Fig. 10.12)	Typically appear as well-circumscribed zones of dense bone with low signal on T1WI, PDWI, T2WI, and FS T2WI. No infiltration is seen into the adjacent soft tissues by osteomas. Zones of bone destruction or associated soft tissue mass-lesions are not associated with osteomas. Periosteal reaction is not associated with osteomas except in cases with coincidental antecedent trauma.	Benign primary bone tumors composed of dense lamellar, woven, and/or compact cortical bone usually located at the surface of bones. Multiple osteomas usually occur in Gardner syndrome, which is an autosomal dominant disorder that is associated with intestinal polyposis, fibromas, and desmoid tumors. Account for less than 1% of primary benign bone tumors. Occur in patients age 16 to 74 years, most frequent in sixth decade.
Parosteal lipoma (▶ Fig. 10.13)	Fatty lesions often have smooth and sometimes lobular margins, and are immediately adjacent to the outer intact surface of adjacent bone. Lesions typically have fat signal on magnetic resonance imaging (MRI), as well as zones of low signal on T1WI and T2WI from fibrous changes and ossification changes that can occur within these lesions and at the junction with bone cortex. Zones with intermediate signal on T1WI and high signal on T2WI can occur in these lesions secondary to cartilaginous contents.	Rare benign slow-growing painless tumors with mature adipose tissue associated with the periosteum of bone. Account for 0.3% of lipomas, typically occur in patients 40 to 60 years of age. Common sites include the femur, proximal radius, tibia, and humerus. Other sites have been reported. May be associated with compression of adjacent nerves causing sensory or motor deficits.

(continued on page 324)

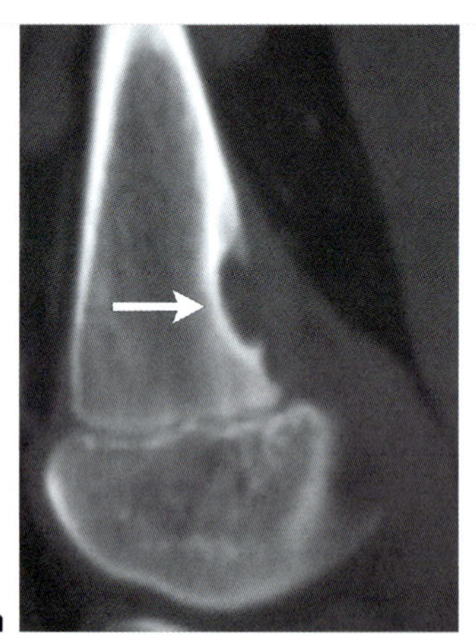

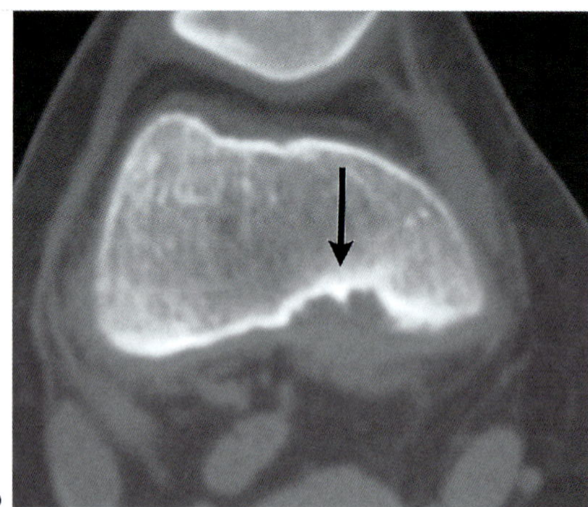

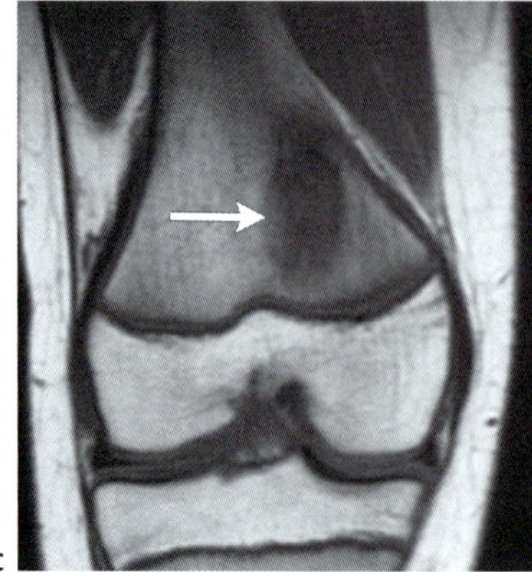

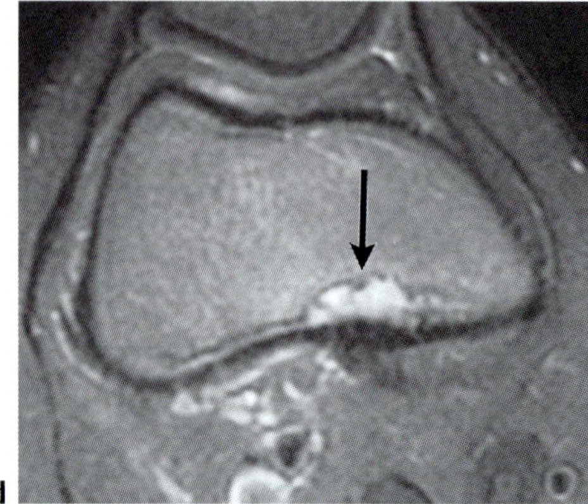

Fig. 10.11 A 10-year-old girl with a cortical desmoid at the distal dorsal aspect of the femur medially adjacent to the insertion of the medial gastrocnemius muscle tendon. Sagittal (a) and axial (b) computed tomographic images show cortical irregularity at cortical desmoid (arrow), which has low-intermediate signal (arrow) on coronal (c) T1-weighted imaging and high signal (arrow) on axial fat-suppressedT2-weighted imaging (d).

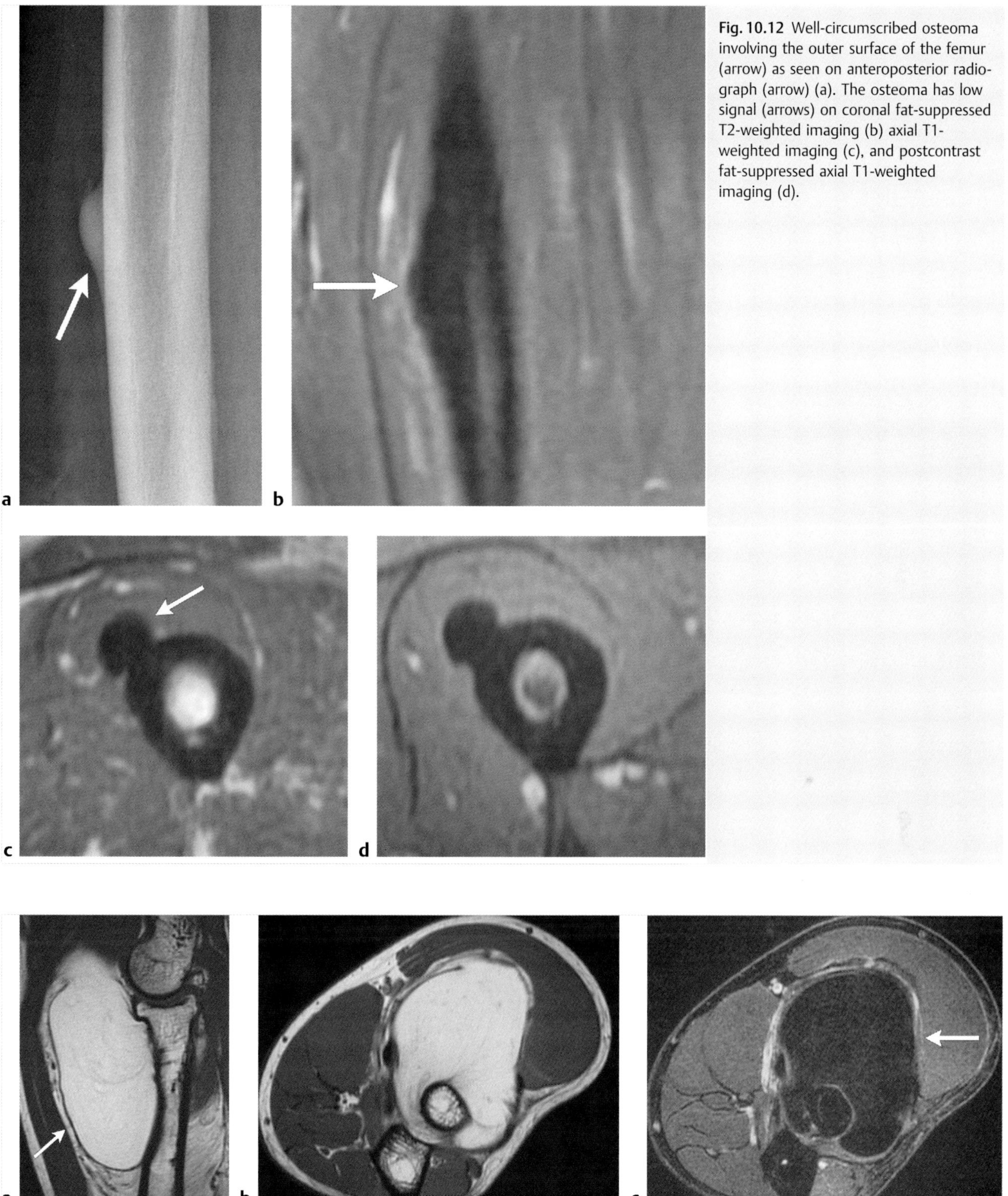

Fig. 10.12 Well-circumscribed osteoma involving the outer surface of the femur (arrow) as seen on anteroposterior radiograph (arrow) (a). The osteoma has low signal (arrows) on coronal fat-suppressed T2-weighted imaging (b) axial T1-weighted imaging (c), and postcontrast fat-suppressed axial T1-weighted imaging (d).

Fig. 10.13 Well-circumscribed parosteal lipoma involving the outer surface of the proximal radius femur (arrow) as seen on sagittal (a) and axial (b) T1-weighted imaging. The fat signal of the lipoma is suppressed on axial fat-suppressed T2-weighted imaging (arrow) (c).

Table 10.1 (Cont.) Lesions involving the outer surface of bone

Abnormalities	MRI findings	Comments
Melorheostosis (▶ Fig. 10.14)	MRI signal varies based on the relative proportions of mineralized osteoid, chondroid, and soft tissue components in these lesions. Mineralized osteoid zones along bone cortex typically have low signal on T1WI and T2WI, no Gd-contrast enhancement. Soft tissue lesions may also occur adjacent to the cortical lesions, which have mixed signal on T1WI and T2WI.	Melorheostosis is a rare bone dysplasia with cortical thickening that has a "flowing candle wax" configuration. Associated soft tissue masses occur in approximately 25%. The soft tissue lesions often contain mixtures of chondroid material, mineralized osteoid, and fibrovascular tissue.
Heterotopic ossification (▶ Fig. 10.15)	Long-standing lesions can have variable low to intermediate signal on T1WI, PDWI, and T2WI depending on the degree of mineralization/ossification, fibrosis, and hemosiderin deposition. Zones of high signal on T1WI and T2WI may occur from fatty marrow metaplasia. Gd-contrast enhancement in old mature lesions is often minimal or absent. Signal abnormalities within bone marrow are usually absent.	Represents localized nonneoplastic reparative lesions in soft tissues separate or adjacent to bone, which are composed of reactive hypercellular fibrous tissue, cartilage, and/or bone. Can arise secondary to trauma (myositis ossificans circumscripta, ossifying hematoma), although may also occur without a history of prior injury (pseudomalignant osseous tumor of the soft tissues).

(continued on page 326)

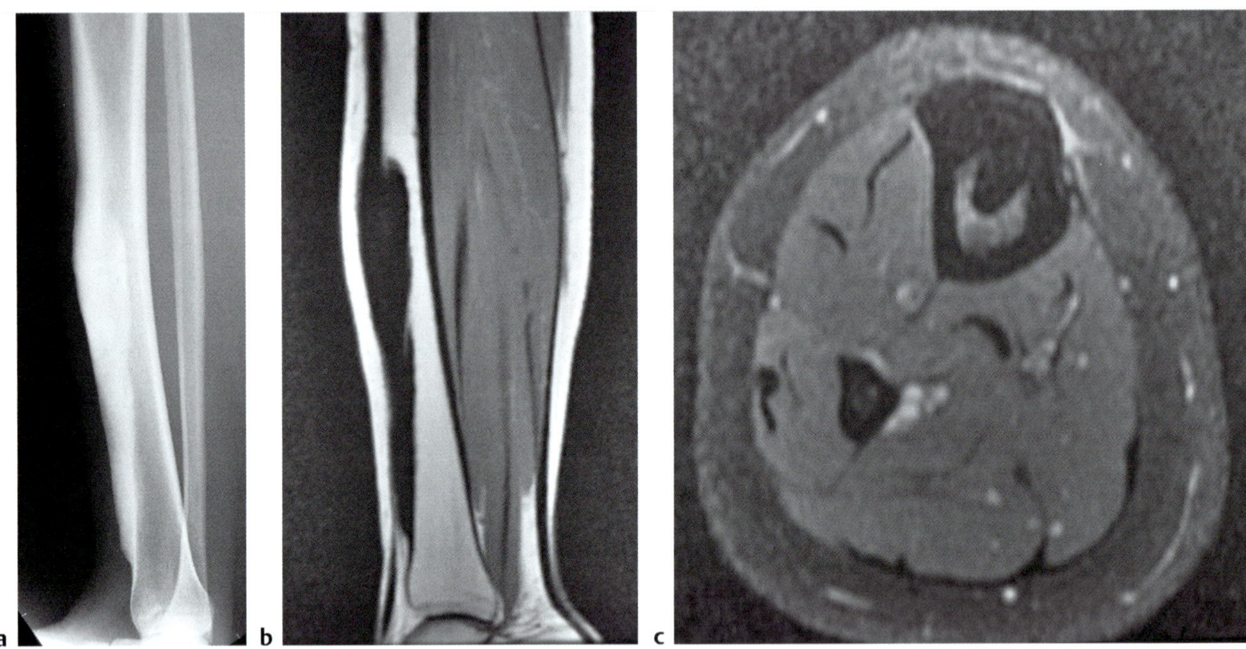

Fig. 10.14 Melorheostosis with cortical bone thickening at the anterior surface of the tibia and endosteal surface as seen on lateral radiograph (a), which has low signal on sagittal T1-weighted imaging (b), and axial fat-suppressed T2-weighted imaging (c).

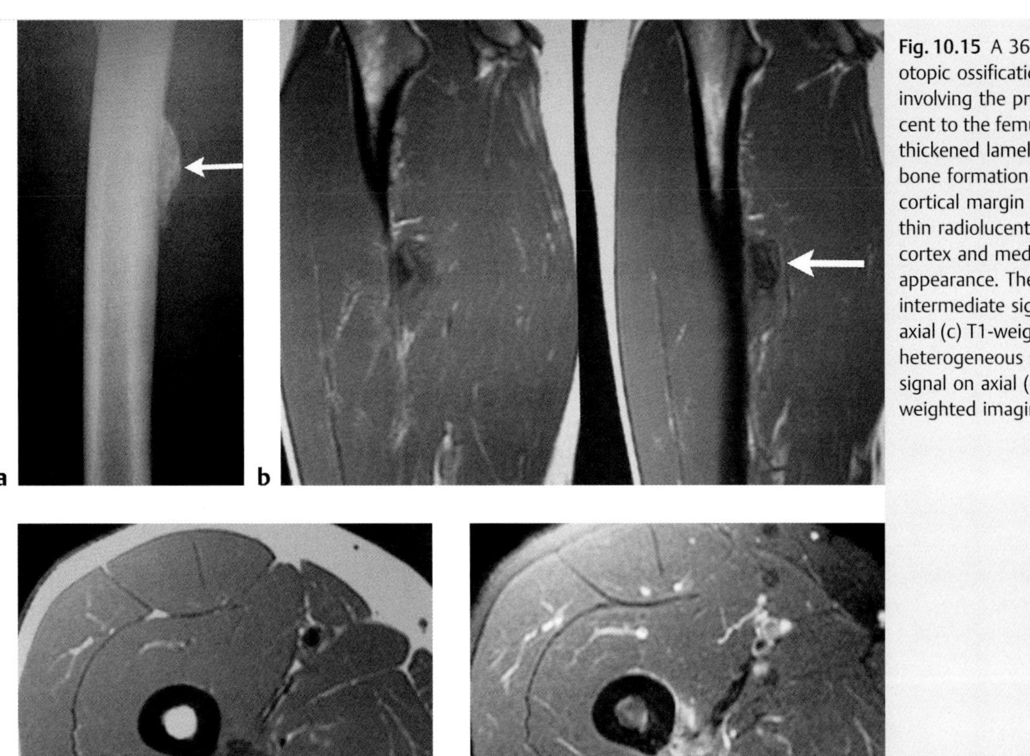

Fig. 10.15 A 36-year-old man with heterotopic ossification/myositis ossificans involving the proximal medial thigh adjacent to the femur. Radiograph (a) shows a thickened lamellar type of extraosseous bone formation adjacent to the outer cortical margin (arrow) separated by a thin radiolucent zone. Adjacent bone cortex and medullary bone are normal in appearance. The lesion has low and intermediate signal on coronal (b) and axial (c) T1-weighted imaging (arrow), and heterogeneous slightly high and high signal on axial (d) fat-suppressed T2-weighted imaging (arrow).

Table 10.1 (Cont.) Lesions involving the outer surface of bone

Abnormalities	MRI findings	Comments
Schwannoma (▸ Fig. 10.16)	Schwannomas are circumscribed ovoid or fusiform lesions with low-intermediate signal on T1WI, intermediate signal on PDWI, and intermediate to high signal on T2WI and FS T2WI. After Gd-contrast administration, lesions typically show moderate to prominent enhancement. Schwannomas involving spinal nerve roots may be associated with chronic erosive changes of adjacent vertebrae. Lesions may show signal heterogeneity on T2WI and heterogeneous Gd-contrast enhancement secondary to cyst formation, hemorrhage, fibrous/collagenous zones, and/or dense cellularity. Signal heterogeneity on T2WI tends to occur frequently in large schwannomas. Malignant schwannomas (malignant peripheral nerve sheath tumors) can be large lesions that have heterogeneous signal on T1WI, T2WI, and FS T2WI; as well as heterogeneous Gd-contrast enhancement because of necrosis and hemorrhage. These tumors can have irregular margins and associated invasion of adjacent structures.	Benign encapsulated tumors that contain differentiated neoplastic Schwann cells. Multiple schwannomas are often associated with neurofibromatosis type 2 (NF2). Account for 5% of benign primary soft-tissue tumors and 3% of all primary soft-tissue tumors. Occurs in patients age 22 to 72 years, mean = 46 years. Peak incidence is in the fourth to sixth decades. With NF2, many patients present in the third decade with bilateral vestibular schwannomas.
Neurofibroma (▸ Fig. 10.17; ▸ Fig. 10.18)	*Localized neurofibromas* are circumscribed ovoid or fusiform lesions with low-intermediate signal on T1WI and intermediate to high signal on T2WI and FS T2WI. After Gd-contrast administration, lesions typically show moderate to prominent enhancement. Large lesions may show signal heterogeneity on T2WI and heterogeneous Gd-contrast enhancement. Neurofibromas involving spinal nerve roots may have a dumbbell shape with or without associated chronic erosive changes of adjacent vertebrae. *Plexiform neurofibromas* appear as curvilinear and multinodular lesions involving multiple nerve branches. Lesions usually have low to intermediate signal on T1WI; and intermediate, slightly high to high signal on T2WI and FS T2WI with or without bands or strands of low signal. On T2WI, lesions may show nodules with high signal surrounding a central region of low signal referred to as a "target sign." Lesions typically show Gd-contrast enhancement in a heterogeneous pattern. Lesions can be associated with remodeling of adjacent bone.	Benign tumors of the peripheral nerve sheath that contain mixtures of Schwann cells, perineural-like cells, and interlacing fascicles of fibroblasts associated with abundant collagen. Unlike schwannomas, neurofibromas lack Antoni A and B regions and cannot be separated pathologically from the underlying nerve. Neurofibromas can be localized lesions (90%), or occur as diffuse or plexiform lesions. The presence of multiple neurofibromas is a typical feature of neurofibromatosis type 1 (NF1), which is an autosomal dominant disorder resulting in mesodermal dysplasia affecting multiple organ systems. Plexiform neurofibromas are associated with an increased risk of malignant transformation into malignant peripheral nerve sheath tumors. Solitary neurofibromas account for 5% of primary benign soft tissue tumors and 3% of all primary soft tissue tumors. Lesions occur in patients 16 to 66 years of age (mean = 37 years). Neurofibromas can also occur in younger children and older adults. NF1 often presents in childhood.

(continued on page 328)

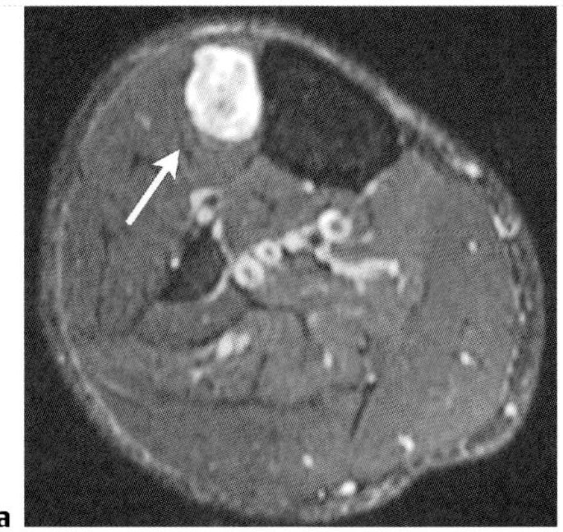

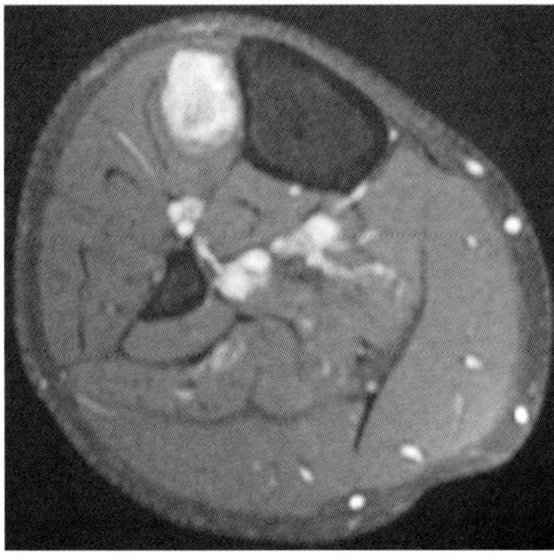

Fig. 10.16 Schwannoma adjacent to the outer surface of the tibia (arrow) as seen on axial fat-suppressed (FS) T2-weighted imaging (a). The lesion shows prominent gadolinium-contrast enhancement on axial FS T1-weighted imaging (b).

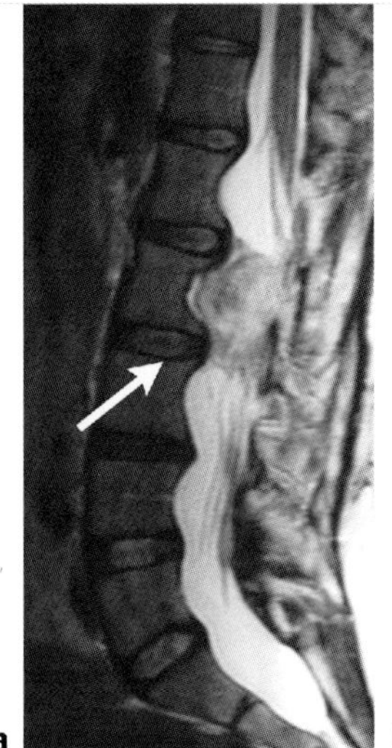

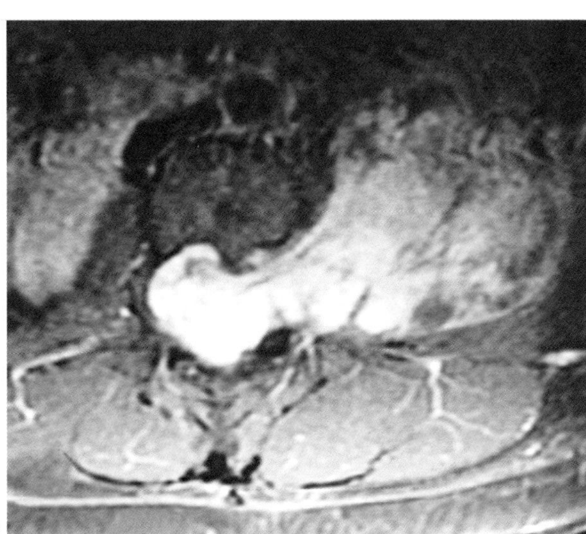

Fig. 10.17 Neurofibroma within the spinal canal at the L2 level resulting in remodeling of the adjacent vertebra (arrow) as seen on sagittal T2-weighted imaging (a) and axial postcontrast fat-suppressed T1-weighted imaging (b).

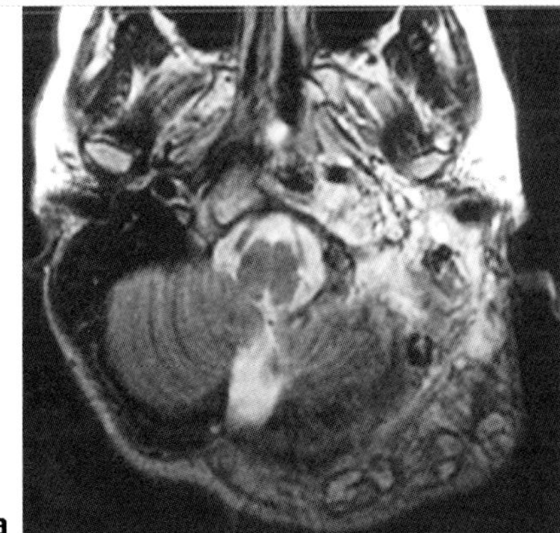

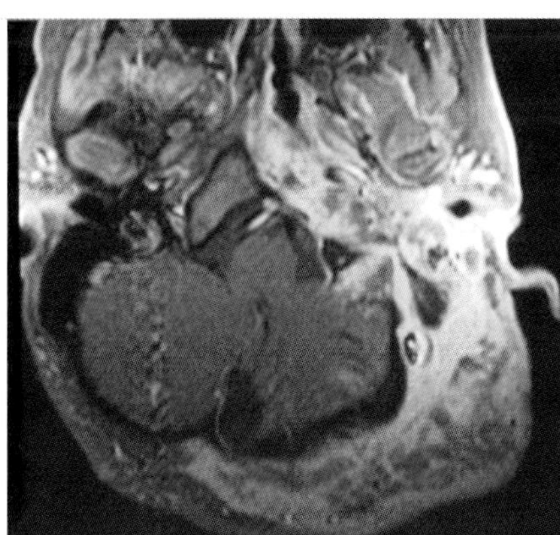

Fig. 10.18 Plexiform neurofibroma in the posterior left scalp and upper neck resulting in remodeling of the occipital bone as seen on axial T2-weighted imaging (a) and axial postcontrast fat-suppressed T1-weighted imaging (b).

Table 10.1 (Cont.) Lesions involving the outer surface of bone

Abnormalities	MRI findings	Comments
Giant cell tumor of tendon sheath (▶ Fig. 10.19)	Lesions usually have well-defined margins and are often adjacent to a tendon/tendon sheath. Lesions can be ovoid or multilobulated and usually have low-intermediate or intermediate signal on T1WI and PDWI that is often similar to or less than that of muscle. On T2WI and FS T2WI, lesions can have mixed low, intermediate, and/or high signal. Zones of low signal on T2WI often correspond to sites of hemosiderin deposition. Lesions often show Gd-contrast enhancement in either a homogeneous or a heterogeneous pattern. Erosions of adjacent bone can be seen with some lesions.	Giant cell tumors of the tendon sheath (also referred to as nodular synovitis) and pigmented villonodular synovitis are benign proliferative lesions of synovium (tendon sheaths, joints, and bursae). Giant cell tumors of the tendon sheaths can occur as localized nodular lesions attached to tendon sheaths outside of joints (hands, feet) or within joints (infrapatellar portion of knee joint); or as a diffuse form near/outside of large joints such as the knee and ankle. Giant cell tumors of the tendon sheath represent 4% of benign soft-tissue tumors and 2% of all soft tissue tumors. Occur in patients age 6 to 71 years, mean = 39 to 46 years with peak ages in third to fourth decades.
Glomus tumor (▶ Fig. 10.20)	Glomus tumors are well-circumscribed ovoid lesions measuring less than 1 cm and are often located under the nail beds at the distal phalanges of fingers and toes. Glomus tumors often have low-intermediate signal on T1WI and PDWI, high signal T2WI and FS T2WI. A thin rim of low signal on T2WI may be seen secondary to a capsule from reactive tissue surrounding the glomus tumor. Lesions typically show Gd-contrast enhancement. MRI can show erosion of the underlying bone.	Benign mesenchymal hamartomas that are composed of round cells derived from the neuromyoarterial apparatus (glomus bodies), which regulate arteriolar blood flow to the skin related to temperature.
Nonmalignant giant cell tumor eroding through bone cortex (▶ Fig. 10.21)	Usually well-defined intraosseous lesions with thin low signal margins on T1WI, PDWI, and T2WI. Solid portions of giant cell tumors often have low to intermediate signal on T1WI and PDWI, intermediate to high signal on T2WI, and high signal on FS PDWI and FS T2WI. Signal heterogeneity on T2WI is not uncommon. Zones of low signal on T2WI and T2*WI imaging may be seen secondary to hemosiderin. Aneurysmal bone cysts can be seen in 14% of giant cell tumors, resulting in cystic zones with variable signal and fluid-fluid levels. After Gd-contrast administration, mild to prominent enhancement of the solid intraosseous portions of the lesions is seen, as well as peripheral rimlike enhancement around cystic zones/aneurysmal bone cysts. Contrast enhancement is usually seen in the extraosseous portions of the tumors. Poorly defined zones of enhancement and high signal on FS T2WI may also be seen in the marrow peripheral to the portions of the lesions associated with radiographic evidence of bone destruction, indicating reactive inflammatory and edematous changes associated with elevated tumor prostaglandin levels.	Aggressive bone tumors composed of neoplastic ovoid mononuclear cells and scattered multinucleated osteoclast-like giant cells (derived from fusion of marrow mononuclear cells). Up to 10% of all giant cell tumors are malignant. Benign giant cell tumors account for approximately 5 to 9.5% of all bone tumors and up to 23% of benign bone tumors. Occurs in patients age 4 to 81 years (median = 30 years), 75% occur in patients between the ages of 15 and 45 years.

(continued on page 330)

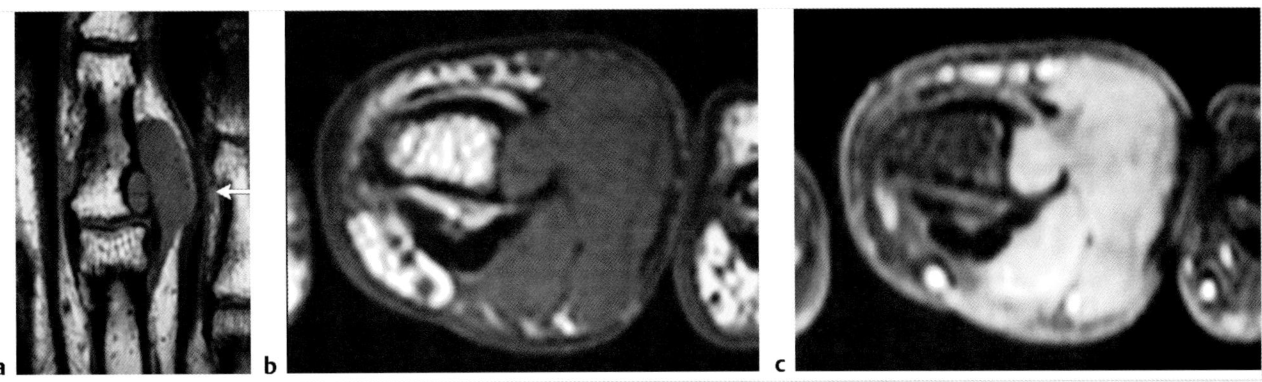

Fig. 10.19 Giant cell tumor of the tendon sheath (nodular synovitis) causing focal erosion of the adjacent phalanx (arrow) as seen on coronal (a) and axial T1-weighted imaging (T1WI) (b) and postcontrast fat-suppressed axial T1WI (c).

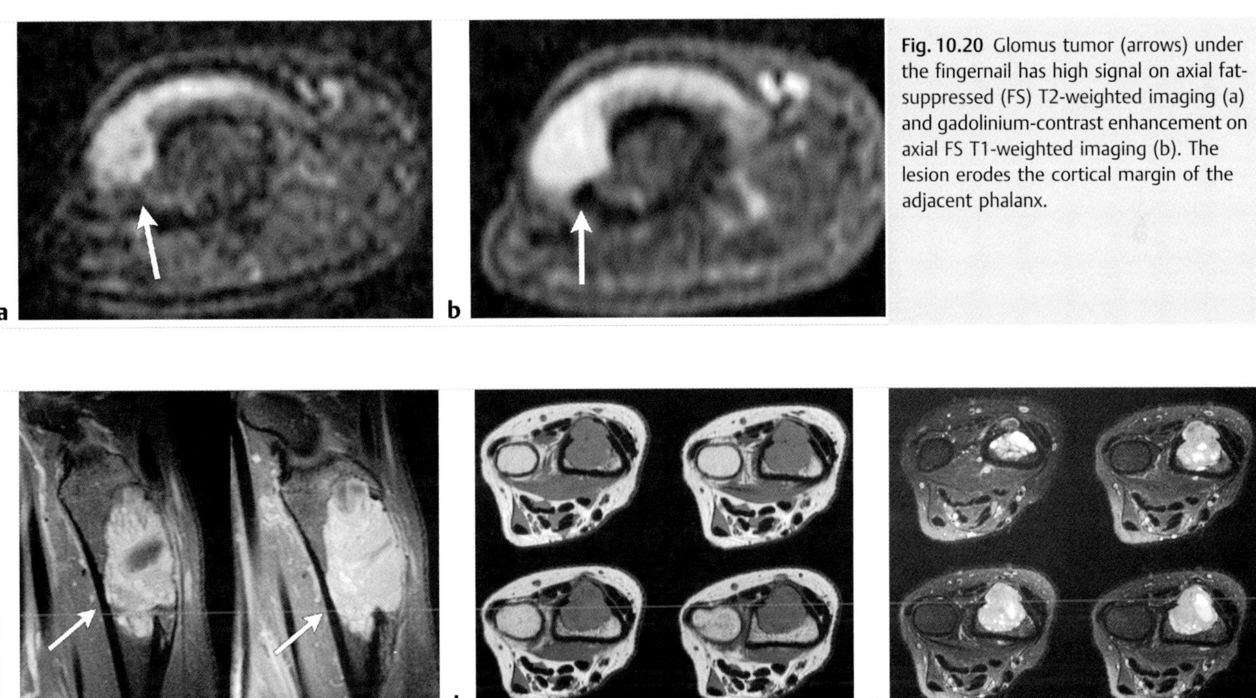

Fig. 10.20 Glomus tumor (arrows) under the fingernail has high signal on axial fat-suppressed (FS) T2-weighted imaging (a) and gadolinium-contrast enhancement on axial FS T1-weighted imaging (b). The lesion erodes the cortical margin of the adjacent phalanx.

Fig. 10.21 Giant cell tumor of bone involving the distal radius. The intramedullary lesion erodes cortical bone and extends into the extraossesous soft tissues (arrows). The lesion shows prominent gadolinium-contrast enhancement on sagittal fat-suppressed T1-weighted imaging (FS T1WI) (a) and has intermediate signal on axial T1WI (b) and high signal on FS T2-weighted imaging (c).

Table 10.1 (Cont.) Lesions involving the outer surface of bone

Abnormalities	MRI findings	Comments
Inflammatory lesions		
Myositis/cellulitis associated with infection of bone (▶ Fig. 10.22)	Irregular poorly defined zones with slightly high to high signal on T2WI and FS T2WI are typically seen with Gd-contrast enhancement. Circumscribed zones with high signal on T2WI and FS T2WI may also be seen with abscess formation.	Infection of soft tissues can result in erosion, destruction, and invasion of adjacent bone.
Osetomyelitis (▶ Fig. 10.23)	Periosteal reaction associated with osteomyelitis is seen as a peripheral rim of high signal on T2WI and FS T2WI and Gd-contrast enhancement on FS T1WI adjacent to the low signal of cortical bone. A periosteal reaction associated with osteomyelitis is seen as a peripheral rim of high signal on T2WI and FS T2WI and Gd-contrast enhancement on FS T1WI adjacent to the low signal of cortical bone. A subperiosteal abscess with high signal on T2WI and FS T2WI can often be seen elevating a single low signal thin band of periosteum. Within the underlying marrow, poorly defined zones with high signal on T2WI and FS T2WI and Gd-contrast enhancement are seen with or without associated zones of cortical destruction.	Osteomyelitis refers to infection of bone and can result from hematogenous spread of micro-organisms, trauma-direct inoculation, extension from adjacent tissues, and complications from surgery. *Staphylococcus aureus* and *Streptococcus pyogenes* are the most common bacterial infections involving bone. Osteomyelitis can also result from other bacteria as well as from tuberculosis, fungi, parasites, and viruses.
Chronic recurrent multifocal osteomyelitis (▶ Fig. 10.24)	Multifocal lesions that occur in metaphyses of tubular bones (distal femur, proximal and distal tibia and fibula), clavicles, and vertebrae. Radiographs show radiolucent and/or sclerotic osseous lesions with proliferative periosteal bone formation. MRI shows heterogeneous abnormal high signal on FS T2WI in marrow and periosteal soft tissues with Gd-contrast enhancement.	Painful inflammatory osseous disorder of unknown cause with histopathology of acute and chronic osteomyelitis without identification of infectious agent, diagnosis of exclusion. Usually occurs in children and adolescents, median age = 10 years, F 85%/M 15%. Multiepisodic skeletal disorder of unknown cause that can occur over 7 to 25 years. Treatment of symptoms with NSAIDS. Can be associated with acne vulgaris or palmoplantaris pustulosis SAPHO (synovitis, acne, pustulosis, hyperostosis, osteitis).
Syndromes of hyperostosis, osteitis, and skin lesions (SAPHO syndrome)	Periosteal elevation with cortical thickening can be seen as well as syndesmophyte formation at one or multiple vertebral levels.	Syndrome that includes abnormalities such as synovitis, acne, pustulosis, hyperostosis with periosteal proliferation (sternum, clavicle, anterior ribs, symphysis pubis, femur, sacrum, iliac bones) and osteitis at the chest wall.

(continued on page 332)

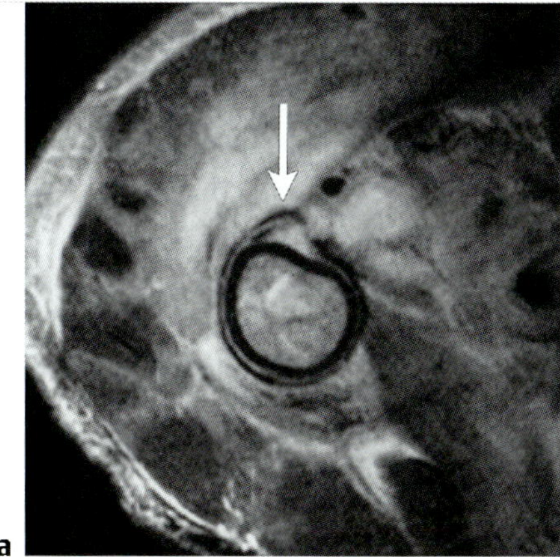
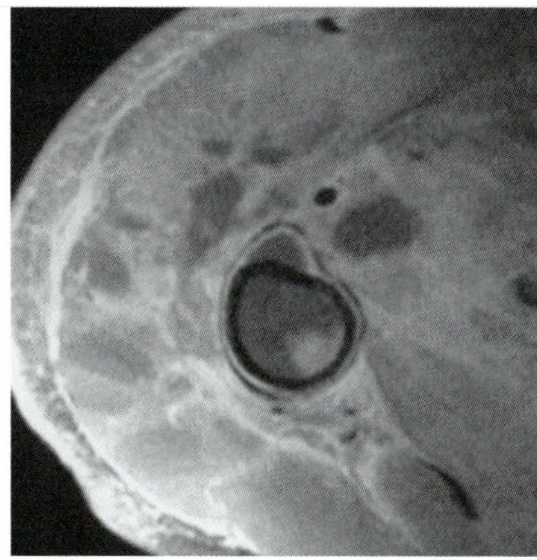

Fig. 10.22 Myositis with abnormal increased signal on T2WI and contrast enhancement of muscles and other soft tissues at the shoulder with erosion of cortical bone, intraosseous extension, periosteal reaction, and subperiosteal abscess (arrow) as seen on axial T2-weighted imaging (a) and postcontrast axial fat-suppressed T1-weighted imaging (b).

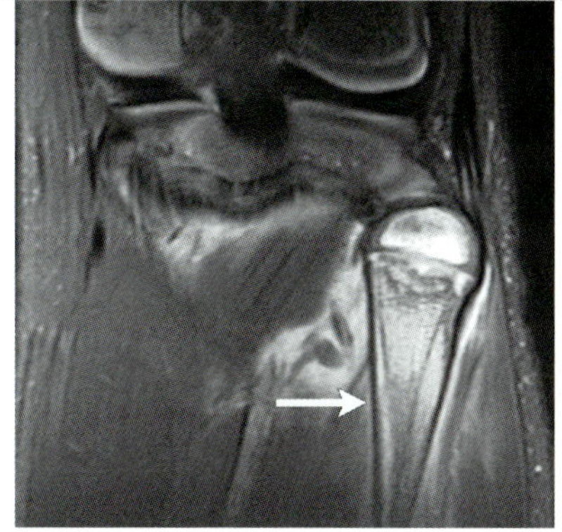
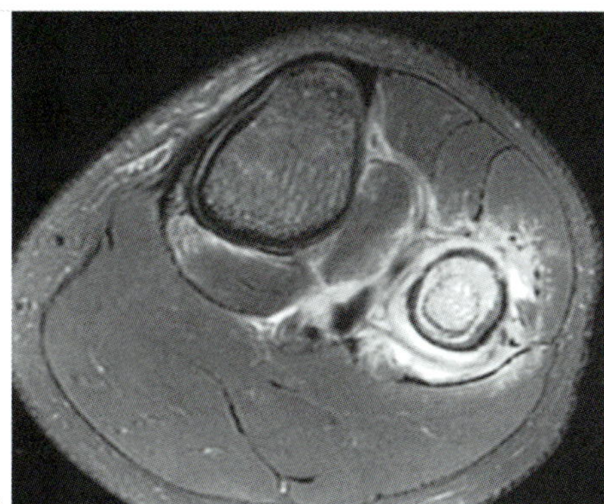

Fig. 10.23 An 11-year-old male with osteomyelitis involving the metadiaphyseal and epiphyseal portions of the proximal fibula. The infection is seen as poorly defined zones of gadolinium-contrast enhancement in the marrow associated with periosteal elevation and poorly defined zones of gadolinium-contrast enhancement in the adjacent soft tissues on coronal (a) and axial fat-suppressed T1-weighted imaging (arrow) (b).

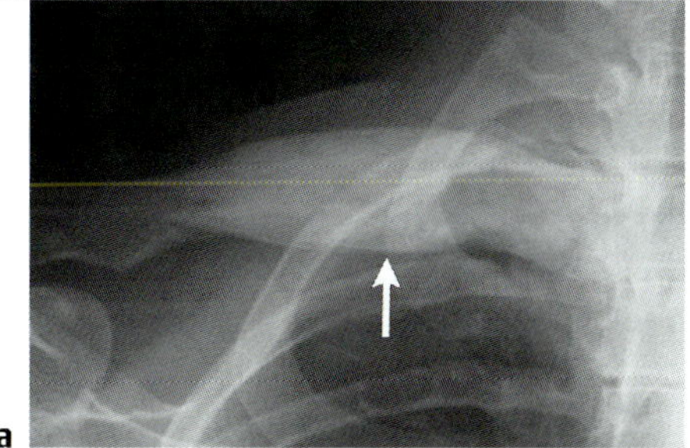
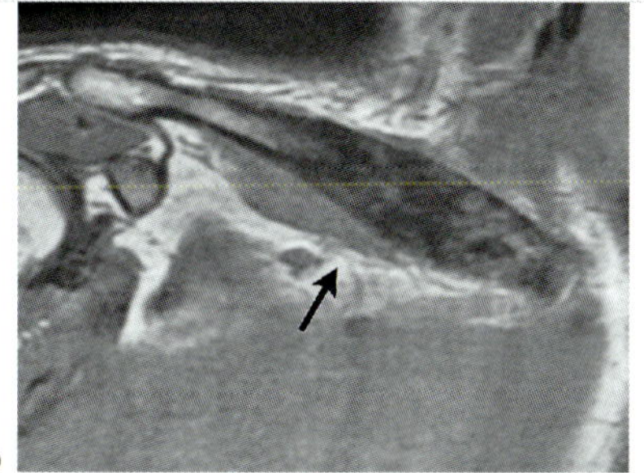
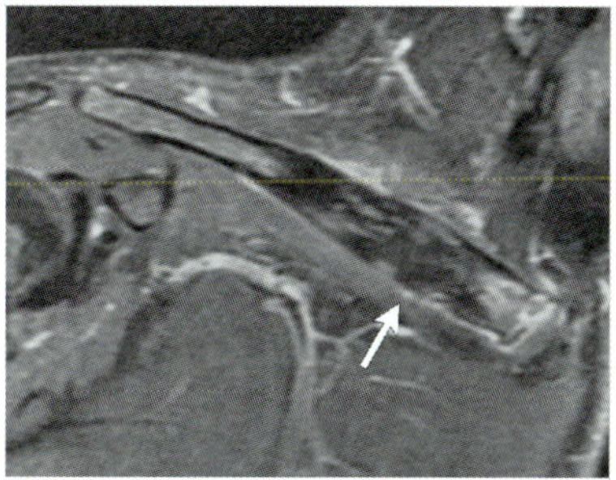

Fig. 10.24 Chronic recurrent multifocal osteomyelitis involving the clavicle. Radiograph shows diffuse cortical thickening (arrow) (a). Heterogeneous low and intermediate signal on T1-weighted imaging (T1WI) (arrow) (b) and heterogenenous gadolinium-contrast enhancement on fat-suppressed T1WI (arrow) (c) are seen involving the cortex and marrow.

Table 10.1 (Cont.) Lesions involving the outer surface of bone

Abnormalities	MRI findings	Comments
Eosinophilic granuloma eroding through bone cortex (▶ Fig. 10.25)	Focal intramedullary lesion(s) associated with trabecular and cortical bone destruction, which typically have low-intermediate signal on T1WI and PDWI; and heterogeneous slightly high to high signal on T2WI. Poorly defined zones of high signal on T2WI are usually seen in the marrow peripheral to the portions of the lesions associated with radiographic evidence of bone destruction, indicating reactive inflammatory and edematous changes. Extension of lesions from the marrow into adjacent soft tissues through areas of cortical disruption are commonly seen as well as linear periosteal zones of high signal on T2WI. Lesions typically show prominent Gd-contrast enhancement in marrow and in extraosseous soft tissue portions of the lesions.	Single or multiple eosinophilic granulomas are benign tumor-like lesions consisting of Langerhans cells (histiocytes) and variable amounts of lymphocytes, polymorphonuclear cells, and eosinophils. Account for 1% of primary bone lesions and 8% of tumor-like lesions, 5 to 20 per 1,000,000 children per year in the United States. Occurs in patients age 1 to 60 years, median = 10 years, average = 13.5 years, peak incidence is between 5 and 10 years, 80 to 85% occur in patients less than 30 years, and 60% occur in children less than 10 years.
Rheumatoid pannus adjacent to and eroding bone (▶ Fig. 10.26)	Erosions of intra-articular bone vertebral endplates, spinous processes, and uncovertebral and apophyseal joints. Irregular enlarged enhancing synovium (pannus low-intermediate signal on T1WI, intermediate-high signal on T2WI and FS T2WI) in joints and at atlanto-dens articulation results in erosions of dens and transverse ligament, ± destruction of transverse ligament with C1 on C2 subluxation and neural compromise.	Most common type of inflammatory arthropathy, which results in synovitis causing destructive/erosive changes of cartilage, ligaments, and bone. Cervical spine involvement in two thirds of patients, juvenile and adult types.

(continued on page 334)

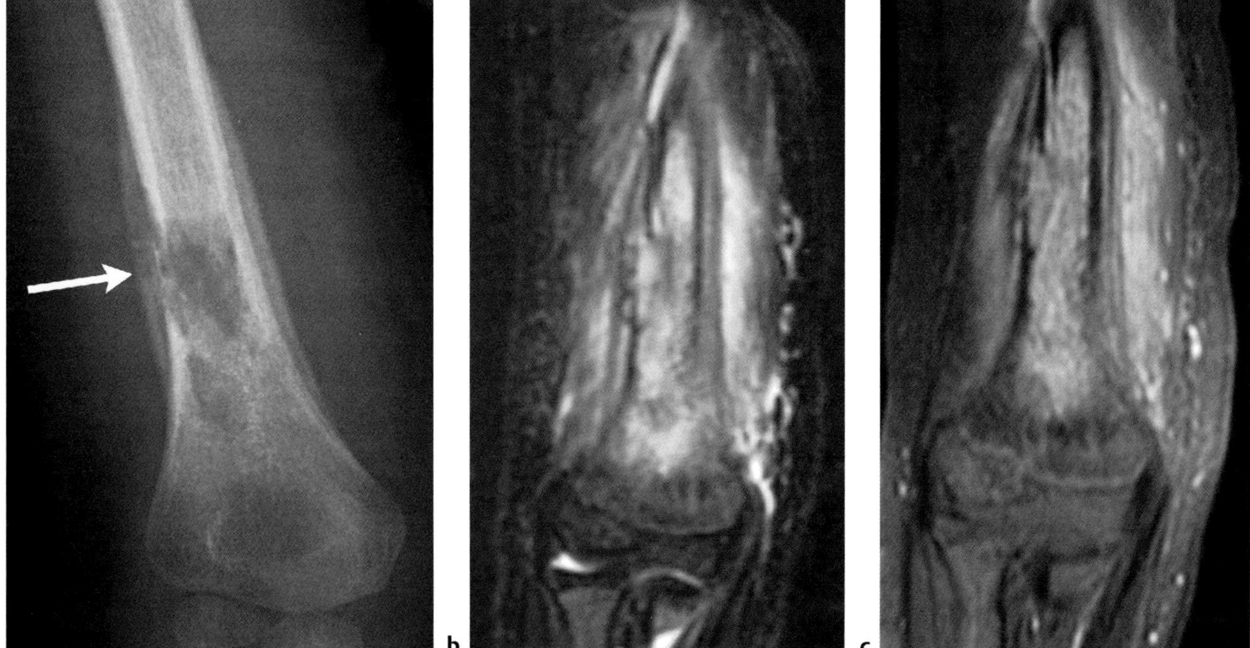

Fig. 10.25 Eosinophilic granuloma involving the distal humerus in a 5-year-old boy. Anteroposterior radiograph shows a radiolucent intramedullary lesion with irregular margins, cortical disruption, and single layer of smooth periosteal reaction (a). A zone of disruption of the periosteum is seen laterally at the radial aspect (arrow). Magnetic resonance imaging shows an intramedullary poorly defined lesion with heterogeneous slightly high to high signal on coronal fat-suppressed T2-weighted imaging (FS T2WI) (b) and corresponding gadolinium-contrast enhancement on coronal FS T1-weighted imaging (c). Extension of the lesion from the marrow into adjacent soft tissues is seen through areas of cortical disruption. Zones of high signal on FS T2WI and gadolinium-contrast enhancement are seen superficial and deep to the elevated periosteum, which is seen as a linear zone of low signal.

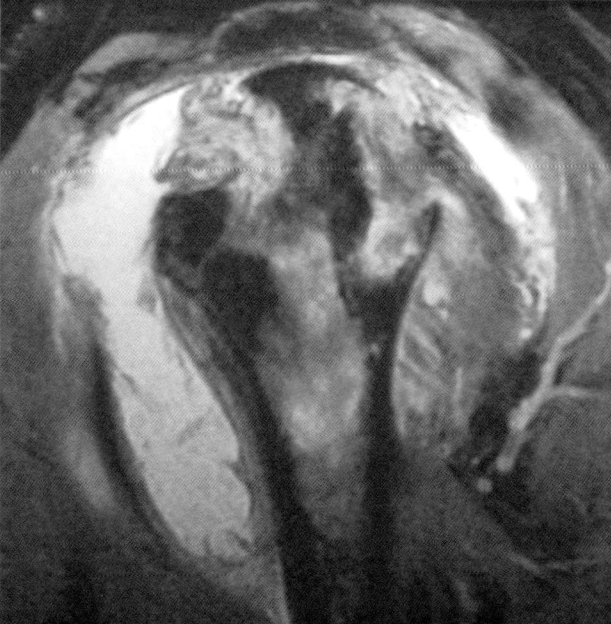

Fig. 10.26 Rheumatoid arthritis at the shoulder with pannus eroding the humerus as seen on sagittal fat-suppressed T2-weighted imaging. Pannus is seen as poorly defined thickened synovium with mixed intermediate, slightly high and low signal. A large joint fluid collection is also present.

Table 10.1 (Cont.) Lesions involving the outer surface of bone

Abnormalities	MRI findings	Comments
Gout (▶ Fig. 10.27)	Tophi have variable sizes and shapes and often have low-intermediate signal on T1WI, FS T2WI, and T2WI. Zones of high signal on T2WI can be seen secondary to regions with increased hydration and proteinaceous zones associated with the deposits of urate crystals. Erosions of bone, synovial pannus, joint effusion, bone marrow and soft tissue edema can be seen with MRI. Tophi may be associated with heterogeneous, diffuse, or peripheral/marginal Gd-contrast enhancement patterns. Contrast enhancement seen with tophi is likely secondary to the hypervascular granulation tissue and reactive inflammatory cells in the synovium and/or adjacent soft tissues.	Inflammatory disease involving synovium resulting from deposition of monosodium urate crystals when serum urate levels exceed its solubility (7 mg/dL in men and 6 mg/dL in women) in various tissues and body fluids. Can be a primary disorder (inherited metabolic defects in purine metabolism or abnormal renal tubular secretion of urate) or secondary disorder (alcohol or medications such as thiazide diuretics, salicylates, cyclosporine) that results from diminished renal excretion of uric acid salts, or from increased metabolic turnover of nucleic acids associated with malignancy, chemotherapy, endocrine, vascular, and/or myeloproliferative diseases. Prevalence of gout ranges from 0.5% to 2.8% of men and between 0.1 to 0.6% of women in the United States. Accounts for 5% of arthritis cases. Usually occurs in middle-aged and elderly patients.
Pigmented villonodular synovitis (PVNS) (▶ Fig. 10.28)	Often appears as irregular, multinodular, and/or irregular thickening of synovium with low or low-intermediate signal on T1WI and T2WI. Solitary nodular lesions can also occur. Areas of low signal on T2WI and T2*WI in lesions are secondary to hemosiderin. Joint effusions are usually present, rarely with fluid-fluid levels. PVNS usually shows Gd-contrast enhancement in homogeneous, heterogeneous, and/or septal patterns.	Benign intra-articular lesions of proliferative synovium containing zones of recent or remote hemorrhage. Similar histopathologic features with giant cell tumors of the tendon sheath. Account for < 1% of benign and all soft-tissue tumors. Mean age = 38 years, median age = 32 years.

(continued on page 336)

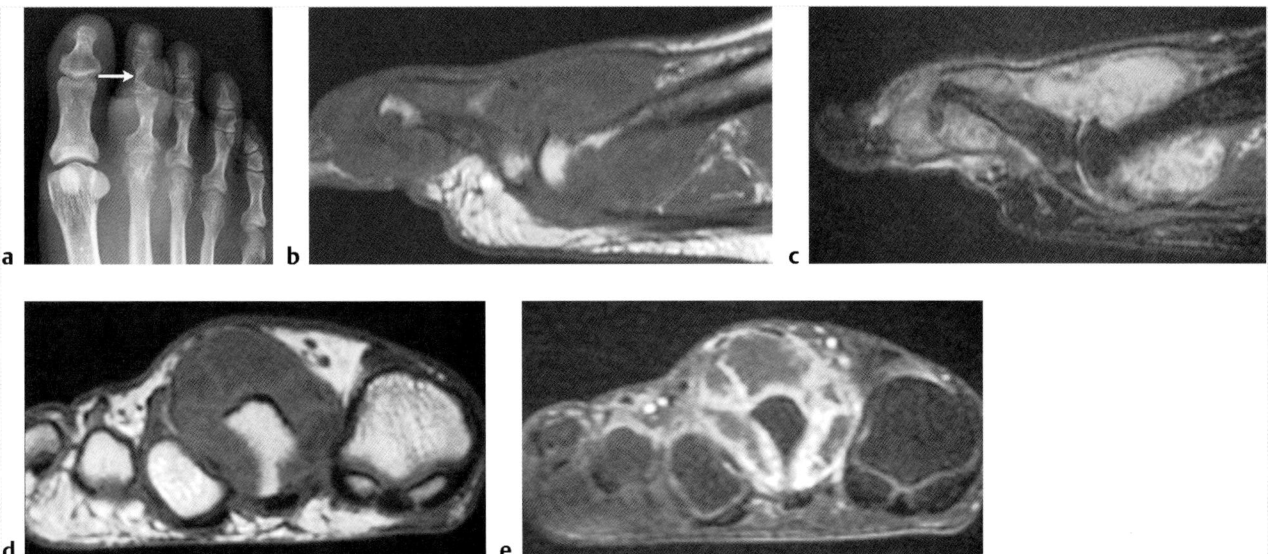

Fig. 10.27 Gout involving a metatarsal–phalangeal joint. Osseous erosions (arrow) are seen on a radiograph (a) from tophi, which have intermediate signal on sagittal (b) and axial T1-weighted imaging (d), heterogeneous intermediate-slightly high and high signal on fat-suppressed (FS) T2-weighted imaging (c). Only peripheral irregular gadolinium-contrast enhancement is seen on coronal FS T1-weighted imaging (e).

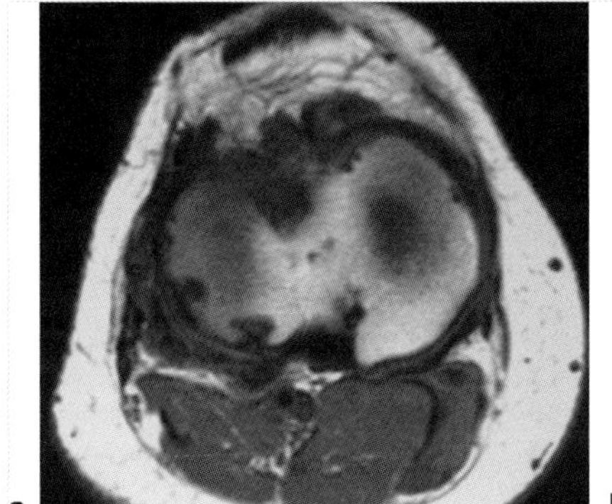

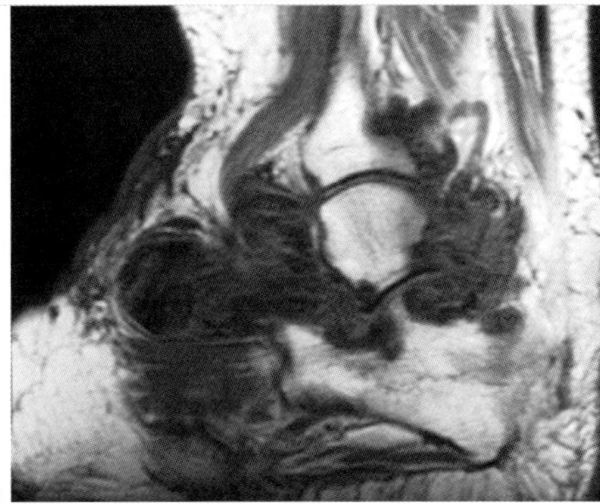

Fig. 10.28 Pigmented villonodular synovitis associated with focal erosions of the tibia on axial T1-weighted imaging (T1WI) (a) in one patient and involving the talus and calcaneus in another on sagittal T1WI (b).

Table 10.1 (Cont.) Lesions involving the outer surface of bone

Abnormalities	MRI findings	Comments
Calcific tendinitis eroding into bone (▶ Fig. 10.29)	Zones with slightly high and low signal on T2WI and FS T2WI are seen in tendons with or without erosion of bone cortex. Intramedullary zones with mixed low, intermediate, and/or high signal on T2WI and FS T2WI may be seen in the adjacent marrow.	Degenerative disorder with amorphous calcificatons in tendons or bursa associated with erosion of adjacent bone cortex, with or without marrow invasion. Most common in humerus and femur in patients 16 to 82 years, average = 50 years.
Abnormalities involving the periosteum		
Noninterrupted periosteal reaction from fracture (▶ Fig. 10.30)	Noninterrupted periosteal reaction from stress fractures and healing traumatic fractures typically appears as a linear thin single 1- to 2-mm band of low signal superficial to bone cortex, which is surrounded by poorlydefined zones with high signal on FS T2WI and Gd-contrast enhancement. Poorly defined intramedullary zones with high signal on FS T2WI and Gd-contrast enhancement are usually seen in the underlying bone marrow. A thin linear radiodense line is seen at the elevated periosteum 7 to 10 days later.	Forty-eight hours after fracture, extravascular red blood cells lyse causing an intense inflammatory reaction followed by granulation tissue in-growth. Periosteal reaction occurs when fibroblasts are induced to form osteoblasts in the outer periosteal layer secondary to trauma. Periosteal reaction occurs earlier in children compared with adults.
Subperiosteal hematoma (▶ Fig. 10.31)	Low signal thin bands of periosteum separated from underlying bone cortex can be seen surrounded by irregular zones with intermediate to high signal on T2WI and FS T2WI, and irregular Gd-contrast enhancement.	Subperiosteal hematomas can result from bone fractures or avulsion of periosteum near sites of tendinous insertions.

(continued on page 338)

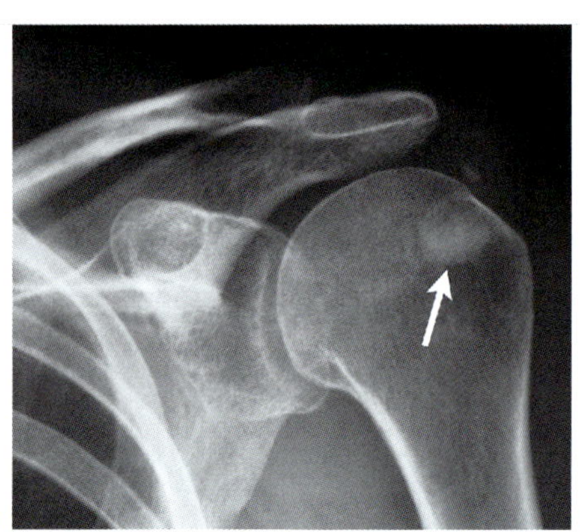
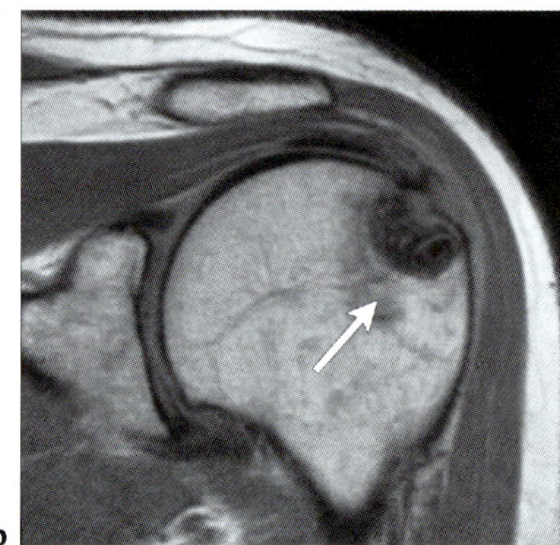
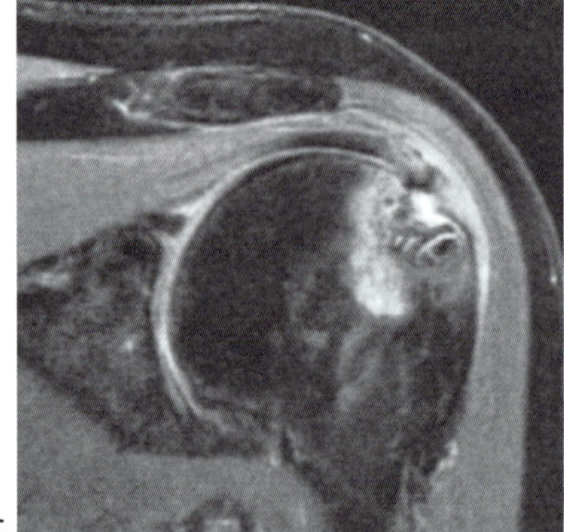
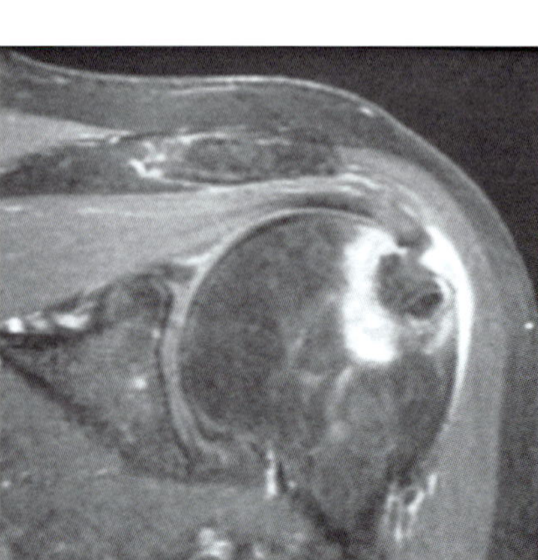

Fig. 10.29 Calcific tendonitis of the supraspinatus eroding into the humerus. Anteroposterior radiograph (a) shows calcifications in the supraspinatus tendon and within the humerus (arrow). Zones with low signal (arrow) on coronal T1-weighted imaging (T1WI) (b) and heterogeneous low, intermediate, and high signal on coronal fat-suppressed T2-weighted imaging (FS T2WI) (c) are seen in the supraspinatus tendon associated with erosion of bone cortex and intramedullary extension. Intramedullary zones with mixed low, intermediate, and/or high signal on FS T2WI are seen in the marrow. Poorly defined zones of gadolinium-contrast enhancement are seen in the marrow and tendon on coronal FS T1WI (d).

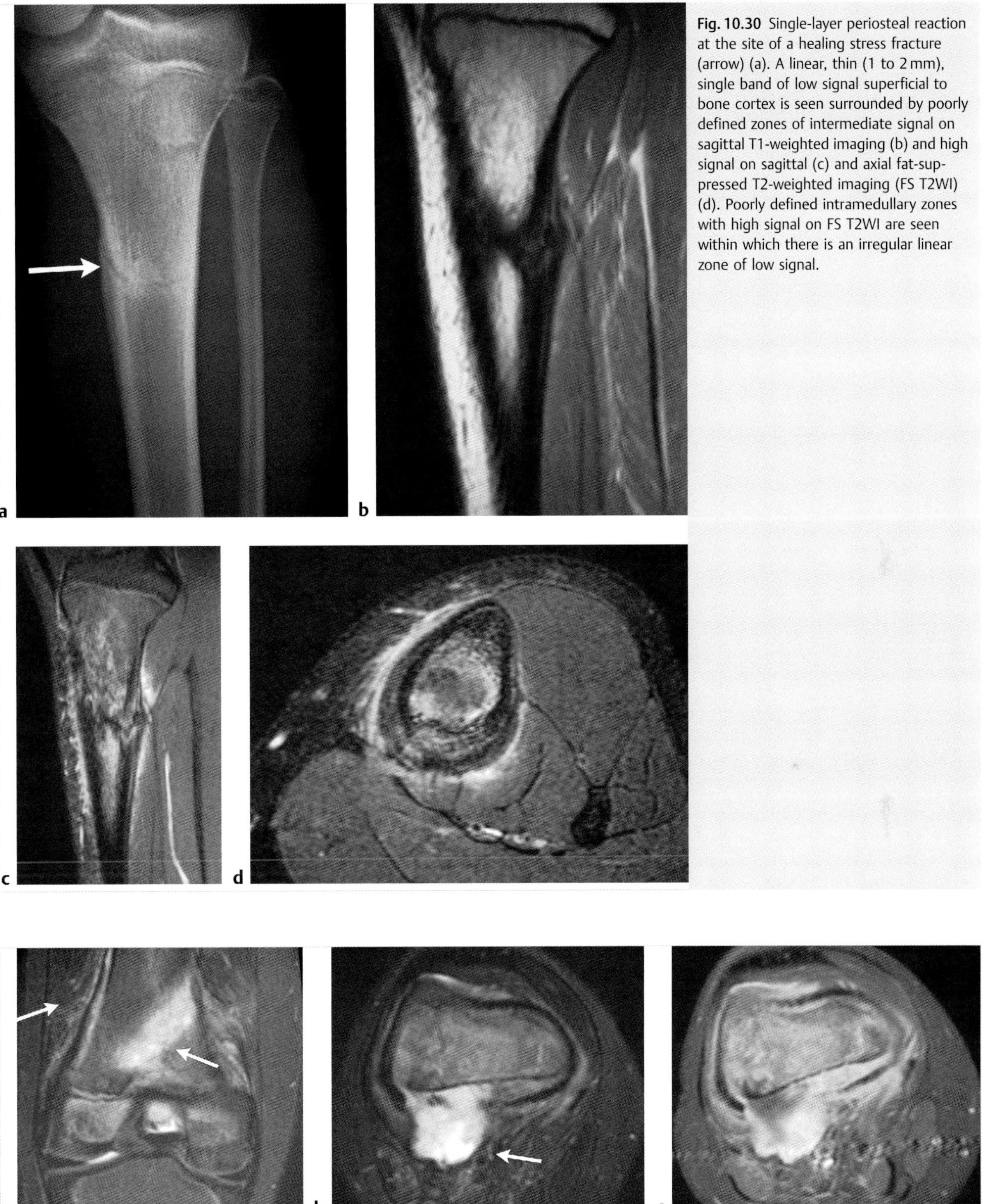

Fig. 10.30 Single-layer periosteal reaction at the site of a healing stress fracture (arrow) (a). A linear, thin (1 to 2 mm), single band of low signal superficial to bone cortex is seen surrounded by poorly defined zones of intermediate signal on sagittal T1-weighted imaging (b) and high signal on sagittal (c) and axial fat-suppressed T2-weighted imaging (FS T2WI) (d). Poorly defined intramedullary zones with high signal on FS T2WI are seen within which there is an irregular linear zone of low signal.

Fig. 10.31 Traumatic fracture of the distal femur with periosteal elevation and subperiosteal hematoma (arrows) as seen on coronal (a) and axial fat-suppressed T2-weighted imaging (FS T2WI) (b). Focal disruption of the periosteum is also seen dorsally on axial FS T2WI and axial post-gadolinium-contrast FS T1-weighted imaging (c).

Table 10.1 (Cont.) Lesions involving the outer surface of bone

Abnormalities	MRI findings	Comments
Hemophilic pseudotumor	Subperiosteal pseudotumors elevate the perisoteum from hemorrhage associated with cortical erosion and periosteal reaction. Lesions usually have mixed low, intermediate and high signal on T1WI and T2WI, as well as fluid-fluid levels.	Lesions can occur within medullary bone or in a subperiosteal location, as well as within soft tissues in 1 to 2% of patients with severe factor VIII or IX deficiency. Enlarging lesions may require surgical resection.
Noninterrupted periosteal reaction from primary hypertrophic osteoarthropathy (pachydermoperiostosis)	Linear and/or irregular periosteal and cortical thickening seen in tubular bones of the extremities bilaterally (tibia, fibula, radius, ulna are common sites, also seen in other bones and skull). Can involve epiphyseal, metaphyseal, and/or diaphyseal portions of long bones.	Rare clinical syndrome in adolescents or adults with swollen painful joints, enlargement of the extremities from osseous proliferation and periostitis, clubbing of digits, thickening of skin of the face and scalp with excessive sweating and sebaceous secretions. Can be hereditary (autosomal dominant with variable expression) or idiopathic.
Noninterrupted periosteal reaction from secondary hypertrophic osteoarthropathy (▶ Fig. 10.32)	Smooth, wavy, and or irregular periosteal and cortical thickening seen in the diaphyseal and metaphyseal portions of long bones of the upper and lower extremities, as well as in other bones.	Clinical syndrome with clubbing of the digits, periostitis, hypertrophic osteoarthropathy, skin thickening, limb swelling, nail bed abnormalities (striations, increased curvature) related to extraskeletal lesions involving the lungs (bronchogenic carcinoma, metastasis, cystic fibrosis, bronchiectasis, infection, lymphoma), pleura (mesothelioma), abdomen (biliary atresia, cirrhosis, tumors, ulcerative colitis, Crohn disease), heart (cyanotic heart disease), and neoplasms at other sites. Regression of hypertrophic osteoarthropathy can occur after thoracotomy in patients with thoracic abnormalities, even in those without complete removal of the intrathoracic lesions.
Noninterrupted periosteal reaction from venous stasis (▶ Fig. 10.33)	Smooth and wavy periosteal and cortical thickening seen in the diaphyseal and metaphyseal portions of long bones of the lower extremities (tibia, fibula, metatarsal bones, phalanges).	Venous stasis is associated with edematous changes in the soft tissues as well as soft tissue ossification, periostitis, and cortical thickening.
Noninterrupted periosteal reaction from infantile cortical hyperostosis (Caffey disease)	Smooth, wavy, and/or irregular periosteal and cortical thickening seen in the diaphyseal and metaphyseal portions of one or multiple bones.	Clinical disorder that affects infants less than 5 months with findings of soft tissue swelling (commonly over the mandible), fever, hyperirritability, and cortical hyperostosis (ribs, ulna, tibia, fibula, humerus, femur, radius, metacarpal and metatarsal bones). The clinical course is variable, but regression of findings can occur over 3 to 4 years.
Noninterrupted periosteal reaction from thyroid acropachy	Asymmetric, irregular, spiculated periosteal thickening seen in the diaphyseal portions of one or multiple bones (metacarpal and metatarsal bones, phalanges, other bones).	This disorder represents an extreme form of autoimmune thyroid disease with clinical manifestations such as swelling of the digits and toes, digital clubbing, and periosteal reaction. Thyroid dermopathy (pretibial myxedema) occurs in 4% of patients with Graves ophthalmopathy. Pronounced cases of thyroid dermopathy can be associated with thyroid acropachy in 1% of patients with Graves opthalmopathy.
Progressive diaphyseal dysplasia (Camurati-Engelmann disease)	Bilateral symmetric thickening of bone cortex (both periosteal and endosteal surfaces) of the diaphyseal portions of long bones (sites of membranous bone formation). The metadiaphyseal portions of long bones are typically not involved because endochondral bone formation occurs in these portions.	Autosomal dominant disorder with abnormal intramembranous (periosteal) bone formation. Mutations involve premature activation of the transforming growth factor-beta 1 (TGF-beta1) gene, which results in hyperostosis involving the periosteal and endosteal portions of long bones.

(continued on page 340)

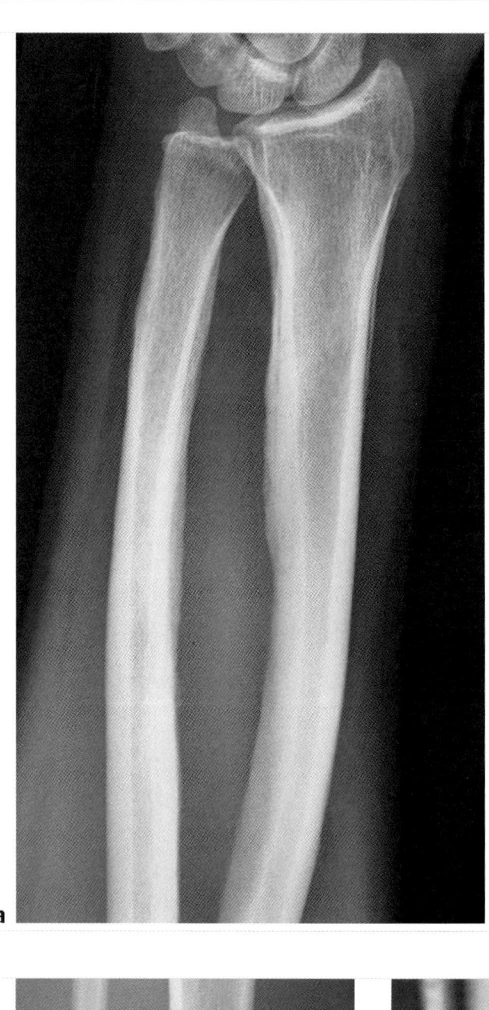

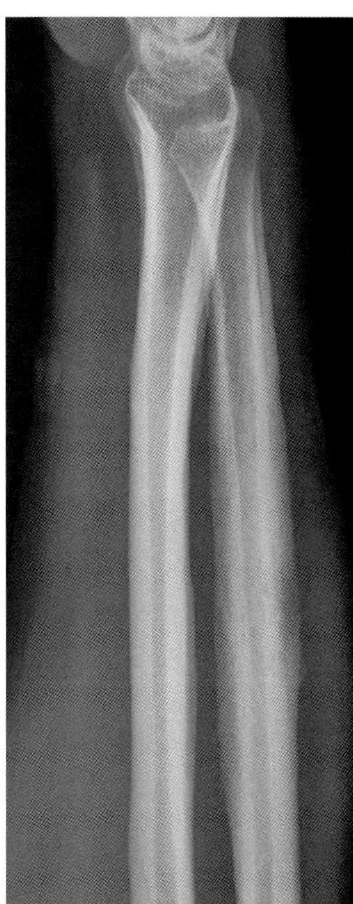

Fig. 10.32 Secondary hypertrophic osteoarthropathy in a 58-year-old man with lung cancer. Anteroposterior (a) and oblique (b) radiographs show smooth, wavy periosteal and cortical thickening involving the diaphyseal and metaphyseal portions of the radius and ulna.

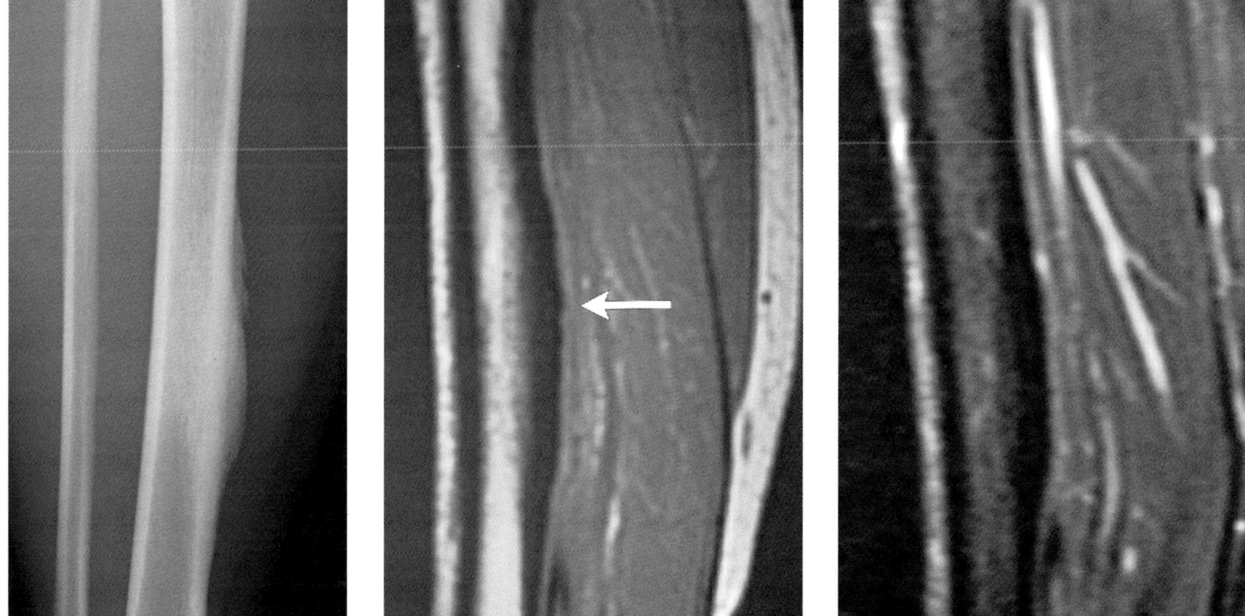

Fig. 10.33 Thickened noninterrupted periosteal reaction from venous stasis as seen on oblique radiograph (a). The periosteal bone formation has low signal (arrow) on sagittal T1-weighted imaging (T1WI) (b) and postcontrast fat-suppressed T1WI (c).

Table 10.1 (Cont.) Lesions involving the outer surface of bone

Abnormalities	MRI findings	Comments
Noninterrupted periosteal reaction from hypervitaminosis A	Smooth and wavy periosteal and cortical thickening seen in the diaphyseal portions of one or multiple bones (ulna, metatarsal bones, clavicle, tibia, fibula, other bones). Damage to the physeal plates can result in irregularities and premature fusion, as well as splaying and cupping deformities of the metaphyses. Smooth and wavy periosteal and cortical thickening seen in the diaphyseal portions of one or multiple bones.	Vitamin A intoxication in children can result in anorexia and dermatologic and osseous disorders. In children, damage to the physeal plates may be irreversible despite cessation of Vitamin A administration. In adults, anorexia, weight loss, and dermatologic disorders are frequently associated with hypervitaminosis A. Vitamin A deficiency can result in anemia, dermatologic (dry and scaly skin), growth retardation, osseous abnormalities, cranial nerve and visual disorders.
Periosteal reaction from hypovitaminosis C (scurvy)	In children, periosteal elevation with new bone formation can be seen in the diaphyseal and metaphyseal portions of one or multiple bones from subperiosteal hemorrhage. Metaphyseal beaklike bone protrusions can occur from the abnormal zones of provisional calcification at the physeal plate, as well as subepiphyseal fractures. In adults, osteopenia with hemarthrosis can be associated with ischemic necrosis and fractures with mild periosteal reaction.	In young children, vitamin C deficiency after 4 to 10 months can result in infantile scurvy with clinical features including failure to thrive, petechial hemorrhages, ulcerated gingiva, hematemesis, melena, hematuria, and anemia. Clinical features associated with adult scurvy include anorexia, fatigue, weakness, petechial hemorrhages involving gingiva and skin, hemarthrosis, osteoporosis, ischemic necrosis, dermatologic disorders (dry and scaly skin), growth retardation, osseous and nerve disorders.
Neurofibromatosis type 1 (▶ Fig. 10.34)	Undulating zones of periosteal bone formation can occur in the lower extremities in patients with NF1.	One of the most common genetic diseases with the involved locus on chromosome 17q12 typically resulting in multiple neurofibromas This autosomal dominant disorder results in mesodermal dysplasia affecting multiple organ systems. Can result in periosteal proliferation in the long bones of the lower extremities.
Periostitis associated with acute/subacute bone infarction (▶ Fig. 10.35)	Acute and subacute bone infarcts typically show intramedullary zones with low-intermediate signal on T1WI and slightly high to high signal on FS T2WI, often with heterogeneous Gd-contrast enhancement. Elevation of the periosteum surrounded by increased signal on FS T2WI and Gd-contrast enhancement on FS T1WI can also occur from associated periostitis.	Acute and subacute intramedullary bone infarcts can be associated with a periostitis that can be seen on MRI.

(continued on page 342)

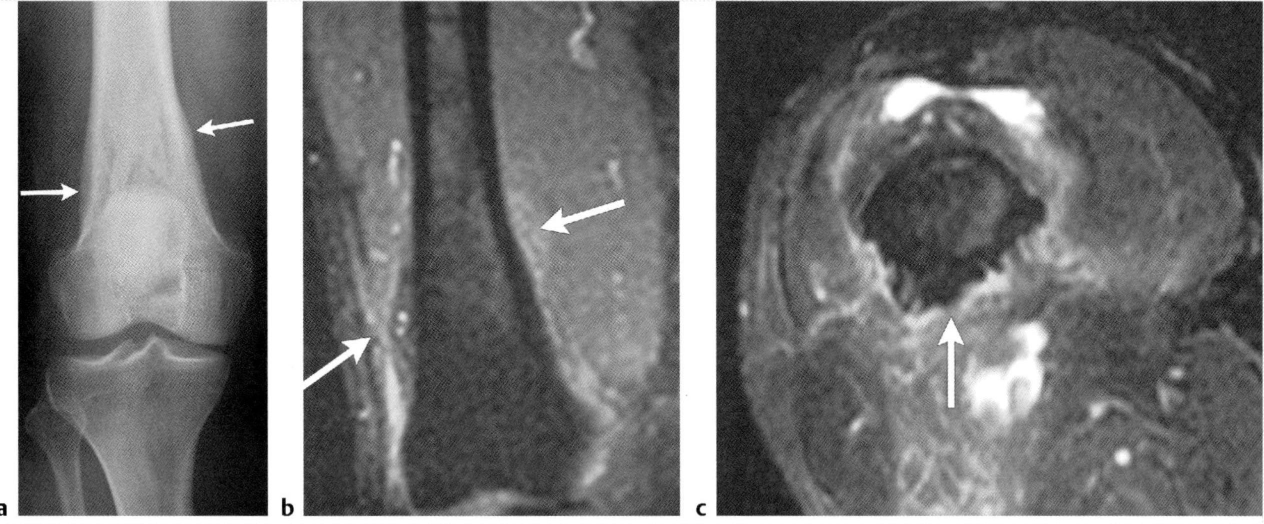

Fig. 10.34 Thickened irregular noninterrupted periosteal reaction (arrows) in a patient with neurofibromatosis type 1 as seen on anteroposterior radiograph (a). The periosteal bone formation has low signal (arrows) on coronal (b) and axial fat-suppressed T2-weighted imaging (c).

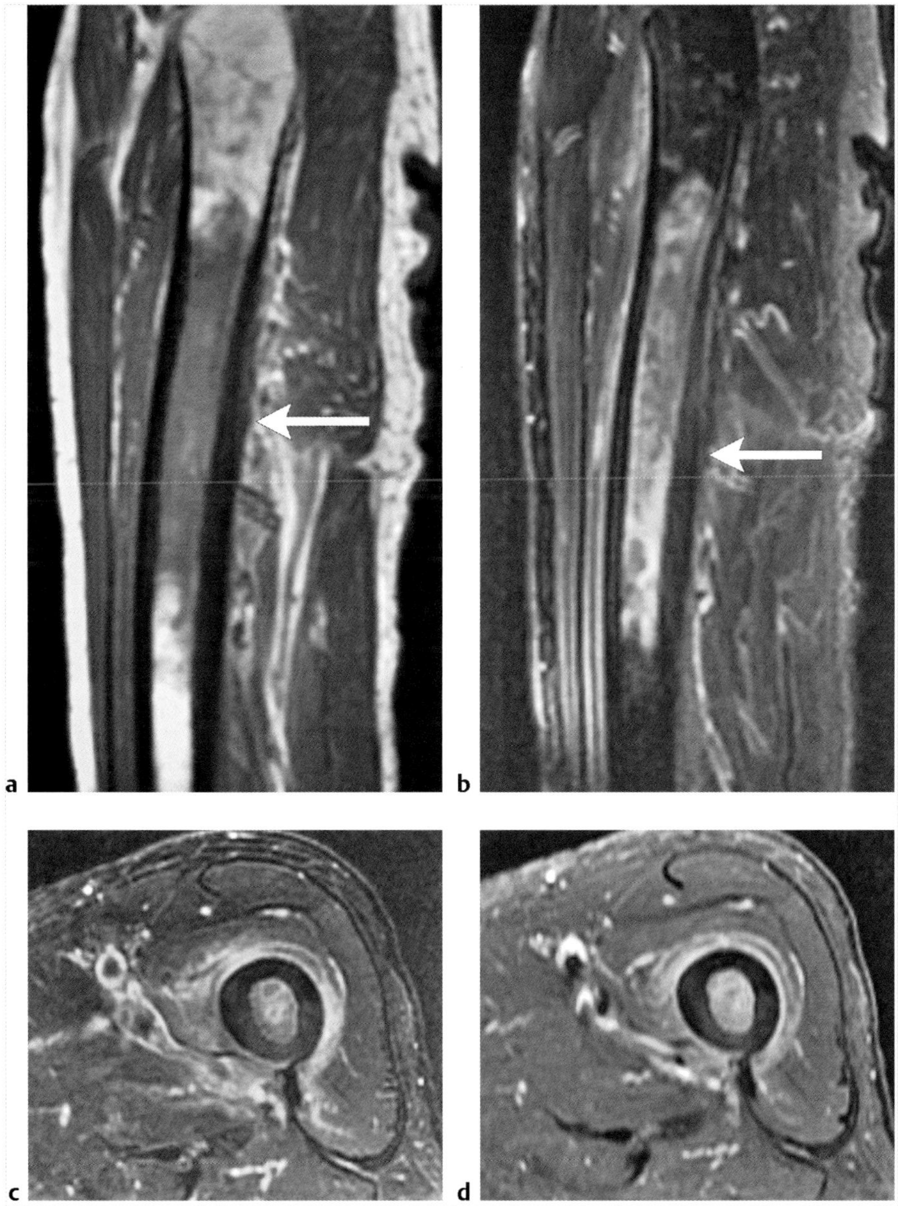

Fig. 10.35 Subacute bone infarct involving the diaphyseal marrow of the femur. The involved marrow (arrows) has heterogeneous intermediate signal on sagittal T1-weighted imaging (T1WI) (a), heterogeneous slightly high and high signal on sagittal (b) and axial fat-suppressed T2-weighted imaging (FS T2WI) (c), and shows gadolinium-contrast enhancement on axial FS T1WI (d). A thin linear zone with low signal is seen superficial to the cortex representing elevated periosteum, which is surrounded by zones of Gd-contrast enhancement and high signal on FS T2WI.

Table 10.1 (Cont.) Lesions involving the outer surface of bone

Abnormalities	MRI findings	Comments
Malignant lesions		
Parosteal osteosarcoma (▶ Fig. 10.36)	Tumors occur at the surface of bone and extend outward with well-defined and/or indistinct margins. Tumors typically have mixed soft tissue and mineralized components. The mineralized portions of these tumors usually have low signal on T1WI, PDWI, T2WI, and FS PDWI and FS T2WI. The soft tissue portions of these tumors often have low-intermediate signal on T1WI, intermediate to slightly high or high signal on T2WI, and high signal on FS PDWI and FS T2WI. Areas of hemorrhage, cystic change, and/or necrosis with or without associated fluid-fluid levels may be present. Tumor extension into the medullary space can be seen in up to 50%. Nonnecrotic or nonmineralized soft tissue portions of these tumors with Gd-contrast usually show enhancement as well as sites of invasion into the medullary space and adjacent soft tissues.	Malignant tumor composed of proliferating neoplastic spindle cells, which produce osteoid and/or immature tumoral bone. Parosteal osteosarcomas arise on the external surface of bone and account for 4 to 6% of osteosarcomas, occur in patients age 6 to 80 years, median = 27 years.
Periosteal osteosarcoma (▶ Fig. 10.37)	Tumors usually involve the diaphyseal regions (femur > tibia > humerus > other bones) with associated cortical thickening manifest as low signal on T1WI and T2WI. Tumors often have a broad base along the outer cortex extending outward toward the adjacent soft tissues. Periosteal reaction, seen as linear zones of low signal on T1WI and T2WI, can be associated with these tumors, as well as Codman triangles). Tumors often have low-intermediate signal on T1WI and heterogeneous slightly high to high signal on T2WI and FS T2WI. Tumor extension into the marrow is uncommon, and when present is usually seen associated with a zone of cortical destruction.	Malignant tumor composed of proliferating neoplastic spindle cells, which produce osteoid and/or immature tumoral bone. Periosteal osteosarcoma has been proposed to represent a variant of parosteal osteogenic sarcoma, which contains cartilaginous zones. Account for 1 to 2% of osteosarcomas, occur in patients age 11 to 57 years, median = 17 to 24 years.
Chondrosarcoma (▶ Fig. 10.38)	MRI can easily demonstrate the thickness of cartilaginous caps of osteochondromas as well as erosive and/or destructive changes involving osteochondromas. Cartilage cap thickness exceeding 2 cm is commonly associated with malignant degeneration or dedifferentiation of osteochondromas into secondary chondrosarcomas. Secondary chondrosarcomas from osteochondromas and periosteal chondrosarcomas have low-intermediate signal on T1WI, intermediate signal on PDWI, and heterogeneous intermediate-high signal on T2WI. Lesions show heterogeneous contrast enhancement, with or without Gd-contrast enhancement of adjacent soft tissues suggesting tumor invasion.	Malignant tumors containing cartilage formed within sarcomatous stroma. Primary chondrosarcomas represent neoplasms that occur without preexistent lesions, whereas secondary chondrosarcomas arise from formerly benign cartilaginous lesions. Periosteal chondrosarcomas are rare malignant cartilage tumors that occur on the surface of bone. Account for 12 to 21% of malignant bone lesions, 21 to 26% of primary sarcomas of bone, 5 to 91 years, mean = 40, median = 26 to 59 years.

(continued on page 344)

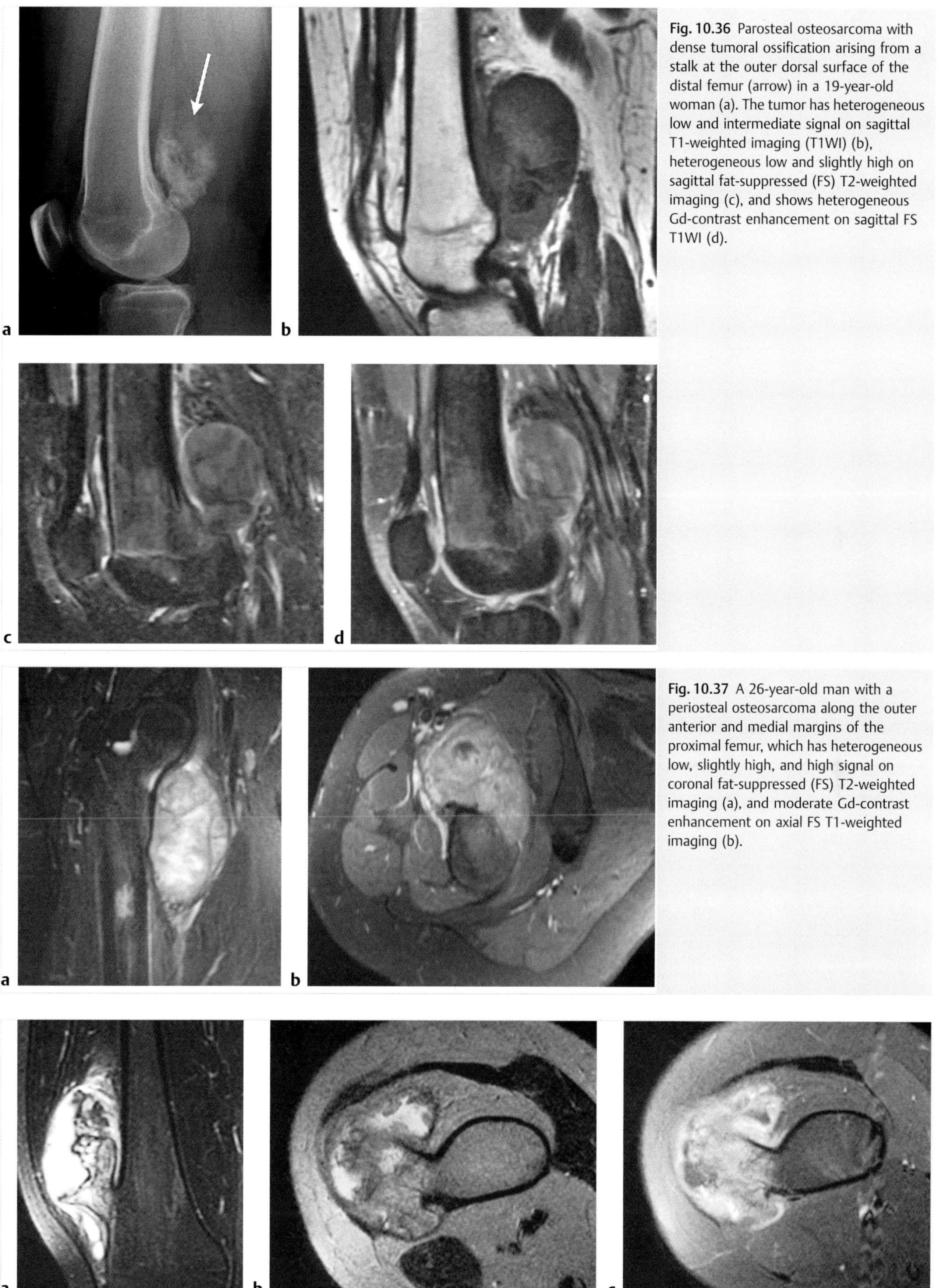

Fig. 10.36 Parosteal osteosarcoma with dense tumoral ossification arising from a stalk at the outer dorsal surface of the distal femur (arrow) in a 19-year-old woman (a). The tumor has heterogeneous low and intermediate signal on sagittal T1-weighted imaging (T1WI) (b), heterogeneous low and slightly high on sagittal fat-suppressed (FS) T2-weighted imaging (c), and shows heterogeneous Gd-contrast enhancement on sagittal FS T1WI (d).

Fig. 10.37 A 26-year-old man with a periosteal osteosarcoma along the outer anterior and medial margins of the proximal femur, which has heterogeneous low, slightly high, and high signal on coronal fat-suppressed (FS) T2-weighted imaging (a), and moderate Gd-contrast enhancement on axial FS T1-weighted imaging (b).

Fig. 10.38 Chondrosarcoma arising from an osteochondroma at the distal femur in an 18-year-old woman. The tumor has heterogeneous slightly high and high signal on coronal fat-suppressed T2-weighted imaging (FS T2WI) (a), heterogeneous intermediate and high signal on axial T2WI (b), and shows heterogeneous Gd-contrast enhancement on axial FS T1-weighted imaging (c). Cortical destruction and intramedullary extension of tumor are also seen.

Table 10.1 (Cont.) Lesions involving the outer surface of bone

Abnormalities	MRI findings	Comments
Hemangioendothelioma (▸ Fig. 10.39)	Intramedullary tumors usually have sharp margins that may be slightly lobulated. Lesions often have low-intermediate and/or high signal on T1WI and PDWI, and heterogeneous intermediate-high signal on T2WI and FS T2WI with or without zones of low signal. Lesions can be multifocal. Extraosseous extension of tumor through zones of cortical destruction commonly occur. Lesions often show prominent heterogeneous Gd-contrast enhancement.	Low grade malignant vasoformative/endothelial neoplasms that are locally aggressive and rarely metastasize, compared with the high-grade endothelial tumors such as angiosarcoma. Account for less than 1% of primary malignant bone tumors. Patients range from 10 to 82 years, median = 36 to 47 years. Patients with multifocal lesions tend to be approximately 10 years younger on average than those with unifocal tumors.
Sarcoma of soft tissue eroding into bone (▸ Fig. 10.40)	Lesions with circumscribed or ill-defined margins may be associated with erosions and/or focal destruction of adjacent cortical bone with or without intraosseous extension of tumor.	Malignant tumors in extraosseous soft tissues can erode adjacent cortex and extend into the marrow.
Intramedullary primary sarcoma eroding through bone cortex (▸ Fig. 10.41)	Poorly defined and/or circumscribed lesions in marrow with low-intermediate signal on T1WI; variable low, intermediate and/or high signal on T2WI and FS T2WI; and variable Gd-contrast enhancement associated with sites of cortical destruction and extraosseous tumor extension.	Malignant primary and metastatic tumors in marrow usually show trabecular bone destruction with frequent eventual cortical destruction and extraosseous tumor extension.

(continued on page 346)

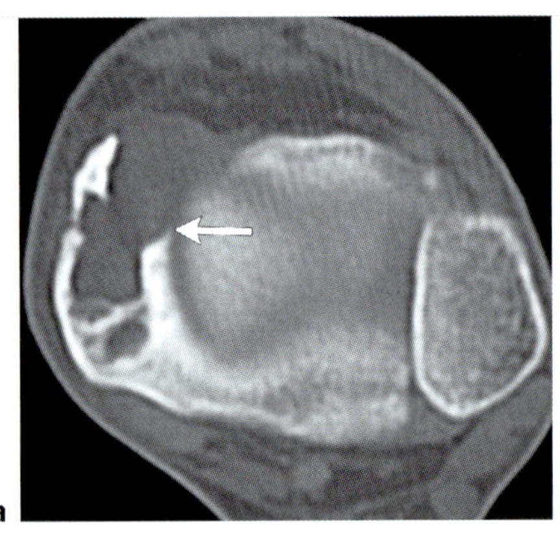
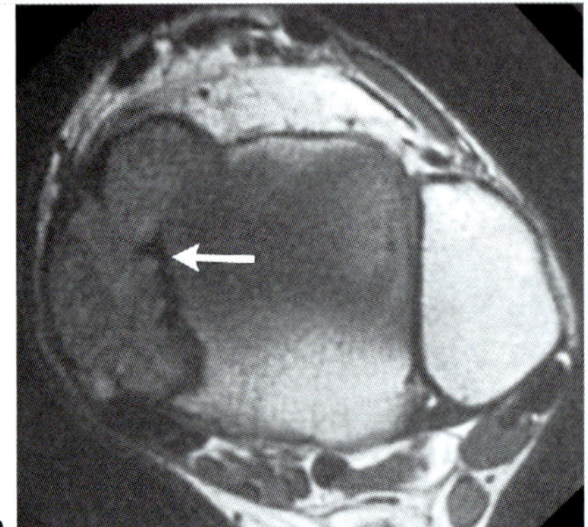
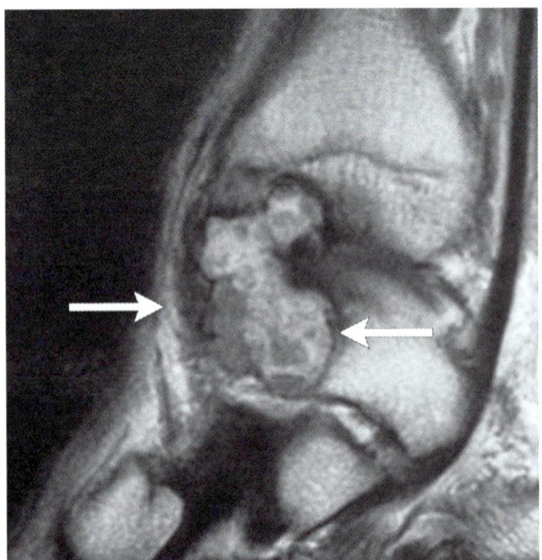
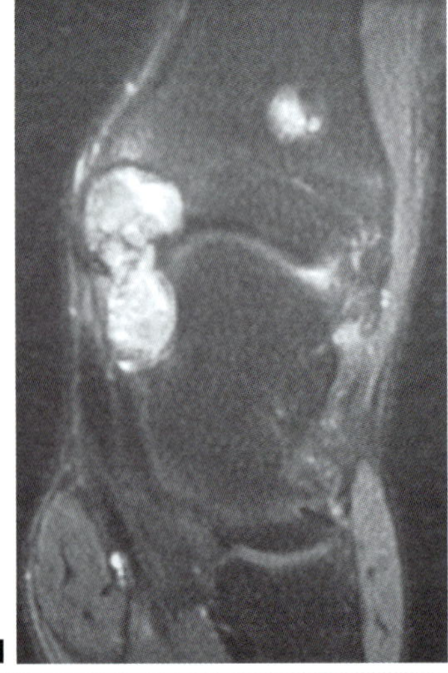

Fig. 10.39 Hemangioendothelioma in an 18-year-old woman that involves the marrow of the distal tibia with cortical destruction, extension into the ankle joint, and invasion of the talus (arrow) as seen on axial computed tomography (a). The tumor has intermediate signal on axial T1-weighted imaging (T1WI) (arrow) (b), heterogeneous slightly high signal (arrows) on sagittal T2-weighted imaging (c), and shows contrast enhancement on coronal fat-suppressed T1WI (d). Note that another focus of tumor is seen in the metaphyseal region.

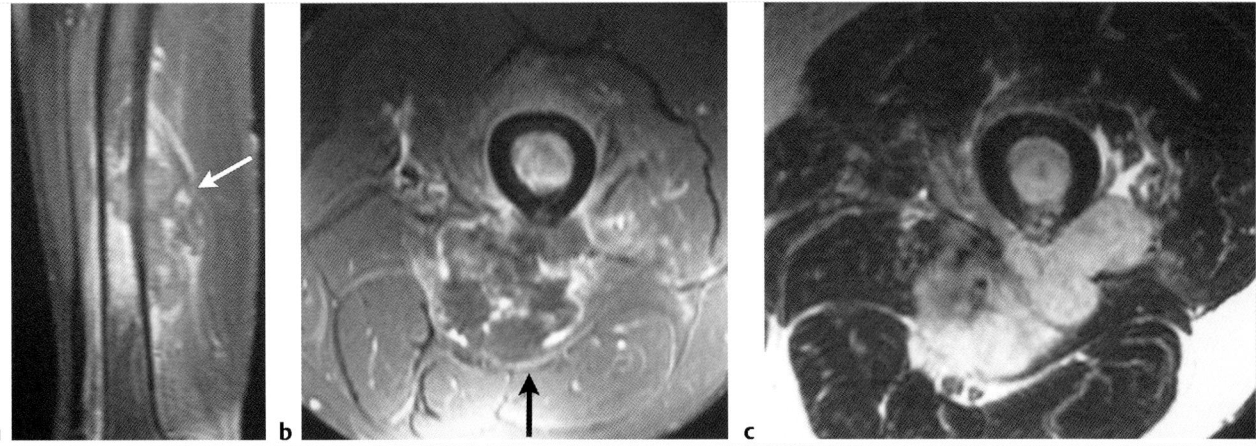

Fig. 10.40 Clear cell sarcoma of soft tissue (formerly called malignant melanoma of soft parts) involving the deep soft tissue of the lower thigh in a 52-year-old man. The tumor shows heterogeneous gadolinium-contrast enhancement on sagittal (a) and axial fat-suppressed T1-weighted imaging (arrows) (b) and has heterogeneous mostly high signal on axial T2-weighted imaging (c). The tumor is associated with cortical destruction and intraosseous extension.

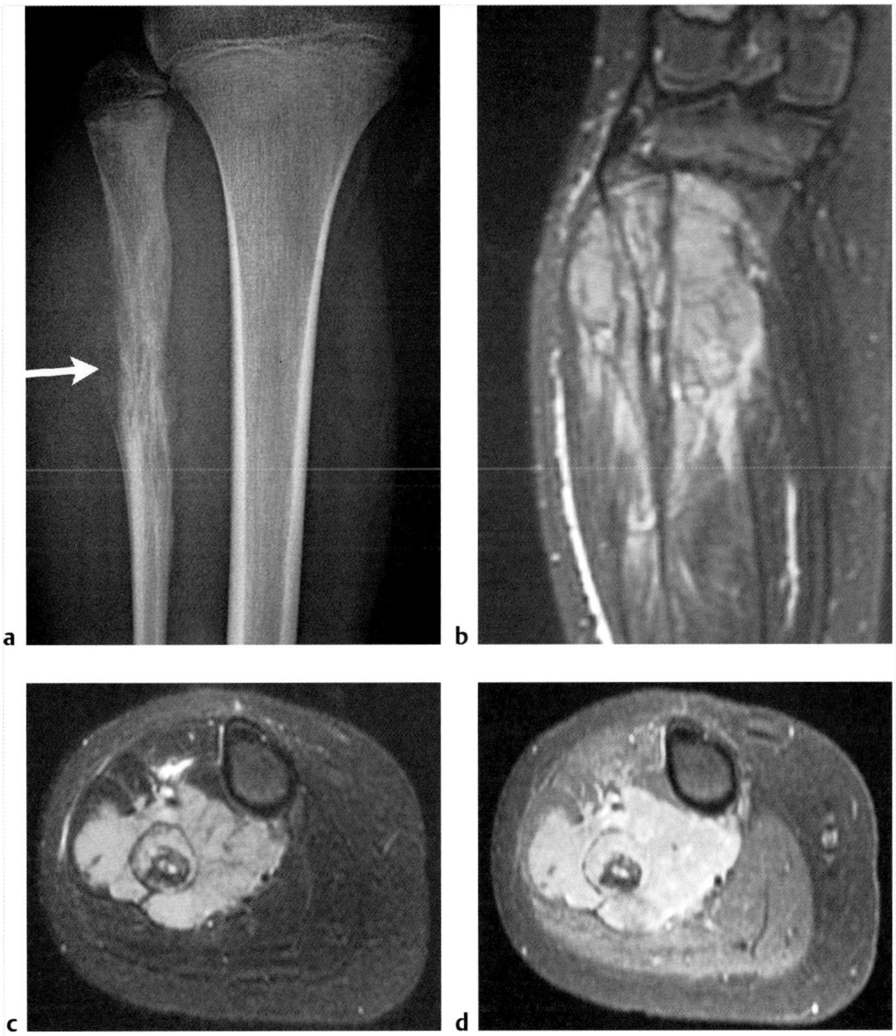

Fig. 10.41 A 10-year-old girl with Ewing sarcoma involving the proximal fibula with permeative medullary and cortical bone destruction, and discontinuous periosteal elevation (arrow) as seen on anteroposterior radiograph. (a) Magnetic resonance imaging shows tumor extension from the marrow through destroyed cortical bone into the adjacent soft tissues and has heterogeneous, slightly high signal on coronal (b) and axial fat-suppressed (FS) T2-weighted imaging (c). The tumor shows heterogeneous Gd-contrast enhancement on axial FS T1-weighted imaging (d).

Table 10.1 (Cont.) Lesions involving the outer surface of bone

Abnormalities	MRI findings	Comments
Metastatic lesions (▶ Fig. 10.42)	Metastatic tumor within bone often appears as intra-medullary zones with low-intermediate signal on T1WI; low-intermediate to slightly-high signal on PDWI; slightly-high to high signal on T2WI and FS T2WI. Sclerotic lesions often have low signal on T1WI and mixed low, intermediate, and/or high signal on T2WI. Cortical destruction and tumor extension into the extraosseous soft tissues frequently occurs. Pathological fractures can be associated with metastatic lesions involving tubular bones and vertebrae. Lesions show varying degrees of Gd-contrast enhancement. Periosteal reaction can occasionally be seen but is uncommon.	Metastatic lesions typically occur in the marrow with or without cortical destruction and extraosseous tumor extension. Metastatic lesions occur rarely in the cortex alone. Metastatic lesions infrequently have associated single or multilayered periosteal reaction (< 15 to 21%).
Myeloma/ plasmacytoma (▶ Fig. 10.43)	Multiple myeloma or single plasma cell neoplasms (plasmacytoma) are well-circumscribed or poorly defined, diffuse infiltrative lesions involving marrow, low-intermediate signal on T1WI, intermediate-high signal on T2WI, usually show Gd-contrast-enhancement, eventual cortical bone destruction, and extraosseous extension.	Malignant tumors composed of proliferating antibody-secreting plasma cells derived from single clones. Most common primary neoplasm of bone in adults. Most patients are older than 40 years, median = 60 years. May have variable destructive or infiltrative changes involving the axial and/or appendicular skeleton.

(continued on page 348)

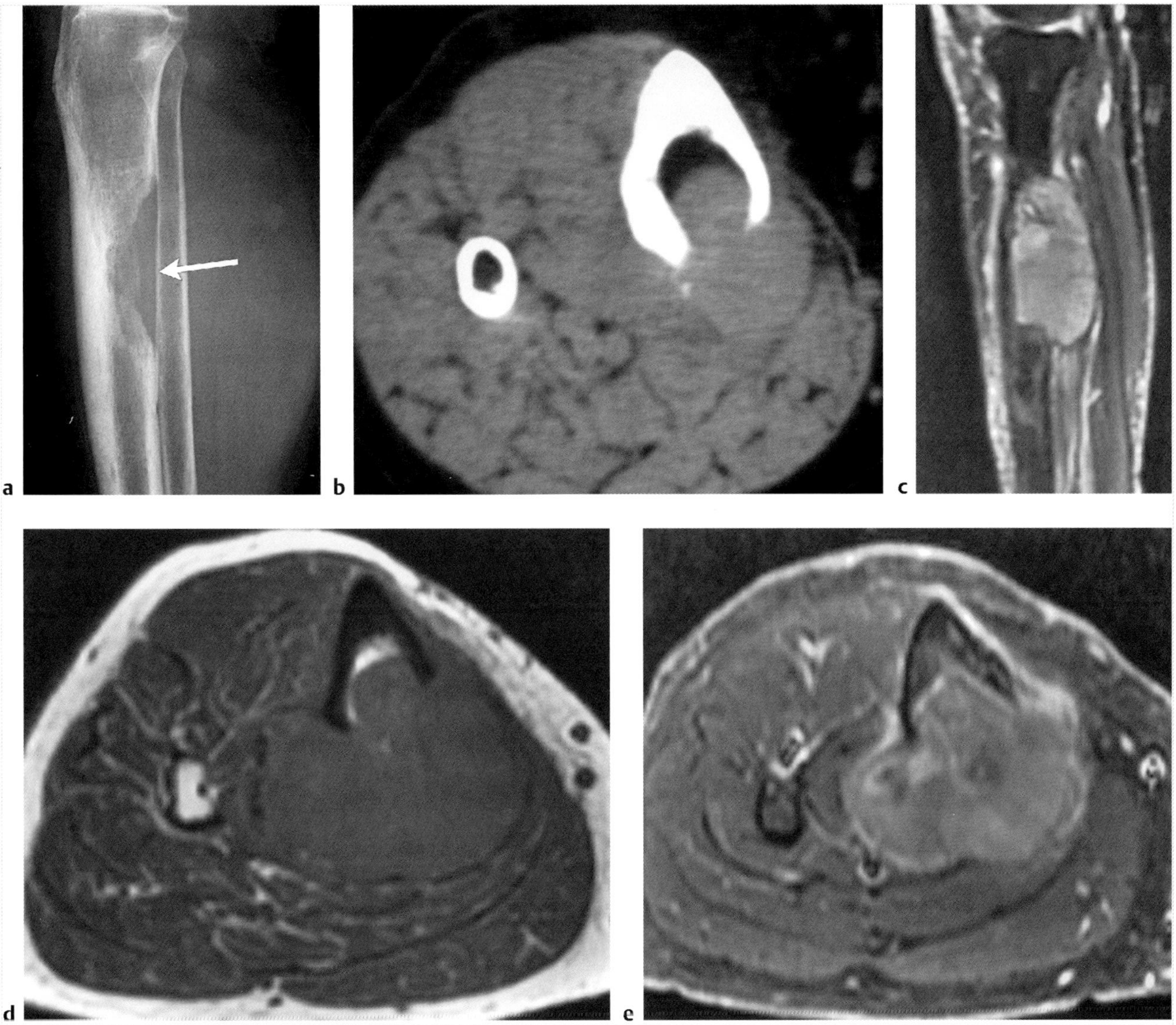

Fig. 10.42 Metastatic lesion from melanoma in the marrow of the tibial diaphysis associated with cortical destruction and extraosseous extension (arrow) as seen on lateral radiograph (a) and axial computed tomography (b). The tumor has slightly high signal on sagittal fat-suppressed (FS) T2-weighted imaging (c), intermediate signal on axial T1-weighted imaging (T1WI) (d), and shows Gd-contrast enhancement on axial FS T1WI (e).

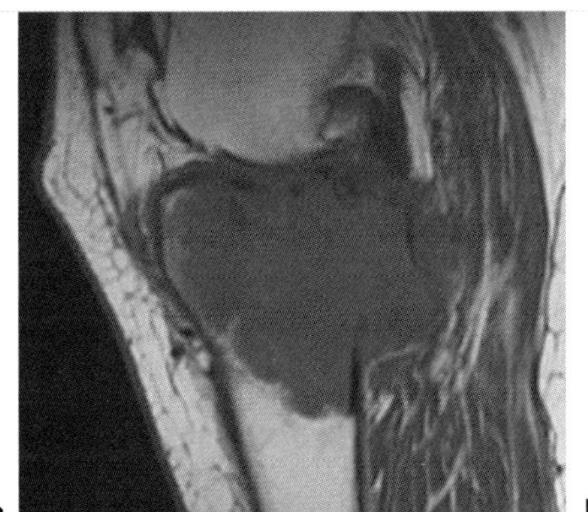

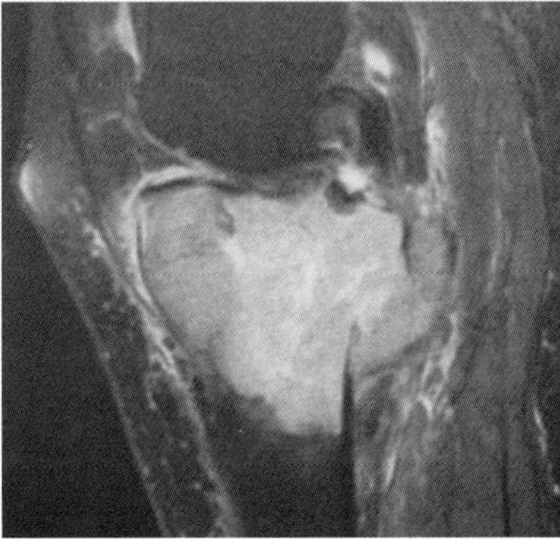

Fig. 10.43 Myeloma involving the marrow of the proximal tibia with intermediate signal on sagittal T1-weighted imaging (a), heterogeneous high signal on fat-suppressed T2-weighted imaging (b), associated with cortical destruction and extraosseous extension dorsally.

Table 10.1 (Cont.) Lesions involving the outer surface of bone

Abnormalities	MRI findings	Comments
Lymphoma (▶ Fig. 10.44)	Single or multiple well-circumscribed or poorly defined, infiltrative lesions involving marrow; low-intermediate signal on T1WI, intermediate-high signal on T2WI and FS T2WI, often shows Gd-contrast enhancement, ± bone destruction and extraosseous extension. Diffuse involvement of vertebra with Hodgkin lymphoma can produce an "ivory vertebra," which has low signal on T1WI and T2WI.	Lymphoid tumors with neoplastic cells typically within lymphoid tissue (lymph nodes and reticuloendothelial organs). Unlike leukemia, lymphoma usually arises as discrete masses. Lymphomas are subdivided into Hodgkin disease (HD) and non-Hodgkin lymphoma (NHL). Almost all primary lymphomas of bone are B cell NHL.
Leukemia (▶ Fig. 10.45)	Single or multiple well-circumscribed or poorly defined infiltrative lesions involving marrow; low-intermediate signal on T1WI, intermediate-high signal on T2WI and FS T2WI, often shows Gd-contrast enhancement, ± bone destruction and extraosseous extension.	Lymphoid neoplasms involving bone marrow with tumor cells also in peripheral blood. In children and adolescents, acute lymphoblastic leukemia (ALL) is the most frequent type. In adults, chronic lymphocytic leukemia (small lymphocytic lymphoma) is the most common type of lymphocytic leukemia. Myelogenous leukemias are neoplasms derived from abnormal myeloid progenitor cells. Acute myelogenous leukemia (AML) occurs in adolescents and young adults and represents approximately 20% of childhood leukemia. Chronic myelogenous leukemia (CML) usually affects adults older than 25 years.
Malignant tumor with interrupted periosteal reaction: sunburst or divergent pattern (▶ Fig. 10.46)	Intramedullary neoplasm can be associated with zones of cortical destruction through which the lesion extends into the extraosseous soft tissues. Zones of reactive and/or tumoral bone formation under the elevated periosteum can have a divergent or "sunburst" appearance with low signal within the extraosseous tumor that often has slightly high to high signal on T2WI and FS T2WI with corresponding Gd-contrast enhancement.	Periosteal elevation by tumor results in formation of a "sunburst or divergent pattern" of underlying bone spicules along vascular channels and fibrous bands (Sharpey fibers), which are stretched out from the outer surface of bone cortex. Typically seen with osteosarcoma, rarely seen with osteoblastoma and osteoblastic metastasis (prostate carcinoma, lung carcinoma, carcinoid, breast carcinoma).

(continued on page 350)

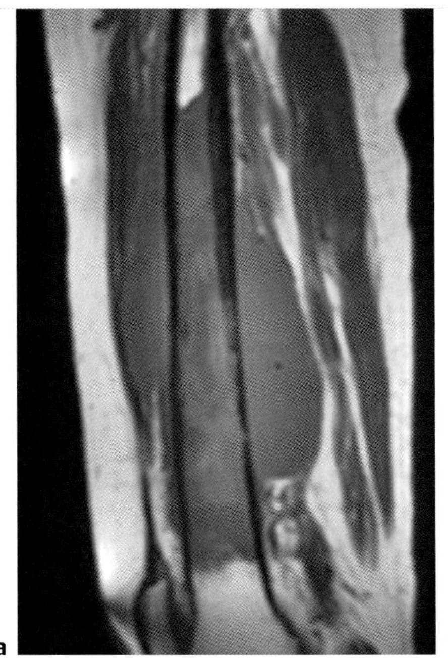
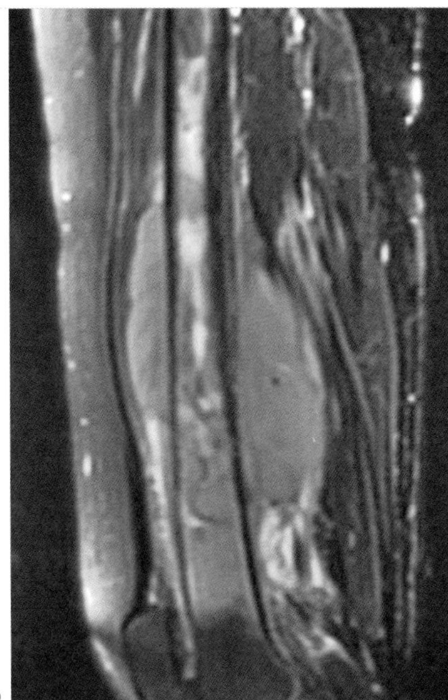

Fig. 10.44 Large B-cell lymphoma involving the diaphyseal marrow of the femur, which has heterogeneous intermediate signal on sagittal T1-weighted imaging (a) and heterogeneous slightly high and high signal on sagittal fat-suppressed T2-weighted imaging (b). The tumor is associated with cortical destruction and extensive extraosseous extension.

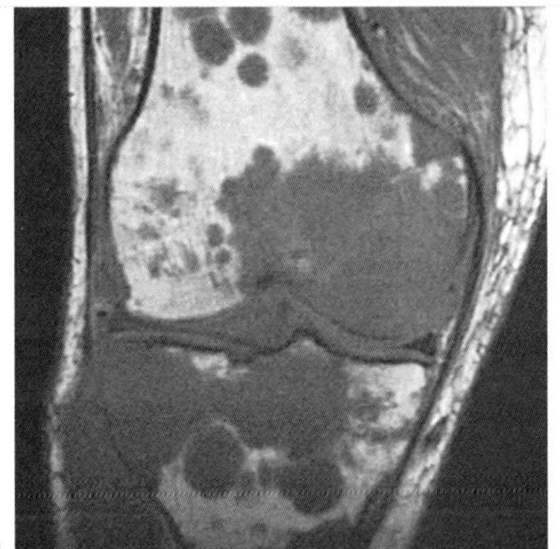
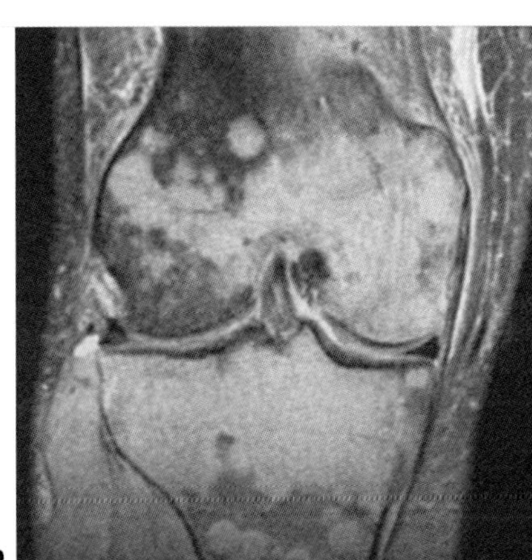

Fig. 10.45 Acute lymphoblastic leukemia involving the marrow of the tibia and fibula associated with cortical destruction and extraosseous extension as seen on coronal T1-weighted imaging (a) and fat-suppressed T2-weighted imaging (b).

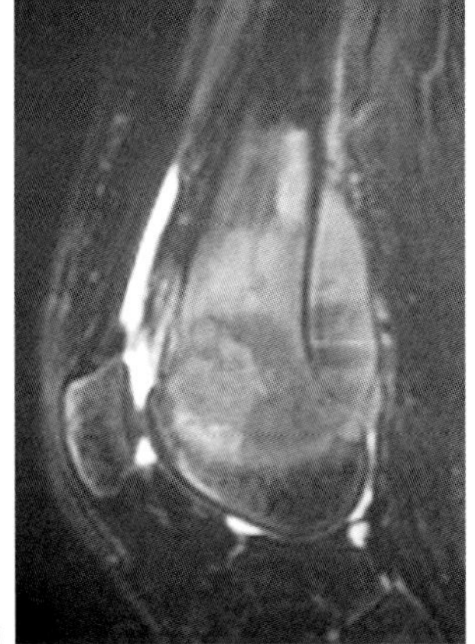
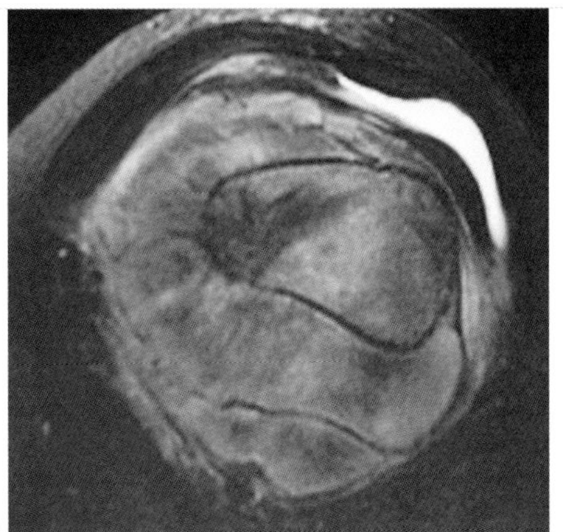
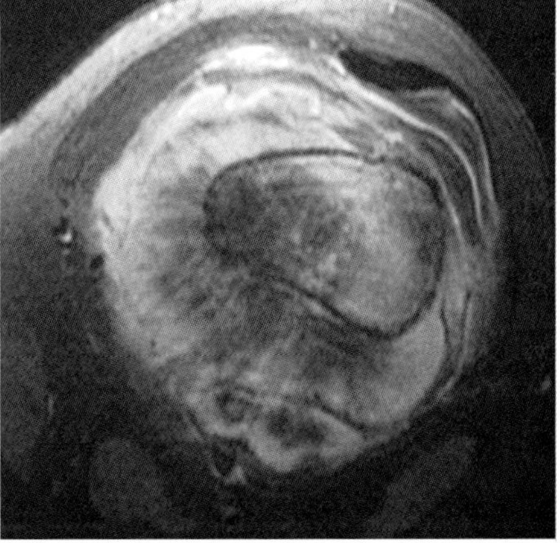

Fig. 10.46 Intramedullary osteogenic sarcoma in a 14-year-old boy. The tumor is associated with cortical destruction and extraosseous extension under an interrupted elevated periosteum. Beneath the elevated periosteum, divergent striated zones of low signal on sagittal (a) and axial fat-suppressed (FS) T2-weighted imaging (b) and post-gadolinium-contrast FS T1-weighted imaging (c) are seen representing divergent or sunburst tumoral bone formation within the extraosseous neoplasm.

Table 10.1 (Cont.) Lesions involving the outer surface of bone

Abnormalities	MRI findings	Comments
Malignant tumor with interrupted periosteal reaction: Codman triangle (▶ Fig. 10.47)	Intramedullary neoplasm or infection can be associated with zones of cortical destruction through which the lesions extend into the extraosseous soft tissues. Lamellated and/or spiculated zones of perisosteal reaction are often seen secondary to tumor invasion and perforation of bone cortex. Low signal from spicules of reactive and tumoral bone formation may have a "sunburst" appearance. Triangular zones of periosteal elevation (Codman triangles) can be seen at the borders of zones of cortical destruction and tumor extension.	Codman triangles are triangular zones of periosteal reaction or reactive bone at the borders of cortical destruction adjacent to extraosseous extension of neoplasms or infections from marrow. Can be seen with malignant primary bone neoplasms and lesions (osteosarcoma, Ewing sarcoma, chondrosarcoma, malignant fibrous histiocytoma, aneurysmal bone cyst, giant cell tumor), metastasis, osteomyelitis, or trauma.
Malignant tumor with interrupted periosteal reaction: disorganized pattern (▶ Fig. 10.48)	Intramedullary neoplasm or infection seen with zones of cortical destruction through which the lesion extends into the extraosseous soft tissues. Irregular disorganized zones of perisosteal reaction can be seen below the elevated periosteum.	Extraosseous extension of tumor or infection results in disorganized thin and/or thick irregular bone spicules under the elevated periosteum. Disorganized periosteal reaction is often seen with highly aggressive osteosarcomas but can also be seen with other benign and malignant tumors that have associated complications of pathological fracture or infection.
Malignant tumor with interrupted periosteal reaction: "hair on end" or perpendicularly oriented spicules of periosteal reaction (▶ Fig. 10.49)	Intramedullary neoplasm or infection seen with zones of cortical destruction through which the lesions extend into the extraosseous soft tissues. Parallel spiculated zones ("hair on end" pattern) of periosteal reaction oriented perpendicular to the long axis of bone can be seen within the extraosseous lesion, often under an elevated periosteum.	Extraosseous extension of tumor or infection results in a perpendicular ("hair on end") pattern of thin bone spicules radially oriented under the elevated periosteum. These bone spicules tend to be thin and oriented along radially oriented blood vessels extending from the cortical surface within the lesions. Most frequently seen with Ewing sarcoma, sometimes with osteosarcoma, and rarely with infection.

(continued on page 352)

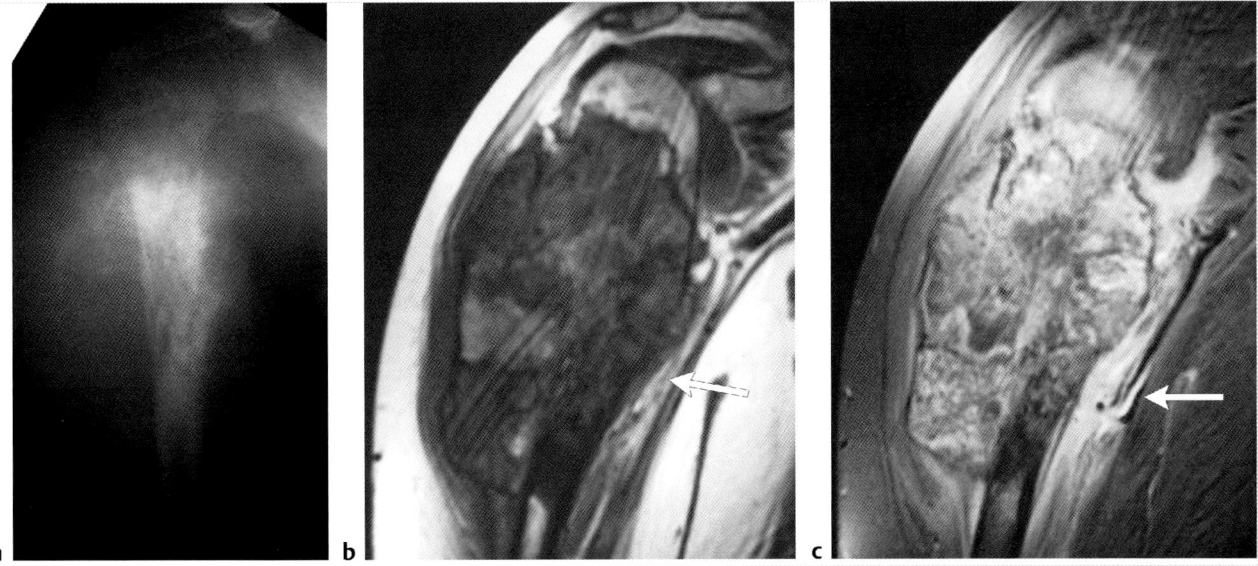

Fig. 10.47 Intramedullary osteogenic osteosarcoma involving the humerus with cortical destruction, extraosseous extension, and interrupted periosteal elevation. Anteroposterior radiograph (a) shows a destructive intraosseous lesion with mineralized ossified matrix, cortical destruction, extraosseous tumor extension with disorganized tumoral bone formation, and a Codman triangle at the medial aspect. The tumor has mixed low, intermediate, and high signal on coronal T1-weighted imaging (T1WI) (arrow) (b) and shows prominent gadolinium-contrast enhancement on coronal fat-suppressed T1WI (arrow) (c).

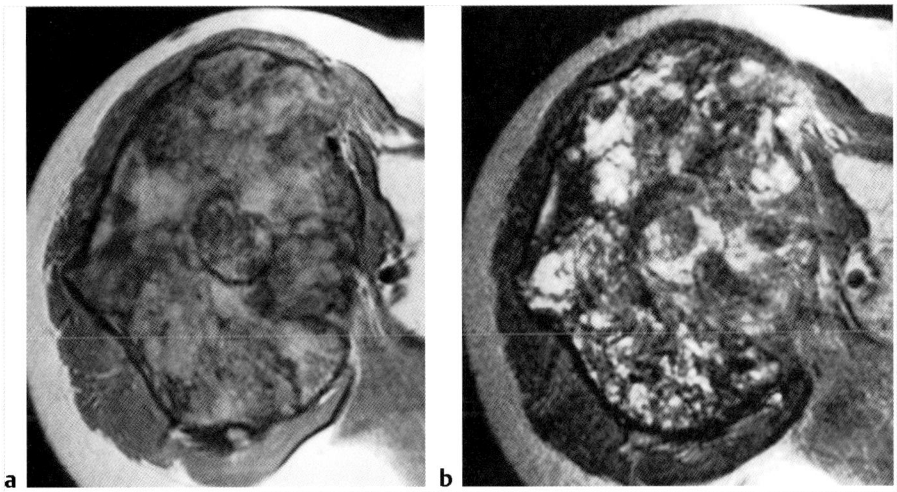

Fig. 10.48 Intramedullary osteogenic osteosarcoma with cortical destruction, extraosseous extension, and interrupted periosteal elevation. The intraosseous tumor is associated with extensive cortical destruction and extraosseous tumor extension containing irregular zones of low signal on axial proton density–weighted imaging (a) and axial T2-weighted imaging (b), representing disorganized tumoral/periosteal bone formation.

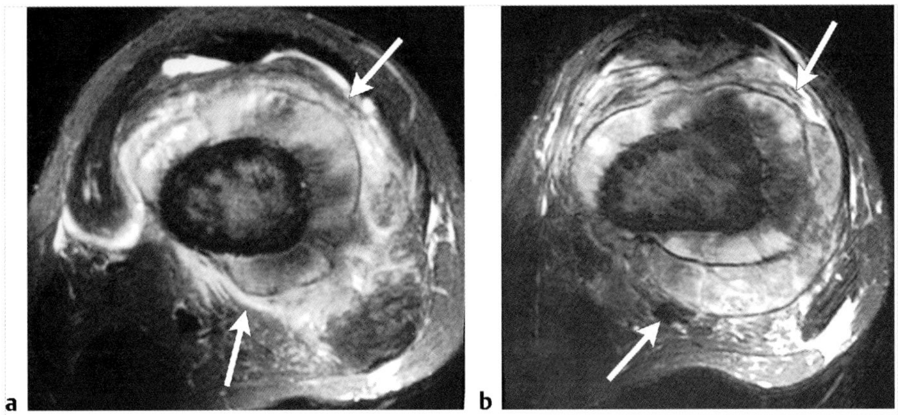

Fig. 10.49 Intramedullary osteogenic sarcoma in a 19-year-old woman. (a,b) The tumor (arrows) is associated with cortical destruction and extraosseous extension under an interrupted elevated periosteum. Beneath the elevated perisoteum, "hair on end" as well as divergent striated/sunburst-type zones of low signal on fat-suppressed T2-weighted imaging are seen representing tumoral bone formation within the extraosseous portions of the neoplasm.

Table 10.1 (Cont.) Lesions involving the outer surface of bone

Abnormalities	MRI findings	Comments
Malignant tumor with interrupted periosteal reaction: "onion skin" multilayered, or multilamellated periosteal reaction oriented parallel to the long axis of bone (▶ Fig. 10.50)	Intramedullary neoplasm, inflammatory lesion, or infection seen with zones of cortical destruction through which the lesions extend into the extraosseous soft tissues. Multiple layers of periosteal reaction oriented parallel to cortical bone ("onion skin" pattern) can be seen within the extraosseous lesion often under an elevated periosteum.	Extraosseous extension of tumor, noninfectious inflammatory lesions, or infection results in a multilayered perisoteal reaction. Most frequently seen with Ewing sarcoma, sometimes with osteosarcoma, lymphoma, and rarely with infection.

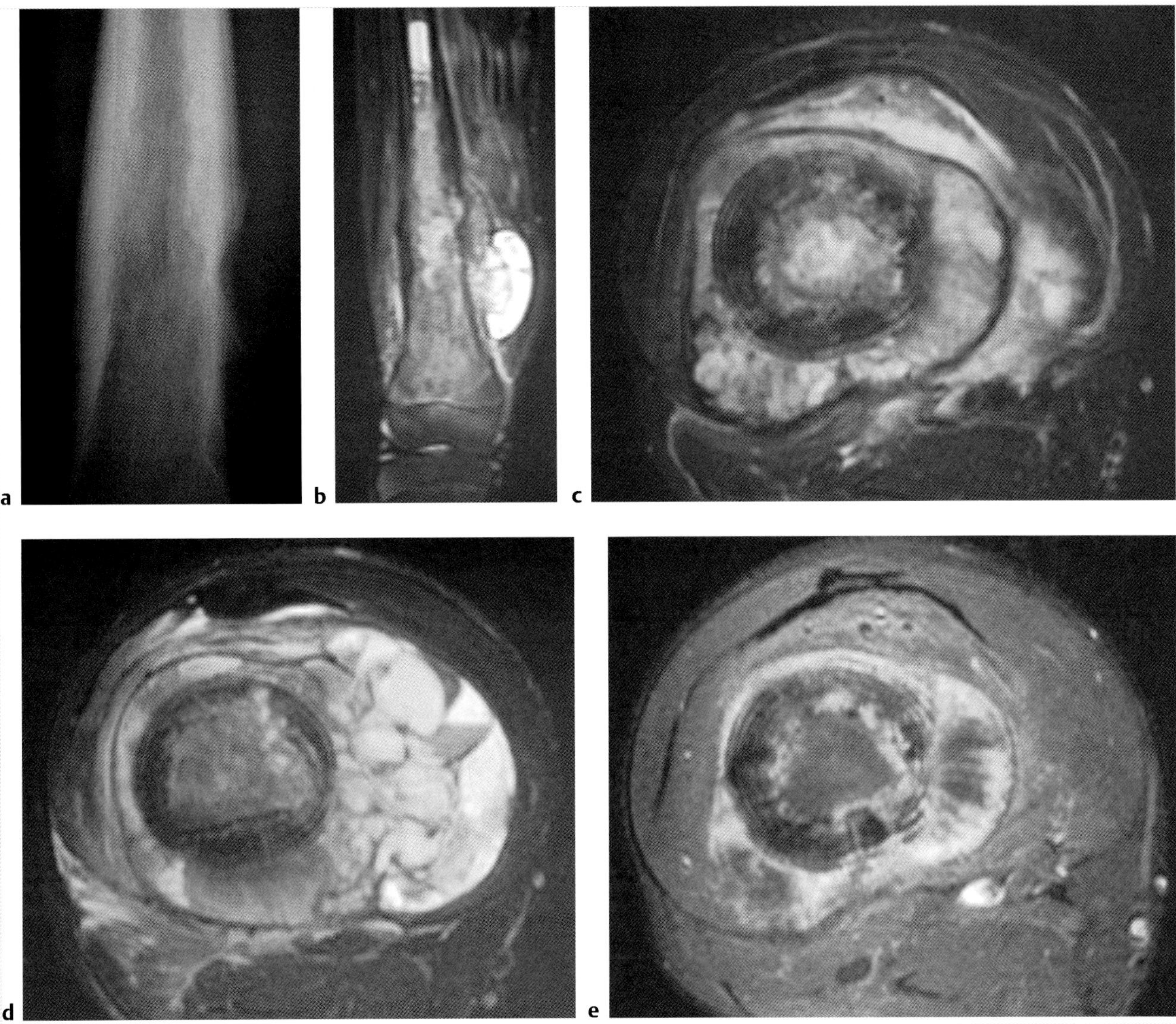

Fig. 10.50 Intramedullary telangiectatic osteosarcoma in the distal femur associated with cortical destruction with extraosseous tumor extension. Multiple layers of periosteal reaction oriented parallel to cortical bone ("onion skin" pattern) and a Codman triangle inferiorly are seen on an anteroposterior radiograph (a). Intraosseous tumor is seen extending through destroyed cortical bone beneath an interrupted periosteum as seen on coronal (b) and axial fat-suppressed T2-weighted imaging (FS T2WI) (c, d), and post-gadolinium-contrast FS T1-weighted imaging (e). Multiple thin layers or periosteal reaction as well as multiple fluid-fluid levels are seen in the extraosseous tumor on axial FS T2WI.

10.2 Lesions Associated with Thickening of Bone Cortex

- Nonmalignant lesions
  - Osteoid osteoma
  - Osteoblastoma
  - Osteoma
  - Juxtacortical chondroma
  - Parosteal lipoma
  - Heterotopic ossification
  - Osteofibrous dysplasia
  - Fibrous dysplasia
  - Focal fibrocartilaginous dysplasia
  - Melorheostosis
  - Healing and healed fractures
  - Paget disease
  - Subacute and acute osteomyelitis
  - Chronic recurrent mutifocal osteomyelitis
  - Syndromes of hyperostosis, osteitis, and skin lesions (SAPHO syndrome)
  - Neurofibromatosis type 1 (NF1)
  - Noninterrupted periosteal reaction and bone formation from primary hypertrophic osteoarthropathy (pachydermoperiostosis)
  - Noninterrupted periosteal reaction and bone formation from secondary hypertrophic osteoarthropathy
  - Noninterrupted periosteal reaction and bone formation from venous stasis
  - Noninterrupted periosteal reaction and bone formation from infantile cortical hyperostosis (Caffey disease)
  - Progressive diaphyseal dysplasia (Camurati-Engelmann disease)
  - Hereditary multiple diaphyseal sclerosis (Ribbing disease)
  - Craniodiaphyseal dysplasia
  - Craniometaphyseal dysplasia
  - Craniometadiaphyseal dysplasia
  - Generalized cortical hyperostosis (van Buchem syndrome)
  - Pyknodysostosis (Maroteaux-Lamy syndrome)
  - Noninterrupted periosteal reaction and bone formation from thyroid acropachy
  - Noninterrupted periosteal reaction from hypervitaminosis A
  - Noninterrupted periosteal reaction from hypovitaminosis C (scurvy)
- Malignant lesions
  - Parosteal osteosarcoma
  - Intraosseous osteosarcoma
  - Adamantinoma

Table 10.2 Lesions associated with thickening of bone cortex

Abnormalities	MRI findings	Comments
Benign lesions		
Osteoid osteoma (▶ Fig. 10.51)	Osteoid osteomas typically show dense fusiform thickening of the cortex, which has low to intermediate signal on T1-weighted imaging (T1WI), proton density–weighted imaging (PDWI), T2-weighted imaging (T2WI), and fat-suppressed (FS) T2WI. Within the thickened cortex, a spheroid or ovoid zone (nidus) measuring less than 1.5 cm is typically seen. The nidus can have irregular, distinct or indistinct margins relative to the adjacent region of cortical thickening. The nidus can have low-intermediate signal on T1WI and PDWI, and low-intermediate or high signal on T2WI and FS T2WI. Calcifications in the nidus can be seen as low signal on T2WI. After gadolinium (Gd)-contrast administration, variable degrees of enhancement are seen at the nidus, adjacent bone cortex, marrow, periosteum, and adjacent soft tissues.	Benign painful osteoblastic lesion composed of a circumscribed nidus less than 1.5 cm usually surrounded by reactive bone formation. Accounts for 11 to 13% of primary benign bone tumors. Occurs in patients age 6 to 30 years, median = 17 years. Approximately 75% occur in patients less than 25 years.
Osteoblastoma (▶ Fig. 10.52)	Lesions appear as spheroid or ovoid zone measuring greater than 1.5 to 2 cm located within medullary and/or cortical bone with low-intermediate signal on T1WI; low-intermediate to slightly high signal on PDWI; and low-intermediate and/or high signal on T2WI and FS T2WI. Calcifications or areas of mineralization can be seen as zones of low signal on T2WI. After Gd-contrast administration, osteoblastomas show variable degrees of enhancement. Zones of thickened cortical bone and medullary sclerosis that are often seen adjacent to osteoblastomas typically show low signal on T1WI, T2WI, and FS T2WI. Poorly defined zones of marrow signal alteration consisting of low-intermediate signal on T1WI, high signal on T2WI and FS T2WI, and corresponding Gd-contrast enhancement can be seen in the marrow adjacent to osteoblastomas as well as within the extraosseous soft tissues.	Rare benign bone-forming tumors, which are histologically related to osteoid osteomas. Osteoblastomas are larger than osteoid osteomas and show progressive enlargement. Account for 3 to 6% of primary benign bone tumors and < 1 to 2% of all primary bone tumors. Occurs in patients age 1 to 30 years, median = 15 years, mean age = 20 years. Approximately 90% of lesions occur in patients less than 30 years.

(continued on page 356)

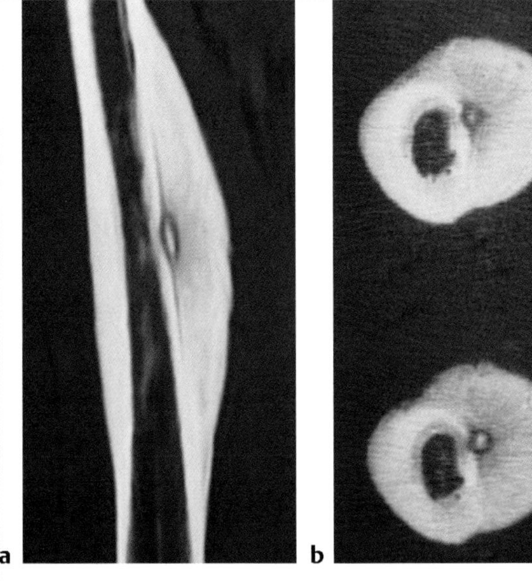

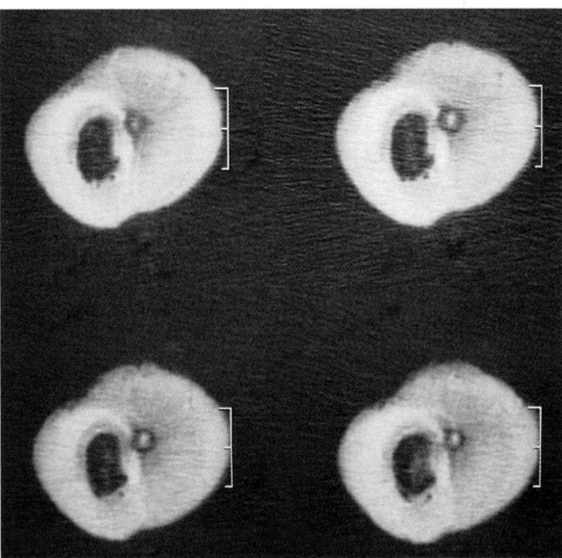

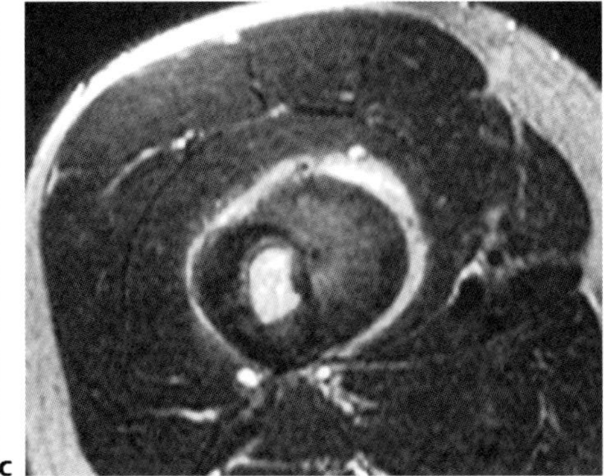

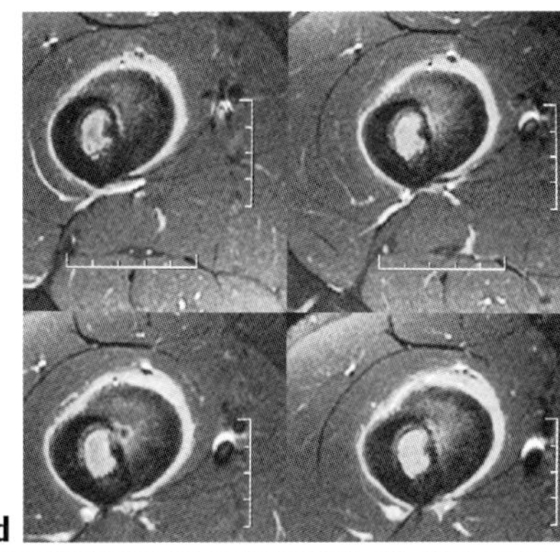

Fig. 10.51 Osteoid osteoma involving the cortex of the proximal femoral shaft in a 15-year-old boy. Coronal (a) and axial (b) computed tomographic images show dense fusiform osteosclerosis surrounding a small radiolucent zone (nidus) with a central calcification. The nidus has slightly high signal on axial T2-weighted imaging (T2WI) (c) and contains a small central calcification with low signal. The thickened cortex has low and slightly high signal on T2WI and is associated with periosteal reaction with high signal. The nidus shows gadolinium (Gd)-contrast enhancement on axial fat-suppressed T1-weighted imaging (FS T1WI) (d). Prominent Gd-contrast enhancement is seen at the periosteal reaction, and mild diffuse enhancement is seen in the cortical thickening adjacent to the nidus. Poorly defined zones of high signal on FS T2WI and corresponding Gd-contrast enhancement on FS T1WI are also seen in the marrow adjacent to the lesion.

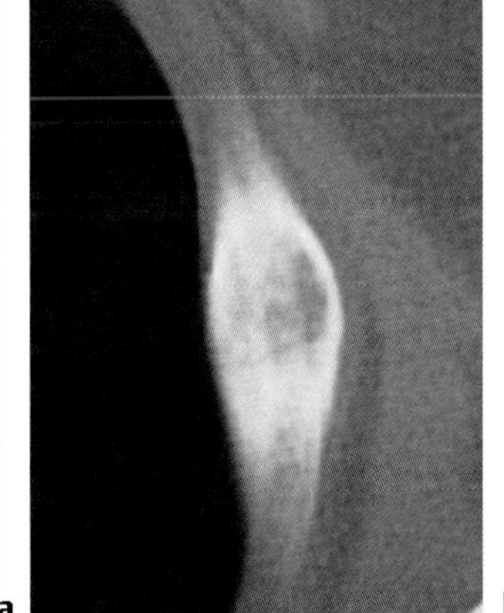

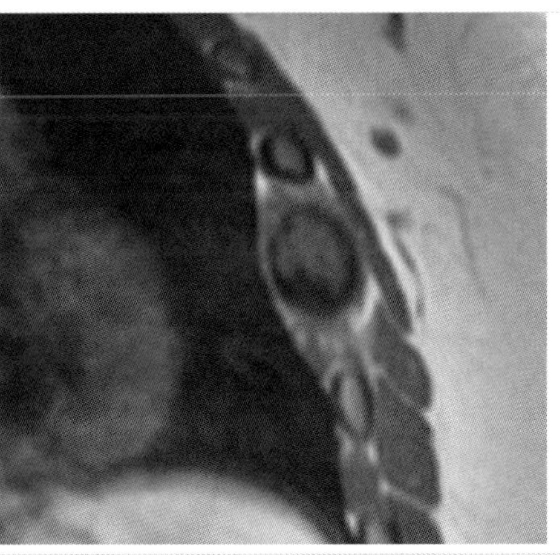

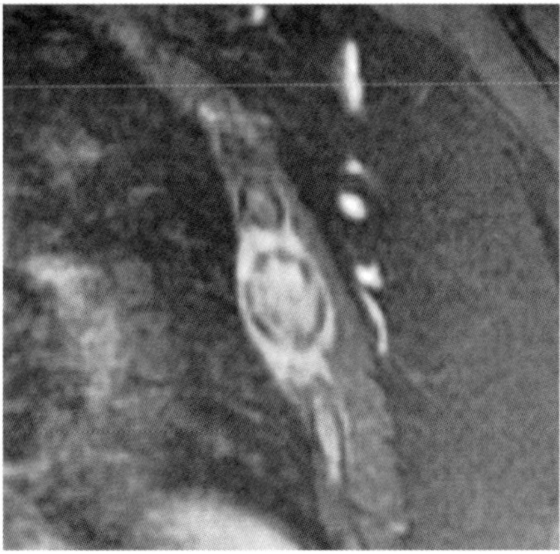

Fig. 10.52 Osteoblastoma involving a rib in a 16-year-old boy. Prominent dense sclerotic reaction is seen involving cortical and medullary bone adjacent to the expansile, mixed radiolucent and radiodense lesion on axial computed tomographic image (a). The lesion has intermediate signal on sagittal T1-weighted imaging (b) and high signal on sagittal fat-suppressed T2-weighted imaging (FS T2WI) (c). Poorly defined zones with high signal on FS T2WI are seen in the marrow and soft tissues adjacent to the lesion.

Table 10.2 (Cont.) Lesions associated with thickening of bone cortex

Abnormalities	MRI findings	Comments
Osteoma (▶ Fig. 10.12)	Lesions typically appear as well-circumscribed zones of dense cortical bone with low signal on T1WI, PDWI, T2WI, and FS T2WI. No infiltration by osteomas is seen into the adjacent soft tissues. Zones of bone destruction or associated soft tissue mass-lesions are not associated with osteomas. Periosteal reaction is not associated with osteomas except in cases with coincidental antecedent trauma.	Benign primary bone lesions composed of dense lamellar, woven, and/or compact cortical bone usually located at the surface of bones. Account for less than 1% of primary benign bone tumors. Occurs in patients age 16 to 74 years, most frequent in sixth decade.
Juxtacortical chondroma (▶ Fig. 10.5)	Lesions are located at the bone surface and are usually lobulated with low-intermediate signal on T1WI, which is hypo- or isointense relative to muscle. Lesions usually have heterogeneous predominantly high signal on T2WI. Lesions are surrounded by low signal borders on T2WI representing thin sclerotic reaction. Areas of low signal on T2WI are secondary to matrix mineralization. Edema is not typically seen in nearby medullary bone. Lesions often show a peripheral pattern of Gd-contrast enhancement, which correlates to fibrovascular bundles surrounding the cartilage lobules.	Benign protuberant hyaline cartilaginous tumors, which arise from the periosteum and superficial to bone cortex. Account for < 1% of bone lesions. Juxtacortical chondromas represent approximately 5 to12% of chondromas. Patient age ranges from 4 to 77 years, median = 26 years.
Parosteal lipoma (▶ Fig. 10.13)	Lesions often have lobular margins and are immediately adjacent to the outer intact surface of adjacent bone. Lesions typically have fat signal on magnetic resonance imaging (MRI), as well as zones of low signal on T1WI and T2WI from ossification changes that can occur within these lesions and at the junction with bone cortex. Zones with intermediate signal on T1WI and high signal on T2WI can occur in these lesions secondary to cartilaginous contents.	Rare benign slow-growing painless tumors with mature adipose tissue associated with the periosteum of bone. Account for 0.3% of lipomas, typically occur in patients 40 to 60 years. Common sites include the femur, proximal radius, tibia, and humerus.
Heterotopic ossification (▶ Fig. 10.15)	Long-standing lesions can have variable low signal on T1WI, PDWI, and T2WI depending on the degree of mineralization/ossification, fibrosis, and hemosiderin deposition. Zones of high signal on T1WI and T2WI may occur from fatty marrow metaplasia. Gd-contrast enhancement in old mature lesions is often minimal or absent. Signal abnormalities within bone marrow are usually absent.	Represents localized nonneoplastic reparative lesions, which are composed of reactive hypercellular fibrous tissue, cartilage, and/or bone. Can arise secondary to trauma (myositis ossificans circumscripta, ossifying hematoma), although may also occur without a history of prior injury (pseudomalignant osseous tumor of the soft tissues).
Osteofibrous dysplasia (▶ Fig. 10.53)	Osteofibrous dysplasia often shows multiple irregular intracortical zones of low-intermediate signal on T1WI, intermediate to slightly high signal on PDWI, and high signal on T2WI and FS T2WI separated by irregular zones of low signal on T1WI and T2WI, the latter representing thickened sclerotic cortical bone. Zones of low signal on T1WI and T2WI of varying thickness are typically seen superficial and deep to the lesions representing sclerotic bone reaction. The outer cortical margins can be expanded and thinned. Intracortical lesions usually show prominent Gd-contrast enhancement. Thin juxtacortical/periosteal enhancement may be seen in lesions with thinned and expanded cortical margins.	Rare self-limited benign fibro-osseous lesion primarily involving the anterior midshaft of the tibial cortex in children and adolescents.

(continued on page 358)

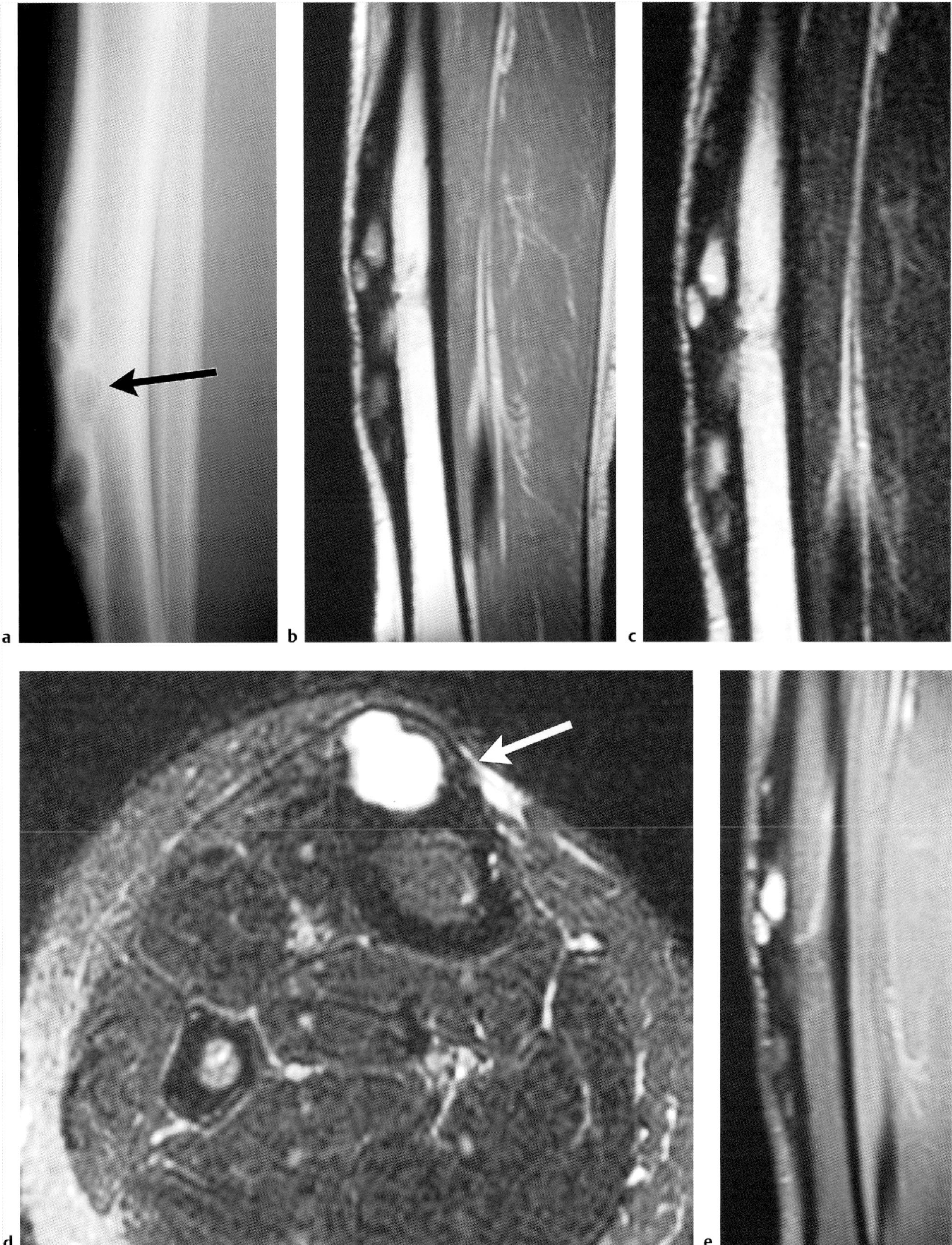

Fig. 10.53 Osteofibrous dysplasia involving the anterior cortex of the proximal shaft of the tibia in a 15-year-old girl. Lateral radiograph (a) shows thickening of bone cortex within which are multiple radiolucent zones (arrow), which have intermediate signal on sagittal proton density–weighted imaging (b) heterogeneous high signal on sagittal T2-weighted imaging (T2WI) (c), high signal (arrow) on axial fat-suppressed (FS) T2WI (d) and which show Gd-contrast enhancement on sagittal FS T1-weighted imaging (e).

Table 10.2 (Cont.) Lesions associated with thickening of bone cortex

Abnormalities	MRI findings	Comments
Fibrous dysplasia (▶ Fig. 10.54; ▶ Fig. 10.55)	MRI features depend on the proportions of bony spicules, collagen, fibroblastic spindle cells, hemorrhagic and/or cystic changes, and associated pathological fracture if present. Lesions are usually well circumscribed and have low or low-intermediate signal on T1WI and PDWI. On T2WI, lesions have variable mixtures of low, intermediate, and/or high signal often surrounded by a low signal rim of variable thickness. Internal septations and cystic changes are seen in a minority of lesions. Bone expansion and cortical thickening can be seen. Lesions show Gd-contrast enhancement that varies in degree and pattern. Periosteal and juxtacortical enhancement can be seen in lesions with associated pathological fractures.	Benign medullary fibro-osseous lesion, which can involve a single site (mono-ostotic) or multiple locations (polyostotic). Thought to occur from developmental failure in the normal process of remodeling primitive bone to mature lamellar bone with resultant zone or zones of immature trabeculae within dysplastic fibrous tissue. Lesions do not mineralize normally and result in loss of mechanical strength predisposing to deformity and pathological fracture. Accounts for approximately 10% of benign bone lesions. Patients range in age from < 1 year to 76 years. Seventy-five percent occur before the age of 30 years.
Focal fibrocartilaginous dysplasia (▶ Fig. 10.56)	Cortical thickening seen along concave side of tibia vara, and asymmetric thickening of the epiphysis medially.	Uncommon benign condition causing deformities of long bones in children. Most frequent at proxial tibia in young children, is typically unilateral, and results in tibia vara. Also occurs less frequently in femur, humerus, and ulna. Lesions show dense collagenous tissue, which may spontaneously regress. Corrective osteomy may be needed for severe and persistent lesions.
Melorheostosis (▶ Fig. 10.14)	MRI signal varies based on the relative proportions of mineralized osteoid, chondroid, and soft tissue components in these lesions. Mineralized osteoid zones involving bone cortex typically have low signal on T1WI and T2WI, no Gd-contrast enhancement. Soft tissue lesions may also occur adjacent to the cortical lesions, which have mixed signal on T1WI and T2WI.	Rare bone dysplasia with cortical thickening that has a "flowing candle wax" configuration. Associated soft tissue masses occur in approximately 25%. The soft tissue lesions often contain mixtures of chondroid material, mineralized osteoid, and fibrovascular tissue.

(continued on page 360)

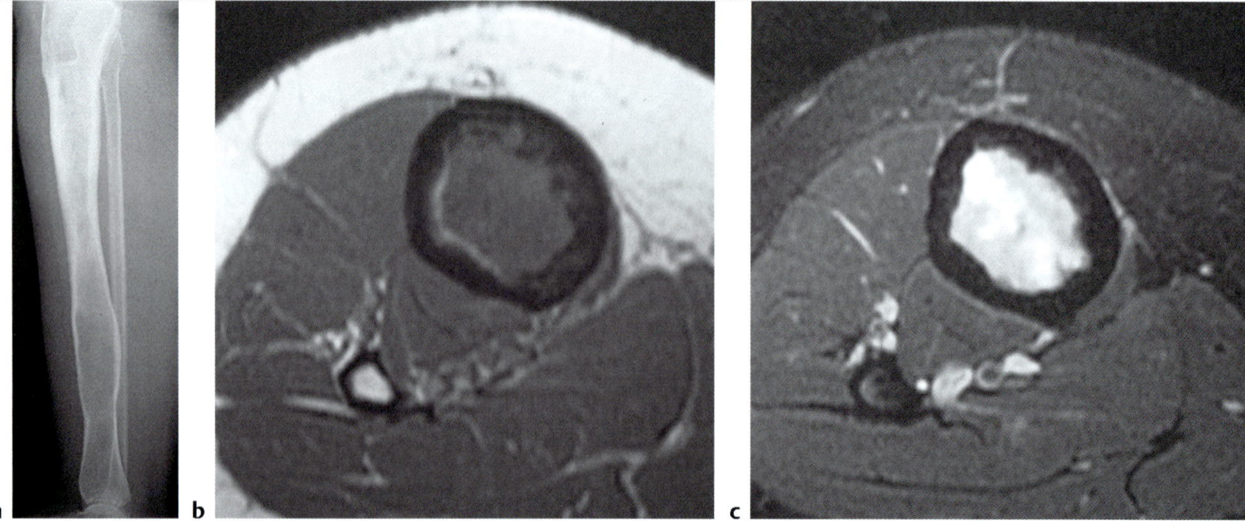

Fig. 10.54 Fibrous dysplasia involving the tibia in a 47-year-old woman. Cortical expansion with mixed thinning and thickening of bone cortex, mixed medullary radiolucency, and ground-glass appearance are seen on lateral radiograph (a). Cortical thickening is seen on axial T1-weighted imaging (T1WI) (b), and axial fat-suppressed T2-weighted imaging (FS T2WI) (c). Also seen is intermediate signal of the lesion within the marrow on axial T1WI and high signal on FS T2WI.

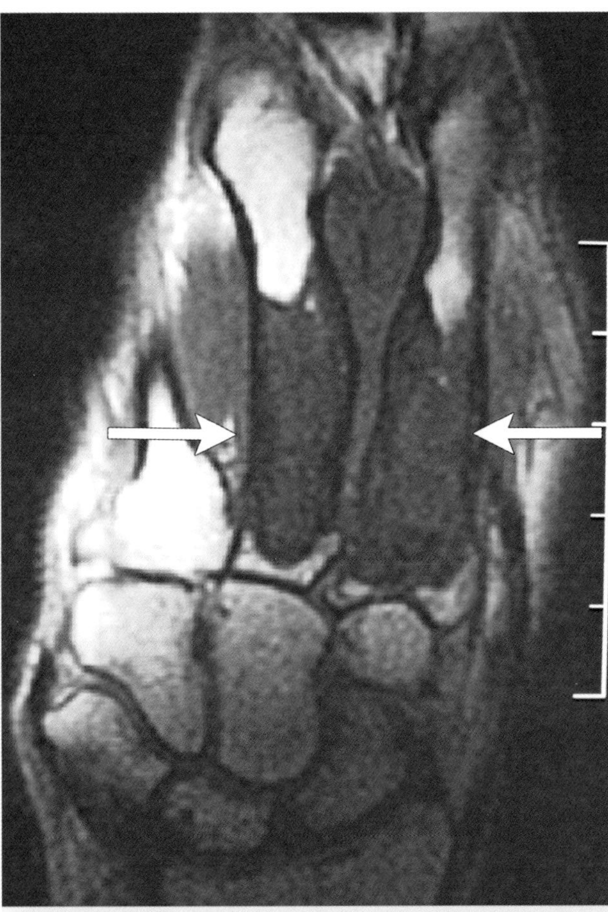

Fig. 10.55 Polyostotic fibrous dysplasia involving adjacent metacarpal bones with cortical thickening and intermediate marrow signal alteration on coronal T1-weighted imaging (arrows).

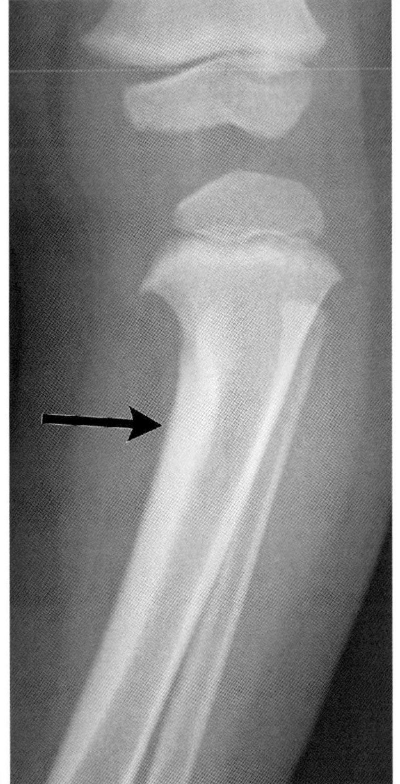

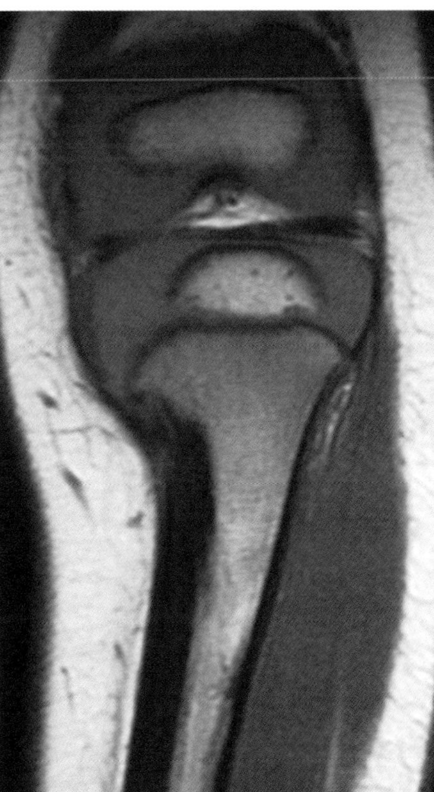

Fig. 10.56 Focal fibrocartilaginous dysplasia with cortical thickening along the concave side of tibia vara, and asymmetric thickening of the epiphysis medially (arrow) on anteroposterior radiograph (a) and coronal T1-weighted imaging (b).

Table 10.2 (Cont.) Lesions associated with thickening of bone cortex

Abnormalities	MRI findings	Comments
Healing and healed fractures (▶ Fig. 10.57; ▶ Fig. 10.58)	Healing stress or traumatic fractures can have periosteal elevation with associated adjacent high signal on T2WI and FS T2WI, as well as poorly defined marrow zones with high signal on T2WI and FS T2WI. Poorly defined zones of Gd-contrast enhancement can be seen in the juxtacortical soft tissues and marrow. Maturation of the periosteal reaction can lead to cortical thickening.	Fracture results in localized hemorrhage followed by an inflammatory response after 48 hours that leads to granulation tissue ingrowth, and activation of the osteoblasts in the periosteum. Periosteal bone formation results in cortical thickening. In addition, endosteal sclerosis with stress fractures can be seen on radiographs, computed tomographic scans, and MRI scans.
Paget disease (▶ Fig. 10.59)	In the late or inactive phases of Paget disease, findings include osseous expansion, cortical thickening, decreased diameter of the medullary canal, and coarsened trabeculae along stress lines. The zones of cortical thickening usually have low signal on T1WI and T2WI. The inner margins of the thickened cortex can be irregular, indistinct, or slightly lobulated.	Chronic skeletal disease in which there is disordered bone resorption and woven bone formation resulting in osseous deformity. Typically occurs in adults, 90% of cases occurring in patients older than 40 years.

(continued on page 362)

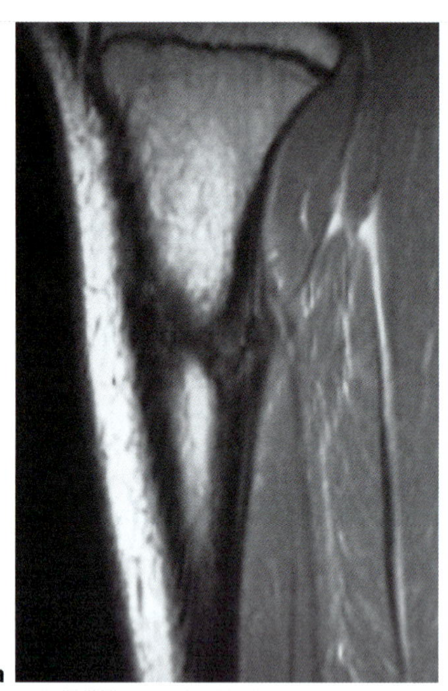

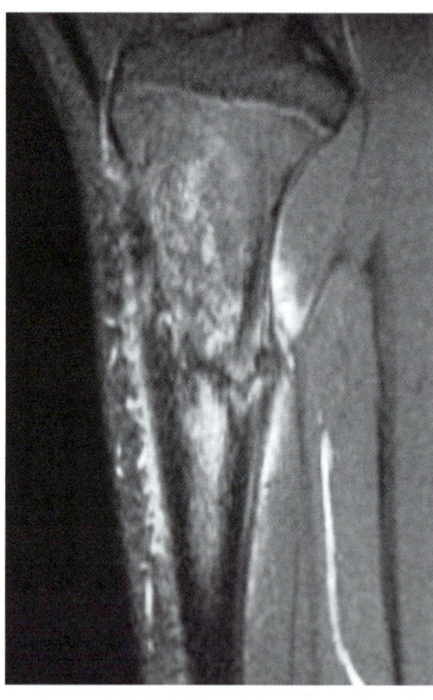

Fig. 10.57 Healing stress fracture involving the proximal tibial diaphysis with cortical thickening and endosteal sclerosis. The cortical thickening has mixed low and intermediate signal on sagittal T1-weighted imaging (a) and mixed slightly high and low signal on sagittal fat-suppressed T2-weighted imaging (FS T2WI) (b). Zones with high signal are seen within the marrow and juxtacortical soft tissues on FS T2WI. A thin zone of low signal is also seen within the marrow.

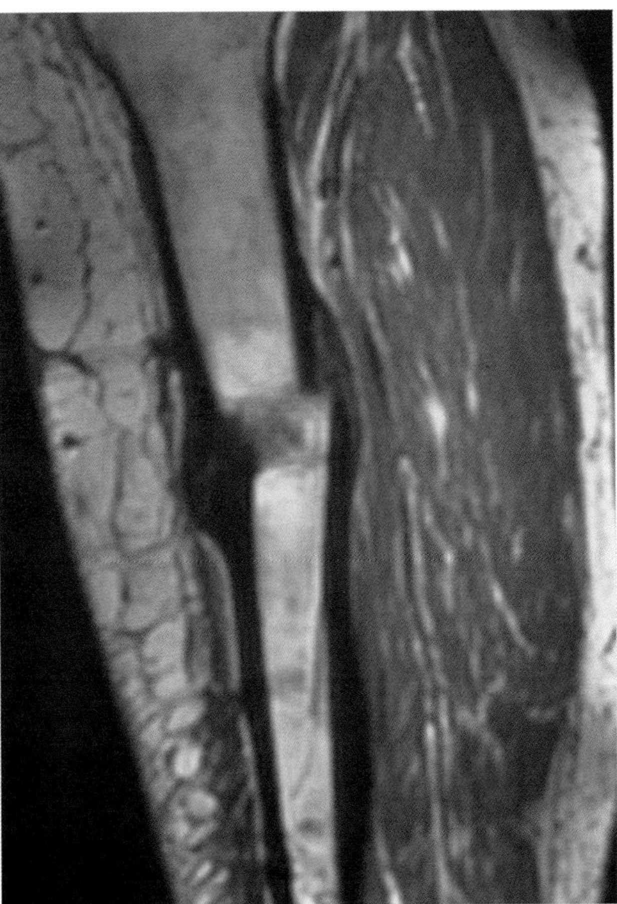

Fig. 10.58 Healed traumatic fracture deformity of the tibial shaft with thickened cortex as seen on sagittal T1-weighted imaging.

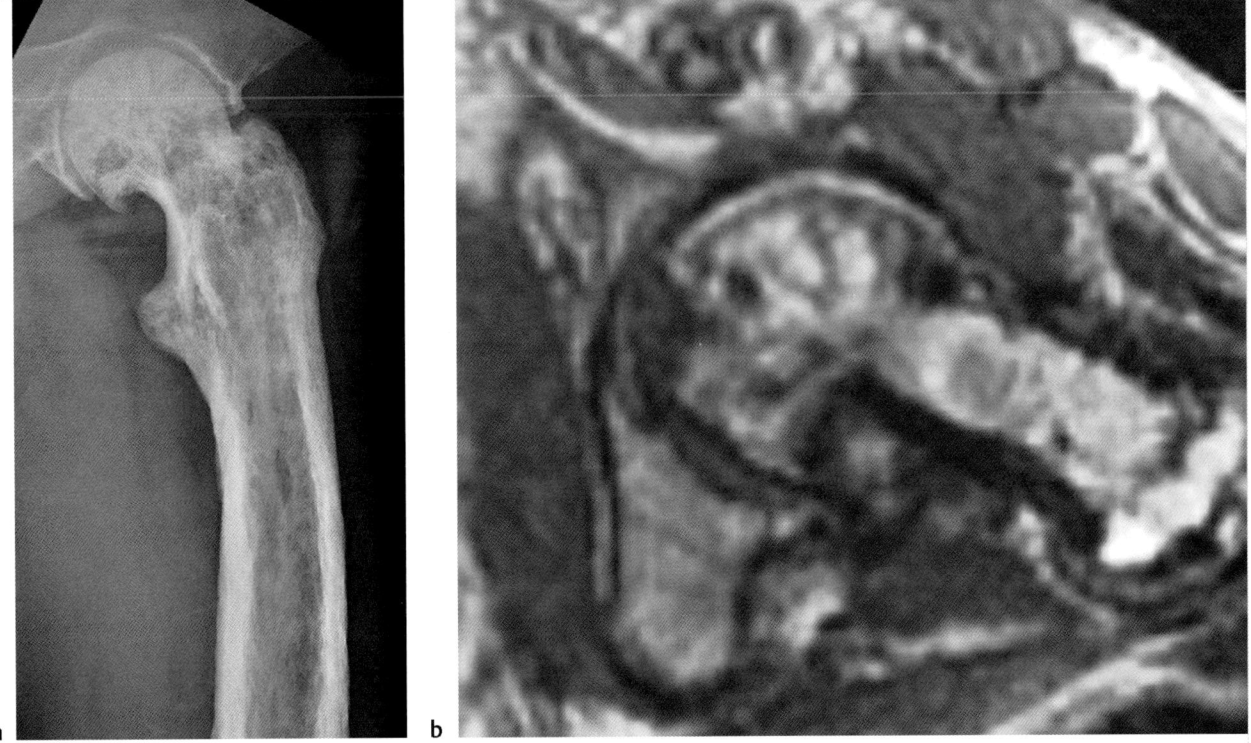

Fig. 10.59 Paget disease involving the proximal femur in a 70-year-old woman with cortical thickening at the medial femoral shaft on radiograph (a). Cortical thickening is seen as irregular zones with low signal on axial T1-weighted imaging (b).

Table 10.2 (Cont.) Lesions associated with thickening of bone cortex

Abnormalities	MRI findings	Comments
Subacute and chronic osteomyelitis (▶ Fig. 10.60)	A Brodie abscess represents a type of subacute osteomyelitis in long bones in which there is an intraosseous lesion (abscess) that can appear as a central zone with low to intermediate signal on T1WI and slightly high to high signal on T2WI surrounded by two rings, and an outer poorly-defined zone or halo with low to intermediate signal on T1WI and high signal on T2WI, FS T2WI, and short TI inversion recovery (STIR). The inner ring surrounding the abscess represents vascularized granulation tissue containing inflammatory cells and connective tissues and usually has low to intermediate signal on T1WI and high signal on T2WI. This inner ring usually shows Gd-contrast enhancement and has been referred to as the "penumbra sign." The outer ring often has low signal on T1WI and T2WI. Peripheral to these two rings, the poorly defined halo representing reactive edema often has low signal on T1WI, and low, intermediate, and/or high signal on T2WI and FS T2WI. The peripheral halo typically shows contrast enhancement. A sinus tract may be seen extending through thickened cortex adjacent to the intraosseous abscess. In chronic active osteomyelitis, findings include intraosseous abscess, sequestra, cloacae, subperiosteal fluid collections, and cortical thickening. A narrow zone or rim of low signal on T1WI and T2WI is often seen separating the site of chronic osteomyelitis from normal adjacent bone marrow. Within this rim, a zone with low-intermediate signal on T1WI and heterogeneous intermediate, slightly high, to high signal is usually seen representing the intraosseous infection or abscess that may contain foci of low signal on T1WI and T2WI from sequestra. Irregular zones of Gd-contrast enhancement may be seen in active chronic osteomyelitis. Cloacae and sinus tracts can appear as linear or curvilinear zones with high signal on T2WI and Gd-contrast enhancement involving thickened cortex and extraosseous soft tissues.	Osteomyelitis refers to infection of bone and can result from hematogenous spread of microorganisms, trauma-direct inoculation, extension from adjacent tissues, and complications from surgery. A Brodie abscess refers to a small metaphyseal or diaphyseal abscess (subacute osteomyelitis) in long bones that are typically walled off by sclerotic bone and often involve the cortex. Sclerosing osteomyelitis of Garré is a chronic bone infection that usually involves the mandible or shafts of long bones, which is associated with extensive new bone formation that often obscures the involved osseous structure.
Chronic recurrent mutifocal osteomyelitis (▶ Fig. 10.24)	Multifocal lesions that occur in metaphyses of tubular bones (distal femur, proximal and distal tibia and fibula), clavicles, and vertebrae. Radiographs show radiolucent and/or sclerotic osseous lesions with proliferative periosteal bone formation. MRI shows heterogeneous abnormal high signal on FS T2WI in marrow and periosteal soft tissues with Gd-contrast enhancement.	Painful inflammatory osseous disorder of unknown cause with histopathology of acute and chronic osteomyelitis without identification of infectious agent, diagnosis of exclusion. Usually occurs in children and adolescents, median age = 10 years, F 85%/M 15%. Multi-episodic skeletal disorder of unknown cause that can occur over 7 to 25 years. Treatment of symptoms with nonsteroidal anti-inflammatory drugs. Can be associated with acne or pustulosis palmoplantaris (SAPHO).
Syndromes of hyperostosis, osteitis, and skin lesions (SAPHO syndrome)	Periosteal elevation with cortical thickening can be seen as well as syndesmophyte formation at one or multiple levels.	Syndrome that includes abnormalities such as synovitis, acne, pustulosis, hyperostosis with periosteal proliferation (sternum, clavicle, anterior ribs, symphysis pubis, femur, sacrum, iliac bones) and osteitis at the chest wall.

(continued on page 364)

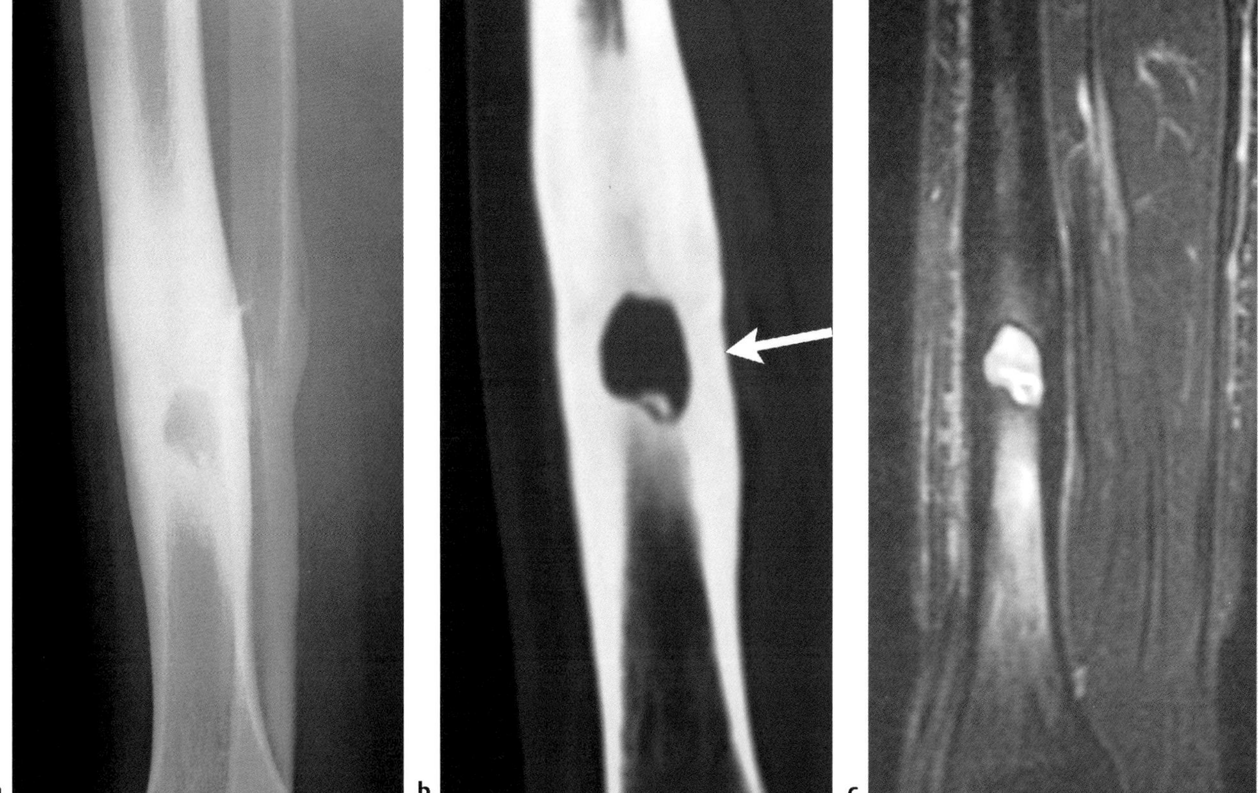

Fig. 10.60 A Brodie abscess in the distal tibial shaft with dense sclerotic thickening of the cortex and medullary bone seen on a radiograph (a) and computed tomographic image (arrow) (b). A radiolucent abscess is also seen in medullary bone. The cortical thickening has mostly low signal on coronal fat-suppressed T2-weighted imaging (FS T2WI) (c). Poorly defined zones with high signal on FS T2WI are seen within the marrow surrounding a circumscribed high signal abscess.

Table 10.2 (Cont.) Lesions associated with thickening of bone cortex

Abnormalities	MRI findings	Comments
Neurofibromatosis type 1 (NF1) (▶ Fig. 10.34)	Irregular periosteal thickening of long bones of the lower extremities can be seen as zones of low signal. Undulating zones of periosteal bone formation can occur in the lower extremities in patients with NF1.	Subperiosteal proliferation of bone can occasionally be seen involving long bones of the lower extremities in patients with NF1. One of the most common genetic diseases with the involved locus on chromosome 17q12 typically resulting in multiple neurofibromas. This autosomal dominant disorder resulting in mesodermal dysplasia affecting multiple organ systems. Can result in periosteal proliferation in the long bones of the lower extremities.
Noninterrupted periosteal reaction and bone formation from primary hypertrophic osteoarthropathy (pachydermoperiostosis) (▶ Fig. 10.61)	Linear and/or irregular periosteal and cortical thickening seen in tubular bones of the extremities bilaterally (tibia, fibula, radius, ulna are common sites, also seen in other bones and skull). Can involve epiphyseal, metaphyseal, and/or diaphyseal portions of long bones.	Rare clinical syndrome in adolescents or adults with swollen painful joints, enlargement of the extremities from osseous proliferation and periostitis, clubbing of digits, thickening of skin of the face and scalp with excessive sweating and sebaceous secretions. Can be hereditary (autosomal dominant with variable expression) or idiopathic.
Noninterrupted periosteal reaction and bone formation from secondary hypertrophic osteoarthropathy (▶ Fig. 10.32)	Smooth, wavy, and or irregular periosteal and cortical thickening seen in the diaphyseal and metaphyseal portions of long bones of the upper and lower extremities, as well as in other bones.	Clinical syndrome with clubbing of the digits, periostitis, hypertrophic osteoarthropathy, skin thickening, limb swelling, nail bed abnormalities (striations, increased curvature) related to extraskeletal lesions involving the lungs (bronchogenic carcinoma, metastasis, cystic fibrosis, bronchiectasis, infection, lymphoma), pleura (mesothelioma), abdomen (biliary atresia, cirrhosis, tumors, ulcerative colitis, Crohn disease), heart (cyanotic heart disease), and neoplasms at other sites. Regression of hypertrophic osteoarthropathy can occur after thoracotomy in patients with thoracic abnormalities, even in those without complete removal of the intrathoracic lesions.
Noninterrupted periosteal reaction and bone formation from venous stasis (▶ Fig. 10.33)	Smooth and wavy periosteal and cortical thickening seen in the diaphyseal and metaphyseal portions of long bones of the lower extremities (tibia, fibula, metatarsal bones, phalanges).	Venous stasis is associated with edematous changes in the soft tissues as well as soft tissue ossification, periostitis, and cortical thickening.
Noninterrupted periosteal reaction and bone formation from infantile cortical hyperostosis (Caffey disease) (▶ Fig. 10.62)	Smooth, wavy, and or irregular periosteal and cortical thickening seen in the diaphyseal and metaphyseal portions of one or multiple bones.	Clinical disorder that affects infants less than 5 months old with findings of soft tissue swelling (commonly over the mandible), fever, hyperirritability, and cortical hyperostosis (ribs, ulna, tibia, fibula, humerus, femur, radius, metacarpal and metatarsal bones). The clinical course is variable but regression of findings can occur over 3 to 4 years.

(continued on page 366)

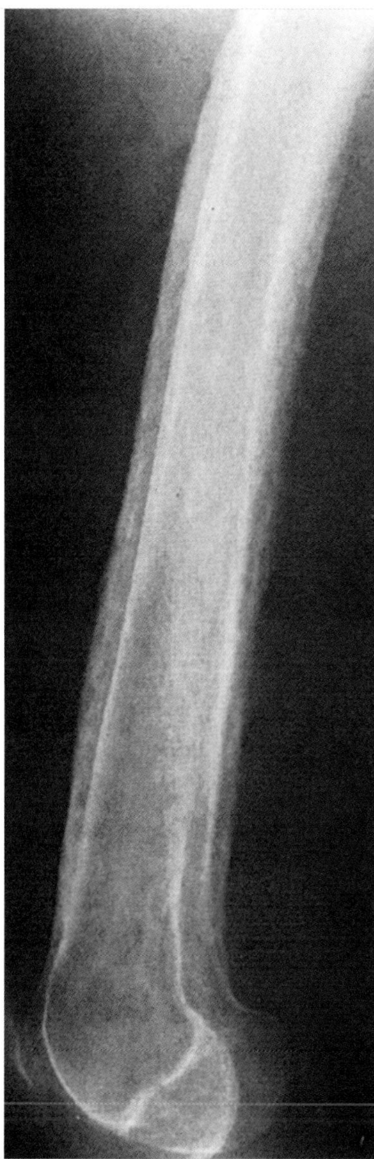

Fig. 10.61 Pachydermoperiostosis. Lateral radiograph shows solid thick and slightly irregular periosteal bone formation.

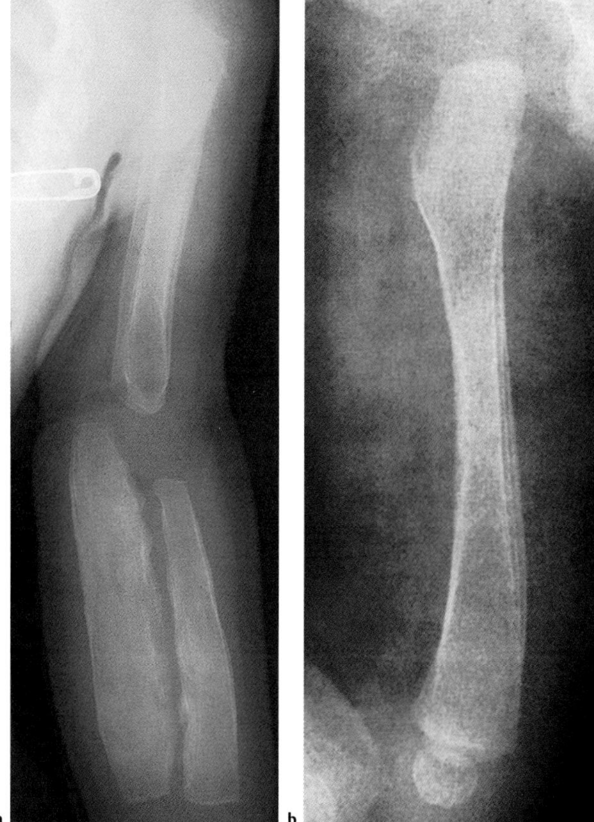

Fig. 10.62 Infantile cortical hyperstosis (Caffey disease) anteroposterior radiograph (a) shows perisoteal thickening with cortical thickening and widened dense diaphyses of long bones of the upper extremity. Lamellated periosteal reaction is seen on radiograph in another patient (b).

Table 10.2 (Cont.) Lesions associated with thickening of bone cortex

Abnormalities	MRI findings	Comments
Progressive diaphyseal dysplasia (Camurati-Engelmann disease) (▶ Fig. 10.63)	Bilateral cortical thickening of both periosteal and endosteal surfaces of long bones (midshafts of diaphyses) in a fusiform pattern with abrupt transition to normal bone. Narrowing of medullary canals. Bones frequently involved: Tibia > femur > fibula > humerus > ulna and radius. Lack of involvement of epiphyses and metaphyses typical. Rarely involves the skull base.	Autosomal dominant neuromuscular disorder involving intramembranous ossification related to mutations of the gene encoding the latency–associated peptide of transforming growth factor-beta1 (TGF-beta1), which mediates bone remodeling. Clinical onset usually 4 to 12 years with muscle weakness, pain, malnutrition, leg weakness, and wide waddling gait.
Hereditary multiple diaphyseal sclerosis (ribbing disease)	Unilateral and/or asymmetric cortical thickening of both periosteal and endosteal surfaces of long bones (midshafts of diaphyses) in a fusiform pattern with abrupt transition to normal bone. Does not involve skull.	Autosomal recessive neuromuscular disorder of unknown genetics involving intramembranous ossification of long bones, clinical onset after puberty with slowly progressive weakness and pain. Symptoms less severe than with Camurati-Engelmann disease.
Craniodiaphyseal dysplasia (▶ Fig. 10.64)	Osteosclerosis of diaphyses of tubular bones in infancy with progressive widened diaphyses and cortical thinning, lack of metaphyseal flaring. Sclerosis of skull base and calvarium, thickened mandible with dental malocclusion, and lack of normal pneumatization of paranasal sinuses and mastoid air cells.	Rare autosomal recessive craniotubular bone dysplasia with progressive hyperostosis of the skull and facial bones, hypertelorism, thickening of cortical bone and lack of normal modeling of short and long tubular bones. Patients often have short stature and have mental retardation.
Craniometaphyseal dysplasia	Hyperostosis of frontal and occipital bones, diaphyseal sclerosis, club-shaped metaphyseal widening of tubular bones.	Rare autosomal dominant craniotubular bone dysplasia. Can be inherited as autosomal dominant from mutations involving the ANKH gene on chromosome 5p15.2–14.1 or autosomal recessive from mutations involving chromosome 6q21–22. Patients usually have normal stature and normal mental function.
Craniometadiaphyseal dysplasia	Large skull with frontal prominence, delayed closure of fontanelles and sutures, dental hypoplasia, wide diaphyses of tubular bones, thinning of cortical bone, wide ribs and clavicles.	Rare autosomal recessive craniotubular bone dysplasia. Patients usually have normal stature and normal mental function.

(continued on page 368)

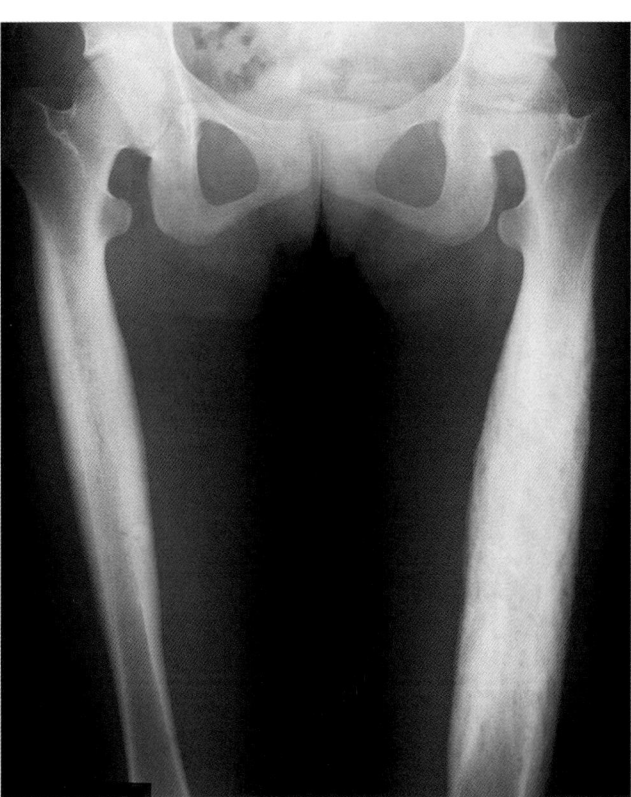

Fig. 10.63 Progressive diaphyseal dysplasia (Camurati-Engelmann disease) radiograph shows bilateral cortical thickening (both periosteal and endosteal surfaces) at the midshafts of the femurs with abrupt transitions to normal bone.

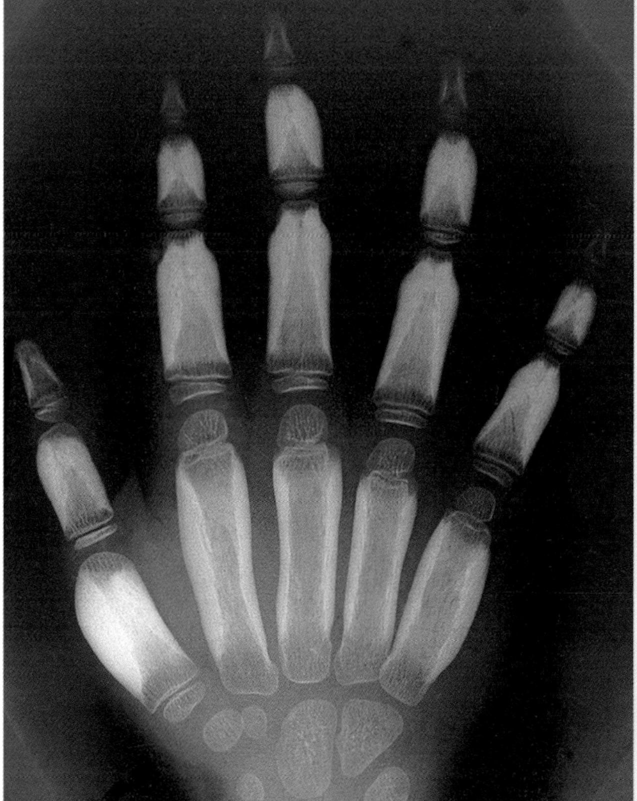

Fig. 10.64 Craniodiaphyseal dysplasia. Radiograph shows thickening of bone cortex of the phalanges and metacarpal bones.

Table 10.2 (Cont.) Lesions associated with thickening of bone cortex

Abnormalities	MRI findings	Comments
Generalized cortical hyperostosis (van Buchem syndrome) (▶ Fig. 10.65)	Bilateral symmetric sclerosis and endosteal cortical bone thickening involving the diaphyses of long bones, as well sclerosis and thickening of the calvarium, skull base, mandible, clavicles, ribs, and spinous processes.Small periosteal excrescences occur in Van Buchem syndrome.	Rare group of intramembranous ossification disorders with endosteal hyperostosis. Four main types, which all involve mutations affecting the Wnt signaling pathway osteoblasts. Van Buchem syndrome is an autosomal recessive disorder that involves mutations of the sclerostin gene on chromosome 17q12-q21; Worth disease has autosomal dominant inheritance related to mutations of the lipoprotein receptor-related protein 5 gene making it unable to normally bind sclerostin; Nakamura disease has autosomal dominant inheritance with enlargement of the mandible and maxillae; and Truswell-Hansen disease is associated with sclerosteosis and syndactyly from mutated gene on chromosome17.
Pyknodysostosis (Maroteaux-Lamy syndrome)	Generalized hyperostsosis of long bones with preservation of medullary canal, sclerosis of calvarium and skull base, wormian bones, little or no pneumatization of paranasal sinuses, mandible hypoplasia.	Autosomal recessive disorder involving osteoclasts resulting from mutations of the cathepsin K gene. Clinical findings include dwarfism, wormian bones, hypoplasia of facial bones, pectus excavatum acro-osteolysis involving fingers.
Noninterrupted periosteal reaction and bone formation from thyroid acropachy (▶ Fig. 10.66)	Asymmetric, irregular, spiculated periosteal thickening seen in the diaphyseal portions of one or multiple bones (metacarpal and metatarsal bones, phalanges, other bones).	This disorder represents an extreme form of autoimmune thyroid disease with clinical manifestations such as swelling of the digits and toes, digital clubbing, and periosteal reaction. Thyroid dermopathy (pretibial myxedema) occurs in 4% of patients with Graves ophthalmopathy. Pronounced cases of thyroid dermopathy can be associated with thyroid acropachy in 1% of patients with Graves ophthalmopathy.
Noninterrupted periosteal reaction from hypervitaminosis A	Smooth and wavy periosteal and cortical thickening seen in the diaphyseal portions of one or multiple bones (ulna, metatarsal bones, clavicle, tibia, fibula, other bones). Damage to the physeal plates can result in irregularities and premature fusion, as well as splaying and cupping deformities of the metaphyses.	Vitamin A intoxication in children can result in anorexia, dermatologic and osseous disorders. In children, damage to the physeal plates may be irreversible despite cessation of vitamin A administration. In adults, anorexia, weight loss, and dermatologic disorders are frequently associated with hypervitaminosis A.
Noninterrupted periosteal reaction from hypovitaminosis A	Smooth and wavy periosteal and cortical thickening seen in the diaphyseal portions of one or multiple bones,	Vitamin A deficiency can result in anemia, dermatologic abnormalities (dry and scaly skin), growth retardation, osseous abnormalities, cranial nerve and visual disorders.

(continued on page 370)

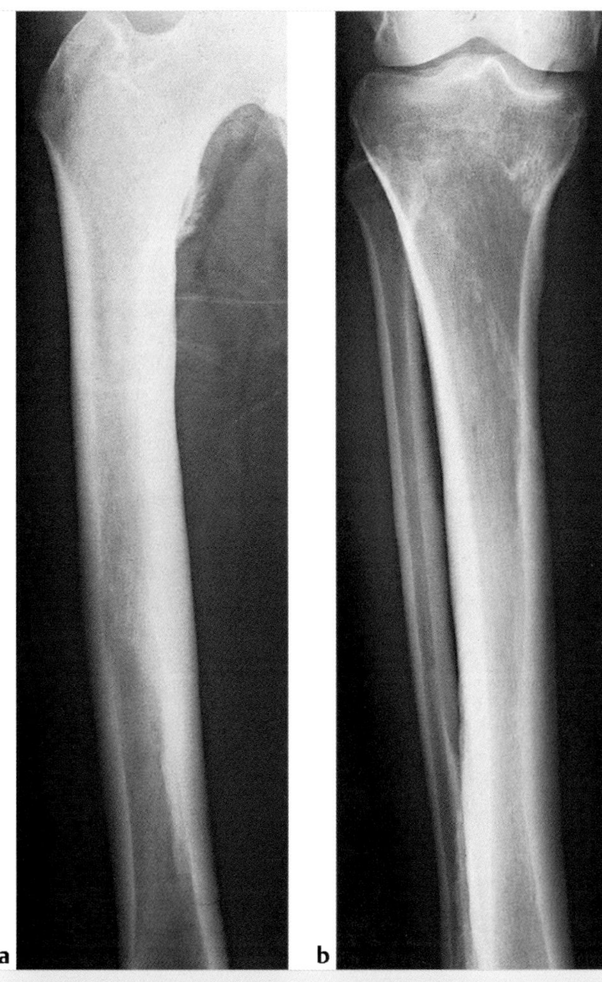

Fig. 10.65 Generalized cortical hyperostosis (van Buchem syndrome). Radiographs show sclerosis and cortical thickening involving the diaphyses of the femur, tibia, and fibula.

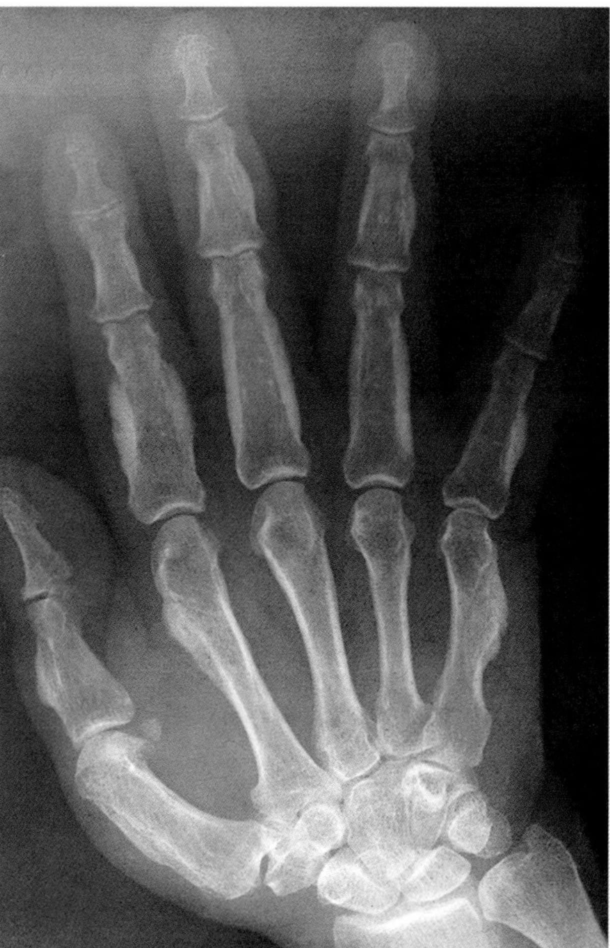

Fig. 10.66 Thyroid acropachy. Radiograph shows asymmetric, irregular, periosteal cortical bone thickening involving the diaphyseal portions of multiple metacarpal bones and phalanges.

Table 10.2 (Cont.) Lesions associated with thickening of bone cortex

Abnormalities	MRI findings	Comments
Noninterrupted periosteal reaction from hypovitaminosis C (scurvy) (▶ Fig. 10.67)	In children, periosteal elevation with new bone formation can be seen in the diaphyseal and metaphyseal portions of one or multiple bones from subperiosteal hemorrhage. Metaphyseal beaklike bone protrusions can occur from the abnormal zones of provisional calcification at the physeal plate, as well as subepiphyseal fractures. In adults, osteopenia with hemarthrosis can be associated with ischemic necrosis and fractures with mild periosteal reaction.	In young children, vitamin C deficiency after 4 to 10 months can result in infantile scurvy with clinical features including failure to thrive, petechial hemorrhages, ulcerated gingiva, hematemesis, melena, hematuria, and anemia. Clinical features associated with adult scurvy include anorexia, fatigue, weakness, petechial hemorrhages involving gingiva and skin, hemarthrosis, osteoporosis, ischemic necrosis, dermatologic disorders (dry and scaly skin), growth retardation, osseous and nerve disorders.
Malignant lesions		
Parosteal osteosarcoma (▶ Fig. 10.68)	These tumors occur at the surface of bone and extend outward with well-defined and/or indistinct margins. Portions of these tumors that extend toward the juxtacortical soft tissues typically have mixed soft tissue and mineralized components. The mineralized portions of these tumors tend to be dense centrally and at the sites of contiguity (broad-based or stalk-like) with the outer cortical margins. The mineralized portions of these tumors usually have low signal on T1WI, PDWI, T2WI, and FS PDWI and FS T2WI. The soft tissue portions of these tumors often have low-intermediate signal on T1WI, intermediate to slightly high or high signal on T2WI, and high signal on FS PDWI and FS T2WI. Tumor extension into the medullary space seen with MRI can occur in up to 50%. After Gd-contrast administration, nonnecrotic or nonmineralized soft tissue portions of these tumors usually show enhancement as well as sites of invasion into the medullary space and adjacent soft tissues.	Malignant tumor composed of proliferating neoplastic spindle cells, which produce osteoid and/or immature tumoral bone. Parosteal osteosarcomas arise on the external surface of bone and account for 4 to 6% of osteosarcomas. They occur in patients age 6 to 80 years, median = 27 years.

(continued on page 372)

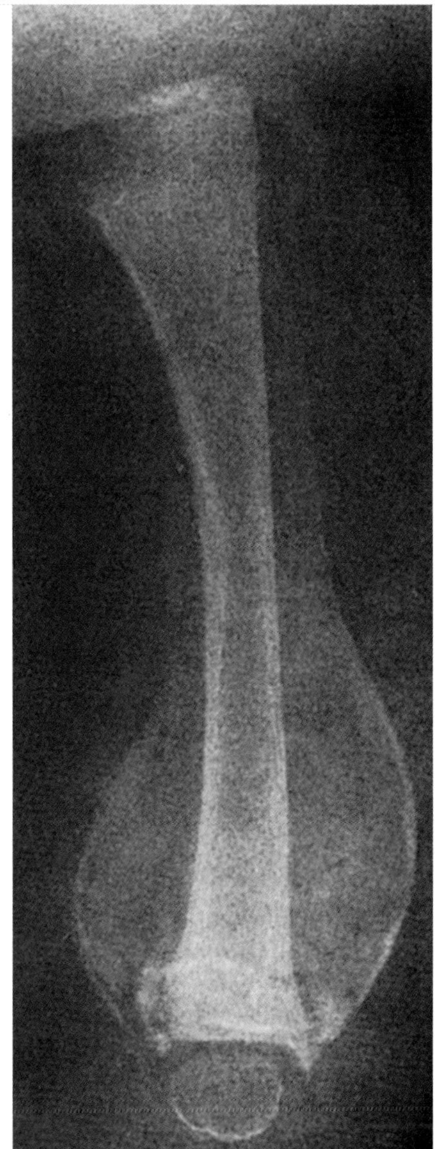

Fig. 10.67 Hypovitaminosis C (scurvy). Radiograph shows periosteal elevation with calcified subperiosteal hemorrhage.

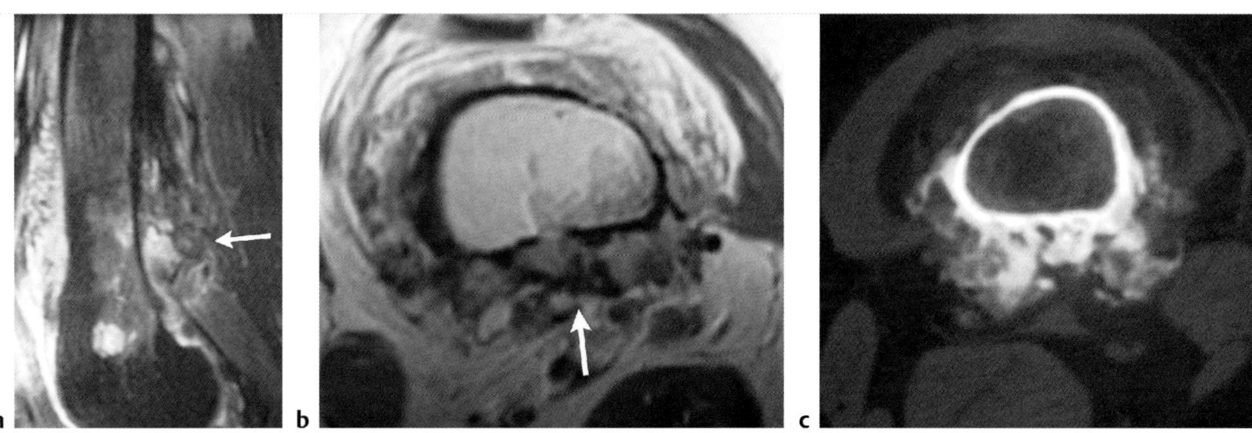

Fig. 10.68 Parosteal osteosarcoma of the dorsal distal portion of the femur in a 45-year-old woman. The tumor has mixed low, intermediate, slightly high, and high signal (arrow) on sagittal fat-suppressed T2-weighted imaging (a) and mixed low and intermediate signal (arrow) on axial proton density–weighted imaging (b). The tumor extends into the marrow through a zone of cortical destruction. The mineralized portions of this tumor have low signal. Axial computed tomographic image (c) shows soft tissue tumor containing mineralized osteoid along the dorsal, medial, and lateral outer margins of the bone cortex.

Table 10.2 (Cont.) Lesions associated with thickening of bone cortex

Abnormalities	MRI findings	Comments
Intraosseous osteosarcoma (▶ Fig. 10.69)	Intramedullary osteosarcomas often have zones of cortical destruction through which tumors extend toward the extraosseous soft tissues under an elevated periosteum. Lamellated and/or spiculated zones of bone formation can occur under the periosteal elevation secondary to tumor invasion and perforation of bone cortex. Low signal from spicules of periosteal, reactive, and tumoral bone formation may have a divergent (sunburst) pattern, perpendicular (hair on end) pattern, or disorganized or complex appearance.	Malignant tumor composed of proliferating neoplastic spindle cells that produce osteoid and/or immature tumoral bone and which most often occur within bone. Intraosseous osteosarcoma accounts for 91 to 95% of osteosarcomas. Osteogenic sarcoma has two age peaks of incidence. The larger peak occurs between the ages of 10 and 20 and accounts for over half of the cases. The second smaller peak occurs in adults over 60 years and accounts for approximately 10% of the cases.
Adamantinoma (▶ Fig. 10.70)	Most frequently appear as a solitary lobulated focus versus a multinodular pattern of signal alteration in thickened bone cortex. More than half involve bone cortex and marrow compared with only cortical involvement. Tumor foci in bone typically have low-intermediate signal on T1WI and PDWI, and slightly high to high signal on T2WI and FS T2WI. Lesions usually show prominent Gd-contrast enhancement. Adamantinomas with a multinodular pattern have enhancing nodules that have high signal on T2WI and FS T2WI separated by zones of low signal from intervening cortical bone.	Rare low-grade malignant bone tumors consisting of epithelial cells surrounded by spindle cells and osteofibrous tissue that often involve the shaft of the tibia and account for < 1% of primary bone tumors. Patients range in age from 3 to 86 years, median = 19 to 25 years, average = 35 years, most common in third and fourth decades.

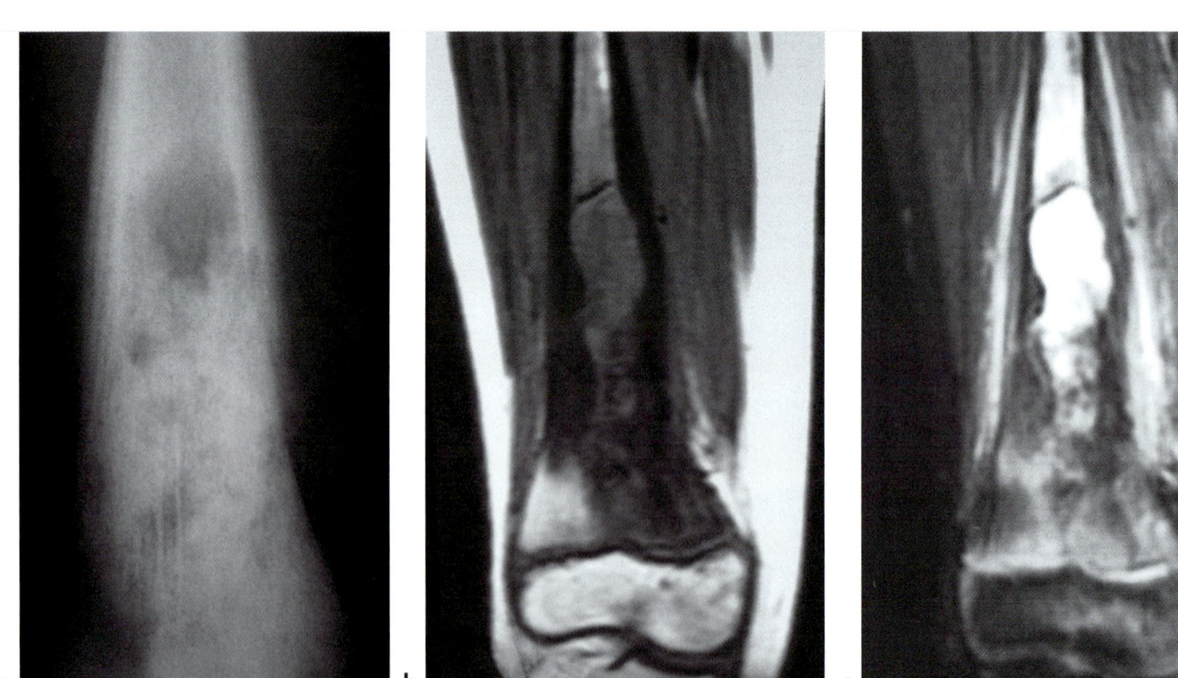

Fig. 10.69 A 10-year-old boy with a conventional intramedullary osteosarcoma in the marrow of the distal dimetaphyseal portion of the femur. The tumor is associated with "onion skin" multilayered tumoral periosteal reaction laterally and interrupted tumoral periosteal reaction with a Codman triangle medially on anteroposterior radiograph (a). The tumor has heterogeneous intermediate signal on coronal T1-weighted imaging (b) and heterogeneous high signal on coronal fat-suppressed T2-weighted imaging (c). The intramedullary tumor is associated with zones of cortical destruction, periosteal elevation, and extraosseous extension.

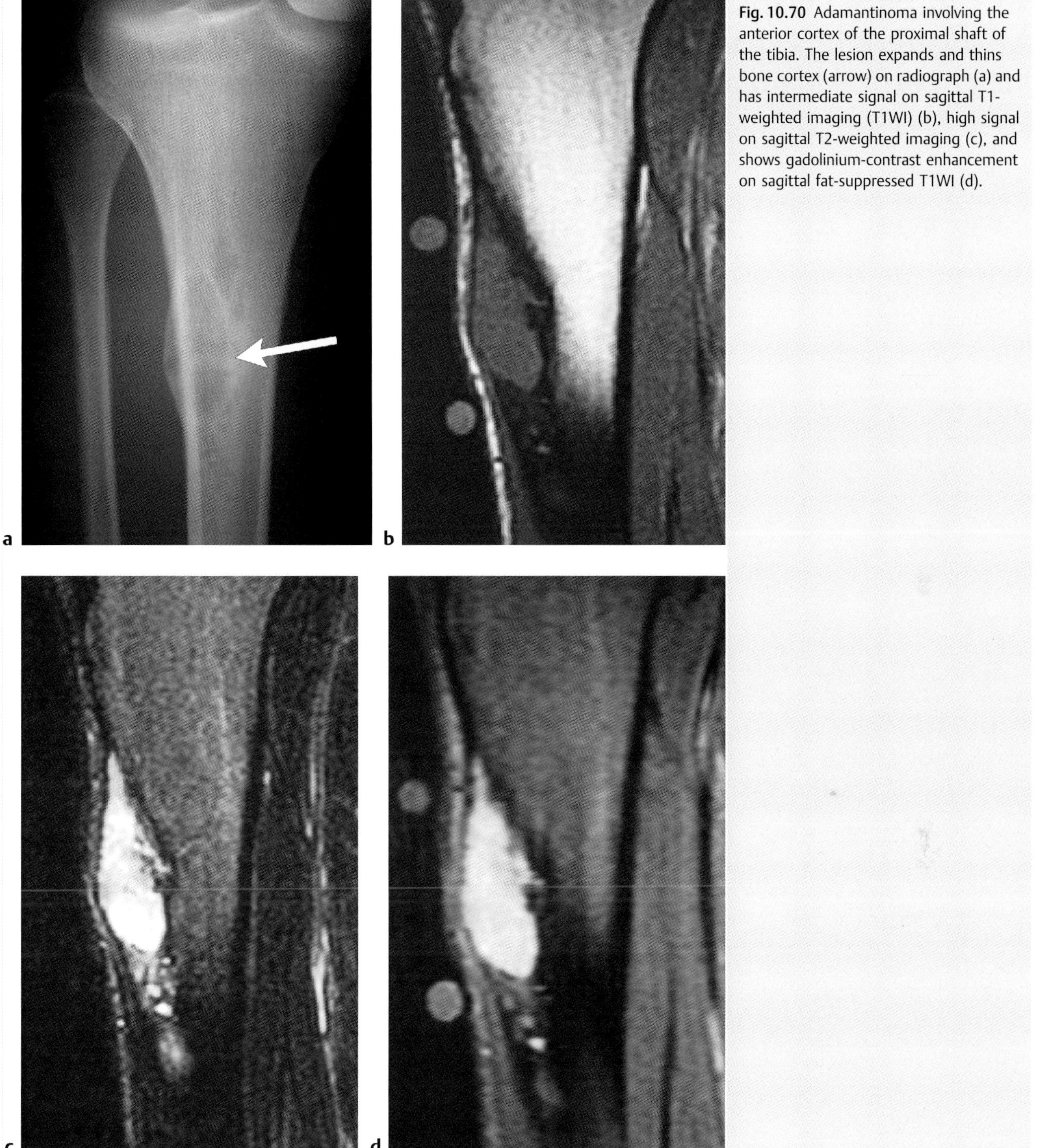

Fig. 10.70 Adamantinoma involving the anterior cortex of the proximal shaft of the tibia. The lesion expands and thins bone cortex (arrow) on radiograph (a) and has intermediate signal on sagittal T1-weighted imaging (T1WI) (b), high signal on sagittal T2-weighted imaging (c), and shows gadolinium-contrast enhancement on sagittal fat-suppressed T1WI (d).

10.3 Intramedullary Lesions Associated with Expansion of Intact Cortical Margins

- Nonmalignant lesions
  - Nonossifying fibroma (fibroxanthoma)
  - Osteochondroma
  - Enchondroma
  - Fibrous dysplasia
  - Unicameral bone cyst (UBC)
  - Aneurysmal bone cyst (ABC)
  - Giant cell reparative granuloma (solid aneurysmal bone cyst)
  - Giant cell tumor of bone
  - Chondromyxoid fibroma
  - Osteoblastoma
  - Hemangioma
  - Chondroblastoma
  - Ameloblastoma
  - Desmoplastic fibroma
  - Osteofibrous dysplasia
  - Gaucher disease
  - Hemophilic pseudotumor
  - Brown tumor
- Malignant lesions
  - Adamantinoma
  - Other malignant lesions

Table 10.3 Intramedullary lesions associated with expansion of intact cortical margins

Abnormalities	MRI findings	Comments
Nonmalignant lesions		
Nonossifying fibroma (fibroxanthoma) (▶ Fig. 10.71)	Well-circumscribed eccentric intramedullary lesions in the dimetaphyseal regions of long bones, which have mixed low-intermediate signal on T1-weighted imaging (T1WI), and mixed low, intermediate, and/or high signal on T2-weighted imaging (T2WI), proton density–weighted imaging (PDWI), and fat-suppressed (FS) T2WI. Zones of low signal on T1WI, PDWI, and T2WI can be seen in the central portions of the lesions. Zones with varying thickness of low signal on T1WI, PDWI, and T2WI are seen at the margins of the lesions representing bone sclerosis. Internal septations are commonly seen as zones of low signal on T2WI in these lesions. Cortical thinning or thickening, and bone expansion can be seen. Lesions can show gadolinium (Gd)-contrast enhancement (heterogeneous > homogeneous patterns). Linear periosteal Gd-contrast enhancement can be seen at lesions with associated fracture or marked cortical expansion/thinning.	Fibrous cortical defects (FCDs) and nonossifying fibromas (NOFs) are well-circumscribed common benign fibrohistiocytic lesions in the metaphyseal portions of long bones, which are composed of whorls of fibroblastic cells combined with smaller amounts of multinucleated giant cells and xanthomatous cells. Both FCDs and NOFs have similar pathological findings, although they differ in size and primary locations in long bones. FCDs are small lesions primarily located in bone cortex, whereas the larger NOFs are located eccentrically in the medullary cavity. FCDs and NOFs are usually asymptomatic and are often detected as incidental findings. The true incidence of these lesions is unknown but may be up to 40% of children; 95% occur between the ages of 5 and 20, median = 14 years.
Osteochondroma (▶ Fig. 10.72)	Circumscribed protruding lesion arising from outer cortex with a central zone with intermediate signal on T1WI and T2WI similar to marrow surrounded by a peripheral zone of low signal on T1WI and T2WI. A cartilaginous cap with high signal on T2WI and FS T2WI is usually present in children and young adults. Increased malignant potential when the cartilaginous cap is > 2 cm thick. The cartilaginous caps regress and involute progressively after skeletal maturation.	Benign cartilaginous tumors arising from defect at periphery of growth plate during bone formation with resultant bone outgrowth covered by a cartilaginous cap. Usually benign lesions unless associated with pain and increasing size of cartilaginous cap. Osteochondromas are common lesions, accounting for 14 to 35% of primary bone tumors. Occur with median age of 20 years, up to 75% of patients are less than 20 years.

(continued on page 376)

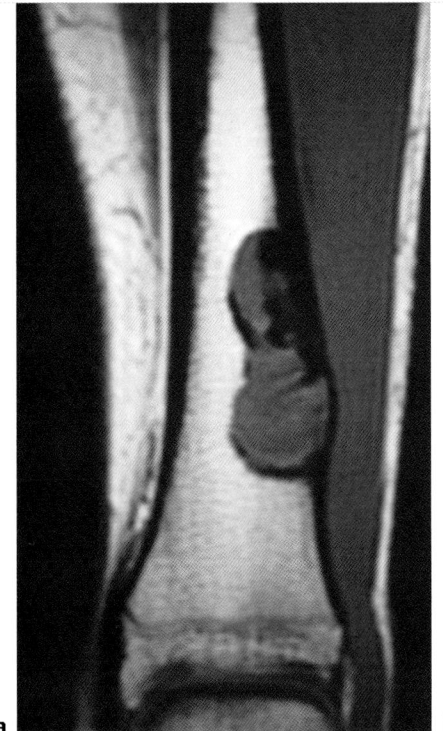

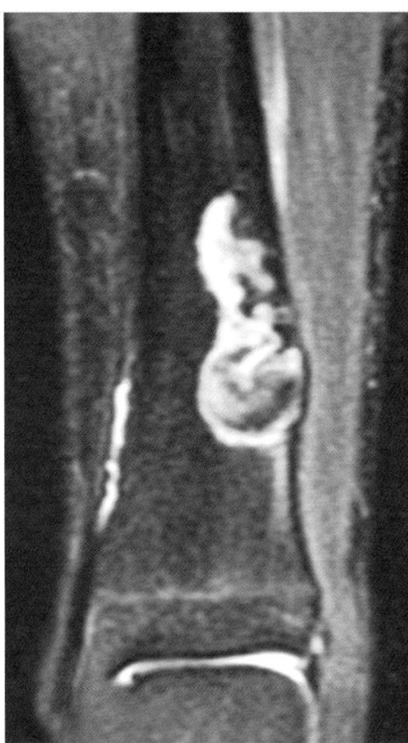

Fig. 10.71 A 16-year-old girl with a non-ossifying fibroma involving the diaphyseal portion of the distal tibia. The lesion has circumscribed margins and has mixed low and intermediate signal on coronal T1-weighted imaging (a) and low and high signal on coronal fat-suppressed T2-weighted imaging (b). Cortical thinning and slight expansion are seen.

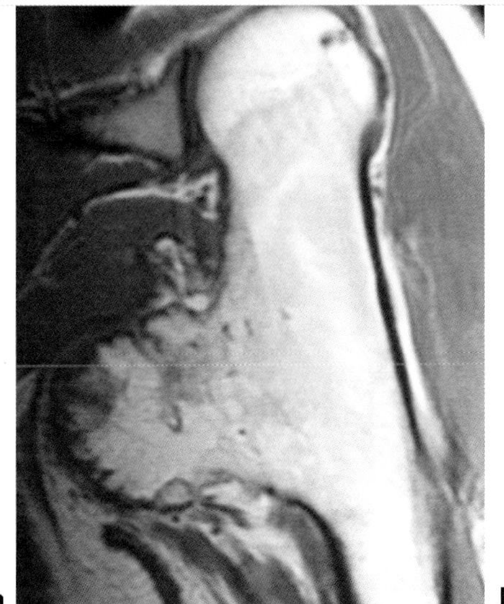

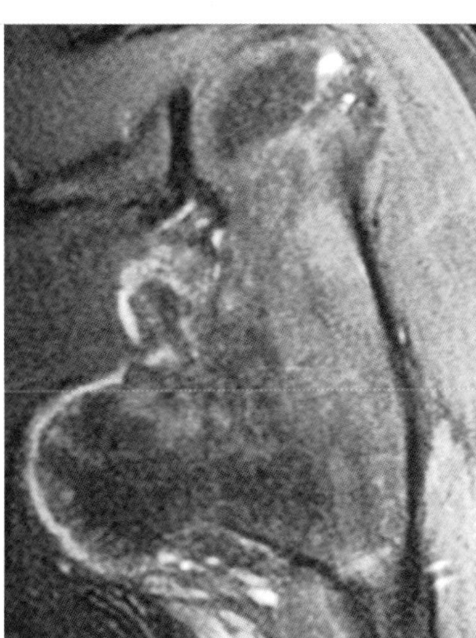

Fig. 10.72 A 22-year-old man with an osteochondroma protruding medially from the proximal humerus as seen on coronal T1-weighted imaging (a) and coronal fat-suppresed T2-weighted imaging (b).

Table 10.3 (Cont.) Intramedullary lesions associated with expansion of intact cortical margins

Abnormalities	MRI findings	Comments
Enchondroma (▸ Fig. 10.73)	Lobulated intramedullary lesions with well-defined borders ranging in size from 3 to 16 cm, mean = 5 cm. Mild endosteal scalloping can be seen. Cortical bone expansion rarely occurs. Lesions usually have low-intermediate signal on T1WI and intermediate signal on PDWI. On T2WI and FS T2WI, lesions usually have predominantly high signal with foci and/or bands of low signal representing areas of matrix mineralization and fibrous strands. No zones of abnormal high signal on T2WI are typically seen in the marrow outside the borders of the lesions. Lesions typically show Gd-contrast enhancement in various patterns (peripheral curvilinear lobular, central nodular/septal and peripheral lobular, or heterogeneous diffuse).	Benign intramedullary lesions composed of hyaline cartilage represent approximately 10% of benign bone tumors. Enchondromas can be solitary (88%) or multiple (12%). Ollier disease is a dyschondroplasia involving endochondral-formed bone resulting in multiple enchondromas (enchondromatosis). Metachondromatosis is a combination of enchondromatosis and osteochondromatosis and is rare. Maffucci syndrome manifests with multiple enchondromas and soft tissue hemangiomas and is very rare. Patients range in age from 3 to 83 years, median = 35 years, mean = 38 to 40 years, peak in third and fourth decades.

(continued on page 378)

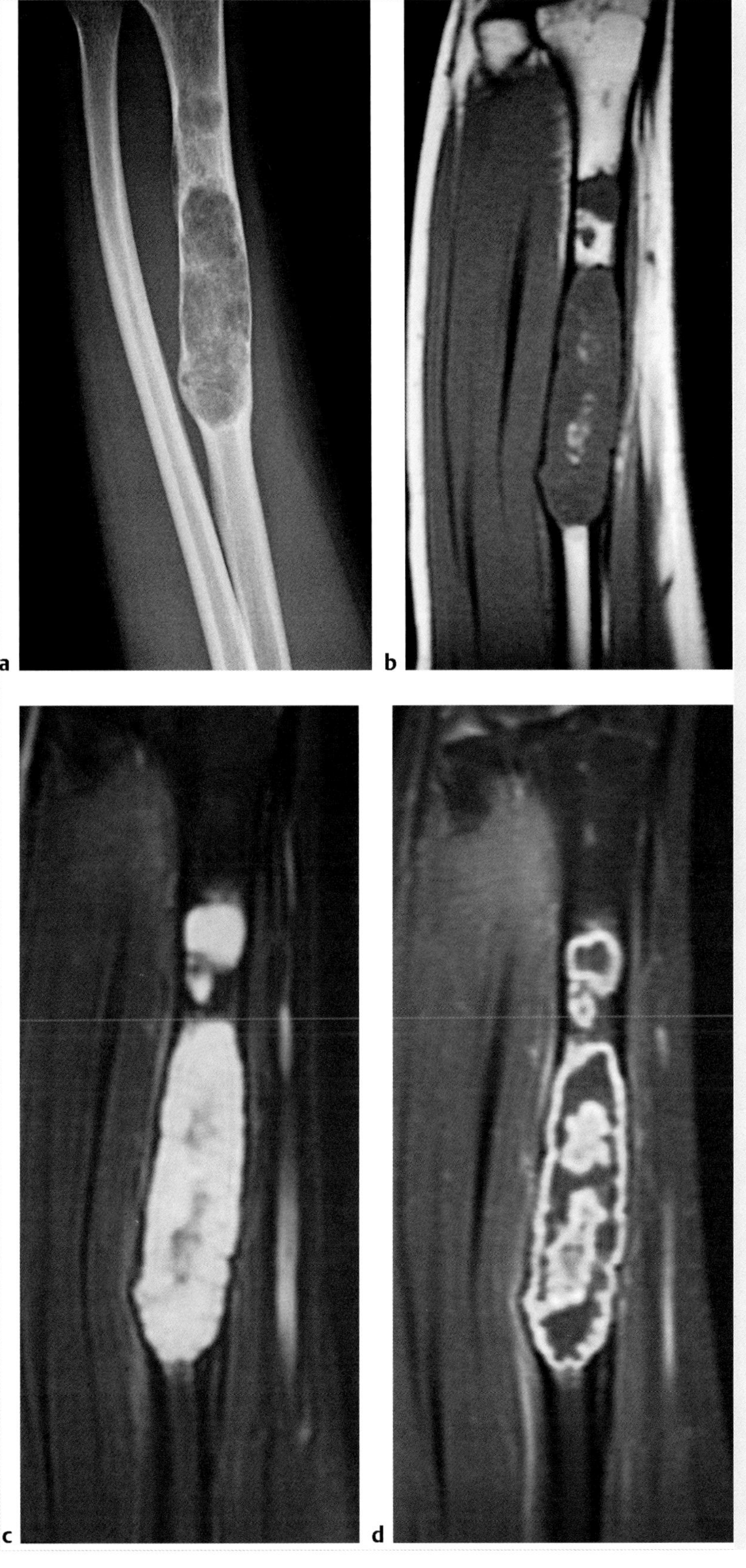

Fig. 10.73 A 16-year-old girl with an enchondroma in the diaphyseal marrow of the radius. The circumscribed radiolucent lesion contains chondroid mineralization and expands and thins bone cortex as seen on radiograph (a). The lesion has intermediate signal on T1-weighted imaging (T1WI) (b) and mostly high signal on fat-suppressed (FS) T2-weighted imaging (c). The lesion shows peripheral and central lobular Gd-contrast enhancement on coronal FS T1WI (d).

Table 10.3 (Cont.) Intramedullary lesions associated with expansion of intact cortical margins

Abnormalities	MRI findings	Comments
Fibrous dysplasia (▶ Fig. 10.74)	MRI features depend on the proportions of bony spicules, collagen, fibroblastic spindle cells, hemorrhagic and/or cystic changes, and associated pathological fracture if present. Lesions are usually well-circumscribed and have low or low-intermediate signal on T1WI and PDWI. On T2WI, lesions have variable mixtures of low, intermediate, and/or high signal often surrounded by a low signal rim of variable thickness. Internal septations and cystic changes are seen in a minority of lesions. Bone expansion with thickened and/or thinned cortex can be seen. Lesions show Gd-contrast enhancement that varies in degree and pattern.	Benign medullary fibro-osseous lesion, which can involve a single site (mono-ostotic) or multiple locations (polyostotic). Thought to occur from developmental failure in the normal process of remodeling primitive bone to mature lamellar bone with resultant zone or zones of immature trabeculae within dysplastic fibrous tissue. Accounts for approximately 10% of benign bone lesions. Patients range in age from < 1 year to 76 years; 75% occur before the age of 30 years.
Unicameral bone cyst (UBC) (▶ Fig. 10.75)	UBCs often have a peripheral rim of low signal on T1 W, PDWI, and T2WI adjacent to normal medullary bone. UBCs usually contain fluid with low to low-intermediate signal on T1WI; low-intermediate, intermediate, or slightly high signal on PDWI; and high signal on T2WI. Fluid-fluid levels may occur. In tubular bones, mild to moderate expansion of bone may occur with variable thinning of the overlying cortex. For UBCs without pathological fracture, thin peripheral Gd-contrast enhancement can be seen at the margins of lesions. UBCs with pathological fracture can have heterogeneous or homogeneous low-intermediate or slightly high signal on T1WI, and heterogeneous or homogeneous high signal on T2WI and FS T2WI. UBCs complicated by fracture can have internal septations and fluid-fluid levels, as well as irregular peripheral Gd-contrast enhancement and at internal septations.	Intramedullary nonneoplastic cavities filled with serous or serosanguinous fluid. Account for 9% of primary tumor-like lesions of bone; 85% occur in the first 2 decades, median = 11 years.

(continued on page 380)

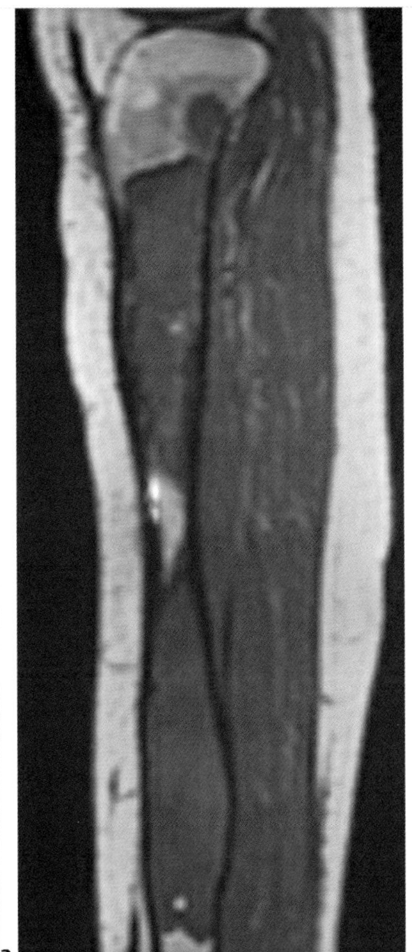

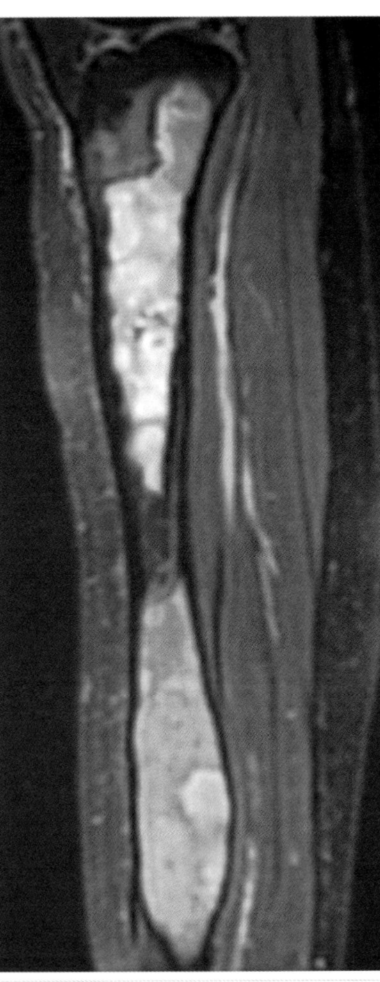

Fig. 10.74 A 46-year-old woman with fibrous dysplasia expanding the metadiaphyseal and diaphyseal portions of the tibia as seen on sagittal T1-weighted imaging (a), and sagittal fat-suppressed T2-weighted imaging (b).

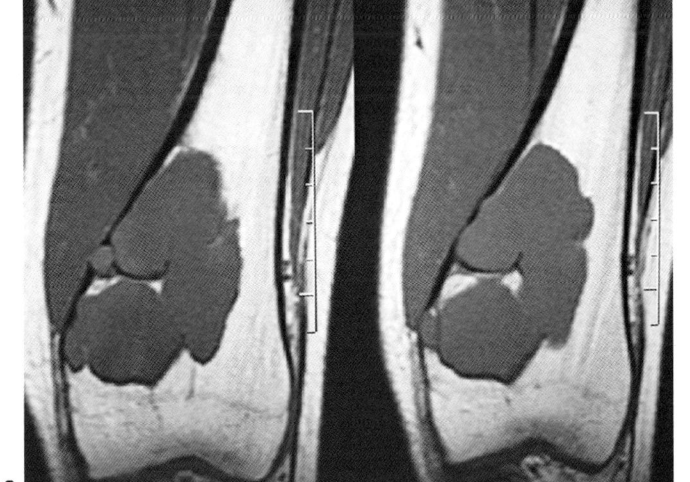

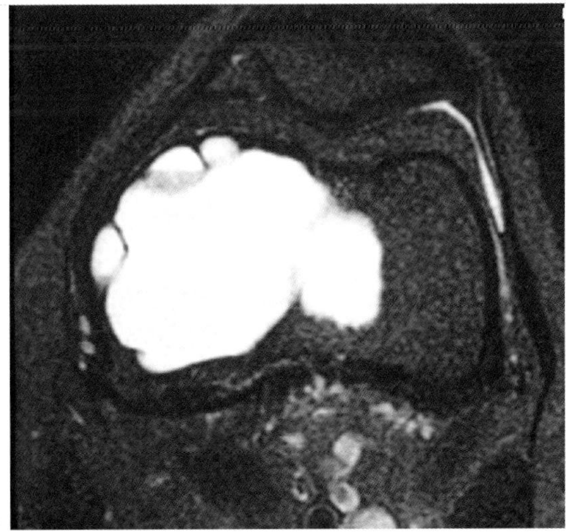

Fig. 10.75 A 17-year-old girl with a unicameral bone cyst within the distal metadiaphyseal portion of the femur as seen on coronal T1-weighted imaging (a) and axial fat-suppressed T2-weighted imaging (b). Cortical thinning and slight expansion are seen.

Table 10.3 (Cont.) Intramedullary lesions associated with expansion of intact cortical margins

Abnormalities	MRI findings	Comments
Aneurysmal bone cyst (ABC) (▶ Fig. 10.76)	ABCs often have a low signal rim on T1WI, PDWI, and T2WI adjacent to normal medullary bone, and between extraosseous soft tissues. Various combinations of low, intermediate, and/or high signal on T1WI, PDWI, and T2WI are usually seen within ABCs as well as fluid-fluid levels. Variable Gd-contrast enhancement is seen at the margins of lesions as well as involving the internal septae.	Tumor-like expansile bone lesions containing cavernous spaces filled with blood. ABCs can be primary bone lesions (2/3) or secondary to other bone lesions/tumors (such as giant cell tumors, chondroblastomas, osteoblastomas, osteosarcomas. chondromyxoid fibromas, nonossifying fibromas, fibrous dysplasia, fibrosarcomas, malignant fibrous histiocytomas, and metastatic disease). Account for approximately 11% of primary tumor-like lesions of bone. Patients usually range in age from 1 to 25 years, median = 14 years.
Giant cell reparative granuloma (solid aneurysmal bone cyst) (▶ Fig. 10.77)	Radiolucent bone lesions on CT, and typically occur in the metaphysis and/or diaphysis. Bone expansion may occur with or without intact thin cortical margins. Extraosseous extension of lesions may occur. Lesions can have heterogeneous low, intermediate, and/or high signal on T1WI, PDWI, and T2WI; as well as peripheral rimlike and central Gd-contrast enhancement on FS T1WI.	Giant cell granulomas (also known as solid aneurysmal bone cysts) are reactive granulomatous lesions that have histological features similar to brown tumors. Lesions contain multinucleated giant cells adjacent to sites of hemorrhage, and fibroblasts. Osteoid formation adjacent to sites of hemorrhage can be seen. Lesions usually occur in patients less than 30 years and are most frequently found in the mandible, maxilla, and small bones of the hands and feet. Lesions in long bones have also been referred to as solid variants of aneurysmal bone cysts.
Giant cell tumor of bone (▶ Fig. 10.78)	Lesions may have expanded and thinned cortical margins on radiographs. Lesions may also show cortical disruption and extraosseous extension on MRI. Solid portions of giant cell tumors often have low to intermediate signal on T1WI and PDWI, intermediate to high signal on T2WI, and high signal on FS PDWI and FS T2WI. Signal heterogeneity on T2WI is common. Aneurysmal bone cysts can be seen in 14% of giant cell tumors. Varying degrees of Gd-contrast enhancement can be seen. Peripheral rim-like Gd-contrast enhancement may be seen around cystic zones/aneurysmal bone cysts.	Aggressive intraosseous tumors composed of neoplastic ovoid mononuclear cells and scattered multinucleated osteoclast-like giant cells (derived from fusion of marrow mononuclear cells). Up to 10% of all giant cell tumors are malignant. Benign giant cell tumors account for approximately 5 to 9.5% of all bone tumors and up to 23% of benign bone tumors. Occurs in patients age 4 to 81 years (median = 30 years); 75% occur in patients between the ages of 15 and 45.

(continued on page 382)

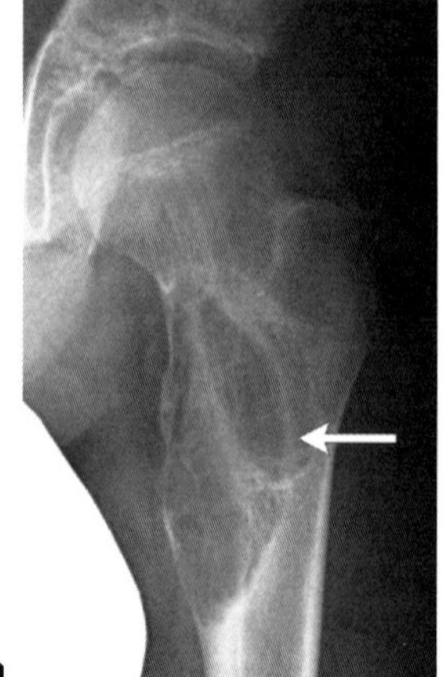

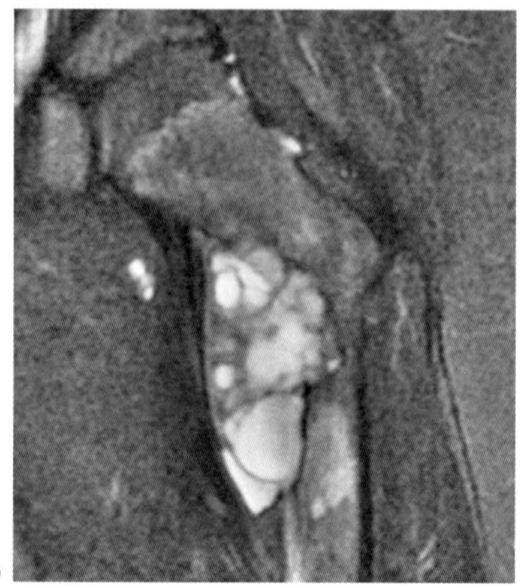

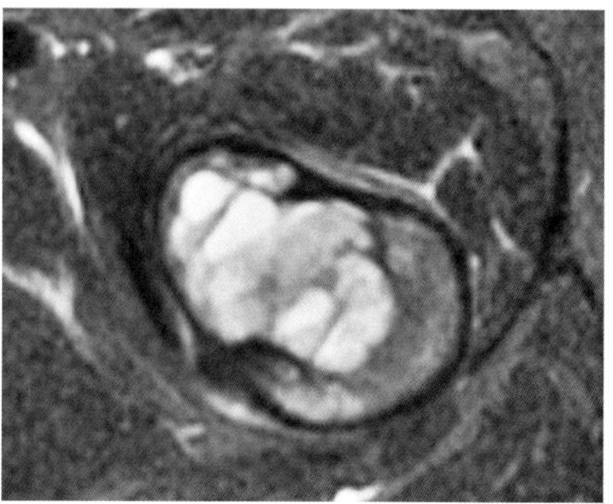

Fig. 10.76 An 11-year-old boy with an aneurysmal bone cyst involving the medial proximal shaft of the femur. Anteroposterior radiograph shows an expansile radiolucent lesion with thinned cortex (arrow) (a). Coronal (b) and axial fat-suppressed T2-weighted imaging (c) shows a multiseptated lesion with fluid-fluid levels containing high and low-intermediate signal.

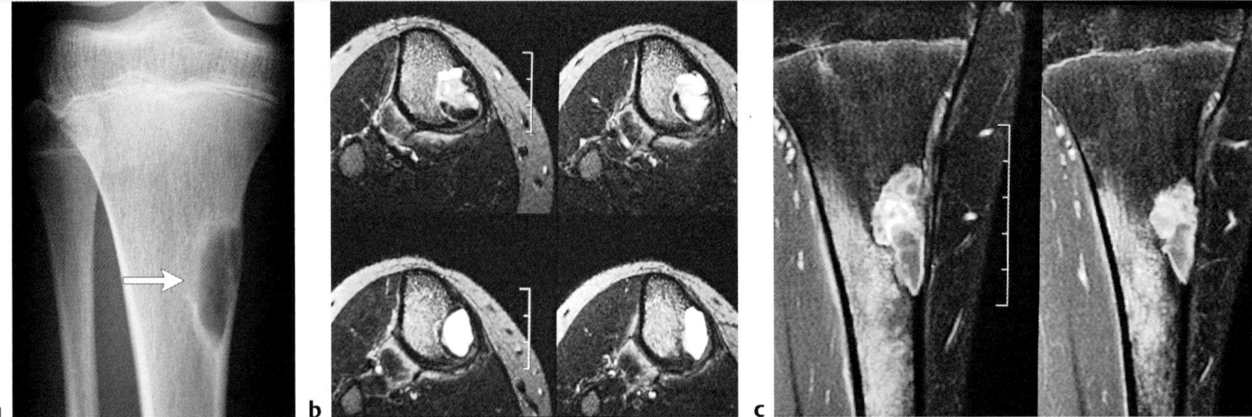

Fig. 10.77 A 14-year-old girl with a giant cell reparative granuloma (solid aneurysmal bone cyst) involving the medial portion of the proximal tibial shaft. Anteroposterior radiograph (a) shows a well-circumscribed radiolucent lesion with thin sclerotic margins, thinning and slight expansion of the bone cortex (arrow). The lesion has mixed low, intermediate, and high signal on axial T2-weighted imaging (b) and shows heterogeneous Gd-contrast enhancement on coronal fat-suppressed T1-weighted imaging (c). Poorly defined contrast enhancement is also seen in the marrow peripheral to the lesion.

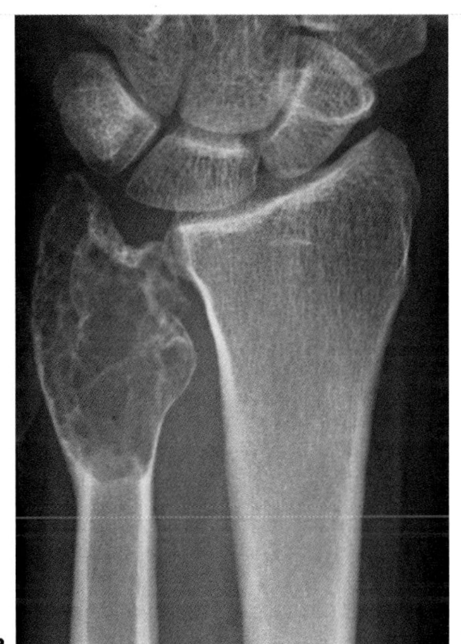

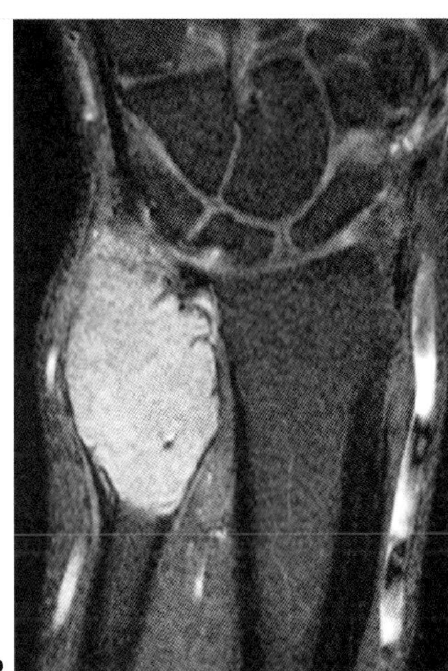

Fig. 10.78 A 52-year-old man with a giant cell tumor involving the distal ulna. The radiolucent lesion expands and thins bone cortex as seen on radiograph (a). The lesion shows Gd-contrast enhancement on coronal fat-suppressed T1-weighted imaging (b).

Table 10.3 (Cont.) Intramedullary lesions associated with expansion of intact cortical margins

Abnormalities	MRI findings	Comments
Chondromyxoid fibroma (▶ Fig. 10.79)	Lesions are often slightly lobulated with low-intermediate signal on T1WI, intermediate signal on PDWI, and heterogeneous predominantly high signal on T2WI. Thin low signal septa within lesions on T2WI are secondary to fibrous strands. Lesions are surrounded by low signal borders representing thin sclerotic reaction. Edema is not typically seen in medullary bone. Lesions show prominent diffuse Gd-contrast enhancement.	Rare benign slow-growing bone lesions that contain chondroid, myxoid, and fibrous components. Chondromyxoid fibromas represent 2 to 4% of primary benign bone lesions, and < 1% of primary bone lesions. Most chondromyxoid fibromas occur between the ages of 1 and 40 years, with a median of 17 years, and peak incidence in the second to third decades.
Osteoblastoma (▶ Fig. 10.80)	Lesions appear as spheroid or ovoid zone measuring greater than 1.5 to 2 cm located within medullary and/or cortical bone with low-intermediate signal on T1WI; low-intermediate to slightly high signal on PDWI; and low-intermediate and/or high signal on T2WI and FS T2WI. After Gd-contrast administration, osteoblastomas show variable degrees of enhancement. Expansion of thinned cortical margins can be seen as well as thickening of cortical bone and medullary sclerosis. Zones of sclerotic bone reaction adjacent to osteoblastomas typically show low signal on T1 W, T2WI, and FS T2WI. Poorly defined zones of marrow signal alteration consisting of low-intermediate signal on T1WI, high signal on T2WI and FS T2WI, and corresponding Gd-contrast enhancement can be seen in the marrow adjacent to osteoblastomas as well as within the extraosseous soft tissues.	Rare benign bone-forming tumors which are histologically related to osteoid osteomas. Osteoblastomas are larger than osteoid osteomas and show progressive enlargement. Account for 3 to 6% of primary benign bone tumors and < 1 to 2% of all primary bone tumors. Occurs in patients age 1 to 30 years, median = 15 years, mean age = 20 years. Approximately 90% of lesions occur in patients less than 30 years.

(continued on page 384)

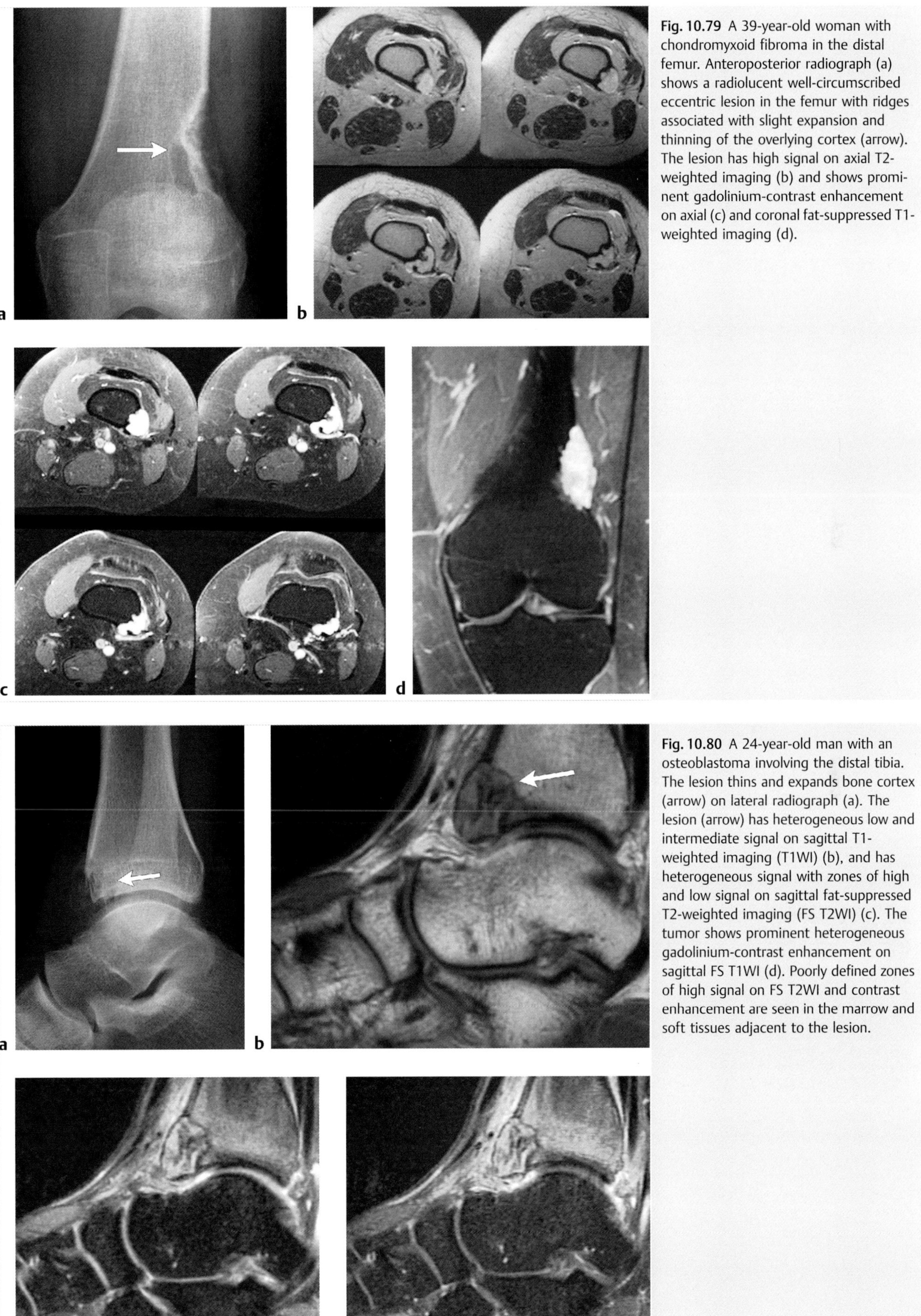

Fig. 10.79 A 39-year-old woman with chondromyxoid fibroma in the distal femur. Anteroposterior radiograph (a) shows a radiolucent well-circumscribed eccentric lesion in the femur with ridges associated with slight expansion and thinning of the overlying cortex (arrow). The lesion has high signal on axial T2-weighted imaging (b) and shows prominent gadolinium-contrast enhancement on axial (c) and coronal fat-suppressed T1-weighted imaging (d).

Fig. 10.80 A 24-year-old man with an osteoblastoma involving the distal tibia. The lesion thins and expands bone cortex (arrow) on lateral radiograph (a). The lesion (arrow) has heterogeneous low and intermediate signal on sagittal T1-weighted imaging (T1WI) (b), and has heterogeneous signal with zones of high and low signal on sagittal fat-suppressed T2-weighted imaging (FS T2WI) (c). The tumor shows prominent heterogeneous gadolinium-contrast enhancement on sagittal FS T1WI (d). Poorly defined zones of high signal on FS T2WI and contrast enhancement are seen in the marrow and soft tissues adjacent to the lesion.

Table 10.3 (Cont.) Intramedullary lesions associated with expansion of intact cortical margins

Abnormalities	MRI findings	Comments
Hemangioma (▶ Fig. 10.81)	Often well-circumscribed lesions, which often have intermediate to high signal on T1WI, PDWI, T2WI, and FS T2WI. Hemangiomas usually show Gd-contrast enhancement (mild to prominent). Expansion of cortical margins can occasionally occur with intraosseous hemangiomas.	Benign lesions of bone and soft tissues composed of capillary, cavernous, and/or malformed venous vessels. Considered to be a hamartomatous disorder, account for 2 to 4% of benign bone tumors and approximately 1% of all bone tumors.
Chondroblastoma (▶ Fig. 10.82)	Tumors often have fine lobular margins and typically have low-intermediate heterogeneous signal on T1WI, and mixed low, intermediate, and/or high signal on T2WI. Areas of low signal on T2WI are secondary to chondroid matrix mineralization, and/or hemosiderin. Lobular, marginal, or septal Gd-contrast enhancement patterns can be seen. Tumors may have thin margins of low signal on T2WI representing sclerotic borders. Bone expansion can occasionally occur. Poorly defined zones of high signal on T2WI and corresponding Gd-contrast enhancement can be seen in the adjacent marrow and extraosseous soft tissues.	Benign cartilaginous tumors with chondroblast-like cells and areas of chondroid matrix formation. Accounts for 5 to 9% of benign bone lesions and 1 to 3% of all primary bone tumors; patients range in age from 10 to 30 years, median = 17 years.
Ameloblastoma (▶ Fig. 10.83)	Lesions are often radiolucent with associated bone expansion and cortical thinning on CT. Tumors often have circumscribed margins and can show mixed low, intermediate, and/or high signal on T1WI, T2WI, and FS T2WI. Lesions can show heterogeneous Gd-contrast enhancement.	Ameloblastomas are slow-growing solid and cystic bone tumors that contain epithelioid cells (basaloid and/or squamous types) associated with regions of spindle cells and fibrous stroma. These tumors occur in the mandible and maxilla and typically lack metastatic potential.
Desmoplastic fibroma (▶ Fig. 10.84)	Lobulated lesions with abrupt zones of transition. Lesions usually have low-intermediate signal on T1WI, intermediate signal on PDWI, heterogeneous intermediate to high signal on T2WI. Lesions may have internal or peripheral zones of low signal on T1WI and T2WI secondary to dense collagenous parts of the lesions and/or foci with high signal onT2WI from cystic zones. Thin curvilinear zones of low signal on T2WI can be seen at the margins of the lesions. Lesions show variable degrees and patterns of Gd-contrast enhancement.	Represent rare intraosseous desmoid tumors, which are composed of benign fibrous tissue with elongated or spindle-shaped cells adjacent to collagen. Account for < 1% of primary bone lesions. Occur in patients age 1 to 71 years, mean = 20 years, median = 34 years, peak second decade.

(continued on page 386)

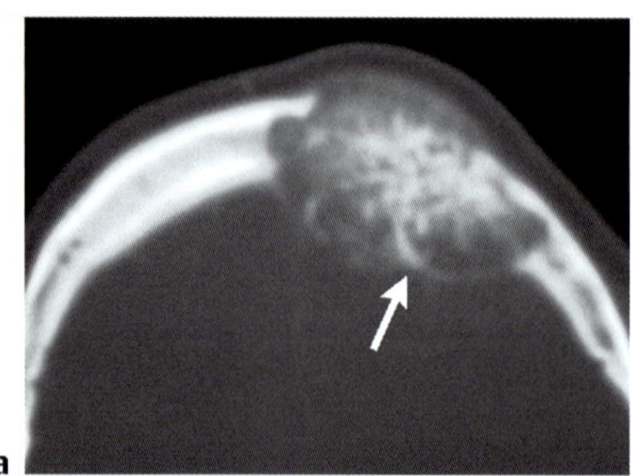

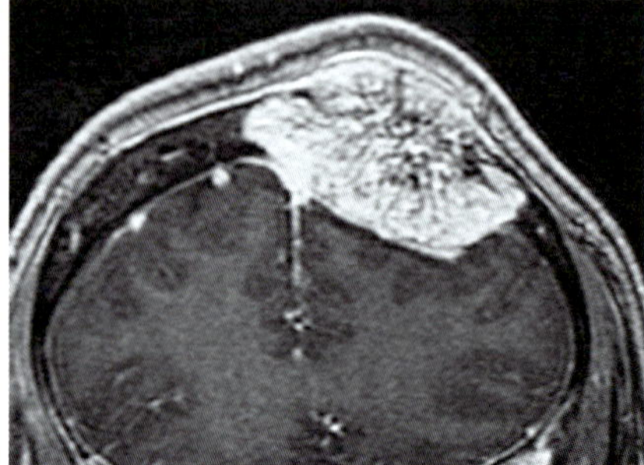

Fig. 10.81 A 33-year-old woman with a hemangioma involving the skull. The circumscribed lesion contains thickened trabeculae in a "spoke-wheel pattern" within a radiolucent zone (arrow). The lesion is associated with expansion and thinning of both the inner and outer tables of the skull on axial computed tomography (a). The lesion shows heterogeneous gadolinium-contrast enhancement on coronal T1-weighted imaging (b).

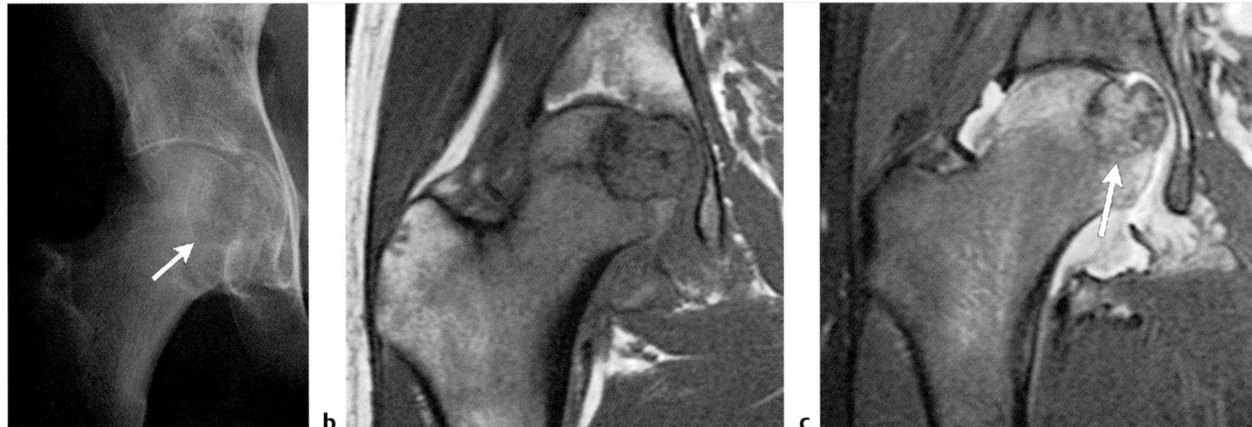

Fig. 10.82 A 17-year-old boy with chondroblastoma involving the epiphysis of the femoral head. The radiolucent lesion expands and thins the medial cortical margin (arrow) as seen on radiograph (a). The lesion has a thin peripheral zone of low signal on coronal T1-weighted imaging (T1WI) (b) and coronal fat-suppressed T2-weighted imaging (FS T2WI) (c). The lesion has low-intermediate signal on T1WI, and has both zones of intermediate and high signal and FS T2WI (arrow), as well as in the adjacent marrow. Thinning and expansion of the cortex are seen as well as a joint fluid collection.

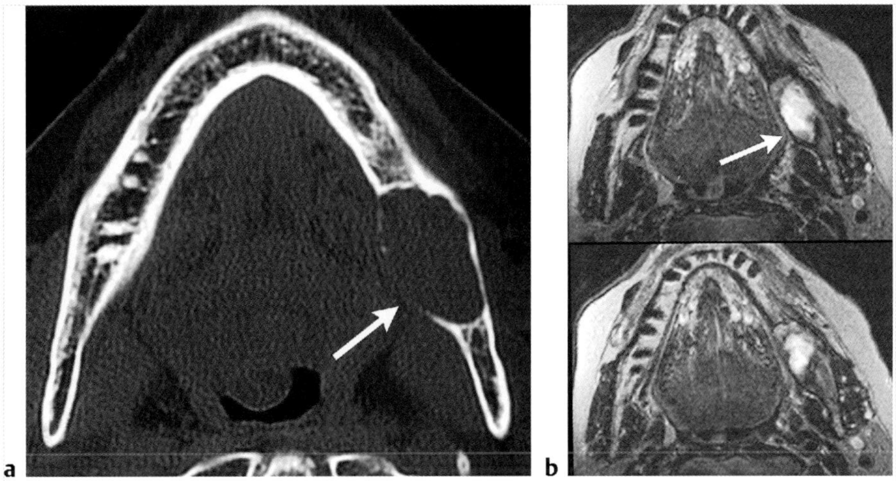

Fig. 10.83 A 70-year-old woman with ameloblastoma involving the right mandible. Axial computed tomographic image shows a radiolucent lesion with expansion and thinning of cortical bone (arrow) (a). The lesion (arrow) has mostly high signal with small zones of low and intermediate signal on axial T2-weighted imaging (b).

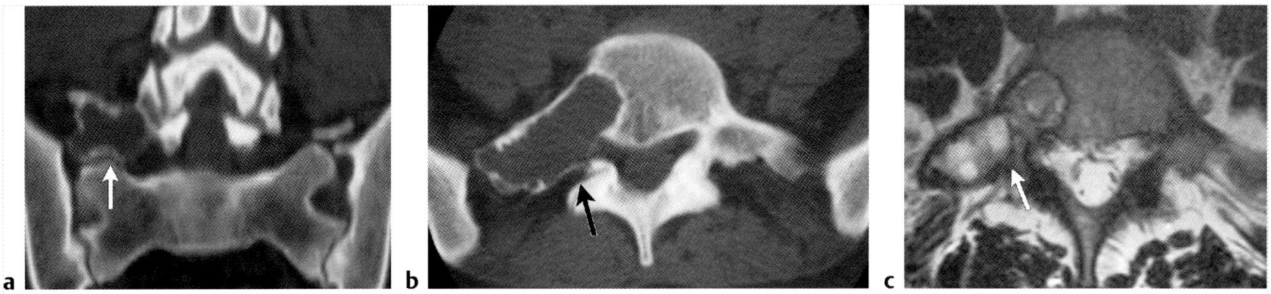

Fig. 10.84 A 33-year-old woman with a desmoplastic fibroma involving the L5 vertebral body, right pedicle, and transverse process. Coronal (a) and axial (b) computed tomographic images show an expansile radiolucent lesion with a thin peripheral shell of bone (arrow). The lesion has mixed signal with zones of intermediate, slightly high, high, and low signal (arrow) on axial T2-weighted imaging (c).

Table 10.3 (Cont.) Intramedullary lesions associated with expansion of intact cortical margins

Abnormalities	MRI findings	Comments
Osteofibrous dysplasia (▶ Fig. 10.85)	Multiple irregular intracortical zones of low-intermediate signal on T1 W images, intermediate to slightly high signal on PDWI, and high signal on T2WI and FS T2WI separated by irregular zones of low signal on T1WI and T2WI, the latter representing thickened sclerotic cortical bone. Zones of low signal on T1WI and T2WI of varying thickness are typically seen superficial and deep to the lesions representing sclerotic bone reaction. The outer cortical margins can be expanded and thinned. The intracortical lesions usually show prominent Gd-contrast enhancement. Thin juxtacortical/periosteal enhancement may be seen in lesions with thinned and expanded cortical margins. Prominent diffuse high signal on T2WI and marrow enhancement are seen for lesions with acute/subacute pathological fractures.	Rare self-limited benign fibro-osseous lesion primarily involving the anterior midshaft of the tibial cortex in children. Osteofibrous dysplasia represents rare bone lesions that typically involve the cortex of the tibia and/or fibula in children and adolescents.
Gaucher disease (▶ Fig. 10.86)	Diffuse and/or patchy heterogeneous zones with low-intermediate signal on T1WI, and heterogeneous intermediate to high signal on T2WI and FS T2WI.	Rare, heritable metabolic disorder with deficient activity of the lysosomal enzyme-hydrolase beta-glucosidase. Results in accumulation of the lipid-glucosylceramide within lysosomes of the monocyte-macrophage system (Gaucher cells) of the bone marrow, liver, and spleen. Marrow infiltration by Gaucher cells often results in zones of ischemia and bone infarction.
Hemophilic pseudotumor	Can appear as expansile radiolucent lesions on radiographs and CT. Lesions usually have mixed low, intermediate, and high signal on T1WI and T2WI, as well as fluid-fluid levels.	Lesions can occur within bone (femur, pelvis, tibia, hand) or soft tissue in 1 to 2% of patients with factor VIII or IX deficiency. Enlarging lesions may require surgical resection.
Brown tumor	Lesions are usually radiolucent on radiographs and CT. Lesions often have low-intermediate signal on T1WI, intermediate to slightly high signal on T2WI, and typically show Gd-contrast enhancement. Zones of low signal on T2WI may occur from hemosiderin. Expansion of cortical margins can occur with or without cortical disruption/destruction.	Lesions in bone contain multinucleated giant cells, fibrous tissue, blood vessels, and zones of hemorrhage/hemosiderin. Histological and imaging features are similar to giant cell reparative granulomas. Most often involves ribs, mandible, clavicle, pelvis, craniofacial bones, and vertebrae. Can result from primary hyperparathyroidism (3 to 7%) (oversecretion of parathyroid hormone [PTH] from parathyroid adenoma associated with hypercalcemia), secondary type (vitamin D deficiency or chronic renal failure with hypocalcemia resulting in secretion of PTH and parathyroid gland hyperplasia) (1 to 2%), or tertiary type in which the secondary type leads to eventual autonomous elevated PTH secretion from parathyroid gland hyperplasia.

(continued on page 388)

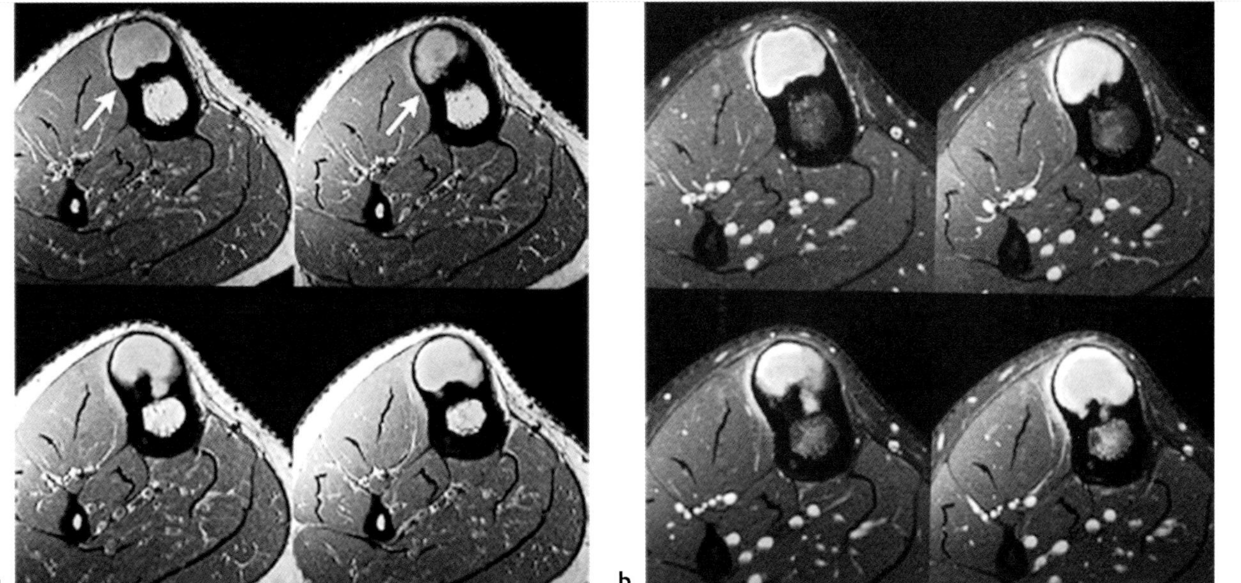

Fig. 10.85 An 18-year-old woman with osteofibrous dysplasia involving the anterior tibial cortex. Intracortical intermediate to slightly high signal (arrows) is seen in the lesion on axial proton density–weighted imaging (a) with corresponding prominent gadolinium-contrast enhancement on axial fat-suppressed T1-weighted imaging (b). The outer cortical margin is expanded and markedly thinned.

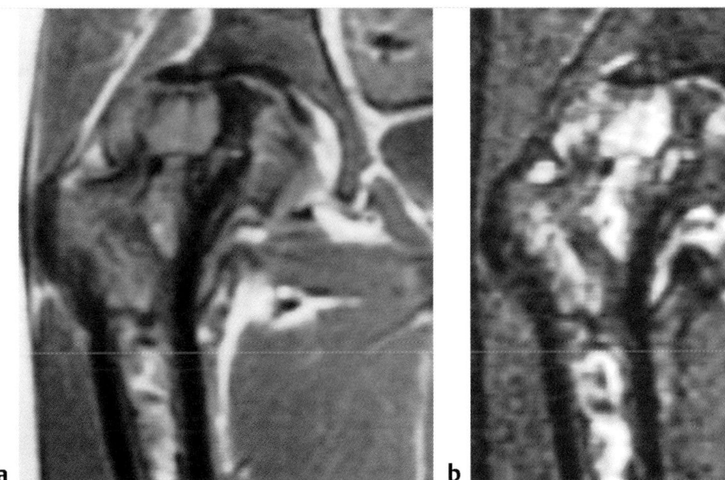

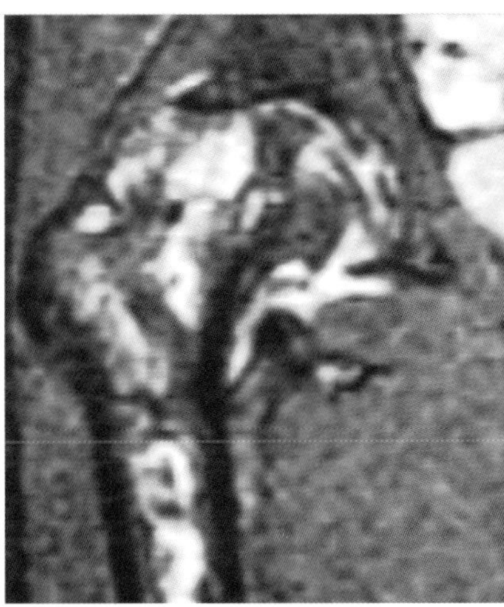

Fig. 10.86 A 34-year-old woman with Gaucher disease. Heterogeneous signal is seen in the marrow of the proximal femur on coronal proton density–weighted imaging (a) and short TI inversion recovery (b), as well as trabecular disruption, and thinning and expansion of cortical bone laterally.

Table 10.3 (Cont.) Intramedullary lesions associated with expansion of intact cortical margins

Abnormalities	MRI findings	Comments
Malignant lesions		
Adamantinoma (▶ Fig. 10.87)	Can appear as a solitary lobulated focus versus multinodular pattern of signal alteration in thickened bone cortex. More than half involve bone cortex and marrow compared with only cortical involvement. Bone cortex can be expanded and thinned. Tumor foci in bone typically have low-intermediate signal on T1WI and PDWI, and slightly high to high signal on T2WI and FS T2WI. Lesions usually show prominent Gd-contrast enhancement. Adamantinomas with a multinodular pattern have enhancing nodules that have high signal on T2WI and FS T2WI separated by zones of low signal from intervening cortical bone.	Rare low-grade malignant bone tumors consisting of epithelial cells surrounded by spindle cells and osteofibrous tissue that often involve the shaft of the tibia. Account for < 1% of primary bone tumors. Patients range in age from 3 to 86 years, median = 19 to 25 years, average = 35 years, most common in third and fourth decades.
Other malignant lesions (▶ Fig. 10.88)	Tumors may have poorly defined or sharp margins and often have low-intermediate signal on T1WI with heterogeneous intermediate-high signal on T2WI and FS T2WI. Lesions often show prominent heterogeneous Gd-contrast enhancement.	Primary and metastatic tumors may initially show expansion of thinned intact cortical margins followed by eventual extraosseous extension of tumor through zones of cortical destruction. Hemangioendotheliomas and metastases from tumors such as renal cell carcinoma, breast, and lung carcinomas can show this pattern.

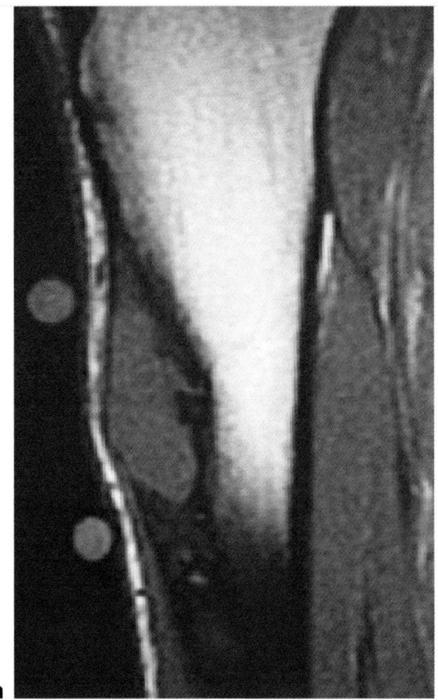
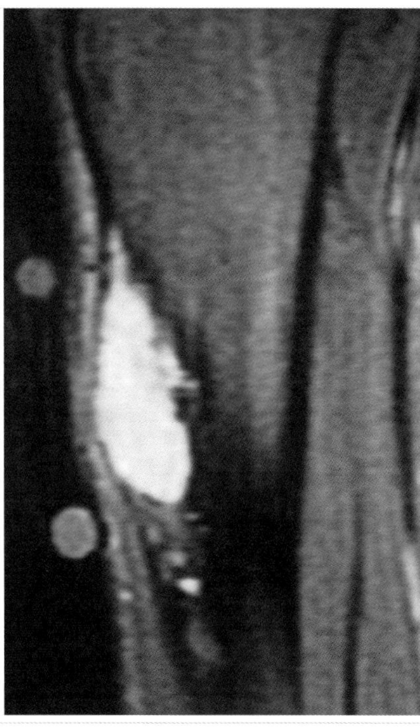

Fig. 10.87 A 23-year-old woman with an adamantinoma of the tibial diaphysis. The lesion has intermediate signal on sagittal proton density–weighted imaging (a) and high signal on sagittal fat-suppressed T2-weighted imaging (b). There is thinning and expansion of cortical bone as well as tumor extension toward the marrow.

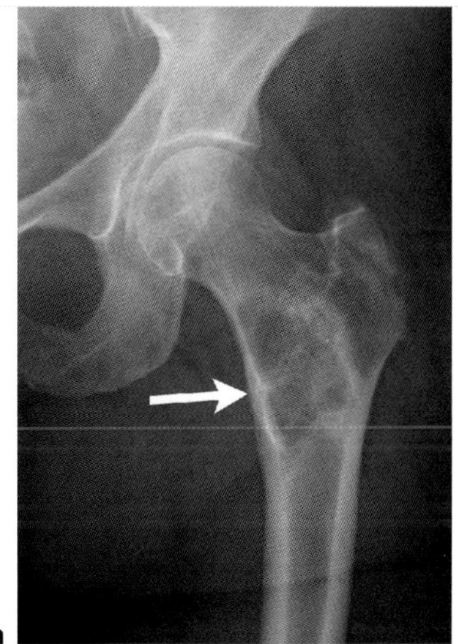
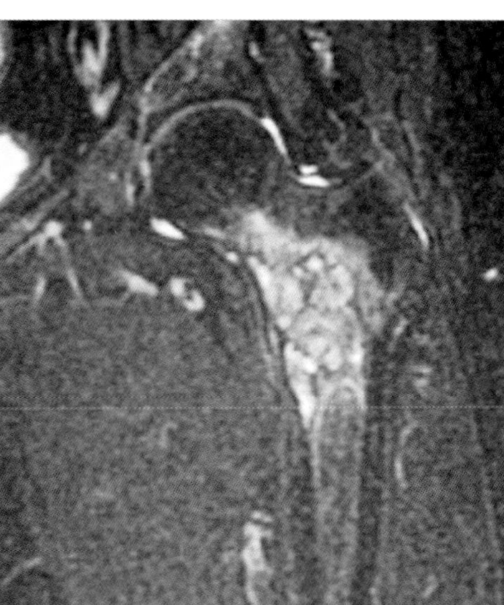

Fig. 10.88 Metastatic lesion in the proximal femur. Anteroposterior radiograph shows a radiolucent lesion with partial sclerotic margins and cortical thinning (arrow) (a). Coronal fat-suppressed T2-weighted imaging (b) shows the lesion to have heterogeneous high signal that extends beyond the sclerotic margins and is associated with thinning and slight expansion of bone cortex medially.

10.4 Intramedullary Lesions Associated with Cortical Destruction and Extraosseous Extension

- Nonmalignant lesions
  - Osteomyelitis
  - Chronic recurrent multifocal osteomyelitis
  - Eosinophilic granuloma
  - Sarcoidosis
  - Nonmalignant giant cell tumor
  - Sickle cell disease with adjacent extramedullary hematopoiesis
  - Brown tumor
  - Atypical hemangioma
- Malignant lesions
  - Metastatic tumor
  - Myeloma/plasmacytoma
  - Leukemia
  - Lymphoma
  - Osteosarcoma
  - Chondrosarcoma
  - Ewing sarcoma
  - Chordoma
  - Fibrosarcoma
  - Malignant fibrous histiocytoma
  - Malignant giant cell tumor
  - Hemangioendothelioma
  - Hemangiopericytoma
  - Liposarcoma
  - Paget sarcoma

Table 10.4 Intramedullary lesions associated with cortical destruction and extraosseous extension

Abnormalities	MRI findings	Comments
Nonmalignant lesions		
Osteomyelitis (▶ Fig. 10.89)	Poorly defined zones with high signal on T2-weighted imaging (T2WI) and fat-suppressed (FS) T2WI and gadolinium (Gd)-contrast enhancement are seen in marrow with associated zones of cortical destruction. Periosteal reaction can be seen as a peripheral rim of high signal on T2WI and FS T2WI and Gd-contrast enhancement on FS T1-weighted imaging adjacent to the low signal of cortical bone. A subperiosteal abscess with high signal on T2WI and FS T2WI can often be seen elevating a single low signal thin band of periosteum.	Infection of bone, which can result from hematogenous spread of microorganisms, trauma-direct inoculation, extension from adjacent tissues, and complications from surgery. *Staphylococcus aureus* and *Streptococcus pyogenes* are the most common bacterial infections involving bone. Osteomyelitis can also result from other bacteria as well as from tuberculosis, fungi, parasites, and viruses.
Chronic recurrent mutifocal osteomyelitis (▶ Fig. 10.90)	Multifocal lesions that occur in metaphyses of tubular bones (distal femur, proximal and distal tibia and fibula), clavicles, and vertebrae. Radiographs show radiolucent and/or sclerotic osseous lesions with proliferative periosteal bone formation. Magnetic resonance imaging (MRI) shows heterogeneous abnormal high signal on FS T2WI in marrow and periosteal soft tissues with Gd-contrast enhancement.	Painful inflammatory osseous disorder of unknown cause with histopathology of acute and chronic osteomyelitis without identification of infectious agent, diagnosis of exclusion. Usually occurs in children and adolescents, median age = 10 years, F 85%/M 15%. Multi-episodic skeletal disorder of unknown cause that can occur over 7 to 25 years. Treatment of symptoms with nonsteroidal anti-inflammatory drugs. Can be associated with acne or pustulosis palmoplantaris (SAPHO).

(continued on page 392)

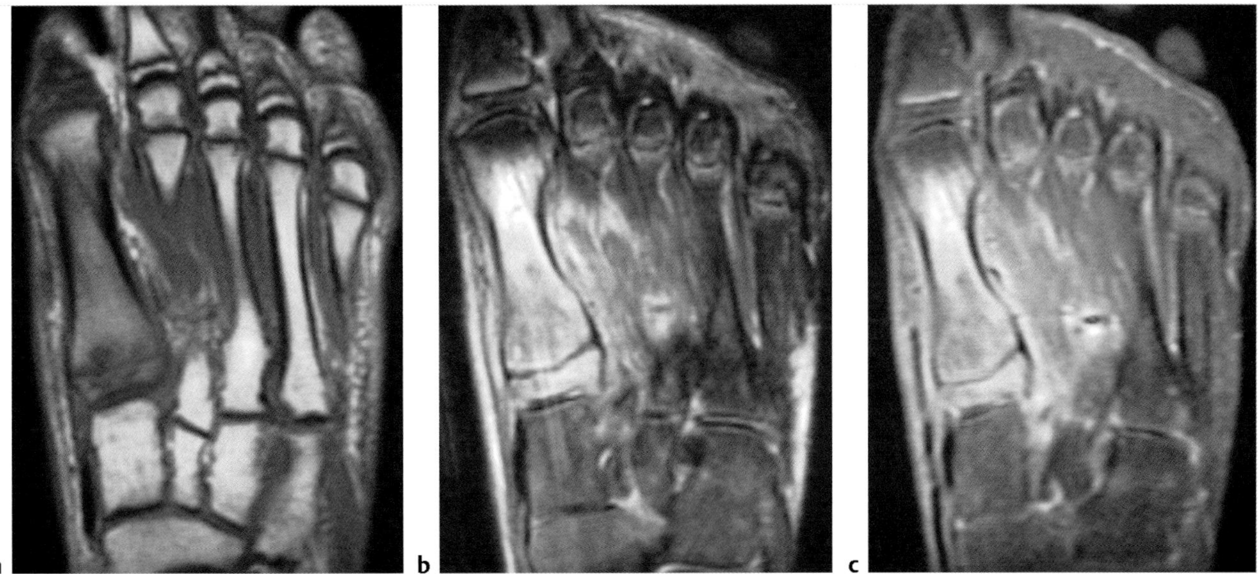

Fig. 10.89 A 14-year-old male with osteomyelitis involving the first metatarsal bone. Poorly defined zones of low-intermediate signal on coronal T1-weighted imaging (T1WI) (a), high signal on coronal fat-suppressed (FS) T2-weighted imaging (FS T2WI) (b) and gadolinium-contrast enhancement on FS T1WI (c) are seen within the marrow and extraosseous soft tissues. Zones of cortical bone disruption are also seen.

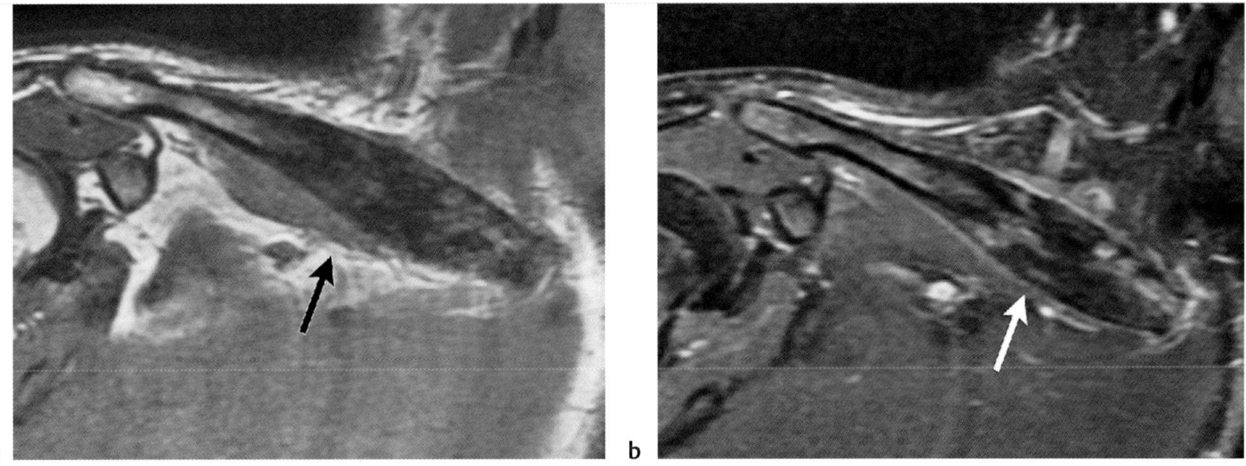

Fig. 10.90 Chronic recurrent multifocal osteomyelitis involving the clavicle. Heterogeneous low and intermediate signal on T1-weighted imaging (T1WI) (a) and heterogenenous contrast enhancement on fat-suppressed T1WI (b) are seen involving thickened bone cortex and within bone marrow (arrows).

Table 10.4 (Cont.) Intramedullary lesions associated with cortical destruction and extraosseous extension

Abnormalities	MRI findings	Comments
Eosinophilic granuloma (▶ Fig. 10.91)	Focal intramedullary lesion(s) associated with trabecular and cortical bone destruction, which typically have low-intermediate signal on T1WI and proton density–weighted imaging (PDWI); and heterogeneous slightly high to high signal on T2WI. Poorly defined zones of high signal on T2WI are usually seen in the marrow peripheral to the lesions secondary to inflammatory changes. Extension of lesions from the marrow into adjacent soft tissues through areas of cortical disruption are commonly seen as well as linear periosteal zones of high signal on T2WI. Lesions typically show prominent Gd-contrast enhancement in marrow and in extraosseous soft tissue portions of the lesions.	Benign tumor-like lesions consisting of Langerhans cells (histiocytes), and variable amounts of lymphocytes, polymorphonuclear cells, and eosinophils. Account for 1% of primary bone lesions, and 8% of tumor-like lesions. Occurs in patients with median age = 10 years, average = 13.5 years, peak incidence is between 5 and 10 years, 80 to 85% occur in patients less than 30 years.
Sarcoidosis (▶ Fig. 10.92)	Lesions usually appear as intramedullary zones with low to intermediate signal on T1WI and slightly high to high signal on T2WI and FS PDWI and FS T2WI. Erosions and zones of destruction involving adjacent bone cortex can occur with or without extraosseous extension of the granulomatous process. After Gd-contrast administration, lesions typically show moderate to prominent enhancement.	Chronic systemic granulomatous disease of unknown etiology in which noncaseating granulomas occur in various tissues and organs including bone.

(continued on page 394)

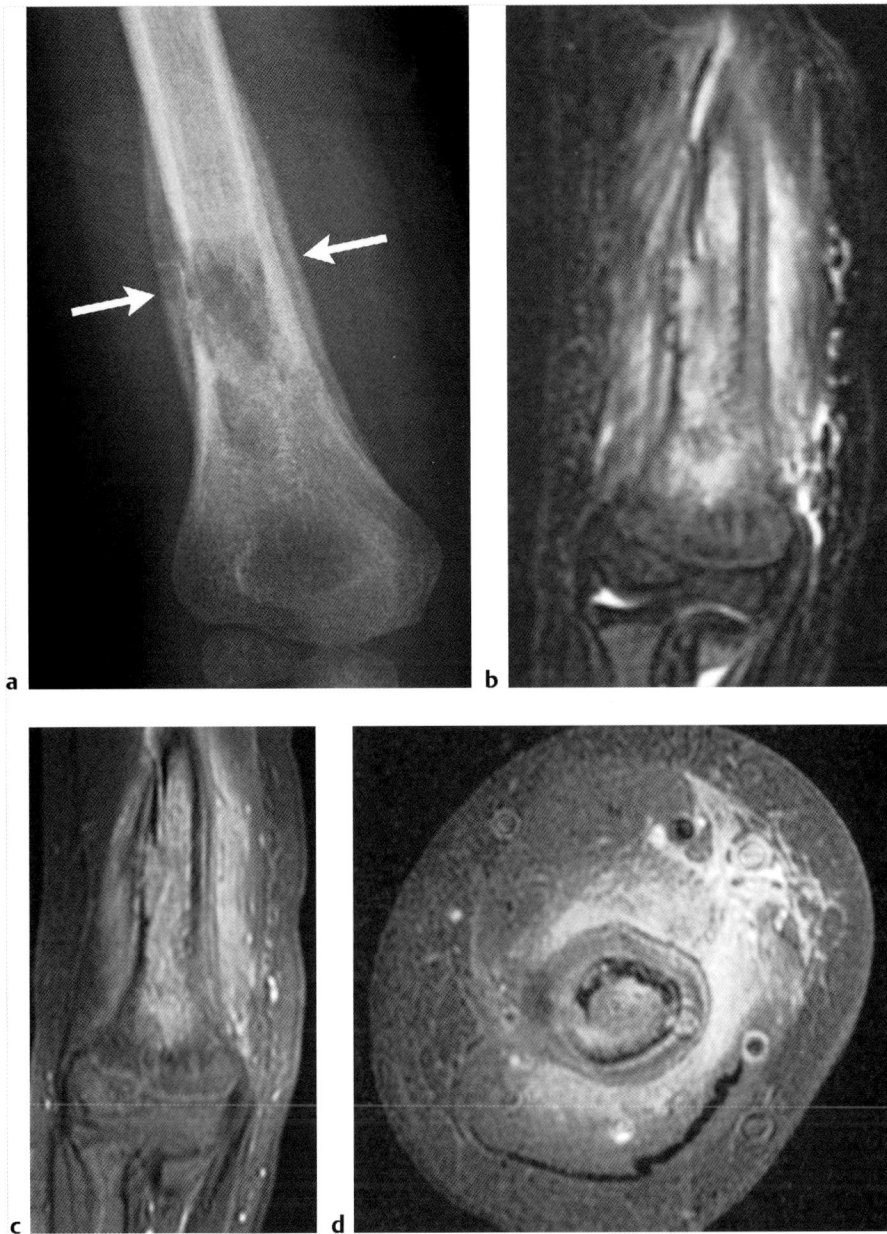

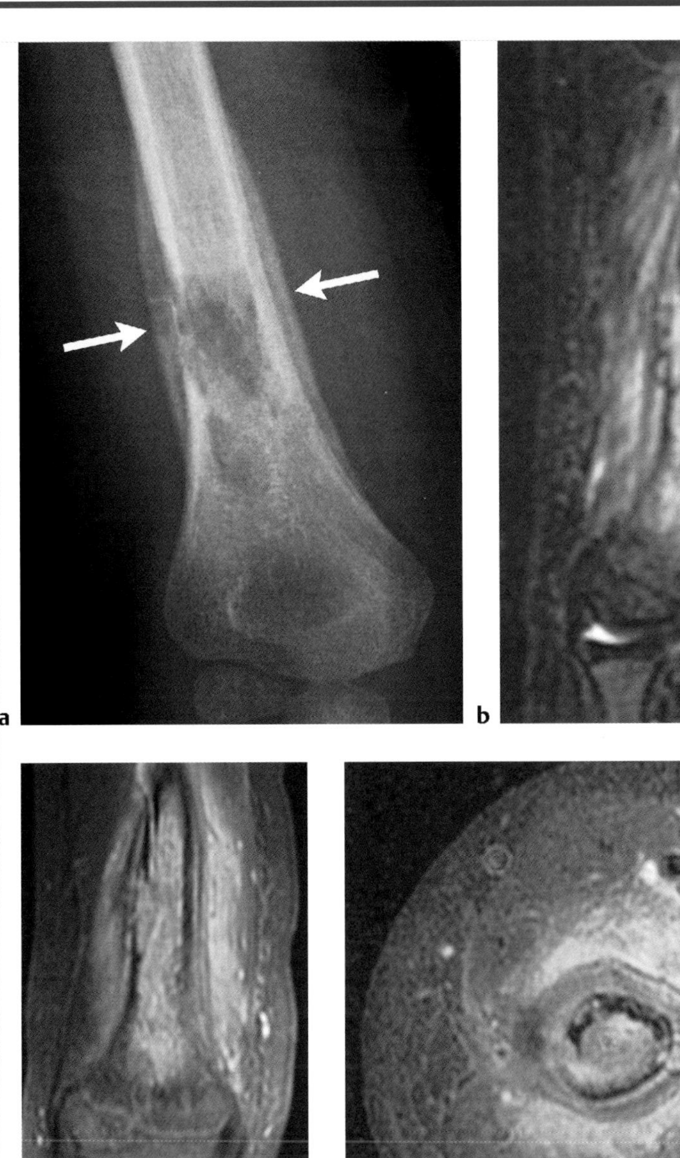

Fig. 10.91 A 5-year-old boy with an eosinophilic granuloma involving the distal humerus. Radiograph shows a radiolucent intramedullary lesion associated with linear periosteal reaction (arrows) (a). The lesion in the marrow has high signal on coronal fat-suppressed (FS) T2-weighted imaging (b) and shows prominent Gd-contrast enhancement on coronal (c) and axial FS T1-weighted imaging (d). The lesion is associated with cortical bone destruction, periosteal elevation, and extraossseous extension into the adjacent soft tissues.

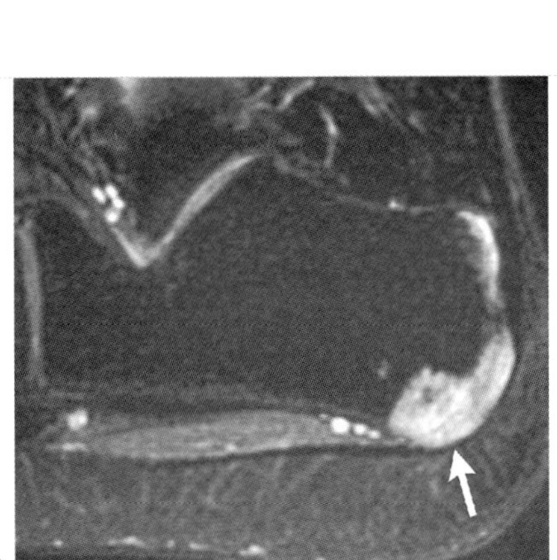

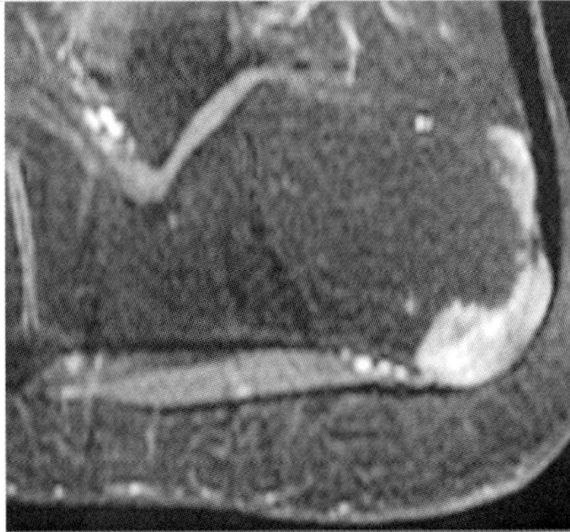

Fig. 10.92 A 31-year-old man with sarcoidosis involving the dorsal inferior portion of the calcaneus. The lesion in the marrow has high signal (arrow) on sagittal fat-suppressed (FS) T2-weighted imaging (a) and shows Gd-contrast enhancement on sagittal FS T1-weighted imaging (b). The lesion is associated with erosion of cortical bone with extension into the adjacent soft tissues.

Table 10.4 (Cont.) Intramedullary lesions associated with cortical destruction and extraosseous extension

Abnormalities	MRI findings	Comments
Nonmalignant giant cell tumor (▶ Fig. 10.93)	Usually well-defined lesions with thin low signal margins on T1WI, PDWI, and T2WI. Solid portions of giant cell tumors often have low to intermediate signal on T1WI and PDWI, intermediate to high signal on T2WI, and high signal on FS PDWI and FS T2WI. Signal heterogeneity on T2WI is common. Aneurysmal bone cysts can be seen in 14% of giant cell tumors. Varying degrees of Gd-contrast enhancement can be seen in the lesions, as well as peripheral rimlike enhancement around cystic zones/aneurysmal bone cysts. Poorly defined zones of enhancement and high signal on FS T2WI may also be seen in the marrow peripheral to the lesions secondary to reactive inflammatory changes from elevated tumor prostaglandin levels.	Aggressive bone tumors composed of neoplastic ovoid mononuclear cells and scattered multinucleated osteoclast-like giant cells (derived from fusion of marrow mononuclear cells). Up to 10% of all giant cell tumors are malignant. Benign giant cell tumors account for approximately 5 to 9.5% of all bone tumors and up to 23% of benign bone tumors. Occurs in patients age 4 to 81 years (median = 30 years), 75% occur in patients between the ages of 15 and 45.
Sickle cell disease with adjacent extramedullary hematopoiesis (▶ Fig. 10.94)	Lesions can have low, intermediate, and/or high signal on T1WI and T2WI depending on the proportions and distribution of fat and red marrow. Lesions may be seen extending from marrow through zones of cortical disruption, or as isolated abnormalities.	Represents proliferation of erythroid precursors outside of medullary bone secondary to physiological compensation for abnormal medullary hematopoiesis from congenital disorders such as hemoglobinopathies (Sickle cell, thalassemia, etc.) as well as acquired disorders such as myelofibrosis, leukemia, lymphoma, myeloma, or metastatic carcinoma.
Brown tumor	Lesions are usually radiolucent on radiographs and computed tomography (CT). Lesions often have low-intermediate signal on T1WI, intermediate to slightly high signal on T2WI, and typically show Gd-contrast enhancement. Zones of low signal on T2WI may occur from hemosiderin. Expansion of cortical margins can occur with or without cortical disruption/destruction.	Lesions in bone containing multinucleated giant cells, fibrous tissue, blood vessels, and zones of hemorrhage/hemosiderin. Histological and imaging features are similar to giant cell reparative granulomas. Can result from primary hyperparathyroidism (3 to 7%) (oversecretion of parathyroid hormone [PTH] from parathyroid adenoma associated with hypercalcemia), secondary type (vitamin D deficiency or chronic renal failure with hypocalcemia resulting in secretion of PTH and parathyroid gland hyperplasia) (1 to 2%), or tertiary type in which the secondary type leads to eventual autonomous elevated PTH secretion from parathyroid gland hyperplasia.

(continued on page 396)

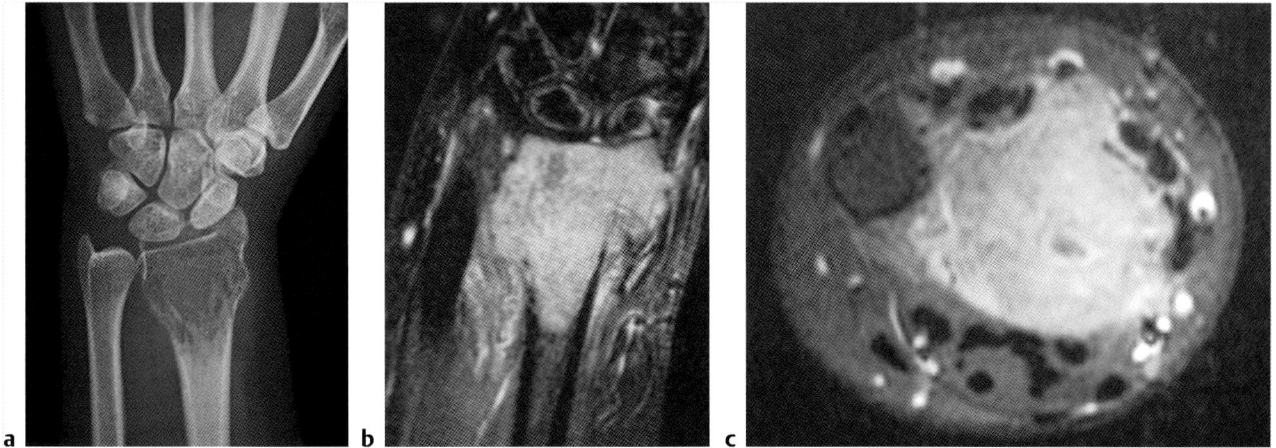

Fig. 10.93 A 19-year-old woman with a giant cell tumor in the distal radius as seen as a radiolucent lesion with ill-defined margins (a), and zones of cortical destruction on radiograph (b). The tumor extends through destroyed bone cortex and has high signal on coronal fat-suppressed (FS) T2-weighted imaging and shows gadolinium-contrast enhancement on axial FS T1-weighted imaging (c).

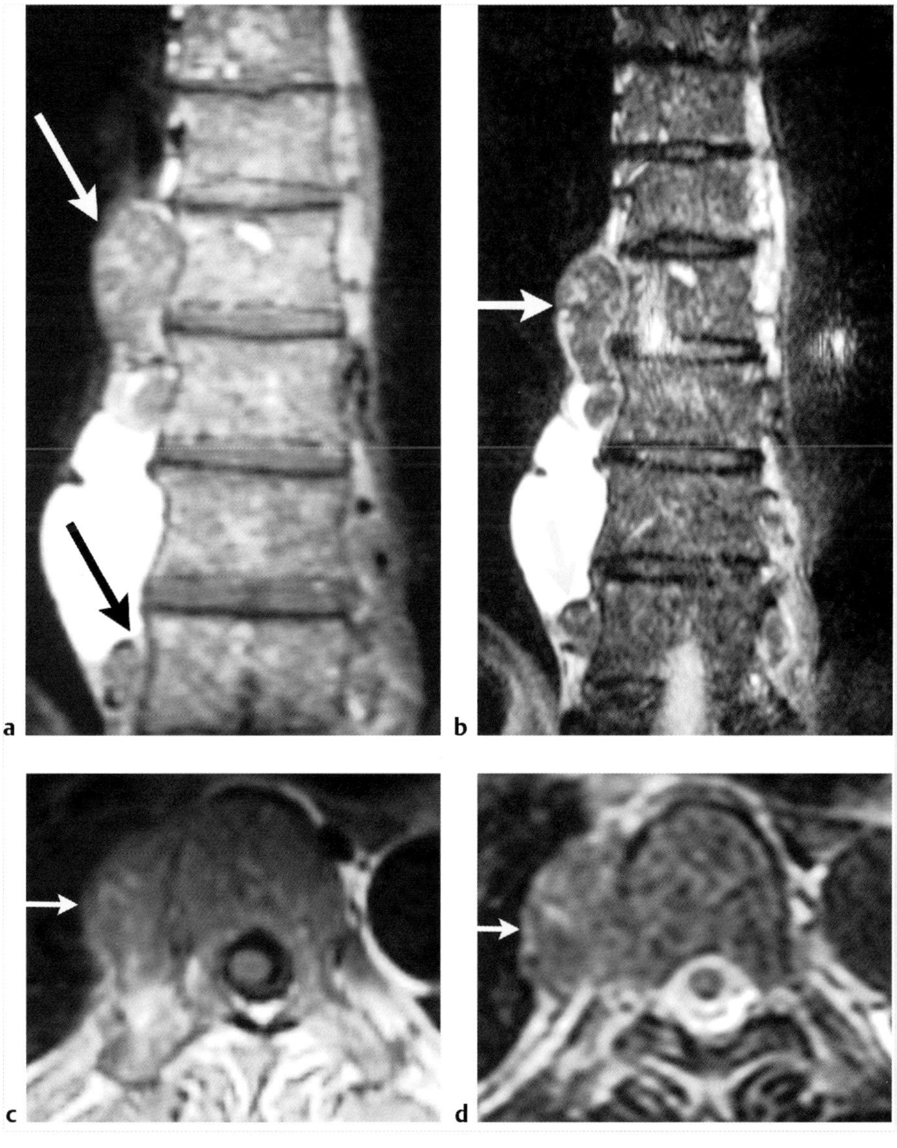

Fig. 10.94 A 56-year-old man with sickle cell disease and extramedullary hematopoiesis. The lesions (arrows) have signal comparable to the intraosseous marrow on coronal (a) and axial T1-weighted imaging (c) and coronal (b) and axial T2-weighted imaging (d). Small sites of cortical disruption are seen on the axial images.

Table 10.4 (Cont.) Intramedullary lesions associated with cortical destruction and extraosseous extension

Abnormalities	MRI findings	Comments
Atypical hemangioma (▶ Fig. 10.95)	Rare intraosseous hemangiomas may be associated with cortical disruption and extraosseous extension. Lesions can have low-intermediate signal on T1WI, and usually have high signal on T2WI and FS T2WI. Lesions typically show prominent Gd-contrast enhancement.	Benign hamartomatous lesions of bone and soft tissues composed of capillary, cavernous, and/or malformed venous vessels. Account for 2 to 4% of benign bone tumors and approximately 1% of all bone tumors.
Malignant lesions		
Metastatic tumor (▶ Fig. 10.96)	Single or multiple well-circumscribed or poorly defined infiltrative lesions involving marrow associated with cortical destruction and extraosseous extension. Lesions often have low-intermediate signal on T1WI, low, intermediate, and/or high signal on T2WI and FS T1WI, usually show Gd-contrast enhancement. Cortical destruction and tumor extension into the extraosseous soft tissues frequently occurs. Pathological fractures can be associated with metastatic lesions involving tubular bones and vertebrae. Periosteal reaction is uncommon.	Metastatic lesions typically occur in the marrow with or without cortical destruction and extraosseous tumor extension.
Myeloma/plasmacytoma (▶ Fig. 10.97)	Multiple myeloma or single plasma cell neoplasms (plasmacytoma) are well-circumscribed or poorly defined diffuse infiltrative lesions involving marrow, low-intermediate signal on T1WI, intermediate-high signal on T2WI and FS T2WI, usually show Gd-contrast-enhancement, eventual cortical bone destruction, and extraosseous extension.	Malignant tumors composed of proliferating antibody-secreting plasma cells derived from single clones. Most common primary neoplasm of bone in adults, median age = 60 years. Most patients are older than 40 years. May have variable destructive or infiltrative changes involving the axial and/or appendicular skeleton.
Leukemia (▶ Fig. 10.98)	Single or multiple well-circumscribed or poorly defined infiltrative lesions involving marrow; low-intermediate signal on T1WI, intermediate-high signal on T2WI and FS T2WI, often shows Gd-contrast enhancement, ± bone destruction and extraosseous extension.	Lymphoid neoplasms with involvement of bone marrow with tumor cells also in peripheral blood. In children and adolescents, acute lymphoblastic leukemia (ALL) is the most frequent type. In adults, chronic lymphocytic leukemia (small lymphocytic lymphoma) is the most common type of lymphocytic leukemia. Myelogenous leukemias are neoplasms derived from abnormal myeloid progenitor cells. Acute myelogenous leukemia (AML) occurs in adolescents and young adults, and represents approximately 20%) of childhood leukemia. Chronic myelogenous leukemia (CML) usually affects adults older than 25 years.

(continued on page 398)

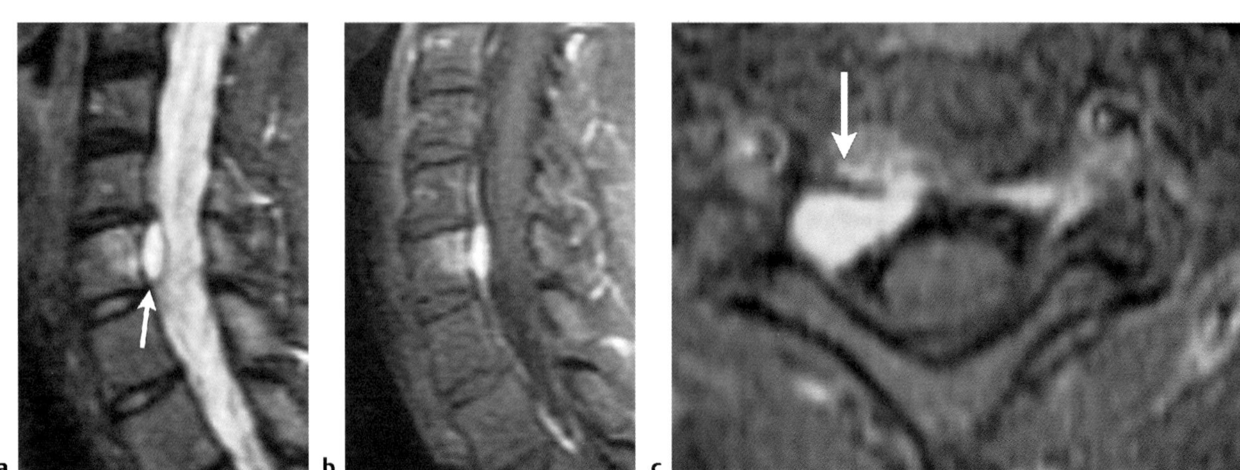

Fig. 10.95 A 43-year-old woman with an atypical hemangioma involving the posterior right marrow of the C6 vertebral body associated with cortical bone disruption and extension into the right anterior epidural soft tissues. The lesion has high signal (arrow) on a sagittal short TI inversion recovery image (a) and shows gadolinium-contrast enhancement on sagittal (b) and axial fat-suppressed T1-weighted imaging (arrow) (c).

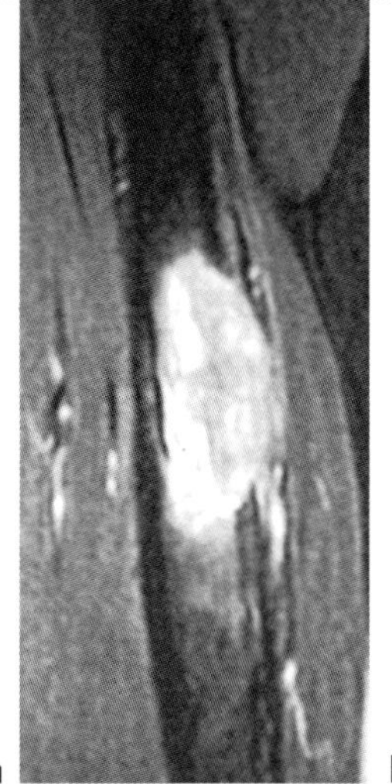

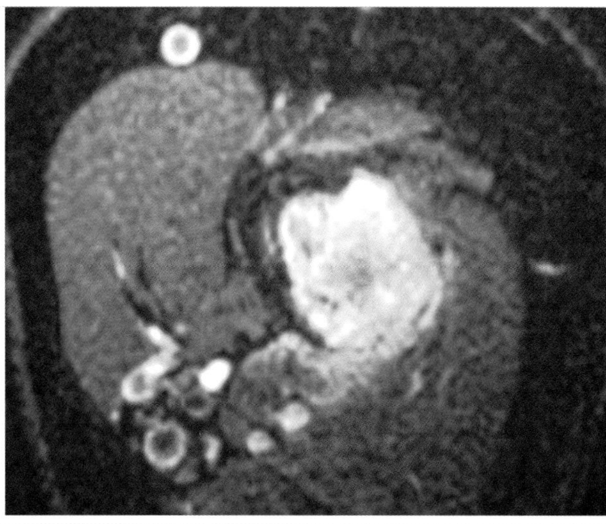

Fig. 10.96 A 63-year-old woman with metastatic lung carcinoma to the diaphyseal portion of the humerus associated with cortical destruction and extraosseous extension as seen on coronal (a) and axial fat-suppressed T2-weighted imaging (b).

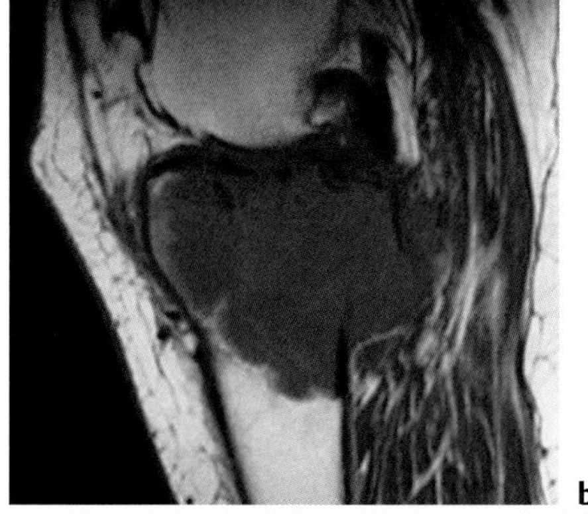

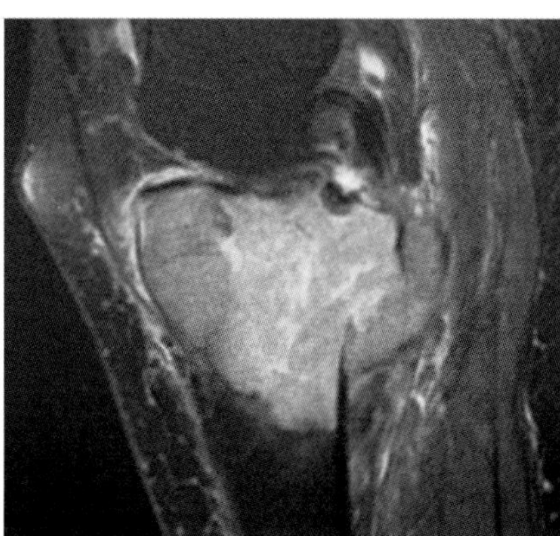

Fig. 10.97 A 77-year-old woman with myeloma in the proximal tibia. The intramedullary tumor has intermediate signal on sagittal T1-weighted imaging (a) and high signal on fat-suppressed T2-weighted imaging (b). Tumor is seen extending through destroyed bone cortex into the adjacent soft tissues.

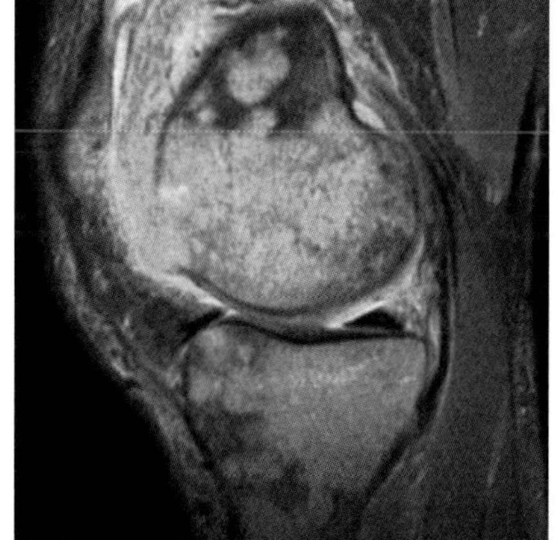

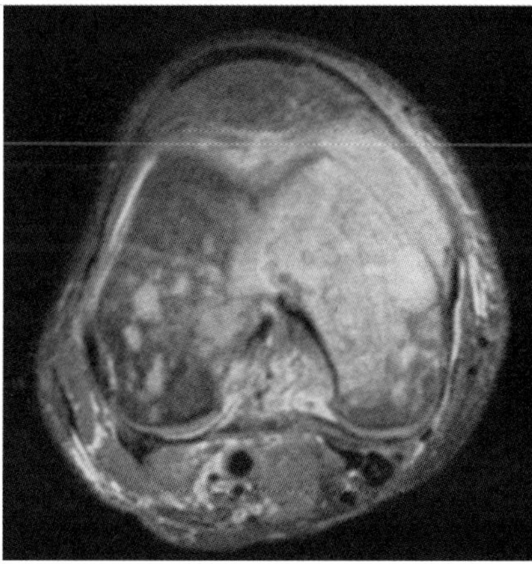

Fig. 10.98 Patient with acute lymphoblastic leukemia within the femoral and tibial marrow associated with cortical destruction and extraosseous extension as seen on sagittal (a) and axial fat-suppressed T2-weighted imaging (b).

Table 10.4 (Cont.) Intramedullary lesions associated with cortical destruction and extraosseous extension

Abnormalities	MRI findings	Comments
Lymphoma (▶ Fig. 10.99)	Non-Hodgkin lymphoma (NHL) and Hodgkin disease (HD) within bone typically appear as single or multifocal poorly defined or circumscribed intramedullary zones with low-intermediate signal on T1WI, and intermediate, slightly high, and/or high signal on T2WI and high signal on FS T2WI; often show Gd-contrast enhancement. Zones of cortical destruction may occur associated with extraosseous soft tissue extension. HD involving bone with associated sclerosis seen on plain films or CT usually have low signal on T1WI and variable/mixed signal on T2WI. In some cases of NHL, intramedullary tumor may be associated with bulky extraosseous lesions without extensive cortical destruction. High-resolution MRI in these cases shows thin penetrating channels of tumor extending through bone cortex into the extraosseous soft tissues.	Lymphoid tumors with neoplastic cells typically within lymphoid tissue (lymph nodes and reticuloendothelial organs). Unlike leukemia, lymphoma usually arises as discrete masses. Lymphomas are subdivided into HD and NHL. Almost all primary lymphomas of bone are B cell NHL. HD, mean age = 32 years. Osseous NHL, median = 35 years.
Osteosarcoma (▶ Fig. 10.100)	Destructive intramedullary malignant lesions, low-intermediate signal on T1WI, mixed low, intermediate, high signal on T2WI, usually with matrix mineralization/ossification-low signal on T2 W images, usually show Gd-contrast enhancement (usually heterogeneous). Zones of cortical destruction are common through which tumors extend into the extraosseous soft tissues under an elevated periosteum. Lamellated and/or spiculated zones of bone formation can occur under the periosteal elevation secondary to tumor invasion and perforation of bone cortex. Low signal from spicules of periosteal, reactive, and tumoral bone formation may have a divergent (sunburst) pattern, perpendicular (hair on end) pattern, or disorganized or complex appearance. Triangular zones of periosteal elevation (Codman triangles) can be seen at the borders of zones of cortical destruction and tumor extension.	Malignant tumor composed of proliferating neoplastic spindle cells that produce osteoid and/or immature tumoral bone and which most frequently arise within medullary bone (metadiaphyseal > metaphyseal > diaphyseal locations). Two age peaks of incidence. The larger peak occurs between the ages of 10 and 20 and accounts for over half of the cases. The second smaller peak occurs in adults over 60 years and accounts for approximately 10% of the cases. Occurs in children as primary tumors and adults (associated with Paget disease, irradiated bone, chronic osteomyelitis, osteoblastoma, giant cell tumor, fibrous dysplasia).

(continued on page 400)

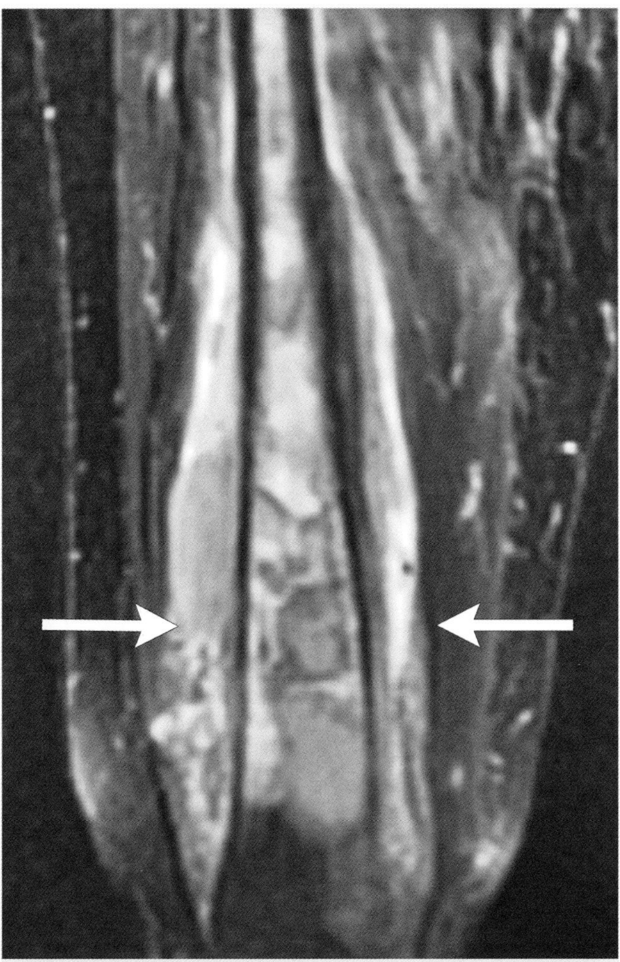

Fig. 10.99 Large B-cell non-Hodgkin lymphoma in the distal femoral marrow associated with cortical destruction and extraosseous extension with periosteal elevation (arrows) as seen on coronal fat-suppressed T2-weighted imaging.

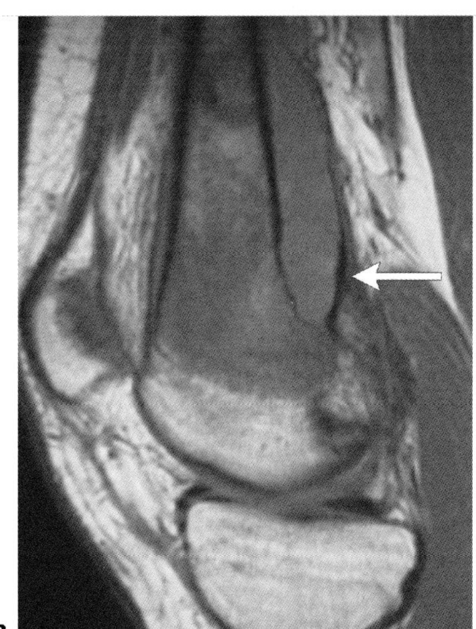

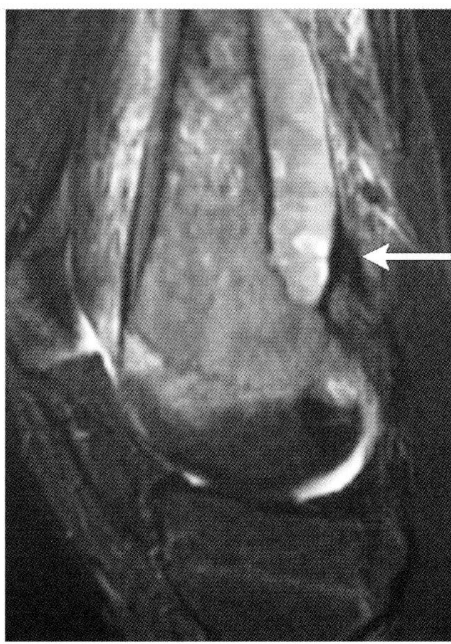

Fig. 10.100 Osteosarcoma in the distal femoral marrow associated with cortical destruction, extraosseous extension, and periosteal elevation (arrows) as seen on sagittal T1-weighted imaging (a) and fat-suppressed T2-weighted imaging (b).

Table 10.4 (Cont.) Intramedullary lesions associated with cortical destruction and extraosseous extension

Abnormalities	MRI findings	Comments
Chondrosarcoma (▶ Fig. 10.101)	Intramedullary tumors often have low-intermediate signal on T1WI, intermediate signal on PDWI, and heterogeneous intermediate-high signal on T2WI. Lesions usually show heterogeneous contrast enhancement. Zones of cortical destruction can be seen with extraosseous extension of tumor.	Chondrosarcomas are malignant tumors containing cartilage formed within sarcomatous stroma. Account for 12 to 21% of malignant bone lesions, 21 to 26% of primary sarcomas of bone, usually occurs between 5 and 91 years of age, mean = 40 years, median = 26 to 59 years.

(continued on page 402)

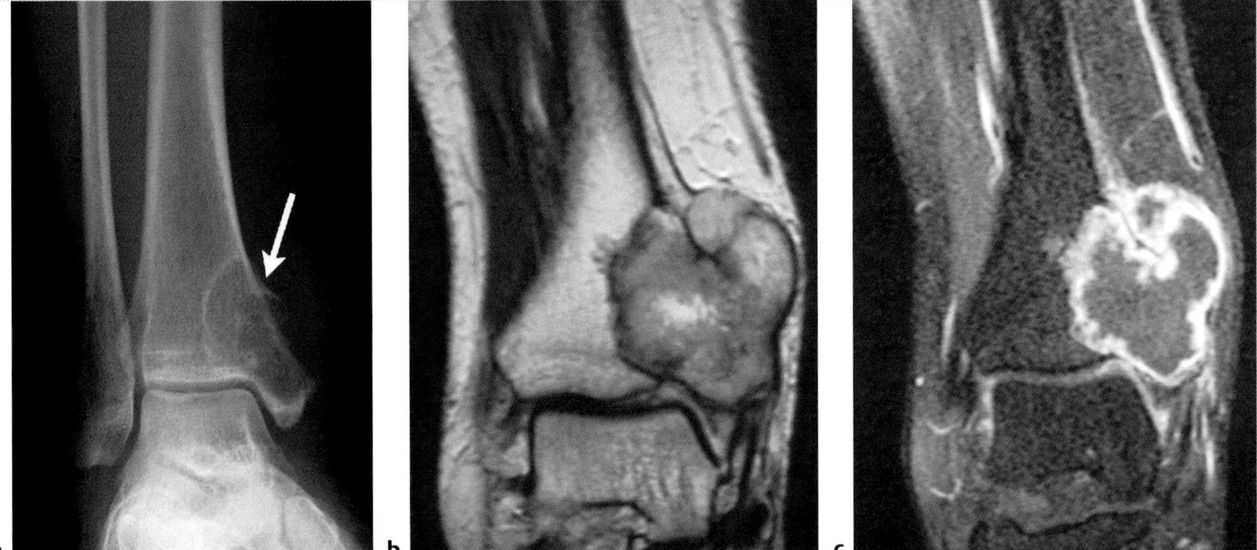

Fig. 10.101 Radiograph of a 44-year-old woman with a chondrosarcoma involving the medial distal tibia shows a zone of medullary and cortical bone destruction (arrow) (a). Intramedullary tumor extends through destroyed bone cortex into the extraosseous soft tissue and has heterogeneous slightly high to high signal on coronal T2-weighted imaging (b) and a peripheral lobular pattern of gadolinium-contrast enhancement on coronal fat-suppressed T1-weighted imaging (c).

Table 10.4 (Cont.) Intramedullary lesions associated with cortical destruction and extraosseous extension

Abnormalities	MRI findings	Comments
Ewing sarcoma (▶ Fig. 10.102)	Destructive malignant lesions involving marrow, low-intermediate signal on T1WI, mixed low, intermediate, and/or high signal on T2WI and FS T2WI, usually shows Gd-contrast enhancement (usually heterogeneous). Extraosseous tumor extension through sites of cortical destruction is commonly seen beneath an elevated periosteum. Thin striated zones of low signal on T2WI can sometimes be seen oriented perpendicular to the long axis of the involved bone under the elevated periosteum representing the hair on end appearance of reactive bone formation secondary to the tumor. In long bones, tumors are most often located in the diaphyseal region, followed by the metadiaphyseal region.	Malignant primitive tumor of bone composed of undifferentiated small cells with round nuclei. Accounts for 6 to 11% of primary malignant bone tumors, 5 to 7% of primary bone tumors. Usually occurs between the ages of 5 and 30, males > females, locally invasive, high metastatic potential.
Chordoma (▶ Fig. 10.103)	Tumors are often midline in location, often have lobulated or slightly lobulated margins. Lesions can involve marrow with associated destruction of trabecular and cortical bone with extrosseous extension. Chondroid chordomas are either midline or off-midline in location. Chordomas typically have low-intermediate signal on T1WI and heterogeneous predominantly high signal on T2WI. Chordomas typically enhance with Gd-contrast often in a heterogeneous pattern.	Rare locally aggressive slow-growing low- to intermediate-grade malignant tumors derived from ectopic notochordal remnants along the axial skeleton. Chordomas account for 2 to 4% of primary malignant bone tumors, 1 to 3% of all primary bone tumors, and less than 1% of intracranial tumors. Patients range in age from 6 to 84 years, median = 58 years.
Fibrosarcoma (▶ Fig. 10.104)	Intramedullary lesions with irregular margins, with or without associated cortical destruction and/or extraosseous soft tissue masses. Lesions usually have low-intermediate signal on T1WI and PDWI, and heterogeneous intermediate, slightly high, and/or high signal on T2WI. Lesions usually show heterogeneous Gd-contrast enhancement.	Fibrosarcomas are uncommon malignant tumors consisting of bundles of neoplastic fibroblasts/ spindle cells with varying proportions of collagen, lacking other tissue differentiating features such as tumor bone, osteoid, or cartilage. Can be primary lesions (75%) or arise as secondary tumors (25%) associated with prior irradiation, Paget disease, bone infarct, chronic osteomyelitis, fibrous dysplasia, giant cell tumor. Accounts for 3 to 5% of primary malignant bone tumors and 2 to 4% of all bone tumors, median age= 43 years.

(continued on page 404)

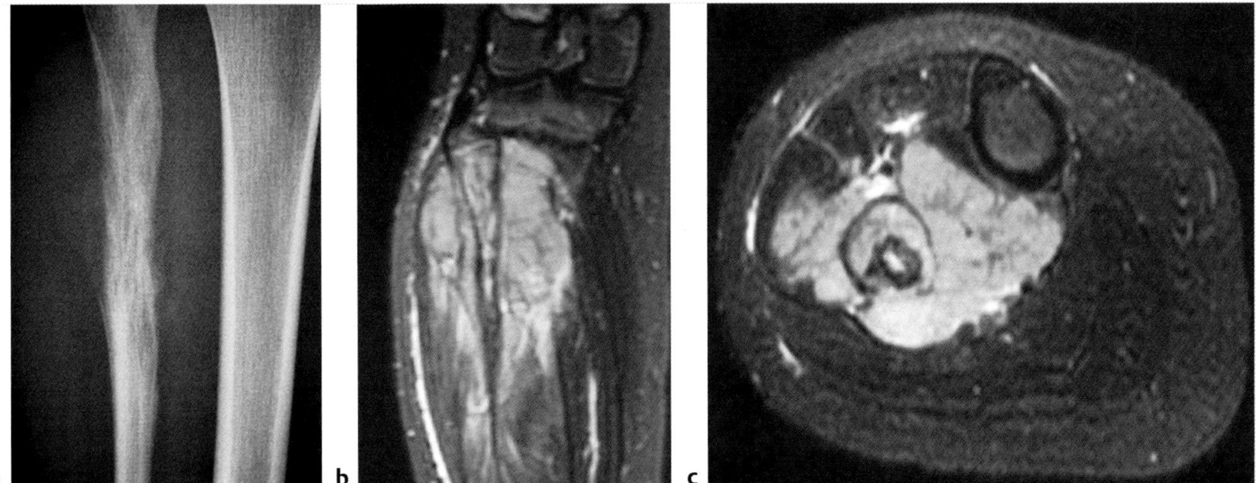

Fig. 10.102 Radiograph of a 10-year-old girl with Ewing sarcoma involving the proximal fibula shows permeative medullary and cortical bone destruction as well as interrupted periosteal reaction (a). Coronal (b) and axial fat-suppressed T2-weighted imaging (c) shows the intramedullary tumor with high signal extending through destroyed bone cortex into the extraosseous soft tissues.

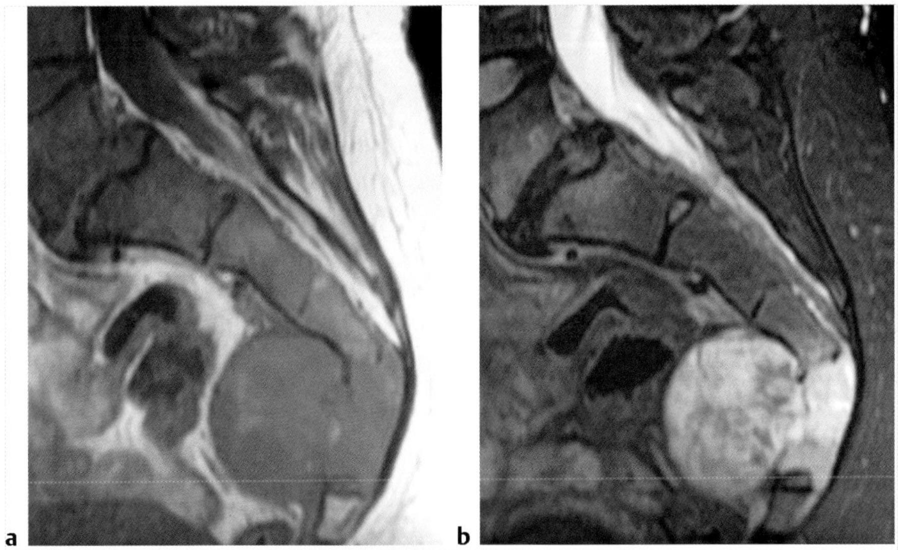

Fig. 10.103 A 30-year-old woman with a chordoma involving the marrow of the lower sacrum associated with cortical bone destruction and tumor extension into the adjacent soft tissues. The tumor has mostly intermediate signal on sagittal T1-weighted imaging (a) and heterogeneous mostly high signal on sagittal fat-suppressed T2-weighted imaging (b).

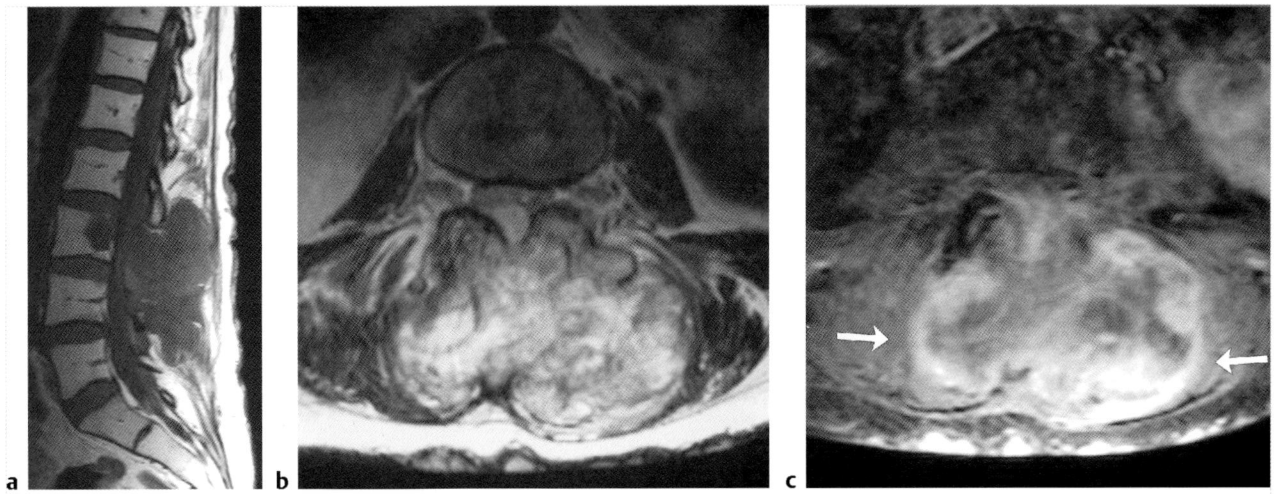

Fig. 10.104 A 25-year-old man with fibrosarcoma extending from the posterior elements of the L3 vertebra into the adjacent soft tissues through destroyed bone cortex. The tumor has intermediate signal on sagittal T1-weighted imaging (T1WI) (a), heterogeneous mostly high signal on axial T2-weighted imaging (b), and shows heterogeneous Gd-contrast enhancement (arrows) on axial fat-suppresed T1WI (c).

Table 10.4 (Cont.) Intramedullary lesions associated with cortical destruction and extraosseous extension

Abnormalities	MRI findings	Comments
Malignant fibrous histiocytoma (▶ Fig. 10.105)	Intramedullary lesions with irregular margins and zones of cortical destruction and extraosseous extension. Tumors often have low-intermediate signal on T1WI; low-intermediate signal on PDWI, and heterogeneous intermediate-high signal on T2WI and FS T2WI. Invasion into joints occurs in 30%. May be associated with bone infarcts, bone cysts, chronic osteomyelitis, Paget disease, and other treated primary bone tumors. Lesions usually show heterogeneous Gd-contrast prominent enhancement.	Malignant tumor involving soft tissue and rarely bone derived from undifferentiated mesenchymal cells. Contains cells with limited cellular differentiation such as mixtures of fibroblasts, myofibroblasts, histiocyte-like cells, anaplastic giant cells, and inflammatory cells. Accounts for 1 to 5% of primary malignant bone tumors and < 1% to 3% of all primary bone tumors, patient ages range from 11 to 80 years, median = 48 years, mean = 55 years.
Malignant giant cell tumor (▶ Fig. 10.106)	Well-defined lesions with or without thin low signal margins on T1WI and T2WI. Solid portions of giant cell tumors often have low to intermediate signal on T1WI and PDWI, intermediate to high signal on T2WI, and high signal on FS PDWI and FS T2WI. Signal heterogeneity on T2WI is not uncommon. Aneurysmal bone cysts are seen with 14% of giant cell tumors. Lesions show mild to prominent variable and often heterogeneous Gd-contrast enhancement. Poorly defined zones of enhancement and high signal on FS T2WI may occasionally be seen in the adjacent marrow secondary to inflammatory reaction from elevated tumor prostaglandin levels. Cortical destruction and extraosseous tumor extension are frequently seen.	Aggressive bone tumors composed of neoplastic ovoid mononuclear cells and scattered multinucleated osteoclast-like giant cells. Up to 10% of all giant cell tumors are malignant. Benign giant cell tumors account for approximately 5 to 9.5% of all bone tumors and up to 23% of benign bone tumors. 75% of malignant giant cell tumors occur in patients between the ages of 15 and 45.
Hemangioendothelioma (▶ Fig. 10.107)	Intramedullary tumors usually with sharp margins that may be slightly lobulated. Lesions often have low-intermediate and/or high signal on T1WI and PDWI, and heterogeneous intermediate-high signal on T2WI and FS T2WI with or without zones of low signal. Lesions can be multifocal. Extraosseous extension of tumor through zones of cortical destruction commonly occur. Lesions often show prominent heterogeneous Gd-contrast enhancement.	Low-grade vasoformative/endothelial malignant neoplasms, which are locally aggressive and rarely metastasize, compared with the high-grade endothelial tumors such as angiosarcoma. Account for less than 1% of primary malignant bone tumors. Patients range from 10 to 82 years, median = 36 to 47 years. Patients with multifocal lesions tend to be approximately 10 years younger on average than those with unifocal tumors.

(continued on page 406)

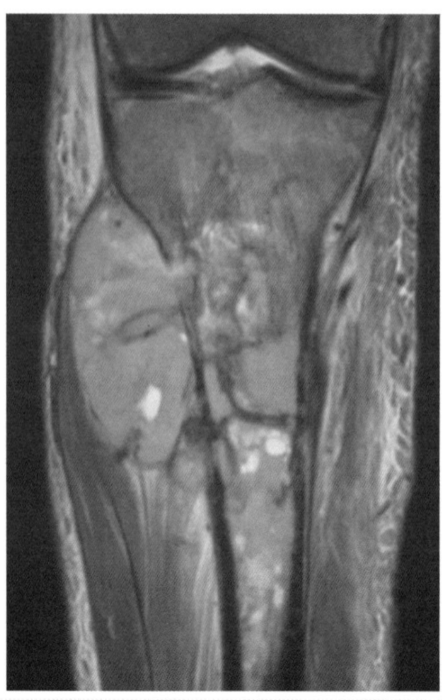
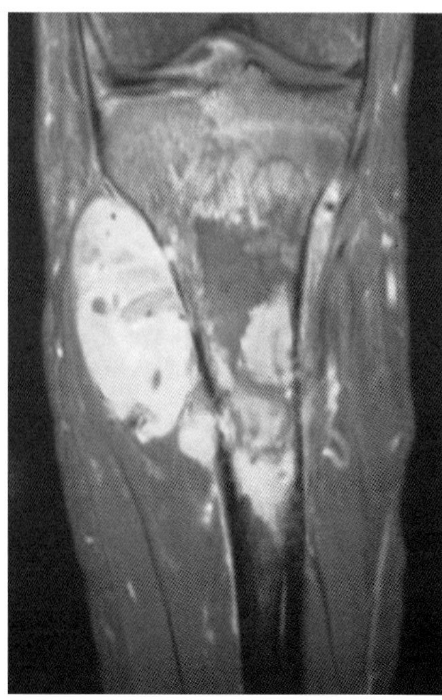

Fig. 10.105 A 27-year-old man with a malignant fibrous histiocytoma involving the proximal tibia. Intramedullary tumor extends through destroyed bone cortex into the extraosseous soft tissues and has heterogeneous mixed signal on coronal T2-weighted imaging (a) and heterogeneous Gd-contrast enhancement on coronal fat-suppressed T1-weighted imaging (b).

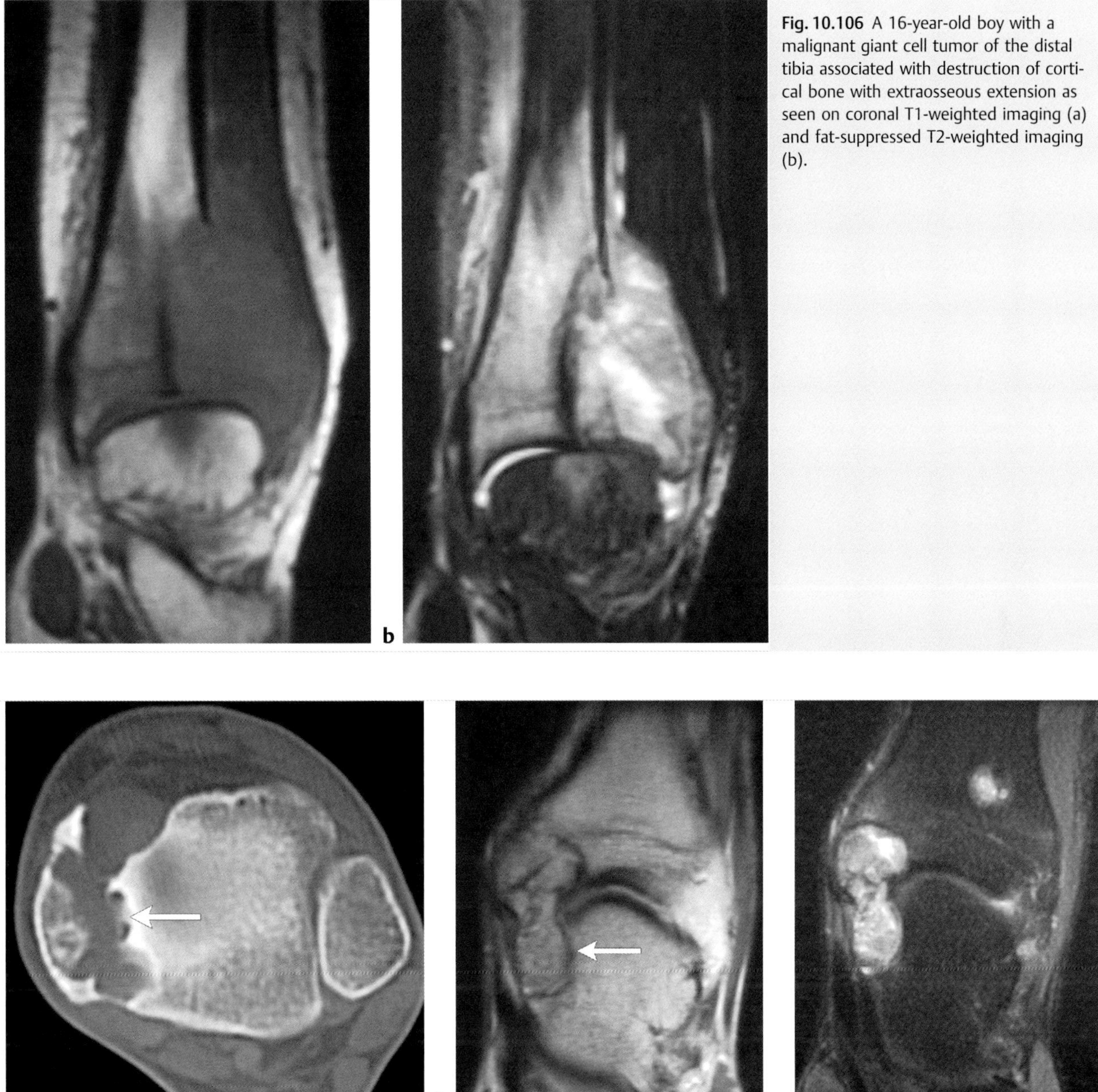

Fig. 10.106 A 16-year-old boy with a malignant giant cell tumor of the distal tibia associated with destruction of cortical bone with extraosseous extension as seen on coronal T1-weighted imaging (a) and fat-suppressed T2-weighted imaging (b).

Fig. 10.107 A 19-year-old man with hemangioendothelioma involving the distal medial tibia. The tumor causes medullary and cortical bone destruction (arrow) on axial computed tomography (a). The tumor has slightly high signal (arrow) on coronal T2-weighted imaging (b) and shows prominent Gd-contrast enhancement on coronal fat-suppressed T1-weighted imaging (c). Intramedullary tumor extends through sites of cortical bone destruction into the ankle joint. Another small hemangendothelioma is also seen in the distal marrow of the tibia more laterally.

Table 10.4 (Cont.) Intramedullary lesions associated with cortical destruction and extraosseous extension

Abnormalities	MRI findings	Comments
Hemangiopericytoma (▶ Fig. 10.108)	Radiolucent intramedullary lesions can have associated cortical destruction and soft tissue extension. Lesions usually have low-intermediate signal on T1WI, intermediate signal on PDWI, and slightly high to high signal on T2WI. On T1WI and T2WI, thin tubular signal voids representing blood vessels may be seen within and/or at the periphery of tumors, as well as being arranged in"spoke-wheel"patterns. Typically show Gd-contrast enhancement.	Rare malignant tumors of presumed pericytic origin that show pericytic/myoid differentiation with variously shaped pericytic cells (oval, round, spindle-like) and adjacent irregular branching vascular spaces lined by endothelial cells. Can occur in soft tissues and less frequently in bone. Account for < 1% of primary bone tumors. Patients range in age from 1 to 90 years, median = 40 years.
Liposarcoma (▶ Fig. 10.109)	Tumors can have intermediate and/or slightly high to high signal on T1WI and T2WI and show Gd-contrast enhancement.	Malignant mesenchymal tumors containing portions showing differentiation into adipose tissue. Primary liposarcoma in bone is very rare. Median age = 31 years.
Paget sarcoma (▶ Fig. 10.110)	Irregular zones of medullary and cortical bone destruction associated with an extraosseous soft-tissue mass-lesion. The involved marrow typically has low to intermediate signal on T1WI and PDWI, and low to high signal on T2WI. Abnormal Gd-contrast enhancement is seen in the marrow as well as in the extraosseous tumor extension.	Paget disease is the most common bone disease in older adults after osteoporosis. Median age = 66 years. Disordered bone resorption and woven bone formation occurs resulting in osseous deformity. Associated with less than 1% risk for developing secondary sarcomatous changes.

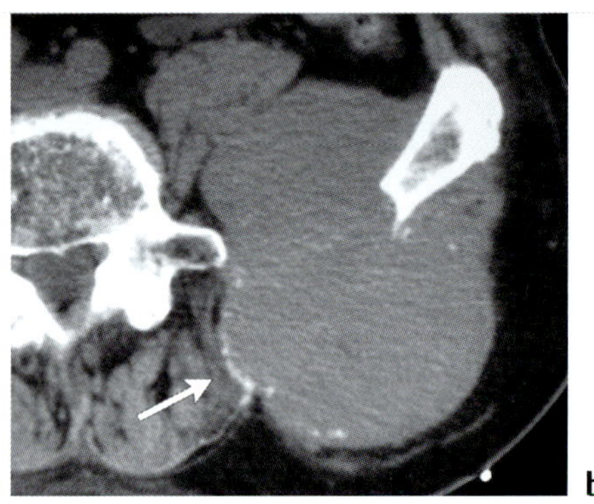

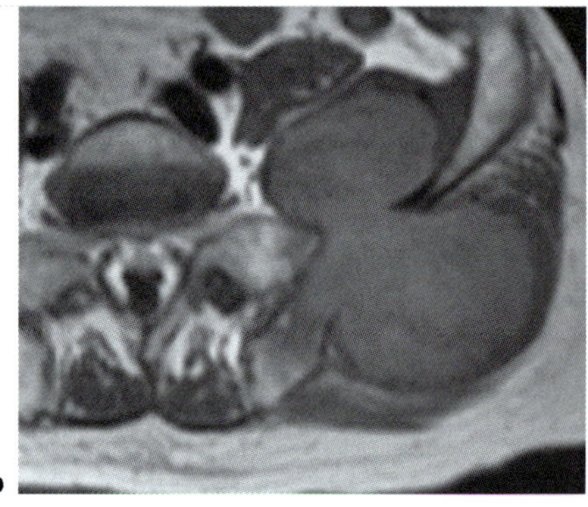

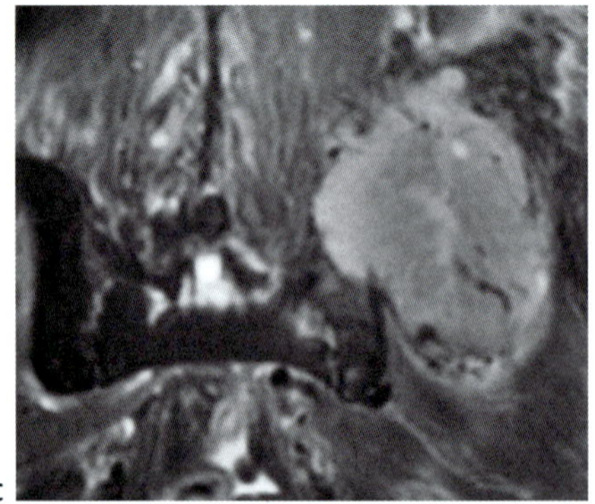

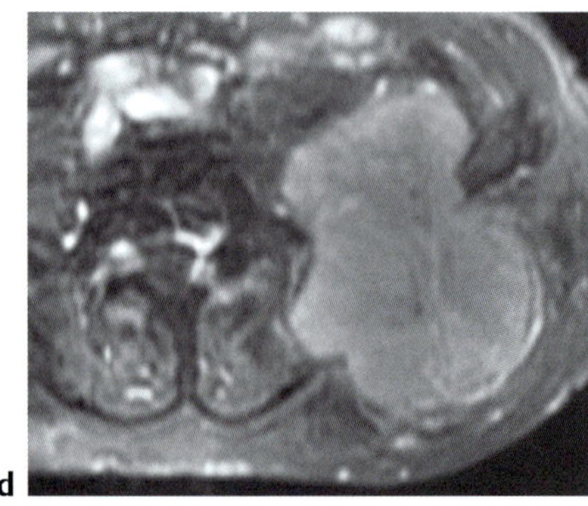

Fig. 10.108 A 78-year-old man with an intraosseous hemangiopericytoma involving the left iliac bone associated with cortical bone destruction and extraosseous tumor extension (arrow) as seen on axial computed tomography (a). Tumor has intermediate signal on axial T1-weighted imaging (T1WI) (b), and slightly high signal on coronal fat-suppressed (FS) T2-weighted imagingl (c). Small flow voids representing blood vessels are seen within the tumor. The tumor shows Gd-contrast enhancement on axial FS T1WI (d).

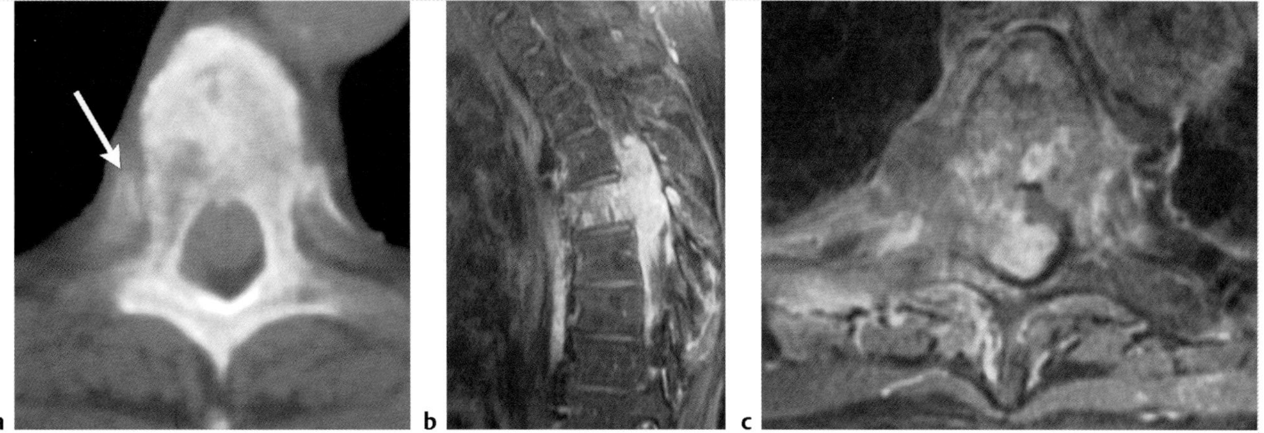

Fig. 10.109 An 81-year-old man with an intraosseous liposarcoma involving a thoracic vertebra. Radiolucent and sclerotic changes (arrow) are seen within the vertebra as well as cortical destruction on axial computed tomography (a). The intraosseous tumor shows gadolinium-contrast enhancement on sagittal (b) and axial fat-suppressed T1-weighted imaging (c). Also seen is cortical destruction with extraosseous tumor extension

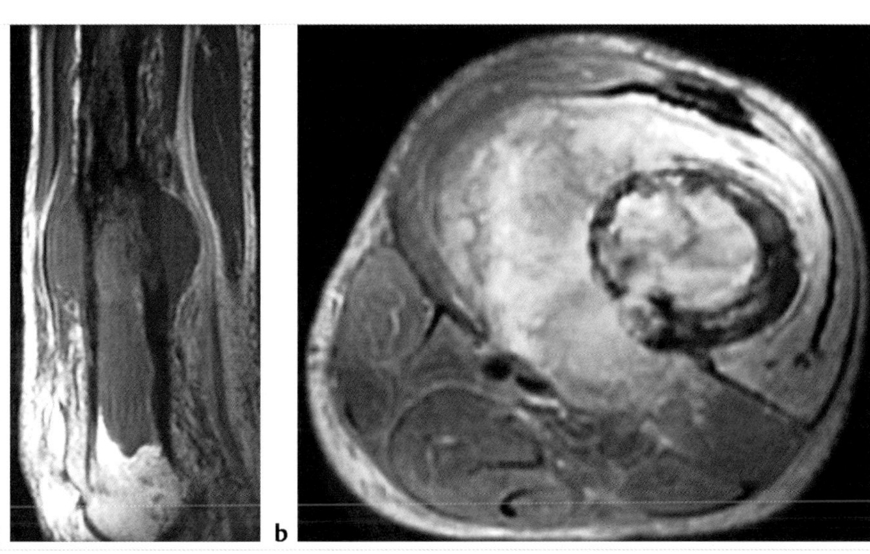

Fig. 10.110 A 71-year-old woman with Paget sarcoma extending from the marrow through destroyed bone cortex into the extraosseous soft tissues as seen on sagittal T1-weighted imaging (a) and axial T2-weighted imaging (b).

10.5 Solitary Intramedullary Lesions with Well-Circumscribed Margins

- Nonmalignant lesions
  - Hemangioma
  - Nonossifying fibroma
  - Enchondroma
  - Fibrous dysplasia
  - Liposclerosing myxofibrous tumor
  - Unicameral bone cyst (UBC)
  - Aneurysmal bone cyst (ABC)
  - Giant cell reparative granuloma
  - Intraosseous lipoma
  - Brown tumor
  - Geode
  - Intraosseous ganglion
  - Bone infarct
  - Enostosis/bone island
  - Giant cell tumor of bone
  - Ameloblastoma
  - Hemophilic pseudotumor
  - Desmoplastic fibroma
- Malignant lesions
  - Metastatic tumor
  - Plasmacytoma
  - Lymphoma
  - Low grade chondrosarcoma
  - Malignant giant cell tumor

Table 10.5 Solitary intramedullary lesions with well-circumscribed margins

Abnormalities	MRI findings	Comments
Nonmalignant lesions		
Hemangioma (▶ Fig. 10.111)	Often well-circumscribed lesions, which typically have intermediate to high signal on T1-weighted imaging (T1WI), proton density–weighted imaging (PDWI), T2-weighted imaging (T2WI), and fat-suppressed (FS) T2WI. On T1WI, hemangiomas usually have signal equal to or greater than adjacent normal marrow secondary to fatty components. Usually show gadolinium (Gd)-contrast enhancement. Pathological fractures associated with intraosseous hemangiomas usually result in low-intermediate marrow signal on T1WI.	Common benign lesions of bone composed of capillary, cavernous, and/or malformed venous vessels. Hemangiomas have been considered to be a hamartomatous disorder. Account for 4% of benign bone tumors and approximately 1% of all bone tumors, likely underestimated. Occurs in all ages, median = 33 years.
Nonossifying fibroma (▶ Fig. 10.112)	Well-circumscribed eccentric intramedullary lesions in the dimetaphyseal regions of long bones that have mixed low-intermediate signal on T1WI, and mixed low, intermediate, and/or high signal on T2WI, PDWI, and FS T2WI. Zones of low signal on T1WI, PDWI, and T2WI can be seen in the central portions of the lesions. Zones with varying thickness of low signal on T1WI, PDWI, and T2WI are seen at the margins of the lesions representing bone sclerosis. Internal septations are commonly seen as zones of low signal on T2WI in these lesions. Lesions can show Gd-contrast enhancement (heterogeneous > homogeneous patterns).	Common benign fibrohistiocytic lesions in the metaphyseal portions of long bones that are composed of whorls of fibroblastic cells combined with smaller amounts of multinucleated giant cells and xanthomatous cells. Usually asymptomatic; 95% occur between the ages of 5 and 20, median = 14 years.
Enchondroma (▶ Fig. 10.113)	Lobulated intramedullary lesions with well-defined borders, mean size = 5 cm. Lesions usually have low-intermediate signal on T1WI and intermediate signal on PDWI. On T2WI and fat-suppressed T2WI, lesions usually have predominantly high signal with foci and/or bands of low signal representing areas of matrix mineralization and fibrous strands. Lesions typically show Gd-contrast enhancement in various patterns (peripheral curvilinear lobular, central nodular/septal and peripheral lobular, or heterogeneous diffuse).	Benign intraosseous lesions composed of hyaline cartilage represent approximately 10% of benign bone tumors. Enchondromas can be solitary (88%) or multiple (12%). Median age = 35 years, peak in third and fourth decades.

(continued on page 410)

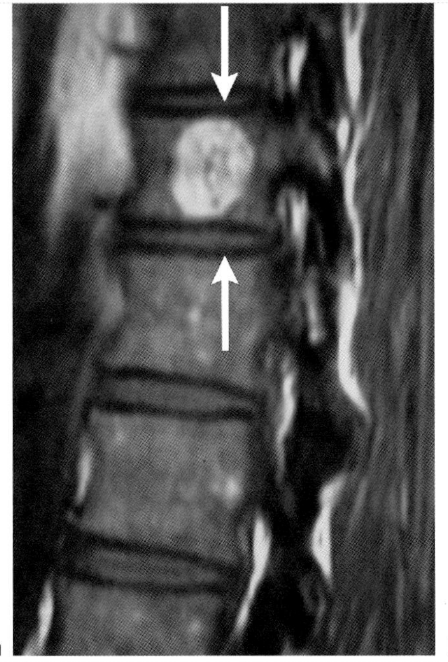

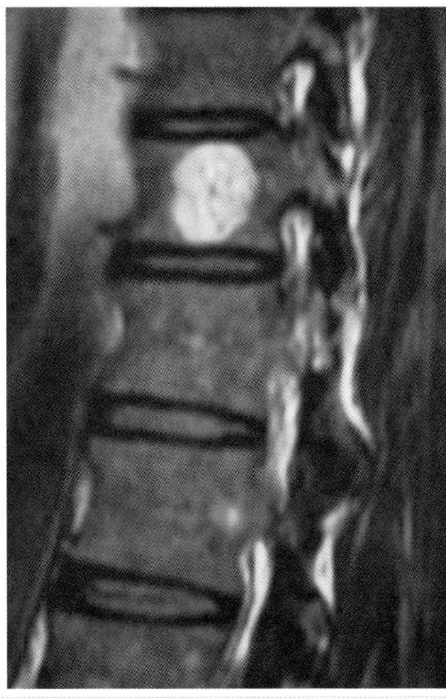

Fig. 10.111 Hemangioma (arrows) within the T12 vertebral body has circumscribed margins and contains high signal on sagittal T1-weighted imaging (a) and T2-weighted imaging (b).

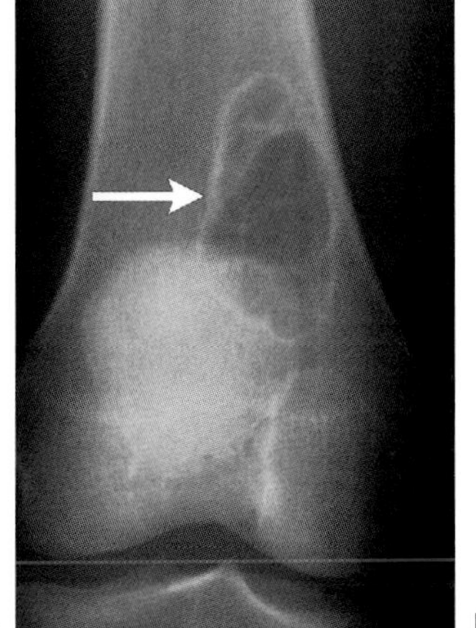

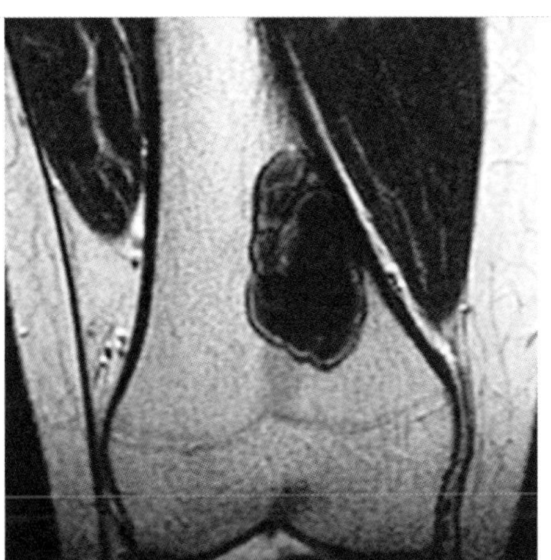

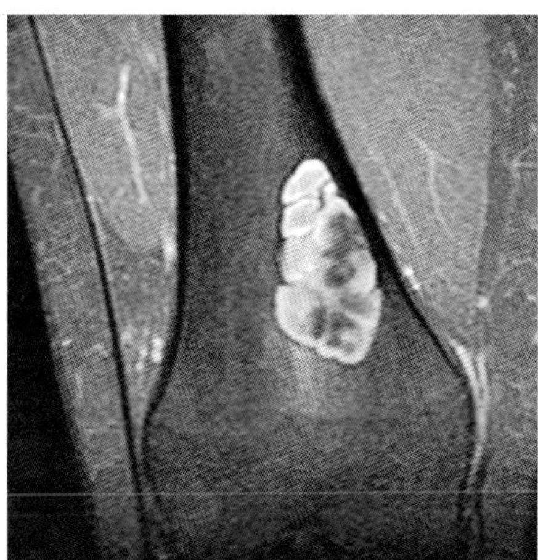

Fig. 10.112 Nonossifying fibroma in the distal femur of a 17-year-old. The radiolucent lesion (arrow) has a thin sclerotic border on anteroposterior radiograph (a) and has heterogeneous mostly low signal on coronal T2-weighted imaging (b). The lesion shows heterogeneous gadolinium-contrast enhancement on coronal fat-suppressed T1-weighted imaging (c).

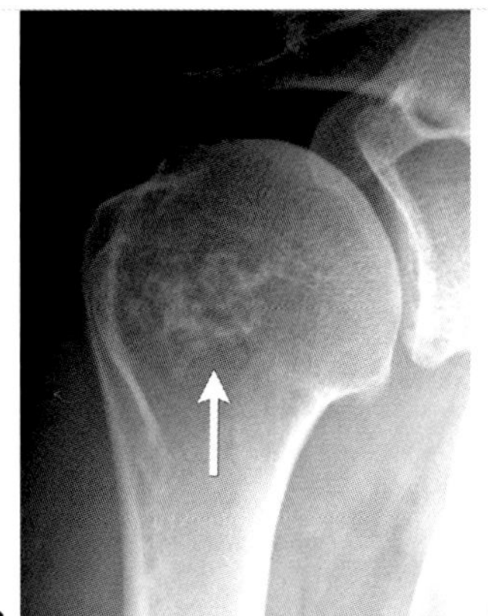

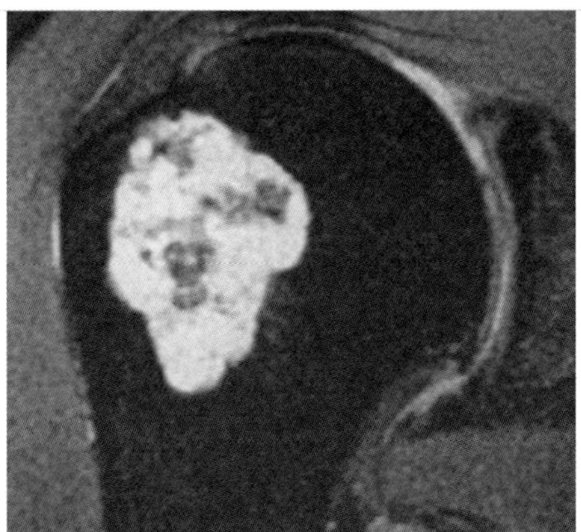

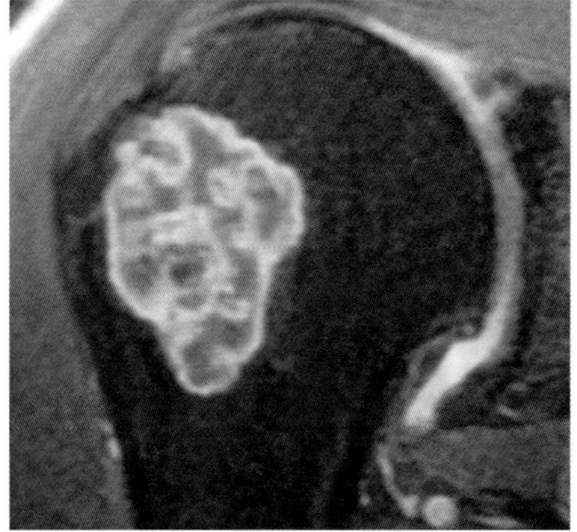

Fig. 10.113 A 47-year-old man with an enchondroma in the proximal humerus, which contains mineralized chondroid matrix on radiograph (a). The lesion has sharp, slightly lobulated margins and has heterogeneous high signal on coronal fat-suppressed (FS) T2-weighted imaging (b); and shows thin peripheral and central gadolinium-contrast enhancement on coronal FS T1-weighted imaging (c).

Table 10.5 (Cont.) Solitary intramedullary lesions with well-circumscribed margins

Abnormalities	MRI findings	Comments
Fibrous dysplasia (▶ Fig. 10.114)	Magnetic resonance imaging (MRI) features depend on the proportions of bony spicules, collagen, fibroblastic spindle cells, hemorrhagic and/or cystic changes, and associated pathological fracture if present. Lesions are usually well circumscribed and have low or low-intermediate signal on T1WI and PDWI. On T2WI, lesions have variable mixtures of low, intermediate, and/or high signal often surrounded by a low signal rim of variable thickness. Internal septations and cystic changes are seen in a minority of lesions. Bone expansion with thickened and/or thinned cortex can be seen. Lesions show Gd-contrast enhancement that varies in degree and pattern.	Benign medullary fibro-osseous lesion, which can involve a single site (mono-ostotic) or multiple locations (polyostotic). Thought to occur from developmental failure in the normal process of remodeling primitive bone to mature lamellar bone with resultant zone or zones of immature trabeculae within dysplastic fibrous tissue. Accounts for approximately 10% of benign bone lesions. Patients range in age from < 1 year to 76 years; 75% occur before the age of 30 years.
Liposclerosing myxofibrous tumor (▶ Fig. 10.115)	Lesions have well-defined margins with variable thickness of low signal borders on T1WI and T2WI. Lesions often have low to intermediate signal on T1WI and intermediate to high signal on T2WI and FS T2WI. Small zones with fat signal may be seen at the periphery of the lesions. Lesions usually lack Gd-contrast enhancement.	Uncommon benign fibro-osseous lesions with mixed histological features of lipoma, fibroxanthoma, myxoma, fibrous dysplasia, bone cyst, myxofibroma, fat necrosis, and/or ischemic ossification. Most of these lesions occur in the intertrochanteric region of the femur. May represent a variant form of fibrous dysplasia. Patients range from 15 to 69 years, mean = 42 years.

(continued on page 412)

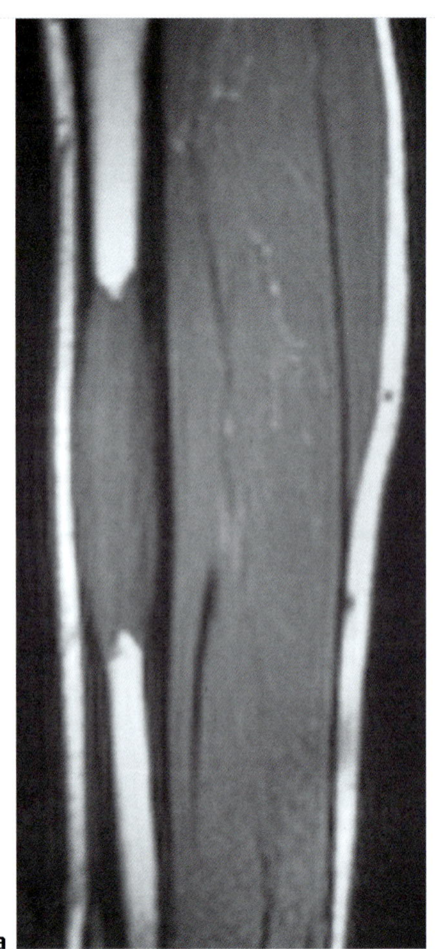

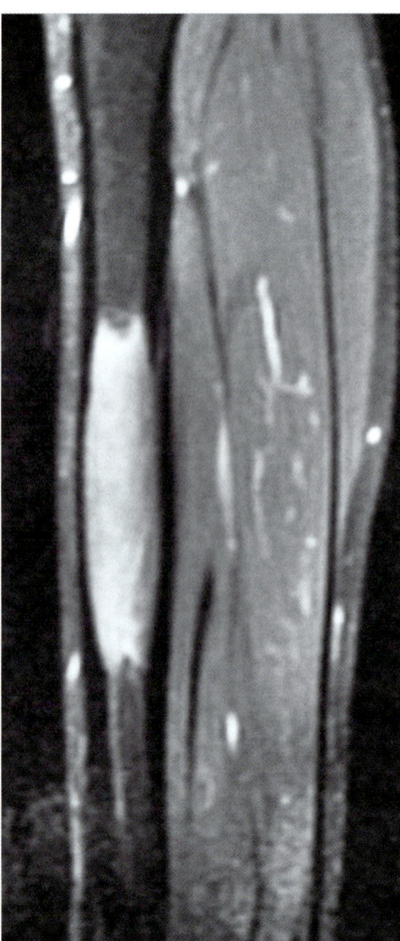

Fig. 10.114 Fibrous dysplasia in the tibia diaphysis of a 19-year-old man, which has intermediate signal on sagittal T1-weighted imaging (T1WI) (a) and shows Gd-contrast enhancement on fat-suppressed T1WI (b).

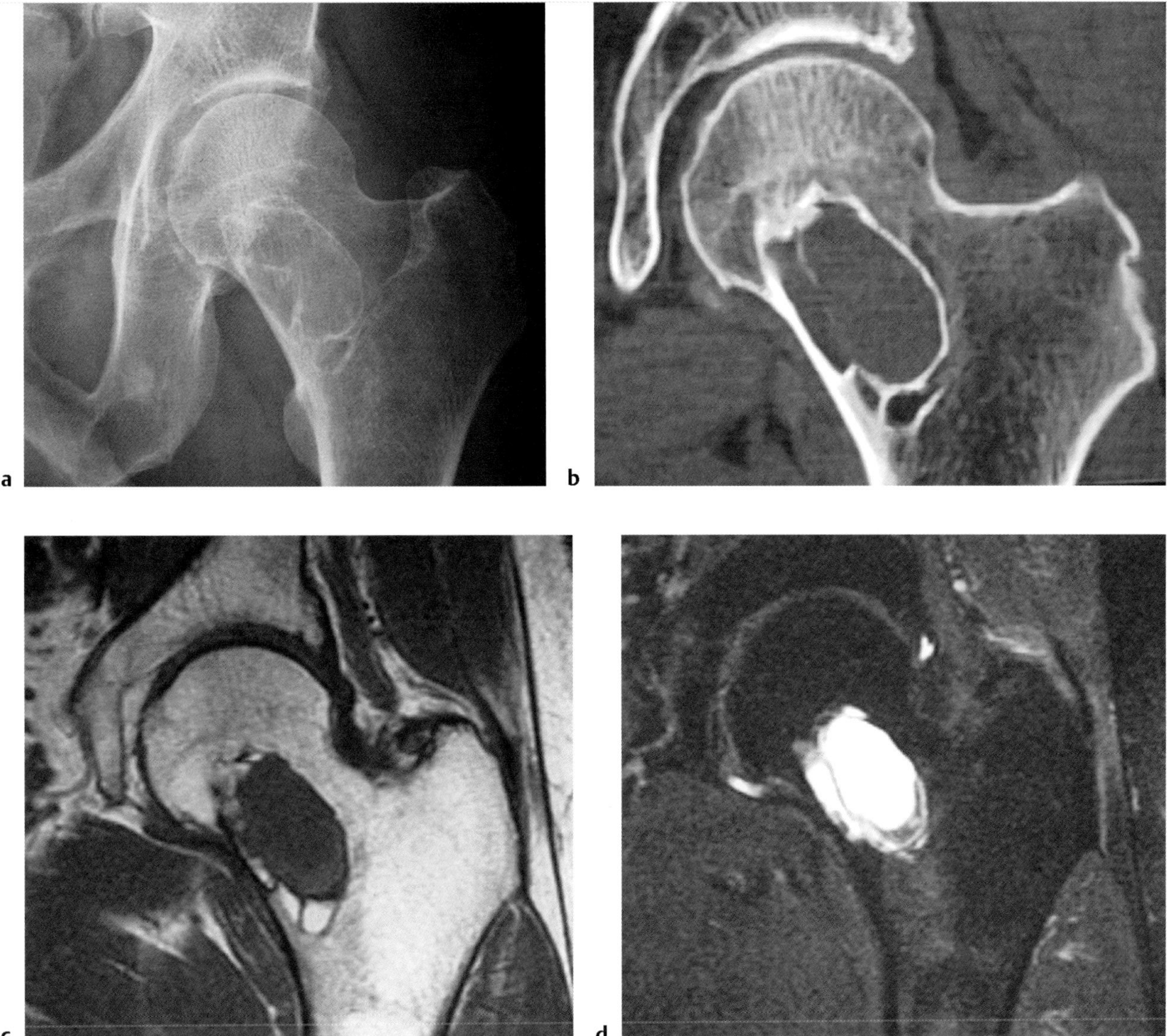

Fig. 10.115 Liposclerosing myxofibrous tumor in the femoral neck of a 61-year-old man. Radiograph (a) and computed tomographic image (b) show a well-defined radiolucent lesion with thin sclerotic margins. The lesion has mostly low signal centrally as well as small peripheral zones with high fat signal on coronal T1-weighted imaging (c) and has mostly high signal on coronal fat-suppressed T2-weighted imaging (d).

Table 10.5 (Cont.) Solitary intramedullary lesions with well-circumscribed margins

Abnormalities	MRI findings	Comments
Unicameral bone cyst (UBC) (▶ Fig. 10.116)	UBCs often have a peripheral rim of low signal on T1WI and T2WI adjacent to normal medullary bone. UBCs usually contain fluid with low to low-intermediate signal on T1WI; high signal on T2WI. Fluid-fluid levels may occur. For UBCs without pathological fracture, thin peripheral Gd-contrast enhancement can be seen at the margins of lesions. UBCs with pathological fracture can have heterogeneous or homogeneous low-intermediate or slightly high signal on T1WI, and heterogeneous or homogeneous high signal on T2WI and FS T2WI. UBCs complicated by fracture can have internal septations and fluid-fluid levels, as well as irregular peripheral Gd-contrast enhancement and at internal septations.	Intramedullary nonneoplastic cavities filled with serous or serosanguinous fluid. Account for 9% of primary tumor-like lesions of bone; 85% occur in the first 2 decades, median = 11 years.
Aneurysmal bone cyst (ABC) (▶ Fig. 10.117)	ABCs often have a low signal rim on T1WI and T2WI adjacent to normal medullary bone and between extraosseous soft tissues. Various combinations of low, intermediate, and/or high signal on T1WI, PDWI, and T2WI are usually seen within aneurysmal bone cysts as well as fluid-fluid levels. Variable Gd-contrast enhancement is seen at the margins of lesions as well as involving the internal septae.	Tumor-like expansile bone lesions containing cavernous spaces filled with blood. ABCs can be primary bone lesions (two thirds) or secondary to other bone lesions/tumors (such as giant cell tumors, chondroblastomas, osteoblastomas, osteosarcomas, chondromyxoid fibromas, nonossifying fibromas, fibrous dysplasia, fibrosarcomas, malignant fibrous histiocytomas, and metastatic disease). Account for approximately 11% of primary tumor-like lesions of bone. Patients usually range in age from 1 to 25 years, median = 14 years.
Giant cell reparative granuloma (▶ Fig. 10.118)	Lesions can have heterogeneous low, intermediate, and/or high signal on T1WI, PDWI, and T2WI; as well as peripheral rimlike and central Gd-contrast enhancement on FS T1WI.	Giant cell reparative granulomas are also referred to as solid ABCs. Histological appearance resembles brown tumors.
Intraosseous lipoma (▶ Fig. 10.119)	Lesions can have heterogeneous low, intermediate, and/or high signal on T1WI, PDWI, and T2WI, as well as peripheral rimlike and central Gd-contrast enhancement on FS T1WI. Intraosseous lipomas. Calcifications, when present, usually appear as zones of low signal or signal void.	Uncommon benign hamartomas composed of mature white adipose tissue without cellular atypia. Osseous or chondroid metaplasia with myxoid changes can be associated with lipomas. Account for approximately 0.1% of bone tumors, likely underreported.

(continued on page 414)

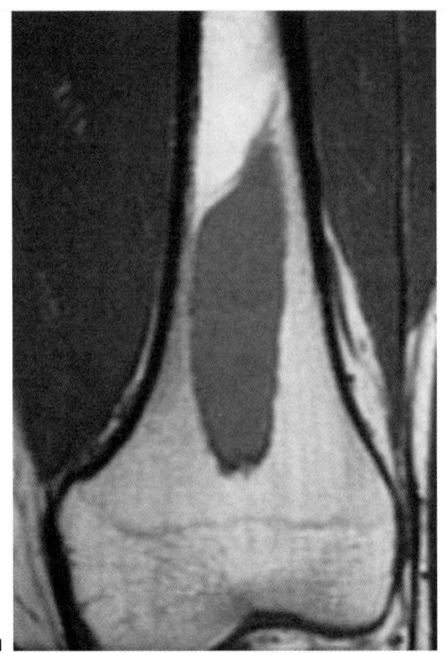

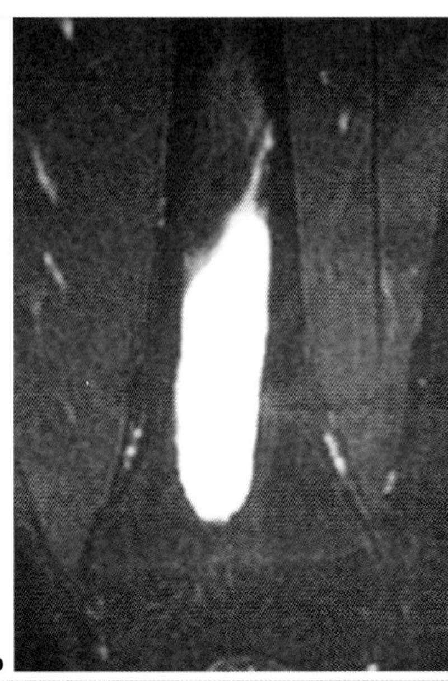

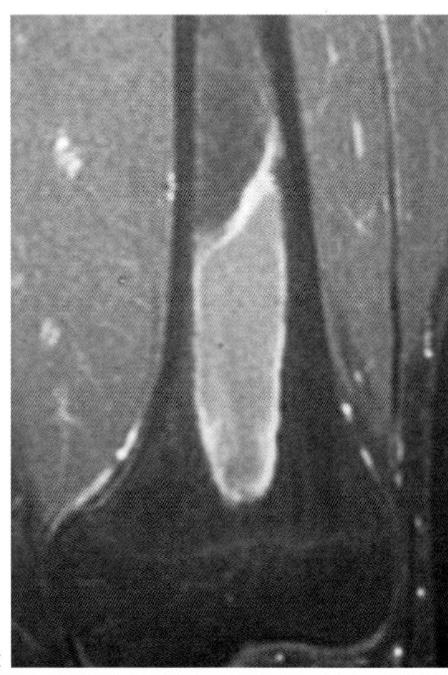

Fig. 10.116 Unicameral bone cyst in the distal femoral shaft of a 16-year-old boy has intermediate signal on coronal proton density–weighted imaging (a), high signal on coronal fat-suppressed (FS) T2-weighted imaging (b), and shows thin peripheral Gd-contrast enhancement on coronal FS T1-weighted imaging (c).

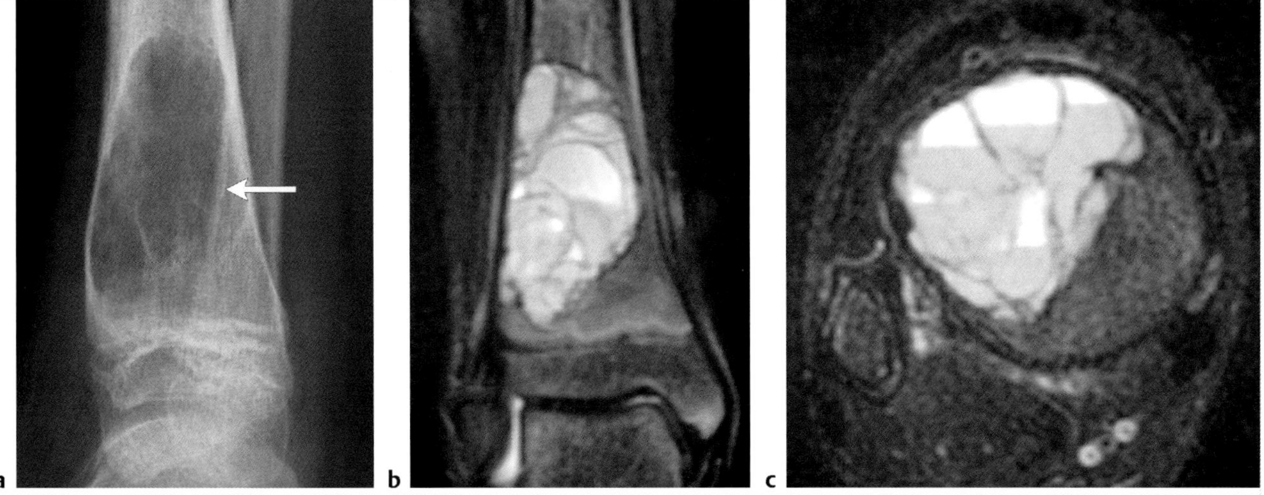

Fig. 10.117 Aneurysmal bone cyst in a 9-year-old girl is seen in the distal tibia. The circumscribed radiolucent lesion (a) (arrow) has a thin margin with low signal and contains multiple fluid-fluid levels as seen on coronal (b) and axial fat-suppressed T2-weighted imaging (c).

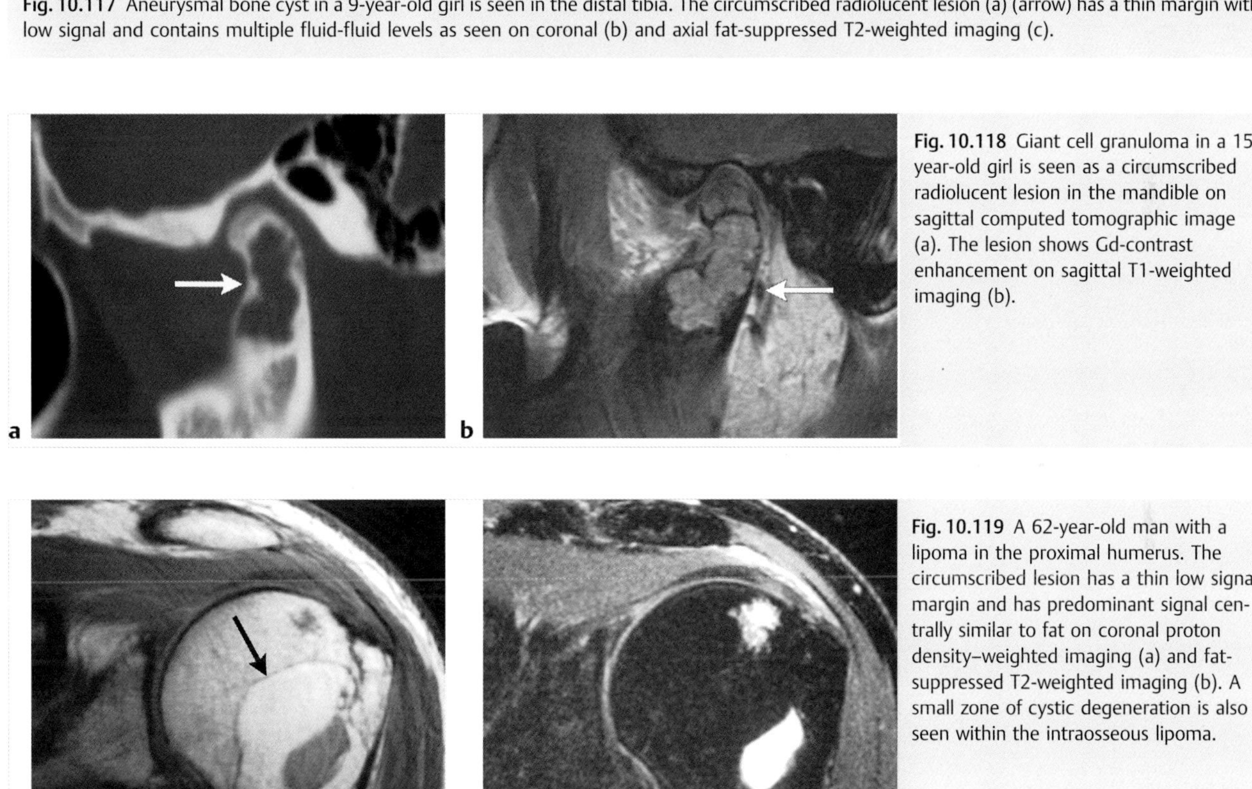

Fig. 10.118 Giant cell granuloma in a 15-year-old girl is seen as a circumscribed radiolucent lesion in the mandible on sagittal computed tomographic image (a). The lesion shows Gd-contrast enhancement on sagittal T1-weighted imaging (b).

Fig. 10.119 A 62-year-old man with a lipoma in the proximal humerus. The circumscribed lesion has a thin low signal margin and has predominant signal centrally similar to fat on coronal proton density–weighted imaging (a) and fat-suppressed T2-weighted imaging (b). A small zone of cystic degeneration is also seen within the intraosseous lipoma.

Table 10.5 (Cont.) Solitary intramedullary lesions with well-circumscribed margins

Abnormalities	MRI findings	Comments
Brown tumor	Lesions are usually radiolucent on radiographs and computed tomography (CT). Lesions often have low-intermediate signal on T1WI, intermediate to slightly high signal on T2WI, and typically show Gd-contrast enhancement. Zones of low signal on T2WI may occur from hemosiderin. Expansion of cortical margins can occur with or without cortical disruption/destruction. Lesions may have circumscribed and/or poorly defined margins.	Lesions in bone contain multinucleated giant cells, fibrous tissue, blood vessels, and zones of hemorrhage/hemosiderin. Histological and imaging features are similar to giant cell reparative granulomas. Most often involves ribs, mandible, clavicle, pelvis, craniofacial bones, and vertebrae. Can result from primary hyperparathyroidism (3 to 7%) (oversecretion of parathyroid hormone [PTH] from parathyroid adenoma associated with hypercalcemia), secondary type (vitamin D deficiency or chronic renal failure with hypocalcemia resulting in secretion of PTH and parathyroid gland hyperplasia) (1 to 2%), or tertiary type in which the secondary type leads to eventual autonomous elevated PTH secretion from parathyroid gland hyperplasia.
Geode (▶ Fig. 10.120)	Typically have sharply defined margins and contain low signal on T1WI, low-intermediate signal on PDWI, and homogeneous high signal on T2WI. Poorly defined zones of Gd-contrast enhancement can be seen in the marrow adjacent to the subchondral cysts on FS T1WI.	A geode or subchondral cyst is a cystic-like lesion located near the end of a long bone where there are changes of degenerative osteoarthropathy. Lesions can result from synovial fluid intrusion and/or bony contusion in the setting of degenerative joint disease.
Intraosseous ganglion (▶ Fig. 10.121)	Can have round, oval, or serpiginous configurations with sharply defined margins. These lesions typically contain low signal on T1WI, low-intermediate signal on PDWI, and high signal on T2WI. Mild thin peripheral Gd-contrast enhancement can be seen.	Benign cystic lesion usually located at or near the ends of long bones, and is not associated with degenerative osteoarthropathy. Lesions can result from intraosseous extension from a ganglion in the soft tissues or from intraosseous mucoid degeneration, synovial rests, or synovial intrusion.
Bone infarct (▶ Fig. 10.122)	A double-line sign (curvilinear adjacent zones of low and high signal on T2WI) is commonly seen at the edges of the infarcts representing the borders of osseous resorption and healing. Irregular Gd-contrast enhancement can be seen from granulation tissue ingrowth.	Zones of ischemic death involving bone trabeculae and marrow, which may be idiopathic or may result from trauma, corticosteroid treatment, chemotherapy, radiation treatment, occlusive vascular disease, collagen vascular and other autoimmune diseases, metabolic storage diseases (e.g., Gaucher disease), sickle cell disease, thalassemia, hyperbaric events/Caisson disease, pregnancy, alcohol abuse, pancreatitis, infections, and lymphoproliferative diseases.
Enostosis/bone island (▶ Fig. 10.123)	Typically appear as well-circumscribed zones of dense bone within marrow with low signal on T1WI, PDWI, T2WI, and FS T2WI. Lesions typically show no Gd-contrast enhancement.	Nonneoplastic intramedullary zone of mature compact bone composed of lamellar bone that is considered to be a developmental anomaly resulting from localized failure of bone resorption during skeletal maturation.

(continued on page 416)

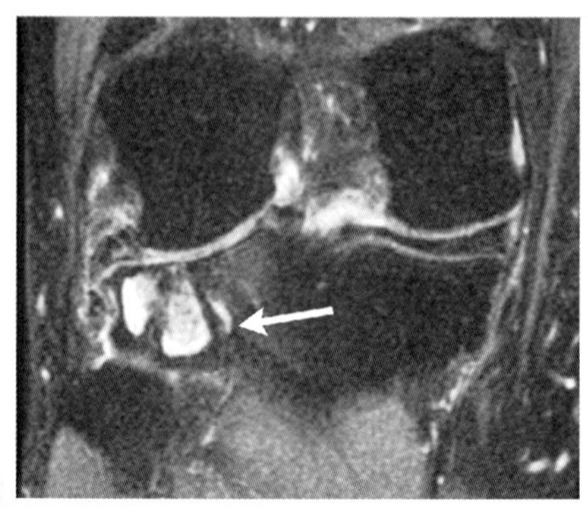
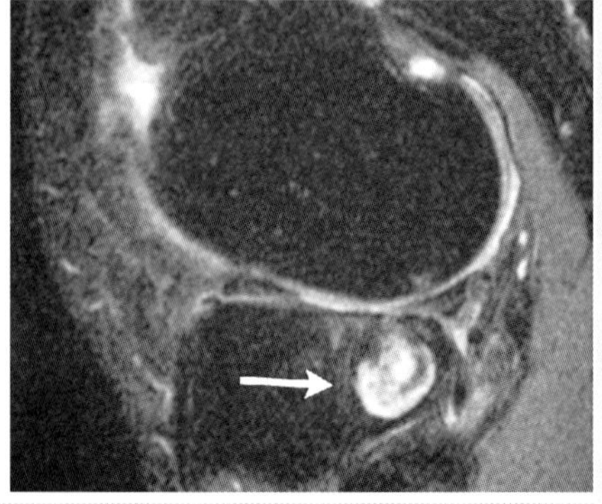

Fig. 10.120 A 50-year-old man with a degenerative cystic lesion (geode) in the subchondral bone of the lateral proximal tibia related to articular damage and focal defects. The circumscribed intraosseous lesion has mostly high signal on coronal (a) and sagittal fat-suppressed T2-weighted imaging (arrows) (b).

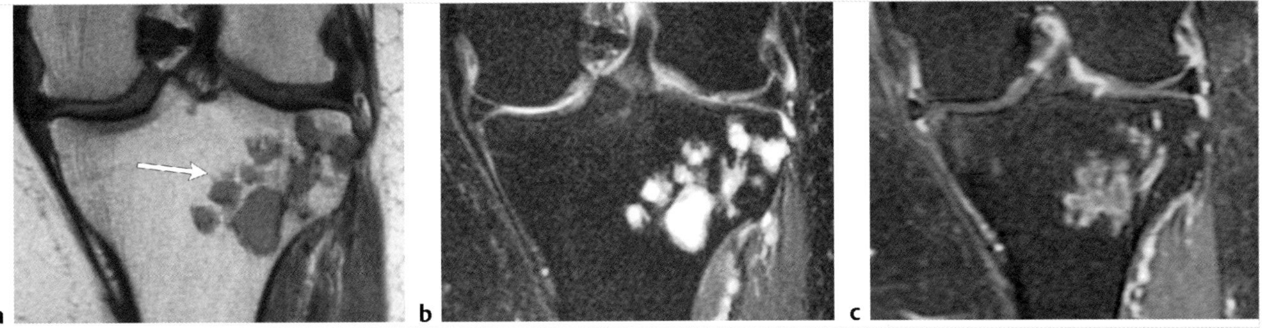

Fig. 10.121 Intraosseous ganglion within the lateral metaphyseal region of the proximal tibia seen on coronal proton density–weighted imaging (a) (arrow) and coronal fat-suppressed T2-weighted imaging (FS T2WI) (b). The lesion has high signal on FS T2WI and is contiguous with an extraosseous ganglion via a small defect in the cortex. Only mild thin peripheral Gd-contrast enhancement is seen on coronal FS T1-weighted imaging (c).

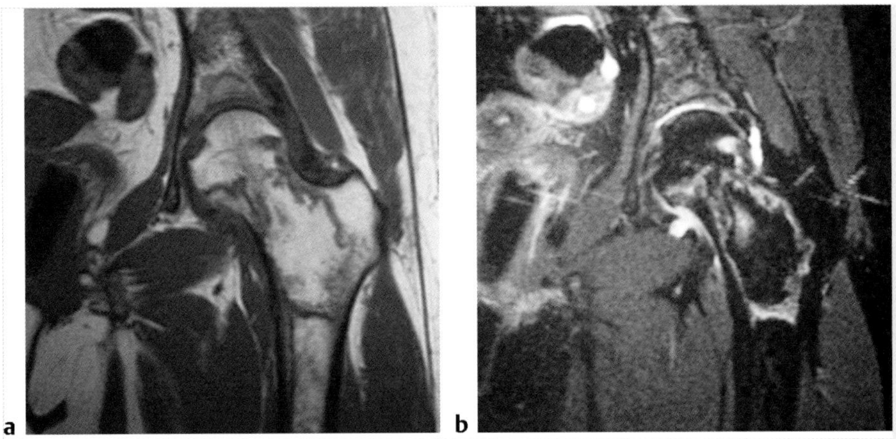

Fig. 10.122 A 29-year-old woman with a nonacute bone infarct in the femoral neck after chemotherapy for leukemia. The circumscribed lesion has thin margins with intermediate signal on coronal T1-weighted imaging (a) and high signal on coronal fat-suppressed T2-weighted imaging (b).

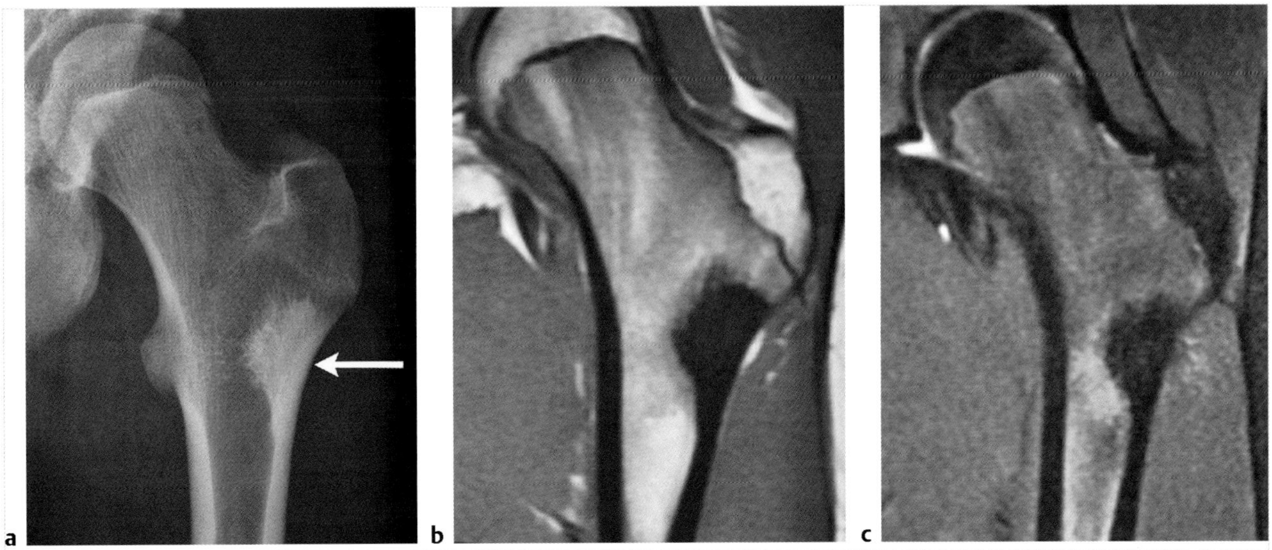

Fig. 10.123 A 12-year-old female with a bone island (arrow) in the proximal femur, which has high attenuation on an anteroposterior radiograph (a). The circumscribed lesion has low signal on coronal T1-weighted imaging (b) and fat-suppressed T2-weighted imaging (c).

Table 10.5 (Cont.) Solitary intramedullary lesions with well-circumscribed margins

Abnormalities	MRI findings	Comments
Giant cell tumor of bone (▶ Fig. 10.124)	Often well-defined lesions with thin low signal margins on T1WI, PDWI, and T2WI. Solid portions of giant cell tumors often have low to intermediate signal on T1WI and PDWI, intermediate to high signal on T2WI, and high signal on FS PDWI and FS T2WI. Zones of low signal on T2WI may be seen secondary to hemosiderin. Aneurysmal bone cysts can be seen in 14% of giant cell tumors. Areas of cortical thinning, expansion, and/or destruction can occur with extraosseous extension. Tumors show varying degrees of Gd-contrast enhancement.	Aggressive bone tumors composed of neoplastic mononuclear cells and scattered multinucleated osteoclast-like giant cells. Accounts for 23% of primary nonmalignant bone tumors and 5 and 9% of all primary bone tumors; median age = 30 years.
Ameloblastoma (▶ Fig. 10.125)	Lesions are often radiolucent with associated bone expansion and cortical thinning on CT. Tumors often have circumscribed margins and can show mixed low, intermediate, and/or high signal on T1WI, T2WI, and FS T2WI. Lesions can show heterogeneous Gd-contrast enhancement.	Ameloblastomas are slow-growing solid and cystic bone tumors that contain epithelioid cells (basaloid and/or squamous types) associated with regions of spindle cells and fibrous stroma. These tumors occur in the mandible and maxilla and typically lack metastatic potential.
Hemophilic pseudotumor	Can appear as expansile radiolucent lesions on radiographs and CT. Lesions usually have mixed low, intermediate, and high signal on T1WI and T2WI, as well as fluid-fluid levels.	Lesions can occur within bone (femur, pelvis, tibia, hand) or soft tissue in 1 to 2% of patients with factor VIII or IX deficiency. Enlarging lesions may require surgical resection.

(continued on page 418)

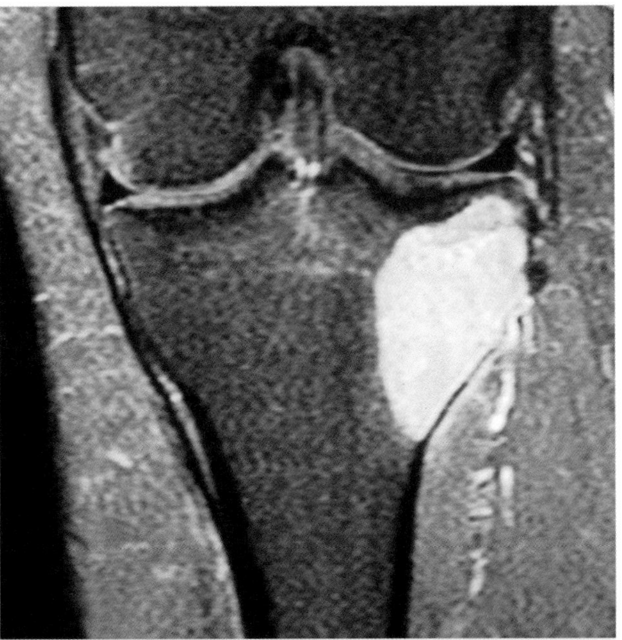

Fig. 10.124 A 22-year-old woman with a giant cell tumor in the proximal tibia, which has circumscribed margins and shows Gd-contrast enhancement on coronal fat-suppressed T1-weighted imaging.

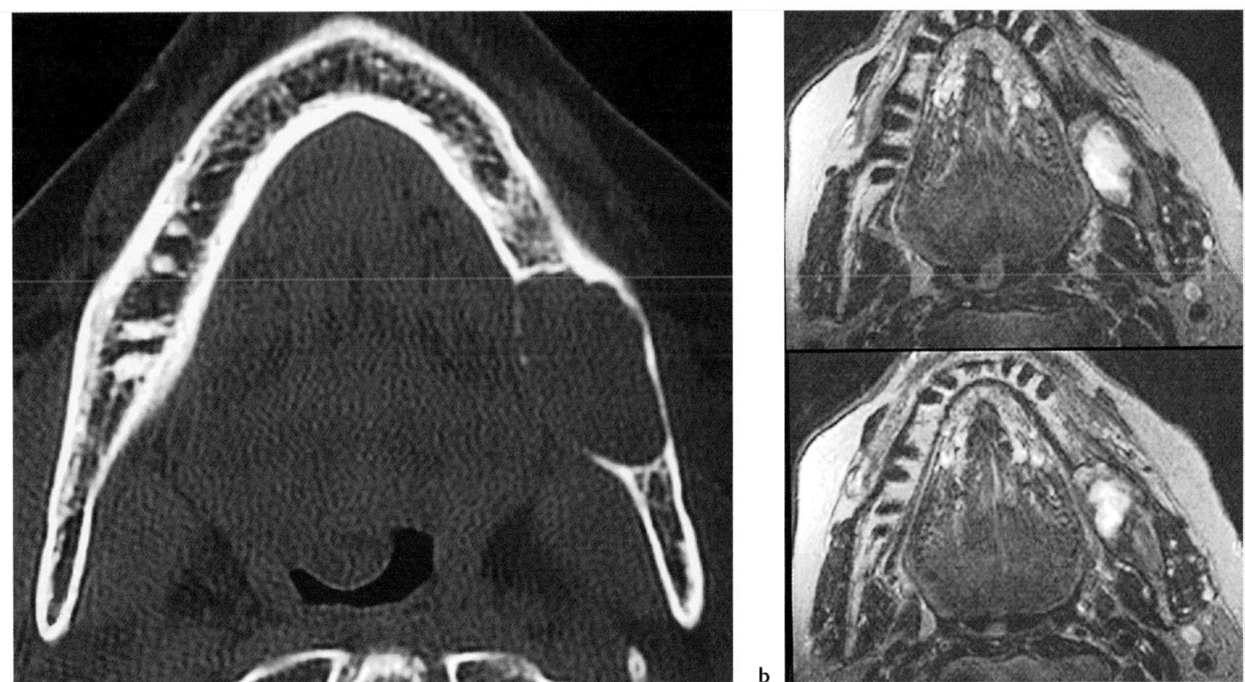

Fig. 10.125 A 70-year-old woman with an ameloblastoma in the mandible, which is seen as a radiolucent expansile lesion on axial computed tomography (a) and has mostly high signal on axial T2-weighted imaging (b).

Table 10.5 (Cont.) Solitary intramedullary lesions with well-circumscribed margins

Abnormalities	MRI findings	Comments
Desmoplastic fibroma (▶ Fig. 10.126)	Lobulated lesions with abrupt zones of transition. Lesions usually have low-intermediate signal on T1WI, intermediate signal on PDWI, heterogeneous intermediate to high signal on T2WI. Lesions may have internal or peripheral zones of low signal on T1WI and T2WI secondary to dense collagenous parts of the lesions and/or foci with high signal on T2WI from cystic zones. Thin curvilinear zones of low signal on T2WI can be seen at the margins of the lesions. Lesions show variable degrees and patterns of Gd-contrast enhancement.	Rare intraosseous desmoid tumors that are composed of benign fibrous tissue with elongated or spindle-shaped cells adjacent to collagen. Account for < 1% of primary bone lesions. Mean age = 20 years, median age = 34 years, peak second decade.
Malignant lesions		
Metastatic tumor (▶ Fig. 10.127)	Single or multiple well-circumscribed or poorly defined infiltrative lesions involving marrow associated with cortical destruction and extraosseous extension. Lesions often have low-intermediate signal on T1WI, low, intermediate, and/or high signal on T2WI and FS T1WI, usually show Gd-contrast enhancement. Cortical destruction and tumor extension into the extraosseous soft tissues can occur. Pathological fractures can be associated with metastatic lesions involving tubular bones and vertebrae. Periosteal reaction is uncommon.	Metastatic lesions typically occur in the marrow with or without cortical destruction and extraosseous tumor extension.
Plasmacytoma (▶ Fig. 10.128)	Well-circumscribed or poorly defined infiltrative lesions involving marrow, low-intermediate signal on T1WI, intermediate-high signal on T2WI and FS T2WI, usually show Gd-contrast enhancement, eventual cortical bone destruction and extraosseous extension.	Malignant tumors composed of proliferating antibody-secreting plasma cells derived from single clones. Most common primary neoplasm of bone in adults. Median age = 60 years. Most patients are older than 40 years. May have variable destructive or infiltrative changes involving the axial and/or appendicular skeleton.

(continued on page 420)

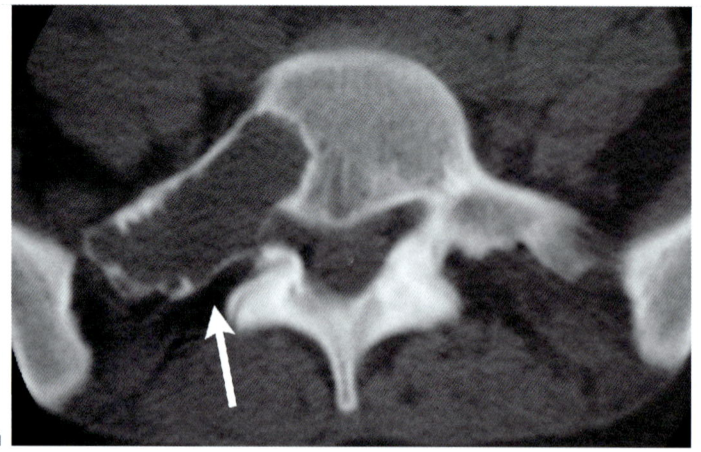

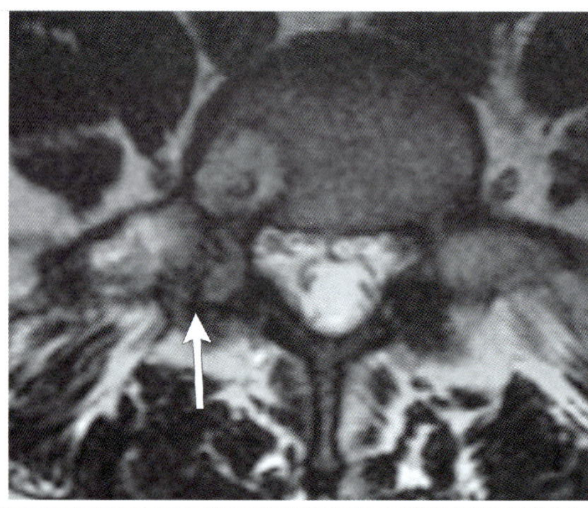

Fig. 10.126 A 32-year-old woman with a desmoplastic fibroma involving the right lateral portion of the L5 vertebra. The radiolucent lesion (arrow) has thinned slightly expanded cortical margins on axial computed tomography (a) and mixed low, intermediate, slightly high, and high signal on axial T2-weighted imaging (arrow) (b).

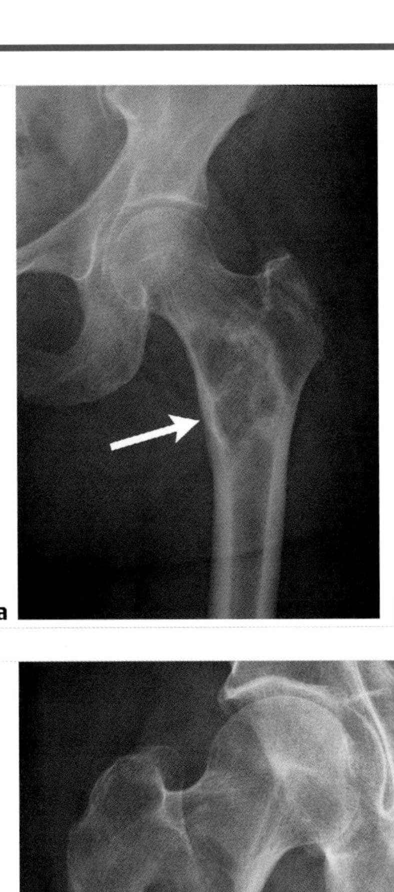

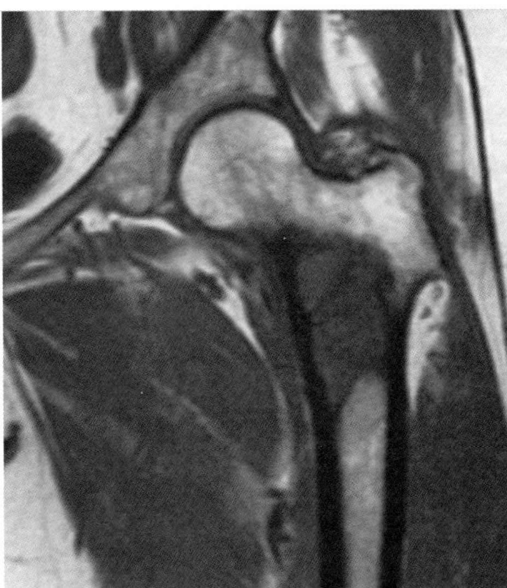

Fig. 10.127 A 56-year-old woman with a metastatic lesion from breast carcinoma involving the proximal shaft of the femur. The radiolucent lesion (arrow) has thick slightly irregular sclerotic margins on radiograph (a) and has low-intermediate signal on coronal T1-weighted imaging (b).

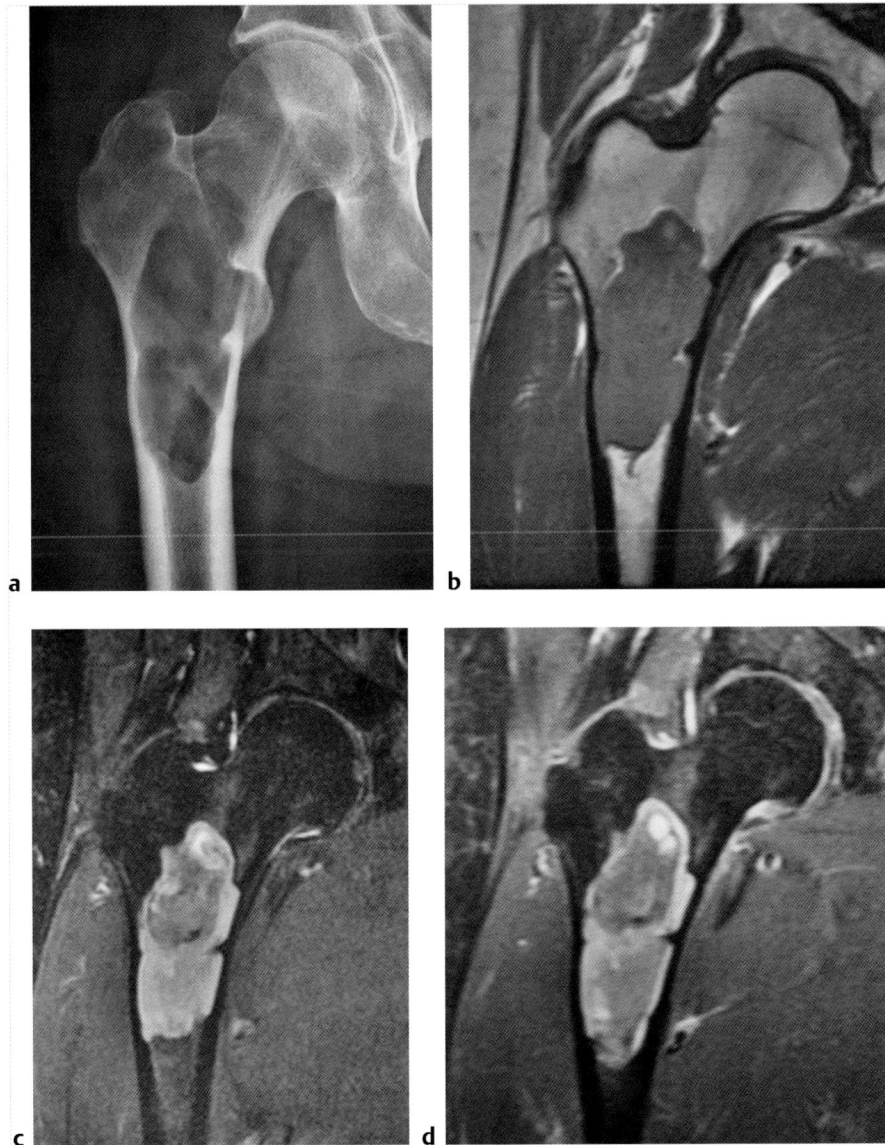

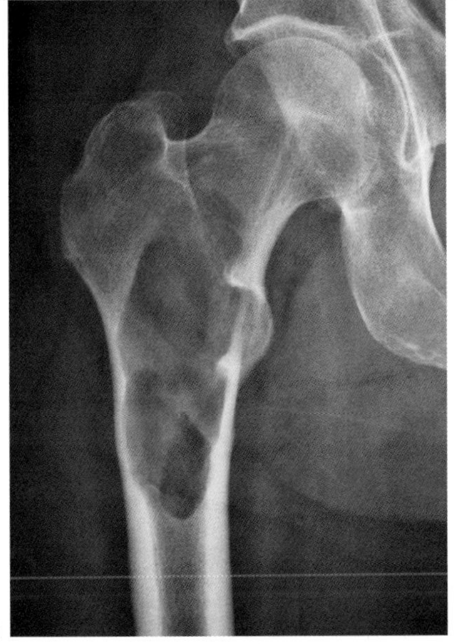

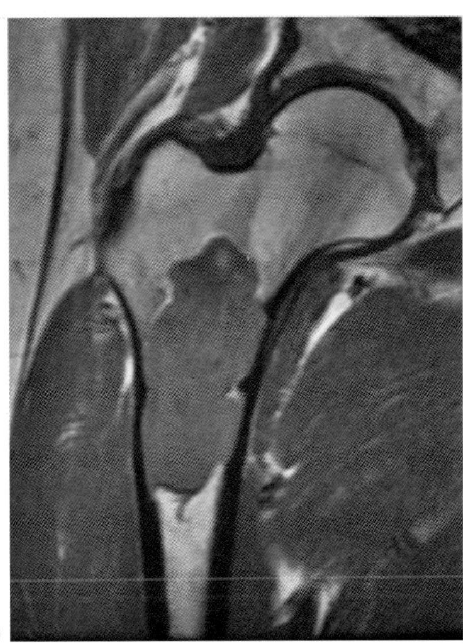

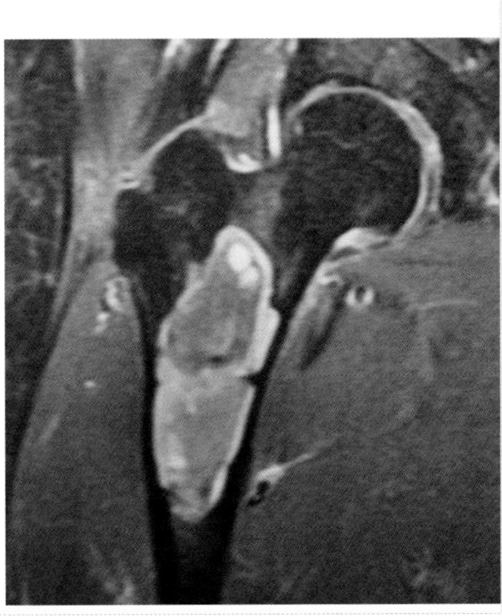

Fig. 10.128 A 56-year-old man with a plasmacytoma involving the proximal shaft of the femur. The radiolucent lesion has sharp margins on radiograph (a). The tumor has low-intermediate signal on coronal T1-weighted imaging (T1WI) (b), high signal on fat-suppressed (FS) T2-weighted imaging (c), and shows Gd-contrast enhancement on coronal FS T1WI (d).

Table 10.5 (Cont.) Solitary intramedullary lesions with well-circumscribed margins

Abnormalities	MRI findings	Comments
Lymphoma (▶ Fig. 10.129)	Non-hodgkin lymphoma (NHL) and Hodgkin disease (HD) within bone typically appears as single or multifocal poorly defined or circumscribed intramedullary zones with low-intermediate signal on T1WI; intermediate, slightly high, and/or high signal on T2WI; and high signal on FS T2WI. Often show Gd-contrast enhancement. Zones of cortical destruction may occur associated with extraosseous soft tissue extension.	Lymphoid tumors with neoplastic cells typically within lymphoid tissue (lymph nodes and reticuloendothelial organs). Unlike leukemia, lymphoma usually arises as discrete masses. Lymphomas are subdivided into HD and NHL. Almost all primary lymphomas of bone are B-cell NHL. HD, mean age = 32 years. Osseous NHL, median = 35 years.
Low grade chondrosarcoma (▶ Fig. 10.130)	Intramedullary tumors often have low-intermediate signal on T1WI, intermediate signal on PDWI, and heterogeneous intermediate-high signal on T2WI. Lesions usually show heterogeneous Gd-contrast enhancement.	Malignant tumors containing cartilage formed within sarcomatous stroma. Account for 12 to 21% of malignant bone lesions, 21 to 26% of primary sarcomas of bone. Mean age = 40 years, median = 26 to 59 years.
Malignant giant cell tumor	Well-defined lesions with or without thin low signal margins on T1WI and T2WI. Solid portions of giant cell tumors often have low to intermediate signal on T1WI and PDWI, intermediate to high signal on T2WI, and high signal on FS PDWI and FS T2WI. Signal heterogeneity on T2WI is not uncommon. Aneurysmal bone cysts are seen with 14% of giant cell tumors. Lesions show mild to prominent variable and often heterogeneous Gd-contrast enhancement. Cortical destruction and extraosseous tumor extension are frequently seen.	Aggressive bone tumors composed of neoplastic ovoid mononuclear cells and scattered multinucleated osteoclast-like giant cells. Up to 10% of all giant cell tumors are malignant. Benign giant cell tumors account for approximately 5 to 9.5% of all bone tumors and up to 23% of benign bone tumors. 75% of malignant giant cell tumors occur in patients between the ages of 15 and 45.

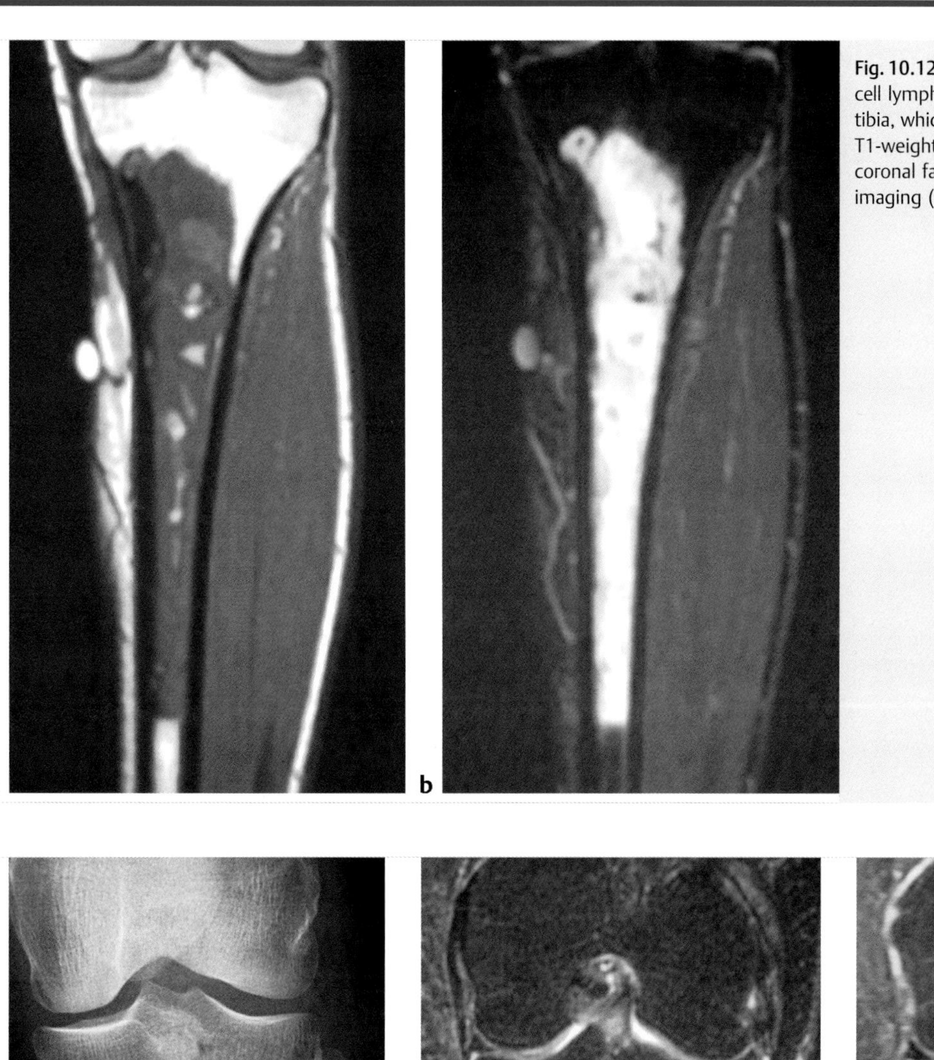

Fig. 10.129 A 19-year-old man with large B-cell lymphoma in the marrow of the proximal tibia, which has intermediate signal on coronal T1-weighted imaging (a) and high signal on coronal fat-suppressed T2-weighted imaging (b).

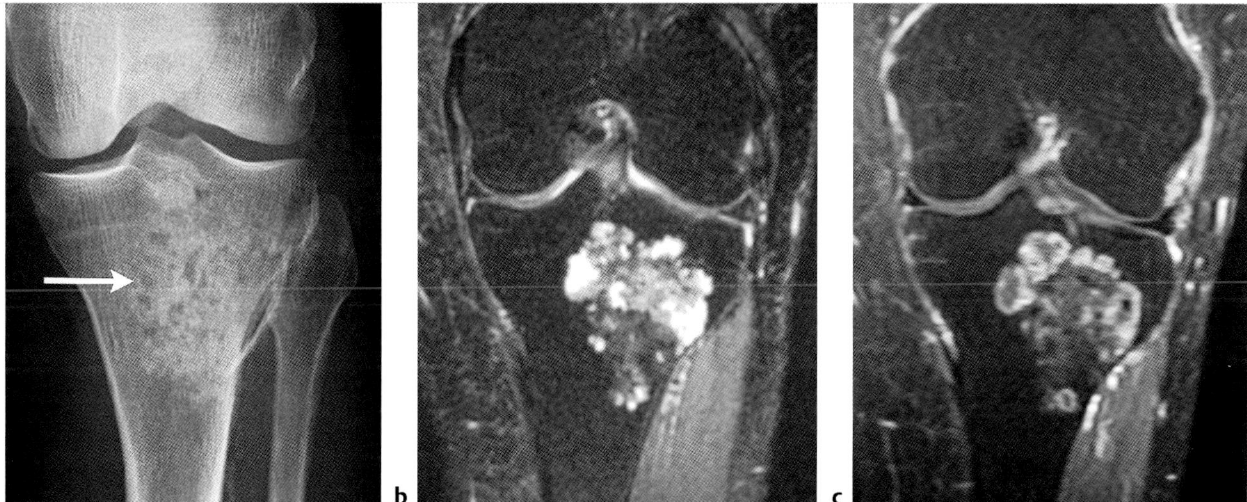

Fig. 10.130 A 46-year-old woman with a low-grade chondrosarcoma involving the proximal tibia. Radiograph shows intraosseous chondroid mineralization (arrow) (a). The lesion has heterogeneous high and low signal on coronal fat-suppressed (FS) T2-weighted imaging (b) and shows peripheral lobular gadolinium-contrast enhancement on coronal FS T1-weighted imaging (c).

10.6 Solitary Intramedullary Lesions with Poorly Defined Margins of Abnormal Marrow Signal

- Nonmalignant lesions
  - Acute and subacute bone ischemia
  - Transient bone marrow edema; also referred to as acute transient bone marrow edema (acute bone marrow edema syndromes [aBMEs], transient osteoporosis of the hip, regional migratory osteoporosis)
  - Bone contusion
  - Fracture
  - Osteomyelitis
  - Eosinophilic granuloma
  - Sarcoidosis
  - Chondroblastoma
  - Giant cell tumor of bone
  - Giant cell reparative granuloma
  - Aneurysmal bone cyst (ABC)
  - Osteoid osteoma
  - Osteoblastoma
  - Brown tumor
- Malignant lesions
  - Metastatic tumor
  - Plasmacytoma
  - Leukemia
  - Lymphoma
  - Chondrosarcoma
  - Osteosarcoma
  - Ewing sarcoma
  - Malignant giant cell tumor
  - Fibrosarcoma
  - Malignant fibrous histiocytoma
  - Paget sarcoma

Table 10.6 Solitary intramedullary lesions with poorly defined margins of abnormal marrow signal

Abnormalities	MRI findings	Comments
Nonmalignant lesions		
Acute and subacute bone ischemia (▶ Fig. 10.131; ▶ Fig. 10.132)	In the early phases of ischemia, diffuse poorly-defined zones of high signal may be seen on fat-suppressed T2-weighted imaging (FS T2WI), which can overlap the magnetic resonance imaging (MRI) features of transient bone marrow edema. In zones of bone infarction, curvilinear zones of low signal on T1-weighted imaging (T1WI) and T2WI may occur in marrow from zones of fibrosis. Irregular zones of low signal on T1WI and high signal on T2WI may occur secondary to zones of fluid from edema, ischemia/infarction, or fracture. Zones with high signal on T1WI and T2WI may also occur from hemorrhage in combination with zones of fibrosis and fluid. A double-line sign (curvilinear adjacent zones of low and high signal on T2WI) is often seen at the edges of the infarcts representing the borders of osseous resorption and healing. Irregular gadolinium (Gd)-contrast enhancement can be seen from granulation tissue ingrowth.	Bone infarcts are zones of ischemic death involving bone trabeculae and marrow, which can be idiopathic or result from trauma, corticosteroid treatment, chemotherapy, radiation treatment, occlusive vascular disease, collagen vascular and other autoimmune diseases, metabolic storage diseases (e.g., Gaucher disease), sickle cell disease, thalassemia, hyperbaric events/Caisson disease, pregnancy, alcohol abuse, pancreatitis, infections, and lymphoproliferative diseases. Osteonecrosis is more common in fatty compared with hematopoietic marrow.

(continued on page 424)

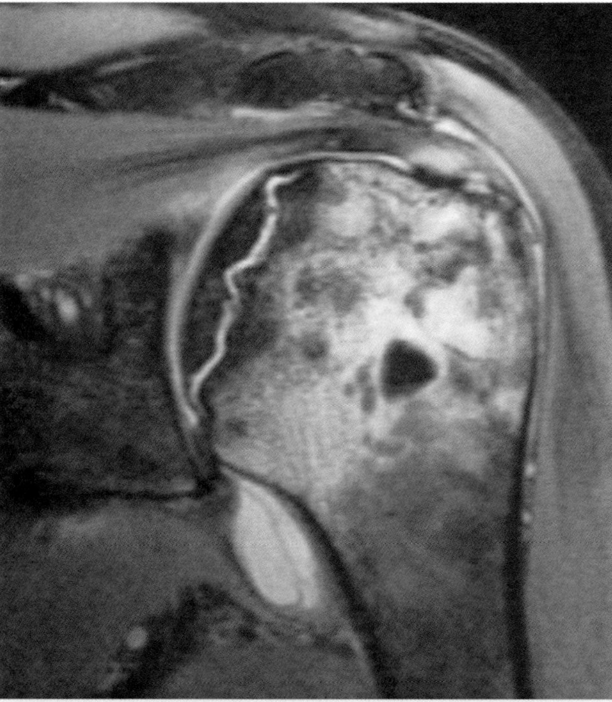

Fig. 10.131 A 50-year-old woman with acute ischemia in the proximal humerus superimposed upon prior ischemia as seen on coronal fat-suppressed proton density–weighted imaging. A poorly defined zone with increased signal is seen in the marrow adjacent to an old bone infarct at the medial aspect of the humeral head.

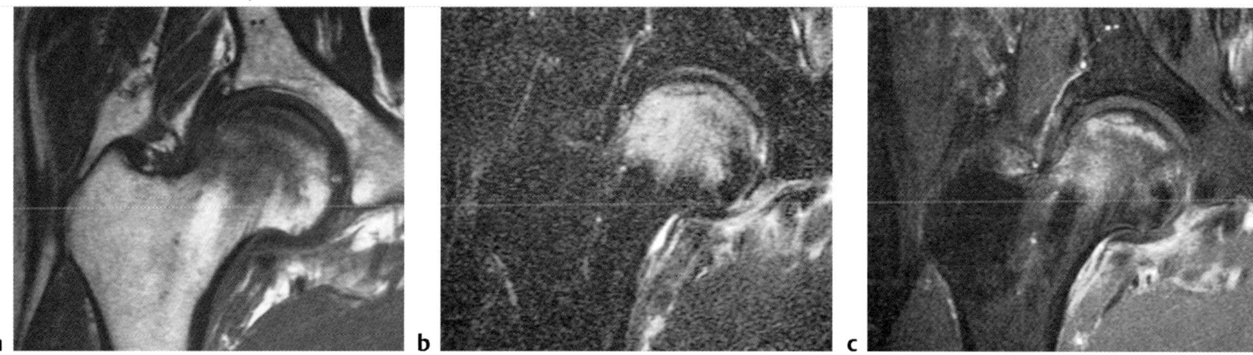

Fig. 10.132 A 50-year-old man with acute and subacute ischemia in the proximal femur. A poorly defined zone with low signal on coronal T1-weighted imaging (T1WI) (a), high signal on coronal fat-suppressed (FS) T2-weighted imaging (b), and corresponding gadolinium (Gd)-contrast enhancement on FS T1WI is seen in the marrow (c). A thin linear zone of low signal is also seen in the subchondral marrow representing bone infarction.

Table 10.6 (Cont.) Solitary intramedullary lesions with poorly defined margins of abnormal marrow signal

Abnormalities	MRI findings	Comments
Transient bone marrow edema; also referred to as acute transient bone marrow edema (acute bone marrow edema syndromes [aBMEs], transient osteoporosis of the hip, regional migratory osteoporosis) (▶ Fig. 10.133)	Poorly defined zones with low-intermediate signal on T1WI and high signal on FS T2WI and short TI inversion recovery (STIR) are seen in the marrow of the proximal hip (femoral head and neck). The signal abnormalities may spare the subchondral marrow. MRI findings can be seen within 48 hours of the onset of symptoms. Joint effusions may be present. With dynamic Gd-contrast administration, delayed peak enhancement can be seen with aBME. With osteonecrosis of the hip, crescentic zones of low signal on T1WI and FS T2WI are seen in the marrow between the necrotic and normal areas. These crescentic zones of low signal on T1WI and FS T2WI are typically absent in aBME.	aBME is an idiopathic spontaneous process with transient edema in bone marrow that is not secondary to trauma and may or may not be associated with osteoporosis. aBME frequently involves the proximal femur in men between 30 and 50 years, and women in the last trimester of pregnancy. aBME is typically associated with pain and limping disability. Biopsies show active osteoblasts and osteoid seams adjacent to thinned disconnected trabeculae, as well as mild fibrosis, edematous changes, vascular congestion with occasional hemorrhage in marrow without osteonecrosis. With conservative therapy such as analgesics, restricted weight-bearing, and antiresortive agents such as bisphosphonates and calcitonin, symptoms resolve in 2 to 9 months. Similar clinical and imaging findings have been reported in other bones, often in juxta-articular locations in the lower extremities, and have been referred to as regional migratory osteoporosis.
Bone contusion (▶ Fig. 10.134)	Contusions usually appear as poorly defined intramedullary zones with low-intermediate signal on T1WI and high signal on FS T2WI, and corresponding Gd-contrast enhancement. Adjacent cortical margins are typically intact.	Also referred to as bone bruises, contusions represent trabecular microfractures without cortical fracture. In the knee, contusions at the lateral femoral condyle and posterolateral proximal tibia are commonly associated with injuries to the anterior cruciate ligament.
Fracture (▶ Fig. 10.135)	Acute/subacute fractures typically have abnormal marrow signal (usually low signal on T1WI, high signal on T2WI and FS T2WI). Gd-contrast enhancement is typically seen in the postfracture period. Angulated cortical margins and periosteal high signal on FS T2WI can be seen with traumatic fractures. A curvilinear zone of low signal on T2WI and FS T2WI may be seen within the marrow edema in stress fractures.	Fractures can result from trauma, primary bone tumors/lesions, metastatic disease, bone infarcts (steroids, chemotherapy, and radiation treatment), osteoporosis, osteomalacia, metabolic (calcium/ phosphate) disorders, vitamin deficiencies, Paget disease, and genetic disorders such as osteogenesis imperfecta, among others.

(continued on page 426)

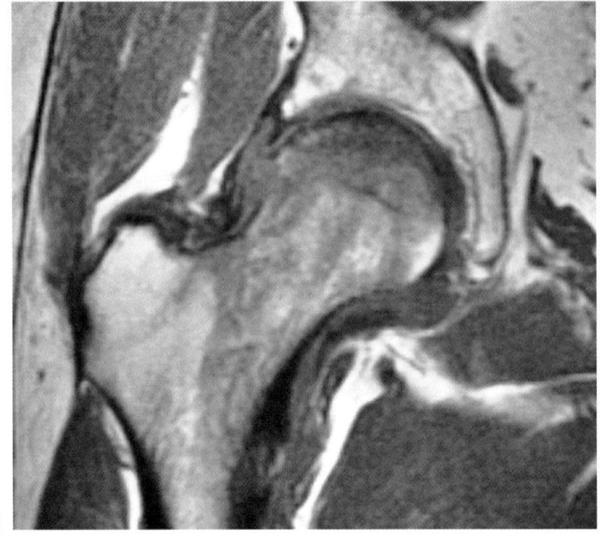

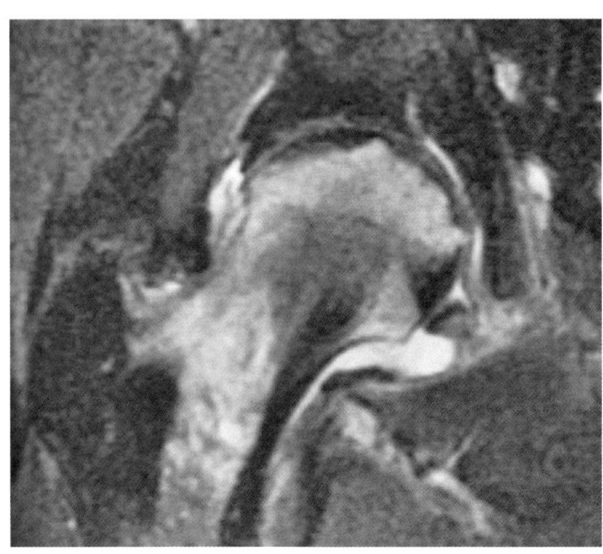

Fig. 10.133 A 53-year-old man with acute bone marrow edema in the proximal femur. A poorly defined zone with low-intermediate signal on coronal T1-weighted imaging (a) and high signal on coronal fat-suppressed T2-weighted imaging (b) is seen in the marrow.

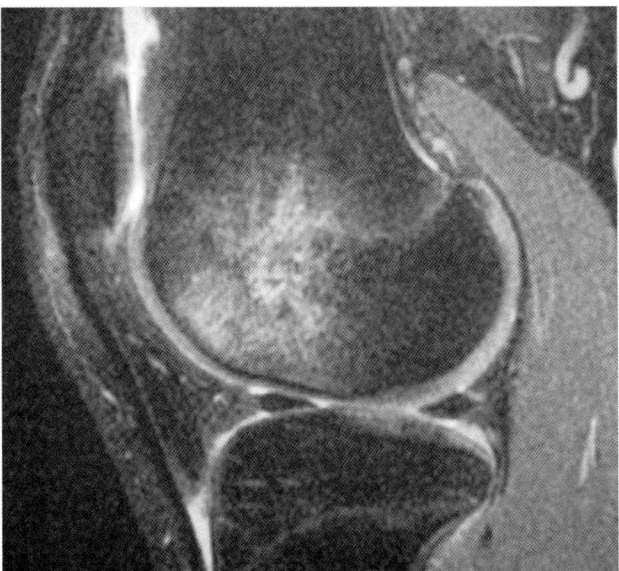

Fig. 10.134 Bone contusion in the distal femur seen as a poorly defined zone with high signal in the subchondral marrow on sagittal fat-suppressed T2-weighted imaging.

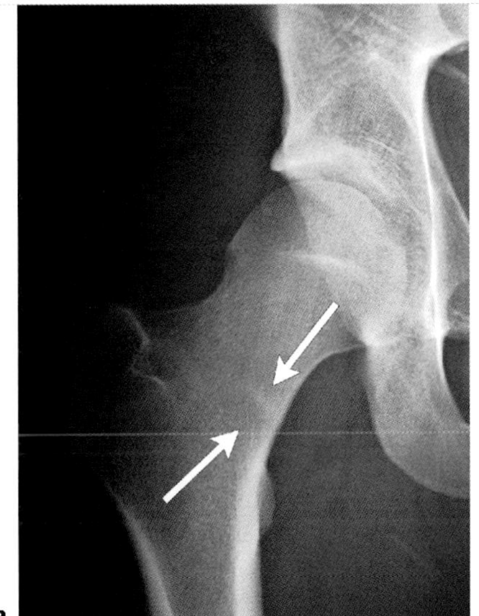

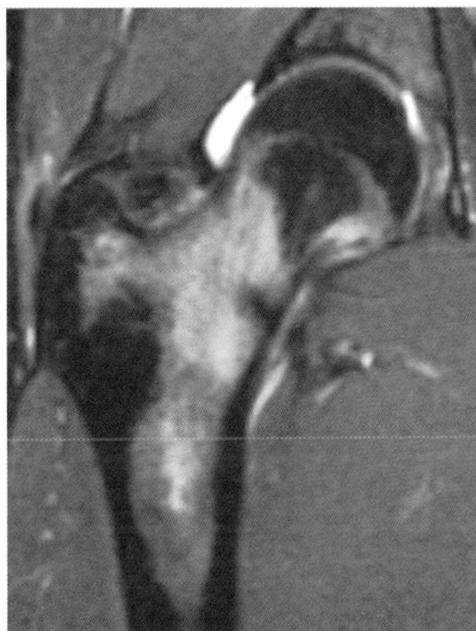

Fig. 10.135 A 17-year-old boy with a fatigue-type stress fracture involving the femoral neck. Anteroposterior radiograph (a) shows a small linear zone of endosteal sclerosis (arrows). A poorly defined zone with high signal is seen in the marrow adjacent to a linear zone of low signal on fat-suppressed T2-weighted imaging (b), as well as thin periosteal reaction with high signal medially.

Table 10.6 (Cont.) Solitary intramedullary lesions with poorly defined margins of abnormal marrow signal

Abnormalities	MRI findings	Comments
Osteomyelitis (▶ Fig. 10.136)	In acute osteomyelitis, poorly defined zones of low or low-intermediate signal on T1WI and high signal on T2WI, STIR, and FS T2WI are seen in the marrow. Loss of definition of the low signal line of the cortical margins is often observed on T1WI, T2WI, STIR, and FS T2WI. After Gd-contrast administration, irregular zones of contrast enhancement are seen in the involved marrow on FS T1WI. In the subacute phase of osteomyelitis, the pyogenic process becomes more localized. The zone of transition between normal and abnormal bone is sharper and more well defined in subacute and chronic osteomyelitis than with acute osteomyelitis.	Osteomyelitis is a disorder in which there is infection of bone and commonly the adjacent soft tissues. Can result from hematogenous spread of micro-organisms as well as from trauma-direct inoculation, extension from adjacent tissues, and complications from surgery. Bacteria such as *Staphylococcus aureus* and *Streptococcus pyogenes* are the most common infectious organisms. Can also result from other bacteria as well as tuberculosis, fungi, parasites, and viruses.
Eosinophilic granuloma (▶ Fig. 10.137)	Focal intramedullary lesions associated with trabecular and cortical bone destruction, which typically have low-intermediate signal on T1WI and proton density–weighted imaging (PDWI) and heterogeneous slightly high to high signal on T2WI. Poorly defined zones of high signal on T2WI are usually seen in the marrow peripheral to the lesions secondary to inflammatory changes. Extension of lesions from the marrow into adjacent soft tissues through areas of cortical disruption are commonly seen as well as linear periosteal zones of high signal on T2WI. Lesions typically show prominent Gd-contrast enhancement in marrow and in extraosseous soft tissue portions of the lesions.	Benign tumor-like lesions consisting of Langerhans cells (histiocytes) and variable amounts of lymphocytes, polymorphonuclear cells, and eosinophils. Account for 1% of primary bone lesions and 8% of tumor-like lesions. Occurs in patients with median age = 10 years, average = 13.5 years, peak incidence is between 5 and 10 years, 80 to 85% occur in patients less than 30 years.
Sarcoidosis	Lesions usually appear as intramedullary zones with low to intermediate signal on T1WI and slightly high to high signal on T2WI and FS PDWI and FS T2WI. Erosions and zones of destruction of adjacent bone cortex as well as periosseous extension of the granulomatous process can occur. Fine perpendicular lines of low signal on T1WI may be seen extending outward from the region of eroded or destroyed cortex. After Gd-contrast administration, lesions typically show moderate to prominent enhancement.	Chronic systemic granulomatous disease of unknown etiology in which noncaseating granulomas occur in various tissues and organs, including bone.
Chondroblastoma (▶ Fig. 10.138)	Tumors often have fine lobular margins and typically have low-intermediate heterogeneous signal on T1WI and mixed low, intermediate, and/or high signal on T2WI. Areas of low signal on T2WI are secondary to chondroid matrix mineralization, and/or hemosiderin. Lobular, marginal, or septal Gd-contrast enhancement patterns can be seen. Poorly defined zones with high signal on T2WI and FS T2WI and corresponding Gd-contrast enhancement are typically seen in the marrow adjacent to the lesions representing inflammatory reaction from prostaglandin synthesis by these tumors.	Benign cartilaginous tumors with chondroblast-like cells and areas of chondroid matrix formation, usually occur in children and adolescents, median = 17 years, mean = 16 years for lesions in long bones, mean = 28 years in other bones. Most cases are diagnosed between the ages of 5 and 25.

(continued on page 428)

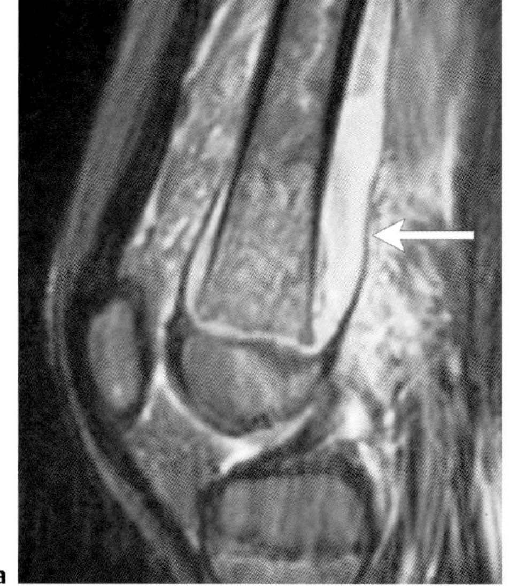

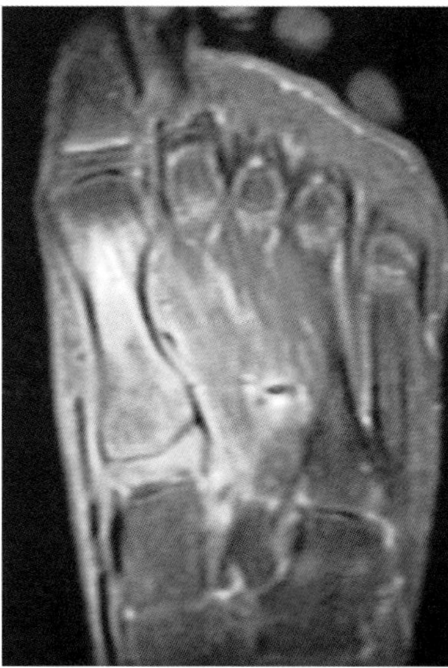

Fig. 10.136 Pyogenic osteomyelitis seen as a poorly defined zone of abnormal high signal on sagittal fat-suppressed (FS) T2-weighted imaging (a) in the marrow of the distal femur of a 6-year-old male. The infection extends through the bone cortex resulting in a subperiosteal abscess (arrow). Osteomyelitis involving the first metatarsal marrow of a 14-year-old boy is seen as a poorly defined zone of Gd-contrast enhancement on coronal FS T1-weighted imaging (b).

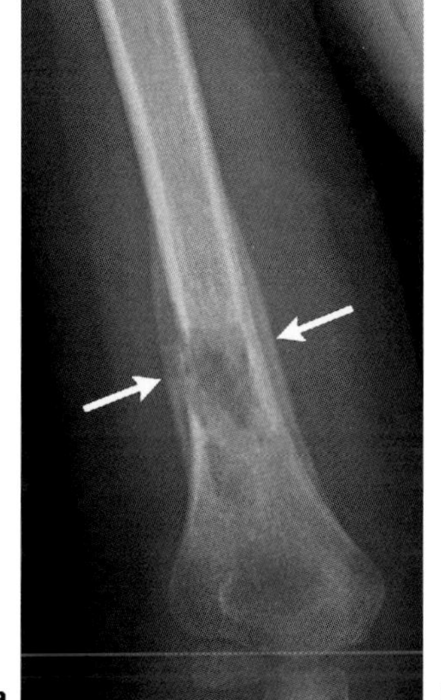

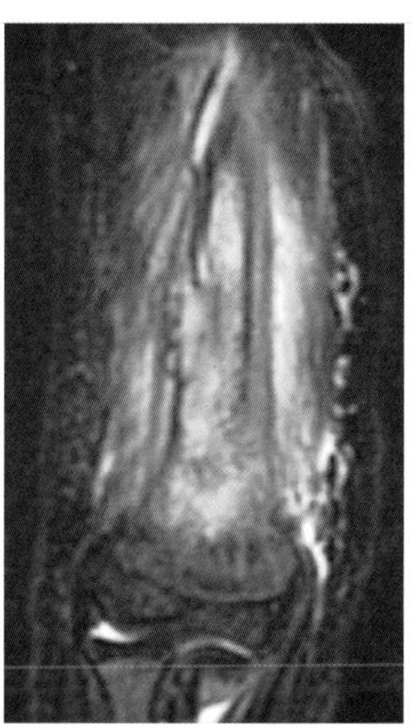

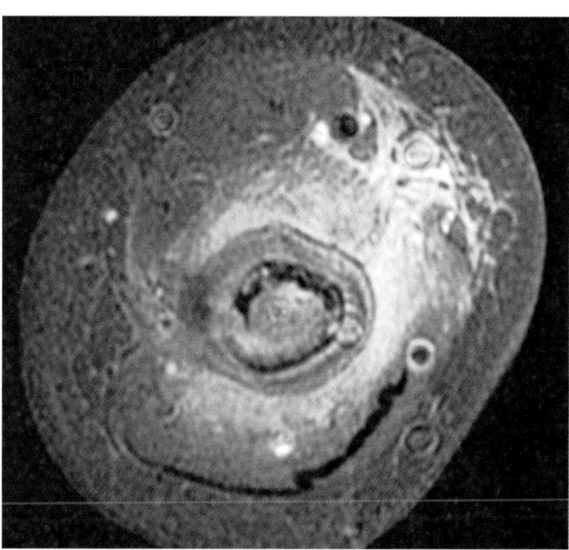

Fig. 10.137 A 5-year-old male with an eosinophilic granuloma in the marrow of the distal humerus seen as a poorly defined radiolucent zone (a), which has high signal on coronal fat-suppressed (FS) T2-weighted imaging (b) and shows prominent gadolinium-contrast enhancement on axial FS T1-weighted imaging (c). The intramedullary lesion extends through the cortex into the adjacent soft tissues. Elevated periosteum is also seen (arrows).

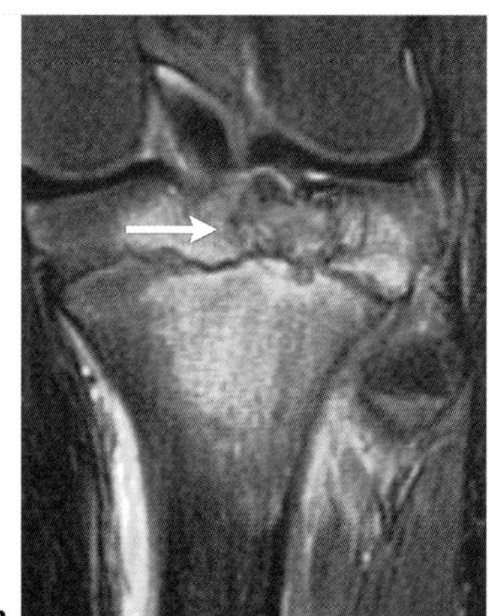

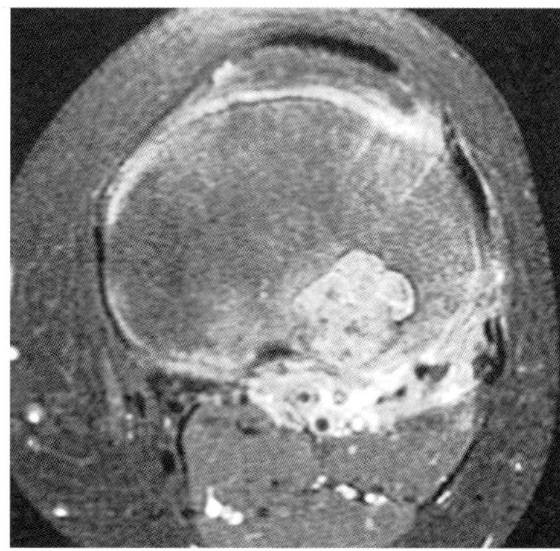

Fig. 10.138 A 13-year-old girl with a chondroblastoma in the epiphysis of the proximal tibia seen as a lesion with thin low signal margins (arrow) surrounding a central zone with low, intermediate, slightly high, and high signal on coronal fat-suppressed T2-weighted imaging (FS T2WI) (a). Poorly defined zones with high signal on FS T2WI and contrast enhancement on axial FS T1-weighted imaging (b) are seen in the epiphyseal and metaphyseal marrow peripheral to the lesion, as well as periosteal zones with high signal and contrast enhancement.

Table 10.6 (Cont.) Solitary intramedullary lesions with poorly defined margins of abnormal marrow signal

Abnormalities	MRI findings	Comments
Giant cell tumor of bone (▶ Fig. 10.139)	Lesions can have thin low signal margins on T1WI, PDWI, and T2WI. Solid portions of giant cell tumors often have low to intermediate signal on T1WI and PDWI, intermediate to high signal on T2WI, and high signal on FS PDWI and FS T2WI. Zones of low signal on T2WI may be seen secondary to hemosiderin. Aneurysmal bone cysts can be seen in 14% of giant cell tumors. Areas of cortical thinning, expansion, and/or destruction can occur with extraosseous extension. Tumors show varying degrees of Gd-contrast enhancement. Poorly defined zones of Gd-contrast enhancement and high signal on FS T2WI may also be seen in the marrow peripheral to the portions of the lesions associated with radiographic evidence of bone destruction, possibly indicating reactive inflammatory and edematous changes associated with elevated tumor prostaglandin levels.	Aggressive bone tumors composed of neoplastic mononuclear cells and scattered multinucleated osteoclast-like giant cells. Accounts for 23% of primary nonmalignant bone tumors and 5 to 9% of all primary bone tumors; median age = 30 years.
Giant cell reparative granuloma (▶ Fig. 10.140)	Lesions can have heterogeneous low, intermediate, and/or high signal on T1WI, PDWI, and T2WI; as well as peripheral rimlike and central Gd-contrast enhancement on FS T1WI. May be surrounded by poorly defined zone of high signal on FS T2WI and Gd-contrast enhancement in the adjacent marrow.	Giant cell reparative granulomas are also referred to as solid aneurysmal bone cysts (ABCs). Histologic appearance resembles brown tumors.
Aneurysmal bone cyst (ABC) (▶ Fig. 10.141)	ABCs often have a low signal rim on T1WI and T2WI adjacent to normal medullary bone, and between extraosseous soft tissues. Various combinations of low, intermediate, and/or high signal on T1 W, PDWI, and T2 W images are usually seen within ABCs as well as fluid-fluid levels. Variable Gd-contrast enhancement is seen at the margins of lesions as well as involving the internal septae. Poorly-defined zones with increased signal on FS T2WI may be seen in marrow adjacent to these lesions.	Tumor-like expansile bone lesions containing cavernous spaces filled with blood. ABCs can be primary bone lesions (two thirds) or secondary to other bone lesions/tumors. Account for approximately 11% of primary tumor-like lesions of bone. Patients usually range in age from 1 to 25 years, median = 14 years.

(continued on page 430)

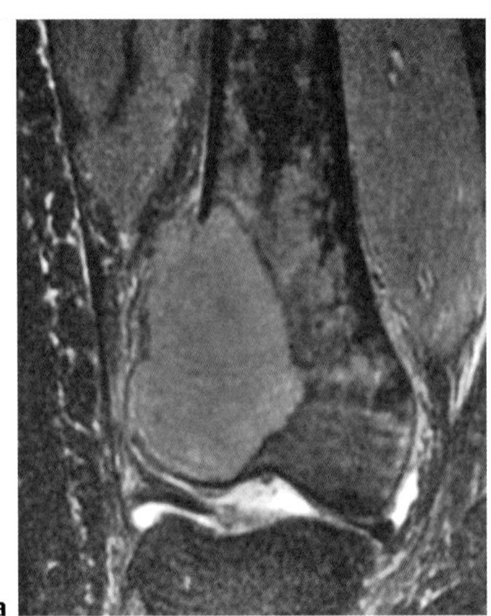

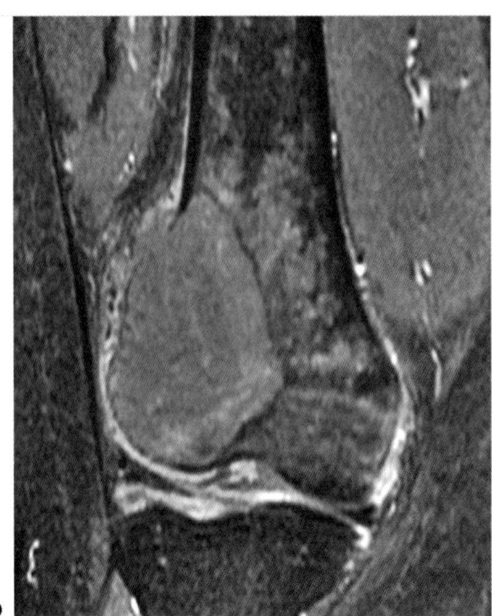

Fig. 10.139 A 34-year-old woman with a giant cell tumor in the distal lateral tibia. Centrally the tumor has high signal on coronal fat-suppressed T2-weighted imaging (FS T2WI) (a) and shows gadolinium-contrast enhancement on coronal FS T1-weighted imaging (b). The tumor is surrounded by a thin rim of low signal and a poorly defined peripheral zone of high signal on FS T2WI and Gd-contrast enhancement in the marrow.

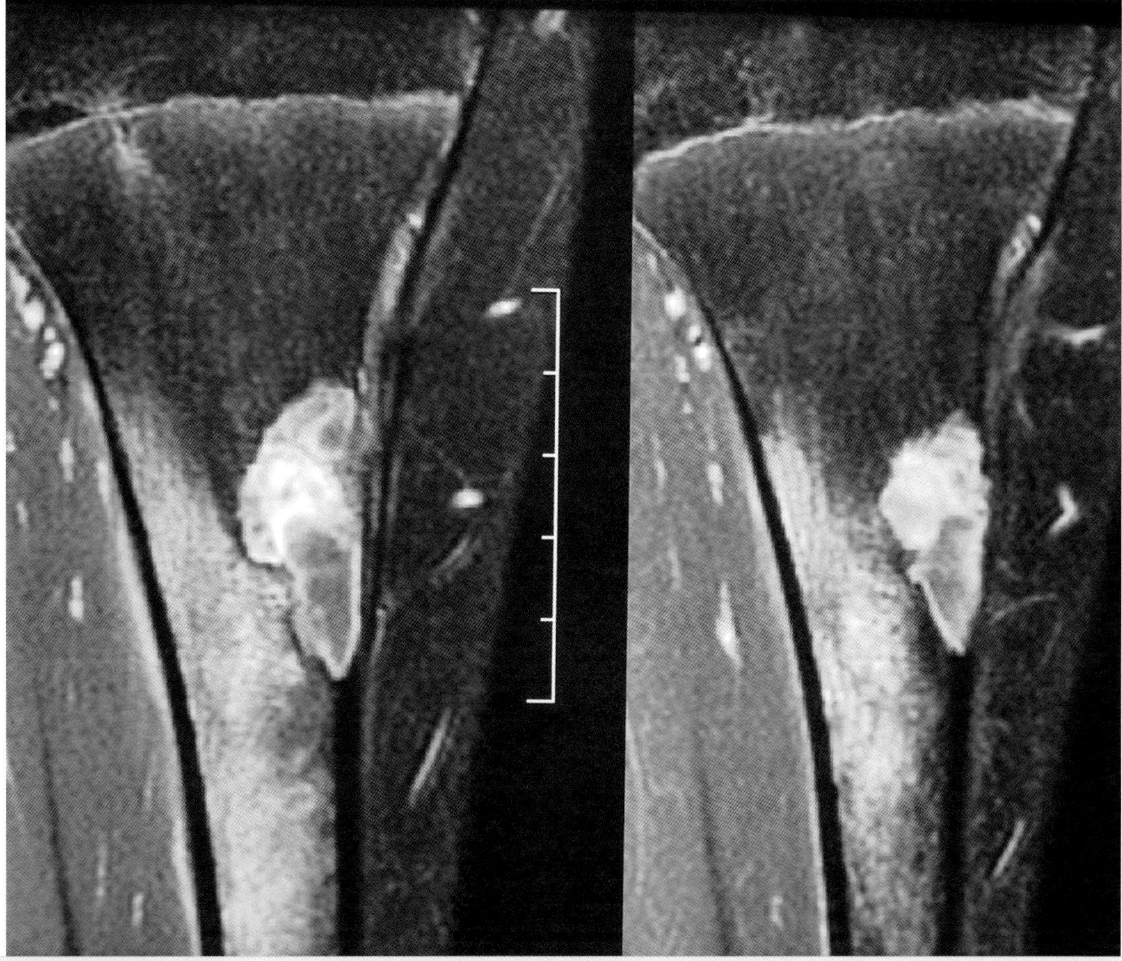

Fig. 10.140 A 14-year-old girl with a giant cell granuloma (solid aneurysmal bone cyst) involving the dimetaphyseal portion of the proximal tibia. The lesion shows a thin peripheral rimlike zone of low signal surrounding a central zone of Gd-contrast enhancement on coronal fat-suppressed T1-weighted imaging. A poorly defined zone of Gd-contrast enhancement is seen in the marrow adjacent to the lesion.

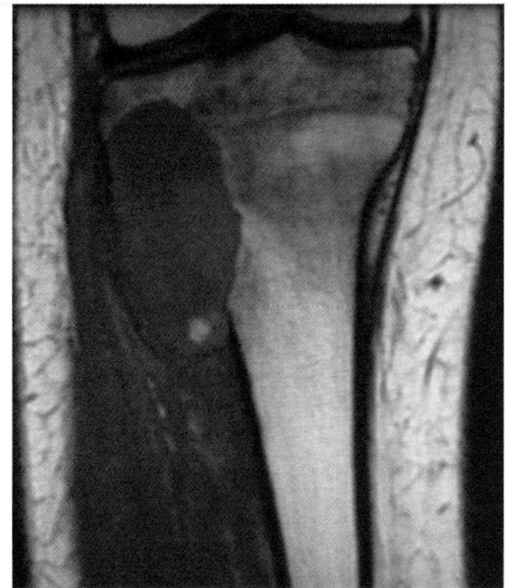

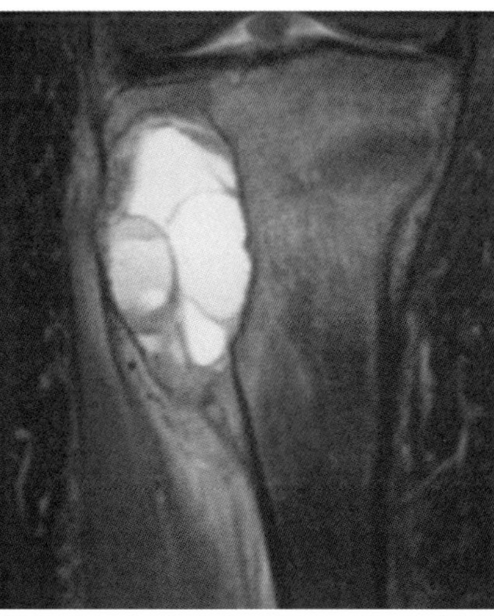

Fig. 10.141 A 14-year-old girl with an aneurysmal bone cyst in the proximal lateral tibia, which has low to intermediate signal as well as a small focus of high signal on coronal T1-weighted imaging (a). The lesion contains multiple fluid-fluid levels on coronal fat-suppressed T2-weighted imaging (FS T2WI) (b). Poorly defined zones with increased signal on FS T2WI are also seen in the adjacent marrow.

Table 10.6 (Cont.) Solitary intramedullary lesions with poorly defined margins of abnormal marrow signal

Abnormalities	MRI findings	Comments
Osteoid osteoma (▶ Fig. 10.142)	Intraosseous circumscribed lesions often less than 1.5 cm in diameter, central zone with low-intermediate signal on T1WI and high signal on T2WI and FS T2WI with prominent Gd-contrast enhancement, surrounded by a peripheral rim of low signal on T1WI and T2WI (sclerosis). Lesions usually have poorly defined zones with high signal on T2WI and FS T2WI and Gd-contrast enhancement in the marrow (edema, inflammation) beyond the zone of sclerosis or in adjacent soft tissues from prostaglandin synthesis by these lesions.	Benign osseous lesion containing a nidus of vascularized osteoid trabeculae surrounded by osteoblastic sclerosis, usually occurs between ages of 5 and 25, males > females. Focal pain and tenderness associated with lesion, which is often worse at night, relieved with aspirin.
Osteoblastoma (▶ Fig. 10.143)	Expansile lesion often greater than 1.5 cm in diameter with low-intermediate signal on T1WI and intermediate-high signal on T2WI and FS T2WI; usually show Gd-contrast enhancement. Lesions usually have poorly defined zones with high signal on T2WI and FS T2WI and Gd-contrast enhancement in the marrow (edema, inflammation) beyond the zone of sclerosis or in adjacent soft tissues from prostaglandin synthesis by these lesions.	Rare benign bone-forming neoplasm (2% of bone tumors) usually occurs in patients aged 6 to 30 years, median = 15 years. Histologically related to osteoid osteomas.
Brown tumor	Lesions are usually radiolucent on radiographs and CT. Lesions often have low-intermediate signal on T1WI, intermediate to slightly high signal on T2WI, and typically show Gd-contrast enhancement. Zones of low signal on T2WI may occur from hemosiderin. Expansion of cortical margins can occur with or without cortical disruption/destruction. Lesions may have circumscribed and/or poorly defined margins.	Most often involves ribs, mandible, clavicle, pelvis, craniofacial bones, and vertebrae. Can result from primary hyperparathyroidism (3 to 7%) (oversecretion of PTH from parathyroid adenoma associated with hypercalcemia), secondary type (vitamin D deficiency or chronic renal failure with hypocalcemia resulting in secretion of PTH and parathyroid gland hyperplasia) (1 to 2%), or tertiary type in which the secondary type leads to eventual autonomous elevated PTH secretion from parathyroid gland hyperplasia.

(continued on page 432)

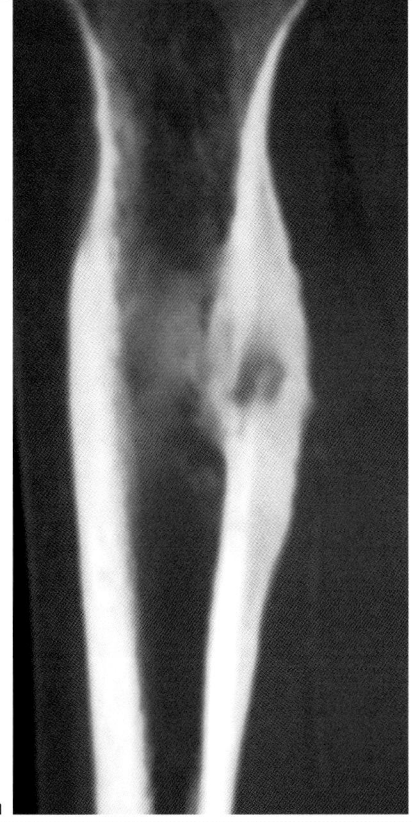
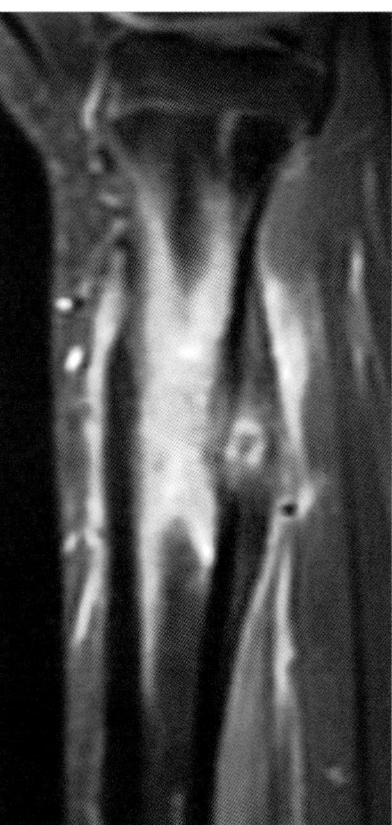

Fig. 10.142 A 15-year-old girl with a subperiosteal osteoid osteoma involving the proximal tibia. The radiolucent nidus of the lesion contains a tiny calcification and is surrounded with endosteal and thick periosteal bone formation on sagittal computed tomographic image (a). The nidus has high signal on sagittal fat-suppression T2-weighted imaging (FS T2WI) (b). Thickened cortex adjacent to the nidus has low and slightly-high signal on FS T2WI and is associated with periosteal reaction with high signal in the marrow and extraosseous soft tissues.

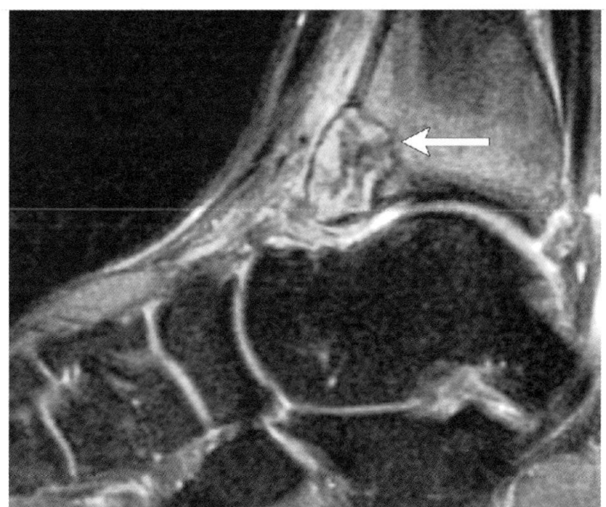
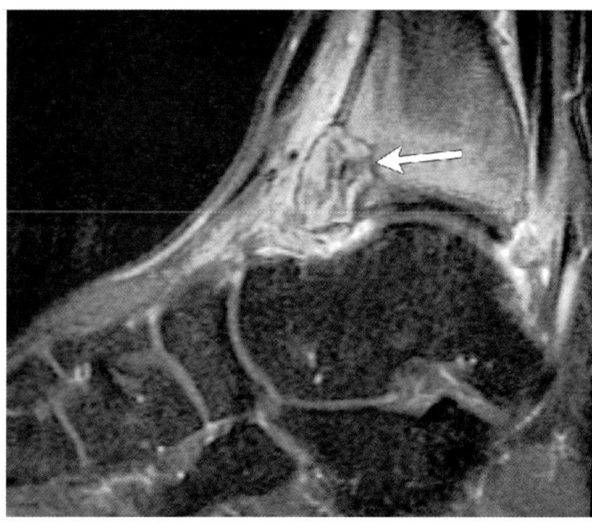

Fig. 10.143 A 24-year-old man with an osteoblastoma (arrow) involving the distal tibia, which has heterogeneous high and low signal on sagittal fat-suppressed T2-weighted imaging (FS T2WI) (a). A thin rim of low signal is seen at the periphery of the tumor and at the border with medullary bone. The tumor causes expansion and irregular thinning of the anterior cortical margin of the distal tibia. The lesion shows prominent heterogeneous gadolinium-contrast enhancement on sagittal FS T1-weighted imaging (arrow) (b). Poorly defined zones of high signal on T2WI and corresponding Gd-contrast enhancement are seen in the marrow and soft tissues adjacent to the osteoblastoma.

Table 10.6 (Cont.) Solitary intramedullary lesions with poorly defined margins of abnormal marrow signal

Abnormalities	MRI findings	Comments
Malignant lesions		
Metastatic tumor (▶ Fig. 10.144)	Single or multiple well-circumscribed or poorly defined infiltrative lesions involving marrow associated with cortical destruction and extraosseous extension. Lesions often have low-intermediate signal on T1WI, low, intermediate, and/or high signal on T2WI and FS T1WI, usually show Gd-contrast enhancement. Cortical destruction and tumor extension into the extraosseous soft tissues can occur. Pathological fractures can be associated with metastatic lesions involving tubular bones and vertebrae. Periosteal reaction is uncommon.	Metastatic lesions typically occur in the marrow with or without cortical destruction and extraosseous tumor extension.
Plasmacytoma (▶ Fig. 10.145)	Multiple myeloma or single plasma cell neoplasms (plasmacytoma) are well-circumscribed or poorly defined infiltrative lesions involving marrow, low-intermediate signal on T1WI, intermediate-high signal on T2WI and FS T2WI; usually show Gd-contrast-enhancement, eventual cortical bone destruction and extraosseous extension.	Malignant tumors composed of proliferating antibody-secreting plasma cells derived from single clones. Most common primary neoplasm of bone in adults, median age = 60 years. Most patients are older than 40 years. May have variable destructive or infiltrative changes involving the axial and/or appendicular skeleton.
Leukemia	Single or multiple well-circumscribed or poorly defined infiltrative lesions involving marrow; low-intermediate signal on T1WI, intermediate-high signal on T2WI and FS T2WI, often shows Gd-contrast enhancement, ± cortical bone destruction and extraosseous extension.	Lymphoid neoplasms with involvement of bone marrow with tumor cells also in peripheral blood. In children and adolescents, acute lymphoblastic leukemia (ALL) is the most frequent type. In adults, chronic lymphocytic leukemia (small lymphocytic lymphoma) is the most common type of lymphocytic leukemia. Myelogenous leukemias are neoplasms derived from abnormal myeloid progenitor cells. Acute myelogenous leukemia (AML) occurs in adolescents and young adults and represents approximately 20% of childhood leukemia. Chronic myelogenous leukemia (CML) usually affects adults older than 25 years.

(continued on page 434)

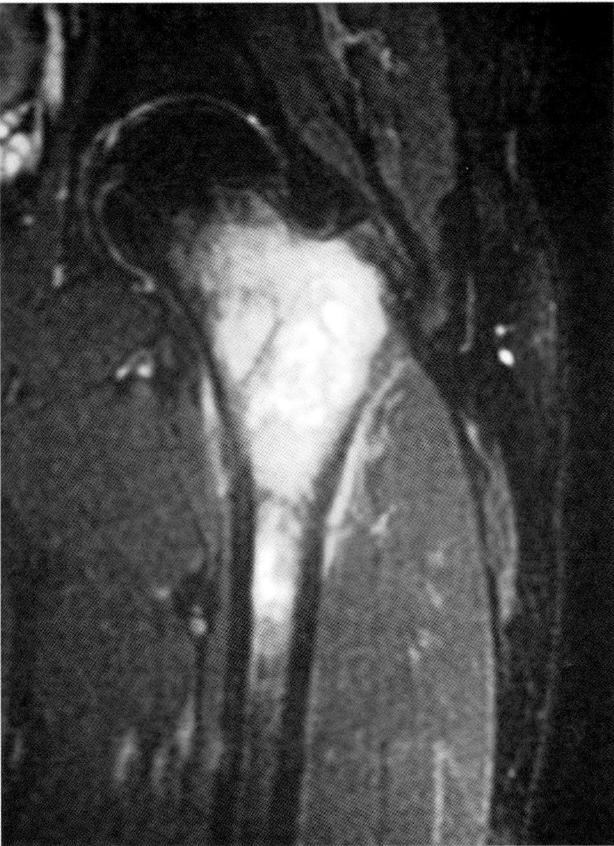

Fig. 10.144 A 26-year-old man with metastatic seminoma in the marrow of the femur seen as a poorly defined zone with slightly high to high signal on coronal fat-suppressed T2-weighted imaging.

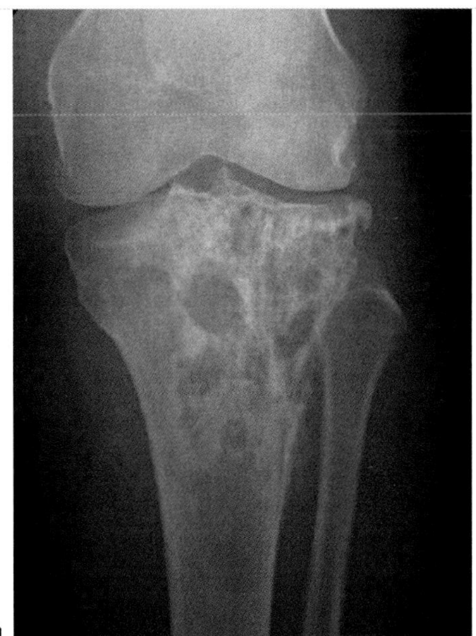

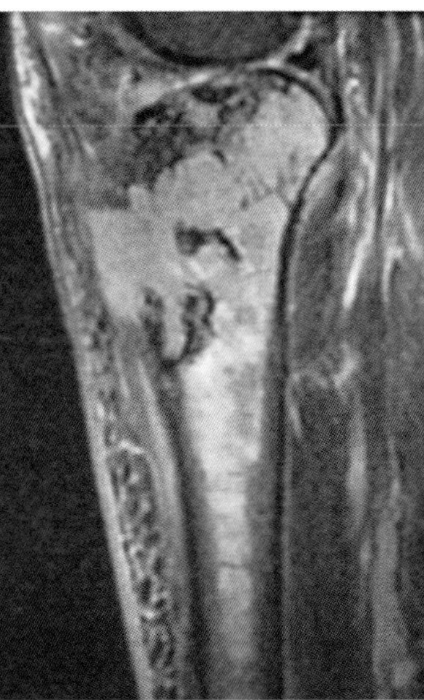

Fig. 10.145 Plasmacytoma in a 75-year-old woman involving the proximal tibia. The radiolucent intramedullary lesion with poorly defined margins and cortical destruction on radiograph (a) has high signal with poorly defined margins in the marrow on sagittal fat-suppressed T2-weighted imaging (b). Tumor extends through destroyed bone cortex into the adjacent soft tissues.

Table 10.6 (Cont.) Solitary intramedullary lesions with poorly defined margins of abnormal marrow signal

Abnormalities	MRI findings	Comments
Lymphoma (▶ Fig. 10.146)	Non-Hodgkin lymphoma (NHL) and Hodgkin disease (HD) within bone typically appears as single or multifocal poorly defined or circumscribed intramedullary zones with low-intermediate signal on T1WI, and intermediate, slightly high, and/or high signal on T2WI and high signal on FS T2WI; often show Gd-contrast enhancement. Zones of cortical destruction may occur associated with extraosseous soft tissue extension.	Lymphoid tumors with neoplastic cells typically within lymphoid tissue (lymph nodes and reticuloendothelial organs). Unlike leukemia, lymphoma usually arises as discrete masses. Lymphomas are subdivided into HD and NHL. Almost all primary lymphomas of bone are B cell NHL. HD, mean age = 32 years. Osseous NHL, median = 35 years.
Chondrosarcoma (▶ Fig. 10.147)	Intramedullary tumors often have low-intermediate signal on T1WI, intermediate signal on PDWI, and heterogeneous intermediate-high signal on T2WI. Lesions usually show heterogeneous contrast enhancement.	Malignant bone tumors containing cartilage formed within sarcomatous stroma. Account for 12 to 21% of malignant bone lesions, 21 to 26% of primary sarcomas of bone. Mean age = 40 years, median = 26 to 59 years.
Osteosarcoma (▶ Fig. 10.148)	Destructive intramedullary malignant lesions, low-intermediate signal on T1WI, mixed low, intermediate, high signal on T2WI, usually with matrix mineralization/ossification-low signal on T2 W images; usually show Gd-contrast enhancement (usually heterogeneous). May have circumscribed and/or ill-defined margins. Zones of cortical destruction are typically seen through which tumors extend into the extraosseous soft tissues under an elevated periosteum. Lamellated and/or spiculated zones of bone formation can occur under the periosteal elevation secondary to tumor invasion and perforation of bone cortex. Low signal from spicules of periosteal, reactive, and tumoral bone formation may have a divergent (sunburst) pattern, perpendicular (hair on end) pattern, or disorganized or complex appearance. Triangular zones of periosteal elevation (Codman triangles) can be seen at the borders of zones of cortical destruction and tumor extension.	Malignant tumor composed of proliferating neoplastic spindle cells that produce osteoid and/or immature tumoral bone, which most frequently arise within medullary bone (metadiaphyseal > metaphyseal > diaphyseal locations). Two age peaks of incidence. The larger peak occurs between the ages of 10 and 20 and accounts for over half of the cases. The second smaller peak occurs in adults over 60 years and accounts for approximately 10% of the cases. Occurs in children as primary tumors and adults (associated with Paget disease, irradiated bone, chronic osteomyelitis, osteoblastoma, giant cell tumor, fibrous dysplasia.

(continued on page 436)

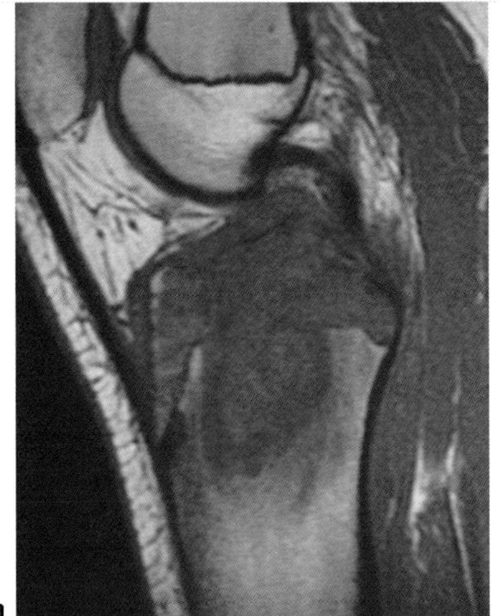

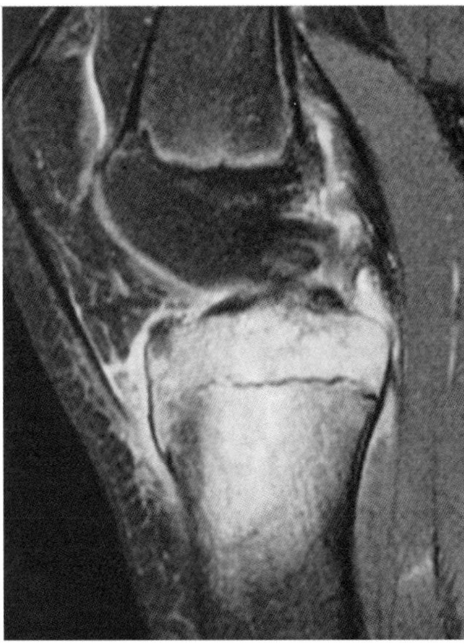

Fig. 10.146 A 13-year-old girl with Burkitt lymphoma involving the marrow of the proximal tibia seen as poorly defined zones with low-intermediate signal on sagittal T1-weighted imaging (a) and high signal on fat-suppressed T2-weighted imaging (b).

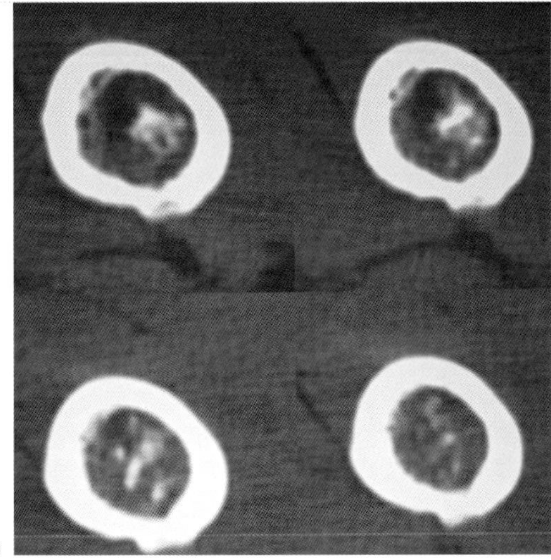

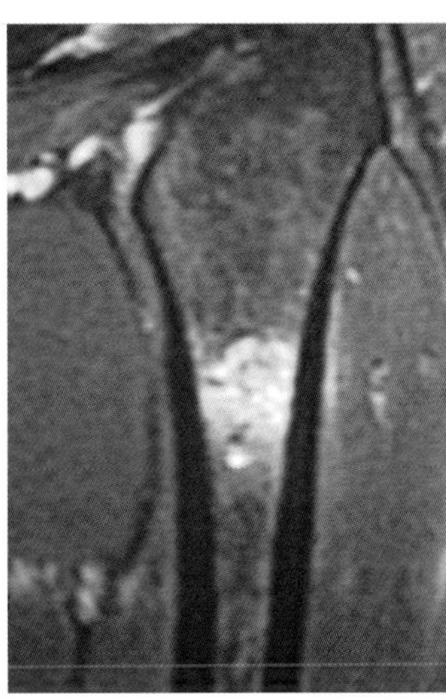

Fig. 10.147 A 44-year-old woman with a chondrosarcoma in the proximal shaft of the femur, which has chondroid mineralization on axial computed tomography (a). The tumor has high signal with poorly defined margins on coronal fat-suppressed T2-weighted imaging (b).

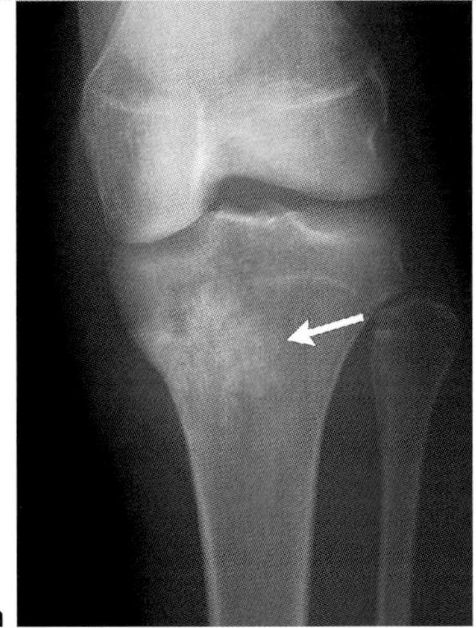

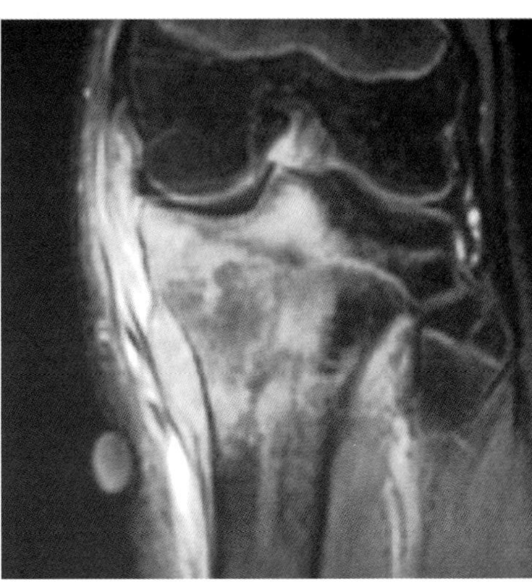

Fig. 10.148 A 9-year-old girl with an osteosarcoma involving proximal epiphyseal and metaphyseal portions of the tibia (arrow) with malignant tumoral ossification (a). The tumor has heterogeneous high signal on coronal fat-suppressed T2-weighted imaging (b) with poorly defined margins and is associated with cortical destruction and periosteal elevation from extraosseous tumor extension.

Table 10.6 (Cont.) Solitary intramedullary lesions with poorly defined margins of abnormal marrow signal

Abnormalities	MRI findings	Comments
Ewing sarcoma (▶ Fig. 10.149)	Destructive malignant lesions involving marrow, low-intermediate signal on T1WI, mixed low, intermediate, and/or high signal on T2WI and FS T2WI, usually shows Gd-contrast enhancement (usually heterogeneous). Extraosseous tumor extension through sites of cortical destruction is commonly seen beneath an elevated periosteum. Thin striated zones of low signal on T2WI can sometimes be seen oriented perpendicular to the long axis of the involved bone under the elevated periosteum representing the hair on end appearance of reactive bone formation secondary to the tumor. In long bones, tumors are most often located in the diaphyseal region, followed by the metadiaphyseal region.	Malignant primitive tumor of bone composed of undifferentiated small cells with round nuclei. Accounts for 6 to 11% of primary malignant bone tumors, 5 to 7% of primary bone tumors. Usually occurs between the ages of 5 and 30, males > females, locally invasive, high metastatic potential.
Malignant giant cell tumor (▶ Fig. 10.150)	Well-defined lesions with or without thin low signal margins on T1WI and T2WI. Solid portions of giant cell tumors often have low to intermediate signal on T1WI and PDWI, intermediate to high signal on T2WI, and high signal on FS PDWI and FS T2WI. Signal heterogeneity on T2WI is not uncommon. Aneurysmal bone cysts are seen with 14% of giant cell tumors. Lesions show mild to prominent variable and often heterogeneous Gd-contrast enhancement. Cortical destruction and extraosseous tumor extension are frequently seen.	Aggressive bone tumors composed of neoplastic ovoid mononuclear cells and scattered multinucleated osteoclast-like giant cells. Up to 10% of all giant cell tumors are malignant. Benign giant cell tumors account for approximately 5 to 9.5% of all bone tumors and up to 23% of benign bone tumors. 75% of malignant giant cell tumors occur in patients between the ages of 15 and 45 years.

(continued on page 438)

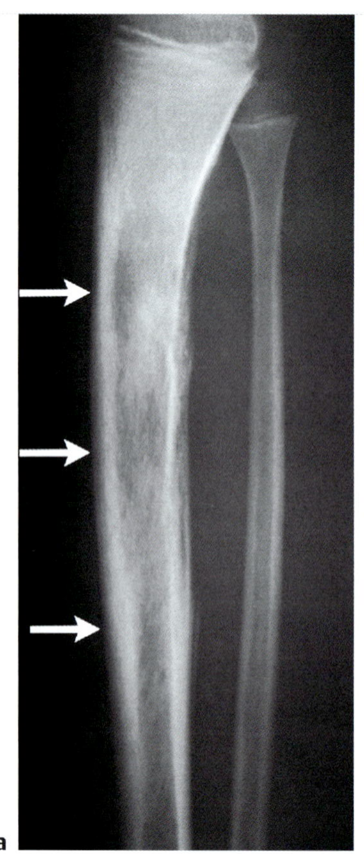

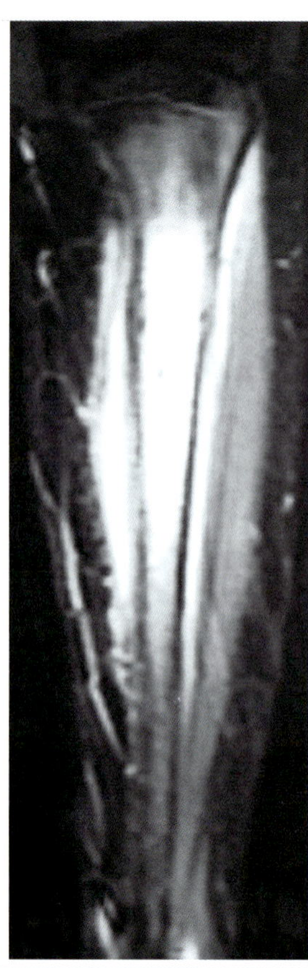

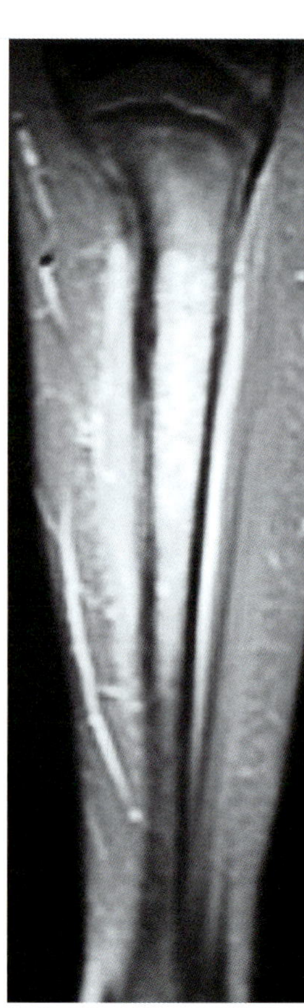

Fig. 10.149 An 11-year-old boy with Ewing sarcoma in the tibia seen as a poorly defined radiolucent intramedullary lesion (arrows) associated with cortical disruption and interrupted periosteal elevation on lateral radiograph (a). The tumor has high signal in the marrow on coronal fat-suppressed (FS) T2-weighted imaging (b) and shows contrast enhancement on coronal FS T1-weighted imaging (c). Tumor extends through destroyed bone cortex with elevation of disrupted periosteum.

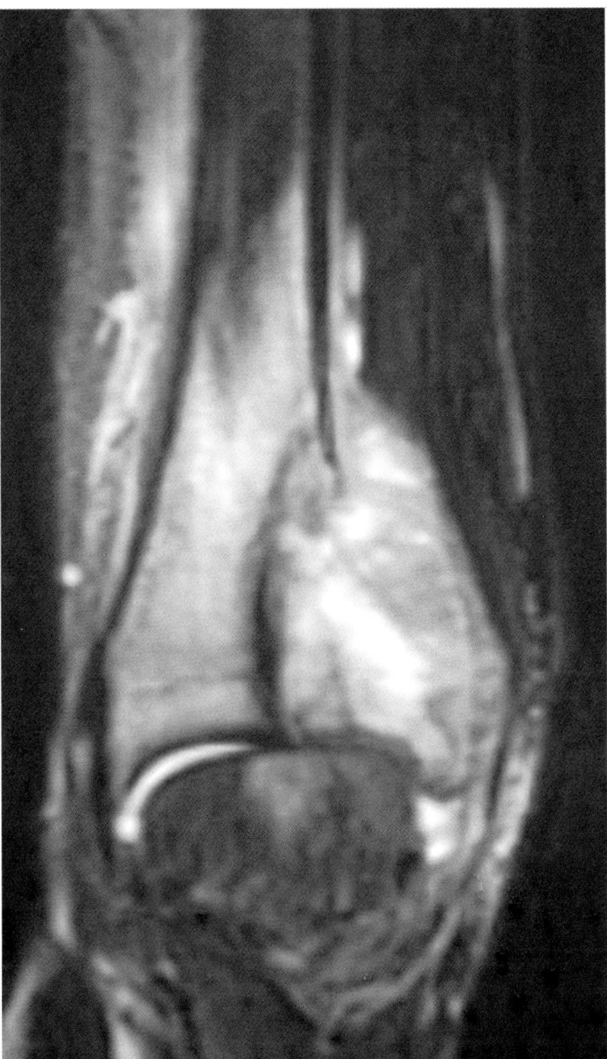

Fig. 10.150 A 16-year-old boy with a malignant giant cell tumor in the marrow of the distal tibia associated with cortical destruction and extraosseous extension. The intramedullary portion of the tumor has high signal centrally on coronal fat-suppressed T2-weighted imaging surrounded by a rim of low signal, and a poorly defined peripheral zone of high signal in the adjacent marrow.

Table 10.6 (Cont.) Solitary intramedullary lesions with poorly defined margins of abnormal marrow signal

Abnormalities	MRI findings	Comments
Fibrosarcoma	Intramedullary lesions with irregular margins, with or without associated cortical destruction and/or extraosseous soft tissue masses. Lesions usually have low-intermediate signal on T1WI and PDWI, and heterogeneous intermediate, slightly high, and/or high signal on T2WI. Lesions usually show heterogeneous Gd-contrast enhancement.	Fibrosarcomas are uncommon malignant tumors consisting of bundles of neoplastic fibroblasts/spindle cells with varying proportions of collagen, lacking other tissue-differentiating features such as tumor bone, osteoid, or cartilage. Can be primary lesions (75%) or arise as secondary tumors (25%) associated with prior irradiation, Paget disease, bone infarct, chronic osteomyelitis, fibrous dysplasia, giant cell tumor. Account for 3 to 5% of primary malignant bone tumors and 2 to 4% of all bone tumors; median age = 43 years.
Malignant fibrous histiocytoma (▶ Fig. 10.151)	Intramedullary lesions with irregular margins with zones of cortical destruction and extraosseous extension. Tumors often have low-intermediate signal on T1WI, low-intermediate signal on PDWI, and heterogeneous intermediate-high signal on T2WI and FS T2WI. Invasion into joints occurs in 30%. May be associated with bone infarcts, bone cysts, chronic osteomyelitis, Paget disease, and other treated primary bone tumors. Lesions usually show heterogeneous Gd-contrast prominent enhancement.	Malignant tumor involving soft tissue and rarely bone derived from undifferentiated mesenchymal cells. Contains cells with limited cellular differentiation such as mixtures of fibroblasts, myofibroblasts, histiocyte-like cells, anaplastic giant cells, and inflammatory cells. Accounts for 1 to 5% of primary malignant bone tumors and < 1% to 3% of all primary bone tumors. Patient ages range from 11 to 80 years, median = 48 years, mean = 55 years.
Paget sarcoma (▶ Fig. 10.152)	Irregular zones of medullary and cortical bone destruction associated with an extraosseous soft-tissue mass-lesion. The involved marrow typically has low to intermediate signal on T1WI and PDWI and low to high signal on T2WI. Abnormal Gd-contrast enhancement is seen in the marrow as well as in the extraosseous tumor extension.	Paget disease is most common bone disease in older adults after osteoporosis. Median age = 66 years. Disordered bone resorption and woven bone formation occurs resulting in osseous deformity. Associated with less than 1% risk for developing secondary sarcomatous changes.

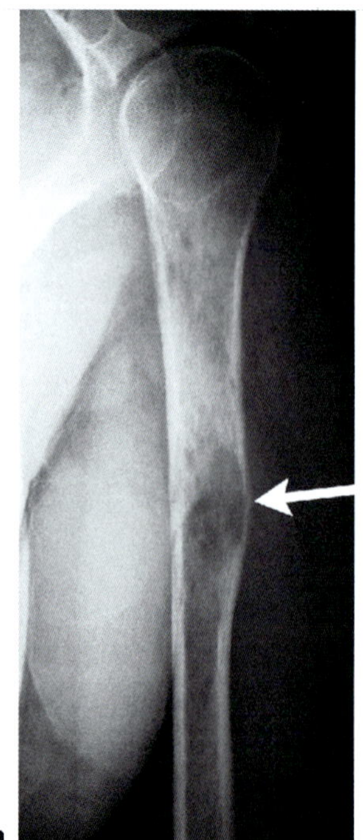

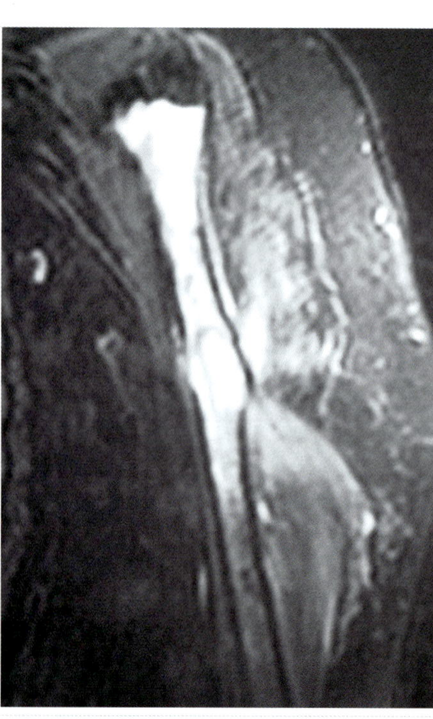

Fig. 10.151 Malignant fibrous histiocytoma involving the humerus in a 55-year-old woman seen as a radiolucent intramedullary lesion (a) (arrow) with poorly defined margins and endosteal erosion, which has high signal with poorly defined margins in the marrow on fat-suppressed T2-weighted imaging (b).

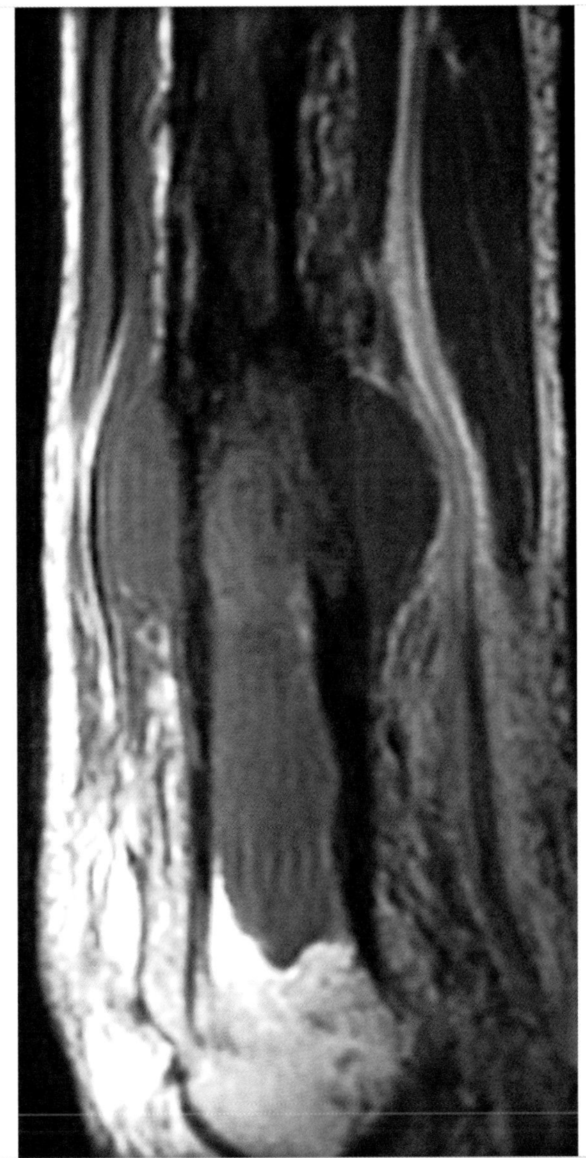

Fig. 10.152 A 71-year-old woman with Paget sarcoma involving the marrow of the distal femur associated with cortical destruction and extraosseous extension as seen on sagittal T1-weighted imaging.

10.7 Solitary Intramedullary Lesions Located Near the Ends of Tubular Bones

- Nonmalignant lesions
  - Enchondroma
  - Giant cell tumor of bone
  - Giant cell reparative granuloma
  - Chondroblastoma
  - Chondromyxoid fibroma
  - Osteoblastoma
  - Intraosseous lipoma
  - Geode/subchondral degenerative cyst
  - Intraosseous ganglion
  - Intraosseous extension of inflammatory synovium/pannus
  - Intraosseous calcific tendinopathy
  - Fracture
  - Bone contusion
  - Osteochondritis dissecans
  - Bone infarct
  - Transient bone marrow edema (acute bone marrow edema syndromes [aBMEs], transient osteoporosis of the hip, regional migratory osteoporosis)
  - Osteomyelitis
  - Eosinophilic granuloma
- Malignant lesions
  - Metastatic lesion
  - Plasmacytoma
  - Lymphoma
  - Leukemia
  - Chondrosarcoma
  - Osteosarcoma
  - Ewing sarcoma
  - Malignant giant cell tumor
  - Fibrosarcoma
  - Malignant fibrous histiocytoma
  - Hemangioendothelioma

Table 10.7 Solitary intramedullary lesions located near the ends of tubular bones

Abnormalities	MRI findings	Comments
Nonmalignant lesions		
Enchondroma (▶ Fig. 10.153; ▶ Fig. 10.154)	Lobulated circumscribed intramedullary lesions, which usually have low-intermediate signal on T1-weighted imaging (T1WI) and intermediate signal on proton density–weighted imaging (PDWI). On T2-weighted imaging (T2WI) and fat-suppressed (FS) T2WI, lesions usually have predominantly high signal with foci and/or bands of low signal representing areas of matrix mineralization and fibrous strands. Lesions typically show gadolinium (Gd)-contrast enhancement in various patterns (peripheral curvilinear lobular, central nodular/septal and peripheral lobular, or heterogeneous diffuse).	Benign intramedullary lesions composed of hyaline cartilage represent approximately 10% of benign bone tumors. Enchondromas can be solitary (88%) or multiple (12%). Median age = 35 years, peak in third and fourth decades.

(continued on page 442)

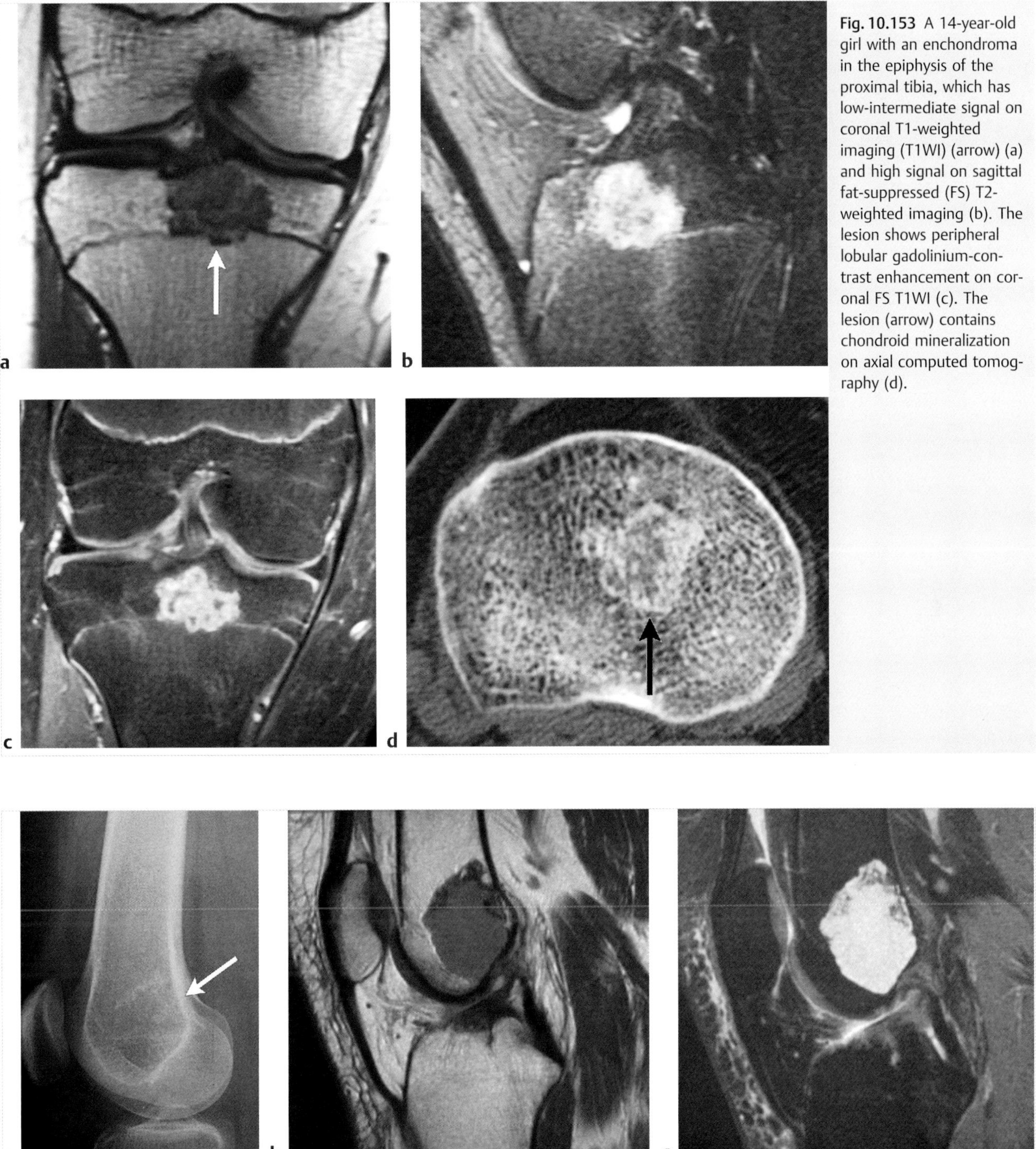

Fig. 10.153 A 14-year-old girl with an enchondroma in the epiphysis of the proximal tibia, which has low-intermediate signal on coronal T1-weighted imaging (T1WI) (arrow) (a) and high signal on sagittal fat-suppressed (FS) T2-weighted imaging (b). The lesion shows peripheral lobular gadolinium-contrast enhancement on coronal FS T1WI (c). The lesion (arrow) contains chondroid mineralization on axial computed tomography (d).

Fig. 10.154 A 39-year-old woman with an enchondroma in the distal femur, which contains chondroid mineralization (arrow) (a). The lesion has low-intermediate signal on sagittal proton density–weighted imaging (b) and high signal on sagittal fat-suppressed T2-weighted imaging (c).

Table 10.7 (Cont.) Solitary intramedullary lesions located near the ends of tubular bones

Abnormalities	MRI findings	Comments
Giant cell tumor of bone (▶ Fig. 10.155)	Often well-defined lesions with thin low signal margins on T1WI, PDWI, and T2WI. Solid portions of giant cell tumors often have low to intermediate signal on T1WI and PDWI, intermediate to high signal on T2WI, and high signal on FS PDWI and FS T2WI. Zones of low signal on T2WI may be seen secondary to hemosiderin. Aneurysmal bone cysts (ABCs) can be seen in 14% of giant cell tumors. Areas of cortical thinning, expansion, and/or destruction can occur with extraosseous extension. Tumors show varying degrees of Gd-contrast enhancement.	Aggressive bone tumors composed of neoplastic mononuclear cells and scattered multinucleated osteoclast-like giant cells. Account for 23% of primary nonmalignant bone tumors and and 5 to 9% of all primary bone tumors. Median age = 30 years.
Giant cell reparative granuloma (▶ Fig. 10.156)	Lesions can have heterogeneous low, intermediate, and/or high signal on T1WI, PDWI, and T2WI as well as peripheral rimlike and central Gd-contrast enhancement on FS T1WI. May be surrounded by poorly defined zone of high signal on FS T2WI and Gd-contrast enhancement in the adjacent marrow.	Giant cell reparative granulomas are also referred to as solid ABCs. Histological appearance resembles brown tumors.
Chondroblastoma (▶ Fig. 10.157)	Tumors often have fine lobular margins and typically have low-intermediate heterogeneous signal on T1WI and mixed low, intermediate, and/or high signal on T2WI. Areas of low signal on T2WI are secondary to chondroid matrix mineralization and/or hemosiderin. Lobular, marginal, or septal Gd-contrast enhancement patterns can be seen. Poorly defined zones with high signal on T2WI and FS T2WI and corresponding Gd-contrast enhancement are typically seen in the marrow adjacent to the lesions representing inflammatory reaction from prostaglandin synthesis by these tumors.	Benign cartilaginous tumors with chondroblast-like cells and areas of chondroid matrix formation, usually occur in children and adolescents, median = 17 years, mean = 16 years for lesions in long bones, mean = 28 years in other bones. Most cases are diagnosed between the ages of 5 and 25 years.

(continued on page 444)

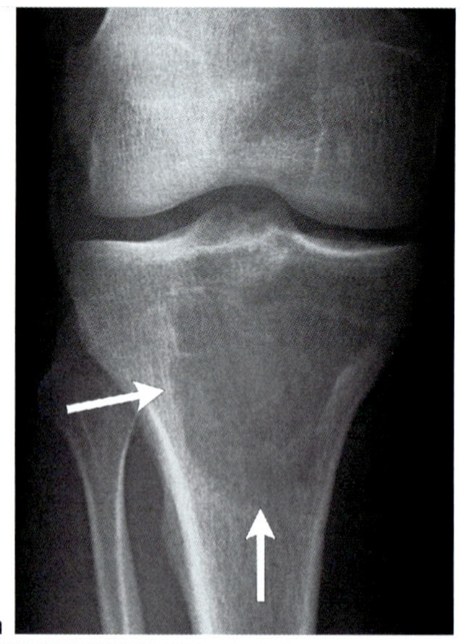

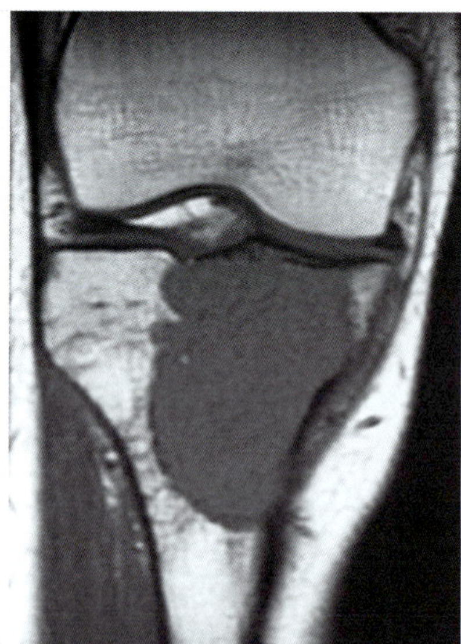

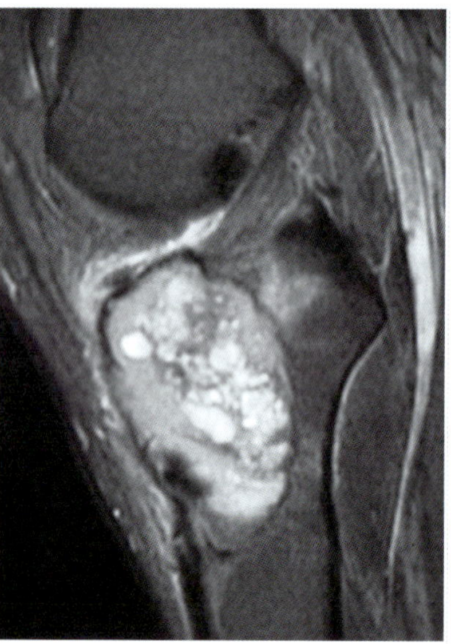

Fig. 10.155 A 28-year-old woman with a giant cell tumor in the proximal tibia. The radiolucent lesion (a) (arrows) with a narrow zone of transition has intermediate signal on coronal T1-weighted imaging (b) and heterogeneous high signal on sagittal fat-suppressed T2-weighted imaging (c).

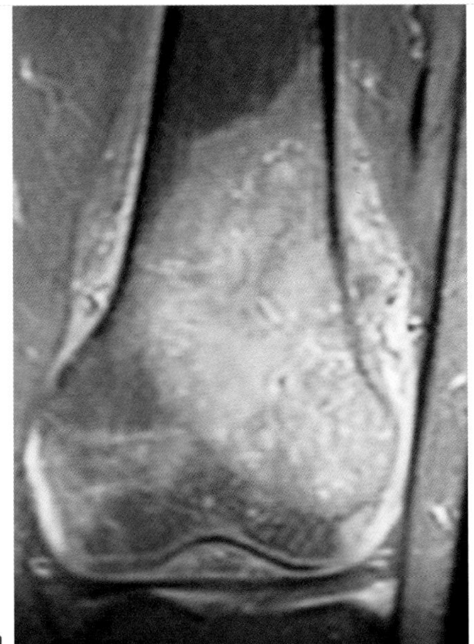

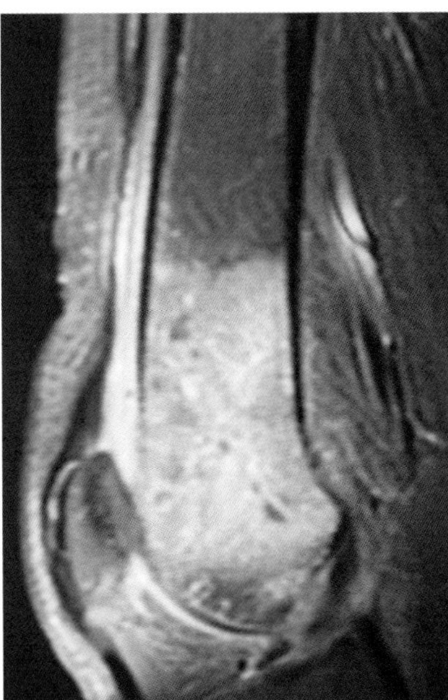

Fig. 10.156 A 33-year-old woman with a giant cell granuloma in the distal femur, which shows gadolinium-contrast enhancement, cortical destruction, and extraosseous extension on coronal (a) and sagittal fat-suppressed T1-weighted imaging (b).

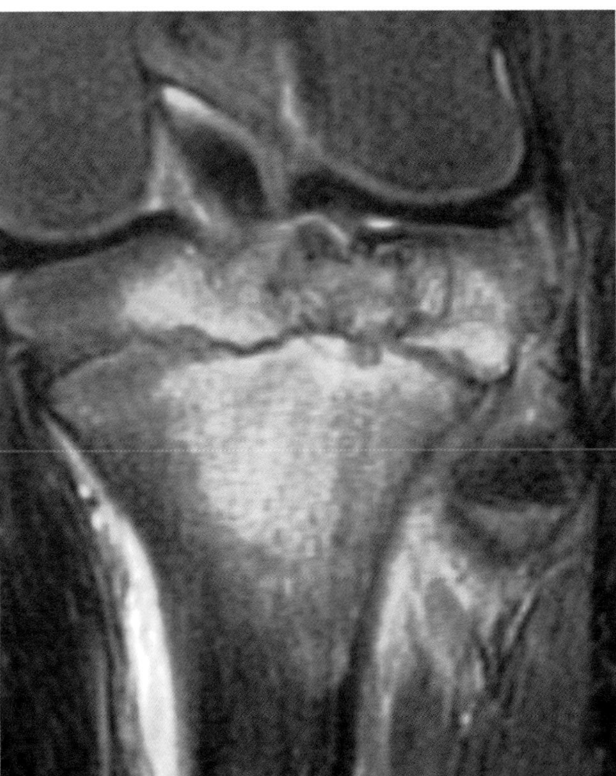

Fig. 10.157 A 13-year-old girl with a chondroblastoma involving the epiphysis of the proximal tibia. The lesion has mixed high and low signal with thin low signal margins on coronal fat-suppressed T2-weighted imaging. Poorly defined zones with high signal are also seen in the adjacent marrow.

Table 10.7 (Cont.) Solitary intramedullary lesions located near the ends of tubular bones

Abnormalities	MRI findings	Comments
Chondromyxoid fibroma (▶ Fig. 10.158)	Lesions are often slightly lobulated with low-intermediate signal on T1WI and heterogeneous predominantly high signal on T2WI. Magnetic resonance (MR) signal heterogeneity on T2WI is related to the proportions of myxoid, chondroid, and fibrous components within the lesions. Thin low signal septa on T2WI can be seen. Lesions are surrounded by low signal borders representing thin sclerotic reaction. Edema is not typically seen in adjacent medullary bone. Lesions show prominent diffuse Gd-contrast enhancement.	Rare, benign, slow-growing bone lesions that contain chondroid, myxoid, and fibrous components. Chondromyxoid fibromas represent 2 to 4% of primary benign bone lesions, and < 1% of primary bone lesions. Most chondromyxoid fibromas occur between the ages of 1 to 40 years, with a median of 17 years, and peak incidence in the second to third decades.
Osteoblastoma (▶ Fig. 10.159)	Expansile lesion often greater than 1.5 cm in diameter with low-intermediate signal on T1WI and intermediate-high signal on T2WI and FS T2WI, typically shows Gd-contrast enhancement. Lesions usually have poorly defined zones with high signal on T2WI and FS T2WI and Gd-contrast enhancement in the marrow (edema, inflammation) beyond zone of sclerosis or in adjacent soft tissues from prostaglandin synthesis by these lesions.	Rare benign bone-forming neoplasm (2% of bone tumors) usually occurs at age 6 to 30 years, median = 15 years.
Intraosseous lipoma (▶ Fig. 10.160)	Lesions can have heterogeneous low, intermediate, and/or high signal on T1WI, PDWI, and T2WI as well as peripheral rimlike and central Gd-contrast enhancement on FS T1WI.	Uncommon benign hamartomas composed of mature white adipose tissue without cellular atypia. Osseous or chondroid metaplasia with myxoid changes can be associated with lipomas. Account for approximately 0.1% of bone tumors; likely underreported.
Geode/subchondral degenerative cyst (▶ Fig. 10.161)	Typically have sharply defined margins and contain low signal on T1WI, low-intermediate signal on PDWI, and homogeneous high signal on T2WI. Poorly defined zones of Gd-contrast enhancement can be seen in the marrow adjacent to the subchondral cysts on FS T1WI.	A geode or subchondral cyst is a cystic lesion located near the end of a long bone where there are changes of degenerative osteoarthropathy. Lesions can result from synovial fluid intrusion and/or bony contusion in the setting of degenerative joint disease.

(continued on page 446)

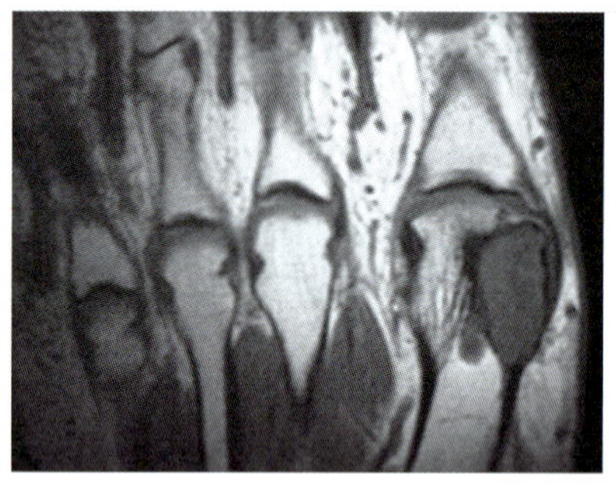
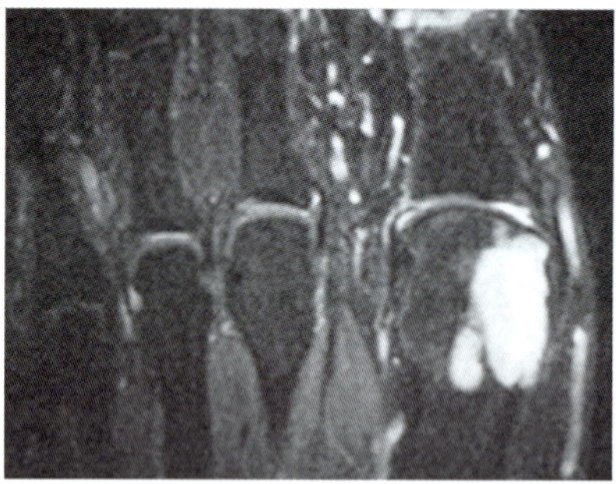
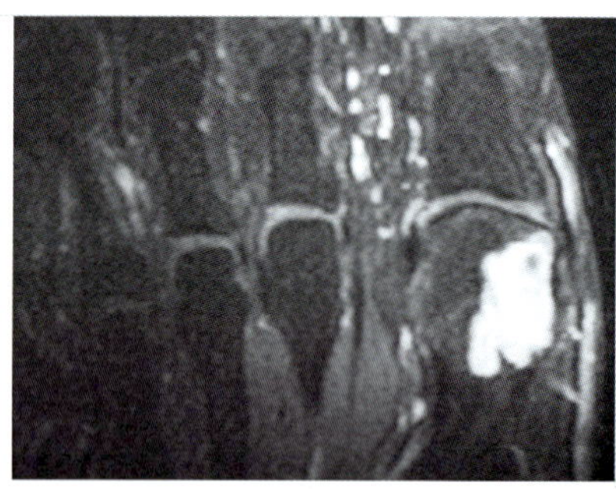

Fig. 10.158 A 34-year-old man with a chondromyxoid fibroma involving the first metatarsal head. The lesion has circumscribed low signal margins and contains intermediate signal on coronal T1-weighted imaging (T1WI) (a) and high signal on coronal fat-suppressed (FS) T2-weighted imaging (b). The lesion shows Gd-contrast enhancement on coronal FS T1WI (c).

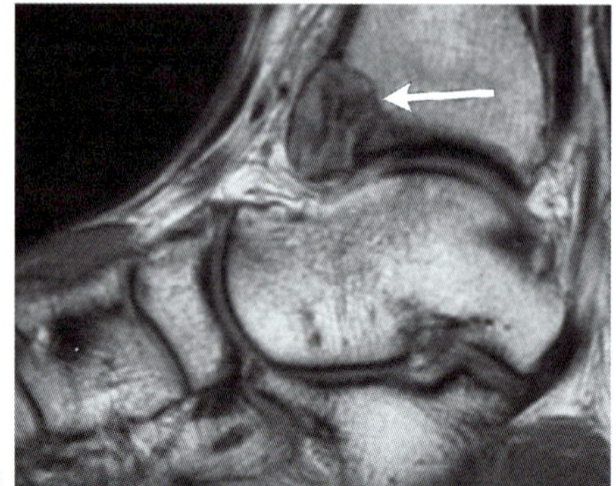
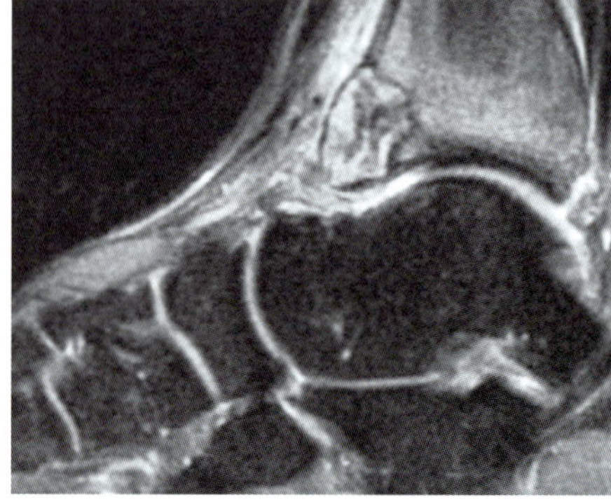

Fig. 10.159 A 24-year-old man with an osteoblastoma in the distal tibia. The lesion (arrow) is associated with cortical thinning and expansion and has low-intermediate signal on sagittal proton density–weighted imaging (a) and heterogeneous high and low signal on sagittal fat-suppressed T2-weighted imaging (FS T2WI) (b). Poorly defined high signal on FS T2WI is also seen in the marrow adjacent to the lesion.

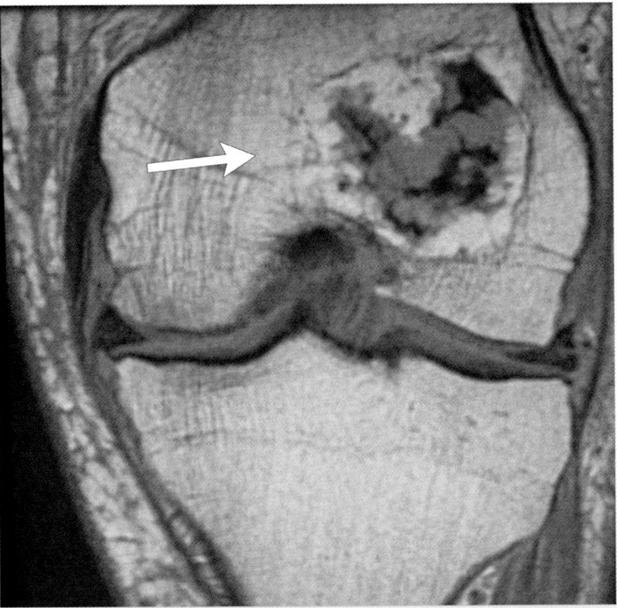

Fig. 10.160 A 74-year-old man with an intraosseous lipoma in the distal portion of the femur (arrow), which has high signal peripherally surrounding a central zone with intermediate and low signal from cystic degeneration and dystrophic calcifications on proton density–weighted imaging.

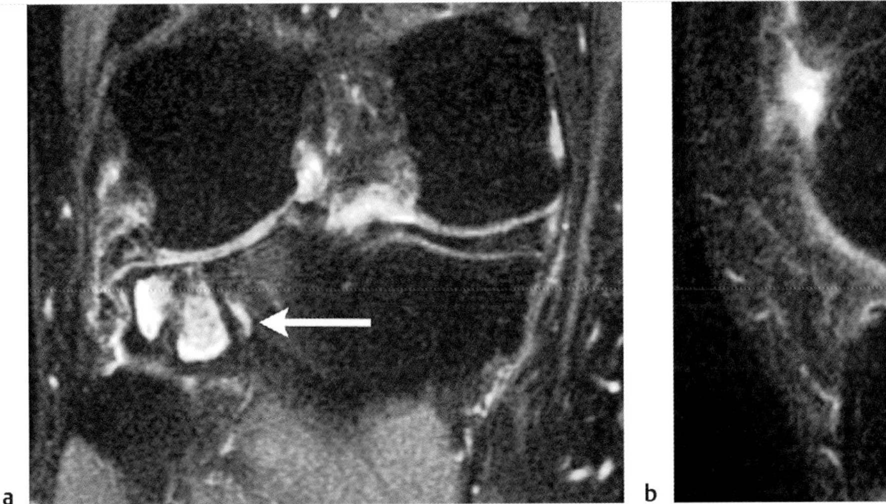

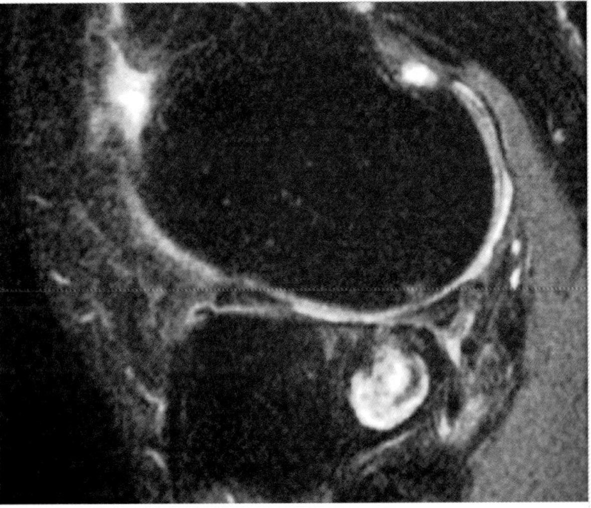

Fig. 10.161 A 50-year-old man with a geode or degenerative-arthritic-subchondral cyst in the proximal lateral tibia beneath a degenerated lateral meniscus and disrupted hyaline cartilage. The lesion (arrow) has circumscribed margins and contains high signal centrally on coronal (a) and sagittal fat-suppressed T2-weighted imaging (b).

Table 10.7 (Cont.) Solitary intramedullary lesions located near the ends of tubular bones

Abnormalities	MRI findings	Comments
Intraosseous ganglion (▶ Fig. 10.162)	Can have round, oval, or serpiginous configurations with sharply defined margins. These lesions typically contain low signal on T1WI, low-intermediate signal on PDWI, and high signal on T2WI.	Benign cystic-like lesion usually located at or near the ends of long bones and not associated with degenerative osteoarthropathy. Lesions can result from intraosseous extension from a ganglion in the soft tissues or from intraosseous mucoid degeneration, synovial rests, or synovial intrusion.
Intraosseous extension of inflammatory synovium/pannus (▶ Fig. 10.163)	Hypertrophied synovium can be diffuse, nodular, and/or villous. Often has low to intermediate or intermediate signal on T1WI and PDWI and low to intermediate, intermediate, and/or slightly high to high signal on T2WI. Erosive changes in subchondral bone appear as zones of low signal on T1WI and high signal on T2WI. Gd-contrast enhancement is often seen within the erosions.	Inflammatory synovitis associated with rheumatoid arthritis can result in progressive destruction of cartilage and cortical bone leading with intraosseous extension and trabecular destruction. Prevalence ranges from 0.3 to 2.1% of the world population; 80% of adult patients present between the ages of 35 and 50. Incidence of juvenile rheumatoid arthritis (JRA) ranges from 6 to 19.6 cases per 100,000. Patients with JRA range in age from 5 to 16 years, mean = 10.2 years.
Intraosseous calcific tendinopathy (▶ Fig. 10.164)	Zones with slightly high and low signal on T2WI and FS T2WI are seen in tendons with or without erosion of bone cortex. Intramedullary zones with mixed low, intermediate, and/or high signal on T2WI and FS T2WI may be seen in the adjacent marrow.	Degenerative disorder with amorphous calcifications in tendons or bursa associated with erosion of adjacent bone cortex, with or without marrow invasion. Most common in humerus and femur in patients aged 16 to 82 years, average = 50 years.

(continued on page 448)

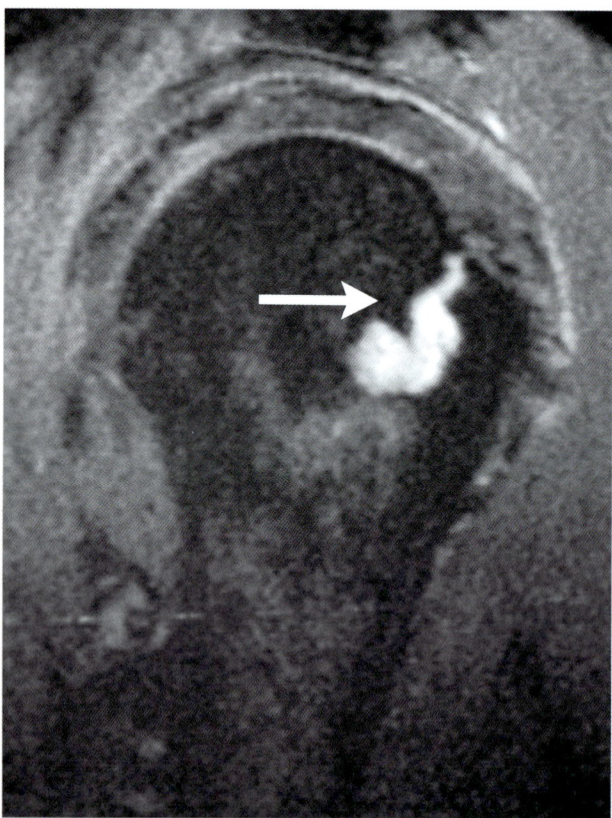

Fig. 10.162 Sagittal fat-suppressed T2-weighted imaging shows an intraosseous ganglion in the proximal humerus, which has high signal (arrow).

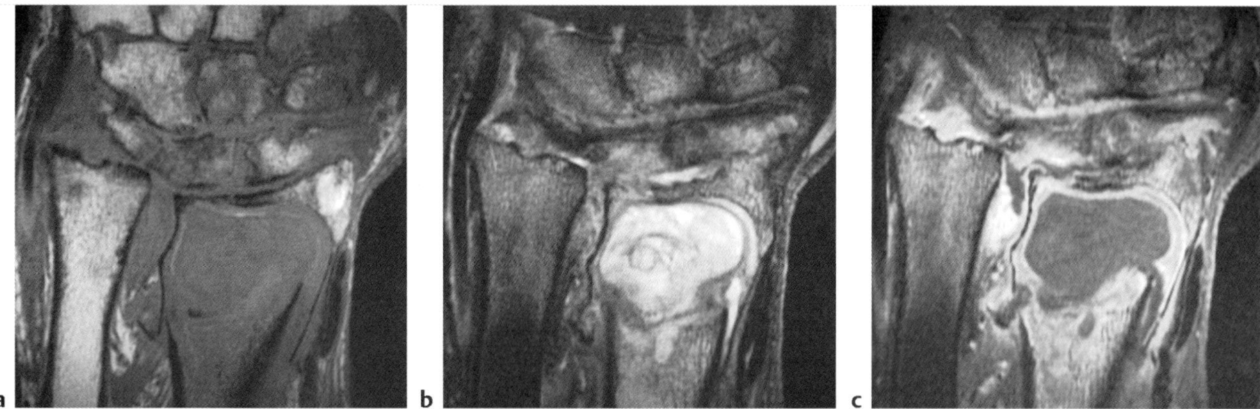

Fig. 10.163 A 71-year-old man with pannus eroding into the distal radius resulting in destruction of trabecular bone and an intraosseous cystlike lesion. The intraosseous lesion has intermediate signal on coronal T1-weighted imaging (T1WI) (a) and heterogeneous high signal on coronal T2-weighted imaging (b). Gadolinium-contrast enhancement is seen at the margins of the intraosseous lesion on coronal fat-suppressed T1WI (c) as well as in the hypertrophied synovium in the wrist. Also seen is destruction of hyaline cartilage at the carpal bones and distal ulna.

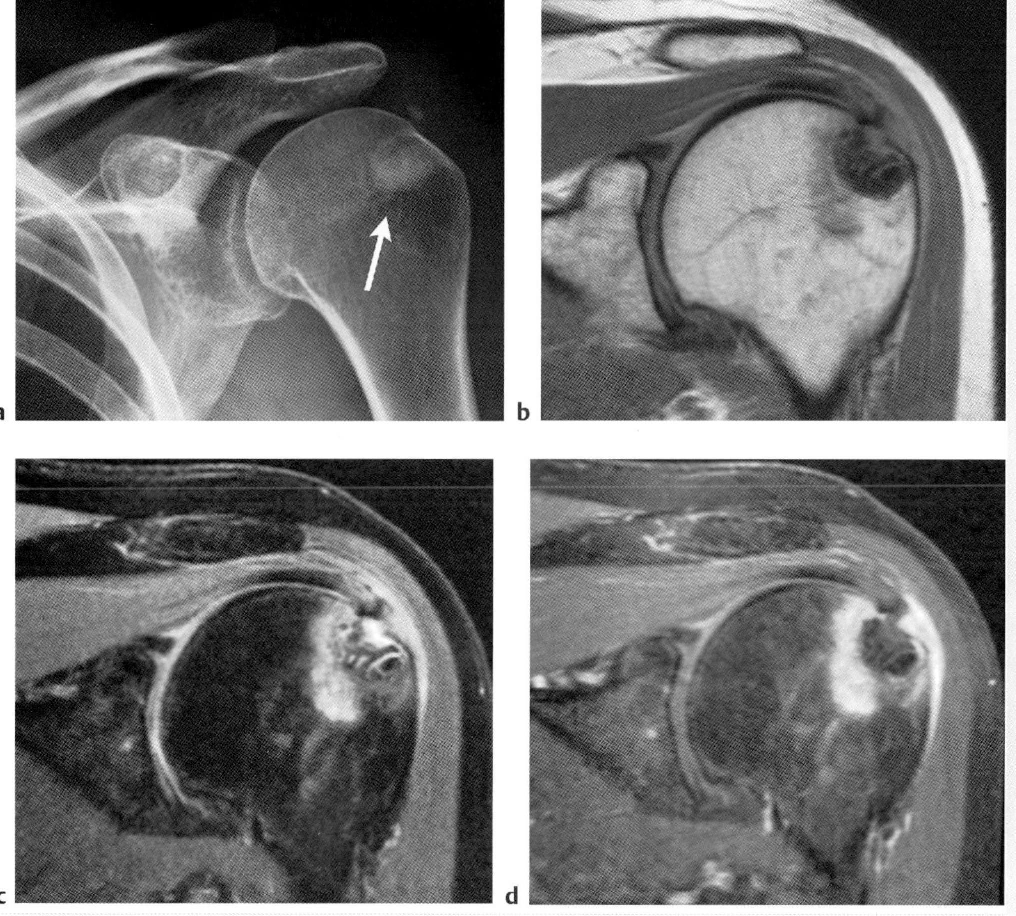

Fig. 10.164 A 57-year-old woman with intraosseous calcific tendinopathy in the humerus. Calcification is seen in the rotator cuff near the insertion site associated with an intraosseous zone of increased attenuation (arrow) on anteroposterior radiograph (a). Coronal proton density–weighted imaging (b) shows a circumscribed intraosseous zone with low and intermediate signal beneath a zone of cortical disruption. The intraosseous lesion has mixed high and low signal on coronal fat-suppressed (FS) T2-weighted imaging (c), as well as a poorly defined zone with high T2 signal in the adjacent marrow. The intraosseous lesion shows marginal Gd-contrast enhancement surrounding the circumscribed lesion, and a poorly defined zone of contrast enhancement is seen in the adjacent bone marrow on FS T1-weighted imaging (d).

Table 10.7 (Cont.) Solitary intramedullary lesions located near the ends of tubular bones

Abnormalities	MRI findings	Comments
Fracture (▶ Fig. 10.165)	Acute/subacute fractures typically have abnormal marrow signal (usually low signal on T1WI, high signal on T2WI and FS T2WI). Gd-contrast enhancement is typically seen in the postfracture period. Angulated cortical margins and periosteal high signal on FS T2WI can be seen with traumatic fractures. A curvilinear zone of low signal on T2WI and FS T2WI may be seen within the marrow edema in stress fractures.	Can result from trauma, primary bone tumors/lesions, metastatic disease, bone infarcts (steroids, chemotherapy, and radiation treatment), osteoporosis, osteomalacia, metabolic (calcium/ phosphate) disorders, vitamin deficiencies, Paget disease, and genetic disorders (e.g., osteogenesis imperfecta).
Bone contusion (▶ Fig. 10.166)	Contusions usually appear as poorly defined intramedullary zones with low-intermediate signal on T1WI and high signal on FS T2WI, and corresponding Gd-contrast enhancement. Adjacent cortical margins are typically intact.	Also referred to as bone bruises, contusions represent trabecular microfractures without cortical fracture. In the knee, contusions at the lateral femoral condyle and posterolateral proximal tibia are commonly associated with injuries to the anterior cruciate ligament.
Osteochondritis dissecans (▶ Fig. 10.167)	Subchondral lesions in marrow ranging from 1 to 3 cm with low-intermediate signal on T1WI and T2WI. Small irregular zones with slightly high to high signal may be seen with FS T2WI. A linear zone with high signal on T2WI along the margins can represent tracking of synovial fluid from a defect in the overlying hyaline cartilage and is associated with an increased risk of fragmentation and separation.	Osteochondrosis in which there is localized necrosis followed by reossification and healing unless there is osteochondral fragmentation and separation. Lesions commonly occur at the lateral surface of the medial femoral condyle as well as the capitellum, talar dome, and femoral head.
Bone infarct (▶ Fig. 10.168)	A double-line sign (curvilinear adjacent zones of low and high signal on T2WI) is commonly seen at the edges of the infarcts representing the borders of osseous resorption and healing. Irregular Gd-contrast enhancement can be seen from granulation tissue ingrowth.	Zones of ischemic death involving bone trabeculae and marrow, which can be idiopathic or result from trauma, corticosteroid treatment, chemotherapy, radiation treatment, occlusive vascular disease, collagen vascular and other autoimmune diseases, metabolic storage diseases (e.g., Gaucher disease), sickle cell disease, thalassemia, hyperbaric events/Caisson disease, pregnancy, alcohol abuse, pancreatitis, infections, and lymphoproliferative diseases.

(continued on page 450)

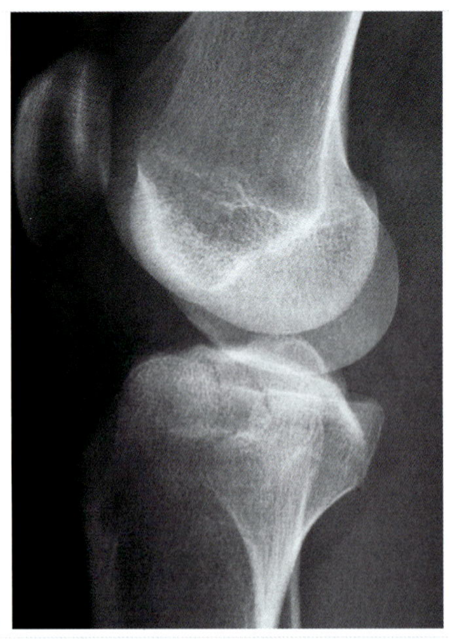

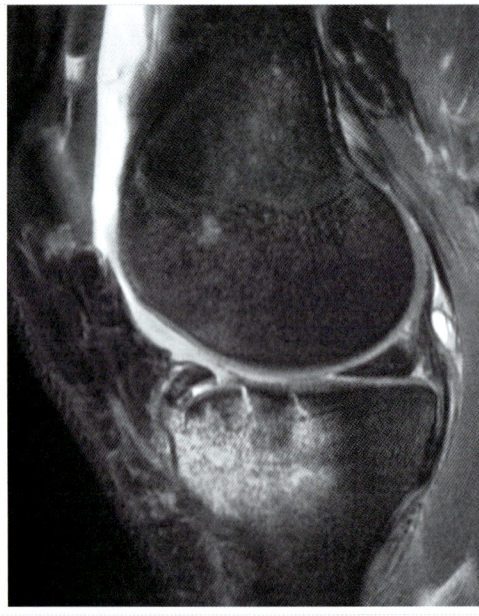

Fig. 10.165 A 20-year-old man with a traumatic fracture of the tibial plateau is seen on lateral radiograph (a). Cortical discontinuity and subjacent poorly defined zones of high signal in the marrow are seen on sagittal fat-suppressed T2-weighted imaging (b).

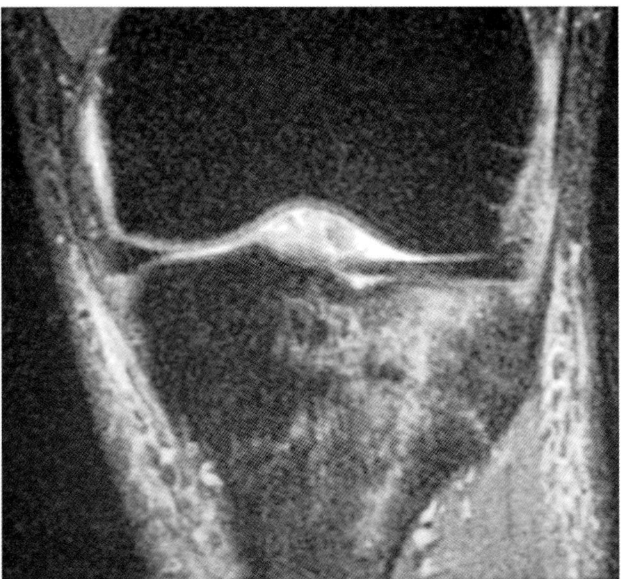

Fig. 10.166 A bone contusion is seen as a poorly defined zone with increased signal on coronal fat-suppressed T2-weighted imaging in the marrow of the proximal tibia with intact overlying bone cortex.

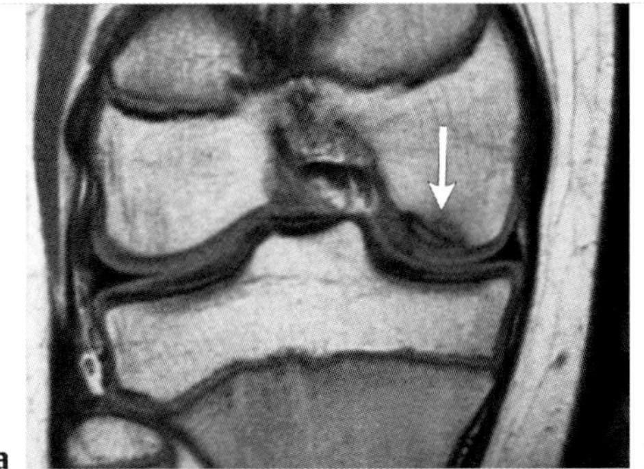

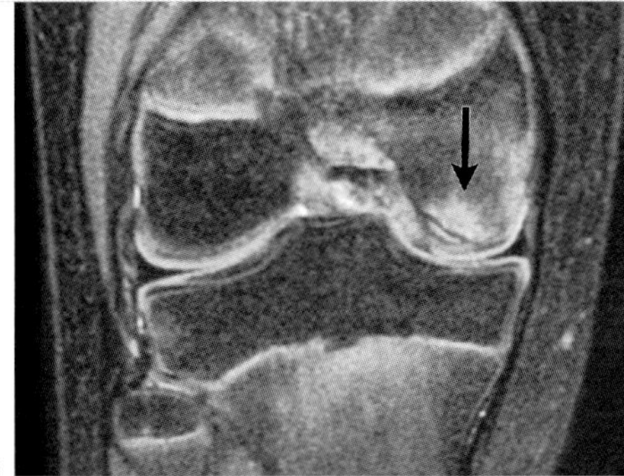

Fig. 10.167 Osteochondritis dissecans involving the lateral aspect of the medial femoral condyle in a 12-year-old boy, which is seen as a poorly defined zone of low-intermediate signal in the subchondral marrow (arrow) on coronal proton density–weighted imaging (a) and high signal (arrow) on coronal fat-suppressed T2-weighted imaging (b).

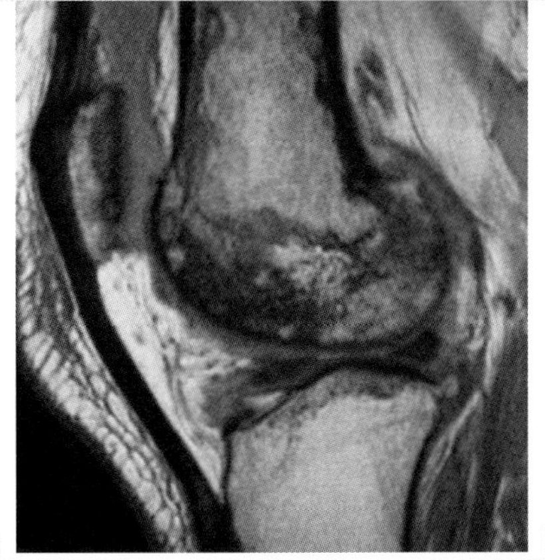

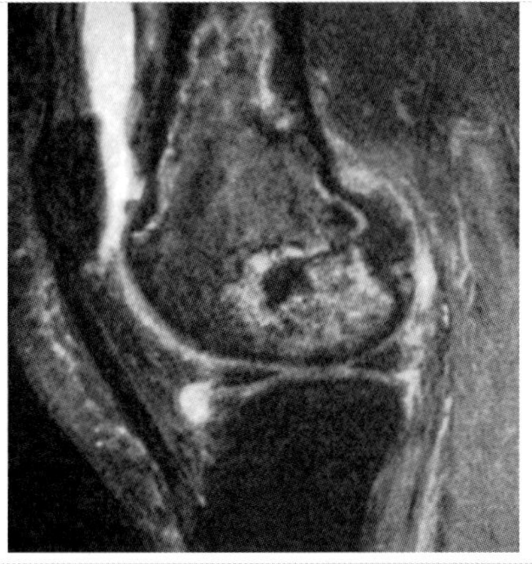

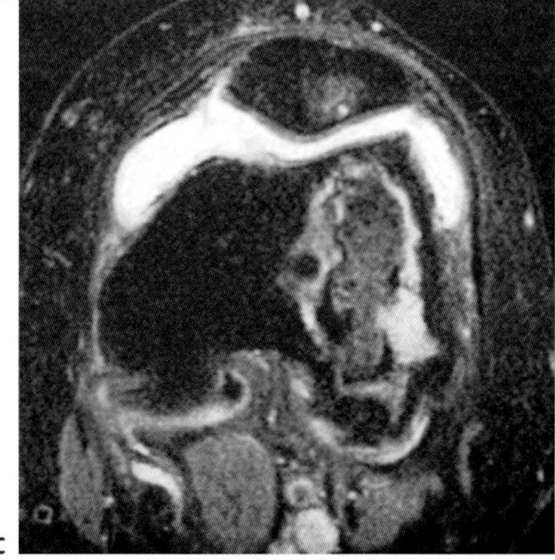

Fig. 10.168 A 49-year-old woman with a bone infarct in the distal femur as seen on sagittal proton density–weighted imaging (a) and sagittal (b) and axial fat-suppressed T2-weighted imaging (c).

Table 10.7 (Cont.) Solitary intramedullary lesions located near the ends of tubular bones

Abnormalities	MRI findings	Comments
Transient bone marrow edema (acute bone marrow edema syndromes [aBMEs], transient osteoporosis of the hip, regional migratory osteoporosis) (▶ Fig. 10.169)	Poorly defined zones with low-intermediate signal on T1WI and high signal on FS T2WI and short TI inversion recovery (STIR) are seen in the marrow of the proximal hip (femoral head and neck). The signal abnormalities may spare the subchondral marrow. Magnetic resonance imaging (MRI) findings can be seen within 48 hours of the onset of symptoms. Joint effusions may be present. With dynamic Gd-contrast administration, delayed peak enhancement can be seen with aBME.	Idiopathic spontaneous process with transient edema in bone marrow that is not secondary to trauma and may or may not be associated with osteoporosis. aBME frequently involves the proximal femur in men between 30 and 50 years and women in the last trimester of pregnancy.
Osteomyelitis (▶ Fig. 10.170)	In acute osteomyelitis, poorly defined zones of low or low-intermediate signal on T1WI and high signal on T2WI, STIR, and FS T2WI are seen in the marrow. Loss of definition of the low signal line of the cortical margins is often observed on T1WI, T2WI, STIR, and FS T2WI. After Gd-contrast administration, irregular zones of contrast enhancement are seen in the involved marrow on FS T1WI. In the subacute phase of osteomyelitis, the pyogenic process becomes more localized. The zone of transition between normal and abnormal bone is sharper and more well defined in subacute and chronic osteomyelitis than with acute osteomyelitis.	Infection of bone, which can result from hematogenous spread of micro-organisms as well as from trauma-direct inoculation, extension from adjacent tissues, and complications from surgery. Bacteria such as *Staphylococcus aureus* and *Streptococcus pyogenes* are the most common infectious organisms. Can also result from other bacteria as well as tuberculosis, fungi, parasites, and viruses.
Eosinophilic granuloma (▶ Fig. 10.171)	Intramedullary lesions associated with trabecular and cortical bone destruction, which typically have low-intermediate signal on T1WI and PDWI and heterogeneous slightly high to high signal on T2WI. Poorly defined zones of high signal on T2WI are usually seen in the marrow peripheral to the lesions secondary to inflammatory changes. Extension of lesions from the marrow into adjacent soft tissues through areas of cortical disruption are commonly seen as well as linear periosteal zones of high signal on T2WI. Lesions typically show prominent Gd-contrast enhancement in marrow and in extraosseous soft tissue portions of the lesions.	Benign tumor-like lesions consisting of Langerhans cells (histiocytes), and variable amounts of lymphocytes, polymorphonuclear cells, and eosinophils. Account for 1% of primary bone lesions and 8% of tumor-like lesions. Occur in patients with median age = 10 years, average = 13.5 years, peak incidence is between 5 and 10 years; 80 to 85% occur in patients less than 30 years.
Malignant lesions		
Metastatic lesion	Single or multiple well-circumscribed or poorly defined infiltrative lesions involving marrow associated with cortical destruction and extraosseous extension. Lesions often have low-intermediate signal on T1WI and low, intermediate, and/or high signal on T2WI and FS T1WI; usually show Gd-contrast enhancement. Pathological fractures can be associated with metastatic lesions involving tubular bones and vertebrae. Periosteal reaction is uncommon.	Metastatic lesions typically occur in the marrow with or without cortical destruction and extraosseous tumor extension.
Plasmacytoma (▶ Fig. 10.172)	Well-circumscribed or poorly defined infiltrative lesions involving marrow, low-intermediate signal on T1WI, intermediate-high signal on T2WI and FS T2WI; usually show Gd-contrast-enhancement, eventual cortical bone destruction, and extraosseous extension.	Malignant tumors composed of proliferating antibody-secreting plasma cells derived from single clones. Most common primary neoplasm of bone in adults, median = 60 years. Most patients are older than 40 years. May have variable destructive or infiltrative changes involving the axial and/or appendicular skeleton.

(continued on page 452)

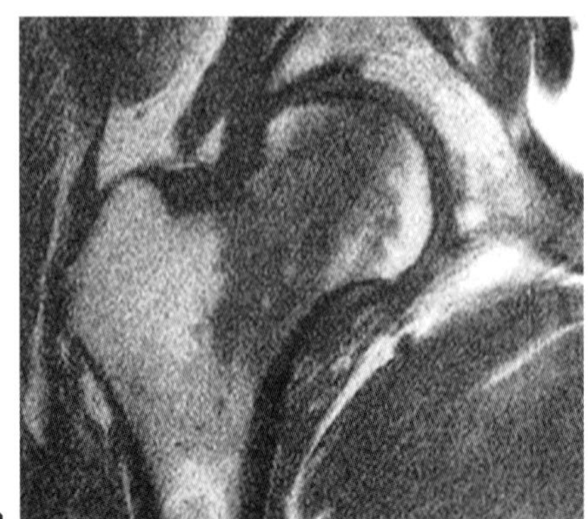
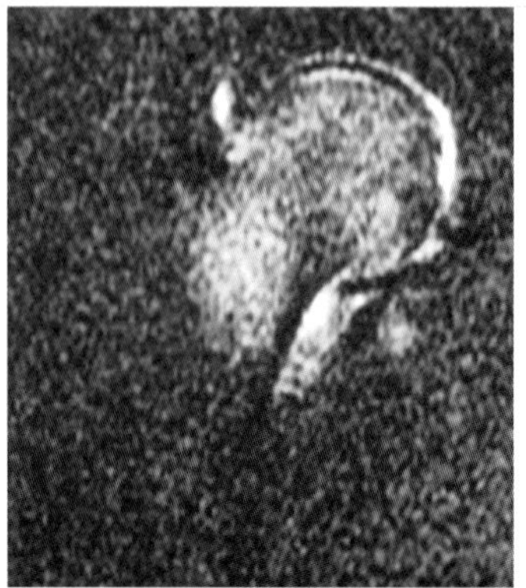
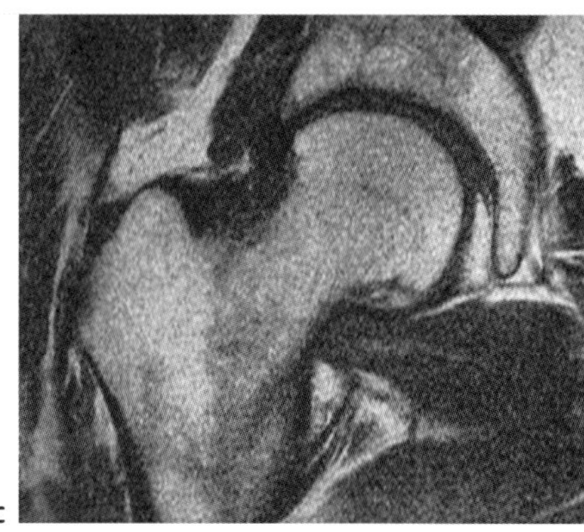

Fig. 10.169 A 51-year-old man with hip pain and magnetic resonance imaging showing acute bone marrow edema with a poorly defined zone with low-intermediate signal in the marrow of the proximal femur on coronal T1-weighted imaging (T1WI) (a) with corresponding high signal on coronal fat-suppressed T2-weighted imaging (b). The abnormal marrow signal resolved 2 months later as seen on coronal T1WI (c).

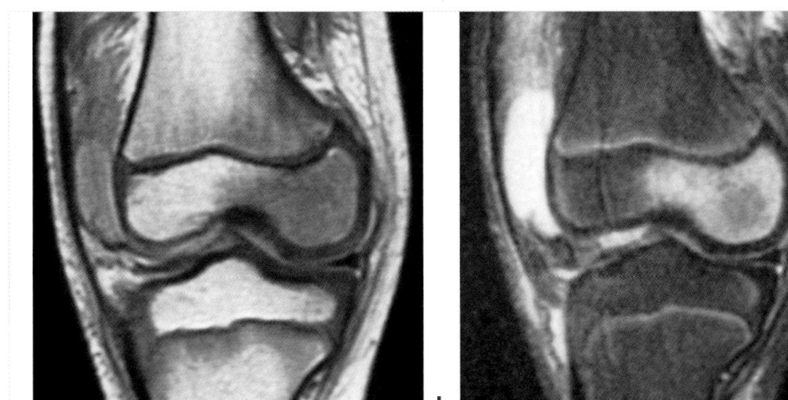
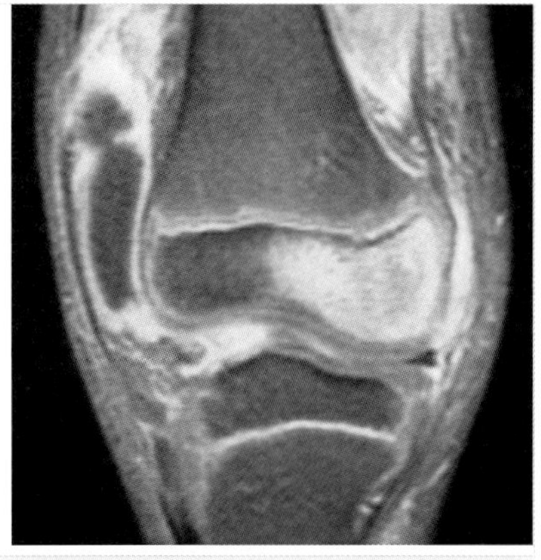

Fig. 10.170 An 11-year-old boy with septic arthritis and pyogenic osteomyelitis from *Staphylococcus aureus* involving the marrow of the femoral epiphysis. A poorly defined zone of intermediate signal is seen in the epiphyseal marrow on coronal T1-weighted imaging (T1WI) (a) with corresponding high signal on coronal fat-suppressed (FS) T2-weighted imaging (b). Abnormal gadolinium-contrast enhancement is seen in the marrow on coronal FS T1WI (c) as well as along the margins of the septic joint collection.

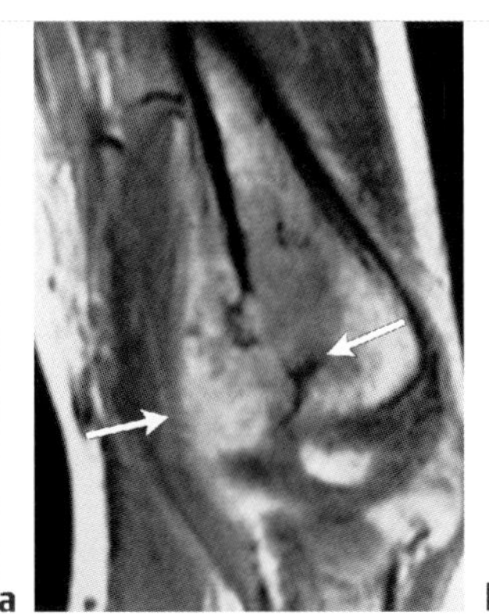
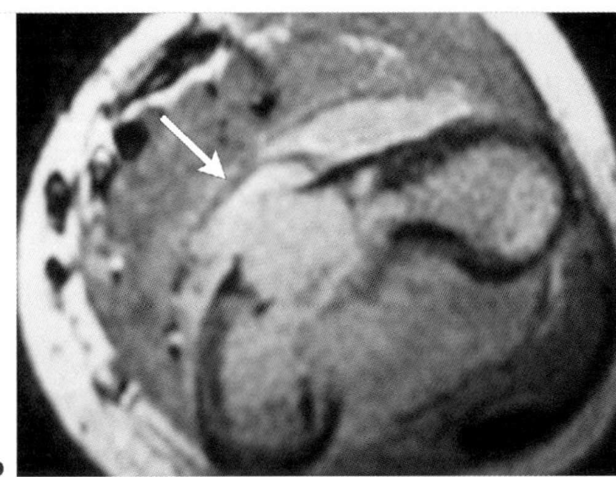

Fig. 10.171 A 5-year-old boy with an eosinophilic granuloma involving the distal humerus. The lesion in the marrow is associated with cortical destruction and extraosseous extension into the adjacent soft tissues (arrows) as seen on sagittal gadolinium-contrast enhanced T1-weighted imaging (a) and axial proton density–weighted imaging (b).

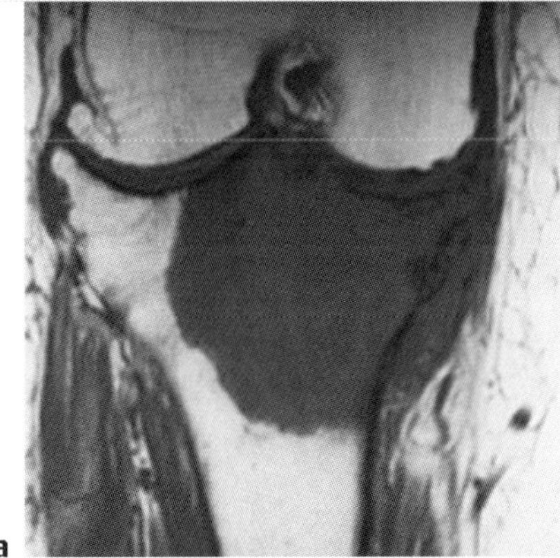
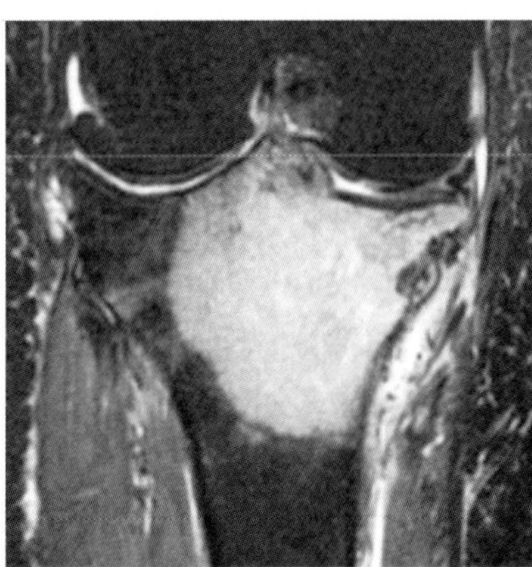
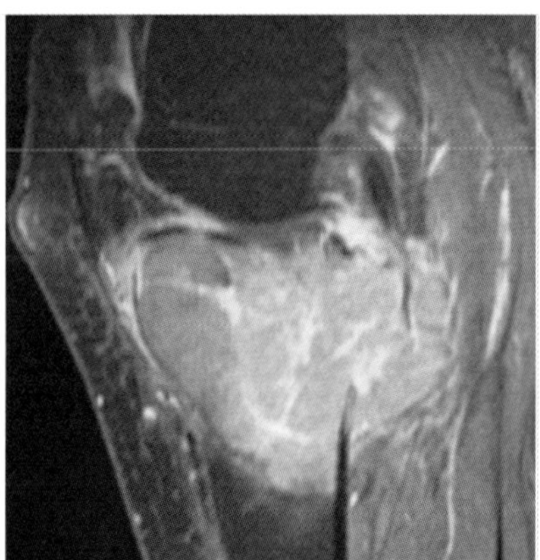

Fig. 10.172 A 77-year-old woman with a plasmacytoma involving the marrow of the proximal tibia, which has low-intermediate signal on coronal T1-weighted imaging (T1WI) (a) and high signal on coronal fat-suppressed (FS) T2-weighted imaging (b). The tumor shows Gd-contrast enhancement on sagittal FS T1WI (c) and extends through destroyed bone cortex into the adjacent soft tissues.

Table 10.7 (Cont.) Solitary intramedullary lesions located near the ends of tubular bones

Abnormalities	MRI findings	Comments
Lymphoma (▶ Fig. 10.173)	Non-Hodgkin lymphoma (NHL) and Hodgkin disease (HD) within bone typically appears as single or multifocal poorly defined or circumscribed intramedullary zones with low-intermediate signal on T1WI; intermediate, slightly high, and/or high signal on T2WI; and high signal on FS T2WI; often show Gd-contrast enhancement. Zones of cortical destruction may occur associated with extraosseous soft tissue extension.	Lymphoid tumors with neoplastic cells typically within lymphoid tissue (lymph nodes and reticuloendothelial organs). Unlike leukemia, lymphoma usually arises as discrete masses. Lymphomas are subdivided into HD and NHL. Almost all primary lymphomas of bone are B-cell NHL. HD, mean age = 32 years. Osseous NHL, median = 35 years.
Leukemia	Single or multiple well-circumscribed or poorly defined infiltrative lesions involving marrow; low-intermediate signal on T1WI, intermediate-high signal on T2WI and FS T2WI; often shows Gd-contrast enhancement, ± cortical bone destruction and extraosseous extension.	Malignant lymphoid neoplasms with involvement of bone marrow as well as tumor cells also in peripheral blood.
Chondrosarcoma (▶ Fig. 10.174)	Intramedullary tumors often have low-intermediate signal on T1WI, intermediate signal on PDWI, and heterogeneous intermediate-high signal on T2WI. Lesions usually show heterogeneous contrast enhancement.	Malignant tumors containing cartilage formed within sarcomatous stroma. Account for12 to 21% of malignant bone lesions, 21 to 26% of primary sarcomas of bone.Mean age = 40 years, median = 26 to 59 years. Clear cell chondrosarcomas are commonly located near the ends of long bones.

(continued on page 454)

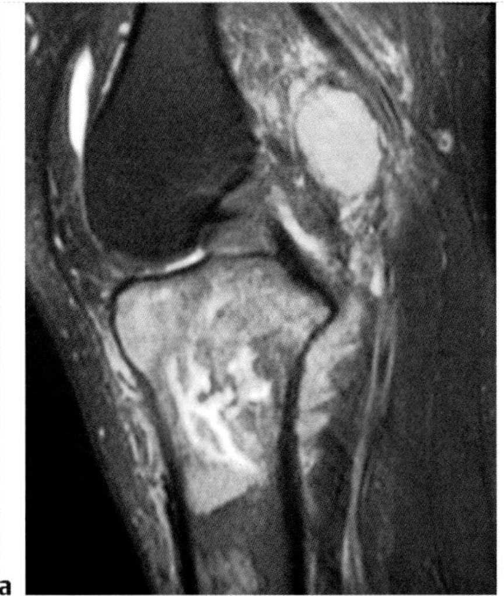

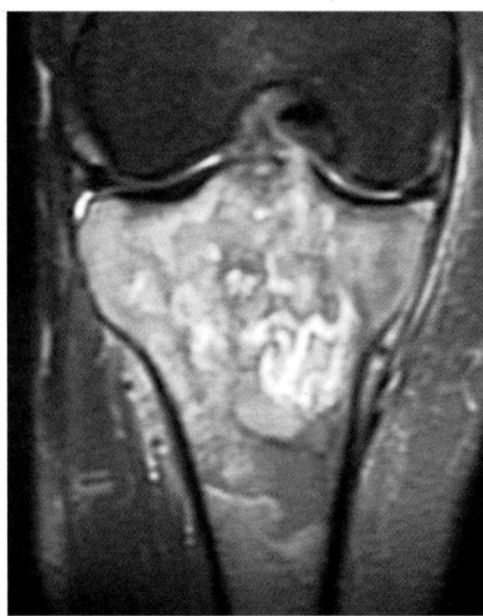

Fig. 10.173 A 32-year-old woman with large B-cell non-Hodgkin lymphoma involving the marrow of the proximal tibia seen as diffuse high signal on sagittal (a) and coronal fat-suppressed T2-weighted imaging (b).

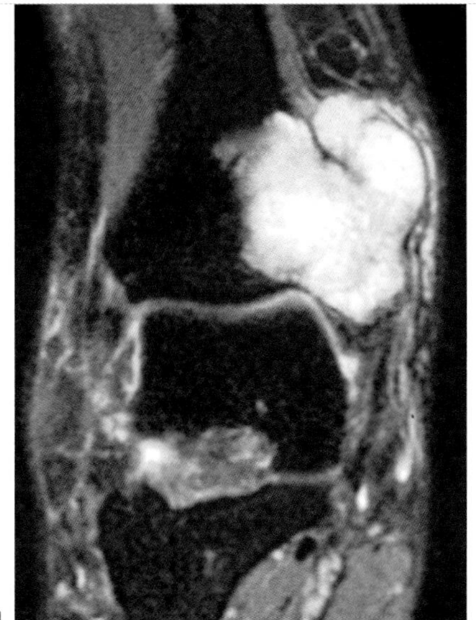

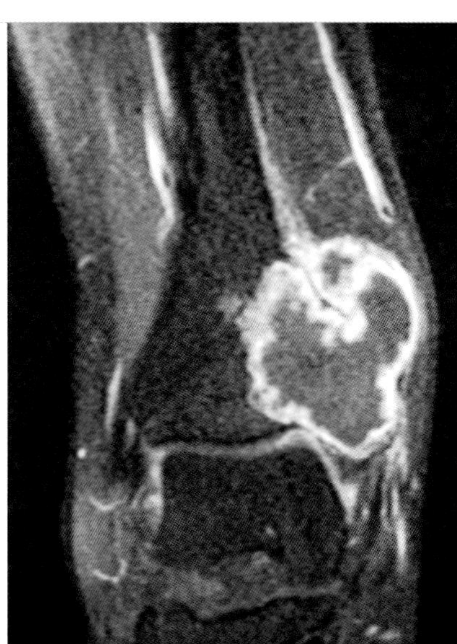

Fig. 10.174 A 44-year-old woman with a chondrosarcoma in the marrow of the distal tibia associated with cortical destruction and extraosseous extension of tumor. The tumor has high signal on coronal fat-suppressed (FS) T2-weighted imaging (a) and shows peripheral lobular Gd-contrast enhancement on FS T1-weighted imaging (b). Tumor extends through the bone cortex into the extraosseous soft tissues.

Table 10.7 (Cont.) Solitary intramedullary lesions located near the ends of tubular bones

Abnormalities	MRI findings	Comments
Osteosarcoma (▶ Fig. 10.175)	Destructive intramedullary malignant lesions, low-intermediate signal on T1WI; mixed low, intermediate, high signal on T2WI, usually with matrix mineralization/ ossification-low signal on T2WI; usually show Gd-contrast enhancement (usually heterogeneous). Zones of cortical destruction are typically seen through which tumors extend into the extraosseous soft tissues under an elevated periosteum. Lamellated and/or spiculated zones of bone formation can occur under the periosteal elevation secondary to tumor invasion and perforation of bone cortex.	Malignant tumor composed of proliferating neoplastic spindle cells, which produce osteoid and/or immature tumoral bone and which most frequently arise within medullary bone. Two age peaks of incidence. The larger peak occurs between the ages of 10 and 20 and accounts for over half of the cases. The second smaller peak occurs in adults over 60 years and accounts for approximately 10% of the cases.
Ewing sarcoma (▶ Fig. 10.176)	Destructive malignant lesions involving marrow. Low-intermediate signal on T1WI; mixed low, intermediate, and/ or high signal on T2WI and FS T2WI; usually shows Gd-contrast enhancement (usually heterogeneous). Extraosseous tumor extension through sites of cortical destruction is commonly seen beneath an elevated periosteum. Thin striated zones of low signal on T2WI can sometimes be seen oriented perpendicular to the long axis of the involved bone under the elevated periosteum representing the hair on end appearance of reactive bone formation secondary to the tumor. In long bones, tumors are most often located in the diaphyseal region, followed by the metadiaphyseal region.	Malignant primitive tumor of bone composed of undifferentiated small cells with round nuclei. Accounts for 6 to 11% of primary malignant bone tumors, 5 to 7% of primary bone tumors. Usually occurs between the ages of 5 and 30, males > females, locally invasive, high metastatic potential.

(continued on page 456)

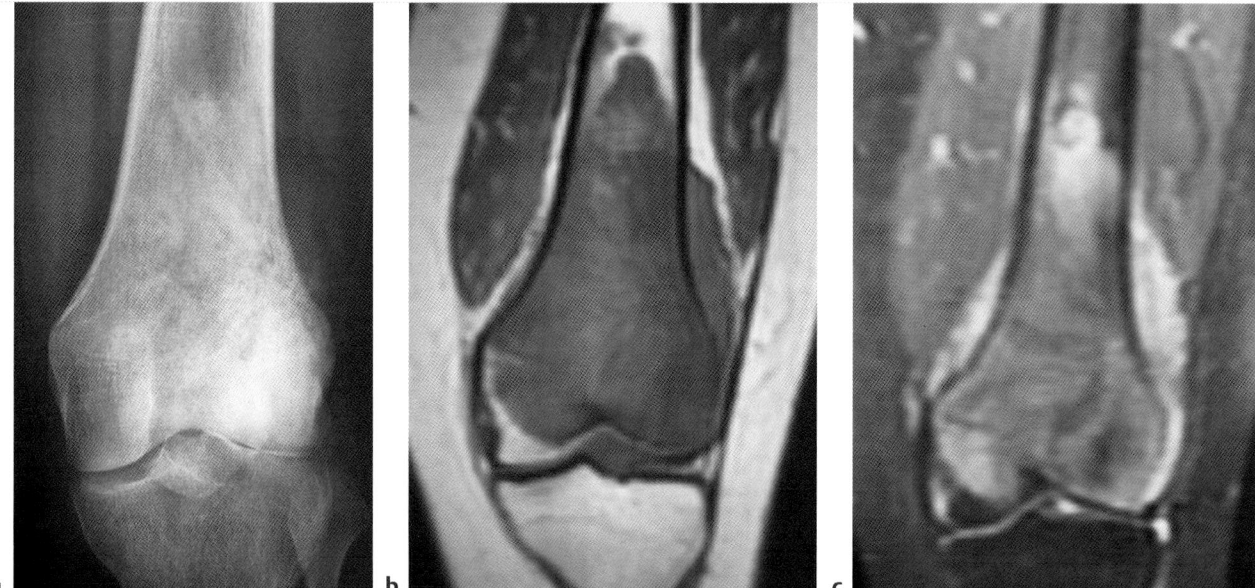

Fig. 10.175 A 16-year-old girl with osteosarcoma in the distal femur associated with malignant osteoid mineralization (a). The tumor has low-intermediate signal on coronal T1-weighted imaging (b) and has heterogeneous slightly high signal on coronal fat-suppressed T2-weighted imaging (c). The tumor is associated with cortical bone destruction and extraosseous extension.

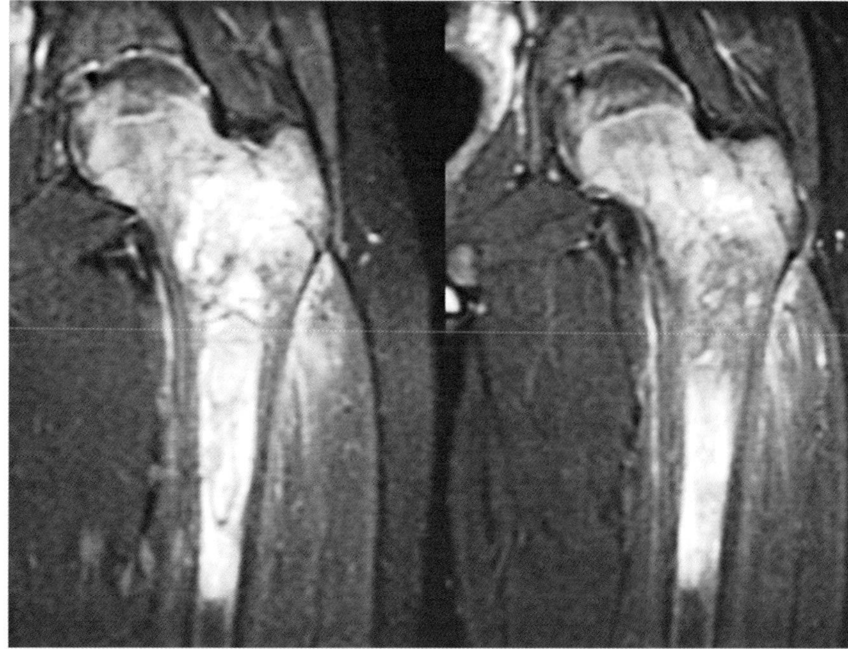

Fig. 10.176 A 15-year-old boy with Ewing sarcoma in the marrow of the proximal femur, which has high signal on coronal fat-suppressed T2-weighted imaging.

Table 10.7 (Cont.) Solitary intramedullary lesions located near the ends of tubular bones

Abnormalities	MRI findings	Comments
Malignant giant cell tumor of bone (▶ Fig. 10.177)	Well-defined lesions with or without thin low signal margins on T1WI and T2WI. Solid portions of giant cell tumors often have low to intermediate signal on T1WI and PDWI, intermediate to high signal on T2WI, and high signal on FS PDWI and FS T2WI. Signal heterogeneity on T2WI is not uncommon. Aneurysmal bone cysts are seen with 14% of giant cell tumors. Lesions show mild to prominent variable and often heterogeneous Gd-contrast enhancement. Cortical destruction and extraosseous tumor extension are frequently seen.	Aggressive bone tumors composed of neoplastic ovoid mononuclear cells and scattered multinucleated osteoclast-like giant cells. Up to 10% of all giant cell tumors are malignant. Benign giant cell tumors account for approximately 5 to 9.5% of all bone tumors and up to 23% of benign bone tumors. 75% of malignant giant cell tumors occur in patients between the ages of 15 and 45 years.
Fibrosarcoma	Intramedullary lesions with irregular margins, with or without associated cortical destruction and/or extraosseous softtissue masses. Lesions usually have low-intermediate signal on T1WI and PDWI and heterogeneous intermediate, slightly high, and/or high signal on T2WI. Lesions usually show heterogeneous Gd-contrast enhancement.	Uncommon malignant tumors consisting of bundles of neoplastic fibroblasts/spindle cells with varying proportions of collagen, lacking other tissue-differentiating features such as tumor bone, osteoid, or cartilage. Can be primary lesions (75%) or arise as secondary tumors (25%) associated with prior irradiation, Paget disease, bone infarct, chronic osteomyelitis, fibrous dysplasia, giant cell tumor. Accounts for 3 to 5% of primary malignant bone tumors and 2 to 4% of all bone tumors. Median age = 43 years.
Malignant fibrous histiocytoma	Intramedullary lesions with irregular margins with zones of cortical destruction and extraosseous extension. Tumors often have low-intermediate signal on T1WI, low-intermediate signal on PDWI, and heterogeneous intermediate-high signal on T2WI and FS T2WI. Invasion into joints occurs in 30%. May be associated with other bone infarcts, bone cysts, chronic osteomyelitis, Paget disease, and other treated primary bone tumors. Lesions usually show heterogeneous Gd-contrast prominent enhancement.	Malignant tumor involving soft tissue and rarely bone derived from undifferentiated mesenchymal cells. Contains cells with limited cellular differentiation such as mixtures of fibroblasts, myofibroblasts, histiocyte-like cells, anaplastic giant cells, and inflammatory cells. Accounts for 1 to 5% of primary malignant bone tumors and < 1% to 3% of all primary bone tumors. Patient ages range from 11 to 80 years, median = 48 years, mean = 55 years.
Hemangioendothelioma (▶ Fig. 10.178)	Intramedullary tumors, which often have low-intermediate and/or high signal on T1WI and heterogeneous intermediate-high signal on T2WI and FS T2WI with or without zones of low signal. Cortical expansion with or without extraosseous extension of tumor through zones of cortical destruction can occur. Lesions often show prominent heterogeneous Gd-contrast enhancement.	Low-grade vasoformative/endothelial malignant neoplasms, which are locally aggressive and rarely metastasize, compared with the high-grade endothelial tumors such as angiosarcoma. Account for less than 1% of primary malignant bone tumors. Patients range from 10 to 82 years, median = 36 to 47 years. Patients with multifocal lesions tend to be approximately 10 years younger on average than those with unifocal tumors.

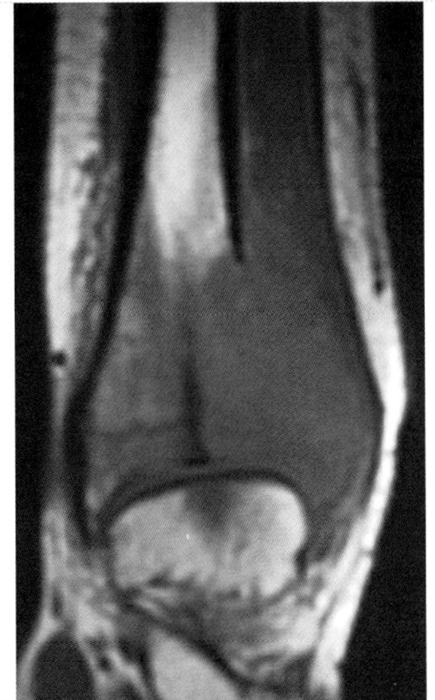

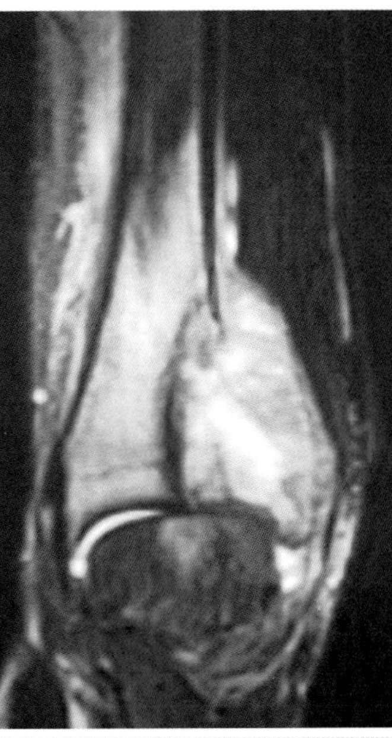

Fig. 10.177 A 16-year-old boy with a malignant giant cell tumor of the distal tibia associated with destruction of cortical bone with extraosseous extension as seen on coronal T1-weighted imaging (a) and fat-suppressed T2-weighted imaging (b).

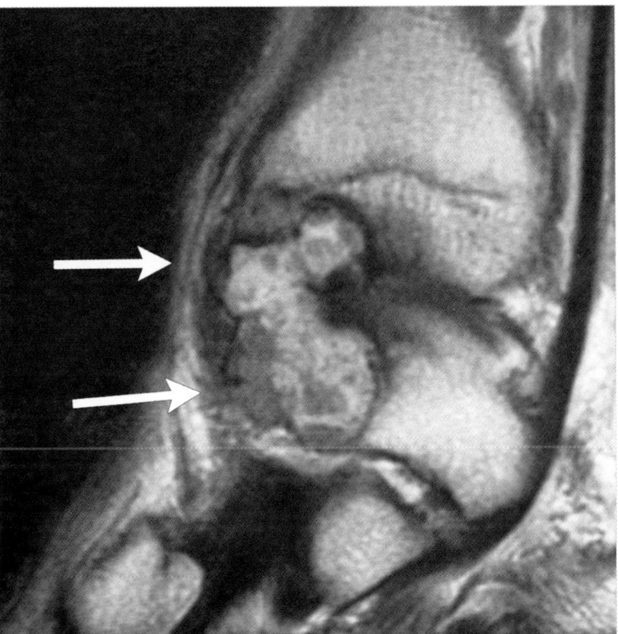

Fig. 10.178 A 19-year-old man with hemangioendothelioma involving the distal tibia with cortical disruption and tumor extension into the ankle joint as seen on sagittal T2-weighted imaging (arrows).

10.8 Solitary Intramedullary Metadiaphyseal Lesions

- Nonmalignant lesions
  - Nonossifying fibroma
  - Enchondroma
  - Unicameral bone cyst (UBC)
  - Aneurysmal bone cyst (ABC)
  - Giant cell tumor (prior to physeal plate closure)
  - Giant cell reparative granuloma
  - Chondromyxoid fibroma
  - Hemangioma
  - Intraosseous lipoma
  - Fibrous dysplasia
  - Liposclerosing myxofibrous tumor
  - Stress fracture
  - Bone infarct
  - Eosinophilic granuloma
  - Osteomyelitis
- Malignant lesions
  - Metastatic lesion
  - Plasmacytoma/myeloma
  - Lymphoma
  - Osteosarcoma
  - Ewing sarcoma
  - Chondrosarcoma
  - Fibrosarcoma
  - Malignant fibrous histiocytoma

Table 10.8 Solitary intramedullary metadiaphyseal lesions

Abnormalities	MRI findings	Comments
Nonmalignant lesions		
Nonossifying fibroma (▶ Fig. 10.179)	Well-circumscribed eccentric intramedullary lesions in the dimetaphyseal regions of long bones, which have mixed low-intermediate signal on T1-weighted imaging (T1WI) and mixed low, intermediate, and/or high signal on T2-weighted imaging (T2WI), proton density–weighted imaging (PDWI), and fat-suppressed (FS) T2WI. Zones of low signal on T1WI, PDWI, and T2WI can be seen in the central portions of the lesions. Zones with varying thickness of low signal on T1WI, PDWI, and T2WI are seen at the margins of the lesions representing bone sclerosis. Internal septations are commonly seen as zones of low signal on T2WI in these lesions. Lesions can show gadolinium (Gd)-contrast enhancement (heterogeneous > homogeneous patterns).	Common benign fibrohistiocytic lesions in the metaphyseal portions of long bones, which are composed of whorls of fibroblastic cells combined with smaller amounts of multinucleated giant cells and xanthomatous cells. Usually asymptomatic, 95% occur between the ages of 5 and 20, median = 14 years.
Enchondroma (▶ Fig. 10.180)	Lobulated intramedullary lesions with well-defined borders, mean size = 5 cm. Lesions usually have low-intermediate signal on T1WI and intermediate signal on PDWI. On T2WI and FS T2WI, lesions usually have predominantly high signal with foci and/or bands of low signal representing areas of matrix mineralization and fibrous strands. Lesions typically show Gd-contrast enhancement in various patterns (peripheral curvilinear lobular, central nodular/septal, and peripheral lobular).	Benign intramedullary lesions composed of hyaline cartilage, represent approximately 10% of benign bone tumors. Enchondromas can be solitary (88%) or multiple (12%). Median age = 35 years, peak in third and fourth decades.

(continued on page 460)

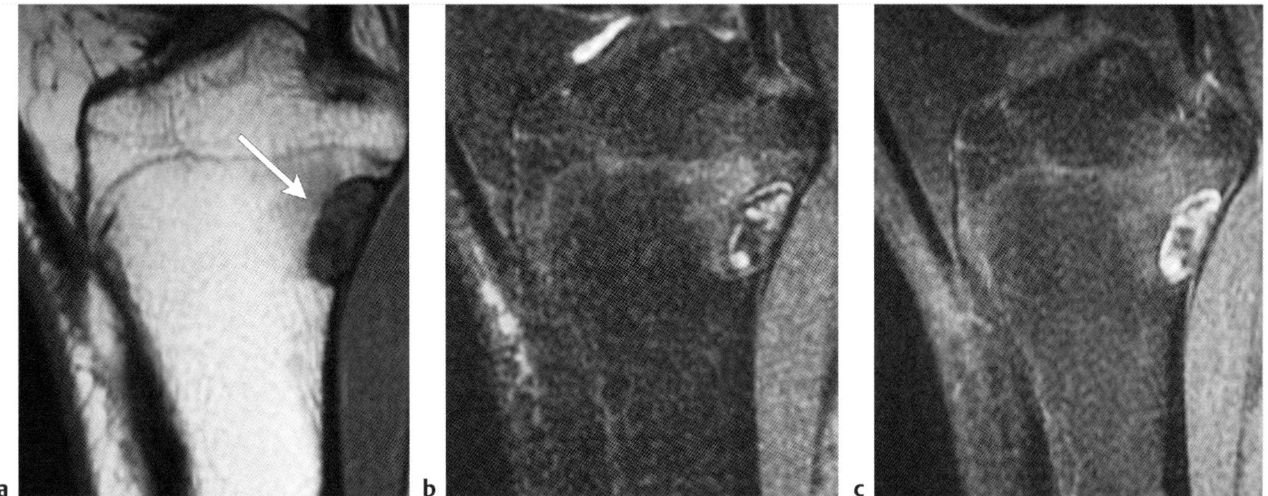

Fig. 10.179 A 15-year-old girl with a nonossifying fibroma in the dorsal proximal tibia (arrow), which has a thin peripheral rim of low signal surrounding a central zone with low-intermediate signal on sagittal T1-weighted imaging (T1WI) (a) and mixed low and high signal on fat-suppressed (FS) T2-weighted imaging (b). The lesion shows thin marginal and central gadolinium-contrast enhancement on sagittal FS T1WI (c).

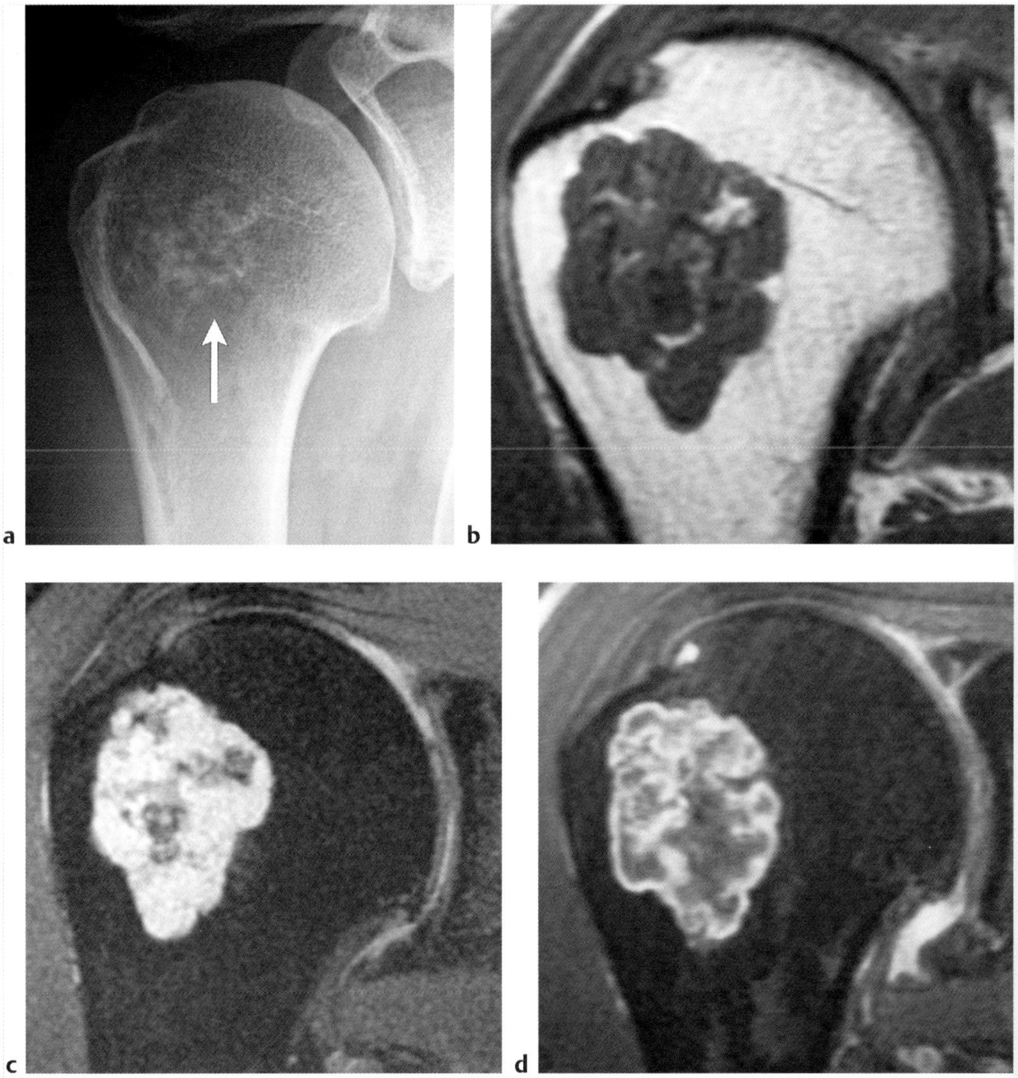

Fig. 10.180 A 46-year-old man with an enchondroma in the metadiaphyseal portion of the proximal humerus, which has chondroid mineralization (arrow) on anteroposterior radiograph (a). The lesion has predominantly intermediate signal on coronal proton density–weighted imaging (b) and high signal on fat-suppressed (FS) T2-weighted imaging (c) as well as zones of low signal corresponding to mineralized chondroid matrix. The lesion shows peripheral lobular contrast enhancement on coronal FS T1-weighted imaging (d).

Table 10.8 (Cont.) Solitary intramedullary metadiaphyseal lesions

Abnormalities	MRI findings	Comments
Unicameral bone cyst (UBC) (▶ Fig. 10.181)	UBCs often have a peripheral rim of low signal on T1WI and T2WI adjacent to normal medullary bone. UBCs usually contain fluid with low to low-intermediate signal on T1WI and low-intermediate and high signal on T2WI. Fluid-fluid levels may occur. For UBCs without pathological fracture, thin peripheral Gd-contrast enhancement can be seen at the margins of lesions. UBCs with pathological fracture can have heterogeneous or homogeneous low-intermediate or slightly high signal on T1WI, and heterogeneous or homogeneous high signal on T2WI and FS T2WI. UBCs complicated by fracture can have internal septations and fluid-fluid levels, as well as irregular peripheral Gd-contrast enhancement and at internal septations.	Intramedullary nonneoplastic cavities filled with serous or serosanguinous fluid. Account for 9% of primary tumor-like lesions of bone; 85% occur in the first 2 decades, median = 11 years.
Aneurysmal bone cyst (ABC) (▶ Fig. 10.182)	ABCs often have a low signal rim on T1WI and T2WI adjacent to normal medullary bone and between extraosseous soft tissues. Various combinations of low, intermediate, and/or high signal on T1WI, PDWI, and T2WI are usually seen within ABCs as well as fluid-fluid levels. Variable Gd-contrast enhancement is seen at the margins of lesions as well as involving the internal septae.	Tumor-like expansile bone lesions containing cavernous spaces filled with blood. ABCs can be primary bone lesions (two thirds) or secondary to other bone lesions/tumors (such as giant cell tumors, chondroblastomas, osteoblastomas, osteosarcomas. chondromyxoid fibromas, nonossifying fibromas, fibrous dysplasia, fibrosarcomas, malignant fibrous histiocytomas, and metastatic disease). Account for approximately 11% of primary tumor-like lesions of bone. Patients usually range in age from 1 to 25 years, median = 14 years.
Giant cell tumor of bone (prior to physeal plate closure) (▶ Fig. 10.183)	Often well-defined lesions with thin low signal margins on T1WI, PDWI, and T2WI. Solid portions of giant cell tumors often have low to intermediate signal on T1WI and PDWI, intermediate to high signal on T2WI, and high signal on FS PDWI and FS T2WI. Zones of low signal on T2WI may be seen secondary to hemosiderin. ABCs can be seen in 14% of giant cell tumors. Areas of cortical thinning, expansion, and/or destruction can occur with extraosseous extension. Tumors show varying degrees of Gd-contrast enhancement.	Aggressive bone tumors composed of neoplastic mononuclear cells and scattered multinucleated osteoclast-like giant cells. Account for 23% of primary nonmalignant bone tumors, and 5 to 9% of all primary bone tumors; median age = 30 years.

(continued on page 462)

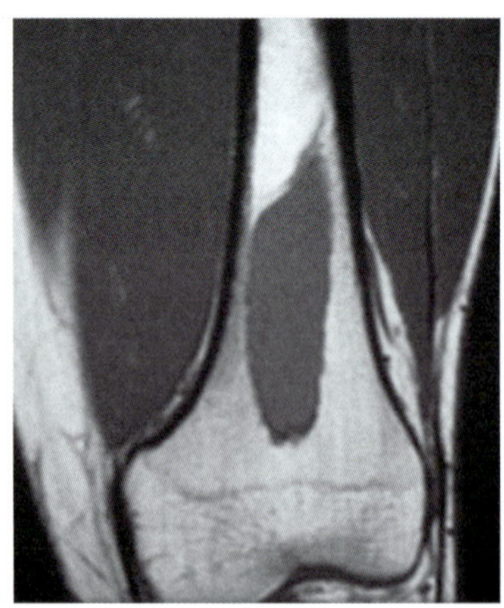

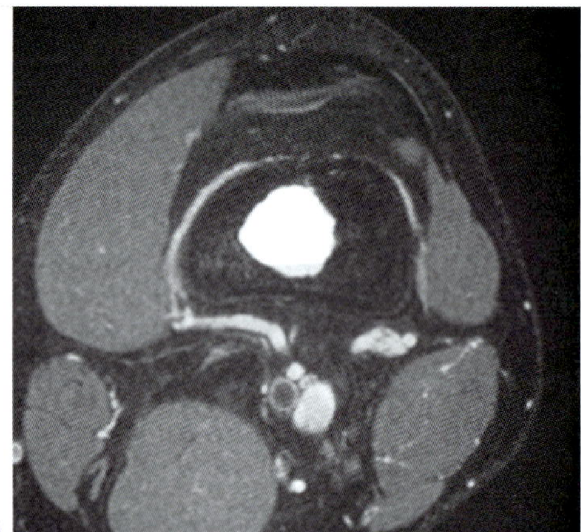

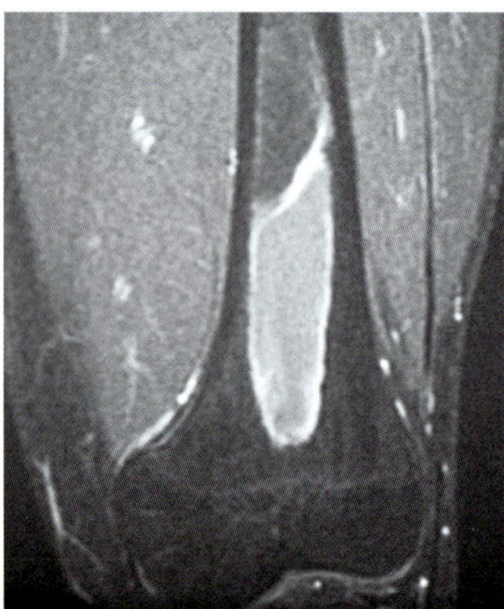

Fig. 10.181 A 16-year-old male with a unicameral bone cyst in the distal femur, which has low-intermediate signal on coronal T1-weighted imaging (T1WI) (a) and high signal on axial fat-suppressed (FS) T2-weighted imaging (b). The lesion shows thin peripheral rim Gd-contrast enhancement on coronal FS T1WI (c).

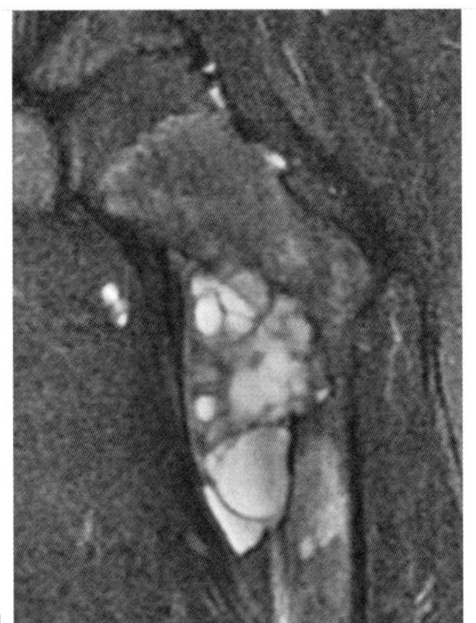

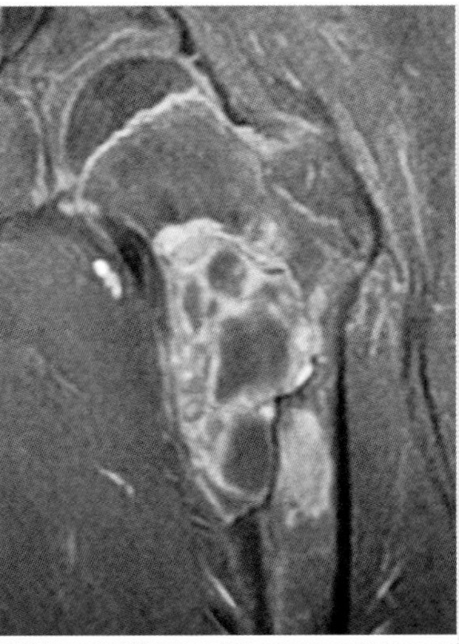

Fig. 10.182 An 11-year-old male with an expansile aneurysmal bone cyst in the proximal femur, which has multiple septations and compartments with high signal on coronal fat-suppressed (FS) T2-weighted imaging (a). Gadolinium-contrast enhancement is seen at the margins and between the fluid zones on coronal FS T1-weighted imaging (b).

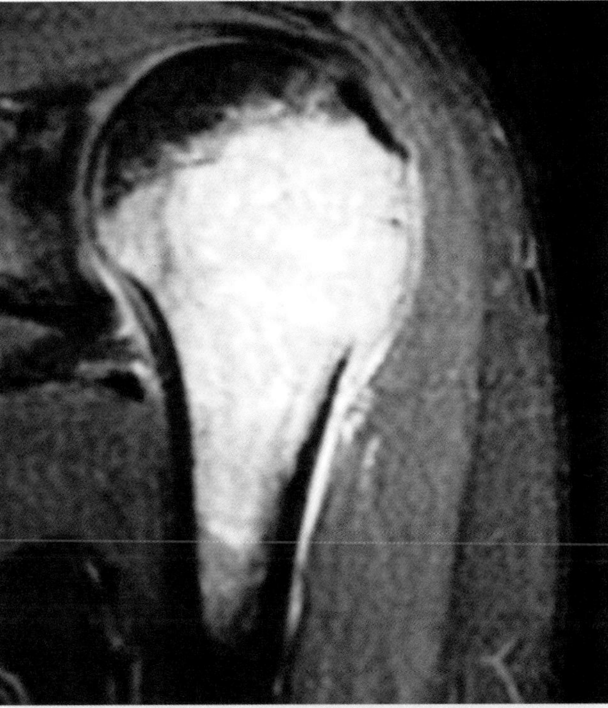

Fig. 10.183 A 14-year-old boy with a giant cell tumor within the metadiaphyseal portion of the proximal humerus, which shows prominent Gd-contrast enhancement on coronal fat-suppressed T1-weighted imaging, as well as cortical destruction and extraosseous extension.

Table 10.8 (Cont.) Solitary intramedullary metadiaphyseal lesions

Abnormalities	MRI findings	Comments
Giant cell reparative granuloma (▶ Fig. 10.184)	Lesions can have heterogeneous low, intermediate, and/or high signal on T1WI, PDWI, and T2WI as well as peripheral rimlike and central Gd-contrast enhancement on FS T1WI. May be surrounded by a poorly defined zone of high signal on FS T2WI and Gd-contrast enhancement in the adjacent marrow.	Giant cell reparative granulomas are also referred to as solid ABCs. Histological appearance resembles brown tumors.
Chondromyxoid fibroma (▶ Fig. 10.185)	Lesions are often slightly lobulated with low-intermediate signal on T1WI, intermediate signal on PDWI, and heterogeneous predominantly high signal on T2WI. Thin low signal septa within lesions on T2WI are secondary to fibrous strands. Lesions are surrounded by low signal borders representing thin sclerotic reaction. Edema is not typically seen in adjacent medullary bone. Lesions show prominent diffuse Gd-contrast enhancement.	Rare, benign, slow-growing bone lesions that contain chondroid, myxoid, and fibrous components. Chondromyxoid fibromas represent 2 to 4% of primary benign bone lesions and < 1% of primary bone lesions. Most chondromyxoid fibromas occur between the ages of 1 to 40 years, with a median of 17 years and peak incidence in the second to third decades.
Hemangioma	Often well-circumscribed lesions that typically have intermediate to high signal on T1WI, PDWI, T2WI, and FS T2WI. On T1WI, hemangiomas usually have signal equal to or greater than adjacent normal marrow secondary to fatty components. Usually show Gd-contrast enhancement. Pathological fractures associated with intraosseous hemangiomas usually result in low-intermediate marrow signal on T1WI.	Common benign lesions of bone composed of capillary, cavernous, and/or malformed venous vessels. Hemangiomas have been considered to be a hamartomatous disorder. Account for 4% of benign bone tumors and approximately 1% of all bone tumors, likely underestimated. Occur in all ages, median = 33 years.
Intraosseous lipoma (▶ Fig. 10.186)	Lesions can have heterogeneous low, intermediate, and/or high signal on T1WI, PDWI, and T2WI as well as peripheral rimlike and central Gd-contrast enhancement on FS T1WI.	Uncommon benign hamartomas composed of mature white adipose tissue without cellular atypia. Osseous or chondroid metaplasia with myxoid changes can be associated with lipomas. Account for approximately 0.1% of bone tumors, likely underreported.

(continued on page 464)

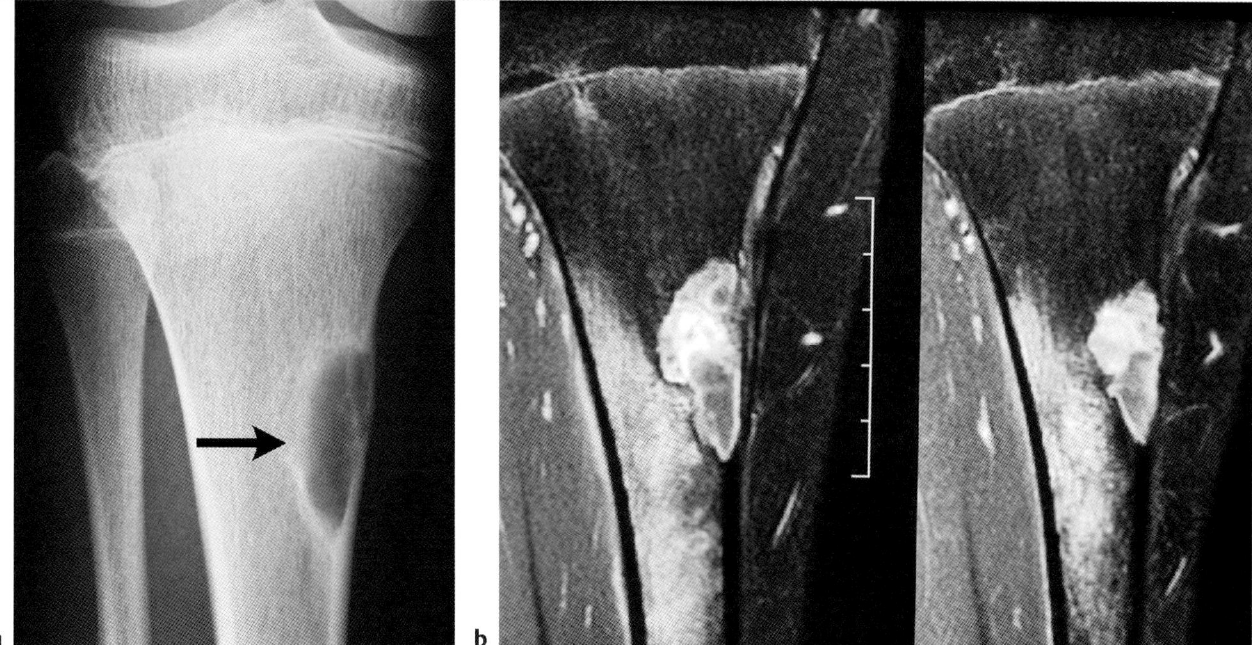

Fig. 10.184 A 14-year-old boy with a giant cell granuloma (also called solid aneurysmal bone cyst) in the metadiaphyseal portion of the proximal tibia, which is seen as a radiolucent lesion with thin sclerotic margins (arrow) on radiograph (a). Gadolinium-contrast enhancement is seen within the lesion as well as in the adjacent marrow on coronal fat-suppressed T1-weighted imaging (b).

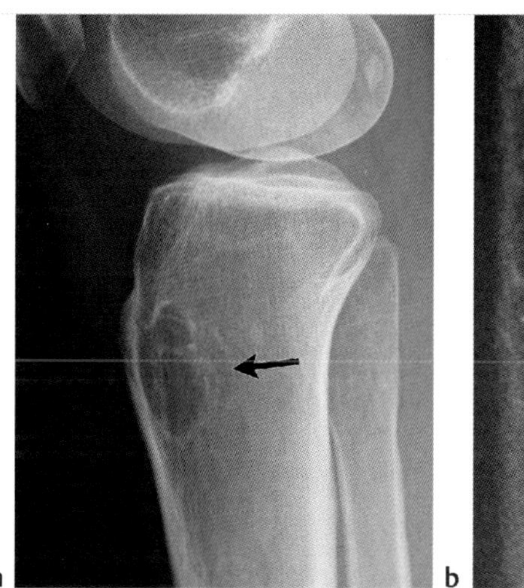

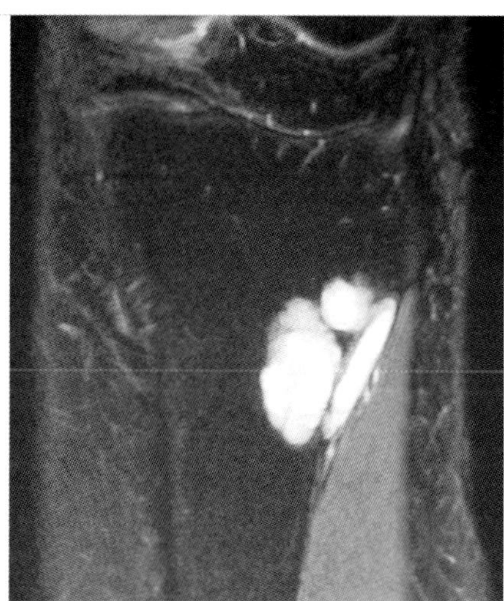

Fig. 10.185 A 48-year-old woman with a chondromyxoid fibroma involving the metadiaphyseal portion of the proximal tibia associated with cortical thinning and expansion. The radiolucent lesion (arrow) (a) has high signal on coronal fat-suppressed T2-weighted imaging (b).

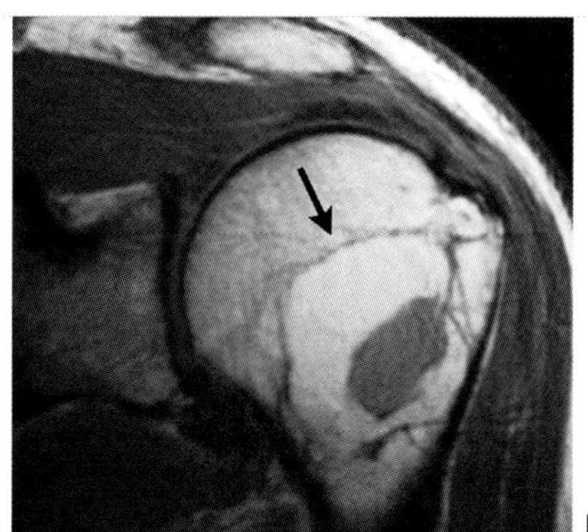

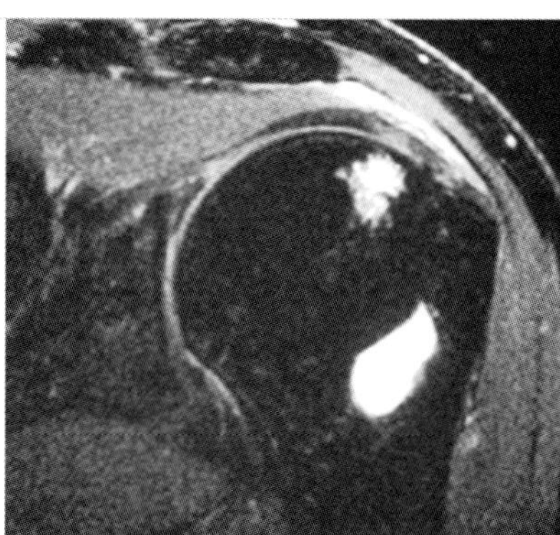

Fig. 10.186 Intraosseous lipoma in the metadiaphyseal portion of the proximal humerus, which has high fat signal peripherally surrounding a central cystlike zone with intermediate signal on coronal proton density–weighted imaging (a) (arrow). The fat signal of the lesion is nulled on coronal fat-suppressed T2-weighted imaging (b), whereas the central cystic region has high signal.

Table 10.8 (Cont.) Solitary intramedullary metadiaphyseal lesions

Abnormalities	MRI findings	Comments
Fibrous dysplasia (▶ Fig. 10.187)	Magnetic resonance imaging (MRI) features depend on the proportions of bony spicules, collagen, fibroblastic spindle cells, hemorrhagic and/or cystic changes, and associated pathological fracture if present. Lesions are usually well circumscribed and have low or low-intermediate signal on T1WI and PDWI. On T2WI, lesions have variable mixtures of low, intermediate, and/or high signal often surrounded by a low signal rim of variable thickness. Internal septations and cystic changes are seen in a minority of lesions. Bone expansion with thickened and/or thinned cortex can be seen. Lesions show Gd-contrast enhancement that varies in degree and pattern.	Benign medullary fibro-osseous lesion, which can involve a single site (mono-ostotic) or multiple locations (polyostotic). Thought to occur from developmental failure in the normal process of remodeling primitive bone to mature lamellar bone with resultant zone or zones of immature trabeculae within dysplastic fibrous tissue. Accounts for approximately 10% of benign bone lesions. Patients range in age from < 1 year to 76 years; 75% occur before the age of 30 years.

(continued on page 466)

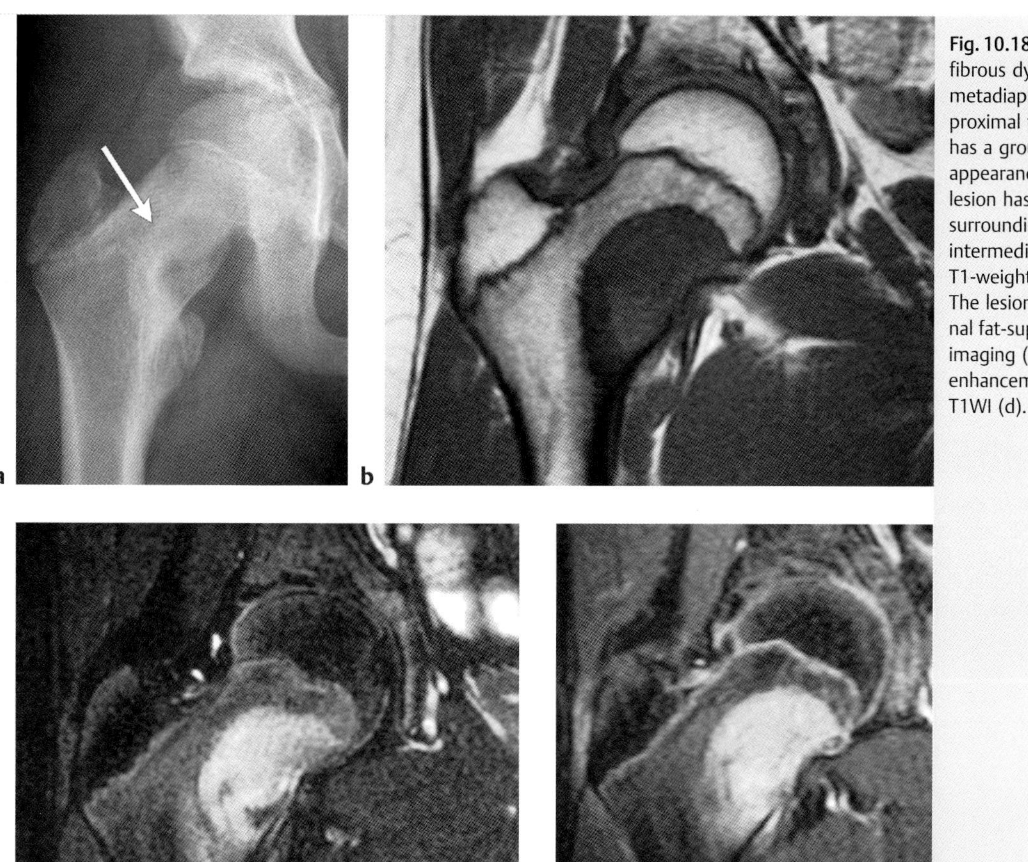

Fig. 10.187 A 14-year-old boy with fibrous dysplasia involving the metadiaphyseal portion of the proximal femur (a) (arrow), which has a ground-glass radiographic appearance. The circumscribed lesion has a margin of low signal surrounding a central zone with intermediate signal on coronal T1-weighted imaging (T1WI) (b). The lesion has high signal on coronal fat-suppressed (FS) T2-weighted imaging (c) and shows Gd-contrast enhancement on coronal FS T1WI (d).

Table 10.8 (Cont.) Solitary intramedullary metadiaphyseal lesions

Abnormalities	MRI findings	Comments
Liposclerosing myxofibrous tumor (▶ Fig. 10.188)	Lesions have well-defined margins with variable thickness of low signal borders on T1WI and T2WI. Lesions often have low to intermediate signal on T1WI and intermediate to high signal on T2WI and FS T2WI. Small zones with fat signal may be seen at the periphery of the lesions. Lesions usually lack Gd-contrast enhancement.	Uncommon benign fibro-osseous lesions with mixed histological features of lipoma, fibroxanthoma, myxoma, fibrous dysplasia, bone cyst, myxofibroma, fat necrosis, and/or ischemic ossification. Most of these lesions occur in the intertrochanteric region of the femur. May represent a variant form of fibrous dysplasia. Patients range from 15 to 69 years, mean = 42 years.
Stress fracture (▶ Fig. 10.189)	Fractures typically have abnormal marrow signal (usually low signal on T1WI, high signal on T2WI and FS T2WI). Gd-contrast enhancement is typically seen in the postfracture period. Angulated cortical margins and periosteal high signal on FS T2WI can be seen. A curvilinear zone of low signal on T2WI and FS T2WI may be seen within the marrow edema, which is often perpendicular or oblique to the long axis of the involved bone.	Stress fractures can result from persistent chronic mechanical overload as well as from osteoporosis or osteomalacia. primary bone tumors/lesions, metastatic disease, and bone infarcts.
Bone infarct (▶ Fig. 10.190)	A double-line sign (curvilinear adjacent zones of low and high signal on T2WI) is commonly seen at the edges of the infarcts representing the borders of osseous resorption and healing. Irregular Gd-contrast enhancement can be seen from granulation tissue ingrowth.	Zones of ischemic death involving bone trabeculae and marrow, which may be idiopathic or result from trauma, corticosteroid treatment, chemotherapy, radiation treatment, occlusive vascular disease, collagen vascular and other autoimmune diseases, metabolic storage diseases (e.g., Gaucher disease), sickle cell disease, thalassemia, hyperbaric events/Caisson disease, pregnancy, alcohol abuse, pancreatitis, infections, and lymphoproliferative diseases.

(continued on page 468)

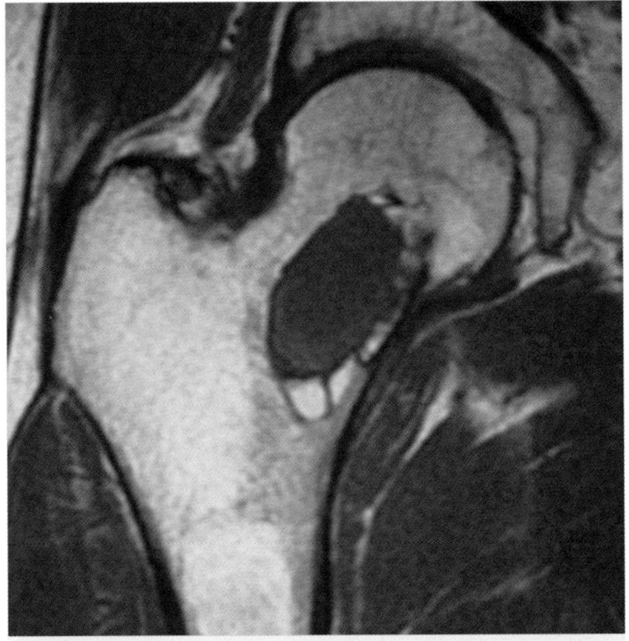

Fig. 10.188 A 61-year-old man with liposclerosing myxofibrous tumor in the metadiaphyseal portion of the proximal femur, which has low-intermediate signal centrally surrounded by foci with fat signal on coronal T1-weighted imaging.

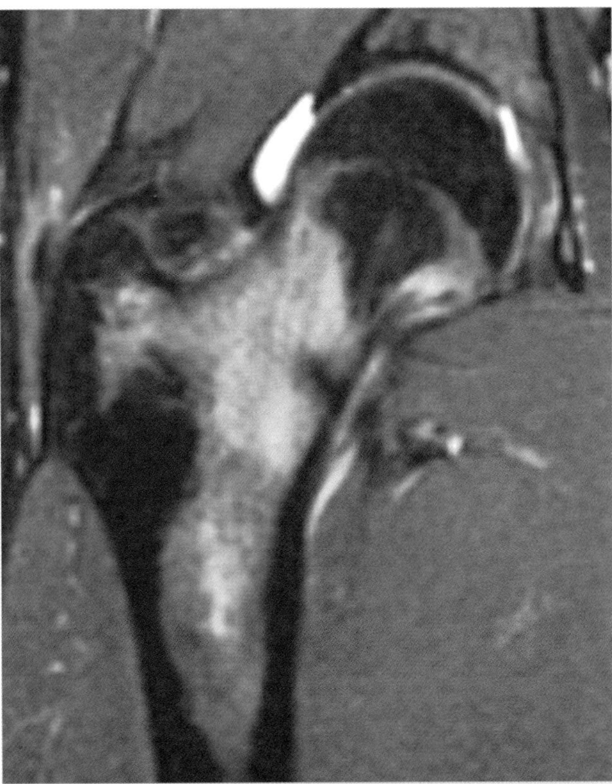

Fig. 10.189 Stress fracture in the proximal femur seen as a poorly defined zone with high signal in the marrow surrounding a linear zone of low signal on coronal fat-suppressed T2-weighted imaging.

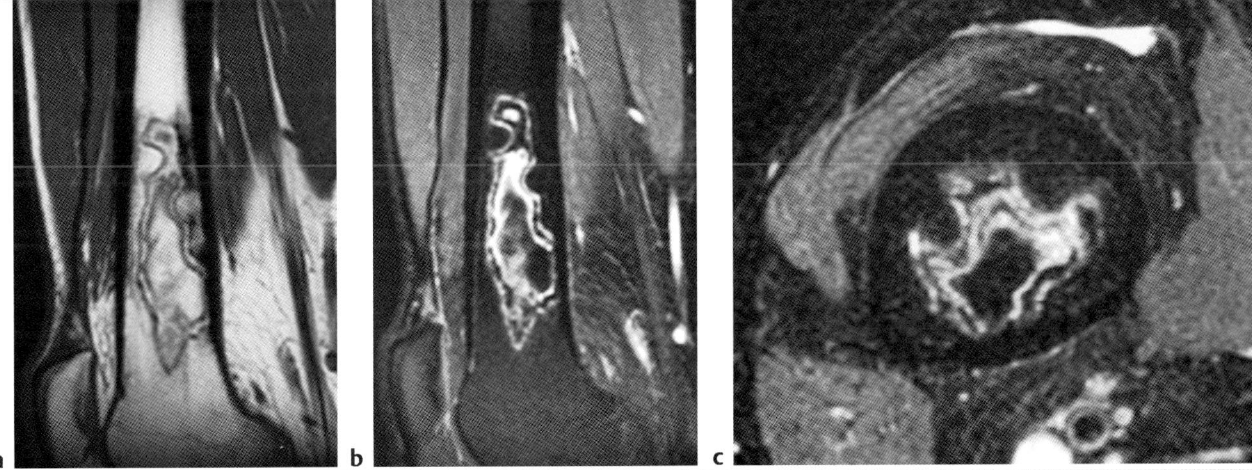

Fig. 10.190 A 38-year-old man with sickle cell trait and a bone infarct in the distal metadiaphyseal portion of the distal femur as seen on sagittal T1-weighted imaging (a) and sagittal (b) and axial fat-suppressedT2-weighted imaging (T2WI) (c). A double-line sign (curvilinear adjacent zones of low and high signal on T2WI) is seen at the edges of the infarct representing the borders of osseous resorption and healing.

Table 10.8 (Cont.) Solitary intramedullary metadiaphyseal lesions

Abnormalities	MRI findings	Comments
Eosinophilic granuloma (▶ Fig. 10.191)	Focal intramedullary lesion(s) associated with trabecular and cortical bone destruction, which typically have low-intermediate signal on T1WI and PDWI and heterogeneous slightly high to high signal on T2WI. Poorly defined zones of high signal on T2WI are usually seen in the marrow peripheral to the lesions secondary to inflammatory changes. Extension of lesions from the marrow into adjacent soft tissues through areas of cortical disruption are commonly seen as well as linear periosteal zones of high signal on T2WI. Lesions typically show prominent Gd-contrast enhancement in marrow and in extraosseous soft tissue portions.	Benign tumor-like lesions consisting of Langerhans cells (histiocytes) and variable amounts of lymphocytes, polymorphonuclear cells, and eosinophils. Account for 1% of primary bone lesions and 8% of tumor-like lesions. Occur in patients with median age = 10 years, average = 13.5 years, peak incidence between 5 and 10 years; 80 to 85% occur in patients less than 30 years.
Osteomyelitis (▶ Fig. 10.192)	Poorly defined zones with high signal on T2WI and FS T2WI and Gd-contrast enhancement are seen in marrow with associated zones of cortical destruction. Periosteal reaction can be seen as a peripheral rim of high signal on T2WI and FS T2WI and Gd-contrast enhancement on FS T1WI adjacent to the low signal of cortical bone. A subperiosteal abscess with high signal on T2WI and FS T2WI can often be seen elevating a single low signal thin band of periosteum.	Infection of bone, which can result from hematogenous spread of microorganisms, trauma-direct inoculation, extension from adjacent tissues, and complications from surgery. *Staphylococcus aureus* and *Streptococcus pyogenes* are the most common bacterial infections involving bone. Osteomyelitis can also result from other bacteria as well as tuberculosis, fungi, parasites, and viruses.
Malignant lesions		
Metastatic lesion (▶ Fig. 10.193)	Single or multiple well-circumscribed or poorly defined infiltrative lesions involving the marrow associated with cortical destruction and extraosseous extension. Lesions often have low-intermediate signal on T1WI; low, intermediate, and/or high signal on T2WI and FS T1WI and usually show Gd-contrast enhancement. Cortical destruction and tumor extension into the extraosseous soft tissues frequently occurs. Pathological fractures can be associated with metastatic lesions involving tubular bones and vertebrae. Periosteal reaction is uncommon.	Metastatic lesions typically occur in the marrow with or without cortical destruction and extraosseous tumor extension.

(continued on page 470)

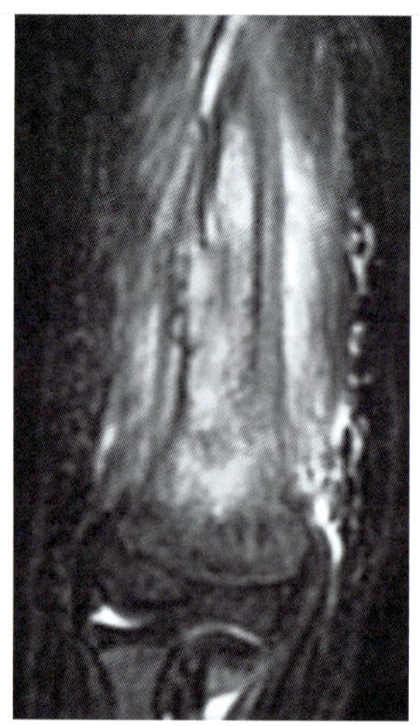

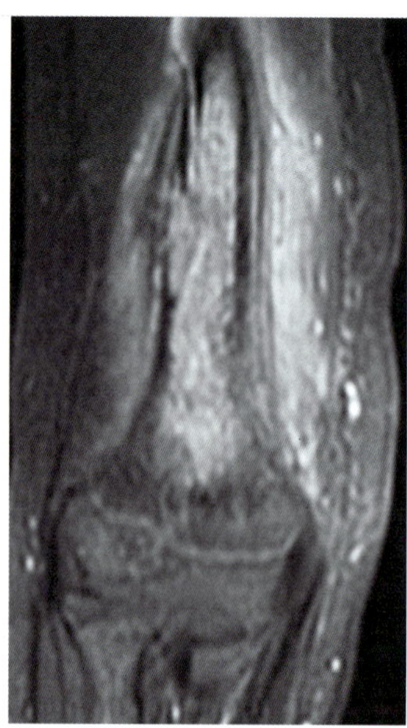

Fig. 10.191 A 5-year-old boy with an eosinophilic granuloma involving the metadiaphyseal portion of the distal humerus. The intramedullary lesion has high signal on coronal fat-suppressed (FS) T2-weighted imaging (a) and is associated with cortical destruction, periosteal elevation, and extraosseous extension with abnormal high signal. The lesion shows prominent gadolinium-contrast enhancement on coronal FS T1-weighted imaging (b).

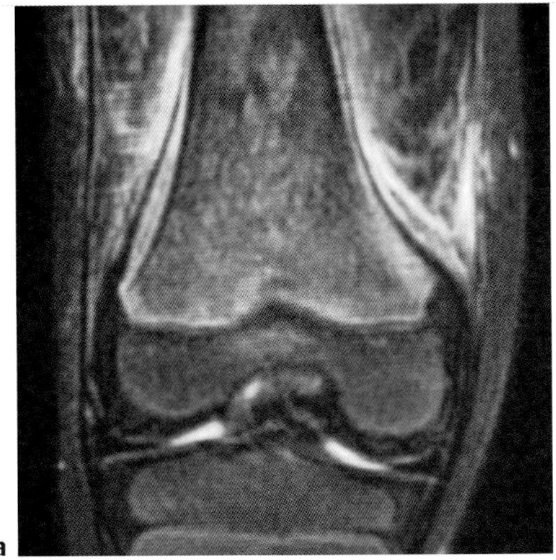

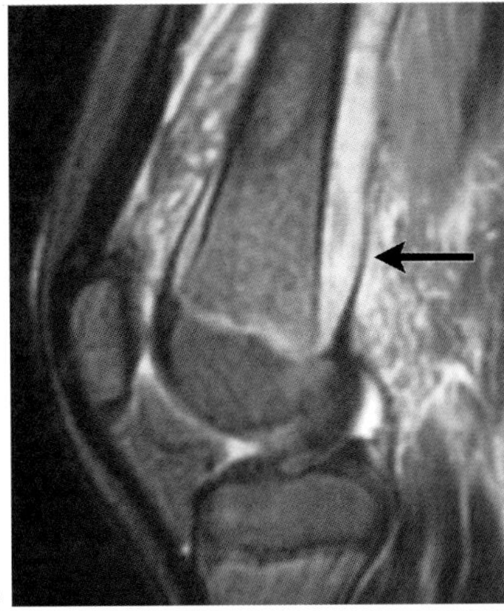

Fig. 10.192 A 6-year-old male with *Staphylococcus aureus* osteomyelitis involving the metadiaphyseal portion of the distal femur, which has heterogeneous slightly high signal on coronal (a) and sagittal fat-suppressed T2-weighted imaging (b). Infection extends through the bone cortex resulting in subperiosteal abscess and infection of adjacent extraosseous soft tissue (arrow).

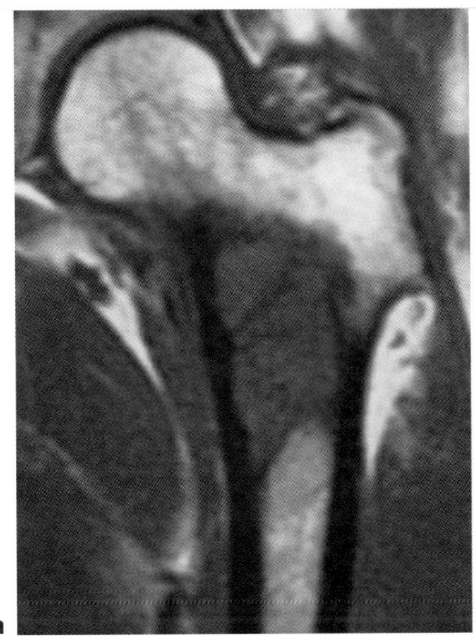

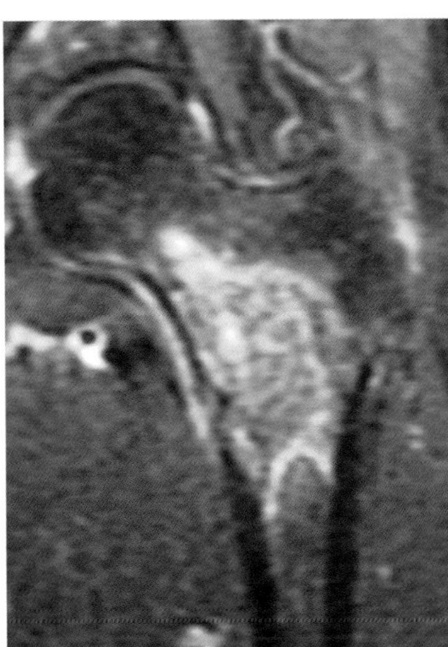

Fig. 10.193 A 56-year-old woman with a metastatic lesion in the metadiaphyseal portion of the proximal femur from breast carcinoma, which has low-intermediate signal on coronal T1-weighted imaging (T1WI) (a) and shows Gd-contrast enhancement on coronal fat-suppressed T1WI (b). A thin zone of periosteal reaction is also seen medially.

Table 10.8 (Cont.) Solitary intramedullary metadiaphyseal lesions

Abnormalities	MRI findings	Comments
Plasmacytoma/myeloma	Multiple (myeloma) or single (plasmacytoma) are well-circumscribed or poorly defined diffuse infiltrative lesions involving marrow, low-intermediate signal on T1WI, intermediate-high signal on T2WI and FS T2WI; usually show Gd-contrast-enhancement, eventual cortical bone destruction, and extraosseous extension.	Malignant tumors composed of proliferating antibody-secreting plasma cells derived from single clones. Most common primary neoplasm of bone in adults; median age = 60 years. Most patients are older than 40 years. May have variable destructive or infiltrative changes involving the axial and/or appendicular skeleton.
Lymphoma (▶ Fig. 10.194)	Non-Hodgkin lymphoma (NHL) and Hodgkin disease (HD) within bone typically appears as single or multifocal poorly defined or circumscribed intramedullary zones with low-intermediate signal on T1WI; intermediate, slightly high, and/or high signal on T2WI; and high signal on FS T2WI; often show Gd-contrast enhancement. Zones of cortical destruction may occur associated with extraosseous soft tissue extension. HD involving bone with associated sclerosis seen on plain films or computed tomography (CT) usually have low signal on T1WI and variable/mixed signal on T2WI. In some cases of NHL, intramedullary tumor may be associated with bulky extraosseous lesions without extensive cortical destruction. High resolution MRI in these cases shows thin penetrating channels of tumor extending through bone cortex into the extraosseous soft tissues.	Lymphoid tumors with neoplastic cells typically within lymphoid tissue (lymph nodes and reticuloendothelial organs). Unlike leukemia, lymphoma usually arises as discrete masses. Lymphomas are subdivided into HD and NHL. Almost all primary lymphomas of bone are B-cell NHL. HD, mean age = 32 years. Osseous NHL, median = 35 years.
Osteosarcoma (▶ Fig. 10.195)	Destructive intramedullary malignant lesions, low-intermediate signal on T1WI; mixed low, intermediate, high signal on T2WI, usually with matrix mineralization/ossification-low signal on T2WI; usually show Gd-contrast enhancement (usually heterogeneous). Zones of cortical destruction are common through which tumors extend into the extraosseous soft tissues under an elevated periosteum. Lamellated and/or spiculated zones of bone formation can occur under the periosteal elevation secondary to tumor invasion and perforation of bone cortex. Low signal from spicules of periosteal, reactive, and tumoral bone formation may have a divergent (sunburst) pattern, perpendicular (hair on end) pattern, or disorganized or complex appearance. Triangular zones of periosteal elevation (Codman triangles) can be seen at the borders of zones of cortical destruction and tumor extension.	Malignant tumor composed of proliferating neoplastic spindle cells, which produce osteoid and/or immature tumoral bone and which most frequently arise within medullary bone (metadiaphyseal > metaphyseal > diaphyseal locations). Two age peaks of incidence. The larger peak occurs between the ages of 10 and 20 and accounts for over half of the cases. The second smaller peak occurs in adults over 60 years and accounts for approximately 10% of the cases. Occurs in children as primary tumors and adults (associated with Paget disease, irradiated bone, chronic osteomyelitis, osteoblastoma, giant cell tumor, fibrous dysplasia).

(continued on page 472)

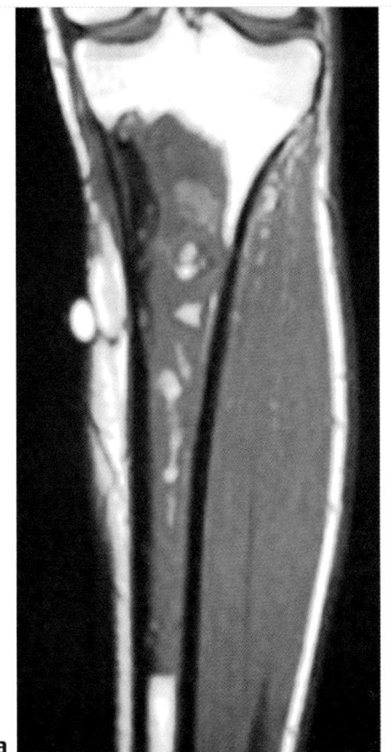

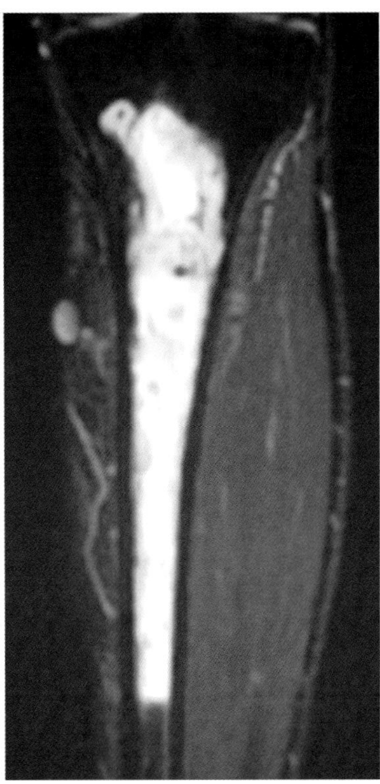

Fig. 10.194 A 19-year-old man with a large B-cell non-Hodgkin lymphoma in the metadiaphyseal marrow of the proximal tibia, which has mostly intermediate signal on coronal T1-weighted imaging (a) and high signal on coronal fat-suppressed T2WI (b).

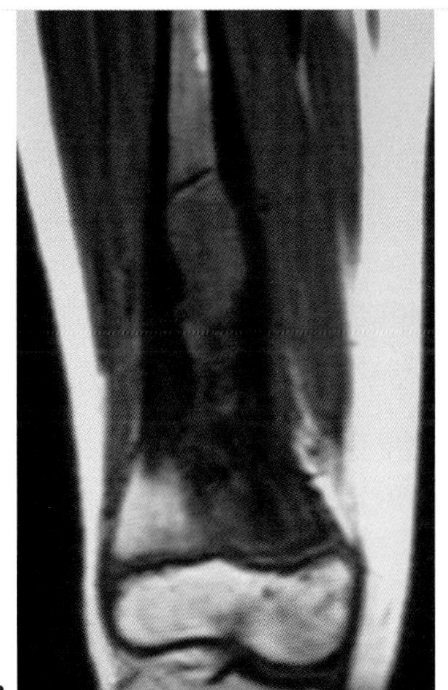

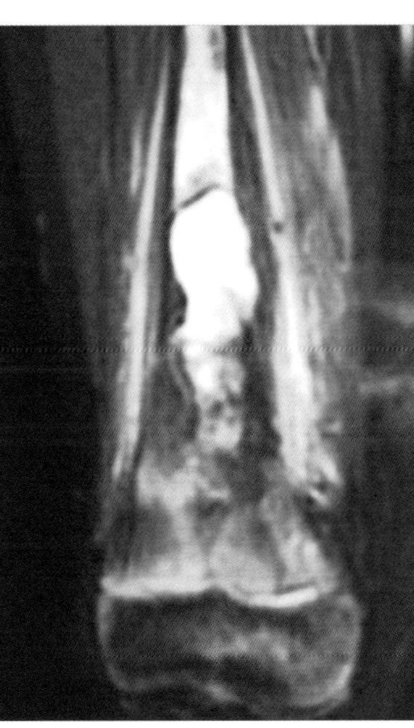

Fig. 10.195 A 9-year-old boy with a chondroblastic osteosarcoma in the metadiaphyseal marrow of the distal femur, which has low and intermediate signal on coronal T1WI (a) and heterogeneous high and low signal on coronal fat-suppressed T2-weighted imaging (b).

Table 10.8 (Cont.) Solitary intramedullary metadiaphyseal lesions

Abnormalities	MRI findings	Comments
Ewing sarcoma (▶ Fig. 10.196)	Destructive malignant lesions involving marrow; low-intermediate signal on T1WI; mixed low, intermediate, and/or high signal on T2WI and FS T2WI; usually shows Gd-contrast enhancement (usually heterogeneous). Extraosseous tumor extension through sites of cortical destruction is commonly seen beneath an elevated periosteum. Thin striated zones of low signal on T2WI can sometimes be seen oriented perpendicular to the long axis of the involved bone under the elevated periosteum representing the hair on end appearance of reactive bone formation secondary to the tumor. In long bones, tumors are most often located in the diaphyseal region, followed by the metadiaphyseal region.	Malignant primitive tumor of bone composed of undifferentiated small cells with round nuclei. Accounts for 6 to 11% of primary malignant bone tumors, 5 to 7% of primary bone tumors. Usually occurs between the ages of 5 and 30, males > females, locally invasive, high metastatic potential.
Chondrosarcoma (▶ Fig. 10.197)	Intramedullary tumors often have low-intermediate signal on T1WI, intermediate signal on PDWI, and heterogeneous intermediate-high signal on T2WI. Lesions usually show heterogeneous contrast enhancement. Zones of cortical destruction can be seen with extraosseous extension of tumor.	Chondrosarcomas are malignant tumors containing cartilage formed within sarcomatous stroma. Account for12 to 21% of malignant bone lesions, 21 to 26% of primary sarcomas of bone.Usually occurs between the ages of 5 and 91, mean = 40 years, median = 26 to 59 years.
Fibrosarcoma	Intramedullary lesions with irregular margins, with or without associated cortical destruction and/or extraosseous soft tissue masses. Lesions usually have low-intermediate signal on T1WI and PDWI, and heterogeneous intermediate, slightly high, and/or high signal on T2WI. Lesions usually show heterogeneous Gd-contrast enhancement.	Fibrosarcomas are uncommon malignant tumors consisting of bundles of neoplastic fibroblasts/spindle cells with varying proportions of collagen, lacking other tissue-differentiating features such as tumor bone, osteoid, or cartilage. Can be primary lesions (75%) or arise as secondary tumors (25%) associated with prior irradiation, Paget disease, bone infarct, chronic osteomyelitis, fibrous dysplasia, giant cell tumor. Accounts for 3 to 5% of primary malignant bone tumors and 2 to 4% of all bone tumors. Median age = 43 years.
Malignant fibrous histiocytoma (▶ Fig. 10.198)	Intramedullary lesions with irregular margins with zones of cortical destruction and extraosseous extension. Tumors often have low-intermediate signal on T1WI, low-intermediate signal on PDWI, and heterogeneous intermediate-high signal on T2WI and FS T2WI. Invasion into joints occurs in 30%. May be associated with bone infarcts, bone cysts, chronic osteomyelitis, Paget disease, and other treated primary bone tumors. Lesions usually show heterogeneous Gd-contrast prominent enhancement.	Malignant tumor involving soft tissue and rarely bone derived from undifferentiated mesenchymal cells. Contains cells with limited cellular differentiation such as mixtures of fibroblasts, myofibroblasts, histiocyte-like cells, anaplastic giant cells, and inflammatory cells. Accounts for 1 to 5% of primary malignant bone tumors and < 1 to 3% of all primary bone tumors. Patient ages range from 11 to 80 years, median = 48 years, mean = 55 years.

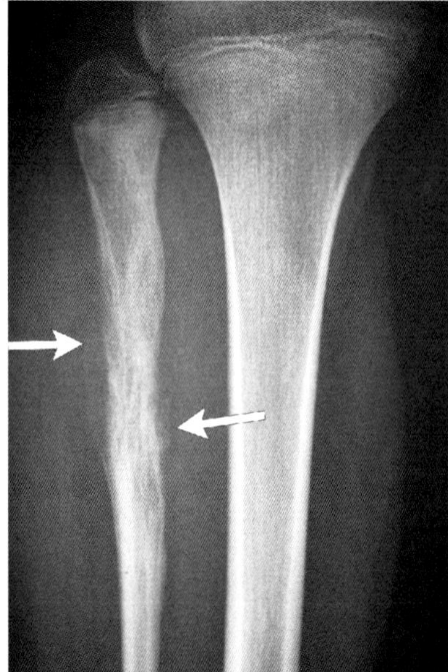

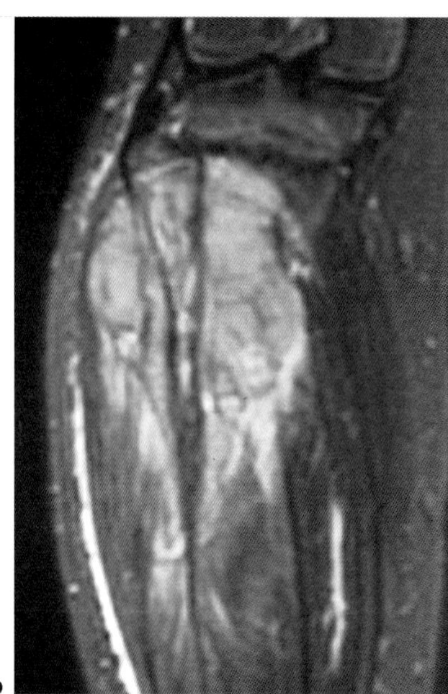

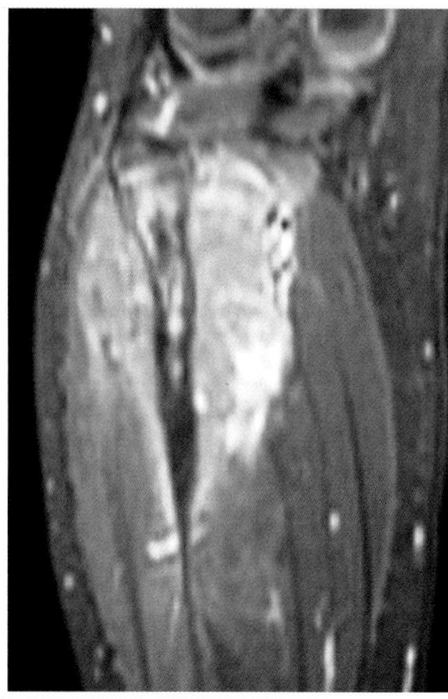

Fig. 10.196 A 10-year-old girl with Ewing sarcoma in the metadiaphyseal portion of the proximal fibula with permeative intramedullary and cortical bone destruction with interrupted periosteal elevation (arrows) (a). The tumor has high signal in the marrow on coronal fat-suppressed T2-weighted imaging (FS T2WI) (b) and shows prominent Gd-contrast enhancement on coronal FS T1WI (c). Intramedullary tumor extends through sites of cortical destruction with periosteal elevation into the adjacent extraosseous soft tissues.

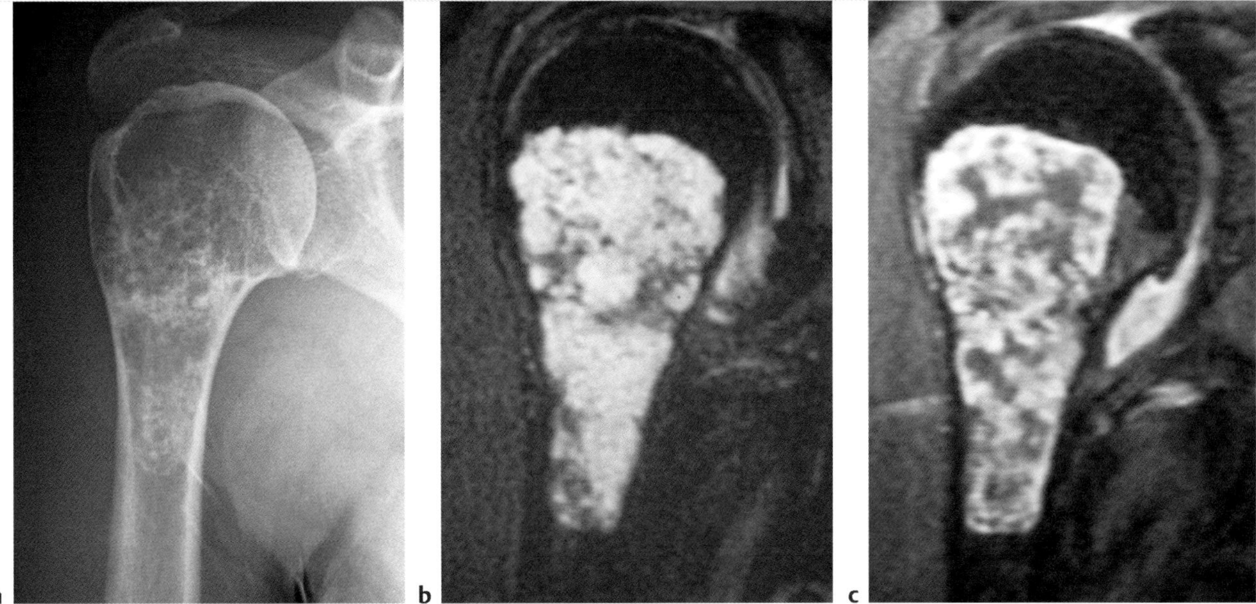

Fig. 10.197 A 46-year-old woman with a low grade chondrosarcoma in the metadiaphyseal portion of the proximal humerus, which contains chondroid mineralization (a). The tumor has high signal on coronal fat-suppression (FS) T2-weighted imaging (b) and shows irregular lobular gadolinium-contrast enhancement on coronal FS T1-weighted imaging (c).

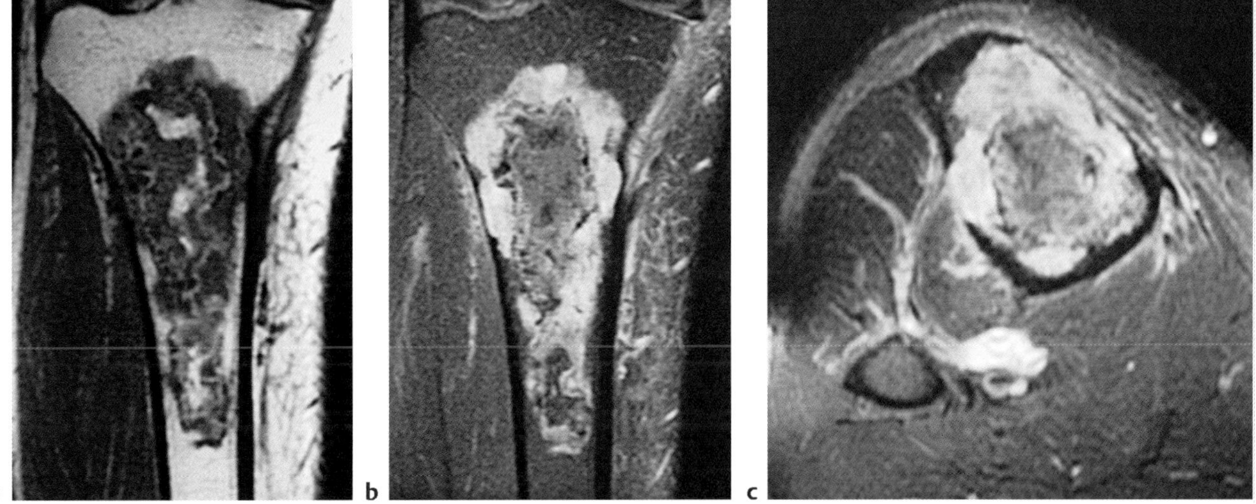

Fig. 10.198 A 53-year-old man with a malignant fibrous histiocytoma in the metadiaphyseal region of the proximal tibia that arose from a bone infarct. The lesion has low, intermediate, and high signal on coronal T1-weighted imaging (T1WI) (a) and shows heterogeneous Gd-contrast enhancement on coronal (b) and axial fat-suppressed T1WI (c). The intramedullary lesion is associated with cortical bone destruction.

10.9 Solitary Intramedullary Diaphyseal Lesions

- Nonmalignant lesions
  - Stress fracture
  - Bone infarct
  - Fibrous dysplasia
  - Fibroxanthoma
  - Enchondroma
  - Eosinophilic granuloma
  - Osteomyelitis
- Malignant lesions
  - Metastatic lesion
  - Plasmacytoma/myeloma
  - Lymphoma
  - Osteosarcoma
  - Ewing sarcoma
  - Chondrosarcoma
  - Fibrosarcoma
  - Malignant fibrous histiocytoma
  - Paget sarcoma

Table 10.9 Solitary intramedullary diaphyseal lesions

Abnormalities	MRI findings	Comments
Nonmalignant lesions		
Stress fracture (▶ Fig. 10.199)	Fractures often have associated poorly defined zones of abnormal marrow signal with low signal on T1-weighted imaging (T1WI), and high signal on T2-weighted imaging (T2WI) and fat-suppressed (FS) T2WI. Gadolinium (Gd)-contrast enhancement is typically seen in the postfracture period. Angulated cortical margins and periosteal high signal on FS T2WI can be seen. A curvilinear zone of low signal on T2WI and FS T2WI may be seen within the marrow edema, which is often perpendicular or oblique to the long axis of the involved bone.	Stress fractures can result from persistent chronic mechanical overload, as well as from osteoporosis or osteomalacia.
Bone infarct (▶ Fig. 10.200)	A double-line sign (curvilinear adjacent zones of low and high signal on T2WI) is commonly seen at the edges of the infarcts representing the borders of osseous resorption and healing. Irregular Gd-contrast enhancement can be seen from granulation tissue ingrowth. Poorly defined zones with high signal on T2WI and Gd-contrast enhancement can be seen in marrow and periosteal soft tissues in acute bone infarcts.	Zones of ischemic death involving bone trabeculae and marrow which can be idiopathic or result from trauma, corticosteroid treatment, chemotherapy, radiation treatment, occlusive vascular disease, collagen vascular and other autoimmune diseases, metabolic storage diseases (e.g., Gaucher disease), sickle cell disease, thalassemia, hyperbaric events/Caisson disease, pregnancy, alcohol abuse, pancreatitis, infections, and lymphoproliferative diseases.

(continued on page 476)

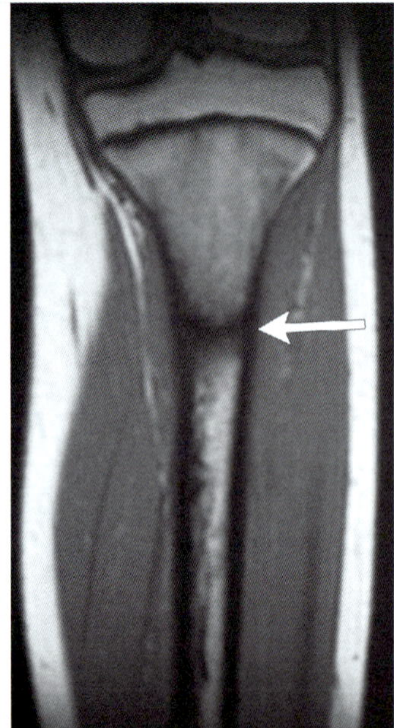

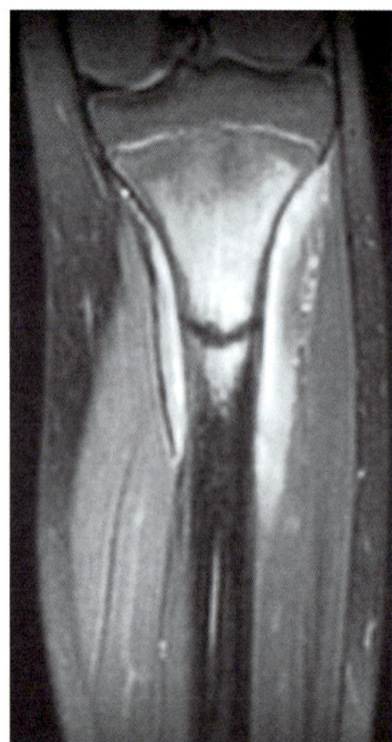

Fig. 10.199 A 12-year-old girl with a fatigue-type stress fracture in the proximal diaphysis of the tibia. A horizontal linear zone of low signal (arrow) is seen within the marrow surrounded by a poorly defined zone of low-intermediate signal on coronal T1-weighted imaging (a) and high signal on coronal fat-suppressed T2-weighted imaging (FS T2WI) (b). The high signal on FS T2WI from edema and/or inflammation extends up into the metaphyseal marrow.

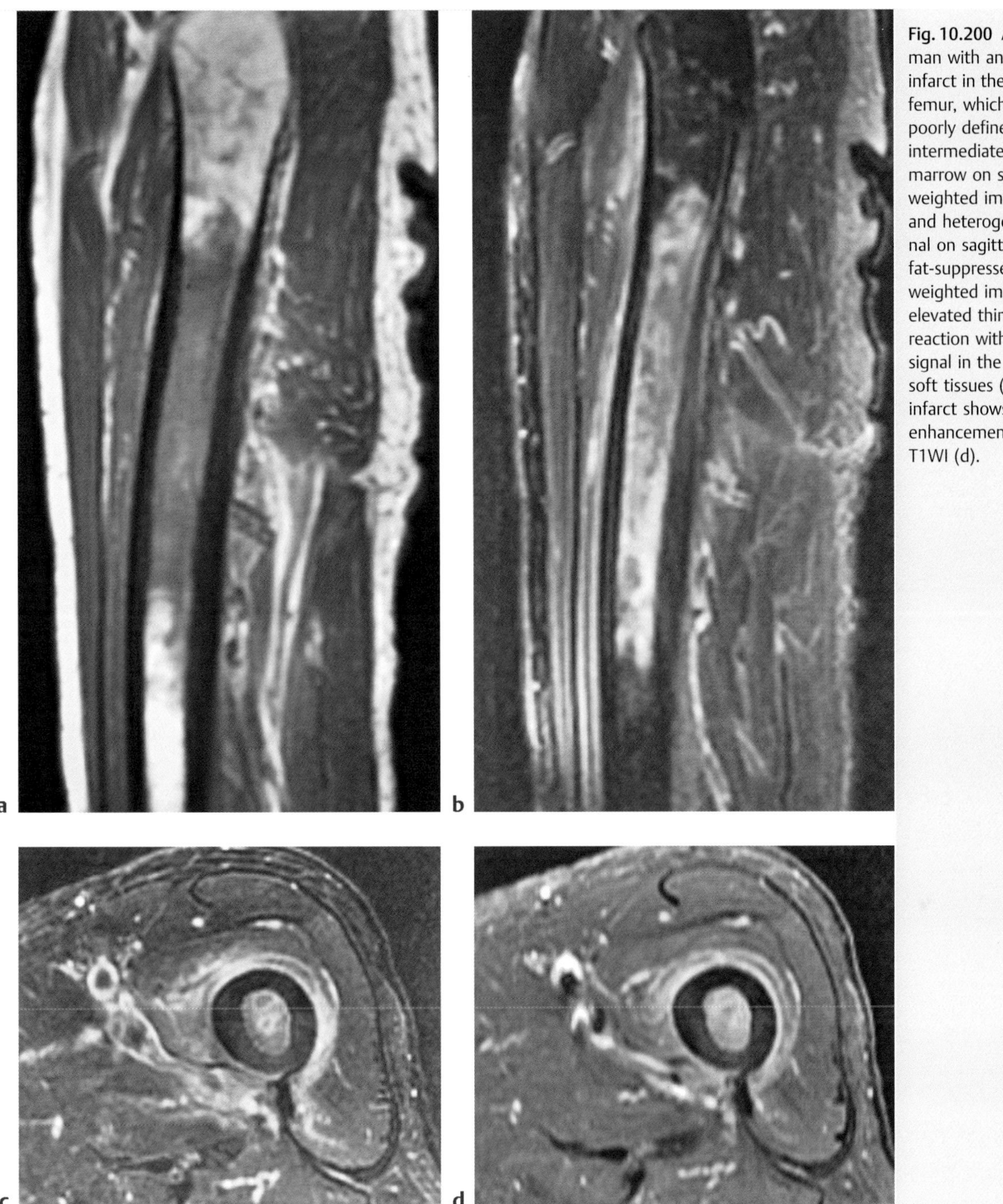

Fig. 10.200 A 76-year-old man with an acute bone infarct in the diaphysis of the femur, which is seen as a poorly defined zone of low-intermediate signal in the marrow on sagittal T1-weighted imaging (T1WI) (a) and heterogeneous high signal on sagittal (b) and axial fat-suppressed (FS) T2-weighted imaging (c) with elevated thin periosteal reaction with adjacent high signal in the extraosseous soft tissues (b). The acute infarct shows Gd-contrast enhancement on axial FS T1WI (d).

Table 10.9 (Cont.) Solitary intramedullary diaphyseal lesions

Abnormalities	MRI findings	Comments
Fibrous dysplasia (▶ Fig. 10.201)	Magnetic resonance imaging (MRI) features depend on the proportions of bony spicules, collagen, fibroblastic spindle cells, hemorrhagic and/or cystic changes, and associated pathological fracture if present. Lesions are usually well-circumscribed and have low or low-intermediate signal on T1WI and PDWI. On T2WI, lesions have variable mixtures of low, intermediate, and/or high signal often surrounded by a low signal rim of variable thickness. Internal septations and cystic changes are seen in a minority of lesions. Bone expansion with thickened and/or thinned cortex can be seen. Lesions show Gd-contrast enhancement that varies in degree and pattern.	Benign medullary fibro-osseous lesion, which can involve a single site (mono-ostotic) or multiple locations (polyostotic). Thought to occur from developmental failure in the normal process of remodeling primitive bone to mature lamellar bone with resultant zone or zones of immature trabeculae within dysplastic fibrous tissue. Accounts for approximately 10% of benign bone lesions. Patients range in age from < 1 year to 76 years; 75% occur before the age of 30 years.
Fibroxanthoma	Well-circumscribed eccentric intramedullary lesions in the diaphyseal regions of long bones, which have mixed low-intermediate signal on T1WI and mixed low, intermediate, and/or high signal on T2WI, PDWI, and FS T2WI. Zones of low signal on T1WI, PDWI, and T2WI can be seen in the central portions of the lesions. Zones with varying thickness of low signal on T1WI, PDWI, and T2WI are seen at the margins of the lesions representing bone sclerosis. Internal septations are commonly seen as zones of low signal on T2WI in these lesions. Lesions can show Gd-contrast enhancement (heterogeneous > homogeneous patterns).	Histologically identical to nonossifying fibromas but occur in diaphyseal portions of long bones. Lesions contain whorls of fibroblastic cells combined with smaller amounts of multi-nucleated giant cells and xanthomatous cells. Patients range in age from 6 to 74 years, 60% of patients are older than 20 years at diagnosis.

(continued on page 478)

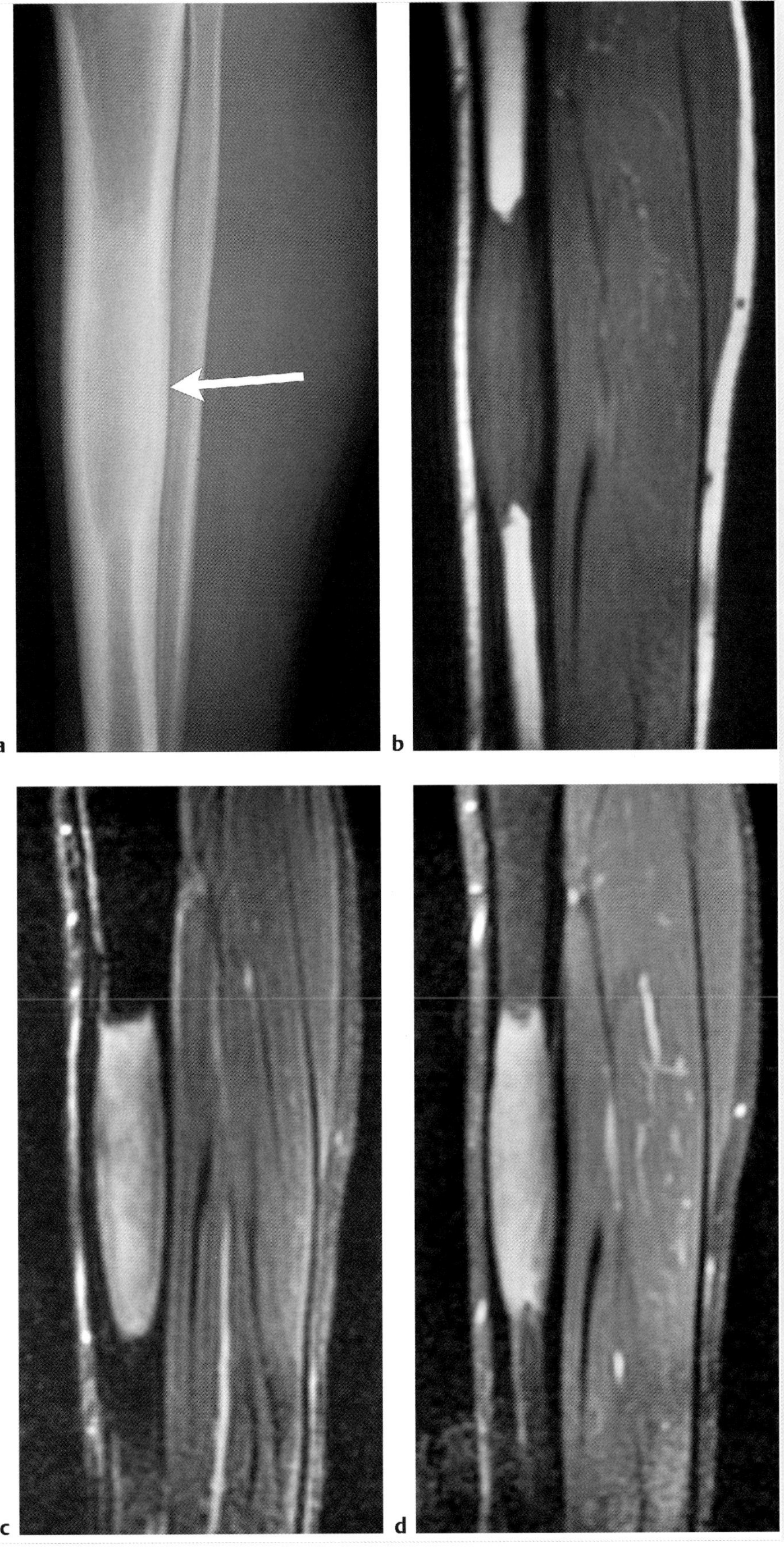

Fig. 10.201 A 19-year-old man with fibrous dysplasia involving the diaphysis of the tibia. The lesion (arrow) has increased attenuation with a ground-glass radiographic appearance and is associated with slight expansion and thinning of adjacent cortical margins (a). The lesion has low-intermediate signal on sagittal T1-weighted imaging (T1WI) (b), slightly high signal on sagittal fat-suppressed (FS) T2-weighted imaging (c), and shows Gd-contrast enhancement on sagittal FS T1WI (d).

Table 10.9 (Cont.) Solitary intramedullary diaphyseal lesions

Abnormalities	MRI findings	Comments
Enchondroma (▶ Fig. 10.202)	Lobulated intramedullary lesions with well-defined borders, which usually have low-intermediate signal on T1WI and intermediate signal on PDWI. On T2WI and FS T2WI, lesions usually have predominantly high signal with foci and/or bands of low signal representing areas of matrix mineralization and fibrous strands. No zones of abnormal high signal on T2WI are typically seen in the marrow outside the borders of the lesions. Lesions typically show Gd-contrast enhancement in various patterns (peripheral curvilinear lobular, central nodular/septal and peripheral lobular, or heterogeneous diffuse).	Benign intramedullary lesions composed of hyaline cartilage, represent approximately 10% of benign bone tumors. Enchondromas can be solitary (88%) or multiple (12%). Ollier disease is a dyschondroplasia involving endochondral-formed bone resulting in multiple enchondromas (enchondromatosis). Metachondromatosis is a combination of enchondromatosis and osteochondromatosis and is rare. Maffucci syndrome refers to a syndrome with multiple enchondromas and soft tissue hemangiomas and is very rare. Patients range in age from 3 to 83 years, median = 35 years, mean = 38 to 40 years, peak in third and fourth decades.
Eosinophilic granuloma (▶ Fig. 10.203)	Focal intramedullary lesion(s) associated with trabecular and cortical bone destruction, which typically have low-intermediate signal on T1WI and PDWI and heterogeneous slightly high to high signal on T2WI. Poorly defined zones of high signal on T2WI are usually seen in the marrow peripheral to the lesions secondary to inflammatory changes. Extension of lesions from the marrow into adjacent soft tissues through areas of cortical disruption are commonly seen as well as linear periosteal zones of high signal on T2WI. Lesions typically show prominent Gd-contrast enhancement in marrow and in extraosseous soft tissue portions.	Benign tumor-like lesions consisting of Langerhans cells (histiocytes), and variable amounts of lymphocytes, polymorphonuclear cells, and eosinophils. Account for 1% of primary bone lesions and 8% of tumor-like lesions. Occur in patients with median age = 10 years, average = 13.5 years, peak incidence is between 5 and 10 years; 80 to 85% occur in patients less than 30 years.

(continued on page 480)

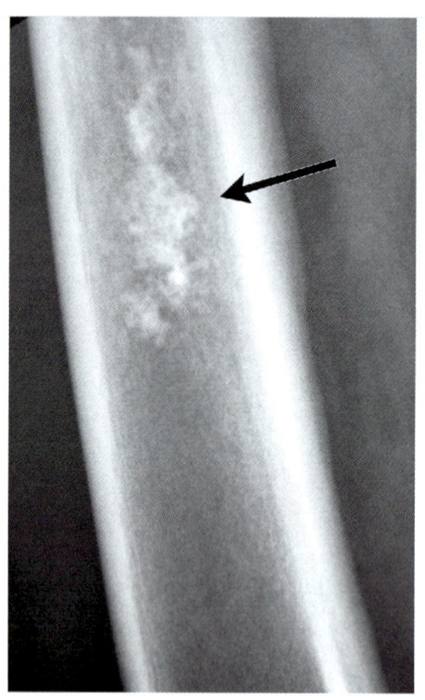

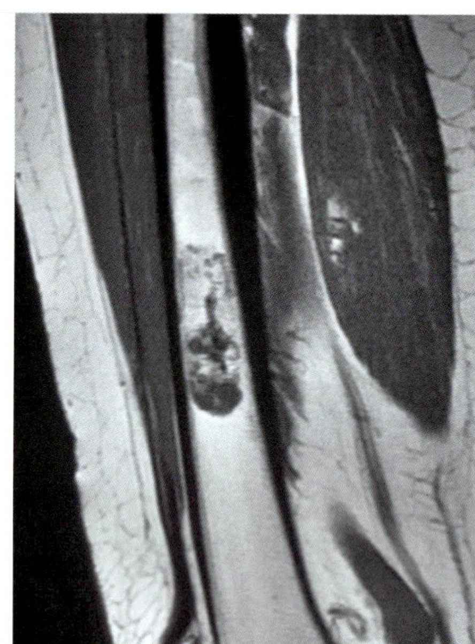

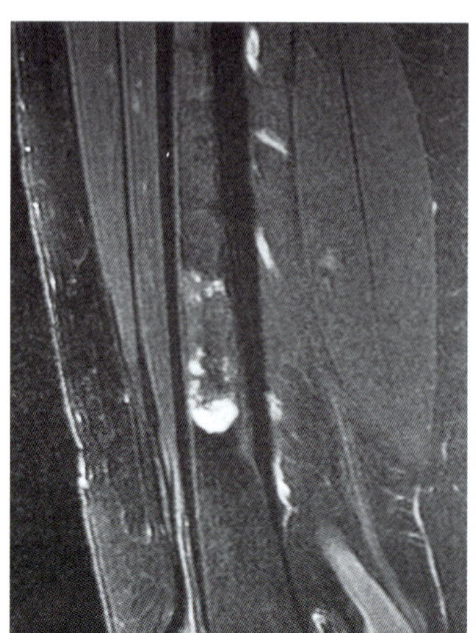

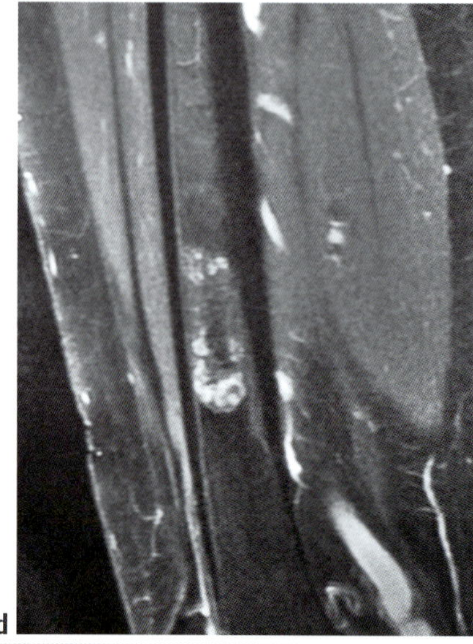

Fig. 10.202 A 47-year-old woman with an enchondroma in the diaphyseal portion of the femur, which contains chondroid matrix mineralization (arrow) on lateral radiograph (a). The lesion has mixed low-intermediate signal on sagittal T1-weighted imaging (T1WI) (b) and high signal on sagittal FS T2-weighted imaging (c). The lesion shows Gd-contrast enhancement on sagittal FS T1WI (d).

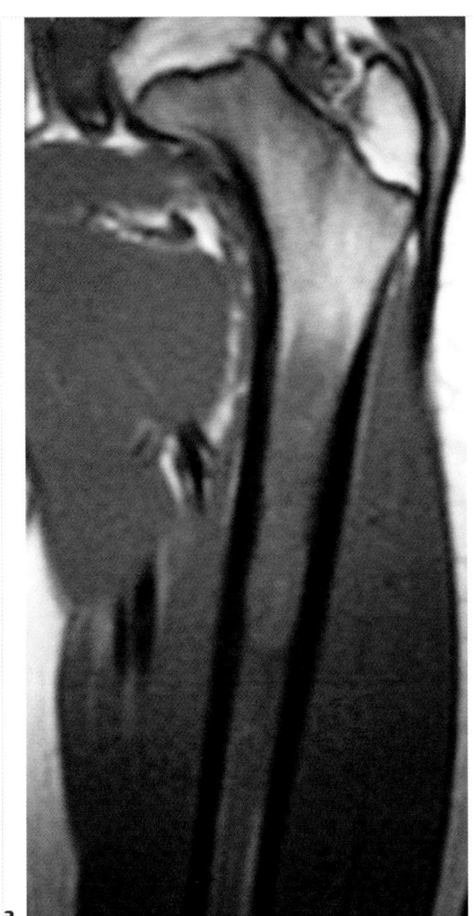
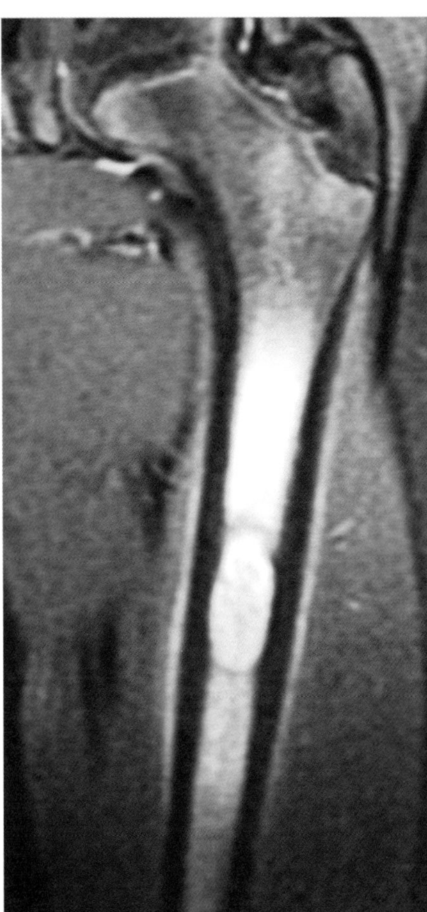

Fig. 10.203 An 18-year-old woman with an eosinophilic granuloma involving the diaphyseal marrow of the femur, which is seen as a poorly defined zone of low-intermediate signal on coronal T1-weighted imaging (a). A thin marginal rim of low signal is seen surrounding a central zone of high signal on coronal fat-suppressed T2-weighted imaging (b), as well as a poorly defined zone of peripheral high signal and thin periosteal reaction with high signal.

Table 10.9 (Cont.) Solitary intramedullary diaphyseal lesions

Abnormalities	MRI findings	Comments
Osteomyelitis (▶ Fig. 10.204; ▶ Fig. 10.205)	Poorly defined zones with high signal on T2WI and FS T2WI and Gd-contrast enhancement are seen in marrow with associated zones of cortical destruction. Periosteal reaction can be seen as a peripheral rim of high signal on T2WI and FS T2WI and Gd-contrast enhancement on FS T1WI adjacent to the low signal of cortical bone. A subperiosteal abscess with high signal on T2WI and FS T2WI can often be seen elevating a single low signal thin band of periosteum. In the subacute phase of pyogenic osteomyelitis, the infection can become localized into an intraosseous (Brodie) abscess with trabecular necrosis, which can be walled off by sclerotic intramedullary and cortical reaction with or without a sinus tract.	Infection of bone that can result from hematogenous spread of micro-organisms, trauma-direct inoculation, extension from adjacent tissues, and complications from surgery. *Staphylococcus aureus* and *Streptococcus pyogenes* are the most common bacterial infections involving bone. Osteomyelitis can also result from other bacteria as well as tuberculosis, fungi, parasites, and viruses.

(continued on page 482)

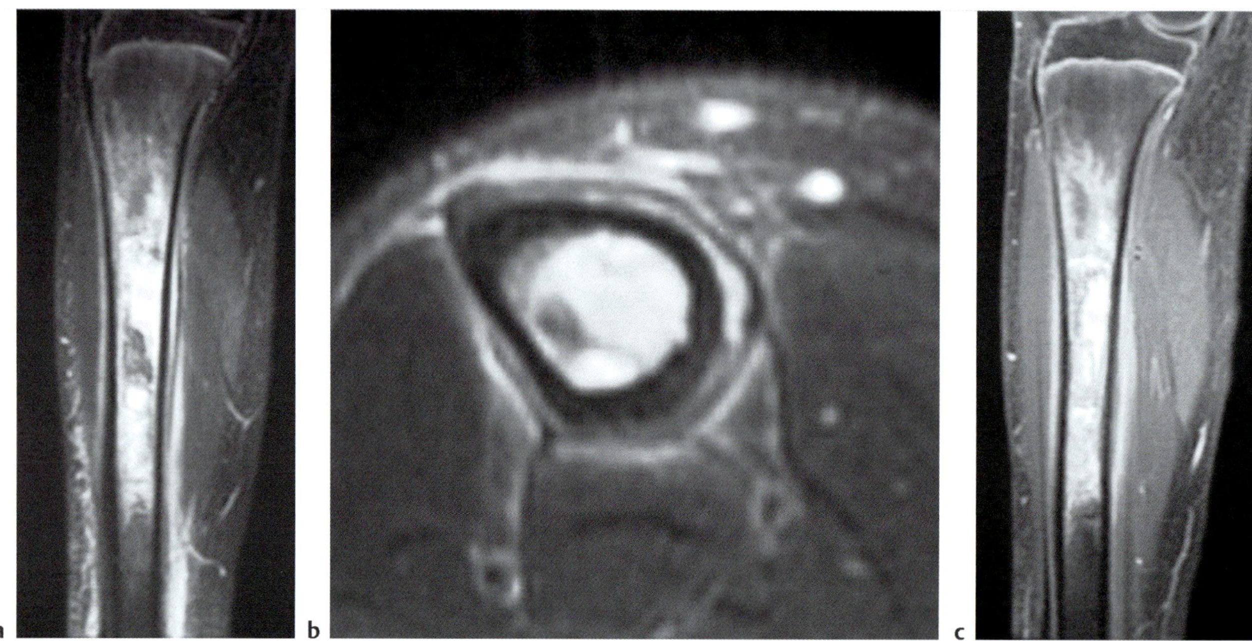

Fig. 10.204 A 13-year-old boy with pyogenic osteomyelitis involving the diaphysis of the tibia, which is seen as a poorly defined zone of high signal on coronal (a) and axial fat-suppressed (FS) T2-weighted imaging (b) in the marrow associated with periosteal elevation, and poorly defined abnormal high T2 signal in the adjacent extraosseous soft tissues. Corresponding abnormal Gd-contrast enhancement is seen in the marrow and adjacent soft tissues on coronal FS T1-weighted imaging (c).

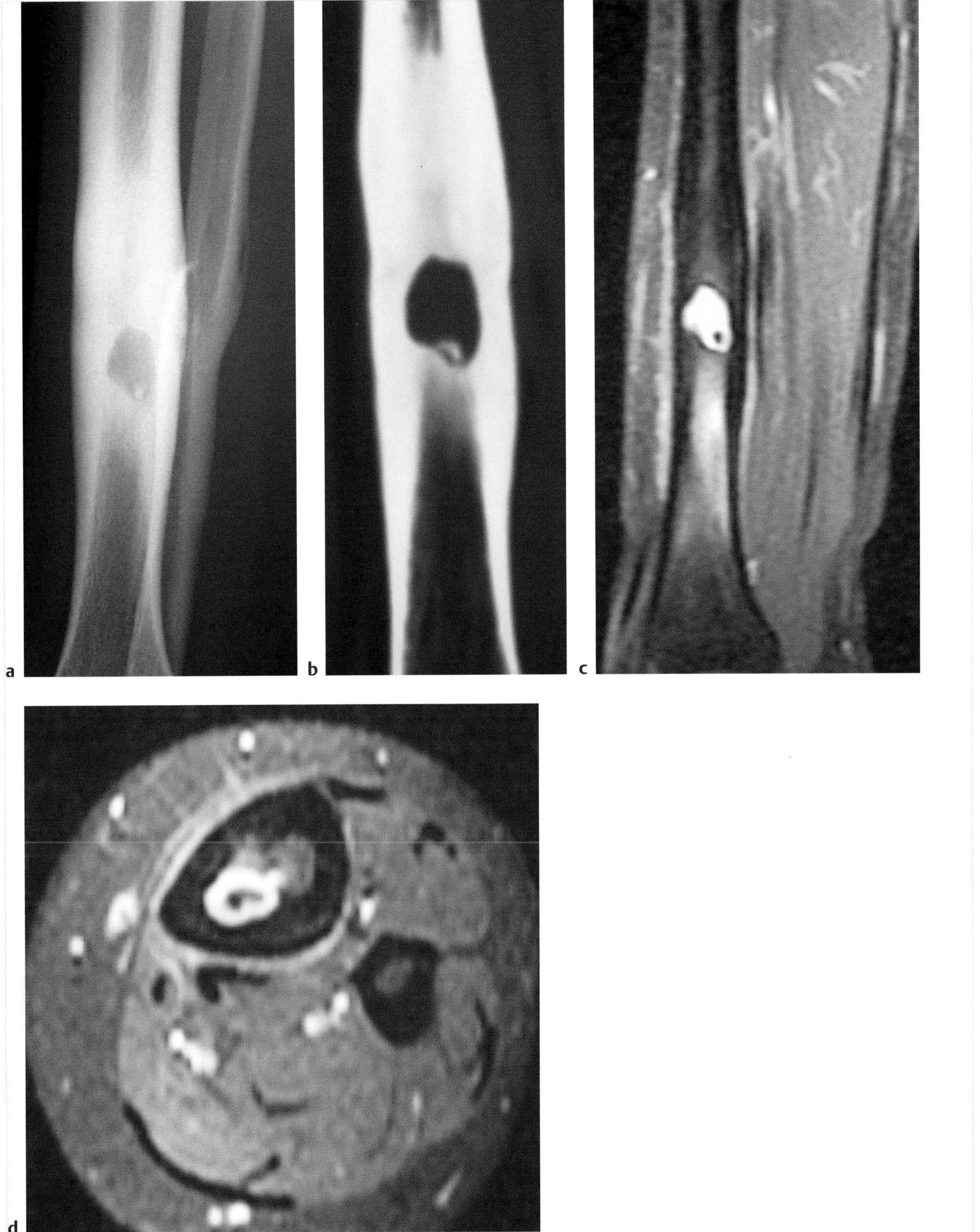

Fig. 10.205 A 21-year-old woman with chronic osteomyelitis involving the diaphysis of the tibia with a Brodie abscess containing a tiny sequestrum, medullary sclerosis, and cortical thickening as seen on radiograph (a) and computed tomography (b). The intramedullary abscess has high signal on coronal fat-suppressed (FS) T2-weighted imaging (c) and is surrounded by a poorly defined zone of high signal in the adjacent marrow. A thin periosteal zone of high signal is also seen. Irregular Gd-contrast enhancement is seen at the periphery of the abscess on axial FS T1-weighted imaging (d).

Table 10.9 (Cont.) Solitary intramedullary diaphyseal lesions

Abnormalities	MRI findings	Comments
Malignant lesions		
Metastatic lesion (▶ Fig. 10.206)	Single or multiple well-circumscribed or poorly defined infiltrative lesions involving the marrow associated with cortical destruction and extraosseous extension. Lesions often have low-intermediate signal on T1WI; low, intermediate, and/or high signal on T2WI and FS T1WI; usually show Gd-contrast enhancement. Cortical destruction and tumor extension into the extraosseous soft tissues frequently occurs. Pathological fractures can be associated with metastatic lesions involving tubular bones and vertebrae. Periosteal reaction is uncommon.	Metastatic lesions typically occur in the marrow with or without cortical destruction and extraosseous tumor extension.
Plasmacytoma/myeloma (▶ Fig. 10.207)	Multiple myeloma or single plasma cell neoplasms (plasmacytoma) are well-circumscribed or poorly defined diffuse infiltrative lesions involving marrow, low-intermediate signal on T1WI, intermediate-high signal on T2WI and FS T2WI; usually show Gd-contrast-enhancement, eventual cortical bone destruction, and extraosseous extension.	Malignant tumors composed of proliferating antibody-secreting plasma cells derived from single clones. Most common primary neoplasm of bone in adults, median age = 60 years. Most patients are older than 40 years. May have variable destructive or infiltrative changes involving the axial and/or appendicular skeleton.

(continued on page 484)

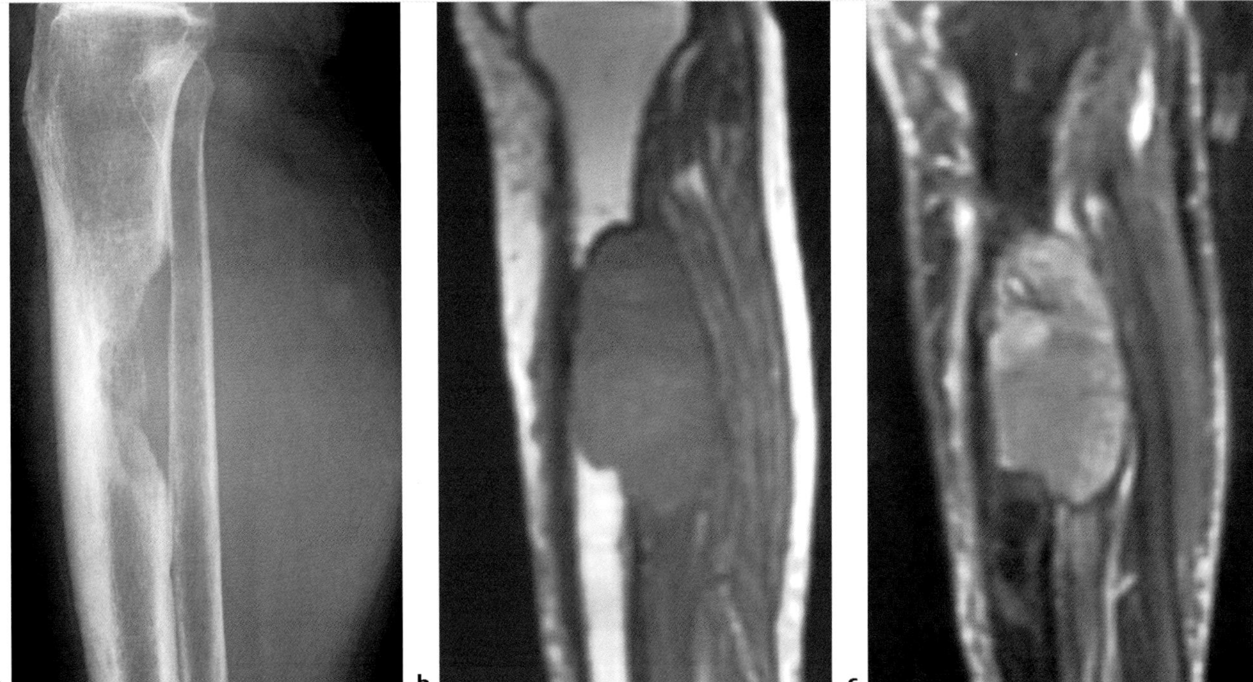

Fig. 10.206 A 74-year-old woman with metastatic melanoma involving the diaphyseal portion of the tibia. The radiolucent intramedullary lesion is associated with cortical bone destruction (a). The tumor has intermediate signal on sagittal T1-weighted imaging (b) and heterogeneous high signal on sagittal fat-suppressed T2-weighted imaging (c). Tumor is seen extending from the marrow into the extraosseous soft tissues through a zone of cortical destruction.

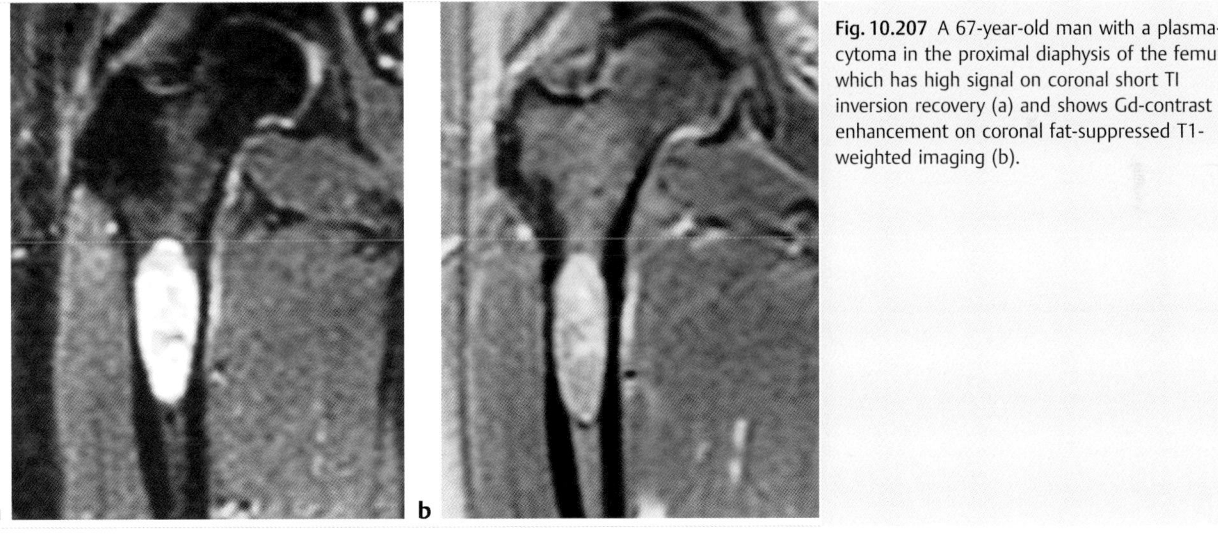

Fig. 10.207 A 67-year-old man with a plasmacytoma in the proximal diaphysis of the femur, which has high signal on coronal short TI inversion recovery (a) and shows Gd-contrast enhancement on coronal fat-suppressed T1-weighted imaging (b).

Table 10.9 (Cont.) Solitary intramedullary diaphyseal lesions

Abnormalities	MRI findings	Comments
Lymphoma (▶ Fig. 10.208)	Non-Hodgkin lymphoma (NHL) and Hodgkin disease (HD) within bone typically appears as single or multifocal poorly defined or circumscribed intramedullary zones with low-intermediate signal on T1WI; intermediate, slightly high, and/or high signal on T2WI; and high signal on FS T2WI; often show Gd-contrast enhancement. Zones of cortical destruction may occur associated with extraosseous soft tissue extension. HD involving bone with associated sclerosis seen on plain films or computed tomography (CT) usually have low signal on T1WI and variable/mixed signal on T2WI. In some cases of NHL, intramedullary tumor may be associated with bulky extraosseous lesions without extensive cortical destruction. High resolution magnetic resonance imaging (MRI) in these cases shows thin penetrating channels of tumor extending through bone cortex into the extraosseous soft tissues.	Lymphoid tumors with neoplastic cells typically within lymphoid tissue (lymph nodes and reticuloendothelial organs). Unlike leukemia, lymphoma usually arises as discrete masses. Lymphomas are subdivided into HD and NHL. Almost all primary lymphomas of bone are B-cell NHL. HD, mean age = 32 years. Osseous NHL, median = 35 years.
Osteosarcoma (▶ Fig. 10.209)	Destructive intramedullary malignant lesions, low-intermediate signal on T1WI; mixed low, intermediate, high signal on T2WI, usually with matrix mineralization/ossification-low signal on T2WI, usually show Gd-contrast enhancement (usually heterogeneous). Zones of cortical destruction are common through which tumors extend into the extraosseous soft tissues under an elevated periosteum. Lamellated and/or spiculated zones of bone formation can occur under the periosteal elevation secondary to tumor invasion and perforation of bone cortex. Low signal from spicules of periosteal, reactive, and tumoral bone formation may have a divergent (sunburst) pattern, perpendicular (hair on end) pattern, or disorganized or complex appearance. Triangular zones of periosteal elevation (Codman triangles) can be seen at the borders of zones of cortical destruction and tumor extension.	Malignant tumor composed of proliferating neoplastic spindle cells, which produce osteoid and/or immature tumoral bone and which most frequently arise within medullary bone (metadiaphyseal > metaphyseal > diaphyseal locations). Two age peaks of incidence. The larger peak occurs between the ages of 10 and 20 and accounts for over half of the cases. The second smaller peak occurs in adults over 60 years and accounts for approximately 10% of the cases. Occurs in children as primary tumors and adults (associated with Paget disease, irradiated bone, chronic osteomyelitis, osteoblastoma, giant cell tumor, fibrous dysplasia).

(continued on page 486)

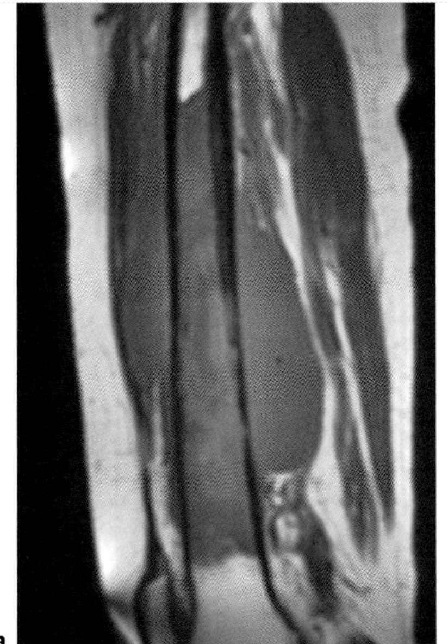

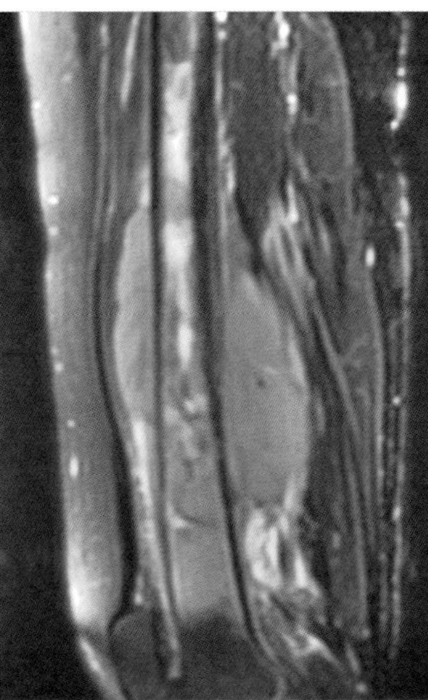

Fig. 10.208 A 36-year-old woman with large B-cell non-Hodgkin lymphoma involving the marrow of the femur, which has slightly indistinct margins and shows extensive extraosseous tumor extension relative to the degree of cortical disruption. The tumor has heterogeneous intermediate signal on sagittal T1-weighted imaging (a) and heterogeneous slightly high and high signal on sagittal fat-suppressed T2-weighted imaging (b).

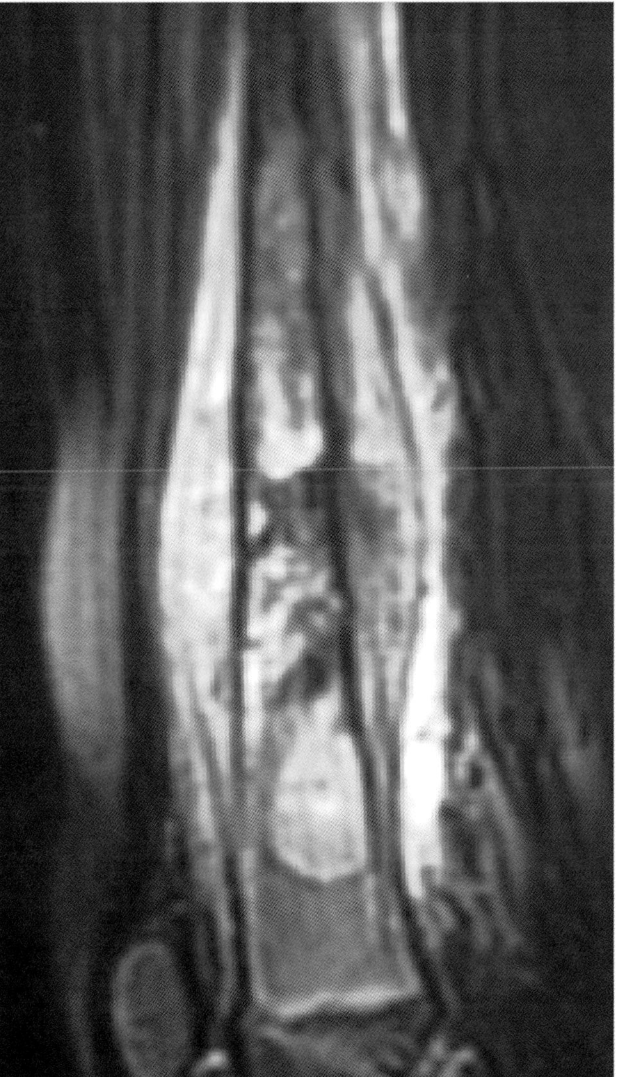

Fig. 10.209 A 16-year-old girl with an osteosarcoma in the marrow of the distal femur, which has high signal on sagittal fat-suppressed T2-weighted imaging. The tumor is associated with cortical bone destruction, extraosseous tumor extension, and periosteal elevation.

Table 10.9 (Cont.) Solitary intramedullary diaphyseal lesions

Abnormalities	MRI findings	Comments
Ewing sarcoma (▸ Fig. 10.210)	Destructive malignant lesions involving marrow; low-intermediate signal on T1WI; mixed low, intermediate, and/or high signal on T2WI and FS T2WI; usually shows Gd-contrast enhancement (usually heterogeneous). Extraosseous tumor extension through sites of cortical destruction is commonly seen beneath an elevated periosteum. Thin striated zones of low signal on T2WI can sometimes be seen oriented perpendicular to the long axis of the involved bone under the elevated periosteum representing the hair on end appearance of reactive bone formation secondary to the tumor. In long bones, tumors are most often located in the diaphyseal region, followed by the metadiaphyseal region.	Malignant primitive tumor of bone composed of undifferentiated small cells with round nuclei. Accounts for 6 to 11% of primary malignant bone tumors, 5 to 7% of primary bone tumors. Usually occurs between the ages of 5 and 30, males > females, locally invasive, high metastatic potential.
Chondrosarcoma (▸ Fig. 10.211)	Intramedullary tumors often have low-intermediate signal on T1WI, intermediate signal on PDWI, and heterogeneous intermediate-high signal on T2WI. Lesions usually show heterogeneous contrast enhancement. Zones of cortical destruction can be seen with extraosseous extension of tumor.	Chondrosarcomas are malignant tumors containing cartilage formed within sarcomatous stroma. Account for 12 to 21% of malignant bone lesions, 21 to 26% of primary sarcomas of bone. Patients range in age from 5 to 91 years, mean = 40 years, median = 26 to 59 years.

(continued on page 488)

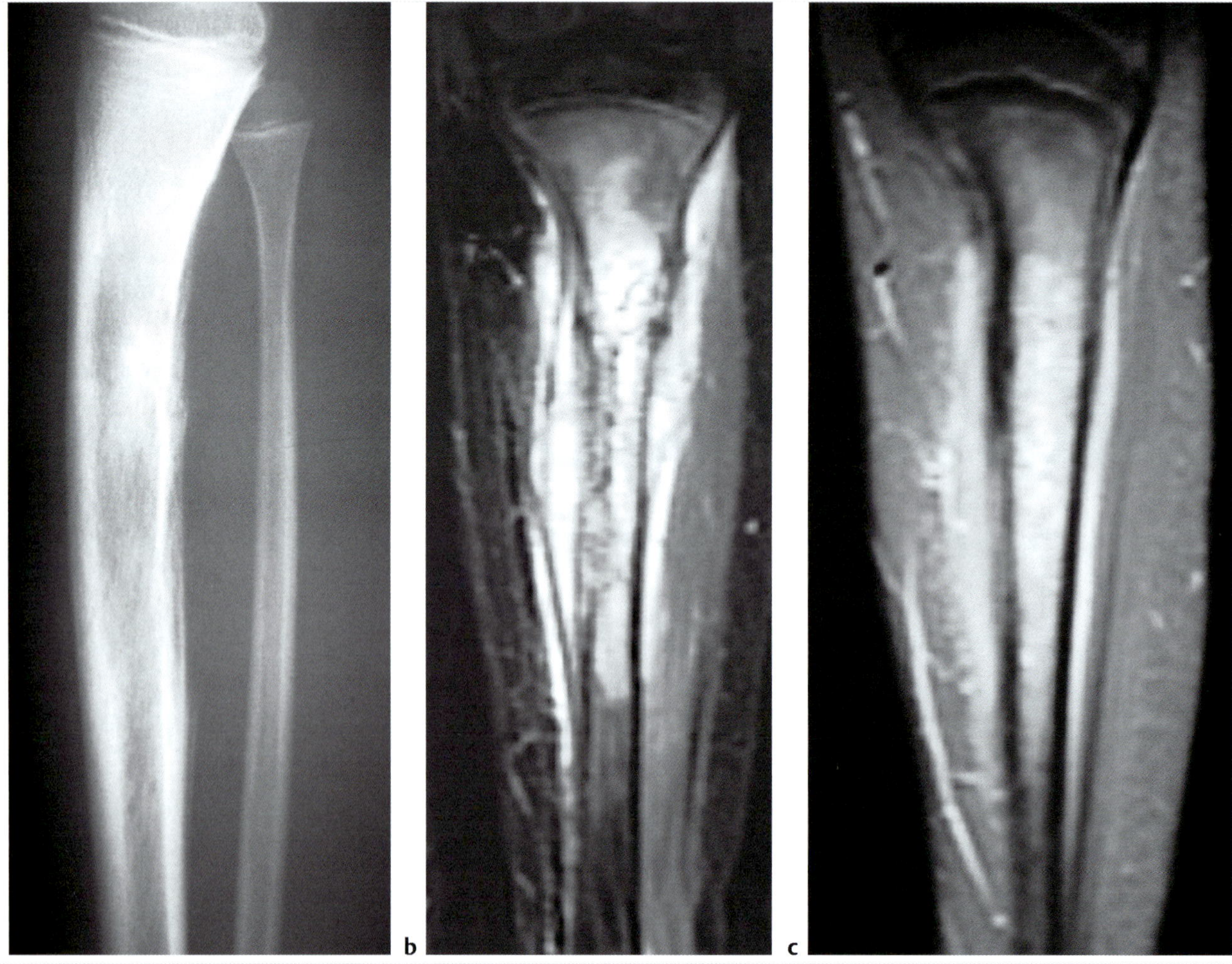

Fig. 10.210 An 11-year-old male with Ewing sarcoma involving the shaft of the tibia. The tumor has permeative radiolucent intramedullary changes, zones of cortical destruction, periosteal elevation, and a Codman triangle inferiorly on radiograph (a). Intramedullary tumor has high signal on coronal fat-suppressed (FS) T2-weighted imaging (b) and shows Gd-contrast enhancement on coronal FS T1-weighted imaging (c). The tumor is associated with cortical bone destruction, extraosseous tumor extension, and periosteal elevation.

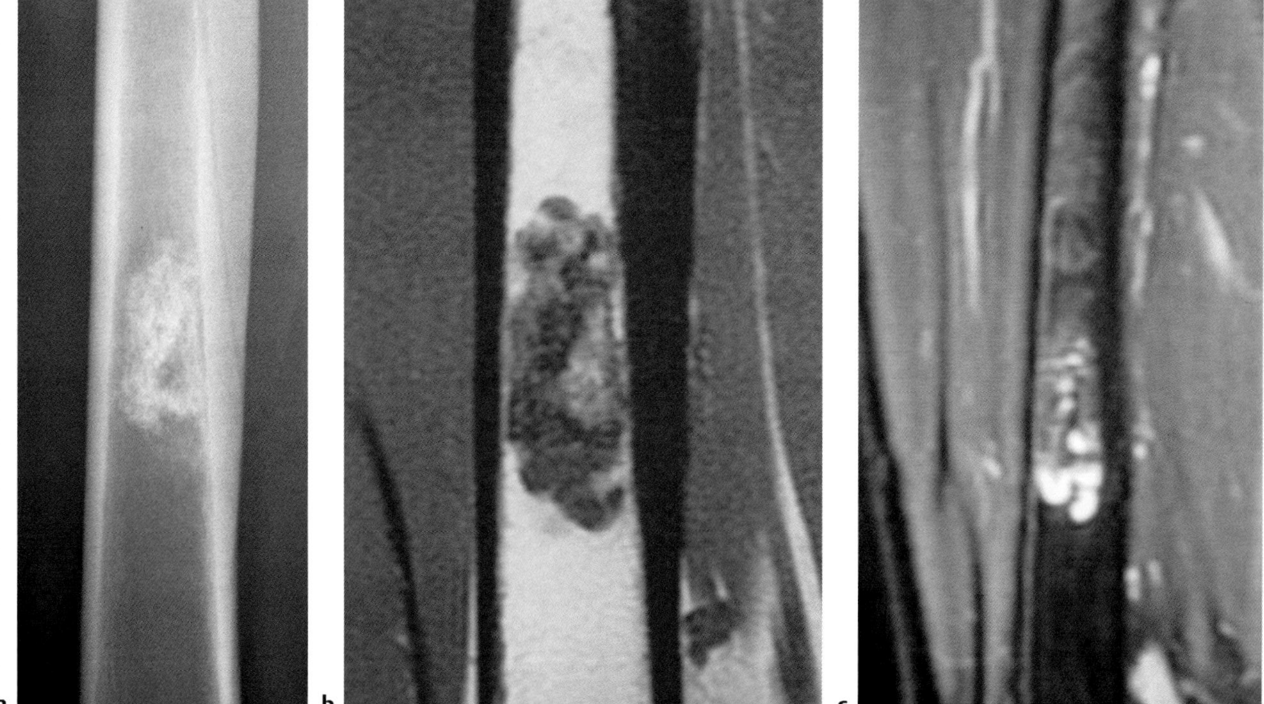

Fig. 10.211 A 39-year-old man with a chondrosarcoma in the marrow of the distal tibial shaft, which has chondroid matrix mineralization on a lateral radiograph (a). The tumor has mixed low and intermediate signal on sagittal T1-weighted imaging (b) and heterogeneous high signal on fat-suppressed T2-weighted imaging (c).

Table 10.9 (Cont.) Solitary intramedullary diaphyseal lesions

Abnormalities	MRI findings	Comments
Fibrosarcoma	Intramedullary lesions with irregular margins, with or without associated cortical destruction and/or extraosseous soft tissue masses. Lesions usually have low-intermediate signal on T1WI and PDWI and heterogeneous intermediate, slightly high, and/or high signal on T2WI. Lesions usually show heterogeneous Gd-contrast enhancement.	Fibrosarcomas are uncommon malignant tumors consisting of bundles of neoplastic fibroblasts/spindle cells with varying proportions of collagen, lacking other tissue-differentiating features such as tumor bone, osteoid, or cartilage. Can be primary lesions (75%) or arise as secondary tumors (25%) associated with prior irradiation, Paget disease, bone infarct, chronic osteomyelitis, fibrous dysplasia, giant cell tumor. Account for 3 to 5% of primary malignant bone tumors and 2 to 4% of all bone tumors. Median age = 43 years.
Malignant fibrous histiocytoma	Intramedullary lesions with irregular margins with zones of cortical destruction and extraosseous extension. Tumors often have low-intermediate signal on T1WI, low-intermediate signal on PDWI, and heterogeneous intermediate-high signal on T2WI and FS T2WI. Invasion into joints occurs in 30%. May be associated with other bone infarcts, bone cysts, chronic osteomyelitis, Paget disease, and other treated primary bone tumors. Lesions usually show heterogeneous Gd-contrast prominent enhancement.	Malignant tumor involving soft tissue and rarely bone derived from undifferentiated mesenchymal cells. Contains cells with limited cellular differentiation such as mixtures of fibroblasts, myofibroblasts, histiocyte-like cells, anaplastic giant cells, and inflammatory cells. Accounts for 1 to 5% of primary malignant bone tumors and < 1 to 3% of all primary bone tumors. Patient ages range from 11 to 80 years, median = 48 years, mean = 55 years.
Paget sarcoma (▶ Fig. 10.212)	Irregular zones of medullary and cortical bone destruction associated with an extraosseous soft-tissue mass-lesion. The involved marrow typically has low to intermediate signal on T1WI and PDWI and low to high signal on T2WI. Abnormal Gd-contrast enhancement is seen in the marrow as well as in the extraosseous tumor extension.	Paget disease is the most common bone disease in older adults after osteoporosis. Median age = 66 years. Disordered bone resorption and woven bone formation occurs, resulting in osseous deformity. Associated with less than 1% risk for developing secondary sarcomatous changes.

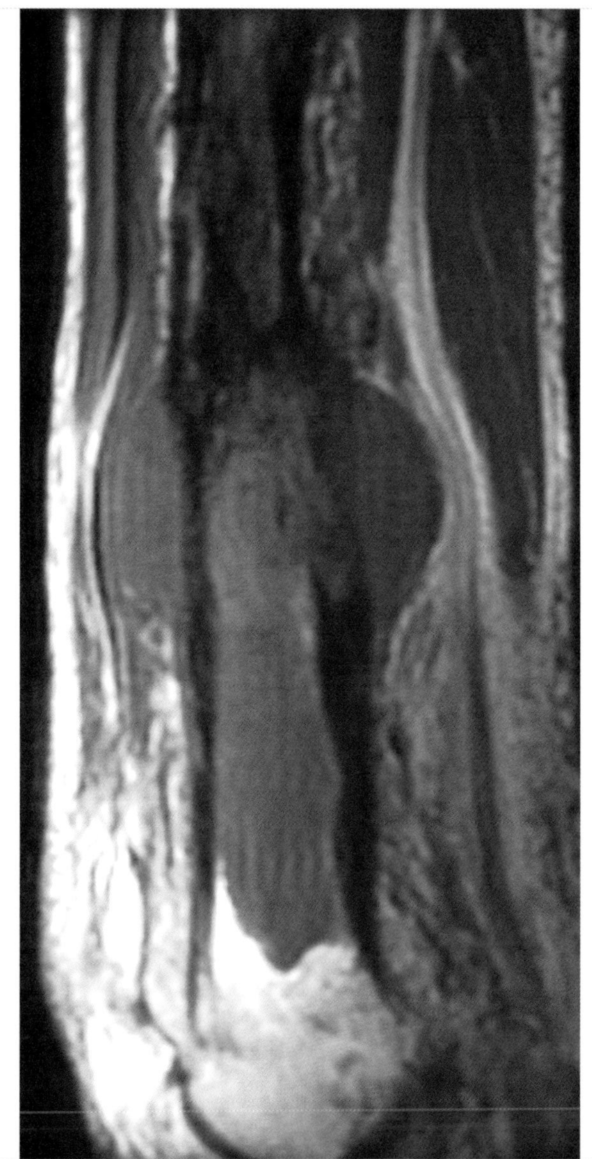

Fig. 10.212 A 71-year-old woman with Paget sarcoma involving the marrow of the distal femur associated with cortical destruction and extraosseous extension as seen on sagittal T1-weighted imaging.

10.10 Osseous Tumors and Tumor-Like Lesions of the Hands and Feet

- Nonmalignant lesions
  - Enchondroma
  - Osteochondroma
  - Bizarre parosteal osteochondromatous proliferation
  - Juxtacortical chondroma
  - Osteoblastoma
  - Osteoid osteoma
  - Chondromyxoid fibroma
  - Lipoma
  - Enostosis/bone island
  - Aneurysmal bone cyst (ABC)
  - Giant cell reparative granuloma
  - Unicameral bone cyst (UBC)
  - Geode
  - Chondroblastoma
  - Hemangioma
  - Glomus body tumor
  - Giant cell tumor
  - Fibrous dysplasia
  - Osteomyelitis
  - Eosinophilic granuloma
  - Sarcoidosis
  - Gout
  - Chronic recurrent multifocal osteomyelitis
  - Bone infarct
- Malignant lesions
  - Metastatic lesion
  - Plasmacytoma/myeloma
  - Chondrosarcoma
  - Osteosarcoma
  - Ewing sarcoma

Table 10.10 Osseous tumors and tumor-like lesions of the hands and feet

Abnormalities	MRI findings	Comments
Nonmalignant lesions		
Enchondroma (▶ Fig. 10.213; ▶ Fig. 10.214)	Lobulated intramedullary lesions with well-defined borders, which usually have low-intermediate signal on T1-weighted imaging (T1WI) and intermediate signal on proton density–weighted imaging (PDWI). On T2-weighted imaging (T2WI) and fat-suppressed T2WI, lesions usually have predominantly high signal. Lesions typically show gadolinium (Gd)-contrast enhancement in various patterns (peripheral curvilinear lobular, central nodular/septal and peripheral lobular, or heterogeneous diffuse).	Benign intramedullary lesions composed of hyaline cartilage, represent approximately 10% of benign bone tumors. Enchondromas can be solitary (88%) or multiple (12%). Ollier disease is a dyschondroplasia involving endochondral-formed bone resulting in multiple enchondromas (enchondromatosis). Maffucci syndrome presents with multiple enchondromas and soft tissue hemangiomas and is very rare. Median age = 35 years, peak in third and fourth decades.
Osteochondroma (▶ Fig. 10.215)	Circumscribed protruding lesion arising from outer cortex with a central zone with intermediate signal on T1WI and T2WI similar to marrow surrounded by a peripheral zone of low signal on T1 W and T2WI. A cartilaginous cap with high signal on T2WI is usually present in children and young adults. Increased malignant potential when cartilaginous cap is > 2 cm thick.	Benign cartilaginous tumors arising from defect at periphery of growth plate during bone formation with resultant bone outgrowth covered by a cartilaginous cap. Usually benign lesions unless associated with pain and increasing size of cartilaginous cap. Osteochondromas are common lesions, accounting for 14 to 35% of primary bone tumors. Occur with median age of 20 years; up to 75% of patients are less than 20 years.

(continued on page 492)

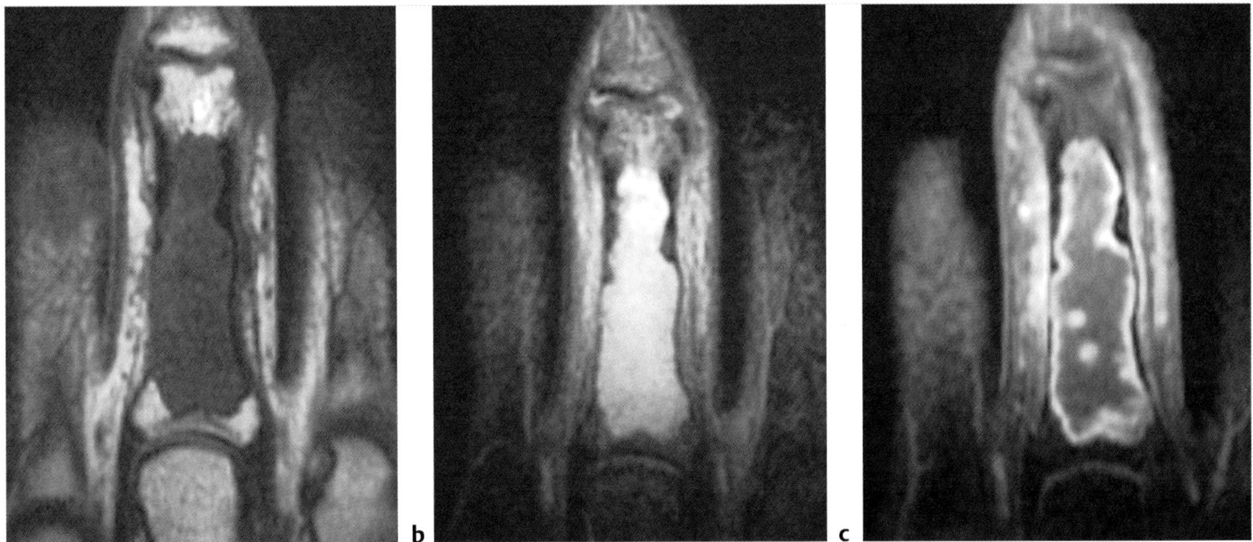

Fig. 10.213 A 39-year-old woman with an enchondroma in a proximal phalanx, which has intermediate signal on coronal T1-weighted imaging (T1WI) (a) and high signal on coronal fat-suppressed (FS) T2-weighted imaging (b). The lesion shows thin peripheral and central nodular gadolinium (Gd)-contrast enhancement on coronal FS T1WI (c). The lesion is associated with thinning and slight expansion of adjacent cortical bone.

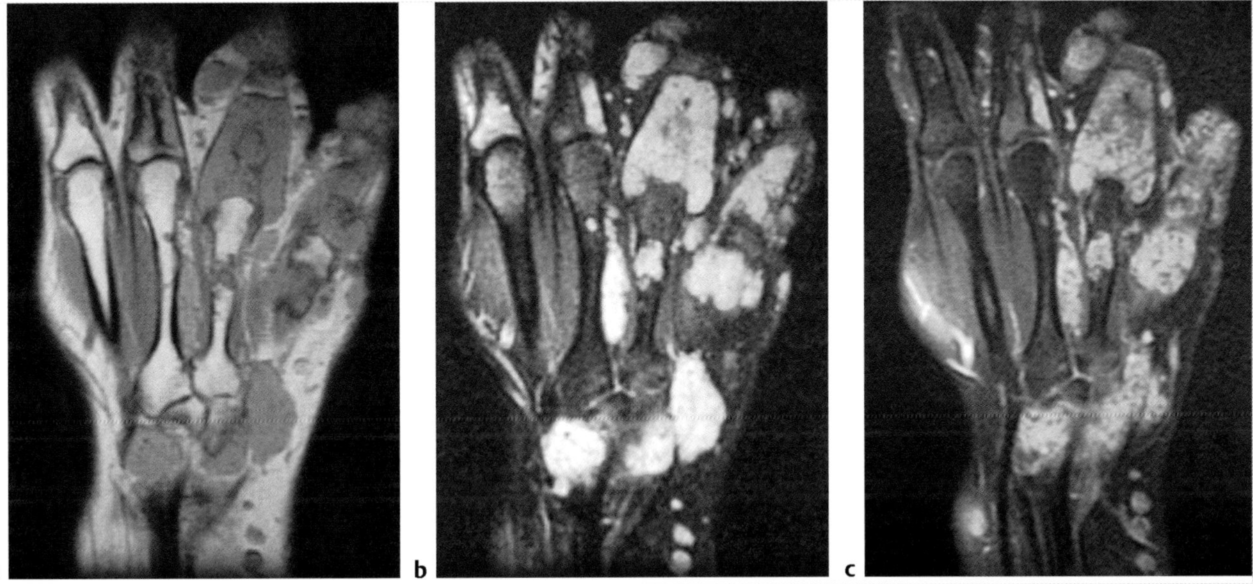

Fig. 10.214 A 20-year-old woman with Maffucci syndrome with multiple enchondromas within bones of the hand, which have intermediate signal on coronal T1-weighted imaging (T1WI) (a) and high signal on coronal fat-suppressed (FS) T2-weighted imaging (b). The enchondromas and soft tissue hemangiomas show Gd-contrast enhancement on coronal FS T1WI (c).

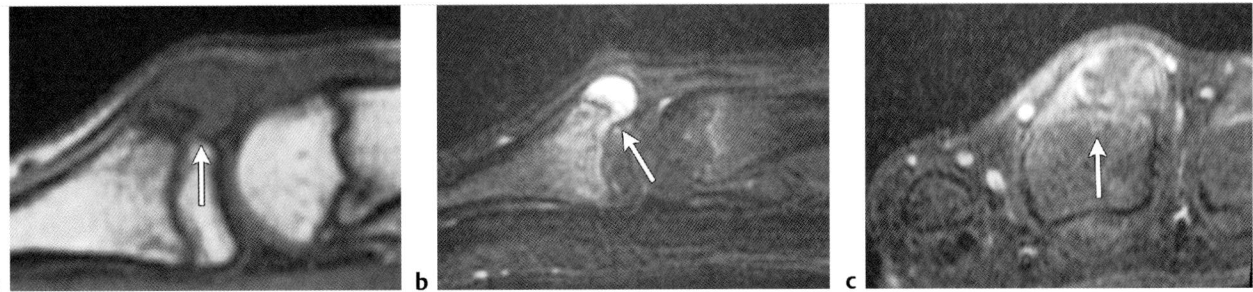

Fig. 10.215 A 14-year-old boy with an osteochondroma involving the proximal metaphyseal surface of a phalanx (arrow), which has intermediate signal on sagittal T1-weighted imaging (T1WI) (a) and high signal (arrow) on sagittal fat-suppressed (FS) T2-weighted imaging (b). The lesion (arrow) shows thin peripheral gadolinium-contrast enhancement on axial FS T1WI (c).

Table 10.10 (Cont.) Osseous tumors and tumor-like lesions of the hands and feet

Abnormalities	MRI findings	Comments
Bizarre parosteal osteochondromatous proliferation (▶ Fig. 10.216)	Smooth and/or lobulated calcified and/or ossified lesions often with a broad base or stalk of attachment to an intact outer cortical surface of bone. Remodeling of adjacent bone cortex can occur. Typically does not invade adjacent extraosseous soft tissues.	Lesions adjacent to or attached to the outer periosteal surface of bone consisting of disorganized conglomerations of bone with short trabeculae, cartilage containing enlarged dysmorphic binucleate chondrocytes, spindle cells, fibrous tissue, and/or myxoid regions. Commonly occurs in the hands and feet (70%), less commonly in long bones. Peak age in fourth decade. May represent a type of heterotopic ossification versus benign tumor. Can be cured by surgical excision, although local recurrence is common.
Juxtacortical chondroma	Lesions are located at the bone surface and are usually lobulated with low-intermediate signal on T1WI, which is hypo- or isointense relative to muscle. Lesions usually have heterogeneous predominantly high signal on T2WI. Lesions are surrounded by low signal borders on T2WI representing thin sclerotic reaction. Areas of low signal on T2WI are secondary to matrix mineralization. Edema is not typically seen in adjacent medullary bone. Lesions often show a peripheral pattern of Gd-contrast enhancement.	Benign protuberant hyaline cartilaginous tumors that arise from the periosteum superficial to bone cortex. Juxtacortical chondromas account for < 1% of bone lesions. Occur with median age of 26 years.

(continued on page 494)

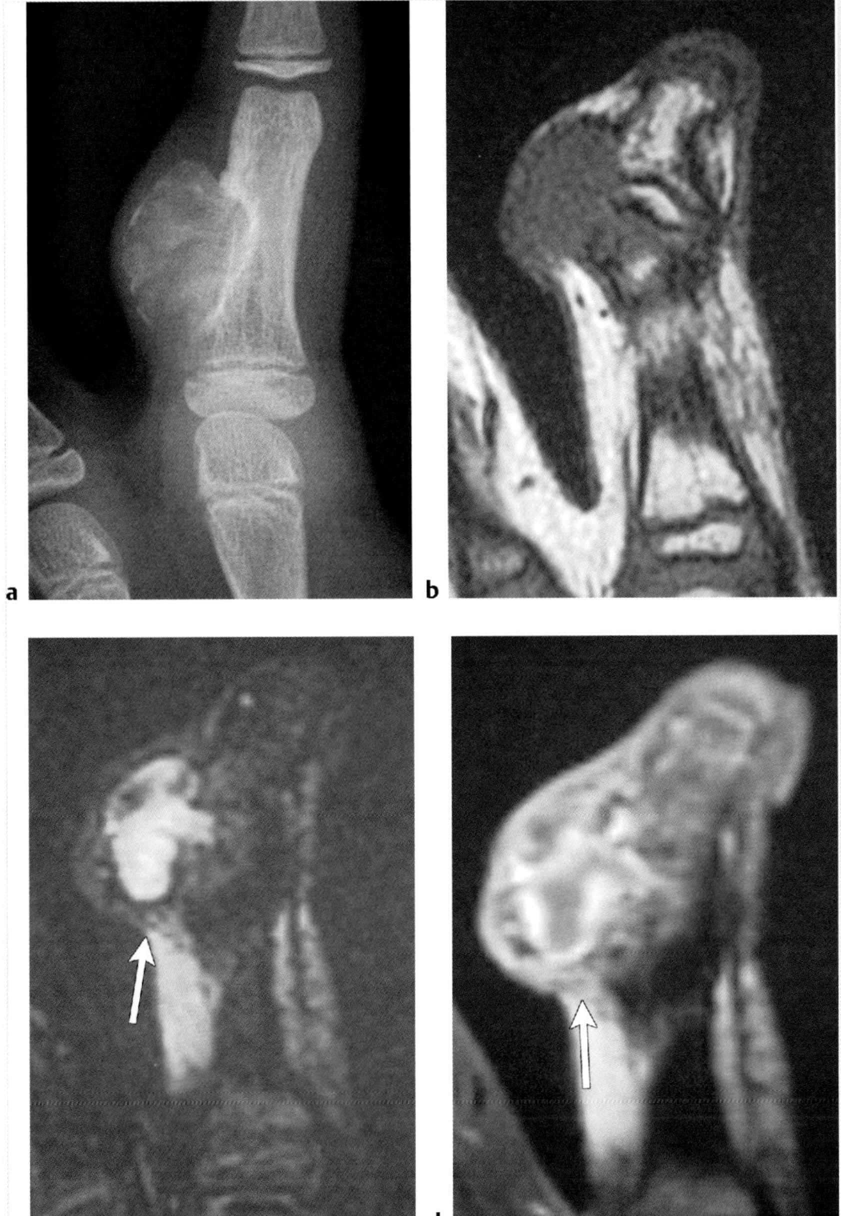

Fig. 10.216 A 10-year-old boy with a bizarre parosteal osteochondromatous proliferation involving a proximal phalanx as seen on a radiograph. The ossified lesion has smooth margins and a broad base along the phalanx (a), and is associated with erosive remodeling of the adjacent cortical bone. The lesion has intermediate signal on coronal T1-weighted imaging (T1WI) (b), and high signal (arrow) on fat-suppressed (FS) T2-weighted imaging (c). The lesion (arrow) shows thin peripheral gadolinium-contrast enhancement on FS T1WI (d).

Table 10.10 (Cont.) Osseous tumors and tumor-like lesions of the hands and feet

Abnormalities	MRI findings	Comments
Osteoblastoma (▶ Fig. 10.217, ▶ Fig. 10.218)	Expansile radiolucent lesions often greater than 1.5 cm in diameter with or without matrix mineralization and peripheral bone sclerosis seen on radiographs and computed tomography (CT). Lesions often have low-intermediate signal on T1WI and intermediate-high signal on T2WI and FS T2WI; usually show Gd-contrast enhancement. Lesions usually have poorly defined zones with high signal on T2WI and FS T2WI and Gd-contrast enhancement in the marrow (edema, inflammation) beyond the zone of sclerosis or in adjacent soft tissues from prostaglandin synthesis by these lesions.	Rare benign bone neoplasm (2% of bone tumors) usually occurs between the ages of 6 and 30 years.
Osteoid osteoma (▶ Fig. 10.219)	Typically shows dense fusiform thickening of the cortex, which has low signal on T1 W, PDWI, T2WI, and FS T2WI. Within the thickened cortex, a spheroid or ovoid zone (nidus) measuring less than 1.5 cm is seen in the region of the original external surface of bone cortex. The nidus can have irregular, distinct, or indistinct margins relative to the adjacent region of cortical thickening. The nidus can have low-intermediate signal on T1WI, and low-intermediate or high signal on T2WI and FS T2WI. Calcifications in the nidus can be seen as low signal on T2WI. After Gd-contrast administration, variable degrees of enhancement are seen at the nidus and adjacent marrow.	Benign osteoblastic lesion composed of a circumscribed nidus less than 1.5 cm and usually surrounded by reactive bone formation. These lesions are usually painful and have limited growth potential. Osteoid osteoma accounts for 11 to 13% of primary benign bone tumors. Occurs in patients age 6 to 30 years, median = 17 years. Approximately 75% occur in patients less than 25 years.
Chondromyxoid fibroma (▶ Fig. 10.220)	Lesions are often slightly lobulated with low-intermediate signal on T1WI, and heterogeneous predominantly high signal on T2WI secondary to myxoid and hyaline chondroid components with high water content. Magnetic resonance (MR) signal heterogeneity on T2WI is related to the proportions of myxoid, chondroid, and fibrous components within the lesions. Thin low signal septa within lesions on T2WI are secondary to fibrous strands. Lesions are surrounded by low signal borders representing thin sclerotic reaction. Lesions show prominent diffuse Gd-contrast enhancement.	Rare benign slow-growing bone lesions that contain chondroid, myxoid, and fibrous components. Chondromyxoid fibromas represent 2 to 4% of primary benign bone lesions, and < 1% of primary bone lesions. Most chondromyxoid fibromas occur between the ages of 1 and 40 years, with a median of 17 years, and peak incidence in the second to third decades.
Lipoma (▶ Fig. 10.221)	Lesions typically have signal of fat and may also contain zones with low, intermediate, and/or high signal on PDWI and T2WI as well as peripheral rimlike and central Gd-contrast enhancement on FS T1WI.	Uncommon benign hamartomas composed of mature white adipose tissue without cellular atypia. Osseous or chondroid metaplasia with myxoid changes can be associated with lipomas. Account for approximately 0.1% of bone tumors, likely underreported.

(continued on page 496)

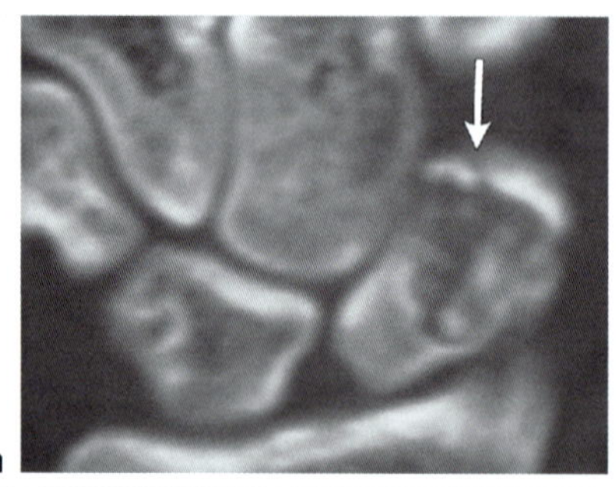

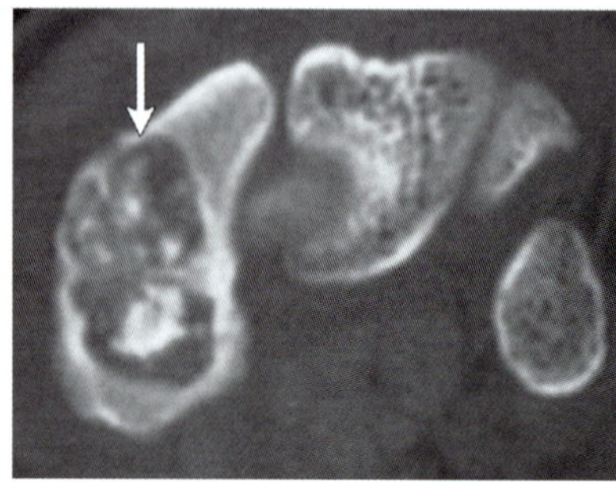

Fig. 10.217 A 16-year-old boy with an osteoblastoma within the scaphoid bone in the wrist, which is seen as a radiolucent lesion containing mineralized matrix on coronal (a) and axial computed tomography (b).

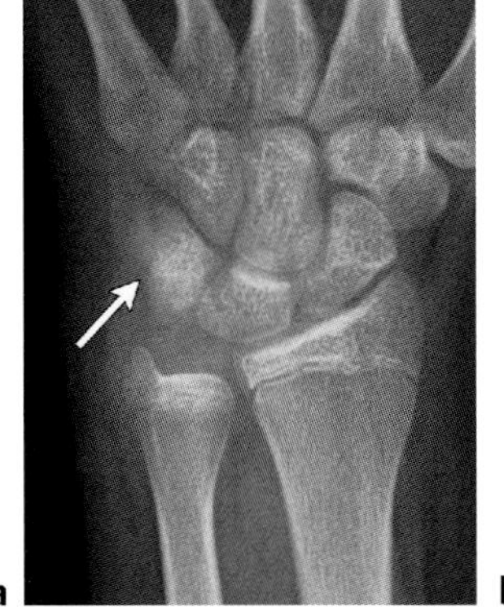
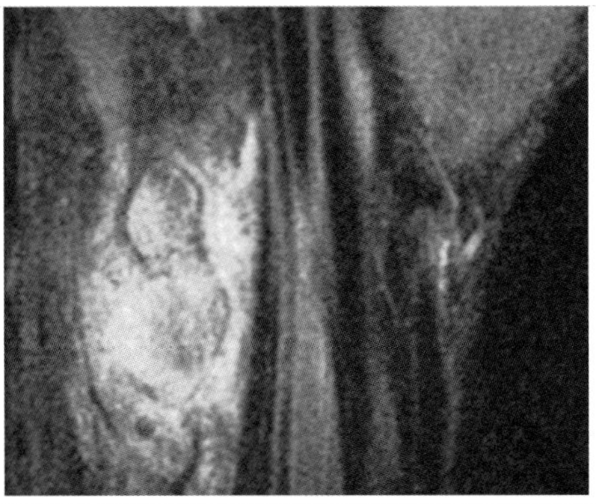
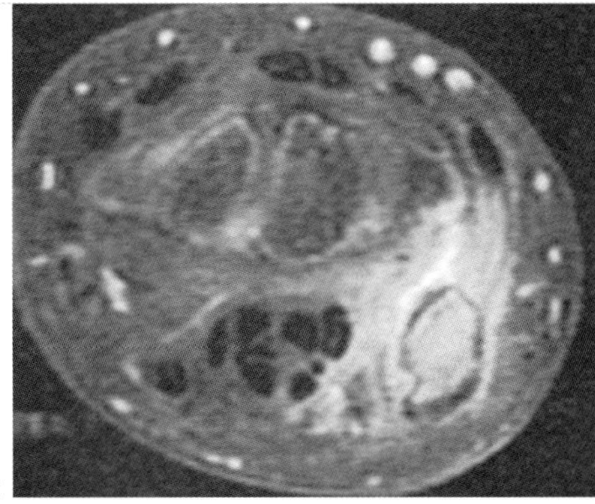

Fig. 10.218 A 13-year-old girl with an osteoblastoma of the pisiform bone, which is a radiolucent lesion (arrow) on radiograph (a). The lesion has high signal on coronal fat-suppressed T2-weighted imaging (FS T2WI) (b) and shows gadolinium-contrast enhancement on axial FS T1-weighted imaging (c). The lesion is associated with cortical bone thinning and destruction with abnormal high signal on FS T2WI and contrast enhancement in the extraosseous soft tissues.

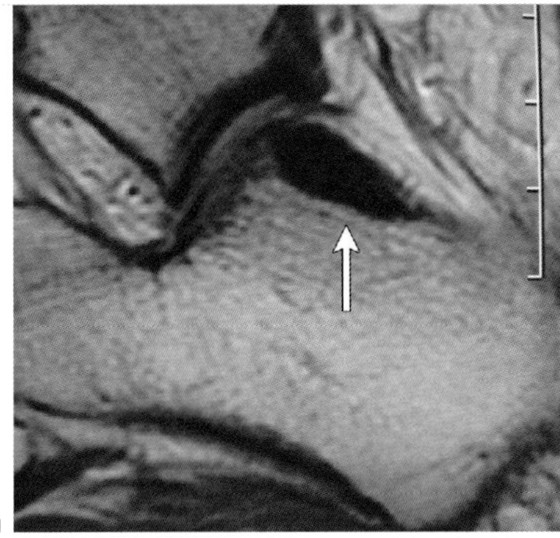
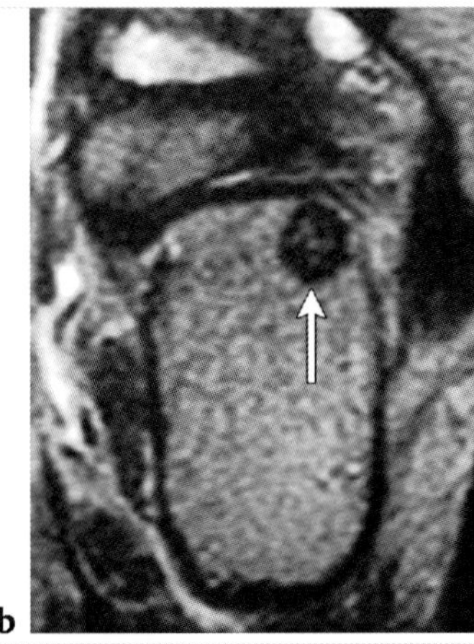

Fig. 10.219 An 18-year-old woman with an osteoid osteoma in the calcaneus. The lesion (arrow) has low signal on sagittal proton density–weighted imaging (a) and low signal peripheral to a central area of intermediate signal (arrow) on axial T2-weighted imaging (b).

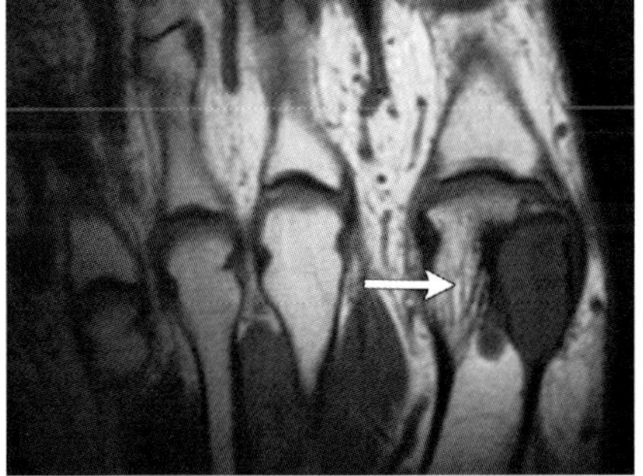
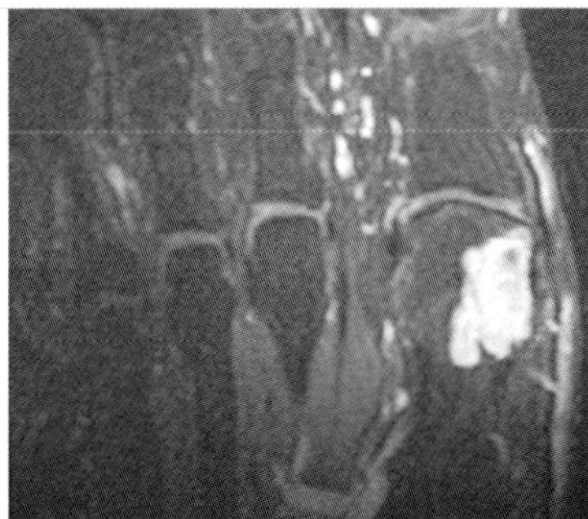

Fig. 10.220 A 34-year-old man with chondromyxoid fibroma in the distal first metatarsal bone. The lesion (arrow) has low-intermediate signal on coronal T1-weighted imaging (a) and heterogeneous high signal on fat-suppressed T2-weighted imaging (b).

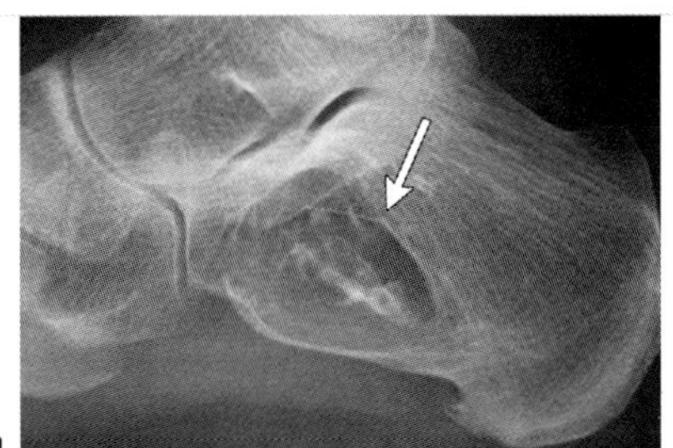
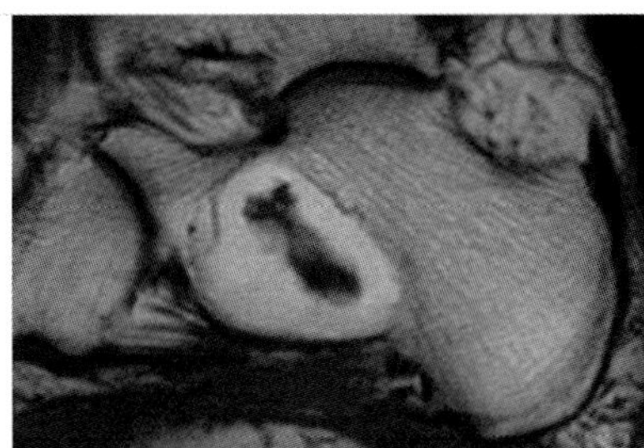

Fig. 10.221 A 47-year-old woman with a radiolucent intraosseous lipoma (arrow) in the calcaneus, which has a central dystrophic calcification on radiograph (a). The lesion has thin low signal margins and mostly high signal on sagittal T1-weighted imaging (b) as well as a central zone of low signal from dystrophic calcification.

Table 10.10 (Cont.) Osseous tumors and tumor-like lesions of the hands and feet

Abnormalities	MRI findings	Comments
Enostosis/bone island	Typically appear as well-circumscribed zones of dense bone with low signal on T1WI, PDWI, T2WI, and FS T2WI. No infiltration into the adjacent soft tissues by ostomas is seen. Zones of bone destruction or associated soft tissue mass-lesions are not associated with osteomas. Periosteal reaction is not associated with osteomas except in cases with coincidental antecedent trauma.	Benign primary bone tumor composed of dense lamellar, woven, and/or compact cortical bone usually located at the surface of bone. Multiple osteomas usually occur in Gardner syndrome, which is an autosomal dominant disorder that is associated with intestinal polyposis, fibromas, and desmoid tumors. Accounts for less than 1% of primary benign bone tumors. Occurs in patients age 16 to 74 years, most frequent in sixth decade.
Aneurysmal bone cyst (ABC) (▶ Fig. 10.222)	ABCs often have a low signal rim on T1 W and T2 W images adjacent to normal medullary bone and between extraosseous soft tissues. Various combinations of low, intermediate, and/or high signal on T1WI, PDWI, and T2WI are usually seen within ABCs as well as fluid-fluid levels. Variable gadolinium-contrast enhancement is seen at the margins of lesions as well as involving the internal septae.	Tumor-like expansile bone lesions containing cavernous spaces filled with blood. ABCs can be primary bone lesions (two thirds) or secondary to other bone lesions/tumors (such as giant cell tumors, chondroblastomas, osteoblastomas, osteosarcomas. chondromyxoid fibromas, nonossifying fibromas, fibrous dysplasia, fibrosarcomas, malignant fibrous histiocytomas, and metastatic disease). Account for approximately 11% of primary tumor-like lesions of bone. Patients usually range in age from 1 to 25 years, median = 14 years.
Giant cell reparative granuloma (▶ Fig. 10.223)	Lesions can have heterogeneous low, intermediate, and/or high signal on T1WI, PDWI, and T2WI as well as peripheral rimlike and central Gd-contrast enhancement on FS T1WI.	Giant cell reparative granulomas are also referred to as solid ABCs. Histological appearance resembles brown tumors.
Unicameral bone cyst (UBC) (▶ Fig. 10.224)	UBCs often have a peripheral rim of low signal on T1 W and T2 W images adjacent to normal medullary bone. Usually contain fluid with low to low-intermediate signal on T1WI, low-intermediate and high signal on T2WI. Fluid-fluid levels may occur. For UBCs without pathological fracture, thin peripheral Gd-contrast enhancement can be seen at the margins of lesions. UBCs with pathological fracture can have heterogeneous or homogeneous low-intermediate or slightly high signal on T1WI, and heterogeneous or homogeneous high signal on T2WI and FS T2WI. UBCs complicated by fracture can have internal septations and fluid-fluid levels, as well as irregular peripheral Gd-contrast enhancement and at internal septations.	Intramedullary nonneoplastic cavities filled with serous or serosanguinous fluid. Account for 9% of primary tumor-like lesions of bone; 85% occur in the first 2 decades, median = 11 years.

(continued on page 498)

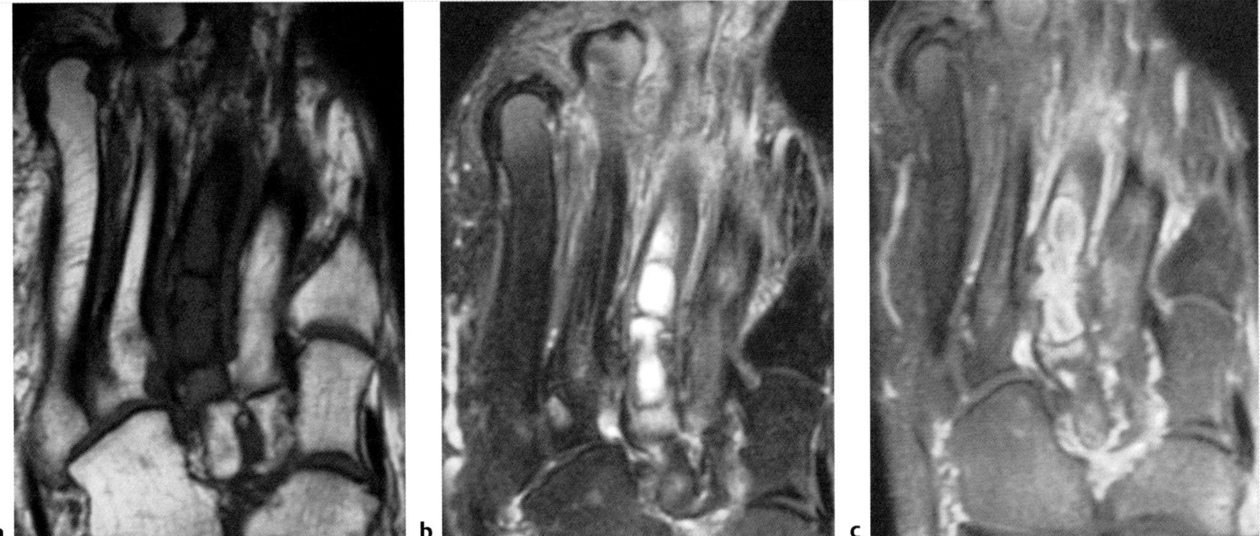

Fig. 10.222 A 48-year-old man with an aneurysmal bone cyst in the proximal portion of the third metatarsal bone, which has low-intermediate signal on coronal T1-weighted imaging (T1WI) (a) and mostly high signal on coronal fat-suppressed T2-weighted imaging (FS T2WI) (b). The lesion shows thin mostly peripheral gadolinium-contrast enhancement on coronal FS T1WI (c). Also seen are slight expansion and thinning of the adjacent cortical margins and poorly defined zones of increased signal on FS T2WI and Gd-contrast enhancement in the adjacent bone marrow.

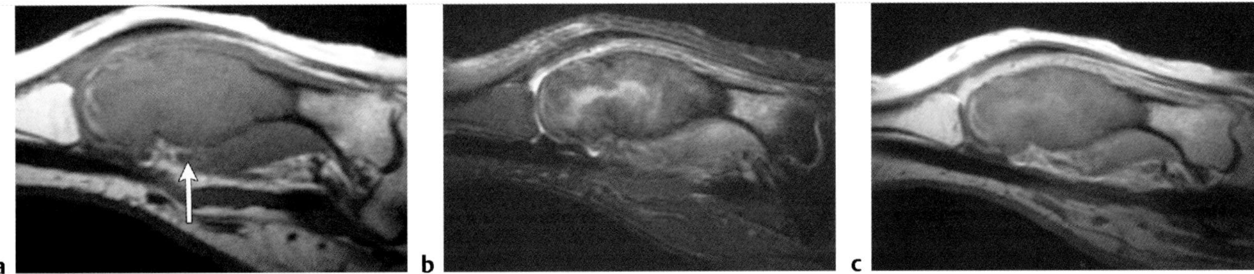

Fig. 10.223 A 39-year-old woman with a giant cell granuloma involving a metacarpal bone. The intramedullary lesion (arrow) expands and thins bone cortex and has intermediate signal on sagittal T1-weighted imaging (T1WI) (a) and heterogeneous low, intermediate, slightly high, and high signal on sagittal fat-suppressed T2-weighted imaging (b). The lesion shows Gd-contrast enhancement on sagittal T1WI (c).

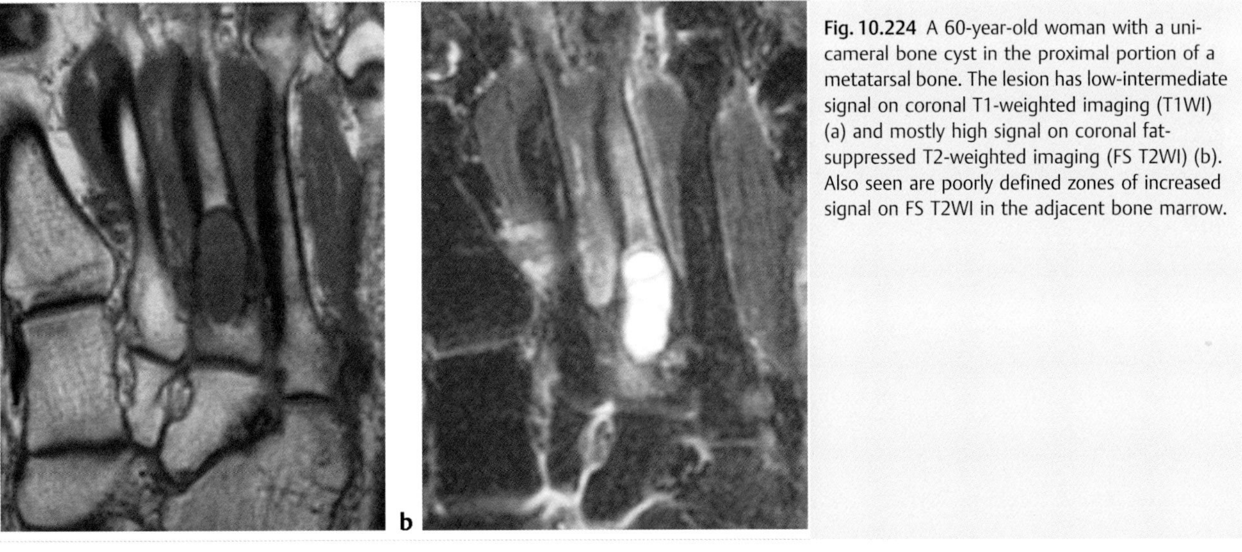

Fig. 10.224 A 60-year-old woman with a unicameral bone cyst in the proximal portion of a metatarsal bone. The lesion has low-intermediate signal on coronal T1-weighted imaging (T1WI) (a) and mostly high signal on coronal fat-suppressed T2-weighted imaging (FS T2WI) (b). Also seen are poorly defined zones of increased signal on FS T2WI in the adjacent bone marrow.

Table 10.10 (Cont.) Osseous tumors and tumor-like lesions of the hands and feet

Abnormalities	MRI findings	Comments
Geode (▶ Fig. 10.225)	Typically have sharply defined margins and contain low signal on T1WI, low-intermediate signal on PDWI, and homogeneous high signal on T2WI. Poorly defined zones of Gd-contrast enhancement can be seen in the marrow adjacent to the subchondral cysts on FS T1WI.	A geode or subchondral cyst is a radiolucent/cystic lesion located near the end of a long bone where there are changes of degenerative osteoarthropathy. Lesions can result from synovial fluid intrusion and/or bony contusion in the setting of degenerative joint disease.
Chondroblastoma (▶ Fig. 10.226; ▶ Fig. 10.227)	Tumors often have fine lobular margins, and typically have low-intermediate heterogeneous signal on T1WI, and mixed low, intermediate, and/or high signal on T2WI. Lobular, marginal, or septal Gd-contrast enhancement patterns can be seen. Poorly defined zones with high signal on T2WI and FS T2WI and corresponding Gd-contrast enhancement are typically seen in the marrow adjacent to the lesions representing inflammatory reaction from prostaglandin synthesis by these tumors. Can have associated secondary ABCs.	Benign cartilaginous tumors with chondroblast-like cells and areas of chondroid matrix formation, usually occur in children and adolescents, median age = 17 years, mean age = 16 years for lesions in long bones, mean age = 28 years in other bones. Most cases are diagnosed between the ages of 5 and 25.
Hemangioma	Often well-circumscribed lesions that typically have intermediate to high signal on T1WI, PDWI, T2WI, and FS T2WI. On T1WI, hemangiomas usually have signal equal to or greater than adjacent normal marrow secondary to fatty components. Usually show Gd-contrast enhancement. Pathological fractures associated with intraosseous hemangiomas usually result in low-intermediate marrow signal on T1WI.	Benign lesions of bone composed of capillary, cavernous, and/or malformed venous vessels. Considered to be a hamartomatous disorder. Account for 4% of benign bone tumors and approximately 1% of all bone tumors, likely underestimated. Occurs in all ages, median = 33 years.

(continued on page 500)

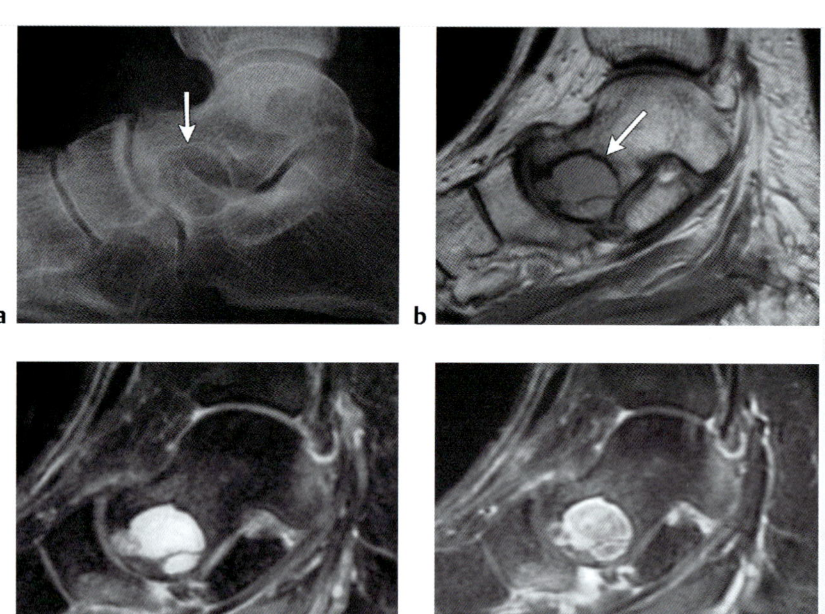

Fig. 10.225 Geode or degenerative-arthritic-subchondral radiolucent "cyst" in the anterior talus adjacent to an arthritic talonavicular joint (arrow) (a). The lesion (arrow) has thin circumscribed low signal margins and contains intermediate signal centrally on sagittal proton density–weighted imaging (b) and high signal centrally on sagittal fat-suppressed T2-weighted imaging (FS T2WI) (c). Peripheral gadolinium-contrast enhancement is seen on sagittal FS T1-weighted imaging (d). Poorly defined zones with slightly increased signal on FS T2WI and minimal contrast enhancement are seen in the adjacent marrow.

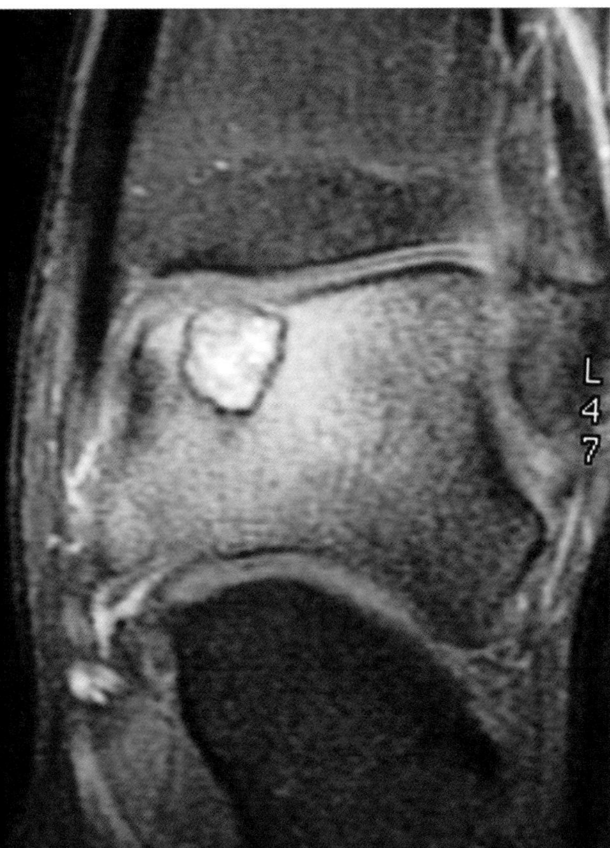

Fig. 10.226 A 15-year-old girl with a chondroblastoma involving the talus, which shows prominent Gd-contrast centrally surrounded by a thin rim of low signal on coronal fat-suppressed T1-weighted imaging. Poorlydefined zones with abnormal contrast enhancement are seen in the marrow adjacent to the lesion.

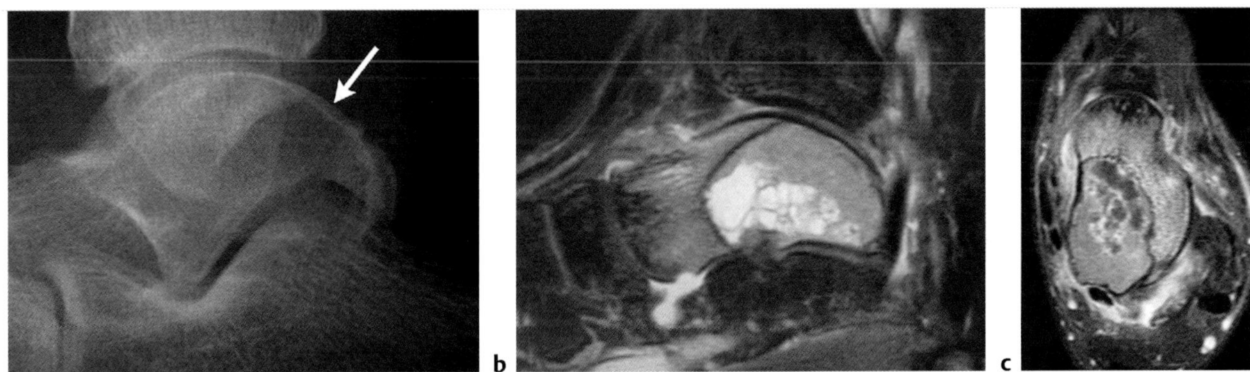

Fig. 10.227 A 20-year-old man with a radiolucent chondroblastoma (arrow) in the talus (a), which has heterogeneous slightly high and high signal on sagittal fat-suppressed T2-weighted imaging (FS T2WI) (b) and heterogeneous Gd-contrast enhancement on axial FS T1-weighted imaging (c) related to the presence of a secondary aneurysmal bone cyst. Poorly defined zones of high signal on FS T2WI and contrast enhancement are also seen in the marrow adjacent to the lesion.

Table 10.10 (Cont.) Osseous tumors and tumor-like lesions of the hands and feet

Abnormalities	MRI findings	Comments
Glomus body tumor (▶ Fig. 10.228)	Glomus body tumors are well-circumscribed ovoid lesions measuring less than 1 cm and are often located under the nail beds at the distal phalanges of fingers and toes. Glomus body tumors often have low-intermediate signal on T1WI and PDWI, although may be hypointense or hyperintense on T1WI relative to the adjacent dermis layers. Glomus tumors usually have high signal T2WI and FS T2WI and typically show Gd-contrast enhancement.	Benign mesenchymal hamartomas derived from the neuromyoarterial apparatus (glomus bodies), which regulate arteriolar blood flow to the skin related to temperature and are normally present throughout the reticular dermis throughout the body. Glomus bodies occur in large numbers under the nail beds of the fingers and toes.
Giant cell tumor (▶ Fig. 10.229; ▶ Fig. 10.230)	Often well-defined lesions with thin low signal margins on T1WI, PDWI, and T2WI. Solid portions of giant cell tumors often have low to intermediate signal on T1WI and PDWI, intermediate to high signal on T2WI, and high signal on FS PDWI and FS T2WI. Zones of low signal on T2WI may be seen secondary to hemosiderin. Aneurysmal bone cysts can be seen in 14% of giant cell tumors. Areas of cortical thinning, expansion, and/or destruction can occur with extraosseous extension. Tumors show varying degrees of Gd-contrast enhancement.	Aggressive bone tumors composed of neoplastic mononuclear cells and scattered multinucleated osteoclast-like giant cells. Account for 23% of primary nonmalignant bone tumors, and 5 to 9% of all primary bone tumors. Median age = 30 years.

(continued on page 502)

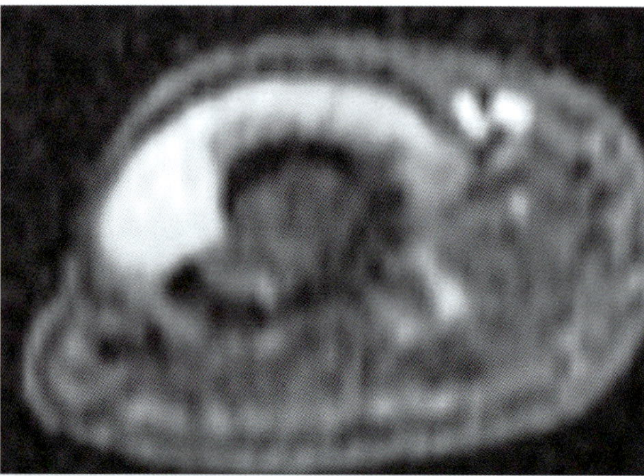

Fig. 10.228 A 24-year-old woman with a glomus tumor under the nail bed laterally associated with erosion of the adjacent cortex of the distal phalanx. The lesion shows prominent Gd-contrast enhancement on coronal fat-suppressed T1-weighted imaging.

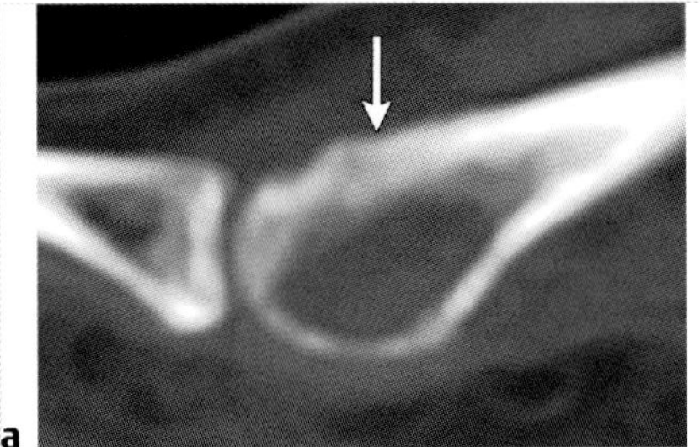

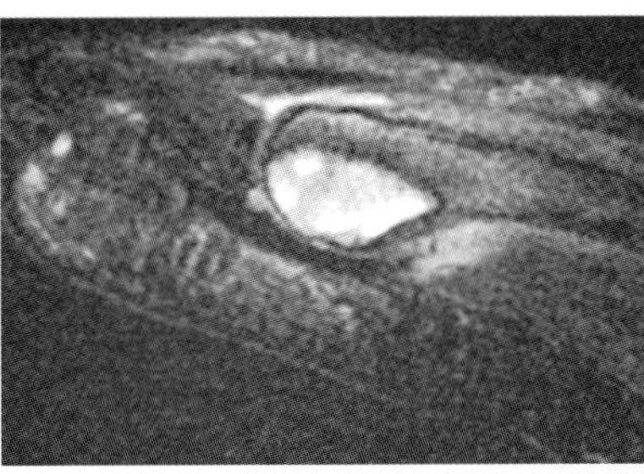

Fig. 10.229 A 29-year-old man with a giant cell tumor involving the distal end of the fourth metatarsal bone. The radiolucent lesion (arrow) is associated with cortical thinning on sagittal computed tomography (a). The lesion has high signal on sagittal fat-suppressed T2-weighted imaging (b).

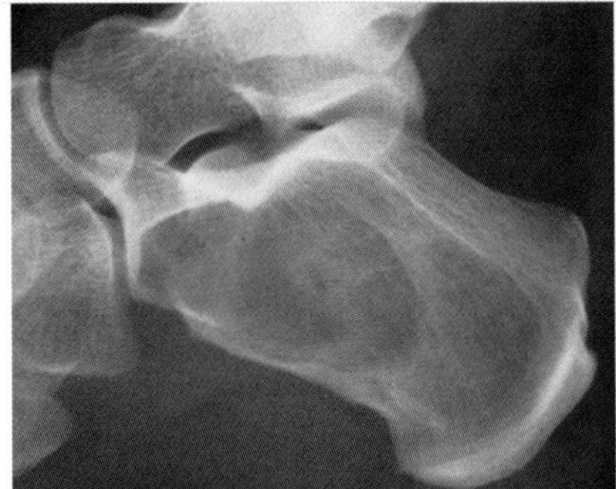

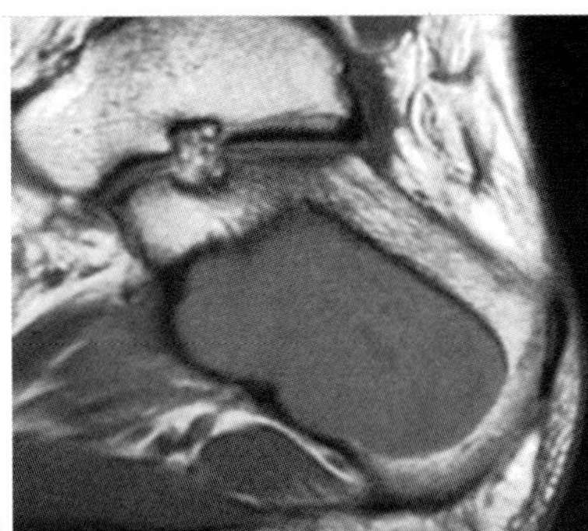

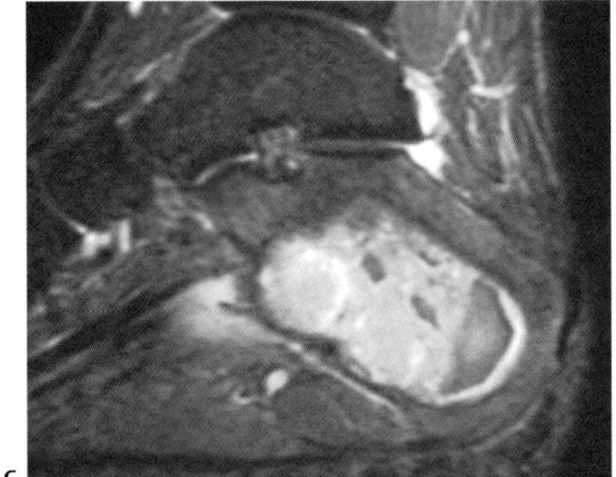

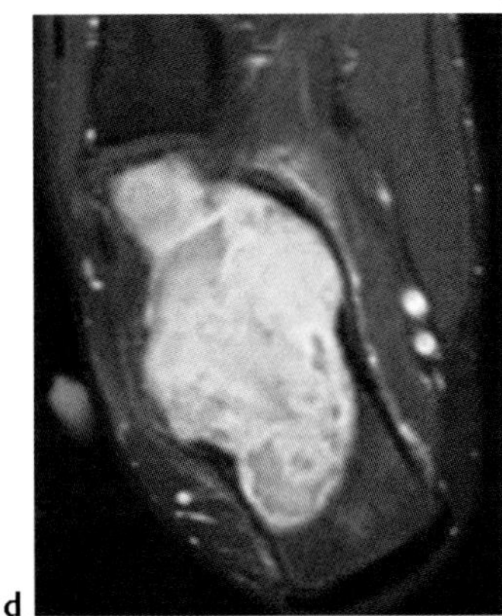

Fig. 10.230 A 25-year-old woman with a radiolucent giant cell tumor in the calcaneus (a). The lesion has intermediate signal on sagittal T1-weighted imaging (T1WI) (b), and high signal on sagittal fat-suppressed (FS) T2-weighted imaging (c). The lesion shows Gd-contrast enhancement on axial FS T1WI (d).

Table 10.10 (Cont.) Osseous tumors and tumor-like lesions of the hands and feet

Abnormalities	MRI findings	Comments
Fibrous dysplasia (▶ Fig. 10.231)	MRI features depend on the proportions of bony spicules, collagen, fibroblastic spindle cells, hemorrhagic and/or cystic changes, and associated pathological fracture if present. Lesions are usually well circumscribed and have low or low-intermediate signal on T1WI and PDWI. On T2WI, lesions have variable mixtures of low, intermediate, and/or high signal often surrounded by a low signal rim of variable thickness. Internal septations and cystic changes are seen in a minority of lesions. Bone expansion with thickened and/or thinned cortex can be seen. Lesions show Gd-contrast enhancement that varies in degree and pattern.	Benign medullary fibro-osseous lesion, which can involve a single site (mono-ostotic) or multiple locations (polyostotic). Thought to occur from developmental failure in the normal process of remodeling primitive bone to mature lamellar bone with resultant zone or zones of immature trabeculae within dysplastic fibrous tissue. Accounts for approximately 10% of benign bone lesions. Patients range in age from < 1 year to 76 years; 75% occur before the age of 30 years.
Osteomyelitis (▶ Fig. 10.232)	In acute osteomyelitis, poorly defined zones of low or low-intermediate signal on T1WI and high signal on T2WI, STIR, and FS T2WI are seen in the marrow. Loss of definition of the low signal line of the cortical margins is often observed on T1WI, T2WI, STIR, and FS T2WI. After Gd-contrast administration, irregular zones of contrast enhancement are seen in the involved marrow on FS T1WI. In the subacute phase of osteomyelitis, the pyogenic process becomes more localized. The zone of transition between normal and abnormal bone is sharper and more well defined in subacute and chronic osteomyelitis than with acute osteomyelitis.	Osteomyelitis is a disorder in which there is infection of bone and commonly the adjacent soft tissues. Can result from hematogenous spread of micro-organisms as well as from trauma-direct inoculation, extension from adjacent tissues, and complications from surgery. Bacteria such as *Staphylococcus aureus* and *Streptococcus pyogenes* are the most common infectious organisms. Can also result from other bacteria as well as tuberculosis, fungi, parasites, and viruses.

(continued on page 504)

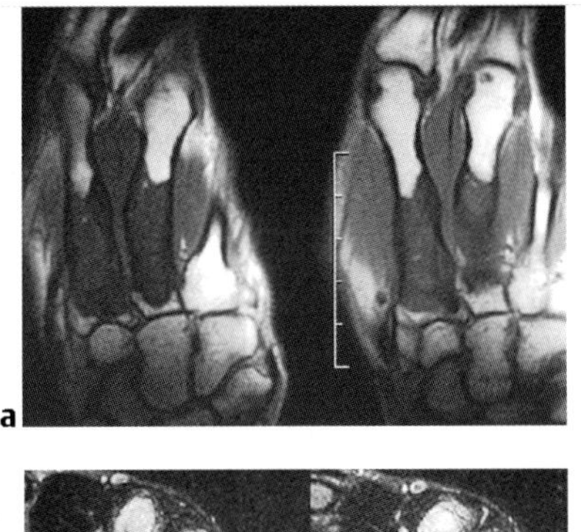

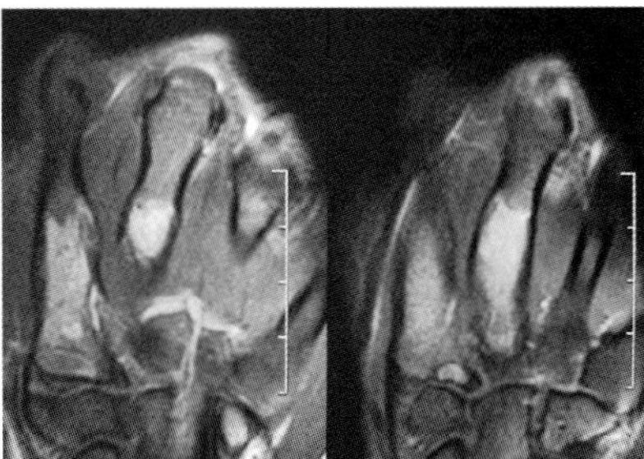

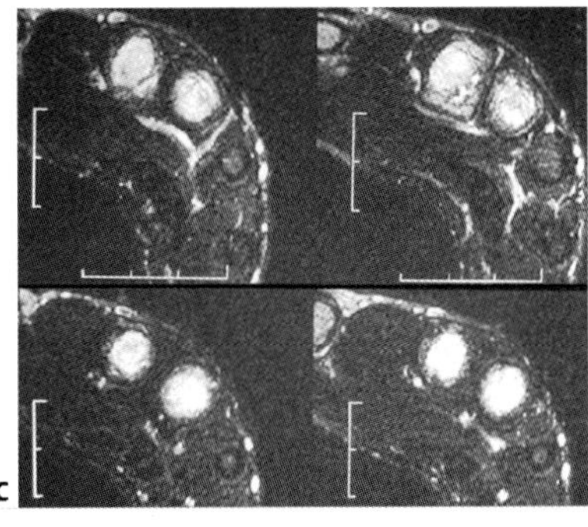

Fig. 10.231 Polyostotic fibrous dysplasia involving two adjacent metacarpal bones. The intramedullary lesions have low-intermediate signal on coronal T1-weighted imaging (T1WI) (a), Gd-contrast enhancement on fat-suppressed T1WI (b), and high signal on axial T2-weighted imaging (c). Slight cortical thickening and expansion are also seen.

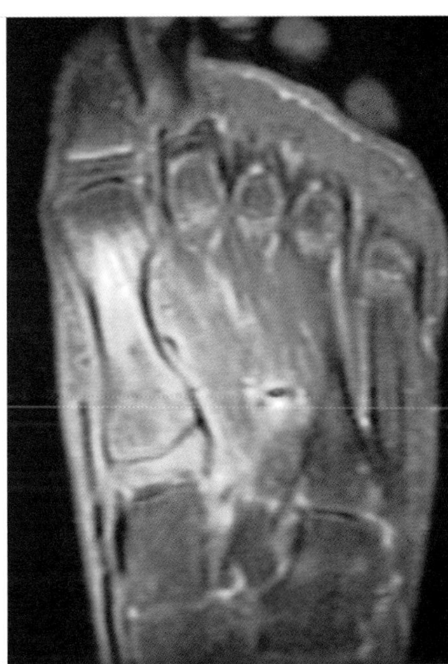

Fig. 10.232 A 54-year-old woman with pyogenic osteomyelitis involving the first metatarsal bone with abnormal Gd-contrast enhancement in the marrow and adjacent soft tissues on coronal fat-suppressed T1-weighted imaging.

Table 10.10 (Cont.) Osseous tumors and tumor-like lesions of the hands and feet

Abnormalities	MRI findings	Comments
Chronic recurrent multifocal osteomyelitis (▶ Fig. 10.233)	Multifocal lesions that occur in metaphyses of tubular bones (distal femur, proximal and distal tibia and fibula), clavicles, and vertebrae. Radiographs show radiolucent and/or sclerotic osseous lesions with proliferative periosteal bone formation. MRI shows heterogeneous abnormal high signal on FS T2WI in marrow and periosteal soft tissues with Gd-contrast enhancement.	Painful inflammatory osseous disorder of unknown cause with histopathology of acute and chronic osteomyelitis without identification of infectious agent, diagnosis of exclusion. Usually occurs in children and adolescents, median age = 10 years, F 85%/M 15%. Multiepisodic skeletal disorder of unknown cause that can occur over 7 to 25 years. Treatment of symptoms with nonsteroidal anti-inflammatory drugs. Can be associated with acne or pustulosis palmoplantaris (SAPHO).
Eosinophilic granuloma	Focal intramedullary lesions associated with trabecular and cortical bone destruction, which typically have low-intermediate signal on T1WI and PDWI and heterogeneous slightly-high to high signal on T2WI. Poorly defined zones. Focal intramedullary lesion associated with trabecular and cortical bone destruction, which typically have low-intermediate signal on T1WI and PDWI; and heterogeneous slightly high to high signal on T2WI. Poorly defined zones of high signal on T2WI are usually seen in the marrow peripheral to the lesions secondary to inflammatory changes. Extension of lesions from the marrow into adjacent soft tissues through areas of cortical disruption are commonly seen as well as linear periosteal zones of high signal on T2WI. Lesions typically show prominent Gd-contrast enhancement in marrow and in extraosseous soft tissue portions of the lesions.	Benign tumor-like lesions consisting of Langerhans cells (histiocytes), and variable amounts of lymphocytes, polymorphonuclear cells, and eosinophils. Account for 1% of primary bone lesions and 8% of tumor-like lesions. Occur in patients with median age = 10 years, average = 13.5 years, peak incidence is between 5 and 10 years; 80 to 85% occur in patients less than 30 years.
Sarcoidosis (▶ Fig. 10.234; ▶ Fig. 10.235)	Lesions usually appear as intramedullary zones with low to intermediate signal on T1WI and slightly high to high signal on T2WI and FS PDWI and FS T2WI. Erosions and zones of destruction of adjacent bone cortex as well as periosseous extension of the granulomatous process can occur. Fine perpendicular lines of low signal on T1WI may be seen extending outward from the region of eroded or destroyed cortex representing collagen separating periosseous extension of granulomas. After Gd-contrast administration, lesions typically show moderate to prominent enhancement.	Chronic systemic granulomatous disease of unknown etiology in which noncaseating granulomas occur in various tissues and organs including bone.

(continued on page 506)

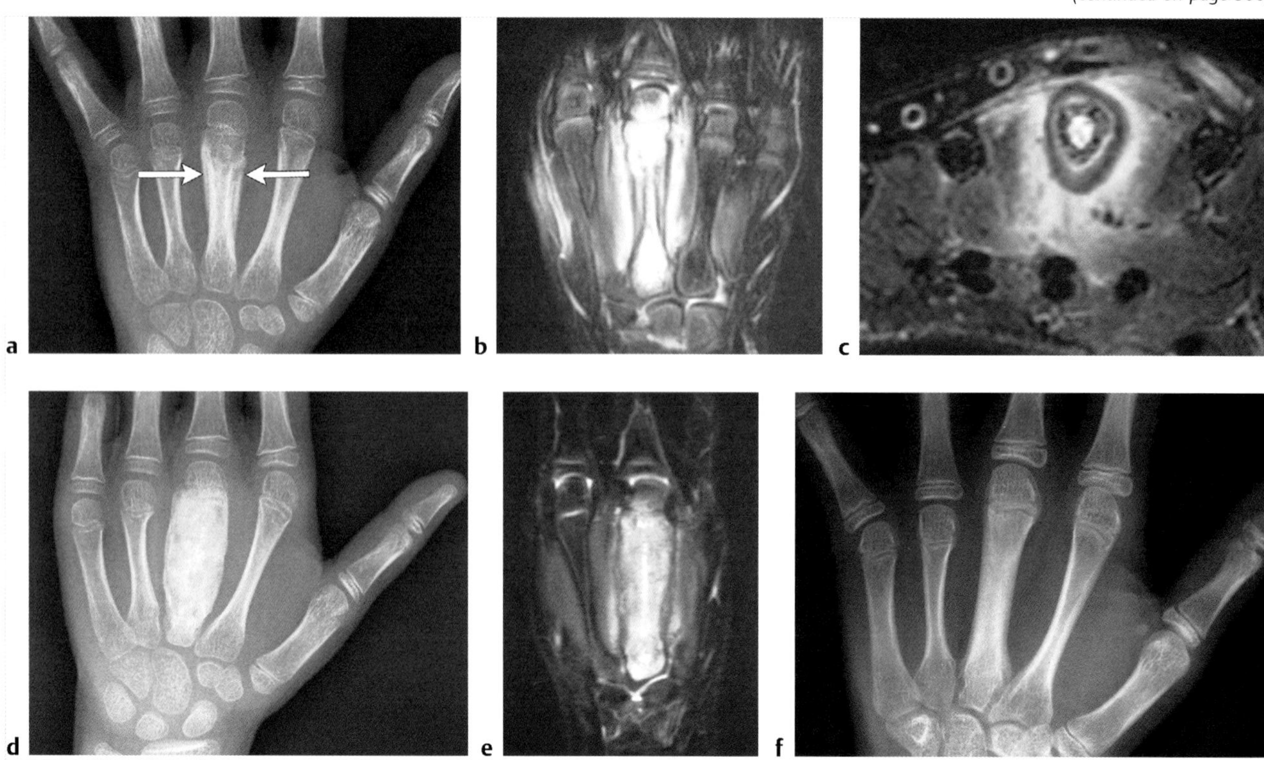

Fig. 10.233 Chronic recurrent multifocal osteomyelitis involving the third metacarpal bone of an 8-year-old female. Radiograph shows intramedullary sclerosis, cortical bone disruption, and thick uninterrupted periosteal reaction (arrow) (a), which has corresponding abnormal high signal in the marrow and periosteal soft tissues on coronal (b) and axial fat-suppressed T2-weighted imaging (FS T2WI) (c). Radiograph obtained 5 months later (d) shows expanded irregular sclerotic bone reaction with corresponding high signal on coronal FS T2WI (e). Radiograph 3 years later (f) shows regression of bone expansion with residual uniform bone sclerosis.

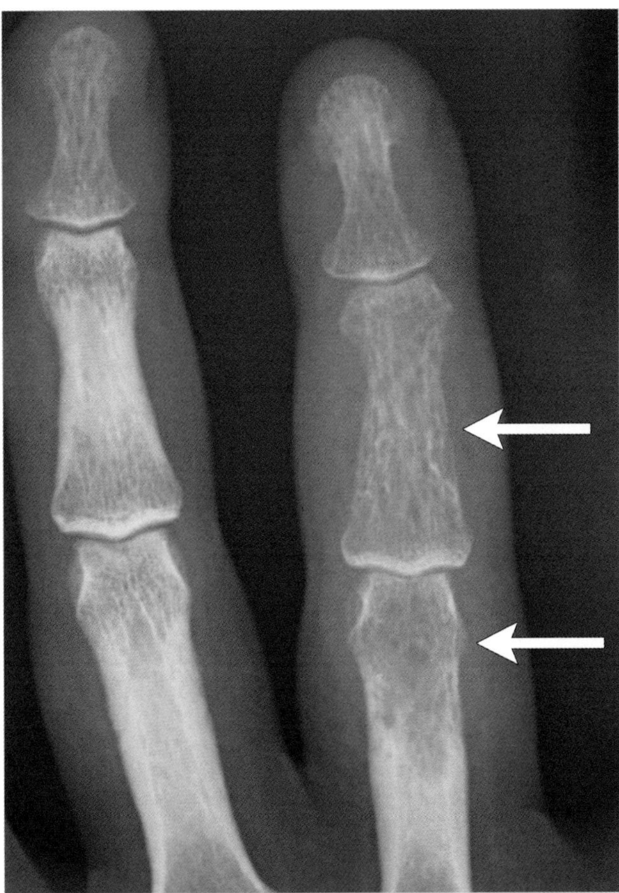

Fig. 10.234 Sarcoid involving bone. Radiograph of a 41-year-old man shows diffuse "lacelike" radiolucent changes involving medullary and cortical bone of the middle phalanx (arrow), distal portion of the proximal phalanx (arrow), and proximal portion of the distal phalanx.

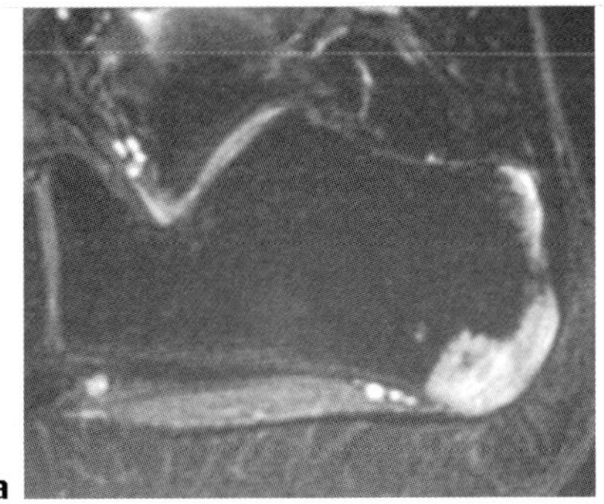

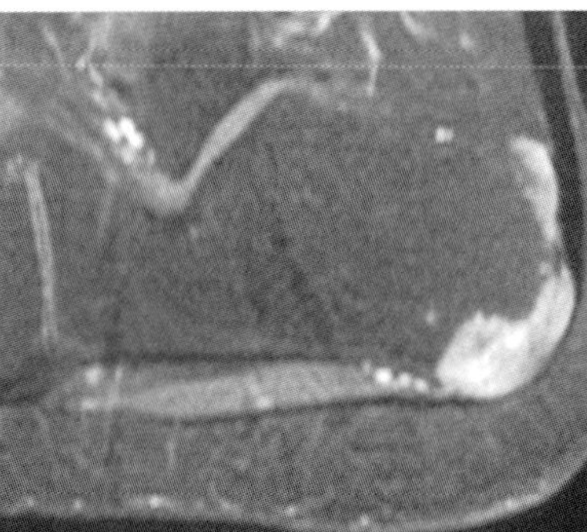

Fig. 10.235 A 31-year-old man with sarcoid involving the dorsal inferior portion of the calcaneus, which has high signal on sagittal fat-suppressed (FS) T2-weighted imaging (a) and gadolinium-contrast enhancement on FS T1-weighted imaging (b).

Table 10.10 (Cont.) Osseous tumors and tumor-like lesions of the hands and feet

Abnormalities	MRI findings	Comments
Gout (▶ Fig. 10.236)	Tophi have variable sizes and shapes, and have low-intermediate signal on T1WI, FS T2WI, and T2WI. Zones of high signal on T2WI can also be seen in tophi. Erosions of bone, synovial pannus, joint effusion, bone marrow, and soft-tissue edema can be seen with MRI. Tophi may show heterogeneous, diffuse, or peripheral/marginal Gd-contrast enhancement patterns.	Gout is an inflammatory disease involving synovium resulting from deposition of monosodium urate crystals and occurs when the serum urate level exceeds its solubility in various tissues and body fluid.
Bone infarct (▶ Fig. 10.237)	A double-line sign (curvilinear adjacent zones of low and high signal on T2WI) is commonly seen at the edges of the infarcts representing the borders of osseous resorption and healing. Irregular Gd-contrast enhancement can be seen from granulation tissue ingrowth.	Zones of ischemic death involving bone trabeculae and marrow, which can be idiopathic or can result from: trauma, corticosteroid treatment, chemotherapy, radiation treatment, occlusive vascular disease, collagen vascular and other autoimmune diseases, metabolic storage diseases (e.g., Gaucher disease), sickle cell disease, thalassemia, hyperbaric events/Caisson disease, pregnancy, alcohol abuse, pancreatitis, infections, and lymphoproliferative diseases.
Malignant lesions		
Metastatic lesion	Single or multiple well-circumscribed or poorly defined infiltrative lesions involving the vertebral marrow associated with cortical destruction and extraosseous extension. Lesions often have low-intermediate signal on T1WI and low, intermediate, and/or high signal on T2WI and FS T1WI; usually show Gd-contrast enhancement. Cortical destruction and tumor extension into the extraosseous soft tissues can occur. Pathological fractures can be associated with metastatic lesions involving tubular bones and vertebrae. Periosteal reaction is uncommon.	Metastatic lesions typically occur in the marrow with or without cortical destruction and extraosseous tumor extension.
Plasmacytoma/ myeloma	Well-circumscribed or poorlydefined infiltrative lesions involving marrow; low-intermediate signal on T1WI, intermediate-high signal on T2WI and FS T2WI; usually show Gd-contrast-enhancement, eventual cortical bone destruction and extraosseous extension.	Malignant tumors composed of proliferating antibody-secreting plasma cells derived from single clones. Most common primary neoplasm of bone in adults, median = 60 years. Most patients are older than 40 years. May have variable destructive or infiltrative changes involving the axial and/or appendicular skeleton.

(continued on page 508)

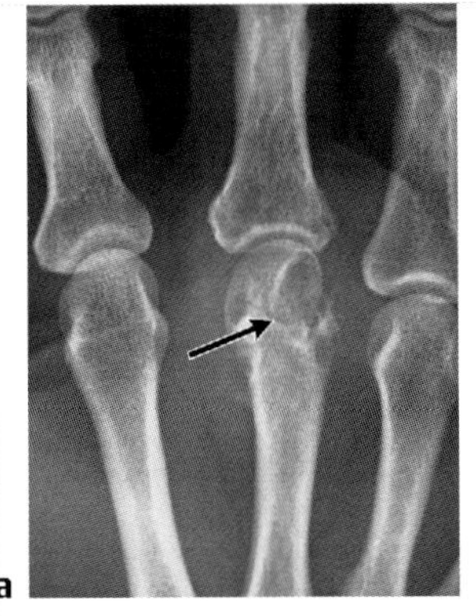

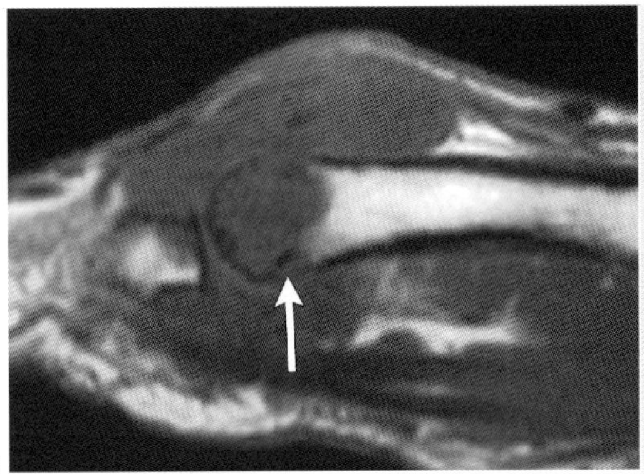

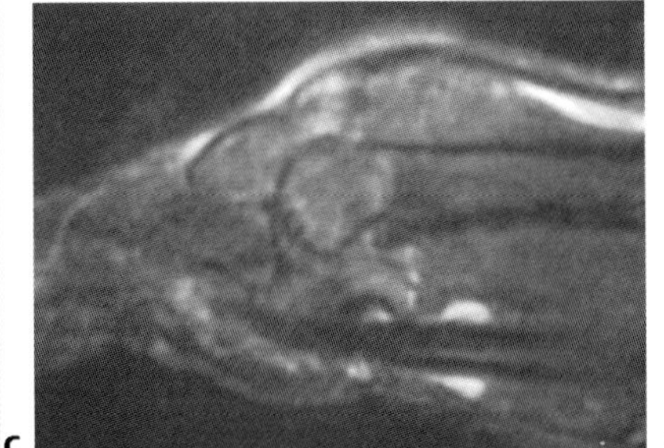

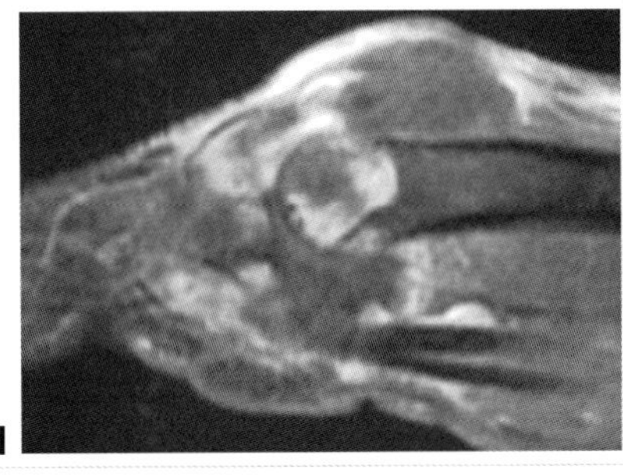

Fig. 10.236 A 53-year-old man with gout involving the metatarsal–phalangeal joint with bone erosions (arrow) seen on radiograph (a). Magnetic resonance imaging shows a soft tissue lesion (tophus) (arrow) with intermediate signal on sagittal T1-weighted imaging (T1WI) (b) and heterogeneous intermediate and slightly high signal on fat-suppressed (FS) T2-weighted imaging (c). The lesion erodes cortical bone and extends into the marrow of the metatarsal head. Only peripheral irregular gadolinium-contrast enhancement is seen with the intraosseous and extraosseous lesions on sagittal FS T1-weighted imaging (d).

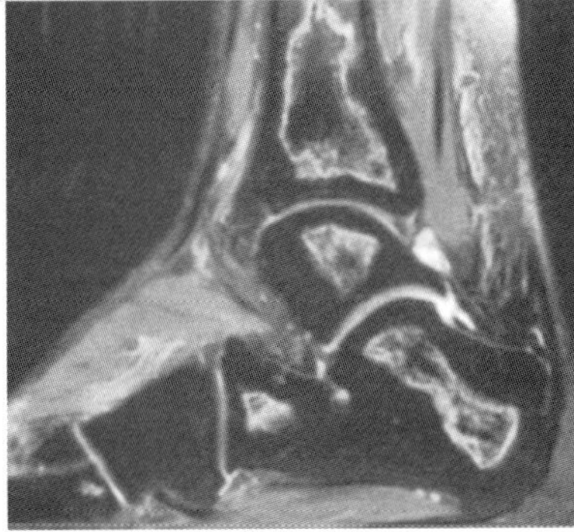

Fig. 10.237 A 36-year-old man with sickle cell trait and bone infarcts in the distal tibia, talus, and calcaneus as seen on sagittal T1-weighted imaging (a) and sagittal fat-suppressed T2-weighted imaging (b).

Table 10.10 (Cont.) Osseous tumors and tumor-like lesions of the hands and feet

Abnormalities	MRI findings	Comments
Chondrosarcoma (▶ Fig. 10.238)	Intramedullary tumors often have low-intermediate signal on T1WI, intermediate signal on PDWI, and heterogeneous intermediate-high signal on T2WI. Lesions usually show heterogeneous contrast enhancement.	Malignant tumors containing cartilage formed within sarcomatous stroma. Account for12 to 21% of malignant bone lesions, 21 to 26% of primary sarcomas of bone. Mean age = 40 years, median = 26 to 59 years.
Osteosarcoma (▶ Fig. 10.239)	Destructive intramedullary malignant lesions, low-intermediate signal on T1WI, mixed low, intermediate, high signal on T2WI, usually with matrix mineralization/ossification-low signal on T2WI; usually show Gd-contrast enhancement. Zones of cortical destruction are typically seen through which tumors extend into the extraosseous soft tissues. Low signal from spicules of periosteal, reactive, and tumoral bone formation may be seen.	Malignant tumor composed of proliferating neoplastic spindle cells, which produce osteoid and/or immature tumoral bone and which most frequently arise within medullary bone. Two age peaks of incidence. The larger peak occurs between the ages of 10 and 20 and accounts for over half of the cases. The second, smaller peak occurs in adults over 60 years and accounts for approximately 10% of the cases. Occurs in children as primary tumors and adults (associated with Paget disease, irradiated bone, chronic osteomyelitis, osteoblastoma, giant cell tumor, fibrous dysplasia.
Ewing sarcoma	Destructive malignant lesions involving marrow; low-intermediate signal on T1WI; mixed low, intermediate, and/or high signal on T2WI and FS T2WI; usually shows Gd-contrast enhancement (usually heterogeneous). Extraosseous tumor extension through sites of cortical destruction is commonly seen. Thin striated zones of low signal on T2WI can sometimes be seen oriented perpendicular to the long axis of the involved bone under the elevated periosteum representing the hair on end appearance of reactive bone formation secondary to the tumor.	Malignant primitive tumor of bone composed of undifferentiated small cells with round nuclei. Accounts for 6 to 11% of primary malignant bone tumors, 5 to 7% of primary bone tumors. Usually occurs between the ages of 5 and 30, males > females, locally invasive, high metastatic potential.

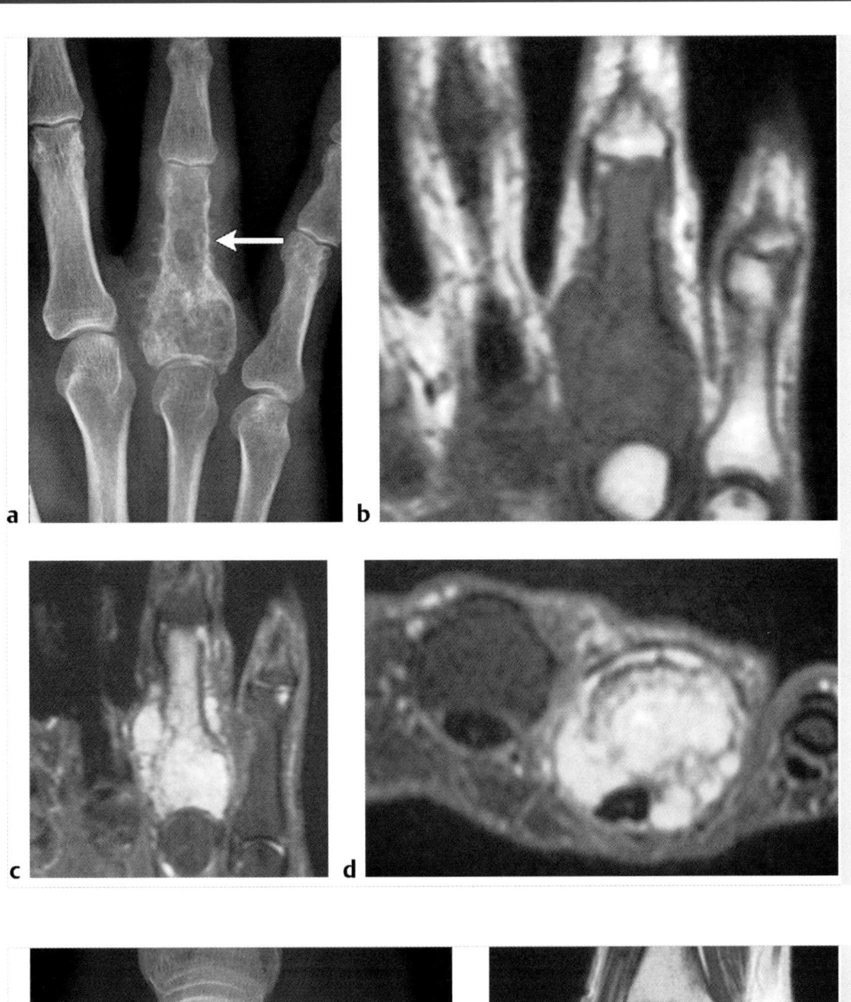

Fig. 10.238 A 56-year-old man with a chondrosarcoma involving a proximal phalanx. Radiograph shows an intramedullary lesion (arrow) with chondroid matrix and cortical destruction (a). The lesion has intermediate signal on coronal T1-weighted imaging (T1WI) (b) and high signal on coronal fat-suppressed (FS) T2-weighted imaging (c). The tumor shows Gd-contrast enhancement on axial FS T1-weighted imaging (d). Cortical destruction and extraosseous tumor extension are seen with magnetic resonance imaging.

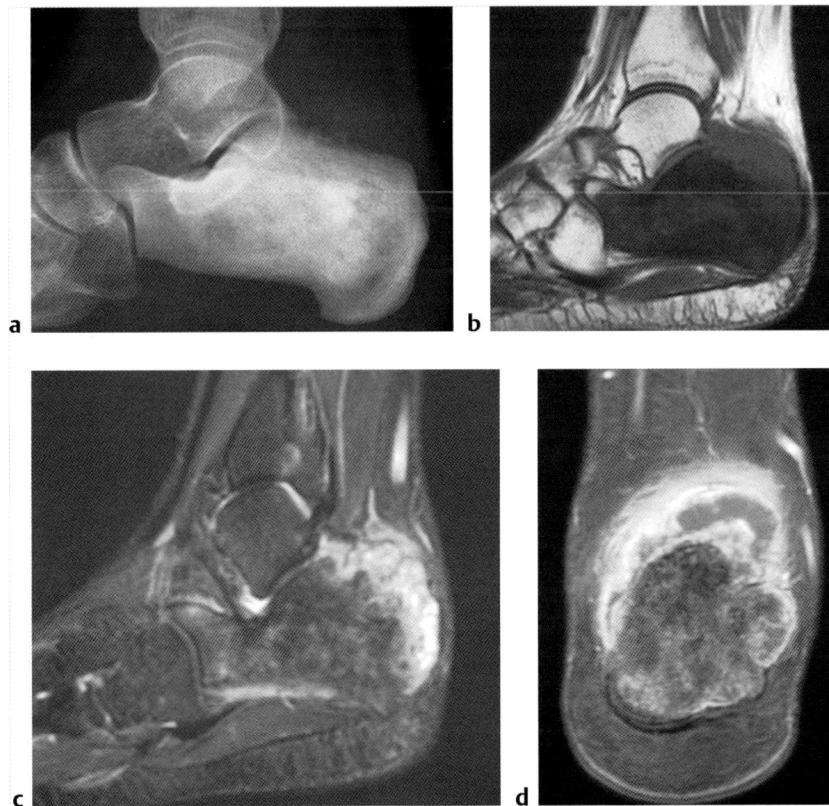

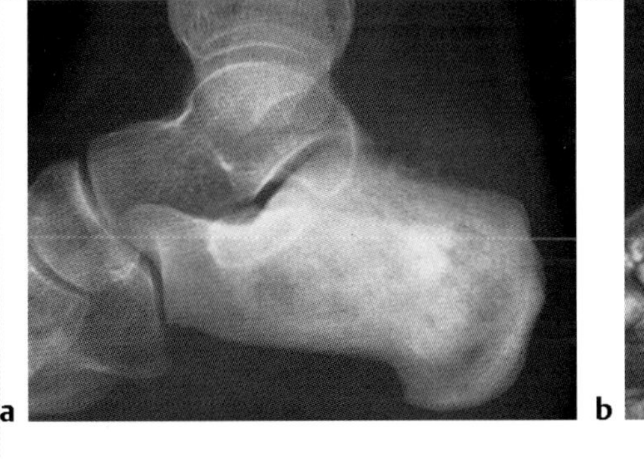

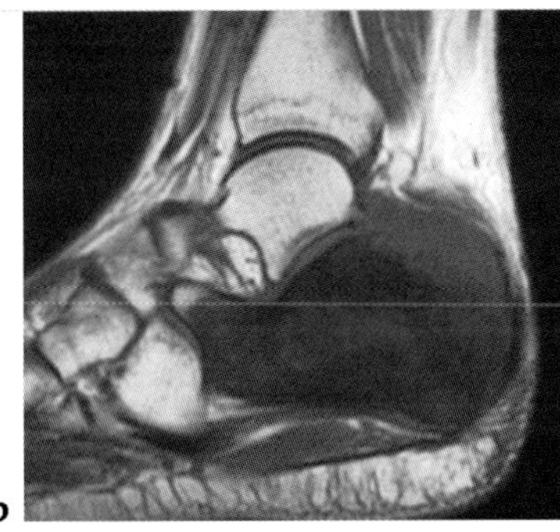

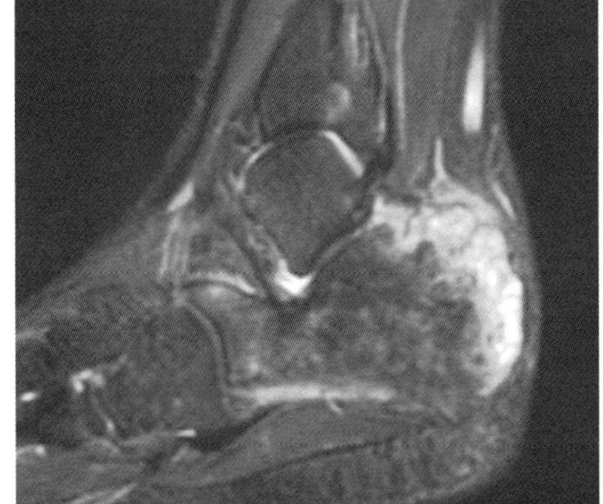

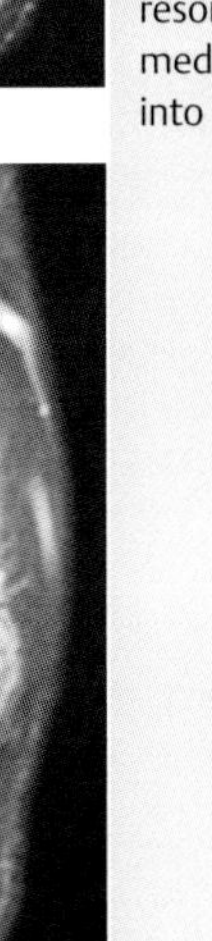

Fig. 10.239 A 17-year-old female with a chondroblastic osteogenic sarcoma of the talus, which has ossified tumor matrix (a), cortical bone destruction, and interrupted periosteal reaction. The tumor has mixed low and intermediate signal on sagittal T1-weighted imaging (T1WI) (b); heterogeneous mixed low, intermediate, and high signal on fat-suppressed (FS) T2-weighted imaging (c); and heterogeneous Gd-contrast enhancement on coronal FS T1WI (d). Magnetic resonance imaging shows extension of intramedullary tumor through destroyed bone cortex into the adjacent soft tissues.

10.11 Diffuse, Multiple, Poorly Defined, and/or Multifocal Zones of Abnormal Marrow Signal

- Nonmalignant abnormalities
  - Hematologic disorders
    - Red marrow reconversion
    - Inherited anemias (sickle cell anemia, thalassemia, sideroblastic anemia)
    - Marrow hyperplasia from exogenous erythropoietin
    - Granulocytemacrophage colony-stimulating factor (GM-CSF)
    - Hemochromatosis and iron deposition from multiple transfusions
    - Age-related vertebral marrow signal changes in adults
  - Metabolic and/or genetic disorders
    - Primary hyperparathyroidism; secondary hyperparathyroidism–renal osteodystrophy
    - Primary oxalosis
    - Hypoparathyroidism
    - Pseudohypoparathyroidism
    - Pseudo-pseudohypoparathyroidism
    - Serous atrophy of marrow from malnutrition
    - Hypervitamosis A and D
    - Fluorosis
    - Gaucher disease
    - Glycogen storage disease type 1B
    - Glycogen storage disease type 1A
    - Mucopolysaccharoidoses
    - Osteogenesis imperfecta
    - Osteopetrosis
  - Inflammatory disorders
    - Osteomyelitis
    - Chronic recurrent multifocal osteomyelitis
    - Eosinophilic granuloma (Langerhans cell histiocytosis)
    - Ankylosing spondylitis
    - Sarcoidosis
    - Erdheim-Chester disease
    - Bilateral sacroiliitis
    - Osteiitis condensans
  - Degenerative/traumatic/posttreatment disorders
    - Bone contusions
    - Bilateral sacral insufficiency fractures
    - Marrow changes related to degenerative disk disease
    - Neuropathic bone and joint disease
    - Reflex sympathetic dystrophy (RSD) (also referred to as Sudek atrophy, algodystrophy, complex regional pain syndromes type I)
    - Regional migratory osteoporosis
    - Radiation injury
    - Bone infarction
    - Bone marrow necrosis
  - Other multifocal nonmalignant bone lesions
    - Hemangiomas
    - Cystic angiomatosis/lymphangiomatosis
    - Hemangioendotheliomas
    - Paget disease
    - Multiple enchondromatosis (Ollier disease, metachondromatosis, and Maffucci syndrome)
    - Poyostotic fibrous dysplasia
    - Osteopoikilosis
- Malignant abnormalities
  - Metastatic disease
  - Multiple myeloma
  - Non-Hodgkin lymphoma
  - Hodgkin lymphoma
  - Leukemia
  - Myelodysplastic syndromes
  - Chronic myeloproliferative disease
  - Waldenström macroglobulinemia (lymphoplasmacytic lymphoma)
  - Mastocytosis

Table 10.11 Diffuse, multiple, poorly defined, and/or multifocal zones of abnormal marrow signal

Abnormalities	MRI findings	Comments
Nonmalignant abnormalities		
Hematologic disorders		
Red marrow reconversion (▶ Fig. 10.240; ▶ Fig. 10.241; ▶ Fig. 10.242)	Involved marrow has slightly to moderately decreased signal relative to fat on T1-weighted imaging (T1WI) and proton density–weighted imaging (PDWI), isointense signal relative to muscle and slightly increased signal relative to fat on fat-suppressed T2-weighted imaging (FS T2WI).	Hyperplasia of normal marrow elements at sites that were previously composed mostly of yellow marrow. May be seen in obese middle-aged patients, tobacco smokers, marathon runners, individuals living at high altitudes.

(continued on page 512)

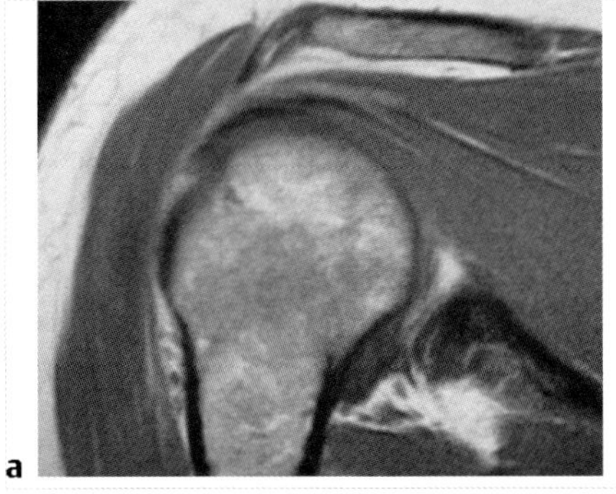

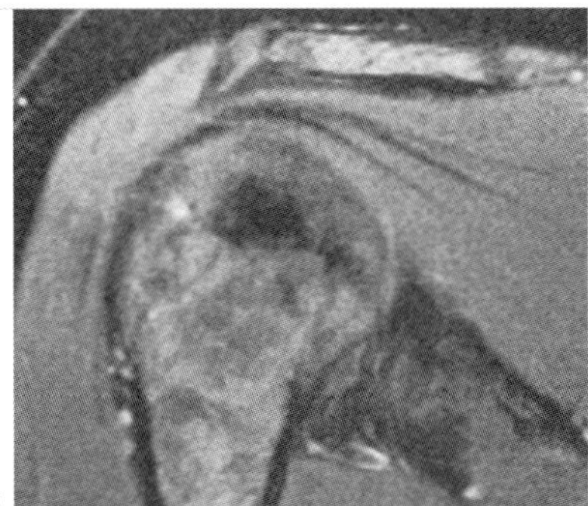

Fig. 10.240 A 51-year-old woman with red marrow reconversion in the proximal humerus as seen by irregular zones with slightly decreased signal relative to fat on sagittal proton density–weighted imaging (a), and isointense signal relative to muscle and slightly increased signal relative to fat on fat-suppressed T2-weighted imaging (b).

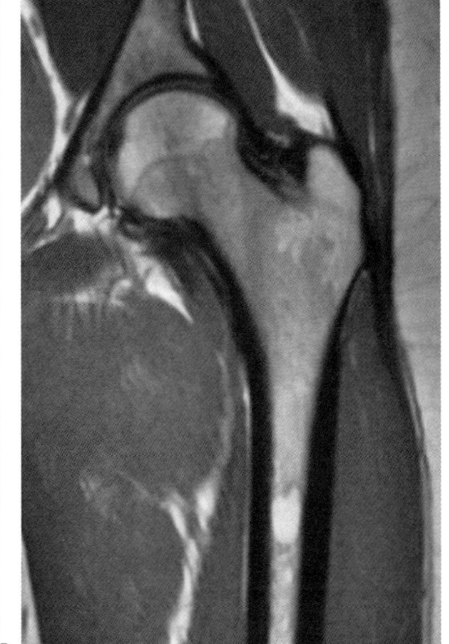

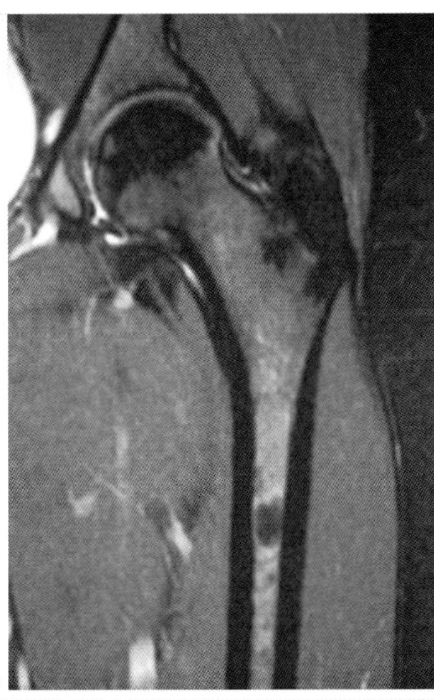

Fig. 10.241 A 40-year-old woman with red marrow reconversion in the metadiaphyseal marrow of the femur as seen on coronal T1-weighted imaging (a) and fat-suppressed T2-weighted imaging (b).

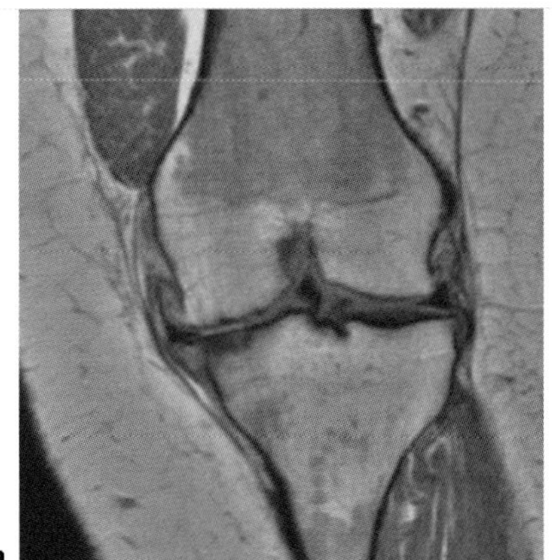

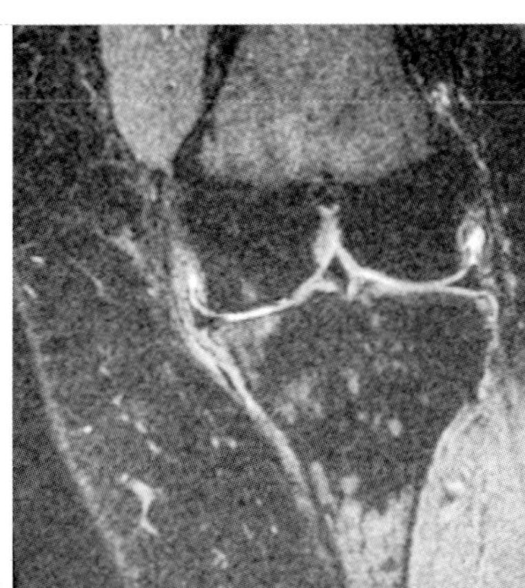

Fig. 10.242 A 36-year-old woman with red marrow reconversion in the metadiaphyseal marrow of the distal femur and proximal tibia as seen on coronal proton density–weighted imaging (a) and coronal fat-suppressed T2-weighted imaging (b).

Table 10.11 (Cont.) Diffuse, multiple, poorly defined, and/or multifocal zones of abnormal marrow signal

Abnormalities	MRI findings	Comments
Inherited anemias (sickle cell anemia, thalassemia, sideroblastic anemia) (▶ Fig. 10.243; ▶ Fig. 10.244; ▶ Fig. 10.245; ▶ Fig. 10.246)	Involved marrow has slightly to moderately decreased signal relative to fat on T1WI and T2WI, isointense to slightly hyperintense signal relative to muscle and increased signal relative to fat on FS T2WI.	Inherited anemias result in hyperplasia of normal marrow elements. Sickle cell disease is the most common hemoglobinopathy in which abnormal hemoglobin S is combined with itself, or other hemoglobin types such as C, D, E, or thalassemia. Hemoglobin SS, SC, and S-thalassemia have the most sickling of erythrocytes. In addition to marrow hyperplasia seen in sickle cell disease, bone infarcts and extramedullary hematopoiesis can also occur. Beta-thalassemia is a disorder in which there is deficient synthesis of beta chains of hemoglobin resulting in excess alpha chains in erythrocytes and erythrocytes causing dysfunctional hematopoiesis and hemolysis. The decrease in beta chains can be severe as in the major type (homozygous), moderate in the intermediate type (heterozygous), or mild in the minor type (heterozygous).

(continued on page 514)

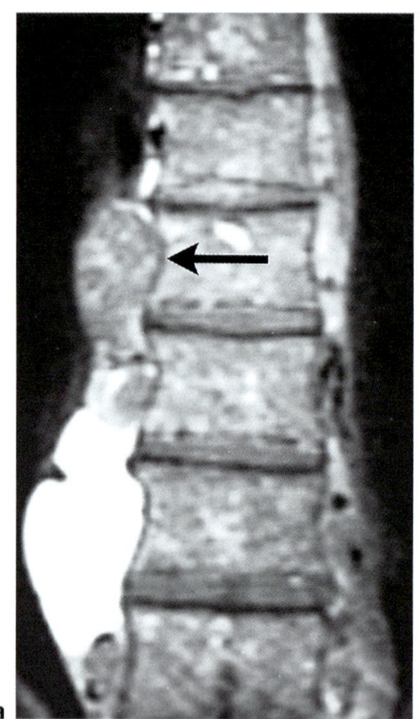

a

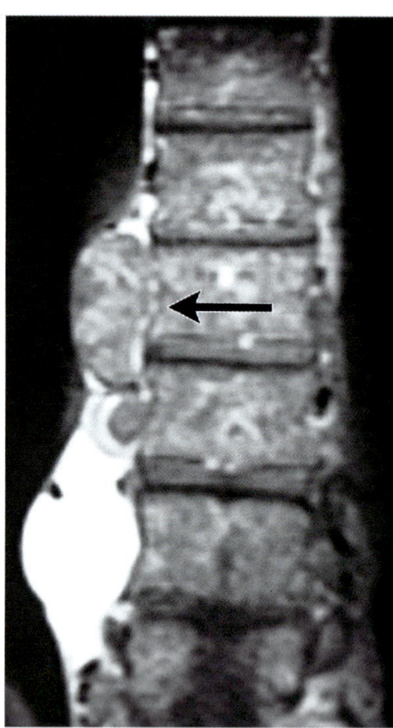

b

Fig. 10.243 A 54-year-old man with sickle cell disease and extramedullary hematopoiesis (arrows). The marrow has heterogeneous intermediate signal and slightly high signal on coronal T1-weighted imaging (a) and coronal T2-weighted imaging (b), which is hypointense to fat.

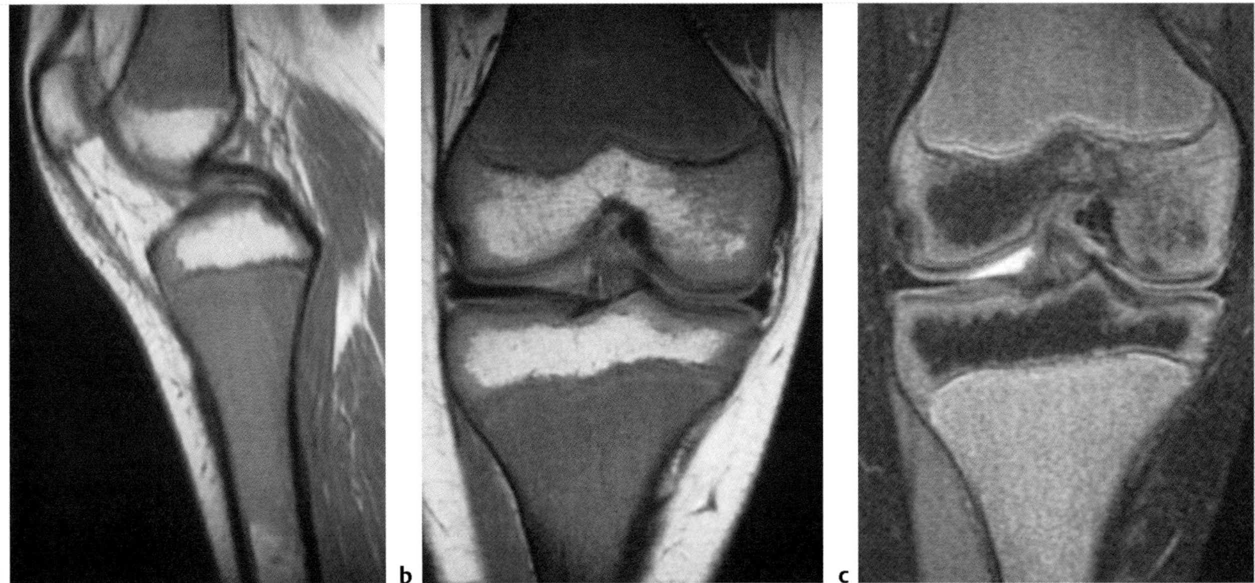

Fig. 10.244 A 14-year-old girl with sickle cell disease with marrow signal alteration in the metaphyseal regions of the knee, and to a lesser extent with epiphyseal marrow. Marrow signal is low-intermediate on sagittal (a) and coronal T1-weighted imaging (b) and hypointense relative to fat. The involved marrow signal is slightly high on coronal fat-suppressed T2-weighted imaging (c), which is hyperintense relative to fat and muscle.

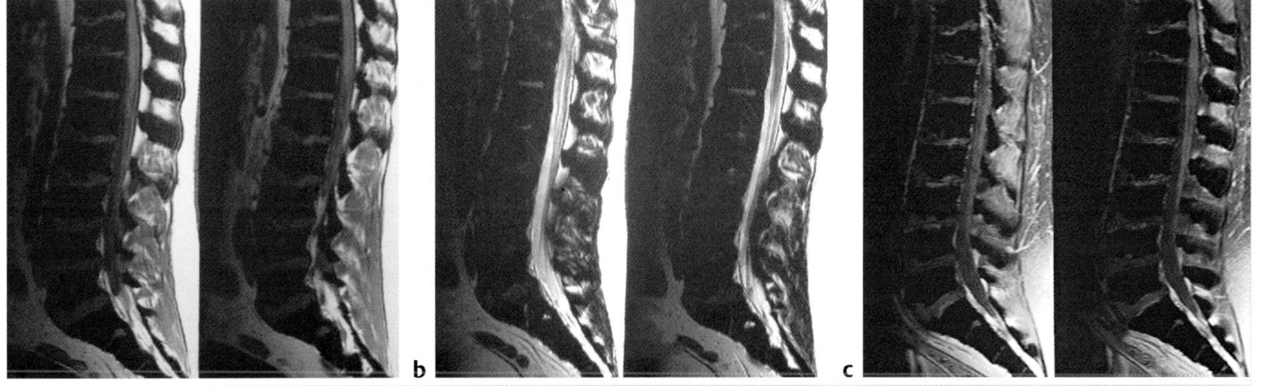

Fig. 10.245 A 22-year-old man with beta thalassemia major. Marrow signal is low on sagittal T1-weighted imaging (T1WI) (a), T2-weighted imaging (b), and post-gadolinium-contrast fat-suppressed T1WI secondary to iron overload (c).

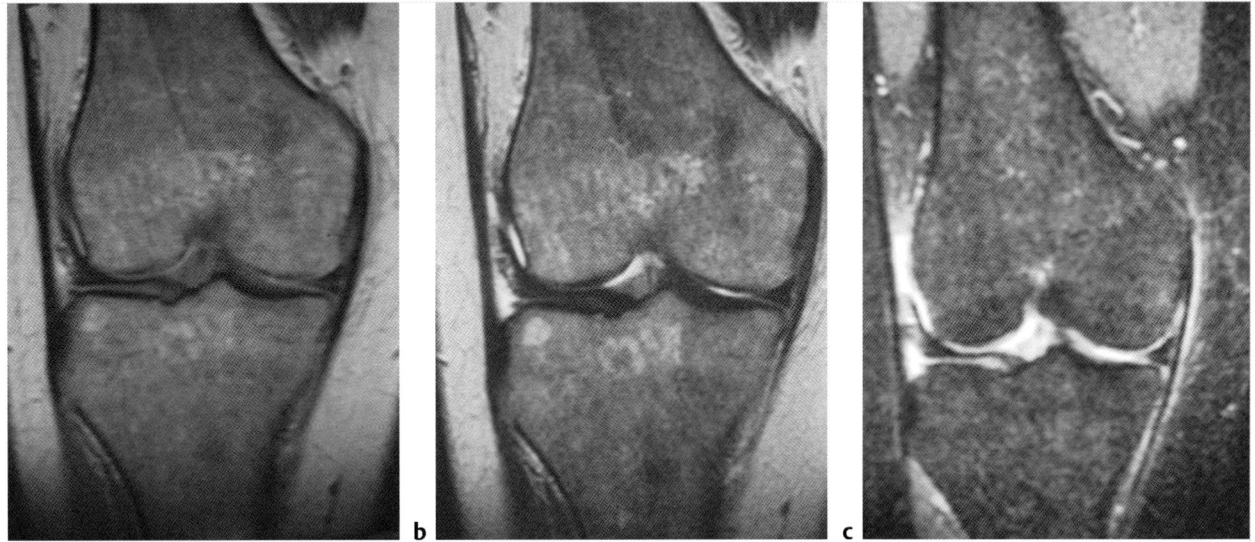

Fig. 10.246 A 49-year-old woman with thalassemia minor. The marrow has heterogeneous mixed low-intermediate signal on coronal proton density–weighted imaging (a) and coronal T2-weighted imaging (T2WI) (b), which is hypointense relative to fat, and slightly high signal on coronal fat-suppressed T2WI (c), which is hyperintense relative to fat.

Table 10.11 (Cont.) Diffuse, multiple, poorly defined, and/or multifocal zones of abnormal marrow signal

Abnormalities	MRI findings	Comments
Marrow hyperplasia from exogenous erythropoietin (▶ Fig. 10.247)	Involved marrow has slightly to moderately decreased signal relative to fat on T1WI and T2WI; isointense signal relative to muscle and slightly increased signal relative to fat on FS T2WI.	Exogenous source (medication) of erythropoietin used for treatment of anemia.
Granulocytemacrophage colony-stimulating factor (GM-CSF) (▶ Fig. 10.248)	Use of these medications induces red marrow reconversion, which occurs more commonly in a diffuse pattern compared with focal sites. Involved marrow has slightly decreased signal relative to fat on T1WI and T2WI; isointense signal relative to muscle and slightly increased signal relative to fat on FS T2WI.	GM-CSF is used as an adjunct for chemotherapy to minimize or correct treatment-related neutropenia by regulating the proliferation and differentiation of hematopoietic progenitor cells.
Hemochromatosis and iron deposition from multiple transfusions (▶ Fig. 10.249)	Involved marrow has low signal on T1WI, PDWI, and T2WI.	Hemochromatosis is an iron storage disorder with abnormal increased deposition of iron in various tissues. Hemochromatosis can be a primary autosomal recessive disorder in which there is increased intestinal absorption of iron resulting in a 10- to 50-fold increase in total body iron. The primary disorder is associated with a gene on chromosome 6 and occurs with an incidence of 3 to 5 per 1,000. Usually presents in adults, and occasionally in children. Secondary hemochromatosis occurs from iron overload from transfusions for sickle cell disease and thalassemia, alcoholic liver disease, and excessive dietary iron.

(continued on page 516)

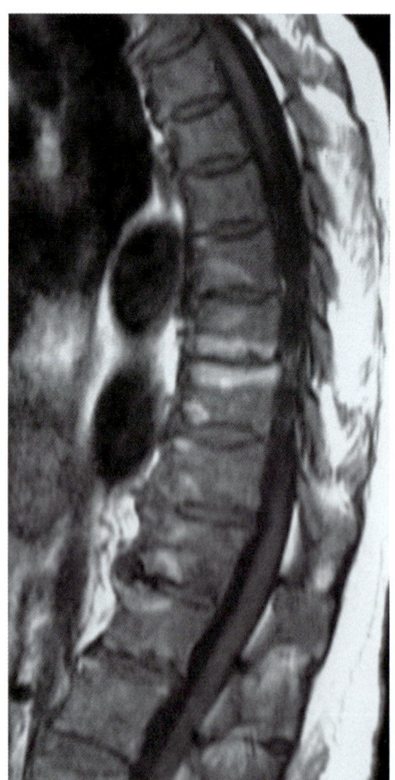

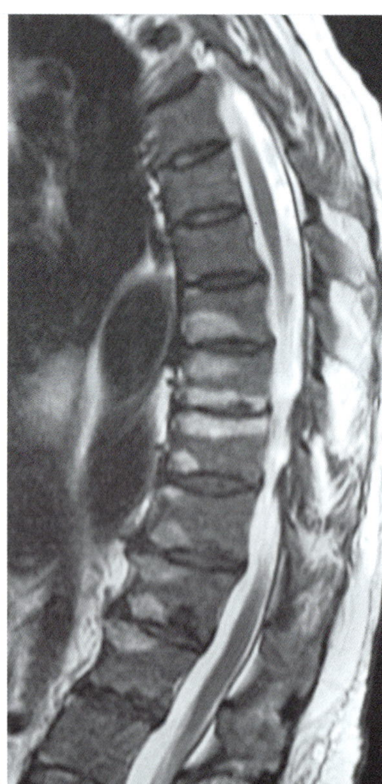

Fig. 10.247 A 60-year-old woman treated with exogeneous erythropoietin for anemia. Marrow has slightly to moderately decreased signal relative to fat on sagittal T1-weighted imaging (a) and sagittal T2-weighted imaging (b).

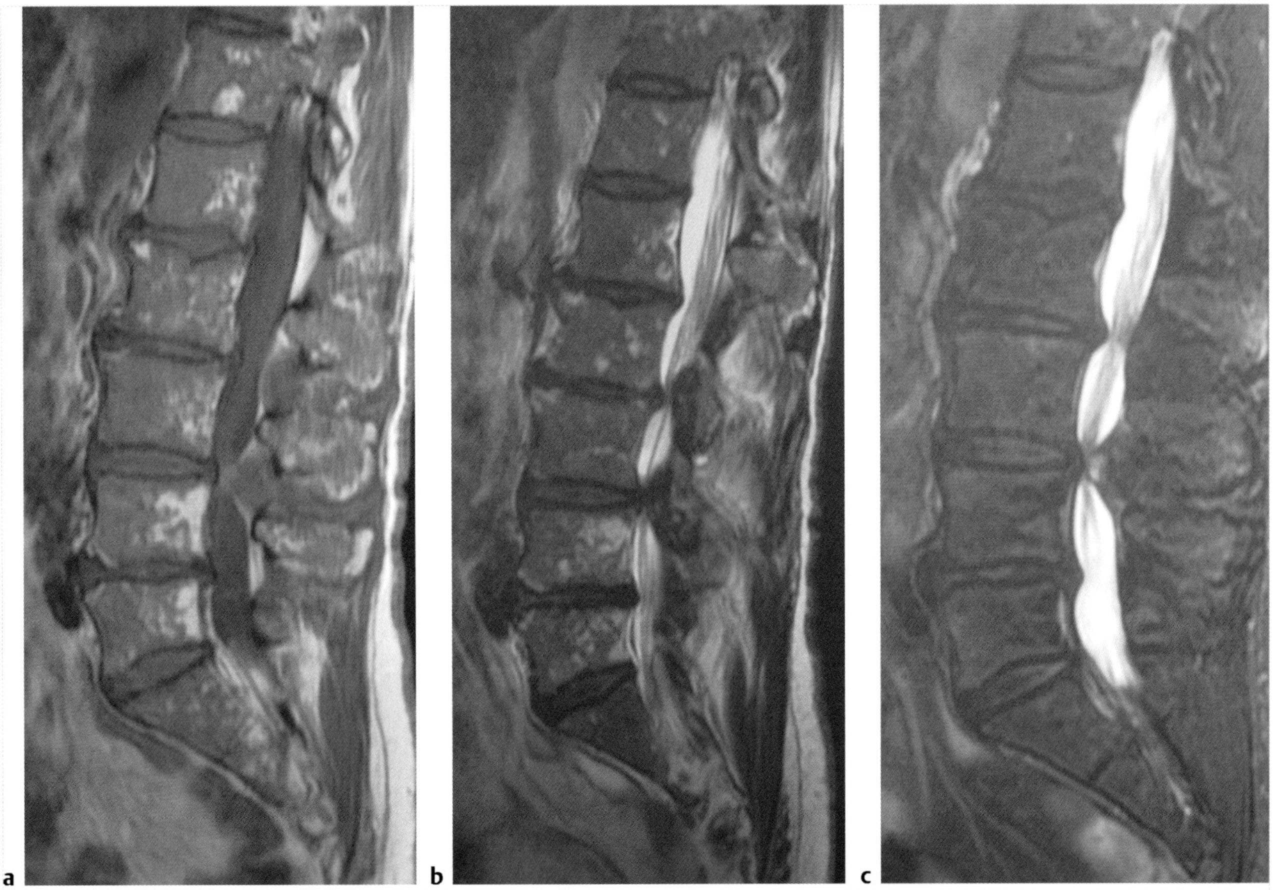

a b c

Fig. 10.248 A 79-year-old woman with neutropenia treated with granulocyte colony-stimulating factor. Marrow has heterogeneous slightly to moderately decreased signal relative to fat on sagittal T1-weighted imaging (a) and sagittal T2-weighted imaging (T2WI) (b). Marrow signal is minimally increased relative to fat on fat-suppressed T2WI (c).

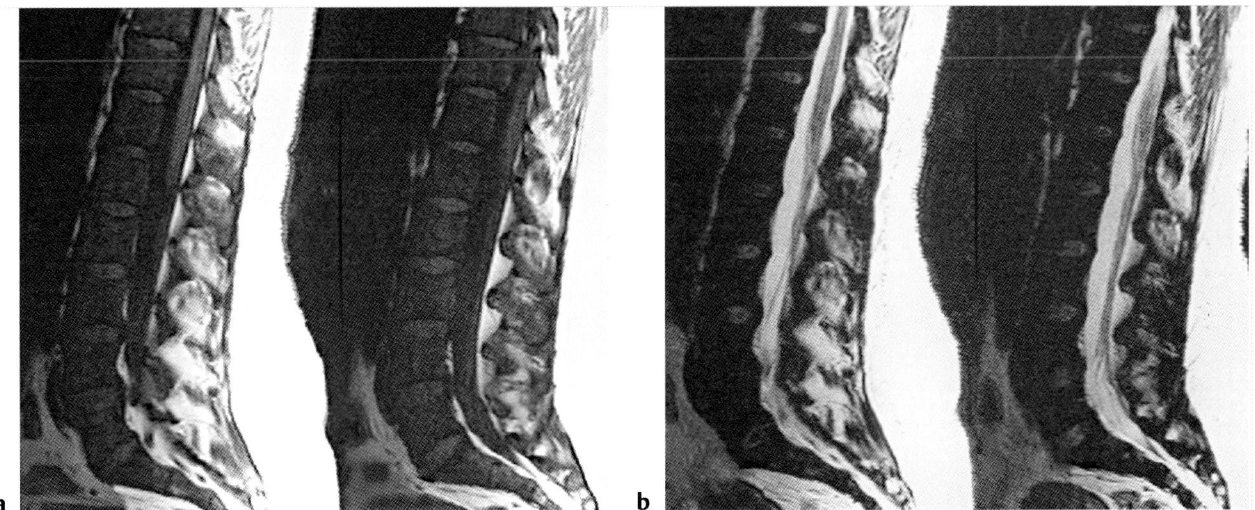

Fig. 10.249 Iron overload in a patient with sickle cell disease from multiple transfusions. Marrow signal is low on sagittal T1-weighted imaging (a) and T2-weighted imaging (b).

Table 10.11 (Cont.) Diffuse, multiple, poorly defined, and/or multifocal zones of abnormal marrow signal

Abnormalities	MRI findings	Comments
Age-related vertebral marrow signal changes in adults (▸ Fig. 10.250)	In vertebral marrow, small nodular or large globular zones with high signal on T1WI and fast spin-echo T2WI are seen. Vertebral marrow typically has uniform low signal on FS T2WI, which is isointense relative to skeletal muscle. No Gd-contast enhancement.	In adults older than 40 years, red marrow in the spine can be progressively replaced by yellow marrow, often in heterogeneous patterns such as with multiple small or globular foci and/or band-like zones of yellow marrow.
Metabolic and/or genetic disorders		
Primary hyperparathyroidism; secondary hyperparathyroidism–renal osteodystrophy (▸ Fig. 10.251)	In secondary hyperparathyroidism, zones of low signal on T1WI and T2WI correspond to regions of bone sclerosis. In the spine bands of low signal on T1WI and T2WI can be seen at bands of sclerosis that occur parallel to endplates ("rugger jersey vertebrae"). Brown tumors are single or multiple radiolucent lesions that can have poorly defined or circumscribed margins; low-intermediate signal on T1WI and high signal on T2WI.	Secondary hyperparathyroidism related to renal failure/end-stage kidney disease is more common than primary hyperparathyroism. Osteoblastic and osteoclastic changes occur in bone as a result of secondary hyperparathyroidism (hyperplasia of parathyroid glands secondary to hypocalcemia in end-stage renal disease related to abnormal vitamin D metabolism; and primary hyperparathyroidism (hypersecretion of parathyroid hormone[PTH] from parathyroid adenoma or hyperplasia). Can result in pathological fractures from osteomalacia. Unlike secondary hyperparathyroidism, diffuse or patchy bone sclerosis infrequently occurs in primary hyperparathyroidism. Brown tumors are more common in primary than in secondary hyperparathyroidism.

(continued on page 518)

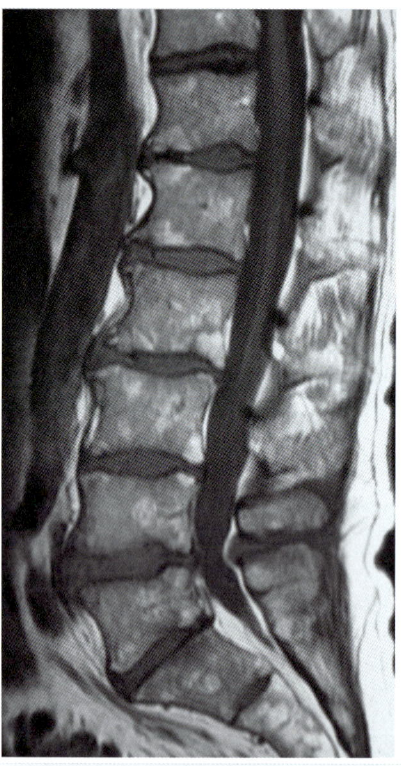

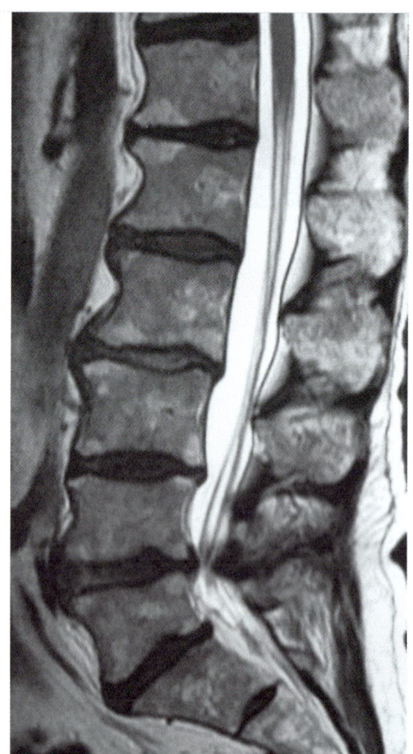

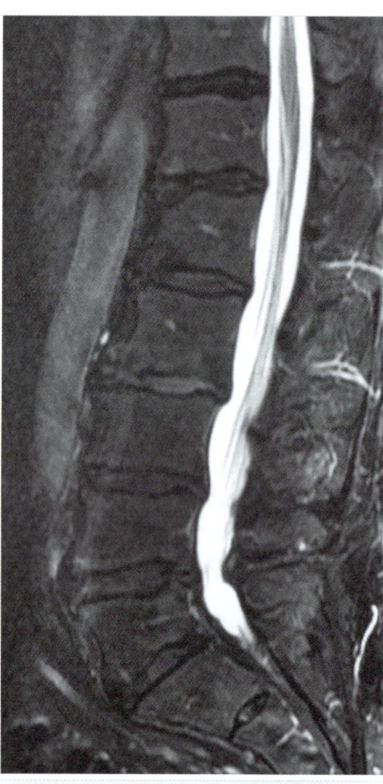

Fig. 10.250 A 75-year-old man with nonpathological age-related replacement of red marrow with zones of yellow marrow as seen as nodular zones with high signal on sagittal T1-weighted imaging (a) and T2-weighted imaging (T2WI) (b), and low signal on fat-suppressed (FS) T2WI (c). The marrow signal on FS T2WI is equal to or lower than that of adjacent skeletal muscle.

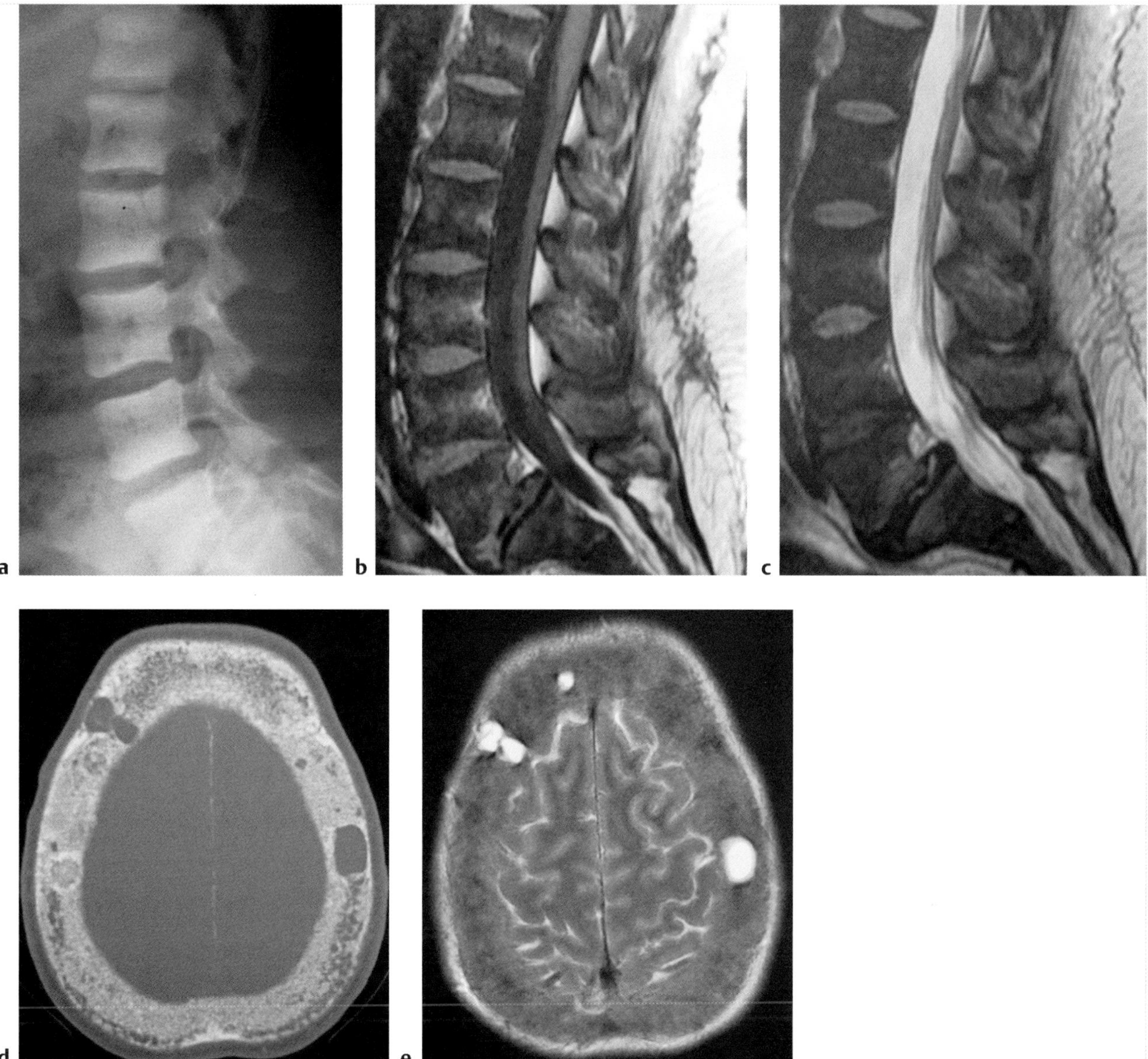

Fig. 10.251 A 34-year-old woman with renal osteodystrophy. Lateral radiograph shows bands of sclerosis parallel to endplates ("rugger jersey vertebrae") (a). Zones of low signal on sagittal T1-weighted imaging (b) and T2-weighted imaging (T2WI) correspond to regions of bone sclerosis (c). A 28-year-old man with renal osteodystrophy (d) who has osteomalacia involving the skull with circumscribed radiolucent zones on computed tomography, which have high signal on T2WI representing brown tumors (e).

Table 10.11 (Cont.) Diffuse, multiple, poorly defined, and/or multifocal zones of abnormal marrow signal

Abnormalities	MRI findings	Comments
Primary oxalosis (▶ Fig. 10.252)	Global medullary and cortical nephrocalcinosis with resultant renal failure. Early radiographic/computed tomographic (CT) findings include osteosclerosis and osteopenia, thin transverse sclerotic bands in long bones and skull. Late findings include osteosclerosis and dense intraossoeus sclerotic bands. Magnetic resonance imaging (MRI): decreased signal on T1WI and T2WI.	Type 1 primary hyperoxaluria is a rare autosomal recessive disorder (1 in 120,000 live births) involving mutations of the AGXT gene, which results in a deficiency of the peroxisomal enzyme: alanine glyoxylate aminotransferase. Systemic oxalate accumulates and precipitates in multiple organs (kidneys, liver, eye, heart, and bone) resulting in organ failure. Fifty percent have end-stage renal failure at 15 years. Treatment is combined liver–kidney transplantation.
Hypoparathyroidism	Localized or generalized osteosclerosis can be seen in bone on radiographs and CT, with corresponding low signal on T1WI and T2WI.	Deficiency in functional parathyroid hormone formation (surgical excision, radiation, trauma, autoimmune disease) results in hypocalcemia and generalized or localized osteosclerosis.
Pseudohypoparathyroidism	Bone density can be normal or diffusely increased or decreased as seen on radiographs. Other features include premature physeal plate closure resulting in short stature; calvarial thickening; shortening of the first, fourth, and fifth metacarpal bones; soft tissue calcifications; and ossification of the posterior longitudinal ligament.	Heritable disorder with end-organ resistance to parathyroid hormone resulting in hypocalcemia, hyperposphatemia with deposition of calcium in soft tissues and basal ganglia in the brain. More common in females, X-linked dominant trait.
Pseudo-pseudohypoparathyroidism	Imaging findings similar to pseudohypoparathyroidism.	Similar clinical and imaging features to pseudohypoparathyroidism except patients are normocalcemic.
Serous atrophy of marrow from malnutrition (▶ Fig. 10.253)	Depending on the severity of the malnutrition, involved marrow can have low-intermediate signal on T1WI and high signal on T2WI and FS T2WI. No Gd-contrast enhancement is usually seen. The marrow signal abnormalities may be localized or diffuse.	In emaciated patients from various causes (malnutrition, malabsorption, anorexia nervosa/bulimia, chronic renal insufficiency, HIV infection, and cancer), decreases in adipose tissue progressively occur in bone marrow and subcutaneous tissue followed by orbital fat. With progression of malnutrition, serous atrophy occurs in marrow in which there is accumulation of extracellular matrix containing hyaluronic acid associated with adipose and hematopoietic cell atrophy. The degree and extent of serous atrophy in marrow are related to body mass index and hemoglobin concentration. The lower limbs are frequent sites of serous atrophy, often being more prominent distally than proximally.
Hypervitaminosis A and D	Hyperostosis and cortical thickening may be seen involving tubular bones of children on plain films and CT.	Intoxication with vitamins A and D can lead to hyperostosis in children from cortical thickening from increased periosteal bone formation.
Fluorosis	Often is seen as dense diffuse osteosclerosis associated with osteophytes involving the spine, thorax, and pelvis. Limited osseous changes are seen in tubular bone of the extremities and the skull. MRI can show corresponding low signal in the spine on T1WI and T2WI.	Disease caused by excessive intake of fluoride via water containing more than 4 ppm. Fluorosis is associated with increased ossification and sclerosis of bone, as well as the posterior longitudinal ligament with resultant myelopathy. Hypertrophy of joints and bones can occur with osteoarthropathy.
Gaucher disease (▶ Fig. 10.254)	Diffuse and/or patchy heterogeneous zones with low-intermediate signal on T1WI, and heterogeneous intermediate to high signal on T2WI and FS T2WI.	Rare, heritable metabolic disorder with deficient activity of the lysosomal enzyme-hydrolase beta-glucosidase. Results in accumulation of the lipid-glucosylceramide within lysosomes of the monocyte-macrophage system (Gaucher cells) of the bone marrow, liver, and spleen. Marrow infiltration by Gaucher cells often results in zones of ischemia and bone infarction.

(continued on page 520)

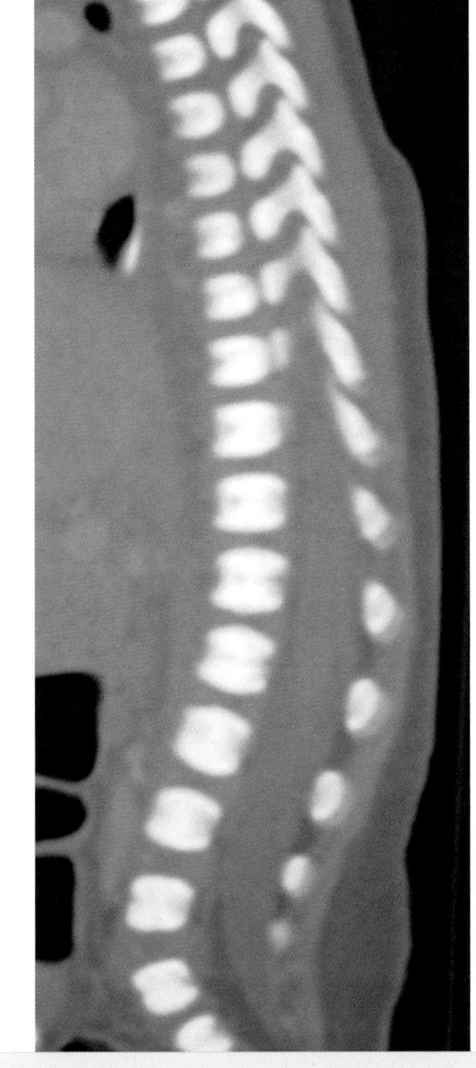

Fig. 10.252 Primary oxalosis in an infant with diffuse osteosclerosis on sagittal computed tomography.

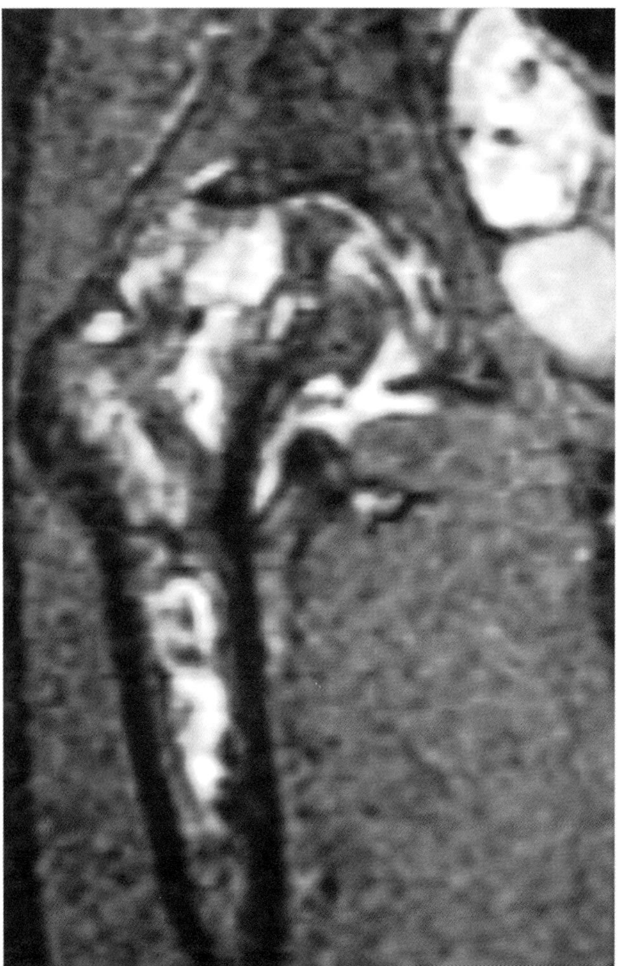

Fig. 10.254 A 34-year-old woman with Gaucher disease with diffuse and patchy heterogeneous zones with intermediate to high signal in the marrow on coronal short TI inversion recovery.

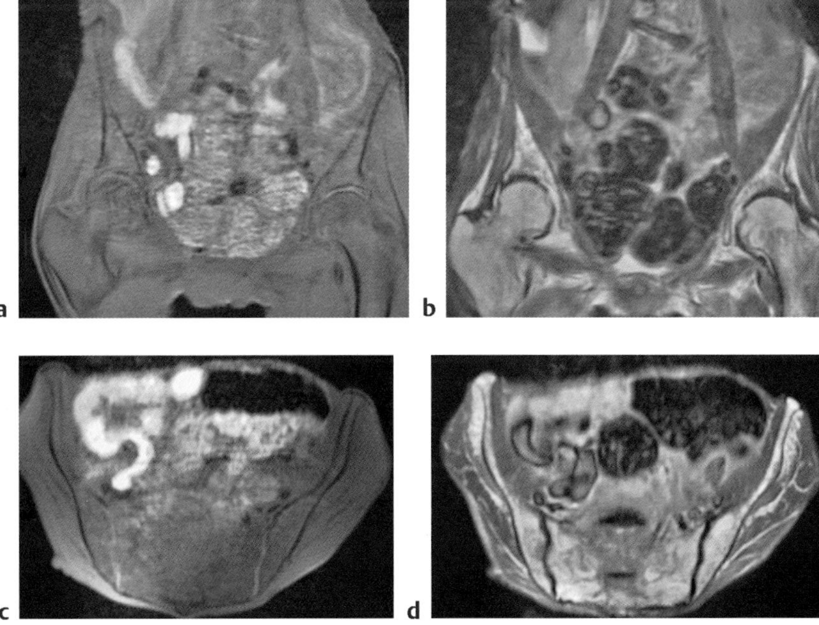

Fig. 10.253 A 66-year-old woman with malabsorption syndrome and cachexia with extensive diffuse serous atrophy of marrow seen as loss of normal fat signal in the soft tissues and marrow on coronal (a) and axial T1-weighted imaging (c). Diffuse abnormal high signal is seen in the marrow on coronal (b) and axial T2-weighted imaging (d).

Table 10.11 (Cont.) Diffuse, multiple, poorly defined, and/or multifocal zones of abnormal marrow signal

Abnormalities	MRI findings	Comments
Glycogen storage disease type 1B	Myeloid hyperplasia in this disorder results in inhomogeneous decreased signal of marrow on T1WI compared with fat, and inhomogeneous hyperintense signal on FS T2WI or short TI inversion recovery (STIR). Marrow signal changes can become more prominent and diffuse during treatment with granulocyte colony-stimulating factor.	Disorder affecting children and young adults in which there is deficiency of functional microsomal glucose-6-phosphatase activity causing impairment of glycogenolysis and gluconeogenesis. As a result, patients suffer from postprandial and fasting hypoglycemia, increased production of lactic acid, uric acid, and triglycerides. Patients have increased susceptibility to bacterial infections secondary to chronic neutropenia, abnormal myeloid maturation, and dysfunction of circulating neutrophils and monocytes. Patients are often treated with granulocyte colony-stimulating factor for neutropenia.
Glycogen storage disease type 1A	Marrow in this disorder is typically fatty.	Disorder affecting children and young adults in which there is deficiency of functional microsomal glucose-6-phosphatase activity causing impairment of glycogenolysis and gluconeogenesis. As a result, patients suffer from postprandial and fasting hypoglycemia, increased production of lactic acid, uric acid, and triglycerides. Unlike glycogen storage disease type 1B, patients do not have increased susceptibility to bacterial infections.
Mucopolysaccharidoses (MPS) (▶ Fig. 10.255)	Imaging findings include wedge-shaped vertebral bodies with anterior beaks (central: Morquio syndrome; anteroinferiorly: Hurler syndrome/Hunter syndrome), decreased heights of vertebral bodies, widened disks, spinal canal stenosis, odontoid hypoplasia, thick clavicles, paddle-shaped ribs, widened symphysis pubis, flared iliac bones, widening of the femoral necks, ± absent femoral heads, coxa valga, shortened metacarpal bones, Madelung deformity, and diaphyseal widening of long bones. Marrow MRI signal may be within normal limits or slightly decreased on T1WI and/or slightly increased on T2WI.	Inherited disorders of glycosaminoglycan catabolism from defects in specific lysosomal enzymes. MPS I (Hurler syndrome, Scheie syndrome)–deficiency of *alpha-L-iduronidase;* MPS II (Hunter syndrome)–X-linked deficiency of iduronate-2-sulfatase; MPS III (Sanfilippo A, B, C, D syndrome, autosomal recessive deficiency of enzymes that break down *heparan sulfate*; MPS IV (Morquio syndrome), autosomal recessive deficiency of *N-acetylgalactosamine-6-sulfatase*; MPS VI (Maroteaux-Lamy syndrome) autosomal deficiency of *N-acetylgalatosamine-4-sulfatase;* MPS VII (Sly syndrome) autosomal recessive deficiency of *beta-glucuronidase;* MPS IX (hyaluronidase deficiency) deficiency of *hyaluronidase*; Disorders result in accumulation of toxic metabolites in lysosomes and in axonal loss and demyelination. Treatments include enzyme replacement and BMT.
Osteogenesis imperfecta	Diffuse osteopenia with predisposition for fractures.	"Brittle bone disease"; 4 to 7 types; hereditary disorder with abnormal type I fibrillar collagen production and osteoporosis resulting from mutations involving the COL1A1 gene on chromosome 17q21.31-q22.05 and the COL1A2 gene on chromosome 7q22.1 (19, 29). Results in fragile bone that is prone to repetitive microfractures and remodeling.
Osteopetrosis (▶ Fig. 10.256)	Radiographs show diffuse and/or bandlike zones of osteosclerosis, which appear as zones of low signal on T1WI and T2WI.	Osteopetrosis consists of four types (precocious type: autosomal recessive form, which is usually lethal; delayed type: autosomal dominant form described by Albers-Schönberg, which can be asymptomatic until there is a pathological fracture or anemia; intermediate recessive type in which patients have short stature, hepatomegaly, and anemia; and tubular acidosis autosomal recessive form in which cerebral calcifications occur as well as renal tubular acidosis, mental retardation, muscle weakness, and hypotonia).

(continued on page 522)

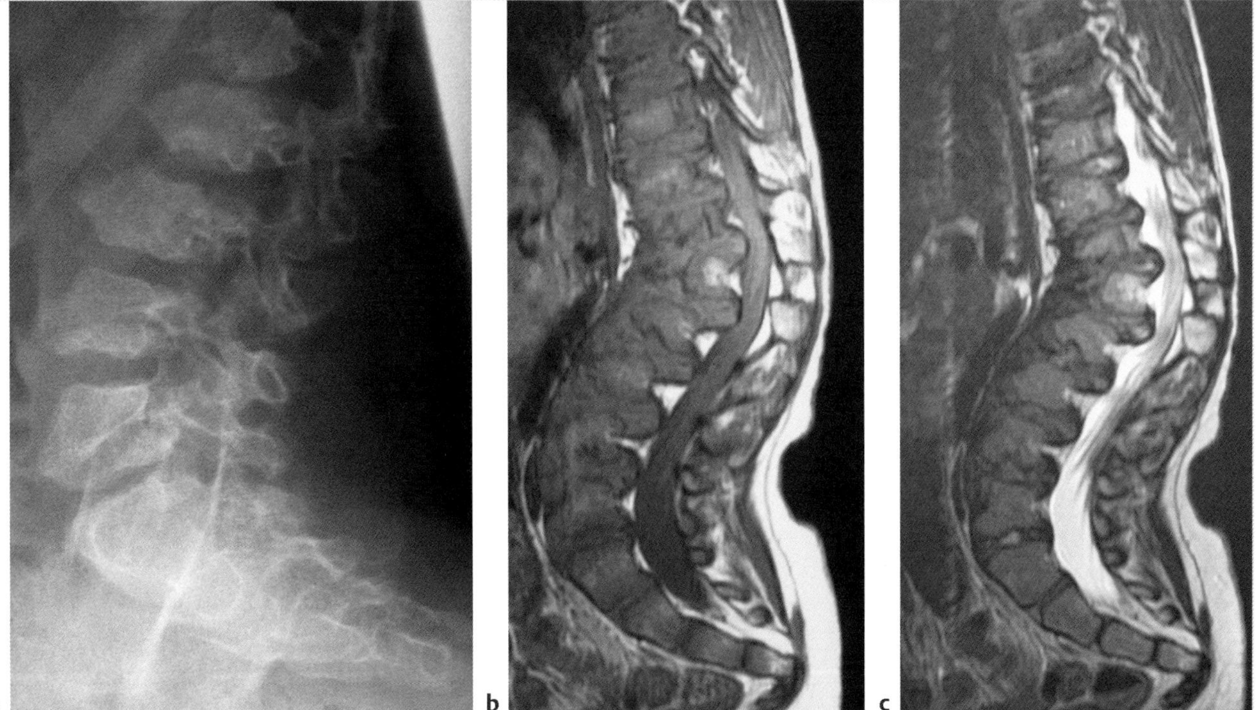

Fig. 10.255 Morquio syndrome. Radiograph shows wedge-shaped vertebral bodies with anterior beaks centrally (a), decreased heights of vertebral bodies, widened disks, and spinal canal stenosis. Marrow magnetic resonance imaging signal is slightly decreased on T1-weighted imaging (b) and slightly increased on T2-weighted imaging (c).

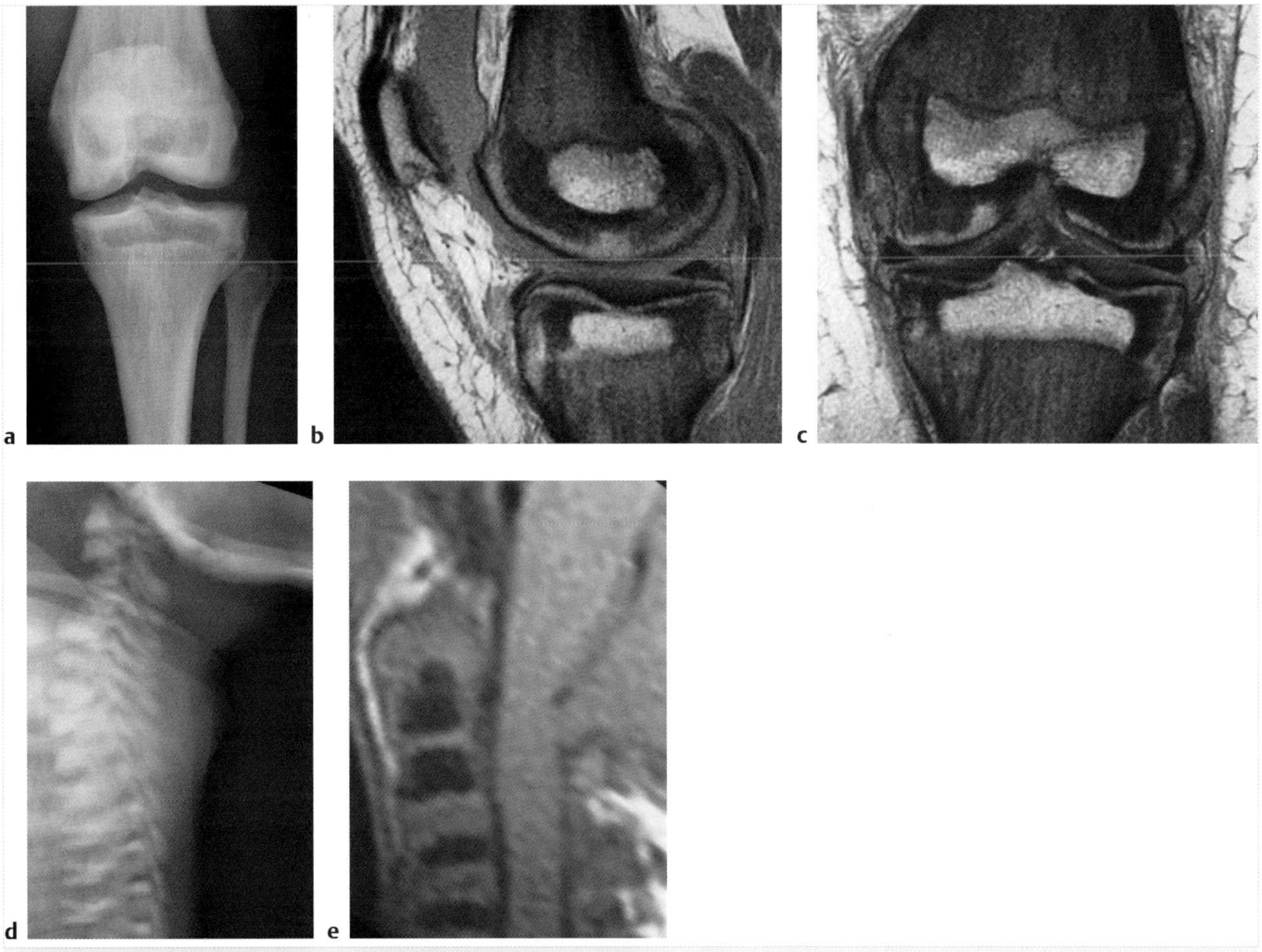

Fig. 10.256 Osteopetrosis. Anteroposterior radiograph (a) of a 28-year-old woman shows diffuse osteosclerosis, which appears as zones with low signal on sagittal (b) and coronal T1-weighted imaging (T1WI) (c). Radiograph of a different patient with infantile osteopetrosis (d) shows dense osteosclerosis with corresponding diffuse low signal in the marrow on sagittal T1WI (e).

Table 10.11 (Cont.) Diffuse, multiple, poorly defined, and/or multifocal zones of abnormal marrow signal

Abnormalities	MRI findings	Comments
Inflammatory disorders		
Osteomyelitis (▶ Fig. 10.257)	In acute osteomyelitis, poorly defined zones of low or low-intermediate signal on T1WI; high signal on T2WI, STIR, and FS T2WI are seen in the marrow. A wide zone of transition between normal bone and edematous and infected bone is typically seen in acute osteomyelitis. Loss of definition of the low signal line of the cortical margins is often observed on T1WI, T2WI, STIR, and FS T2WI. After Gd-contrast administration, irregular zones of contrast enhancement are seen in the involved marrow on FS T1WI.	Osteomyelitis is a disorder in which there is infection of bone and commonly the adjacent soft tissues. Can result from hematogenous spread of micro-organisms as well as from trauma-direct inoculation, extension from adjacent tissues, and complications from surgery. Bacteria such as *Staphylococcus aureus* and *Streptococcus pyogenes* are the most common infectious organisms. Can also result from other bacteria as well as tuberculosis, fungi, parasites, and viruses.
Chronic recurrent multifocal osteomyelitis	Multifocal lesions that occur in metaphyses of tubular bones (distal femur, proximal and distal tibia and fibula), clavicles, and vertebrae. Radiographs show radiolucent and/or sclerotic osseous lesions with proliferative periosteal bone formation. Magnetic resonance imaging (MRI) shows heterogeneous abnormal high signal on FS T2WI in marrow and periosteal soft tissues with Gd-contrast enhancement.	Painful inflammatory osseous disorder of unknown cause with histopathology of acute and chronic osteomyelitis without identification of infectious agent, diagnosis of exclusion. Usually occurs in children and adolescents, median age = 10 years, F 85%/M 15%. Multiepisodic skeletal disorder of unknown cause that can occur over 7 to 25 years. Treatment of symptoms with nonsteroidal anti-inflammatory drugs. Can be associated with acne or pustulosis palmoplantaris (SAPHO).
Eosinophilic granuloma (Langerhans cell histiocytosis)	Focal intramedullary lesion(s) associated with trabecular and cortical bone destruction, which typically have low-intermediate signal on T1WI and PDWI and heterogeneous slightly-high to high signal on T2WI. Poorly defined zones of high signal on T2WI are usually seen in the marrow peripheral to the lesions secondary to inflammatory changes. Extension of lesions from the marrow into adjacent soft tissues through areas of cortical disruption is commonly seen as well as linear periosteal zones of high signal on T2WI. Lesions typically show prominent Gd-contrast enhancement in marrow and in extraosseous soft tissue portions of the lesions.	Benign tumor-like lesions consisting of Langerhans cells (histiocytes) and variable amounts of lymphocytes, polymorphonuclear cells, and eosinophils. Account for 1% of primary bone lesions and 8% of tumor-like lesions. Occur in patients with median age = 10 years, average = 13.5 years, peak incidence is between 5 and 10 years; 80 to 85% occur in patients less than 30 years. Multifocal subtypes (Letterer-Siwe disease and Hand-Schüller-Christian disease) account for 30% of cases.
Ankylosing spondylitis	Inflammation occurs at entheses (sites of attachment of ligaments, tendons, and joint capsules to bone). Zones with high signal on T2WI and contrast enhancement can be seen in marrow at sites of active inflammation at corners of vertebral bodies, sacroiliac joints, and other bones. Progression of inflammation leads to squaring of vertebral bodies with mineralized syndesmophytes across disks, osteopenia, and erosions at sacroiliac joints with eventual fusion across these joints and facets.	Chronic progressive autoimmune inflammatory disease involving the spine and sacroiliac joints. Associated with human leukocyte antigen (HLA)-B27 antigen. In 90%, onset in patients 20 to 30 years, male:female ratio 3:1.
Sarcoidosis (▶ Fig. 10.258)	In small bones, lesions usually appear as intramedullary zones with low to intermediate signal on T1WI and slightly high to high signal on T2WI and FS PDWI and FS T2WI. After Gd-contrast administration, lesions typically show moderate to prominent enhancement. In long bones and axial skeleton, sarcoid lesions are often multiple with variable sizes or solitary within marrow. Zones of cortical destruction associated with intramedullary lesions are uncommon, unlike with sarcoid involving small bones. Lesions can have circumscribed and/or indistinct margins within marrow. Irregular confluent or patchy zones as well as a diffuse stippled patterns of signal alteration in marrow have also been described for skeletal sarcoid. Lesions usually have low to intermediate signal on T1WI and PDWI, and often have slightly high to high signal on T2WI and FS T2WI. Occasional lesions may also have low or intermediate signal on T2WI. Focal areas with MRI signal similar to fat are seen in some lesions in long bones. Lesions with low signal on T2WI correspond to plain film and CT findings of osteosclerosis. After Gd-contrast administration, variable enhancement can be seen.	Sarcoidosis is a chronic systemic granulomatous disease of unknown etiology in which noncaseating granulomas occur in various tissues and organs. Sarcoidosis appears to be related to an abnormal or exaggerated T-helper-induced cellular immune response to antigens or self-antigens resulting in the collection of large numbers of activated T cells in the affected tissue. Bones of the hands and feet are common sites of involvement, but any bone can be affected.

(continued on page 524)

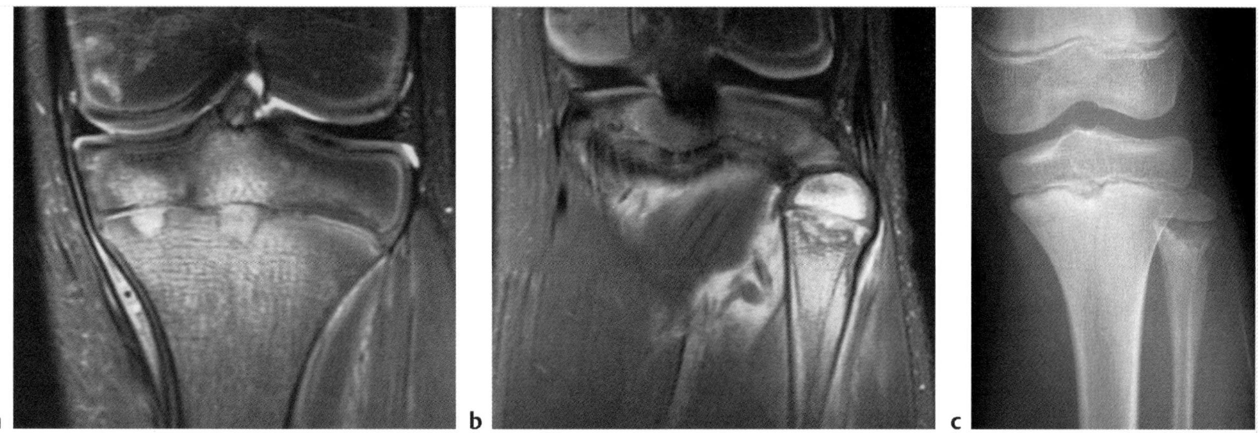

Fig. 10.257 An 11-year-old boy with mulifocal pyogenic osteomyelitis involving the proximal portions of the tibia and fibula. Poorly defined zones with high signal on coronal fat-suppressed T2-weighted imaging (FS T2WI) (a,b) are seen in the marrow. Cortical destruction with extraosseous extension of the infection with periosteal elevation is seen involving the fibula on FS T2WI (c) with corresponding findings on radiograph.

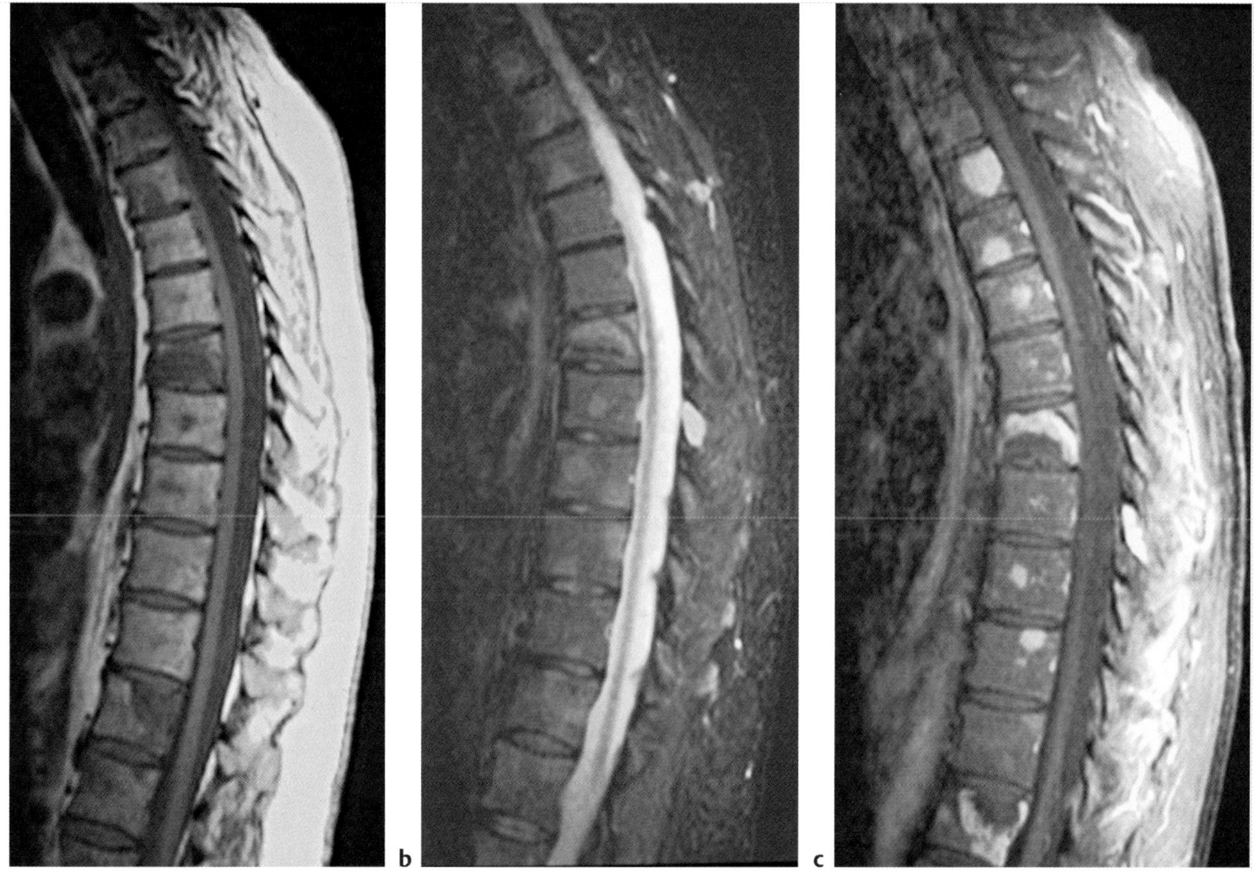

Fig. 10.258 A 50-year-old man with sarcoidosis and multiple intraosseous spinal lesions, which have low-intermediate signal on sagittal T1-weighted imaging (T1WI) (a) and slightly high signal on sagittal fat-suppressed (FS) T2-weighted imaging (b). The lesions show prominent gadolinium-contrast enhancement on sagittal FS T1WI (c).

Table 10.11 (Cont.) Diffuse, multiple, poorly defined, and/or multifocal zones of abnormal marrow signal

Abnormalities	MRI findings	Comments
Erdheim-Chester disease (▶ Fig. 10.259)	Lesions can appear as irregular zones with low and/or intermediate signal on T1WI and PDWI, and mixed low, intermediate, and/or high signal on T2WI and FS T2WI within marrow. Zones of cortical destruction with or without extraosseous lesion extension may be seen occasionally with lesions in long bones. After Gd-contrast administration, heterogeneous enhancement may be seen in the involved marrow and zones of extraosseous extension if present.	Erdheim-Chester disease is a rare multisystem non-Langerhans cell histiocytic disorder of unknown etiology that usually affects adults. Collections of foamy macrophages can be seen within various tissues and organs of the musculoskeletal, pulmonary, cardiac, gastrointestinal, and central nervous systems.
Bilateral sacroiliitis (▶ Fig. 10.260)	Asymmetric or symmetric poorly defined zones with high signal on T2WI and FS T2WI and corresponding Gd-contrast enhancement in the subchondral marrow of the iliac and sacral bones adjacent to the sacroiliac joints.	Commonly occurs in ankylosing spondylitis, which is an autoimmune inflammatory disorder associated with HLA-B27 that frequently involves both sacroiliac joints in most patients, as well as the hips in 35% of patients.
Osteiitis condensans (▶ Fig. 10.261)	Zones of subchondral osteosclerosis usually have corresponding zones of low signal on T1WI and T2WI. In addition, small irregular zones of slightly high signal may be seen in the marrow on FS T2WI, as well as mild irregular Gd-contrast enhancement.	Unilateral or asymmetric or symmetric bilateral osteosclerotic process in the subchondral marrow adjacent to the sacroiliac joints (iliac bone more pronounced than the sacral marrow) and/or pubic symphysis, usually occurs in women and is often associated with pregnancy. The subchondral bone is usually well defined, and the sacroiliac joint is typically intact. Findings may persist or regress.

(continued on page 526)

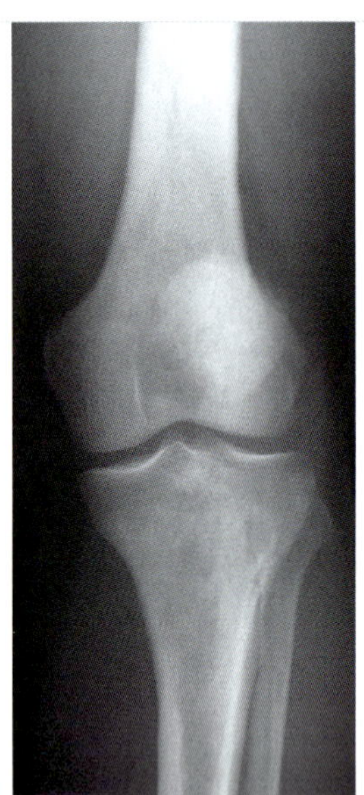

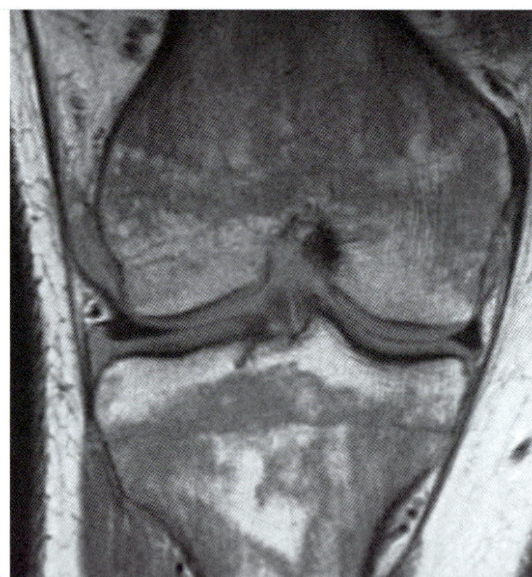

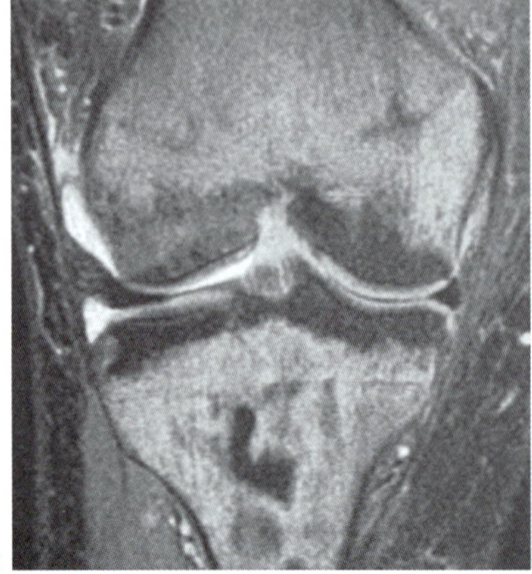

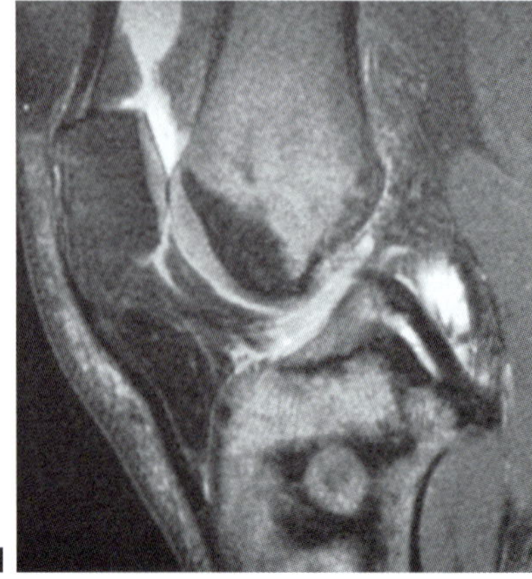

Fig. 10.259 A 39-year-old man with Erdheim-Chester disease with bone marrow involvement. Anteroposterior radiograph (a) shows increased medullary density, coarsened trabecular thickening, and cortical thickening. Irregular zones with intermediate signal on coronal proton density–weighted imaging (b), and slightly high signal on coronal (c) and sagittal fat-suppressed T2-weighted imaging (d) are seen within the marrow of the femur and tibia.

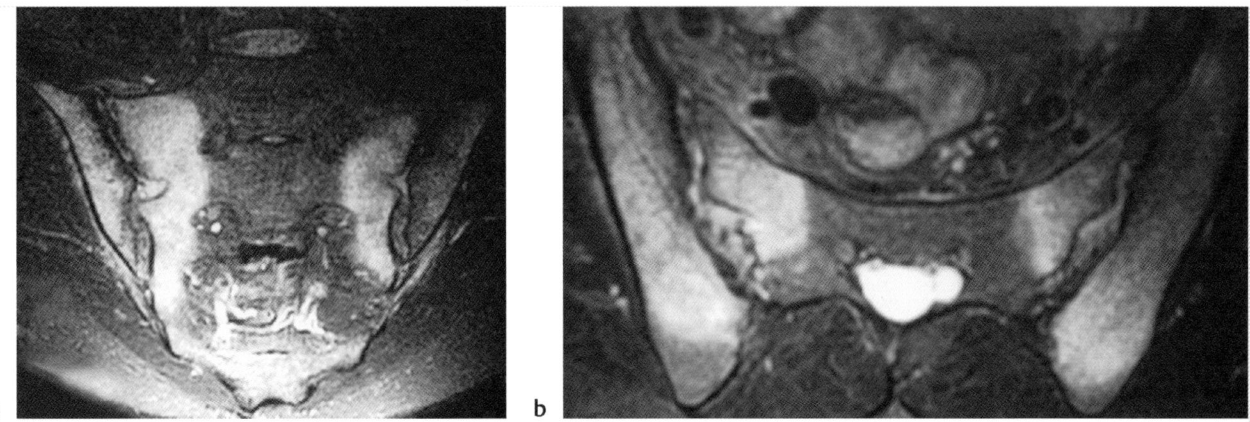

Fig. 10.260 A 35-year-old woman with bilateral sacroiliitis seen as symmetric poorly defined zones with high signal on coronal (a) and axial fat-suppressed T2-weighted imaging (b). Zones with high signal are also seen in the sacroiliac joints.

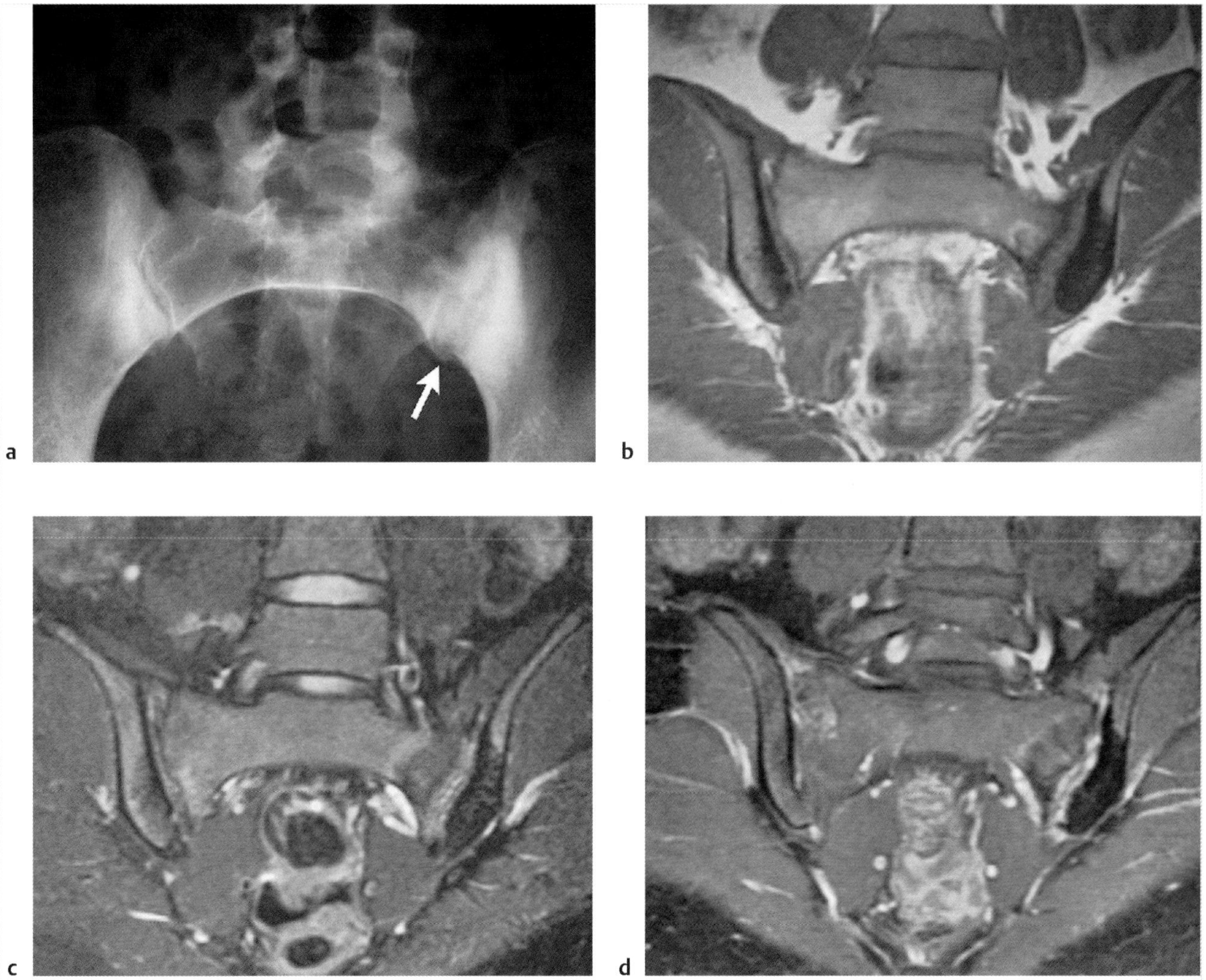

Fig. 10.261 A 35-year-old woman with osteitis condensans ilii at both sacroiliac joints. Zones of subchondral osteosclerosis (arrow) are seen on anteroposterior radiograph (a) at both sacroliliac joints, which have corresponding zones of mostly low signal on coronal T1-weighted imaging (T1WI) (b) and fat-suppressed T2-weighted imaging (FS T2WI) (c). Small irregular zones of slightly high signal are seen in the subchondral marrow on FS T2WI, which show mild irregular Gd-contrast enhancement on coronal FS T1WI (d).

Table 10.11 (Cont.) Diffuse, multiple, poorly defined, and/or multifocal zones of abnormal marrow signal

Abnormalities	MRI findings	Comments
Degenerative/traumatic/posttreatment disorders		
Bone contusions	Contusions usually appear as poorly defined intramedullary zones with low-intermediate signal on T1WI and high signal on FS T2WI, and corresponding Gd-contrast enhancement. Adjacent cortical margins are typically intact.	Also referred to as bone bruises, contusions represent trabecular microfractures without cortical fracture. In the knee, contusions at the lateral femoral condyle and posterolateral proximal tibia are commonly associated with injuries to the anterior cruciate ligament.
Bilateral sacral insufficiency fractures (▶ Fig. 10.262)	Asymmetric or symmetric poorly defined zones with low signal on T1WI, high signal on T2WI and FS T2WI, and corresponding Gd-contrast enhancement are seen in the marrow of both sacral ala within which may be serpiginous curvilinear zones of low signal. No zones with abnormal signal are typically seen in the iliac bones or sacroiliac joints.	Axial forces to sacral bone can result in insufficiency-type stress fractures in osteopenic bone in older patients or from osteomalacia, or fatigue-type stress fractures in athletes (runners, gymnasts, etc). May be associated with pubic bone fractures. Patients can have point tenderness, pain with weight bearing and movement.
Marrow changes related to degenerative disk disease (▶ Fig. 10.263)	Type 1: Poorly defined zones with low-intermediate signal on T1WI (decreased relative to normal marrow), slightly high signal on T2WI (increased relative to normal marrow), and high signal on FS T2WI in marrow next to intact endplates, often associated with Gd-contrast enhancement, intervening disk usually with degenerative changes. Type 2: Poorly defined zones with intermediate-slightly high signal on T1WI (increased relative to normal marrow), intermediate-slightly high signal on T2WI (isointense or increased relative to normal marrow), and low or intermediate signal on FS T2WI in marrow next to intact endplates, ± Gd-contrast enhancement, intervening disk usually with degenerative changes.	Reactive changes in marrow from degenerative disk disease can result from fissuring of endplates with edematous changes and/or replacement with fibrovascular tissue in the subjacent marrow. The endplate margins typically appear intact as thin linear zones of low signal on T1WI and T2WI adjacent to a degenerated disk with low signal on T2WI. These latter two findings differ from the MRI features of vertebral osteomyelitis where there is often destruction of the endplates and annulus, as well as high signal on T2WI within the disk.
Neuropathic bone and joint disease (▶ Fig. 10.264)	Joint effusions with peripheral rim patterns of Gd-contrast enhancement; bone proliferation and fragmentation with intra-articular loose bodies; abnormal increased signal in bone marrow on FS T2WI with Gd-contrast enhancement; subluxation; and degenerative sunchondral radiolucent bone cysts. In the periarticular soft tissues, common features include edema and Gd-contrast enhancement. Superimposed infections involving neuropathic joints often have associated soft tissue abnormalities such as abscesses, ulcers, and/or sinus tracts.	Occurs in patients with dense neuropathy with impaired perception to trauma and pain and often associated peripheral vascular disease. Neuropathic osteoarthropathy occurs from chronic repetitive trauma to bones, cartilage, joints, tendons, and ligaments and results in joint instability, cartilage damage, subchondral degenerative bone changes, poor healing response, ischemic bone changes, deformities, and increased new bone formation. Superimposed infections commonly occur in diabetic patients with neuropathic osteoarthropathy.

(continued on page 528)

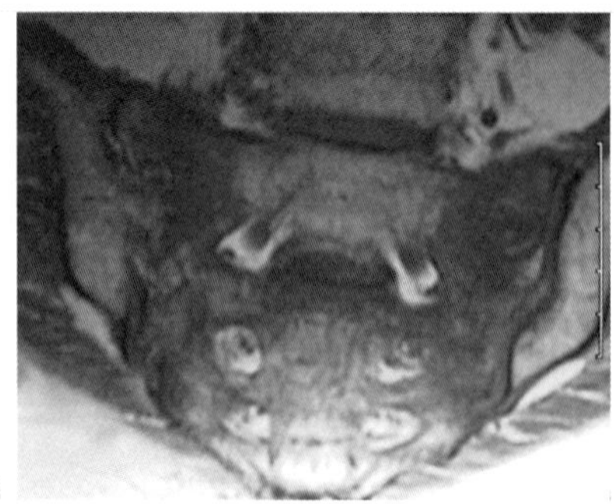

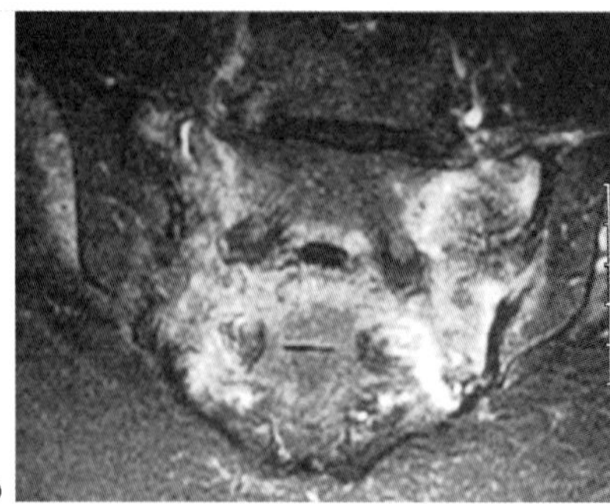

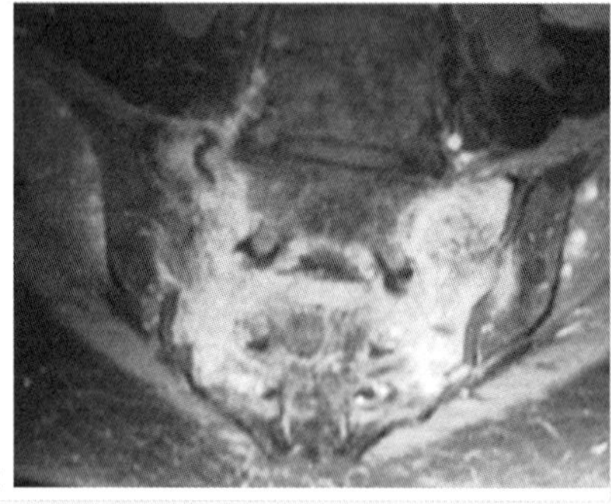

Fig. 10.262 An 85-year-old woman with bilateral sacral insufficiency fractures, which have poorly defined zones of abnormal marrow signal consisting of low signal on coronal T1-weighted imaging (T1WI) (a), and high signal on fat-suppressed T2-weighted imaging (FS T2WI) (b), with corresponding Gd-contrast enhancement on coronal FS T1WI. Serpiginous thin curvilinear zones of low signal are also seen at the fracture sites on FS T2WI (c).

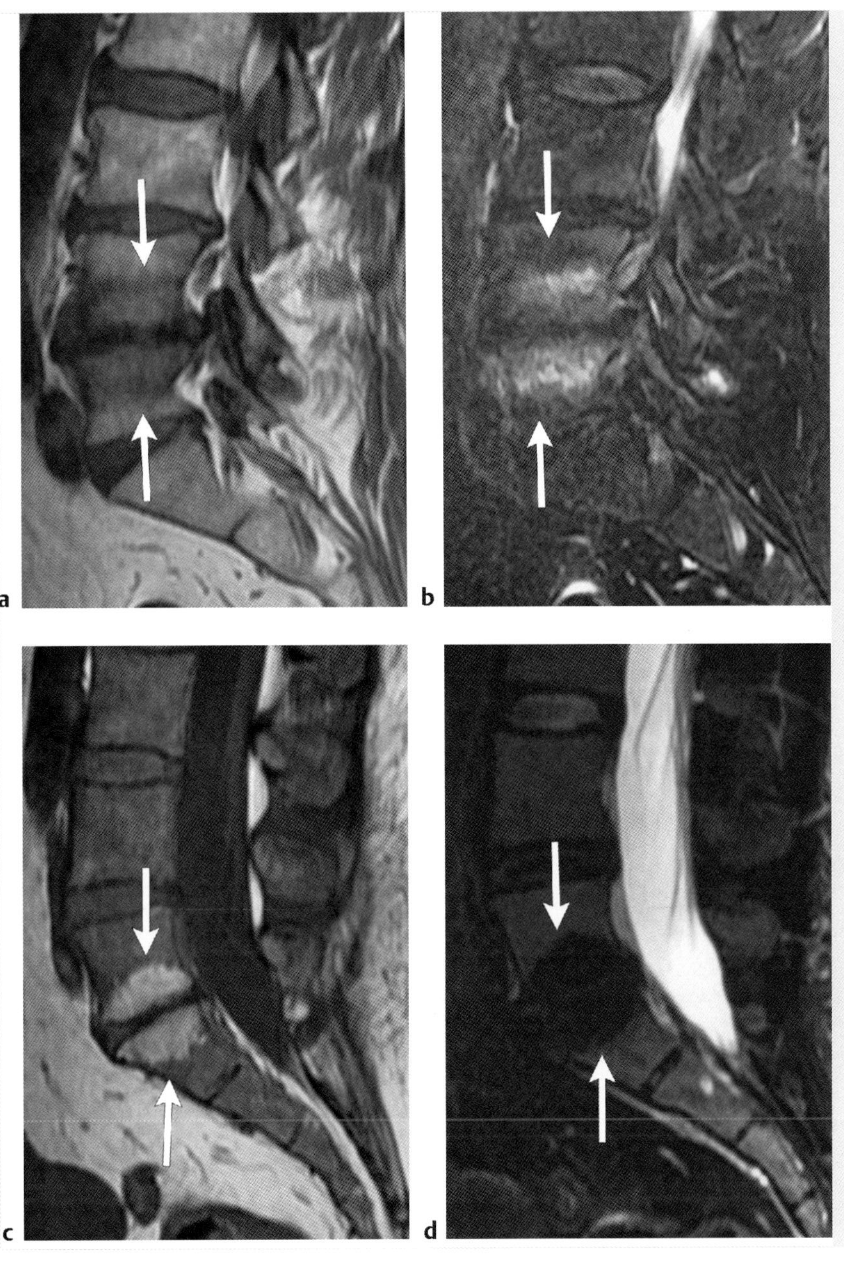

Fig. 10.263 Poorly defined zones with low-intermediate signal on T1-weighted imaging (T1WI) (a) are seen in the marrow adjacent to the intact vertebral body endplates and degenerated disk at the L4–L5 level (arrows), which have high signal (arrows) on fat-suppressed T2-weighted imaging (FS T2WI) (b). Poorly defined zones with fat signal (arrows) on T1-weighted imaging (c) and FS T2WI (d) are seen in the marrow adjacent to the intact endplates and degenerated disk at the L5–S1 level.

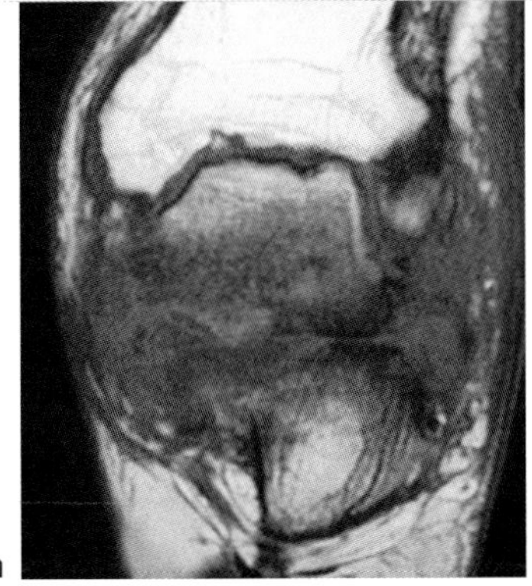

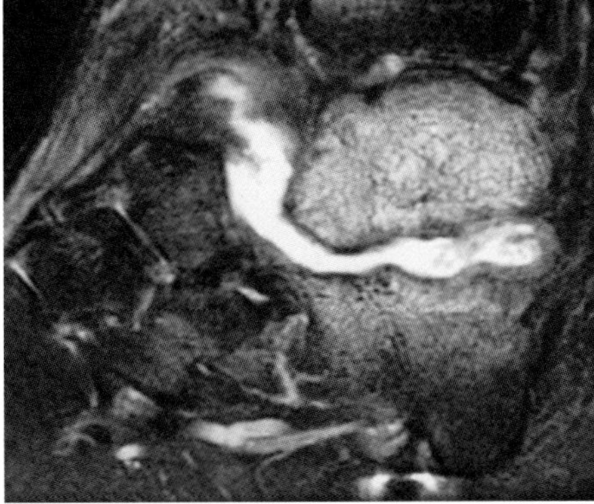

Fig. 10.264 Neuropathic joint disease involving the ankle resulting in bone fragmentation with intra-articular loose bodies; poorly defined zones with abnormal decreased signal on T1-weighted imaging (a) and increased signal on sagittal fat-suppressed T2-weighted imaging (b) in the bone marrow, and joint effusion are seen.

Table 10.11 (Cont.) Diffuse, multiple, poorly defined, and/or multifocal zones of abnormal marrow signal

Abnormalities	MRI findings	Comments
Reflex sympathetic dystrophy (RSD) (also referred to as Sudek atrophy, algodystrophy, complex regional pain syndromes types 1 and 2) (▶ Fig. 10.265)	Poorly defined zones with increased signal on FS T2WI may be seen in the bone marrow of one or more bones in some cases during the warm phase of RSD, but signal abnormalities are typically absent in the dystrophic cold phases of this disorder. Findings of increased signal on FS T2WI may also occur in the adjacent soft tissues in some cases.	Syndromes in which there are clinical findings such as abnormal sensation (continuing pain in the absence of external stimuli, hyperesthesia), and altered vasomotor (skin temperature asymmetry, skin color asymmetry) and autonomic function (edema, sweating changes or sweating asymmetry). In chronic regional pain syndrome type 1 (RSD), no nerve damage can be detected. RSD can occur in a limb after fracture or other injury, or in immobilized limbs of patients who have had cerebral infarcts. Chronic regional pain syndrome type 2 (causalgia) differs from type 1 (RSD) in that the former is associated with nerve damage detectable with electromyography.
Regional migratory osteoporosis	Poorly defined zones with increased signal on FS T2WI may be seen in the bone marrow of one or more periarticular bones of the lower extremities and rarely the spine. Findings of periarticular osteopenia/osteopeorosis are typical 3–6 weeks after onset of symptoms.	Uncommon migrating and transient arthralgia involving the lower extremities and spine, affects middle-aged males (fifth to sixth decades). May be a variant of algodystrophy. Pain is maximal at 2 months, with progressive resolution from 3 to 9 months with or without recurrence or onset of symptoms in other joints.
Radiation injury (▶ Fig. 10.266)	Involved marrow has signal similar to fat. Bone infarcts may be present.	Radiation treatment or exposure typically converts red marrow to yellow due to damage to myeloid- and erythroid-producing cells.
Bone infarction (▶ Fig. 10.267)	In the early phases of ischemia, diffuse poorly defined zones of high signal may be seen on FS T2WI, which can overlap the MRI features of transient painful bone marrow edema. In zones of bone infarction, curvilinear zones of low signal on T1WI and T2WI representing zones of fibrosis are usually seen in the marrow. In addition to the above findings, irregular zones of low signal on T1WI and high signal on T2WI and FS T2WI may be seen in the marrow representing zones of fluid from edema, ischemia/infarction, or fracture if present. Irregular zones with high signal on T1WI and T2WI can occasionally be seen resulting from hemorrhage in combination with zones of fibrosis and fluid. A double-line sign (curvilinear adjacent zones of low and high signal on T2WI) is often seen at the edges of the infarcts representing the borders of osseous resorption and healing. After Gd-contrast administration, irregular enhancement can be seen from granulation tissue ingrowth.	Bone infarcts are zones of ischemic death involving bone trabeculae and marrow, which may be idiopathic or may result from trauma, corticosteroid treatment, chemotherapy, radiation treatment, occlusive vascular disease, collagen vascular and other autoimmune diseases, metabolic storage diseases (e.g., Gaucher disease), sickle cell disease, thalassemia, hyperbaric events/Caisson disease, pregnancy, alcohol abuse, pancreatitis, infections, and lymphoproliferative diseases. Osteonecrosis is more common in fatty compared with hematopoietic marrow. Avascular necrosis involving specific bones may have names such as Legg-Calvé-Perthes disease (femoral head), Kienböck disease (lunate), Preiser disease (scaphoid), Köhler disease (tarsal navicular), Freiberg infraction (metatarsal head), Panner disease (capitulum of humerus), and Thiemann disease (phalanges of hand).

(continued on page 530)

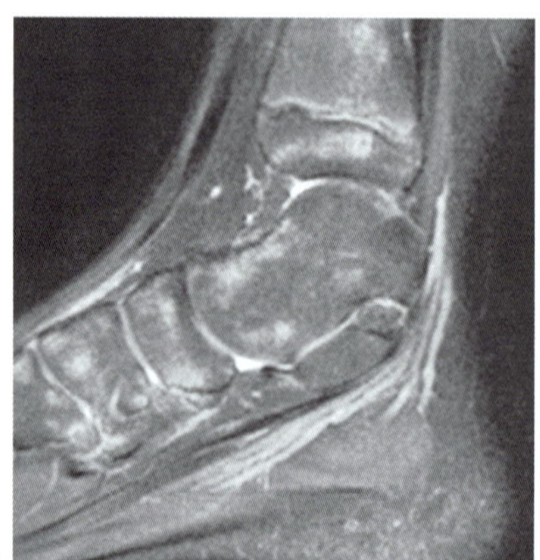
a

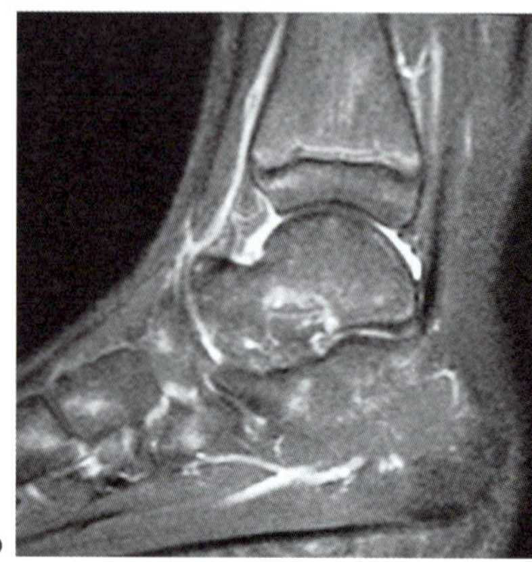
b

Fig. 10.265 Reflex sympathetic dystrophy in a 13-year-old girl. Poorly defined zones with high signal on fat-suppressed T2-weighted imaging are seen in the bone marrow of multiple bones of the foot and ankle without cortical erosion or destruction.

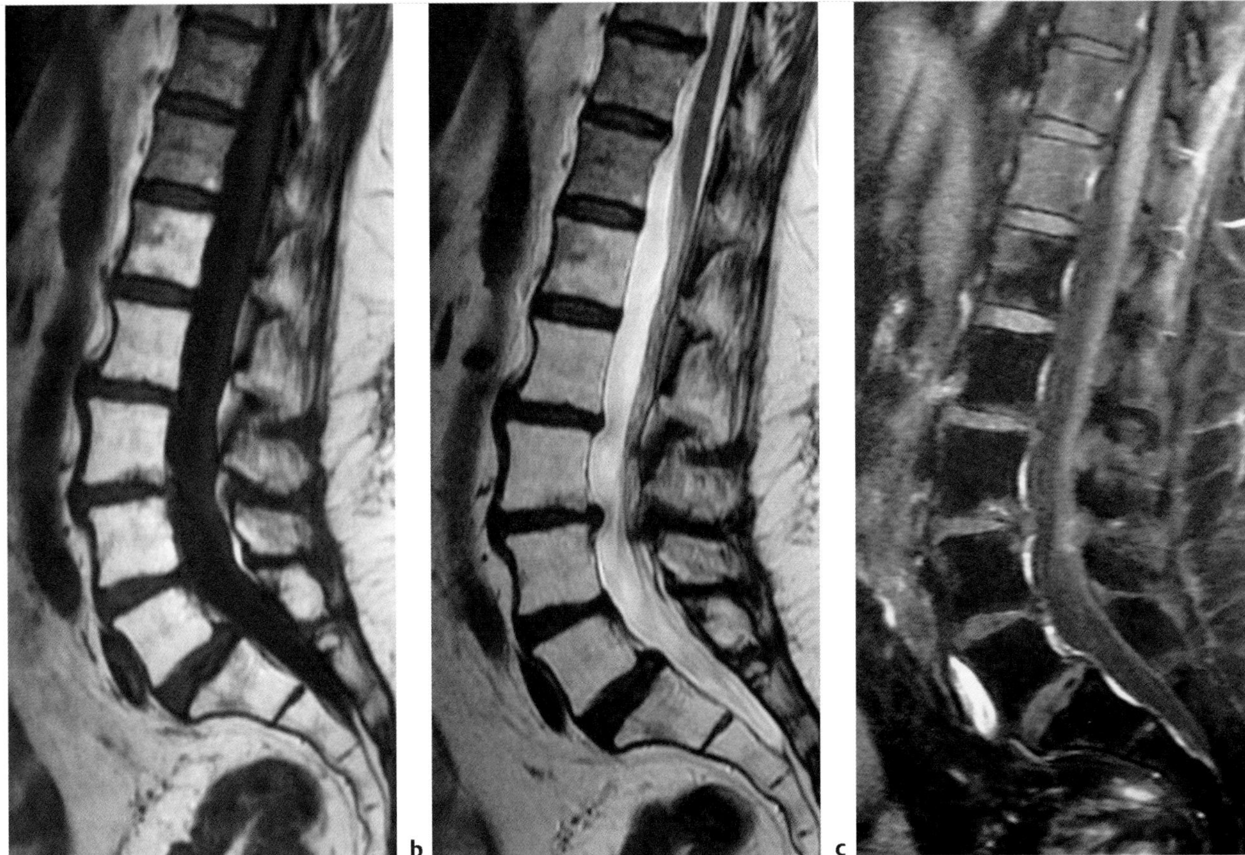

Fig. 10.266 Fatty marrow changes resulting from radiation treatment for pelvic tumor are seen as zones with high signal on T1-weighted imaging (T1WI) (a) and T2-weighted imaging (b) and low signal on post-gadolinium-contrast enhanced fat-suppressed T1WI (c).

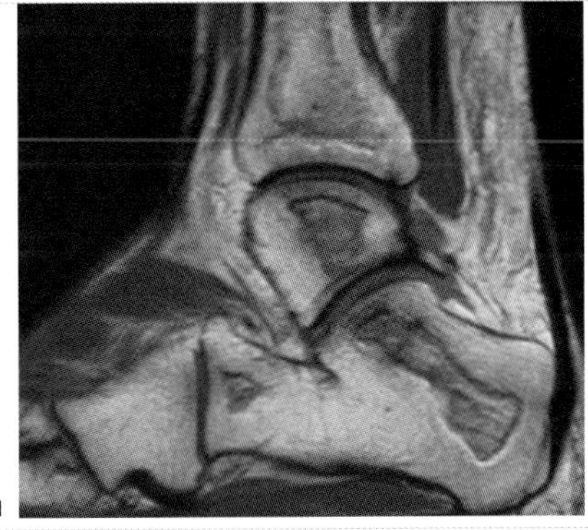

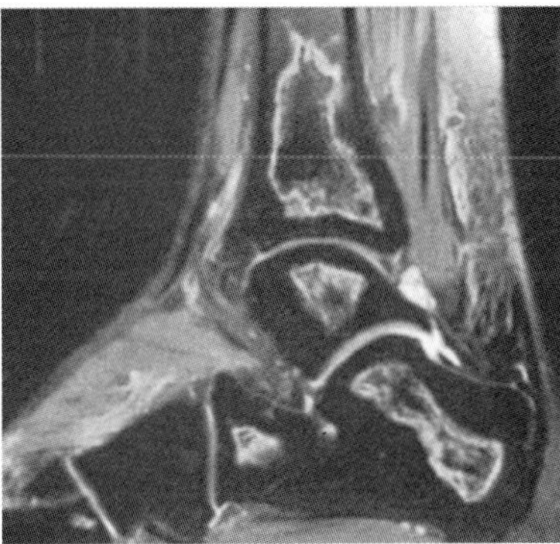

Fig. 10.267 Bone infarction. A 36-year-old man with bone infarcts in the distal tibia, talus, and calcaneus seen as serpiginous zones of low signal on sagittal proton density-weighted imaging (a) and high signal on fat-suppressed T2-weighted imaging (b).

Table 10.11 (Cont.) Diffuse, multiple, poorly defined, and/or multifocal zones of abnormal marrow signal

Abnormalities	MRI findings	Comments
Bone marrow necrosis (▶ Fig. 10.268)	Multifocal zones in bone marrow of spine and pelvis with low-intermediate or decreased signal on T1WI and T2WI surrounded by rims of low signal, which can show irregular Gd-contrast enhancement. Peripheral zones with high signal on FS T2WI and STIR may also occur. These findings can overlap those of bone infarcts. Unlike avascular necrosis, collapse of the vertebral bodies is uncommon in bone marrow necrosis.	Disorder with necrosis of myeloid tissue and medullary stroma within amorphous eosinophilic material, and zones with loss of marrow fat. Occurs in association with hematologic malignancies, postchemotherapy, medications, sickle cell disease, and infection. Differs from avascular necrosis because there is preservation of spicular intramedullary bone in bone marrow necrosis. Differs from aplastic anemia in that the reticular bone marrow structure is destroyed in bone marrow necrosis. Patients present with bone pain (80%), fever (70%), and fatigue. Prognosis is usually poor and is related to the severity of the underlying causative disorder.

(continued on page 532)

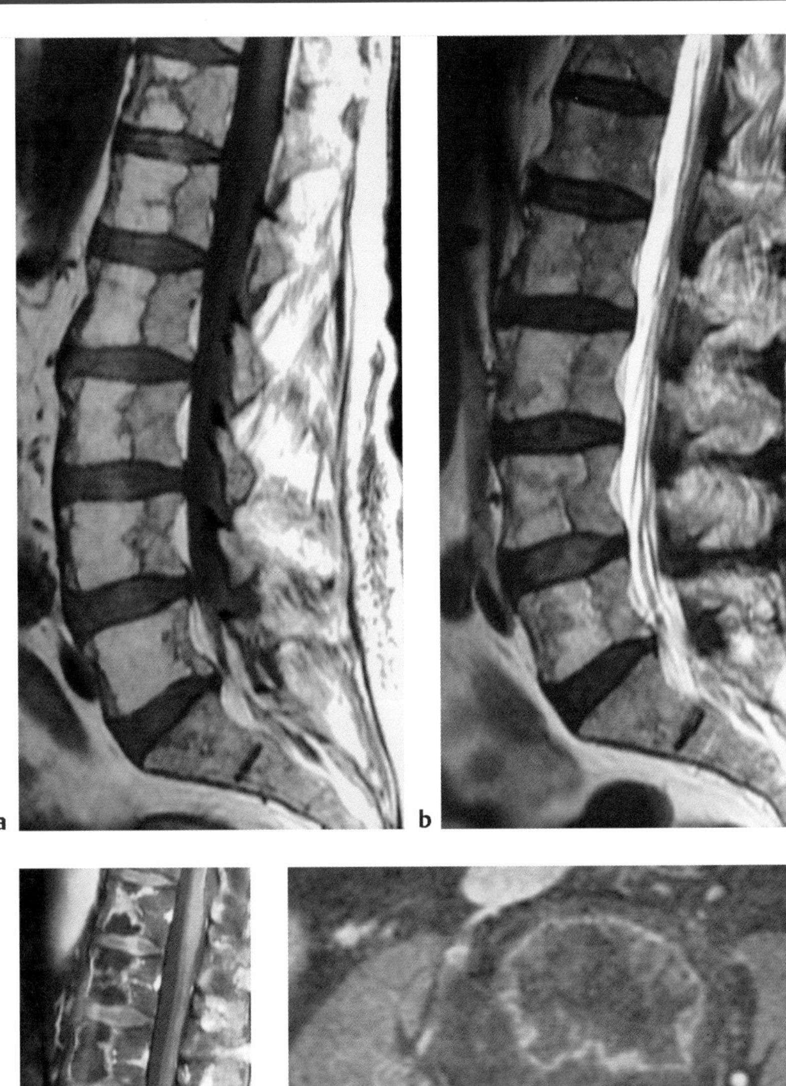

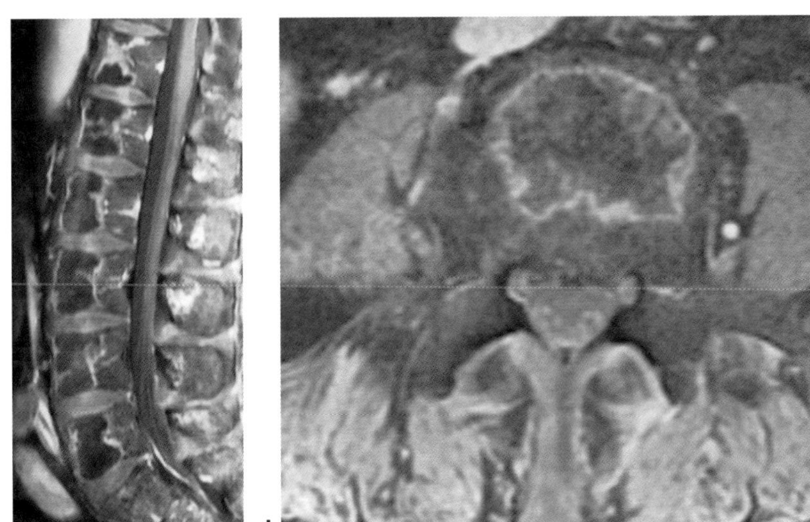

Fig. 10.268 A 68-year-old woman with bone marrow necrosis after high dose chemotherapy for lymphoma. Multiple zones in bone marrow with low-intermediate signal on T1-weighted imaging (T1WI) (a) and T2-weighted imaging (b) surrounded by peripheral rims of low signal are seen, which show irregular Gd-contrast enhancement on sagittal (c) and axial fat-suppressed T1WI (d).

Table 10.11 (Cont.) Diffuse, multiple, poorly defined, and/or multifocal zones of abnormal marrow signal

Abnormalities	MRI findings	Comments
Other multifocal, nonmalignant bone lesions		
Hemangiomas (▶ Fig. 10.269)	Circumscribed or diffuse vertebral lesion usually located in the vertebral body ± extension into the pedicle or isolated within the pedicle, typically have intermediate-high signal on T1WI, high signal on T2WI and FS T2 W, associated with thickened vertical trabeculae; usually show Gd-contrast enhancement, multiple in 30%, thoracic (60%) > lumbar (30%) > cervical (10%).	Most common benign lesions involving vertebral column, women > men, composed of endothelial-lined capillary and cavernous spaces within marrow associated with thickened vertical trabeculae and decreased secondary trabeculae; seen in 11% of autopsies. Usually asymptomatic, rarely cause bone expansion and epidural extension resulting in neural compression (usually in thoracic region), increased potential for fracture with epidural hematoma.

(continued on page 534)

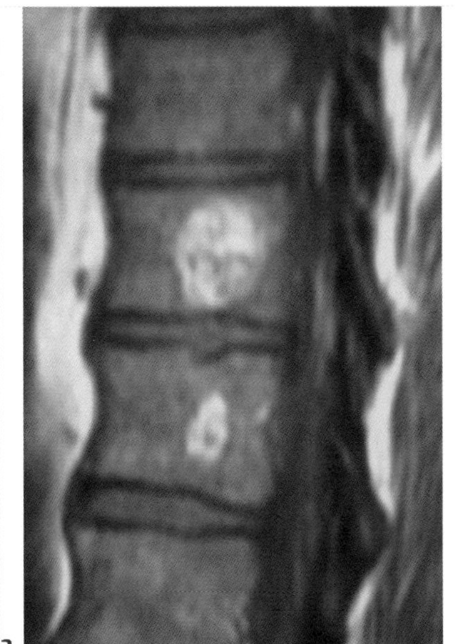

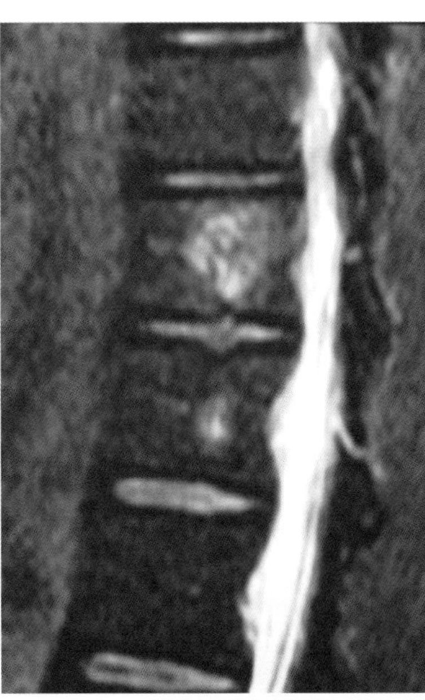

Fig. 10.269 Hemangiomas are seen as circumscribed lesions in two adjacent vertebral bodies that have high signal on sagittal T1-weighted imaging (a) and high signal on fat-suppressed T2-weighted imaging (b).

Table 10.11 (Cont.) Diffuse, multiple, poorly defined, and/or multifocal zones of abnormal marrow signal

Abnormalities	MRI findings	Comments
Cystic angiomatosis/ lymphangiomatosis (▶ Fig. 10.270)	On CT, multiple ovoid radiolucent lesions that can have a "honeycomb" or "soap-bubble"appearance. On MRI: circumscribed, poorly defined or diffuse vertebral lesions usually located in the vertebral body ± extension into pedicle or isolated within the pedicle; typically have mixed low-intermediate and/or high signal on T1WI, high signal on T2WI and FS T2W; associated with thickened vertical trabeculae; usually show Gd-contrast enhancement.	Rare disorder with multiple intraosseous or soft-tissue lesions containing endothelial-lined spaces with delicate walls not surrounded by neoplastic or reactive tissue.

(continued on page 536)

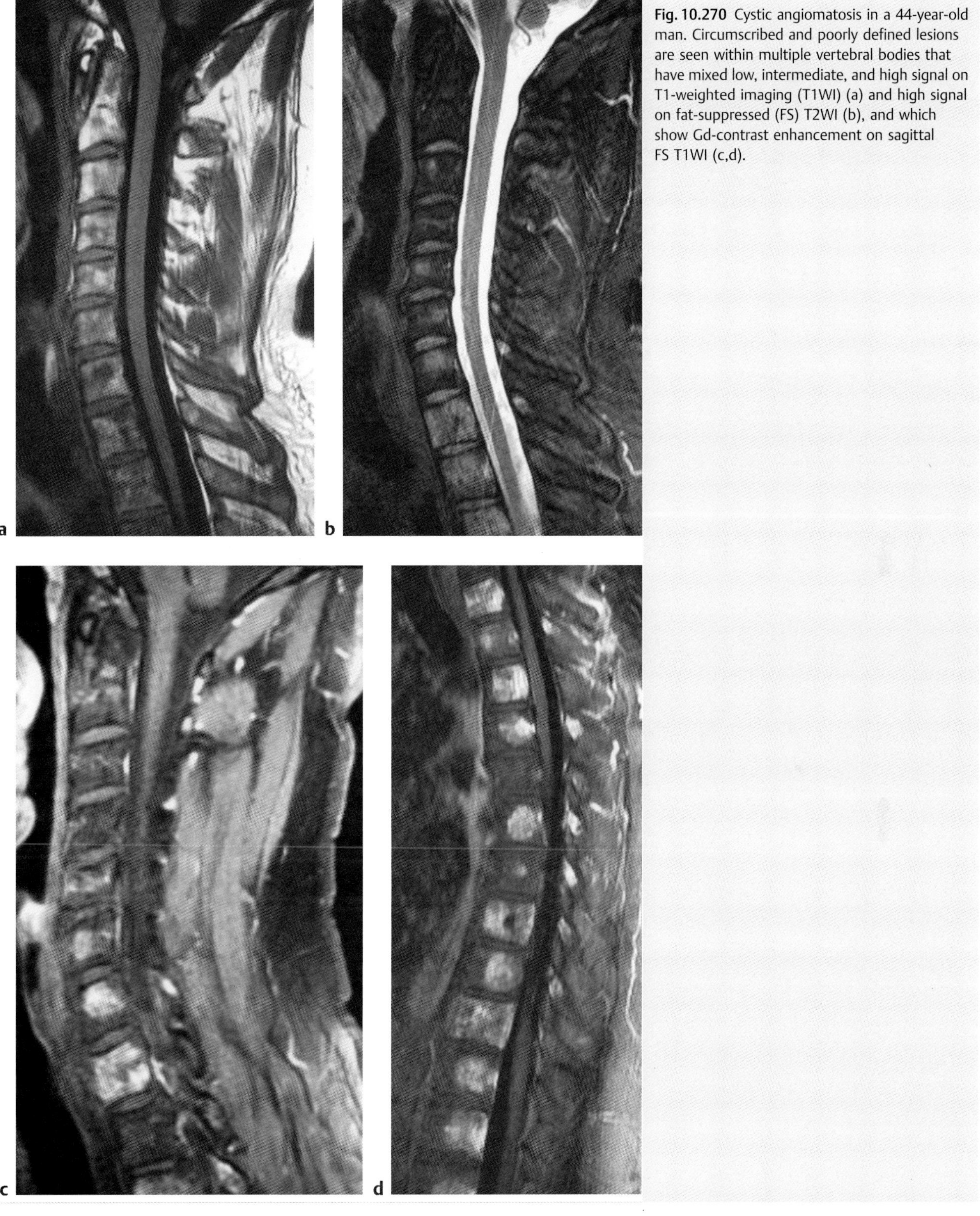

Fig. 10.270 Cystic angiomatosis in a 44-year-old man. Circumscribed and poorly defined lesions are seen within multiple vertebral bodies that have mixed low, intermediate, and high signal on T1-weighted imaging (T1WI) (a) and high signal on fat-suppressed (FS) T2WI (b), and which show Gd-contrast enhancement on sagittal FS T1WI (c,d).

Table 10.11 (Cont.) Diffuse, multiple, poorly defined, and/or multifocal zones of abnormal marrow signal

Abnormalities	MRI findings	Comments
Hemangioendothelioma (▶ Fig. 10.271)	Lesions usually have sharp margins that may be slightly lobulated and often have low-intermediate signal on T1WI, and heterogeneous intermediate-high signal on T2WI and FS T2WI with zones of low signal. Lesions can be multifocal. Extraosseous extension of tumor through zones of cortical destruction can be seen. Lesions often show prominent heterogeneous Gd-contrast enhancement.	Vasoformative/endothelial low-grade malignant neoplasms, which are locally aggressive and rarely metastasize compared with high-grade angiosarcoma.

(continued on page 538)

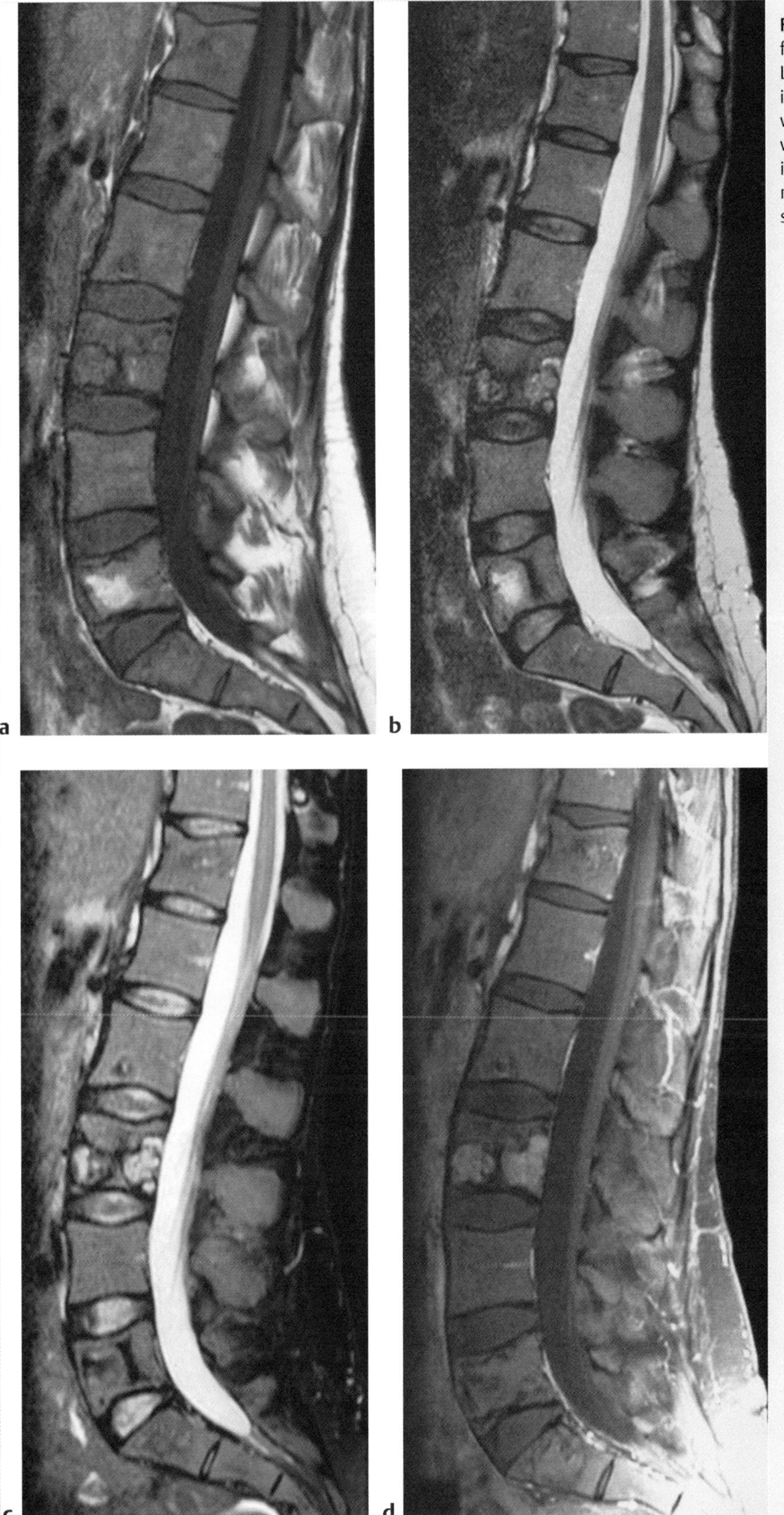

Fig. 10.271 A 42-year-old woman with multifocal hemangioendotheliomas involving the L2, L3, and L5 vertebrae. Tumors have mixed low, intermediate, and high signal on sagittal T1-weighted imaging (T1WI) (a), sagittal T2-weighted imaging (b), and sagittal short TI inversion recovery (c). Lesions show heterogeneous Gd-contrast enhancement on sagittal fat-suppressed T1WI (d).

Table 10.11 (Cont.) Diffuse, multiple, poorly defined, and/or multifocal zones of abnormal marrow signal

Abnormalities	MRI findings	Comments
Paget disease (▶ Fig. 10.272)	In the initial phases, thickening of the involved cortex is seen, which has low to intermediate signal on T1WI and PDWI and often has various combinations of low, intermediate, slightly high, and/or high signal on T2WI and FS T2WI. Irregular Gd-contrast enhancement can be seen in the thickened cortex. Marrow signal during the initial phases of Paget disease can be within normal limits or slightly increased in a V-shape on FS T2WI secondary to fibrovascular tissue replacement of normal marrow, and/or dilated blood vessels with slow flow. In the late or inactive phases of the disease, findings include osseous expansion, cortical thickening, decreased diameter of the medullary canal, and coarsened trabeculae along stress lines. Zones of cortical thickening usually have low signal on T1WI and T2WI. Thick linear intramedullary zones of low signal on T1WI and T2WI can be seen secondary to thickened bone trabeculae. Marrow in late or inactive phases of Paget disease can (1) have signal similar to normal marrow, (2) contain focal areas of fat signal, (3) have low signal on T1WI and T2WI secondary to regions of sclerosis, (4) have areas of high signal on FS T2WI from edema or persistent fibrovascular tissue, or (5) have various combinations of the aforementioned.	Paget disease is a chronic skeletal disease in which there is disordered bone resorption and woven bone formation resulting in osseous deformity. A paramyxovirus may be an etiologic agent for Paget disease. Can be polyostotic in up to 66% of patients. Paget disease is associated with a risk of less than 1% for developing secondary sarcomatous changes.

(continued on page 540)

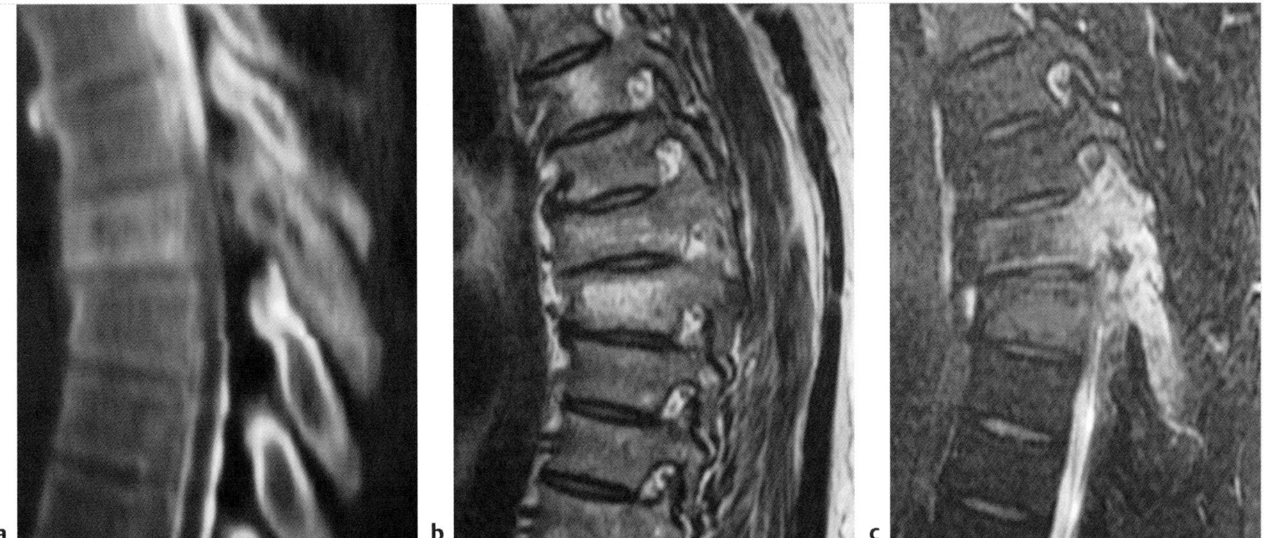

Fig. 10.272 Paget disease involving two adjacent thoracic vertebrae. Sagittal postmyelographic computed tomography (a) shows expansile osteosclerotic changes with mixed intermediate and high attenuation. The involved marrow has heterogeneous slightly high signal on sagittal T2-weighted imaging (T2WI) (b) and heterogeneous slightly high and high signal on fat-suppressed T2WI (c).

Table 10.11 (Cont.) Diffuse, multiple, poorly defined, and/or multifocal zones of abnormal marrow signal

Abnormalities	MRI findings	Comments
Multiple enchondromatosis (Ollier disease, metachondromatosis, and Maffucci syndrome) (▶ Fig. 10.273; ▶ Fig. 10.274)	Lobulated intramedullary lesions with well-defined borders ranging in size, with mean size = 5 cm. Mild endosteal scalloping can be seen. Lesions usually have low-intermediate signal on T1WI and intermediate signal on PDWI. On T2WI and fat-suppressed T2WI, lesions usually have predominantly high signal with foci and/or bands of low signal representing areas of matrix mineralization and fibrous strands. No zones of abnormal high signal on T2WI are typically seen in the marrow outside the borders of the lesions. Lesions typically show Gd-contrast enhancement in various patterns.	Ollier disease results from anomalies of endochondral bone formation with multiple enchondromas located predominantly or only in limbs on one side. Short and long tubular bones of the limbs are primarily affected. Median age = 12 years. Metachondromatosis is a rare disorder that includes the combination of enchondromatosis and osteochondromatosis. Maffucci syndrome is a very rare disease that occurs in children and adults with simultaneous occurrence of multiple enchondromas and soft-tissue cutaneous or visceral hemangiomas.
Polyostotic fibrous dysplasia (▶ Fig. 10.275)	MRI features depend on the proportions of bony spicules, collagen, fibroblastic spindle cells, hemorrhagic and/or cystic changes, and pathological fracture if present. Lesions are usually well circumscribed and have low or low-intermediate signal on T1WI and PDWI. On T2WI, lesions have variable mixtures of low, intermediate, and/or high signal often surrounded by a low signal rim of variable thickness. Internal septations and cystic changes are seen in a minority of lesions. Bone expansion is commonly seen. All or portions of the lesions can show Gd-contrast enhancement that varies from mild to marked in degree.	Benign medullary fibro-osseous lesion of bone, which can occur as solitary lesion (mono-ostotic type, 80 to 85%); or as multiple lesions (polyostotic fibrous dysplasia type). Results from developmental failure in the normal process of remodeling primitive bone to mature lamellar bone with resultant zone or zones of immature trabeculae within dysplastic fibrous tissue. Lesions do not mineralize normally, with predisposition to pathological fracture.

(continued on page 542)

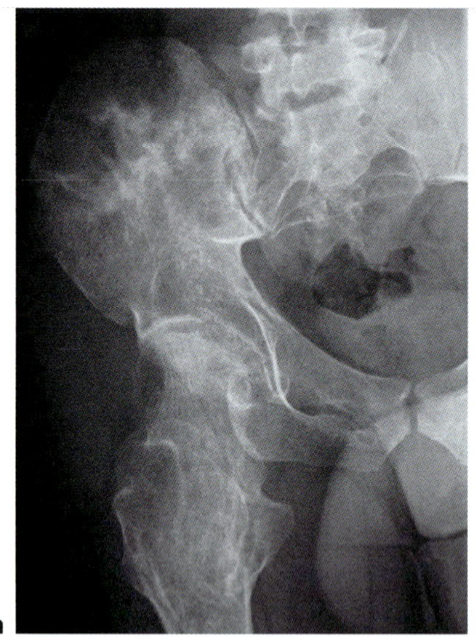

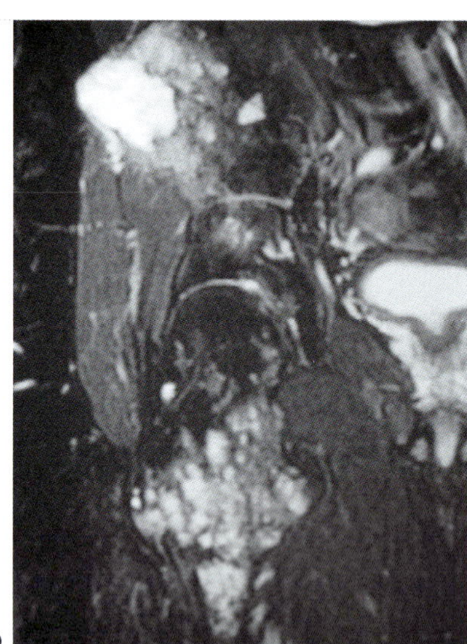

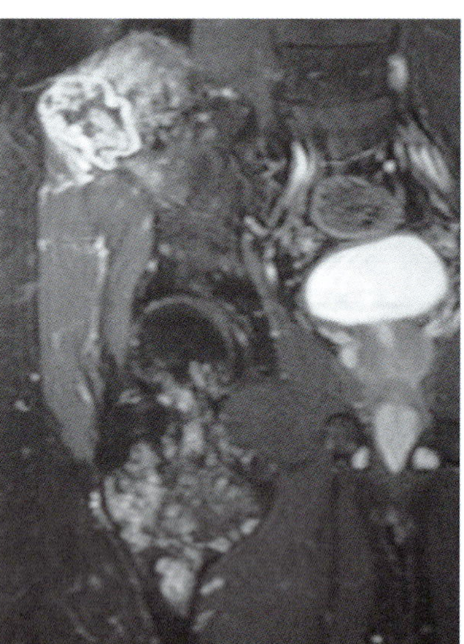

Fig. 10.273 A 29-year-old man with Ollier disease. Anteroposterior radiograph (a) shows multiple enchondromas involving the iliac bone, ischium, pubic bone, and femur. The lesions have high signal on coronal fat-suppressed (FS) T2-weighted imaging (b). The lesions show nodular and lobulated peripheral gadolinium-contrast enhancement on coronal FS T1-weighted imaging (c).

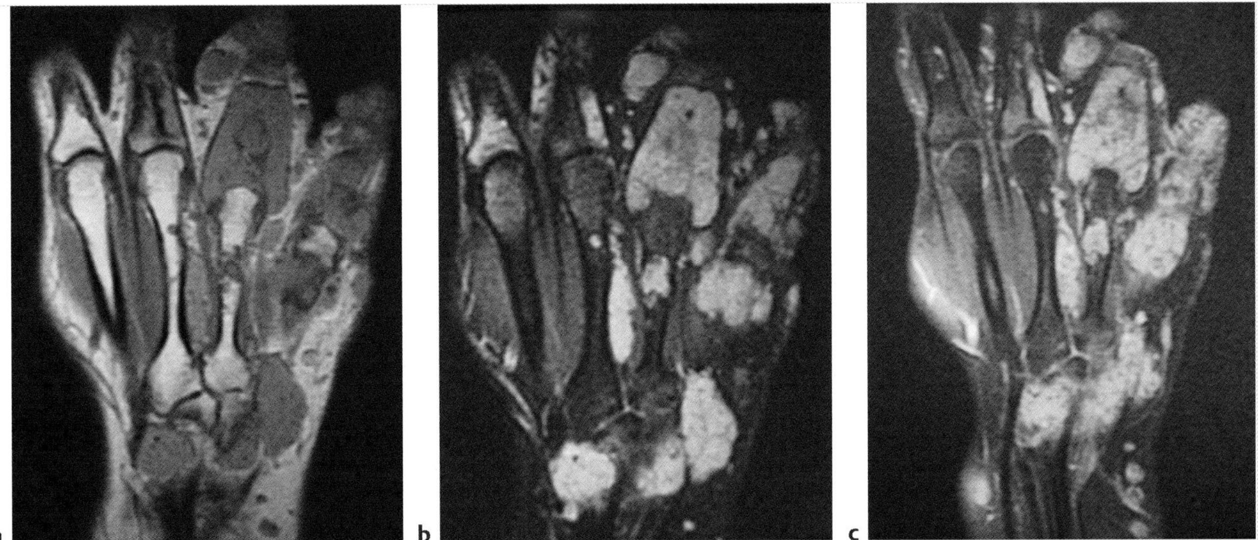

Fig. 10.274 A 20-year-old woman with Maffucci syndrome who has multiple intraosseous enchondromas and soft-tissue hemangiomas involving the wrist and hand. The intra- and extraosseous lesions have mostly intermediate signal on coronal proton density–weighted imaging (a) and high signal on coronal fat-suppressed (FS) T2-weighted imaging (b). Some of the intraosseous lesions are associated with cortical expansion. The lesions show prominent Gd-contrast enhancement on coronal FS T1-weighted imaging (c).

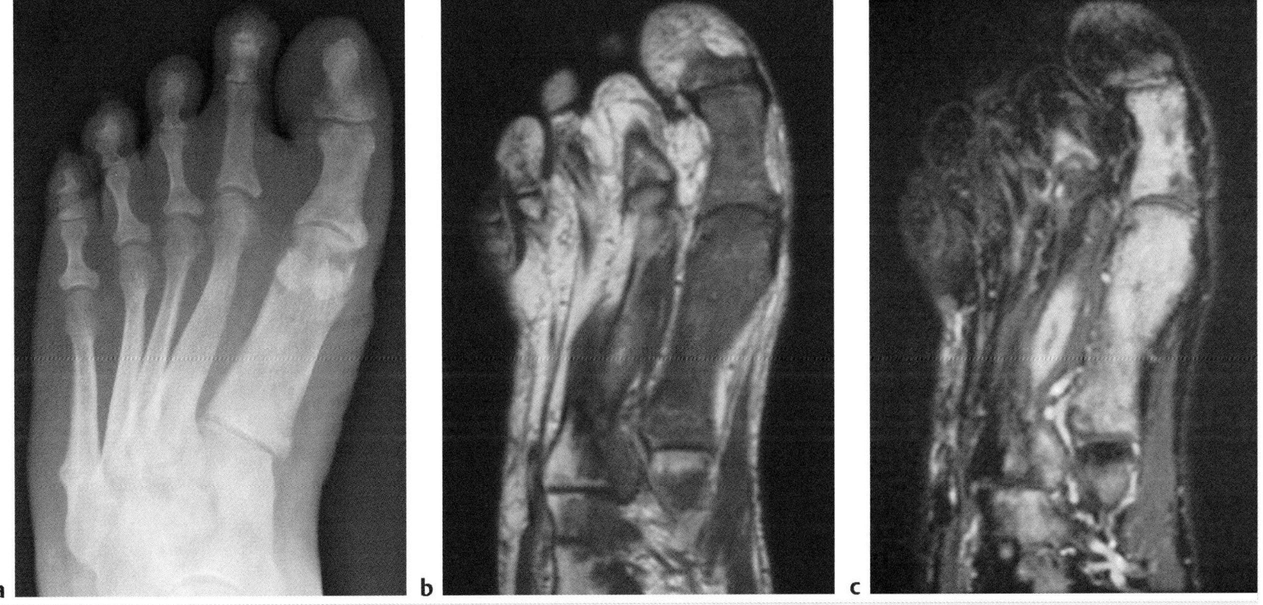

Fig. 10.275 A 45-year-old woman with polyostotic fibrous dysplasia. Radiograph (a) shows multiple lesions involving the metatarsal bones and phalanges, which have an expansile ground-glass appearance. The lesions have low-intermediate signal on T1-weighted imaging (b) and high signal on fat-suppressed T2-weighted imaging (c).

Table 10.11 (Cont.) Diffuse, multiple, poorly defined, and/or multifocal zones of abnormal marrow signal

Abnormalities	MRI findings	Comments
Osteopoikilosis (▶ Fig. 10.276)	Multiple foci with low signal comparable to cortical bone are seen on all pulse sequences within marrow.	Osteopoikilosis (osteopathia condensans disseminate or spotted bone disease) is a sclerosing bone dsyplasia in which numerous small round or oval radiodense foci are seen in medullary bone, giving the appearance of multiple bone islands.
Malignant abnormalities		
Metastatic disease (▶ Fig. 10.277; ▶ Fig. 10.278)	Metastatic tumor within bone often appears as intramedullary zones with low-intermediate signal on T1WI; low-intermediate to slightly high signal on PDWI; slightly-high to high signal on T2WI and FS T2WI. Sclerotic lesions often have low signal on T1WI and mixed low, intermediate and/or high signal on T2WI. Metastatic spinal lesions may be focal or involve most of a vertebra. In tubular bones, metastatic lesions are usually intramedullary with frequent cortical destruction and tumor extension into the extraosseous soft tissues. Metastatic skeletal lesions usually show varying degrees of Gd-contrast enhancement.	Metastatic lesions represent proliferating neoplastic cells that are located in sites or organs separated or distant from their origins. Metastatic lesions can disseminate hematogenously via arteries or veins, along cerebrospinal fluid (CSF) pathways, along surgical tracts, and along lymphatic structures. Metastatic carcinoma is the most frequent malignant tumor involving bone. In adults, metastatic lesions to bone occur most frequently from carcinomas of the lung, breast, prostate, kidney, and thyroid, as well as from sarcomas. Primary malignancies of the lung, breast, and prostate account for 80% of bone metastases.

(continued on page 544)

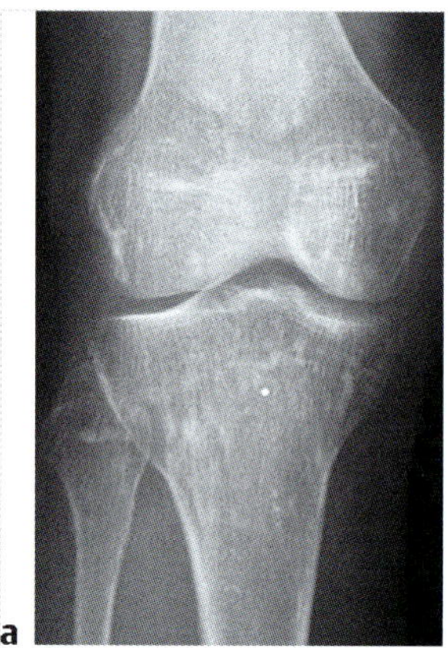
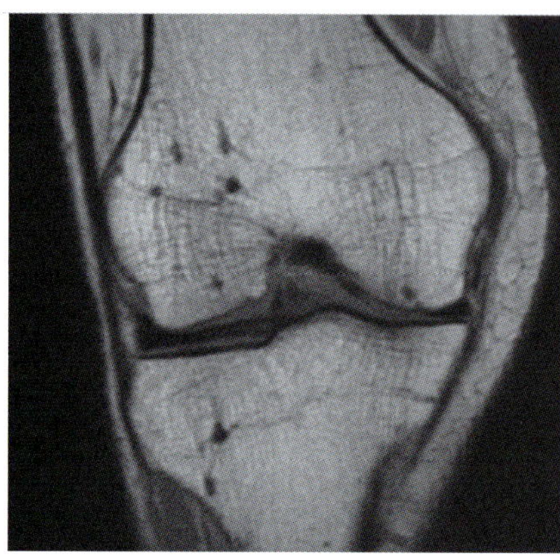
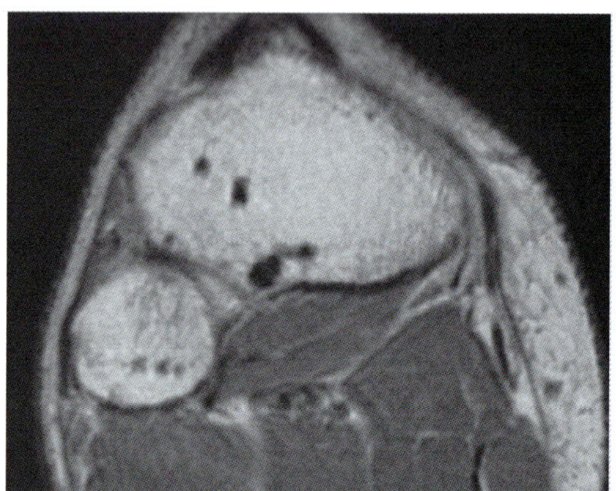

Fig. 10.276 A 41-year-old woman with osteopoikilosis seen as multiple foci with high attenuation in the marrow of the distal femur, proximal tibia, and fibula on anteroposterior radiograph (a), which have corresponding low signal on coronal (b) and axial T1-weighted imaging (c).

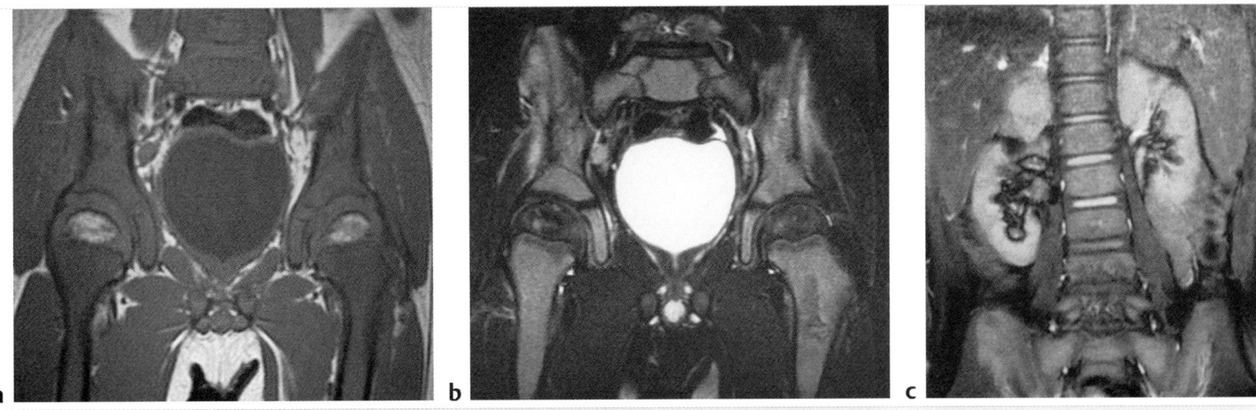

Fig. 10.277 A 2-year-old boy with extensive metastatic neuroblastoma involving the marrow of the spine, pelvis, and femurs seen as diffuse low-intermediate signal on coronal T1-weighted imaging (T1WI) (a), abnormal high signal on coronal fat-suppressed (FS) T2-weighted imaging (b), and Gd-contrast enhancement on FS T1WI (c).

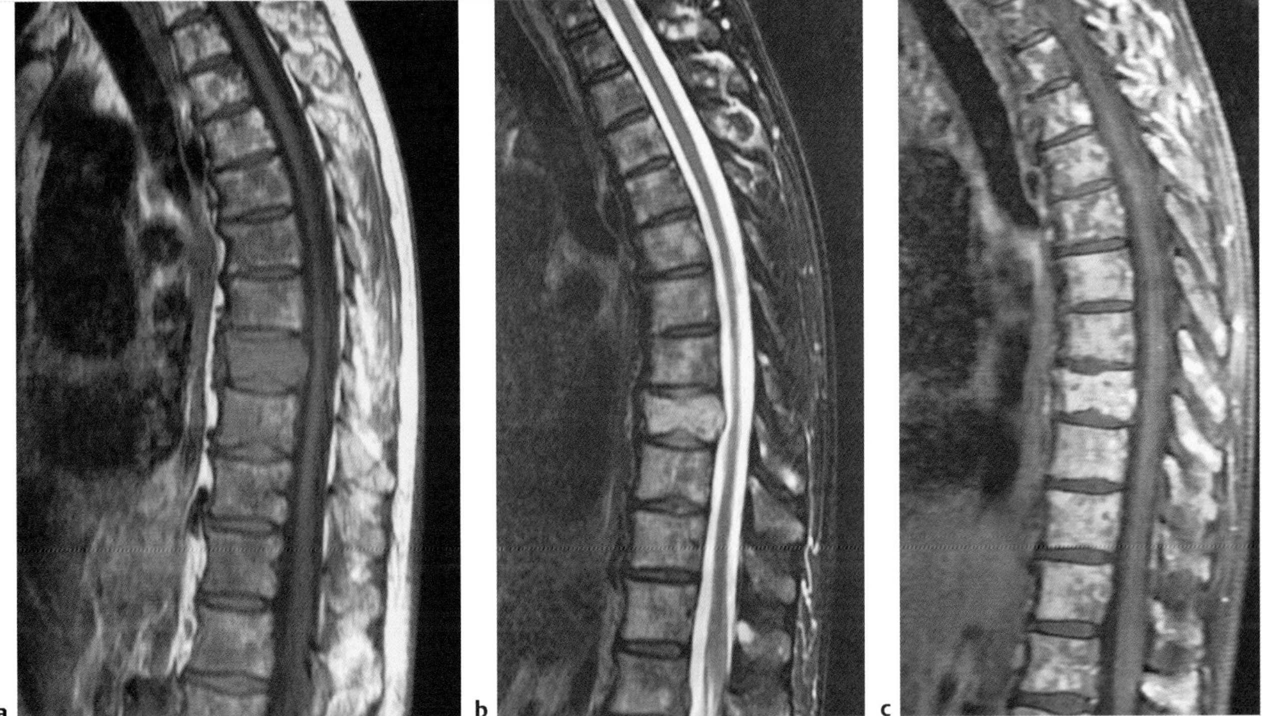

Fig. 10.278 A 63-year-old woman with extensive metastatic breast carcinoma involving the marrow of the spine seen as multiple poorly defined zones with low-intermediate signal on sagittal T1-weighted imaging (T1WI) (a), slightly high signal on sagittal fat-suppressed (FS) T2-weighted imaging (b), and gadolinium-contrast enhancement on FS T1WI (c).

Table 10.11 (Cont.) Diffuse, multiple, poorly defined, and/or multifocal zones of abnormal marrow signal

Abnormalities	MRI findings	Comments
Multiple myeloma (▶ Fig. 10.279)	Multiple myeloma typically appears as multiple intramedullary zones with low-intermediate signal on T1WI and PDWI; intermediate, slightly-high to high signal on T2WI; and slightly-high to high signal on FS T2WI. FS T2WI is important for detecting myeloma because intermediate and high signal heterogeneity on T1WI from red and yellow marrow, respectively, can be seen in normal vertebral marrow in elderly patients. Intramedullary lesions and corresponding signal abnormalities may be diffuse, focal with poorly defined or distinct margins, and/or in an extensive variegated pattern. Multifocal lesions can be seen in long bones. Zones of cortical destruction may occur associated with extraosseous soft tissue lesions. Lesions usually show Gd-contrast enhancement.	Multiple myelomas are malignant tumors composed of proliferating antibody-secreting plasma cells derived from single clones. Multiple myeloma is primarily located in bone marrow. A solitary myeloma or plasmacytoma is an infrequent variant in which a neoplastic mass of plasma cells occurs at a single site of bone or soft tissues.
Non-Hodgkin lymphoma (▶ Fig. 10.280)	Non-Hodgkin lymphoma (NHL) within bone typically appears as intramedullary zones with low-intermediate signal on T1WI and PDWI, slightly high to high signal on T2WI, and high signal on FS T2WI. Zones of low signal on T1WI and T2WI may be secondary to fibrosis. Zones of cortical destruction may occur associated with extraosseous soft tissue lesions. NHL typically shows Gd-contrast enhancement. Destruction of cortical and medullary bone may also occur as a result of invasion from adjacent extraosseous NHL.	Lymphoma represents a group of lymphoid tumors whose neoplastic cells typically arise within lymphoid tissue (lymph nodes and reticuloendothelial organs). Unlike leukemia, lymphoma usually arises as discrete masses. Almost all primary lymphomas of bone are B-cell NHL. Frequently originates at extranodal sites and spreads in an unpredictable pattern.

(continued on page 546)

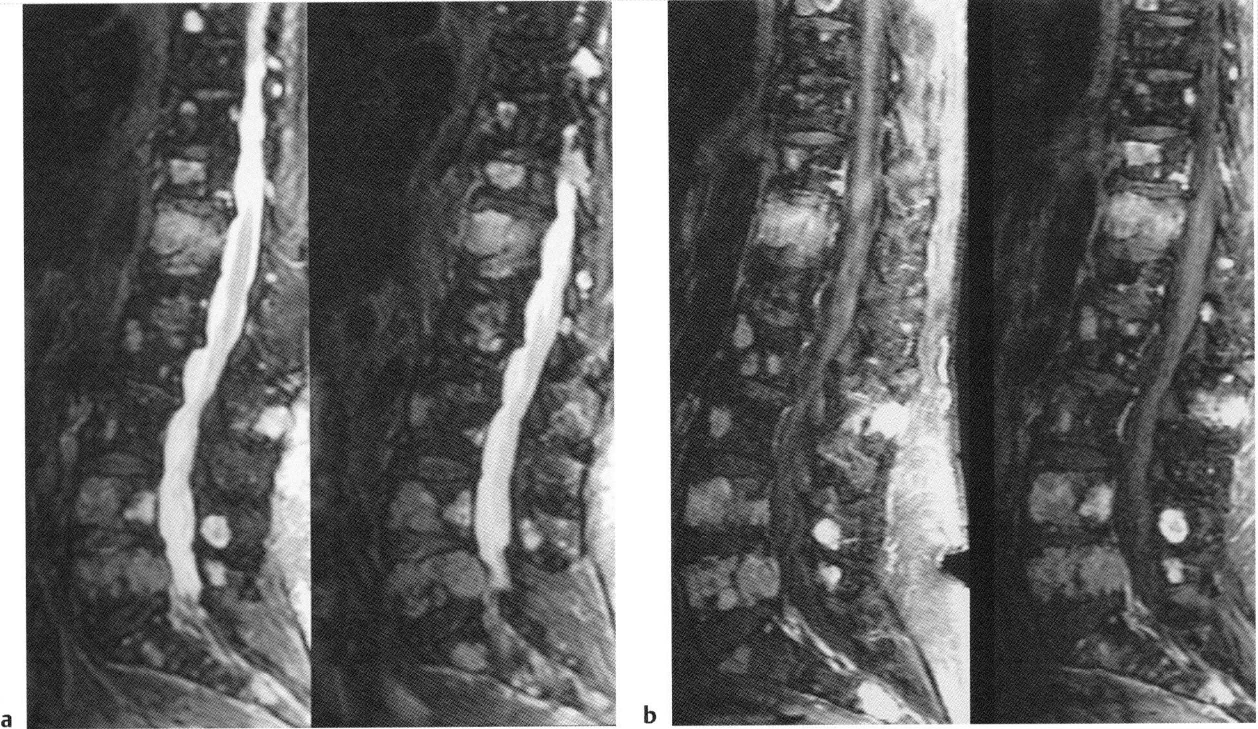

Fig. 10.279 Multiple myelomas seen as numerous lesions in the vertebral marrow with high signal on sagittal fat-suppressed (FS) T2-weighted imaging (a) and gadolinium-contrast enhancement on FS T1-weighted imaging (b).

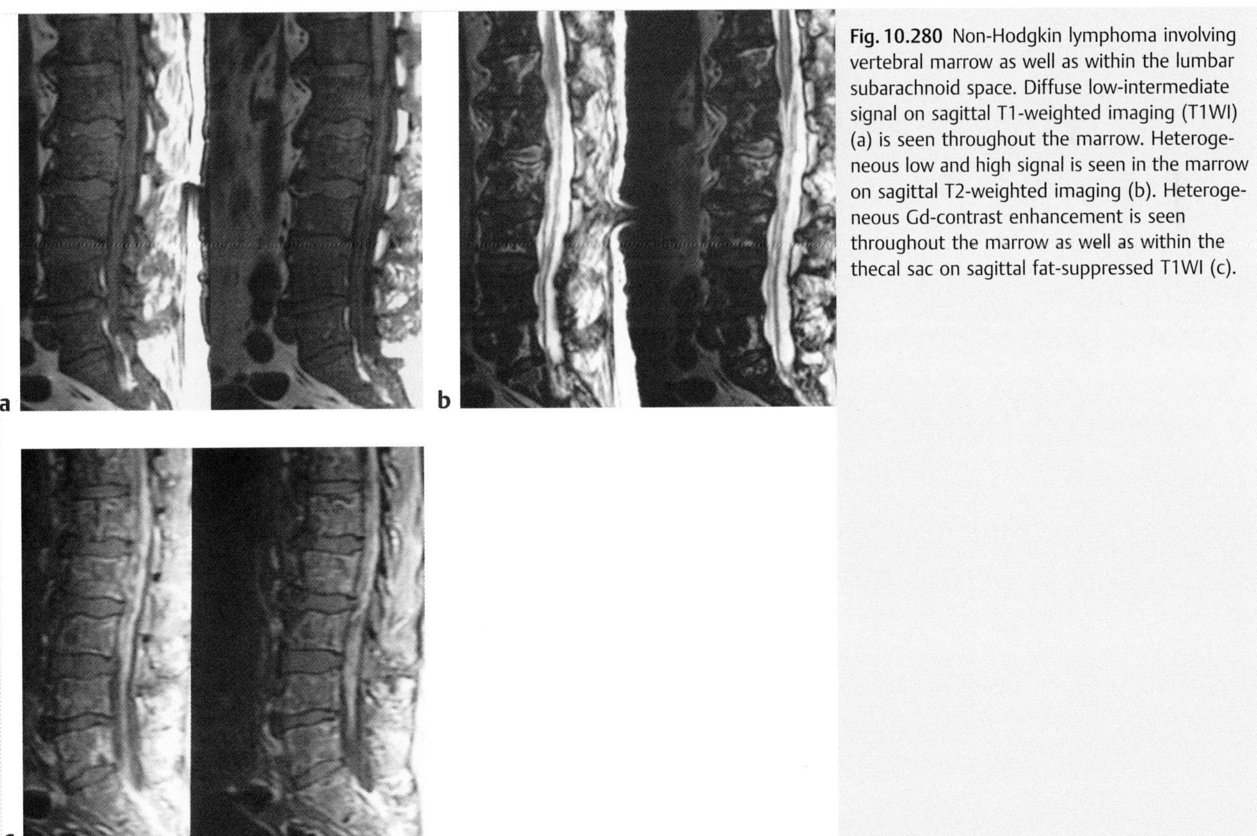

Fig. 10.280 Non-Hodgkin lymphoma involving vertebral marrow as well as within the lumbar subarachnoid space. Diffuse low-intermediate signal on sagittal T1-weighted imaging (T1WI) (a) is seen throughout the marrow. Heterogeneous low and high signal is seen in the marrow on sagittal T2-weighted imaging (b). Heterogeneous Gd-contrast enhancement is seen throughout the marrow as well as within the thecal sac on sagittal fat-suppressed T1WI (c).

Table 10.11 (Cont.) Diffuse, multiple, poorly defined, and/or multifocal zones of abnormal marrow signal

Abnormalities	MRI findings	Comments
Hodgkin lymphoma (▶ Fig. 10.281)	Hodgkin disease (HD) within bone typically appears as intramedullary zones with low-intermediate signal on T1WI; intermediate, slightly high, and/or high signal on T2WI; and high signal on FS T2WI. Intramedullary lesions may have poorly defined or distinct margins. Multifocal lesions can be seen in long bones and vertebrae. Zones of cortical destruction may occur associated with extraosseous soft tissue lesions. Most lesions show Gd-contrast enhancement. HD involving bone with associated sclerosis seen on plain films or CT usually have low signal on T1WI and variable/mixed signal on T2WI. Destruction of cortical and medullary bone may also occur as a result of invasion from adjacent extraosseous lymphadenopathy from HD.	Lymphoma represents a group of lymphoid tumors whose neoplastic cells typically arise within lymphoid tissue (lymph nodes and reticuloendothelial organs). Unlike leukemia, lymphoma usually arises as discrete masses. HD typically arises in lymph nodes and often spreads along nodal chains.

(continued on page 548)

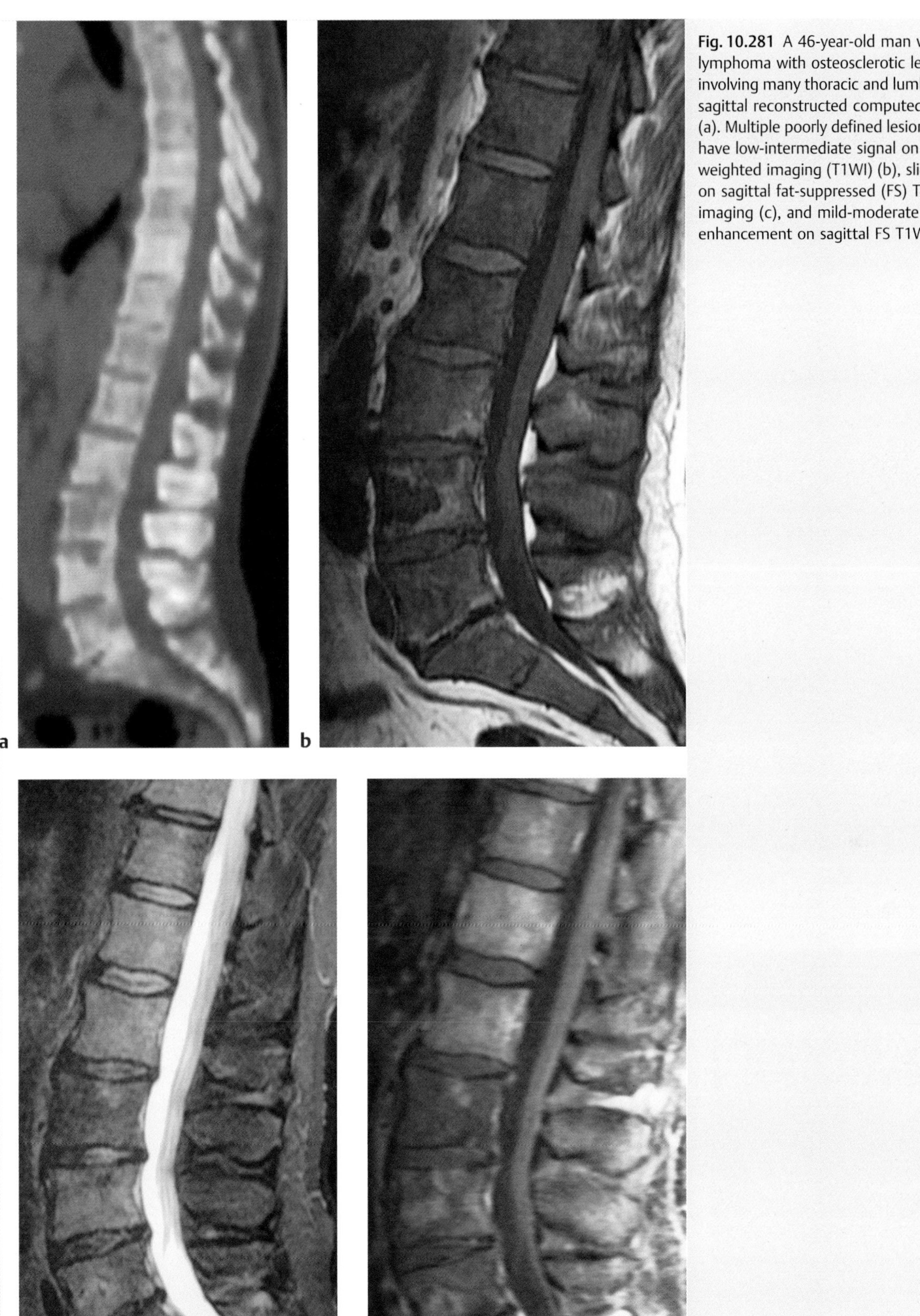

Fig. 10.281 A 46-year-old man with Hodgkin lymphoma with osteosclerotic lesions seen involving many thoracic and lumbar vertebrae on sagittal reconstructed computed tomography (a). Multiple poorly defined lesions in the marrow have low-intermediate signal on sagittal T1-weighted imaging (T1WI) (b), slightly high signal on sagittal fat-suppressed (FS) T2-weighted imaging (c), and mild-moderate Gd-contrast enhancement on sagittal FS T1WI (d).

Table 10.11 (Cont.) Diffuse, multiple, poorly defined, and/or multifocal zones of abnormal marrow signal

Abnormalities	MRI findings	Comments
Leukemia (▶ Fig. 10.282; ▶ Fig. 10.283)	Acute lymphoblastic anemia (ALL), chronic lymphycytic leukemia (CLL), acute myelogenous leukemia (AML), and chronic myelogenous leukemia (CML) infiltration in marrow can appear as diffuse or poorly defined zones of low-intermediate signal on T1WI and PDWI and intermediate-slightly high to high signal on FS T2WI. Focal or geographic regions with similar signal alteration can also be seen. After Gd-contrast administration, ALL, CLL, AML, and CML may show Gd-contrast enhancement on T1WI and FS T1WI. Note should be made that Gd-contrast enhancement may be seen in normal vertebral marrow in children less than 7 years.	Lymphoid neoplasms, which have widespread involvement of the bone marrow as well as tumor cells in peripheral blood. ALL is the most frequent type in children and adolescents. In adults, CLL is the most common type. Myelogenous leukemias represent neoplasms derived from abnormal myeloid progenitor cells that, if normal, would form erythrocytes, monocytes, granulocytes, and platelets. AML usually occurs in adolescents and young adults, and accounts for approximately 20% of childhood leukemia. CML occurs in adults older than 25 years.
Myelodysplastic syndromes (▶ Fig. 10.284)	Marrow signal on FS T2WI and STIR can be isointense or hyperintense to muscle depending on the degree of cellular hyperplasia in the marrow and stage of disease. Can progress to myelofibrosis and myelosclerosis.	Myelodysplastic syndromes (MDSs) are clonal hematopoietic stem cell diseases associated with dysplasias of myeloid cell lines resulting in decreased functional hematopoiesis. Myeloblasts can occur up to 20% in MDS. Progressive marrow failure occurs in MDS as well as eventual progression to acute myeloid leukemia. Usually occurs in older adults over the age of 60 years, incidence up to 30 per million. MDS includes chronic myelomonocytic leukemia, atypical chronic myeloid leukemia, juvenile myelomonocytic leukemia, and myelodysplastic/myeloproliferative disease, unclassifiable.

(continued on page 550)

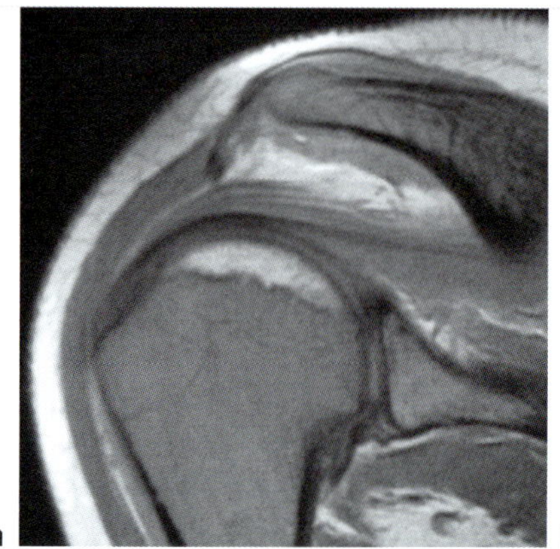
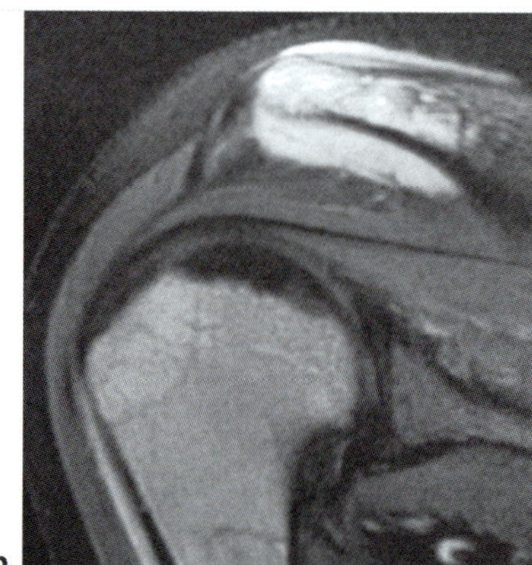
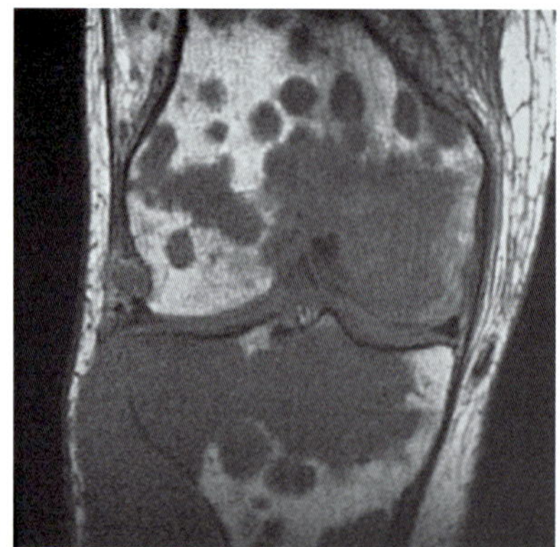
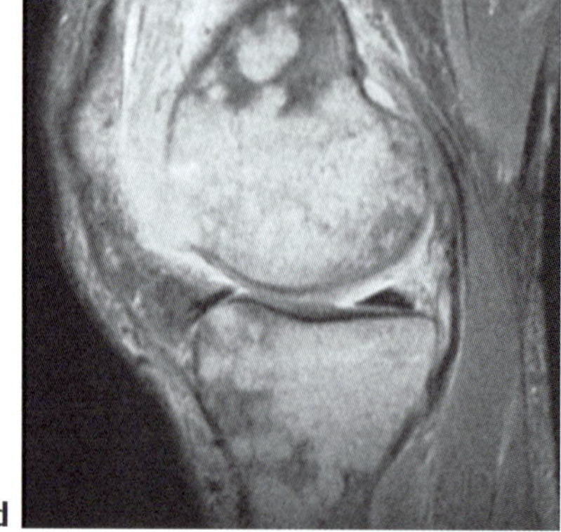

Fig. 10.282 Acute lymphoblastic leukemia in an 18-year-old woman (a,b) and a 58-year-old man (c,d). Leukemic infiltration of marrow has low-intermediate signal on coronal T1-weighted imaging (a,c) and high signal on coronal fat-suppressed T2-weighted imaging (b,d). Intramedullary tumor is seen extending through bone cortex of the clavicle and femur into the extraosseous soft tissues.

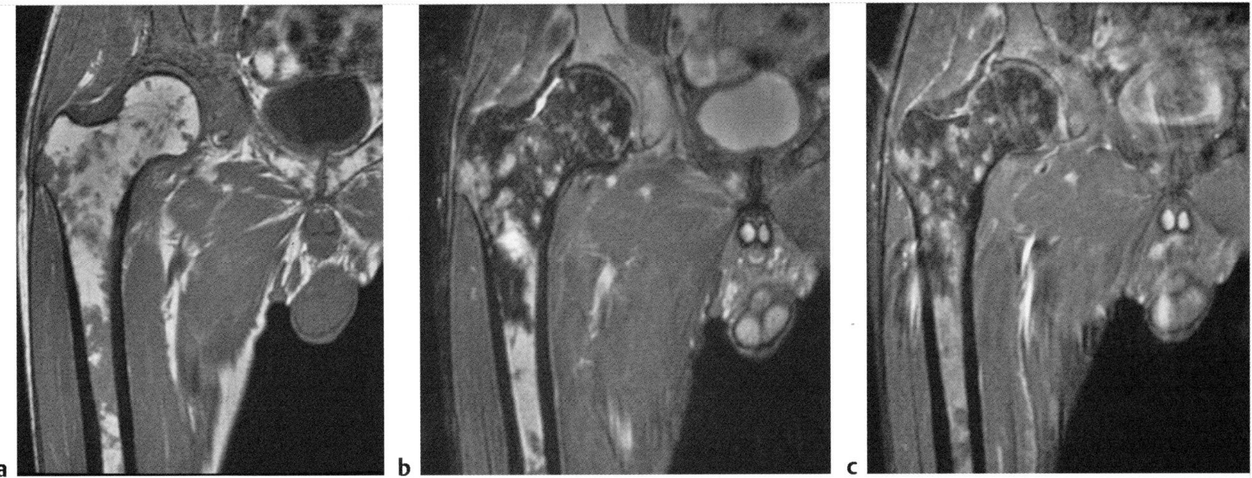

Fig. 10.283 Chronic lymphocytic leukemia involving the marrow of a 61-year-old man. Leukemic deposits are seen as irregular zones with low-intermediate signal on coronal T1-weighted imaging (T1WI) (a) and slightly high or high signal on coronal fat-suppressed (FS) T2-weighted imaging (b). Lesions show Gd-contrast enhancement on coronal FS T1WI (c).

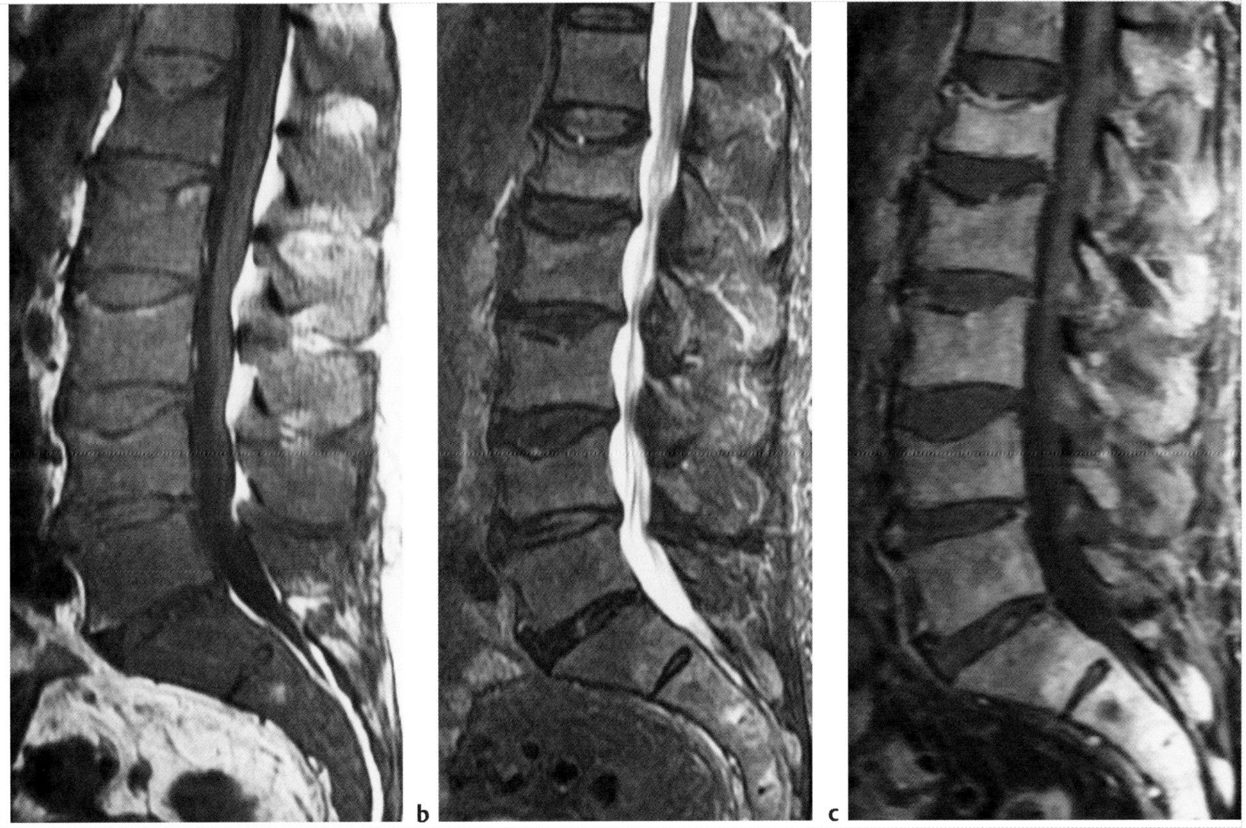

Fig. 10.284 A 74-year-old man with chronic myelodysplastic syndrome with diffuse low-intermediate signal in the vertebral marrow on sagittal T1-weighted imaging (T1WI) (a), intermediate to slightly increased signal on fat-suppressed (FS) T2-weighted imaging (b), with mild diffuse Gd-contrast enhancement on FS T1WI (c).

Table 10.11 (Cont.) Diffuse, multiple, poorly defined, and/or multifocal zones of abnormal marrow signal

Abnormalities	MRI findings	Comments
Chronic myeloproliferative disease (CPMD) (▶ Fig. 10.285)	Involved bone marrow often has low or low-intermediate signal on T1WI and slightly high signal on T2WI and FS T2WI. CPMDs typically have an insidious onset but can progress to myelofibrosis, myelosclerosis, and acute leukemia.	CMPDs represent bone marrow disorders in which there is proliferation of one or more hematopoietic stem cells (granulocytic, erythrocytic, and/or megakaryocytic). Unlike myelodysplastic syndromes, there is relatively normal maturation of the blood cells and platelets along with increased numbers of the cells from the derivatives from the abnormal clonal proliferations in CMPD. Incidence of CMPD is 90 per million, usually involves adults older than 40 years. Percent of marrow blasts is less than 10%. CPMD includes polycythemia rubra vera (PRV), chronic idiopathic myelofibrosis, essential thrombocytopenia, chronic eosinophilic leukemia, chronic neutrophilic leukemia, and chronic early phases of myelogenous leukemia (Philadelphia chromosome t(9;22)(q34;q11), BCR/ABL positive). PCV occurs in up to 13 per million per year and results from proliferation of a clonal hematopoietic stem cell lacking the normal regulatory mechanism for erythropoiesis. Other myeloid clonal proliferations can occur concurrently. PCV occurs in two phases. The initial phase is followed by a postpolycythemic phase that is associated with anemia and cytopenia, myelofibrosis, and potential development of acute leukemia.
Waldenström macroglobulinemia (lymphoplasmacytic lymphoma) (▶ Fig. 10.286)	Marrow may have no associated abnormal signal or have irregular and/or diffuse findings similar to red marrow reconversion. Signal changes in the marrow may become more prominent as well as Gd-contrast enhancement with increasing lymphoplasmacytoid infiltration of bone marrow.	Waldenström macroglobulinemia, also referred to as lymphoplasmacytic lymphoma, is a rare neoplasm of plasmacytoid lymphocytes, plasma cells, and small B lymphocytes, which usually involves bone marrow, spleen, and lymph nodes. Typically associated with a serum monoclonal immunoglobulin M (IgM) protein in concentrations > 3 gm/dL, often with hyperviscosity and cryoglobulinemia. Occurs in older adults, mean age = 63 years. Median survival is approximately 5 years.
Mastocytosis (▶ Fig. 10.287)	Radiographs and CT can show indistinctly marginated sclerotic lesions, radiolucent zones, or mixed sclerotic and radiolucent lesions in medullary bone. Sclerotic lesions usually have low signal on T1WI and T2WI, whereas radiolucent lesions may have intermediate, slightly high to high signal on T2WI and FS T2WI. Marrow signal abnormalities also include varying degrees of nonfatty homogeneous or heterogeneous zones of low signal on T1WI and intermediate, slightly high, and/or high signal on FS T2WI or STIR. In some cases, marrow signal may be normal or have intermediate signal on T1WI and FS T2WI or STIR.	Heterogeneous uncommon disorders with pathological accumulation of mast cells in various tissues (age ranges from first to seventh decades, mean in fourth decade) and can be classified into four clinical categories. Category 1 is the most common and includes 1A, which involves the skin (cutaneous mastocytosis or urticaria pigmentosa), and 1B or systemic mastocytosis with mast cells occurring in various tissues (bone marrow, spleen, gastroinesinal tract, and lymph nodes). Category 1 usually has a favorable prognosis. Category 2 includes mastocytosis associated with a myeloproliferative or myelodysplastic disorder. Prognosis depends on the associated degree of myelodysplasia. Category 3 (lymphadenopathic mastocytosis with eosinophilia or aggressive mastocytosis) is associated with a poor prognosis related to large mast cell burdens. Category 4 results from mast cell leukemia and has a very poor prognosis.

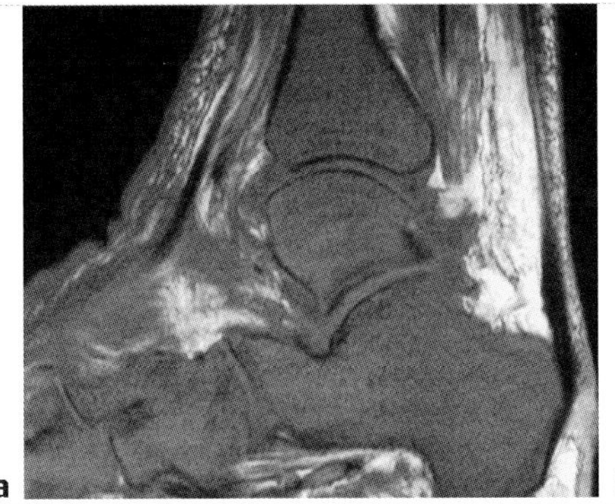
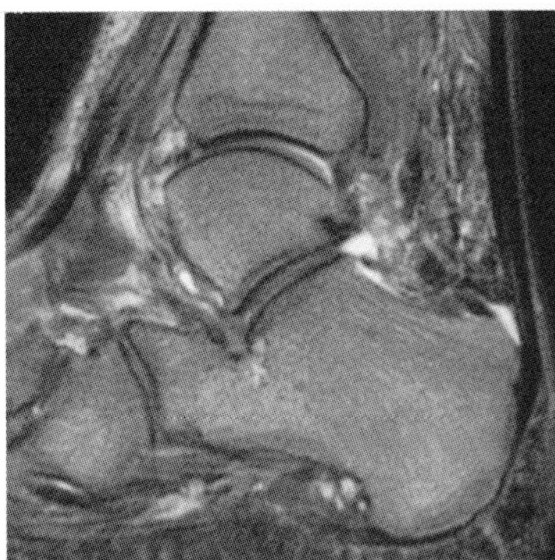

Fig. 10.285 A 49-year-old man with polycythemia rubra vera with diffuse low-intermediate signal in the marrow on sagittal T1-weighted imaging (a) and slightly high signal on sagittal T2-weighted imaging (b) that is slightly hyperintense relative to muscle.

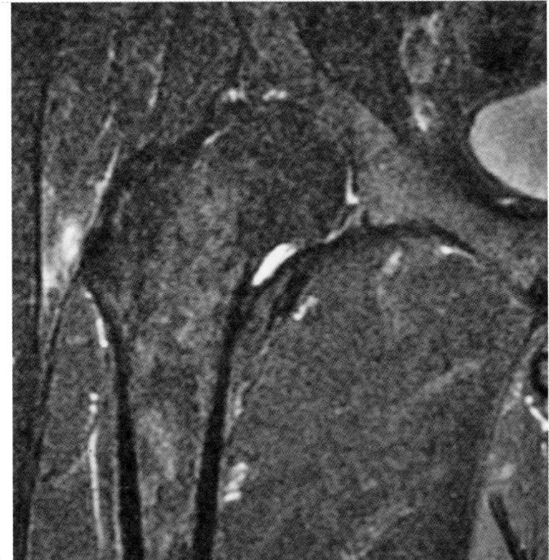
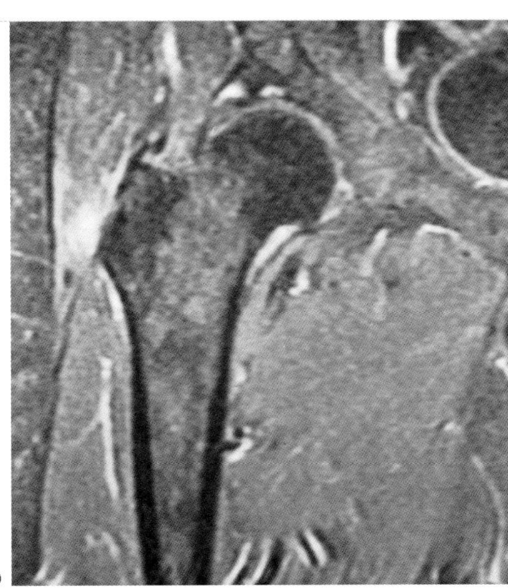
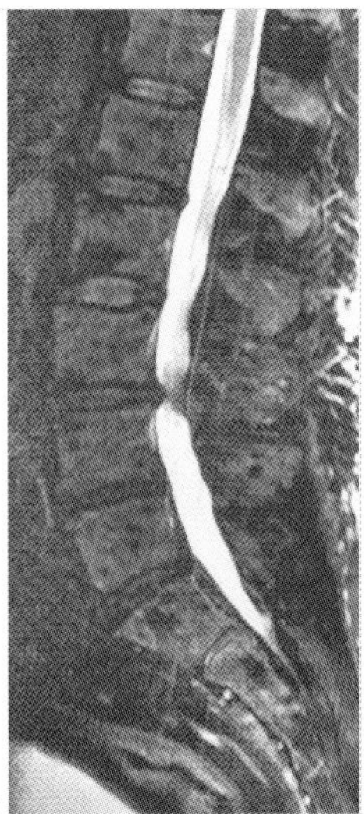

Fig. 10.286 A 61-year-old man with Waldenström macroglobulinemia with irregular zones of intermediate signal in the metadiaphyseal marrow on coronal fat-suppressed T2-weighted imaging (FS T2WI) (a) and mild Gd-contrast enhancement on coronal FS T1-weighted imaging (b). A variegated pattern with slightly high signal on FS T2WI (c) is seen in the vertebral marrow in a 71-year-old patient.

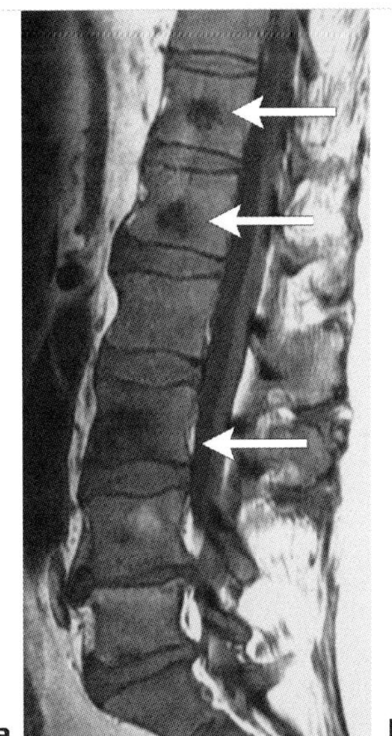
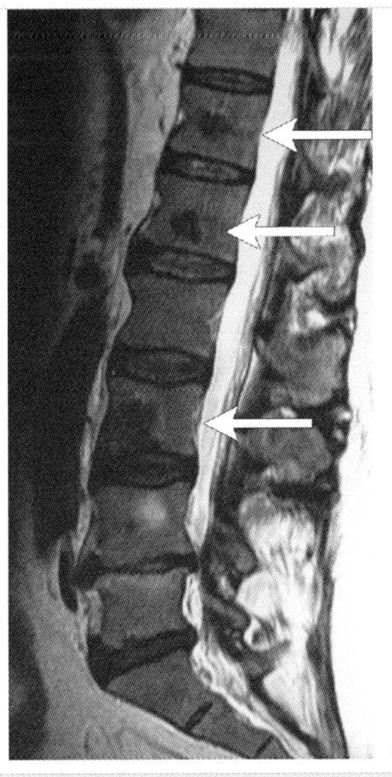
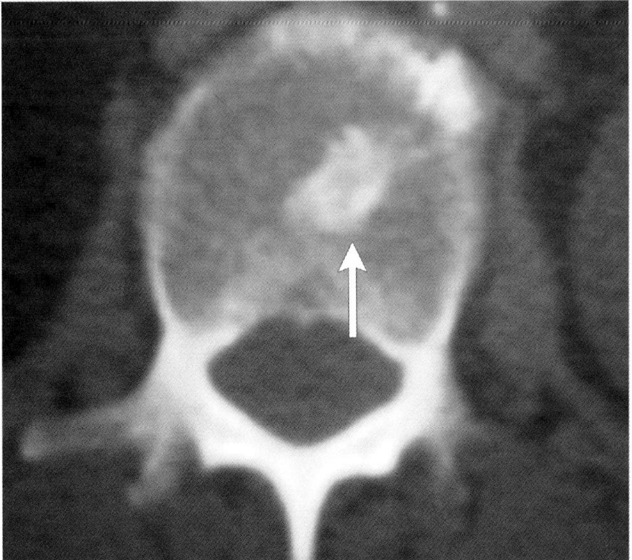

Fig. 10.287 A 68-year-old man with mastocytosis seen as multifocal zones with low signal (arrows) on sagittal T1-weighted imaging (a) and T2-weighted imaging (b), which are osteosclerotic (arrow) on axial computed tomography (c).

10.12 Suggested Reading: Lesions Involving Bones

▶ Adamantinoma

[1] Hogendoorn PCW, Hashimoto H. Adamantinoma. In: Fletcher CDM, Unni KK, Mertens F, eds. World Health Organization Classification of Tumours. Pathology and Genetics of Tumours of Soft Tissue and Bone. Lyon, France: IARC Press; 2002:333–334

[2] Judmaier W, Peer S, Krejzi T, Dessl A, Kühberger R. MR findings in tibial adamantinoma. A case report. Acta Radiol 1998; 39: 276–278

[3] Khanna M, Delaney D, Tirabosco R, Saifuddin A. Osteofibrous dysplasia, osteofibrous dysplasia-like adamantinoma and adamantinoma: correlation of radiological imaging features with surgical histology and assessment of the use of radiology in contributing to needle biopsy diagnosis. Skeletal Radiol 2008; 37: 1077–1084

[4] Kumar D, Mulligan ME, Levine AM, Dorfman HD. Classic adamantinoma in a 3-year-old. Skeletal Radiol 1998; 27: 406–409

[5] Meyers SP. Adamantinoma. In: MRI of Bone and Soft Tissue Tumors and Tumorlike Lesions. Stuttgart, Germany: Thieme; 2008:325–327

[6] Van der Woude HJ, Hazelbag HM, Bloem JL, Taminiau AHM, Hogendoorn PCW. MRI of adamantinoma of long bones in correlation with histopathology. AJR Am J Roentgenol 2004; 183: 1737–1744

[7] Van Rijn R, Bras J, Schaap G, van den Berg H, Maas M. Adamantinoma in childhood: report of six cases and review of the literature. Pediatr Radiol 2006; 36: 1068–1074

▶ Amyloid

[8] Escobedo EM, Hunter JC, Zink-Brody GC, Andress DL. Magnetic resonance imaging of dialysis-related amyloidosis of the shoulder and hip. Skeletal Radiol 1996; 25: 41–48

[9] Meyers SP, Mullins KJ, Kazee AM. Unifocal primary amyloidoma of the spine causing compression of the cervical spinal cord: MR findings. J Comput Assist Tomogr 1996; 20: 592–593

[10] Unal A, Sütlap PN, Kýyýk M. Primary solitary amyloidoma of thoracic spine: a case report and review of the literature. Clin Neurol Neurosurg 2003; 105: 167–169

▶ Aneurysmal Bone Cyst

[11] Bollini G, Jouve JL, Cottalorda J, Petit P, Panuel M, Jacquemier M. Aneurysmal bone cyst in children: analysis of twenty-seven patients. J Pediatr Orthop B 1998; 7: 274–285

[12] Ilaslan H, Sundaram M, Unni KK. Solid variant of aneurysmal bone cysts in long tubular bones: giant cell reparative granuloma. AJR Am J Roentgenol 2003; 180: 1681–1687

[13] Kransdorf MJ, Sweet DE. Aneurysmal bone cyst: concept, controversy, clinical presentation, and imaging. AJR Am J Roentgenol 1995; 164: 573–580

[14] Martinez V, Sissons HA. Aneurysmal bone cyst. A review of 123 cases including primary lesions and those secondary to other bone pathology. Cancer 1988; 61: 2291–2304

[15] Meyers SP. Aneurysmal bone cyst. In: MRI of Bone and Soft Tissue Tumors and Tumorlike Lesions. Stuttgart, Germany: Thieme; 2008:328–333

[16] Rosenberg AE, Nielsen GP, Fletcher JA. Aneurysmal bone cyst. In: Fletcher CDM, Unni KK, Mertens F, eds. World Health Organization Classification of Tumours. Pathology and Genetics of Tumours of Soft Tissue and Bone. Lyon, France: IARC Press; 2002:338–339

[17] Sullivan RJ, Meyer JS, Dormans JP, Davidson RS. Diagnosing aneurysmal and unicameral bone cysts with magnetic resonance imaging. Clin Orthop Relat Res 1999; 366: 186–190

[18] Tsai JC, Dalinka MK, Fallon MD, Zlatkin MB, Kressel HY. Fluid-fluid level: a nonspecific finding in tumors of bone and soft tissue. Radiology 1990; 175: 779–782

▶ Angiosarcoma

[19] Abdelwahab IF, Klein MJ, Hermann G, Springfield D. Angiosarcomas associated with bone infarcts. Skeletal Radiol 1998; 27: 546–551

[20] Meyers SP. Angiosarcoma. In: MRI of Bone and Soft Tissue Tumors and Tumorlike Lesions. Stuttgart, Germany: Thieme; 2008:344–346

[21] Roessner A, Boehling T. Angiosarcoma. In: Fletcher CDM, Unni KK, Mertens F, eds. World Health Organization Classification of Tumours. Pathology and Genetics of Tumours of Soft Tissue and Bone. Lyon, France: IARC Press; 2002:322–323

▶ Bilateral Sacroiliitis

[22] Bredella MA, Steinbach LS, Morgan S, Ward M, Davis JC. MRI of the sacroiliac joints in patients with moderate to severe ankylosing spondylitis. AJR Am J Roentgenol 2006; 187: 1420–1426

[23] Oostveen J, Prevo R, den Boer J, van de Laar M. Early detection of sacroiliitis on magnetic resonance imaging and subsequent development of sacroiliitis on plain radiography. A prospective, longitudinal study. J Rheumatol 1999; 26: 1953–1958

[24] Heuft-Dorenbosch L, Landewé R, Weijers R, et al. Combining information obtained from magnetic resonance imaging and conventional radiographs to detect sacroiliitis in patients with recent onset inflammatory back pain. Ann Rheum Dis 2006; 65: 804–808

[25] Levine DS, Forbat SM, Saifuddin A. MRI of the axial skeletal manifestations of ankylosing spondylitis. Clin Radiol 2004; 59: 400–413

[26] Bennett DL, Ohashi K, El-Khoury GY. Spondyloarthropathies: ankylosing spondylitis and psoriatic arthritis. Radiol Clin North Am 2004; 42: 121–134

[27] Puhakka KB, Jurik AG, Egund N, et al. Imaging of sacroiliitis in early seronegative spondylarthropathy. Assessment of abnormalities by MR in comparison with radiography and CT. Acta Radiol 2003; 44: 218–229

▶ Bizarre Parosteal Osteochondromatous Proliferation

[28] Abramovici L, Steiner GC. Bizarre parosteal osteochondromatous proliferation (Nora's lesion): a retrospective study of 12 cases, 2 arising in long bones. Hum Pathol 2002; 33: 1205–1210

[29] Michelsen H, Abramovici L, Steiner G, Posner MA. Bizarre parosteal osteochondromatous proliferation (Nora's lesion) in the hand. J Hand Surg Am 2004; 29: 520–525

[30] Orui H, Ishikawa A, Tsuchiya T, Ogino T. Magnetic resonance imaging characteristics of bizarre parosteal osteochondromatous proliferation of the hand: a case report. J Hand Surg Am 2002; 27: 1104–1108

[31] Sakamoto A, Imamura S, Matsumoto Y, et al. Bizarre parosteal osteochondromatous proliferation with an inversion of chromosome 7. Skeletal Radiol 2011; 40: 1487–1490

[32] Torreggiani WC, Munk PL, Al-Ismail K, et al. MR imaging features of bizarre parosteal osteochondromatous proliferation of bone (Nora's lesion). Eur J Radiol 2001; 40: 224–231

▶ Bone Cyst

[33] Haims AH, Desai P, Present D, Beltran J. Epiphyseal extension of a unicameral bone cyst. Skeletal Radiol 1997; 26: 51–54

[34] Kalil RK, Araujo ES. Simple bone cyst. In: Fletcher CDM, Unni KK, Mertens F, eds. World Health Organization Classification of Tumours. Pathology and Genetics of Tumours of Soft Tissue and Bone. Lyon, France: IARC Press; 2002: 340

[35] Lee JH, Reinus WR, Wilson AJ. Quantitative analysis of the plain radiographic appearance of unicameral bone cysts. Invest Radiol 1999; 34: 28–37

[36] Margau R, Babyn P, Cole W, Smith C, Lee F. MR imaging of simple bone cysts in children: not so simple. Pediatr Radiol 2000; 30: 551–557

[37] Meyers SP. Bone Cyst. In: MRI of Bone and Soft Tissue Tumors and Tumorlike Lesions. Stuttgart, Germany: Thieme; 2008:334–339

[38] Sullivan RJ, Meyer JS, Dormans JP, Davidson RS. Diagnosing aneurysmal and unicameral bone cysts with magnetic resonance imaging. Clin Orthop Relat Res 1999; 366: 186–190

[39] Wilkins RM. Unicameral bone cysts. J Am Acad Orthop Surg 2000; 8: 217–224

▶ Bone Contusion

[40] Boks SS, Vroegindeweij D, Koes BW, Hunink MGM, Bierma-Zeinstra SMA. Follow-up of occult bone lesions detected at MR imaging: systematic review. Radiology 2006; 238: 853–862

[41] Davies NH, Niall D, King LJ, Lavelle J, Healy JC. Magnetic resonance imaging of bone bruising in the acutely injured knee—short-term outcome. Clin Radiol 2004; 59: 439–445

▶ Bone and Muscle Infarct

[42] Andrews CL. From the RSNA Refresher Courses. Radiological Society of North America. Evaluation of the marrow space in the adult hip. Radiographics 2000; 20 Spec No: S27–S42

[43] Assouline-Dayan Y, Chang C, Greenspan A, Shoenfeld Y, Gershwin ME. Pathogenesis and natural history of osteonecrosis. Semin Arthritis Rheum 2002; 32: 94–124

[44] Balakrishnan A, Schemitsch EH, Pearce D, McKee MD. Distinguishing transient osteoporosis of the hip from avascular necrosis. Can J Surg 2003; 46: 187–192

[45] Bluemke DA, Zerhouni EA. MRI of avascular necrosis of bone. Top Magn Reson Imaging 1996; 8: 231–246

[46] Coates PT, Tie M, Russ GR, Mathew TH. Transient bone marrow edema in renal transplantation: a distinct post-transplantation syndrome with a characteristic MRI appearance. Am J Transplant 2002; 2: 467–470

[47] Fernandez-Canton G, Casado O, Capelastegui A, Astigarraga E, Larena JA, Merino A. Bone marrow edema syndrome of the foot: one year follow-up with MR imaging. Skeletal Radiol 2003; 32: 273–278

[48] Golimbu CN, Firooznia H, Rafii M. Avascular necrosis of carpal bones. Magn Reson Imaging Clin N Am 1995; 3: 281–303

[49] Huang GS, Chan WP, Chang YC, Chang CY, Chen CY, Yu JS. MR imaging of bone marrow edema and joint effusion in patients with osteonecrosis of the femoral head: relationship to pain. AJR Am J Roentgenol 2003; 181: 545–549

[50] Meyers SP. Bone and muscle infarct. In: MRI of Bone and Soft Tissue Tumors and Tumorlike Lesions. Stuttgart, Germany: Thieme; 2008:512–518

[51] Terk MR, Esplin J, Lee K, Magre G, Colletti PM. MR imaging of patients with type 1 Gaucher's disease: relationship between bone and visceral changes. AJR Am J Roentgenol 1995; 165: 599–604

[52] Umans H, Haramati N, Flusser G. The diagnostic role of gadolinium enhanced MRI in distinguishing between acute medullary bone infarct and osteomyelitis. Magn Reson Imaging 2000; 18: 255–262

▸ Bone Marrow Necrosis

[53] Chim CS, Ooi C, Ma SK, Lam C. Bone marrow necrosis in bone marrow transplantation: the role of MR imaging. Bone Marrow Transplant 1998; 22: 1125–1128

[54] Janssens AM, Offner FC, Van Hove WZ. Bone marrow necrosis. Cancer 2000; 88: 1769–1780

[55] Paydas S, Ergin M, Baslamisli F, et al. Bone marrow necrosis: clinicopathologic analysis of 20 cases and review of the literature. Am J Hematol 2002; 70: 300–305

[56] Tang YM, Jeavons S, Stuckey S, Middleton H, Gill D. MRI features of bone marrow necrosis. AJR Am J Roentgenol 2007; 188: 509–514

▸ Calcific Tendinitis

[57] Flemming DJ, Murphey MD, Shekitka KM, Temple HT, Jelinek JJ, Kransdorf MJ. Osseous involvement in calcific tendinitis: a retrospective review of 50 cases. AJR Am J Roentgenol 2003; 181: 965–972

[58] Porcellini G, Paladini P, Campi F, Pegreffi F. Osteolytic lesion of greater tuberosity in calcific tendinitis of the shoulder. J Shoulder Elbow Surg 2009; 18: 210–215

▸ Chondroblastoma

[59] Jee WH, Park YK, McCauley TR, et al. Chondroblastoma: MR characteristics with pathologic correlation. J Comput Assist Tomogr 1999; 23: 721–726

[60] Kaim AH, Hügli R, Bonél HM, Jundt G. Chondroblastoma and clear cell chondrosarcoma: radiological and MRI characteristics with histopathological correlation. Skeletal Radiol 2002; 31: 88–95

[61] Kilpatrick SE, Parisien M, Bridge JA. Chondroblastoma. In: Fletcher CDM, Unni KK, Mertens F, eds. World Health Organization Classification of Tumours. Pathology and Genetics of Tumours of Soft Tissue and Bone. Lyon, France: IARC Press; 2002:241–242

[62] Ly JQ, LaGatta LM, Beall DP. Calcaneal chondroblastoma with secondary aneurysmal bone cyst. AJR Am J Roentgenol 2004; 182: 130

[63] Meyers SP. Chondroblastoma. In: MRI of Bone and Soft Tissue Tumors and Tumorlike Lesions. Stuttgart, Germany: Thieme; 2008:347–351

[64] Weatherall PT, Maale GE, Mendelsohn DB, Sherry CS, Erdman WE, Pascoe HR. Chondroblastoma: classic and confusing appearance at MR imaging. Radiology 1994; 190: 467–474

[65] Yamamura S, Sato K, Sugiura H, et al. Prostaglandin levels of primary bone tumor tissues correlate with peritumoral edema demonstrated by magnetic resonance imaging. Cancer 1997; 79: 255–261

▸ Chondroma, Intramedullary Type (Enchondroma)

[66] Aoki J, Sone S, Fujioka F, et al. MR of enchondroma and chondrosarcoma: rings and arcs of Gd-DTPA enhancement. J Comput Assist Tomogr 1991; 15: 1011–1016

[67] Geirnaerdt MJ, Hogendoorn PC, Bloem JL, Taminiau AH, van der Woude HJ. Cartilaginous tumors: fast contrast-enhanced MR imaging. Radiology 2000; 214: 539–546

[68] Lucas DR, Bridge JA. Chondromas, enchondroma, periosteal chondroma, and enchondromatosis. In: Fletcher CDM, Unni KK, Mertens F, eds. World Health Organization Classification of Tumours. Pathology and Genetics of Tumours of Soft Tissue and Bone. Lyon, France: IARC Press; 2002:237–240

[69] Mertens F, Unni KK. Enchondromatosis: Ollier's disease and Maffucci syndrome. In: Fletcher CDM, Unni KK, Mertens F, eds. World Health Organization Classification of Tumours. Pathology and Genetics of Tumours of Soft Tissue and Bone. Lyon, France: IARC Press; 2002:356–357

[70] Meyers SP. Chondroma, intramedullary type: enchondroma. In: MRI of Bone and Soft Tissue Tumors and Tumorlike Lesions. Stuttgart, Germany: Thieme; 2008:352–358

[71] Murphey MD, Flemming DJ, Boyea SR, Bojescul JA, Sweet DE, Temple HT. Enchondroma versus chondrosarcoma in the appendicular skeleton: differentiating features. Radiographics 1998; 18: 1213–1237, quiz 1244–1245

▸ Chondroma, Periosteal or Juxtacortical Type

[72] Brien EW, Mirra JM, Luck JV. Benign and malignant cartilage tumors of bone and joint: their anatomic and theoretical basis with an emphasis on radiology, pathology and clinical biology. II. Juxtacortical cartilage tumors. Skeletal Radiol 1999; 28: 1–20

[73] Lucas DR, Bridge JA. Chondromas: enchondroma, periosteal chondroma, and enchondromatosis. In: Fletcher CDM, Unni KK, Mertens F, eds. World Health Organization Classification of Tumours. Pathology and Genetics of Tumours of Soft Tissue and Bone. Lyon, France: IARC Press; 2002:237–240

[74] Meyers SP. Chondroma, periosteal or juxtacortical type. In: MRI of Bone and Soft Tissue Tumors and Tumorlike Lesions. Stuttgart, Germany: Thieme; 2008:359–363

[75] Robinson P, White LM, Sundaram M, et al. Periosteal chondroid tumors: radiologic evaluation with pathologic correlation. AJR Am J Roentgenol 2001; 177: 1183–1188

[76] Tillich M, Lindbichler F, Reittner P, Weybora W, Linhart W, Fotter R. Childhood periosteal chondroma: femoral neck thickening and remote hyperostosis as clues to plain film diagnosis. Pediatr Radiol 1998; 28: 899

[77] Woertler K, Blasius S, Brinkschmidt C, Hillmann A, Link TM, Heindel W. Periosteal chondroma: MR characteristics. J Comput Assist Tomogr 2001; 25: 425–430

▸ Chondromyxoid Fibroma

[78] Kim HS, Jee WH, Ryu KN, et al. MRI of chondromyxoid fibroma. Acta Radiol 2011; 52: 875–880

[79] Macdonald D, Fornasier V, Holtby R. Chondromyxoid fibroma of the acromium with soft tissue extension. Skeletal Radiol 2000; 29: 168–170

[80] Marin C, Gallego C, Manjón P, Martinez-Tello FJ. Juxtacortical chondromyxoid fibroma: imaging findings in three cases and a review of the literature. Skeletal Radiol 1997; 26: 642–649

[81] Mehta S, Szklaruk J, Faria SC, Raymond AK, Whitman GJ. Radiologic-pathologic conferences of the University of Texas M. D. Anderson Cancer Center: chondromyxoid fibroma of the sacrum and iliac bone. AJR Am J Roentgenol 2006; 186: 467–469

[82] Meyers SP. Chondromyxoid fibroma. In: MRI of Bone and Soft Tissue Tumors and Tumorlike Lesions. Stuttgart, Germany: Thieme; 2008:364–367

[83] O'Connor PJ, Gibbon WW, Hardy G, Butt WP. Chondromyxoid fibroma of the foot. Skeletal Radiol 1996; 25: 143–148

[84] Ostrowski ML, Spjut HJ, Bridge JA. Chondromyxoid fibroma. In: Fletcher CDM, Unni KK, Mertens F, eds. World Health Organization Classification of Tumours. Pathology and Genetics of Tumours of Soft Tissue and Bone. Lyon, France: IARC Press; 2002; 243–245

[85] Park SH, Kong KY, Chung HW, Kim CJ, Lee SH, Kang HS. Juxtacortical chondromyxoid fibroma arising in an apophysis. Skeletal Radiol 2000; 29: 466–469

[86] Soler R, Rodríguez E, Suárez I, Gayol A. Magnetic resonance imaging of chondromyxoid fibroma of the fibula. Eur J Radiol 1994; 18: 210–211

[87] Wu CT, Inwards CY, O'Laughlin S, Rock MG, Beabout JW, Unni KK. Chondromyxoid fibroma of bone: a clinicopathologic review of 278 cases. Hum Pathol 1998; 29: 438–446

▸ Chondrosarcoma

[88] Geirnaerdt MJ, Hogendoorn PC, Bloem JL, Taminiau AH, van der Woude HJ. Cartilaginous tumors: fast contrast-enhanced MR imaging. Radiology 2000; 214: 539–546

[89] Bertoni F, Bacchini P, Hogendoorn PCW. Chondrosarcoma. In: Fletcher CDM, Unni KK, Mertens F, eds. World Health Organization Classification of Tumours. Pathology and Genetics of Tumours of Soft Tissue and Bone. Lyon, France: IARC Press; 2002:247–251

[90] Brien EW, Mirra JM, Kerr R. Benign and malignant cartilage tumors of bone and joint: their anatomic and theoretical basis with an emphasis on radiology, pathology and clinical biology, I: The intramedullary cartilage tumors. Skeletal Radiol 1997; 26: 325–353

[91] Cannon CP, Nelson SD, Seeger LL, Eckardt JJ. Clear cell chondrosarcoma mimicking chondroblastoma in a skeletally immature patient. Skeletal Radiol 2002; 31: 369–372

[92] Collins MS, Koyama T, Swee RG, Inwards CY. Clear cell chondrosarcoma: radiographic, computed tomographic, and magnetic resonance findings in 34 patients with pathologic correlation. Skeletal Radiol 2003; 32: 687–694

[93] Janzen L, Logan PM, O'Connell JX, Connell DG, Munk PL. Intramedullary chondroid tumors of bone: correlation of abnormal peritumoral marrow and soft-tissue MRI signal with tumor type. Skeletal Radiol 1997; 26: 100–106

[94] Kaim AH, Hügli R, Bonél HM, Jundt G. Chondroblastoma and clear cell chondrosarcoma: radiological and MRI characteristics with histopathological correlation. Skeletal Radiol 2002; 31: 88–95

[95] McCarthy EF, Freemont A, Hogendoorn PCW. Clear cell chondrosarcoma. In: Fletcher CDM, Unni KK, Mertens F, eds. World Health Organization Classification of Tumours. Pathology and Genetics of Tumours of Soft Tissue and Bone. Lyon, France: IARC Press; 2002:257–258

[96] Meyers SP. Chondrosarcoma. In: MRI of Bone and Soft Tissue Tumors and Tumorlike Lesions. Stuttgart, Germany: Thieme; 2008:368–378

[97] Meyers SP, Hirsch WL, Curtin HD, Barnes L, Sekhar LN, Sen C. Chondrosarcomas of the skull base: MR imaging features. Radiology 1992; 184: 103–108

[98] Milchgrub S, Hogendoorn PCW. Dedifferentiated chondrosarcoma. In: Fletcher CDM, Unni KK, Mertens F, eds. World Health Organization Classification of Tumours. Pathology and Genetics of Tumours of Soft Tissue and Bone. Lyon, France: IARC Press; 2002:252–254

[99] Murphey MD, Walker EA, Wilson AJ, Kransdorf MJ, Temple HT, Gannon FH. From the archives of the AFIP: imaging of primary chondrosarcoma: radiologic-pathologic correlation. Radiographics 2003; 23: 1245–1278

[100] Nakashima Y, Park YK, Sugano O. Mesenchymal chondrosarcoma. In: Fletcher CDM, Unni KK, Mertens F, eds. World Health Organization Classification of Tumours. Pathology and Genetics of Tumours of Soft Tissue and Bone. Lyon, France: IARC Press; 2002:255–256

[101] Vanel D, De Paolis M, Monti C, Mercuri M, Picci P. Radiological features of 24 periosteal chondrosarcomas. Skeletal Radiol 2001; 30: 208–212

▸ Chordoma

[102] Diel J, Ortiz O, Losada RA, Price DB, Hayt MW, Katz DS. The sacrum: pathologic spectrum, multimodality imaging, and subspecialty approach. Radiographics 2001; 21: 83–104

[103] Erdem E, Angtuaco EC, Van Hemert R, Park JS, Al-Mefty O. Comprehensive review of intracranial chordoma. Radiographics 2003; 23: 995–1009

[104] Heffelfinger MJ, Dahlin DC, MacCarty CS, Beabout JW. Chordomas and cartilaginous tumors at the skull base. Cancer 1973; 32: 410–420

[105] Meyers SP, Hirsch WL, Curtin HD, Barnes L, Sekhar LN, Sen C. Chordomas of the skull base: MR features. AJNR Am J Neuroradiol 1992; 13: 1627–1636

[106] Meyers SP. Chordomas. In: MRI of Bone and Soft Tissue Tumors and Tumorlike Lesions. Stuttgart, Germany: Thieme; 2008:379–382

[107] Smolders D, Wang X, Drevelengas A, Vanhoenacker F, De Schepper AM. Value of MRI in the diagnosis of non-clival, non-sacral chordoma. Skeletal Radiol 2003; 32: 343–350

▸ Chronic Myeloproliferative Disease

[108] Amano Y, Onda M, Amano M, Kumazaki T. Magnetic resonance imaging of myelofibrosis. STIR and gadolinium-enhanced MR images. Clin Imaging 1997; 21: 264–268

[109] Bock O, Loch G, Schade U, et al. Osteosclerosis in advanced chronic idiopathic myelofibrosis is associated with endothelial overexpression of osteoprotegerin. Br J Haematol 2005; 130: 76–82

[110] Moulopoulos LA, Dimopoulos MA. Magnetic resonance imaging of the bone marrow in hematologic malignancies. Blood 1997; 90: 2127–2147

[111] Sale GE, Deeg HJ, Porter BA. Regression of myelofibrosis and osteosclerosis following hematopoietic cell transplantation assessed by magnetic resonance imaging and histologic grading. Biol Blood Marrow Transplant 2006; 12: 1285–1294

[112] Sideris P, Tassiopoulos S, Sakellaropoulos N, et al. Unusual radiological findings in a case of myelofibrosis secondary to polycythemia vera. Ann Hematol 2006; 85: 555–556

[113] Thiele J, Pierre R, Imbert M, Vardiman JW, Brunning RD, Flandrin G. Chronic idiopathic myelofibrosis. In: Jaffe ES, Harris NL, Sein H, Vardiman JW, eds. World Health Organization Classification of Tumours. Pathology and Genetics of Tumours. Tumours of Haematopoeitic and Lymphoid Tissues. Lyon, France: IARC Press; 2001:35–38

▸ Clear Cell Sarcoma

[114] De Beuckeleer LH, De Schepper AM, Vandevenne JE, et al. MR imaging of clear cell sarcoma (malignant melanoma of the soft parts): a multicenter correlative MRI-pathology study of 21 cases and literature review. Skeletal Radiol 2000; 29: 187–195

▸ Desmoplastic Fibroma

[115] Böhm P, Kröber S, Greschniok A, Laniado M, Kaiserling E. Desmoplastic fibroma of the bone: a report of two patients, review of the literature, and therapeutic implications. Cancer 1996; 78: 1011–1023

[116] Fornasier V, Pritzker KPH, Bridge JA. Desmoplastic fibroma of bone. In: Goldblum J, Fletcher JA. Superficial fibromatoses. In: Fletcher CDM, Unni KK, Mertens F, eds. World Health Organization Classification of Tumours. Pathology and Genetics of Tumours of Soft Tissue and Bone. Lyon, France: IARC Press; 2002:288

[117] Frick MA, Sundaram M, Unni KK, et al. Imaging findings in desmoplastic fibroma of bone: distinctive T2 characteristics. AJR Am J Roentgenol 2005; 184: 1762–1767

[118] Goldblum J, Fletcher JA. Desmoid-type fibromatoses. In: Fletcher CDM, Unni KK, Mertens F, eds. World Health Organization Classification of Tumours. Pathology and Genetics of Tumours of Soft Tissue and Bone. Lyon, France: IARC Press; 2002:83–84

[119] Mahnken AH, Nolte-Ernsting CC, Wildberger JE, Wirtz DC, Günther RW. Cross-sectional imaging patterns of desmoplastic fibroma. Eur Radiol 2001; 11: 1105–1110

[120] Meyers SP. Desmoid tumors. In: MRI of Bone and Soft Tissue Tumors and Tumorlike Lesions. Stuttgart, Germany: Thieme; 2008:396–403

[121] Shuto R, Kiyosue H, Hori Y, Miyake H, Kawano K, Mori HCT. CT and MR imaging of desmoplastic fibroblastoma. Eur Radiol 2002; 12: 2474–2476

[122] Vanhoenacker FM, Hauben E, De Beuckeleer LH, Willemen D, Van Marck E, De Schepper AM. Desmoplastic fibroma of bone: MRI features. Skeletal Radiol 2000; 29: 171–175

▸ Eosinophilic Granuloma/Langerhans Cell Histiocytosis

[123] Beltran J, Aparisi F, Bonmati LM, Rosenberg ZS, Present D, Steiner GC. Eosinophilic granuloma: MRI manifestations. Skeletal Radiol 1993; 22: 157–161

[124] Davies AM, Pikoulas C, Griffith J. MRI of eosinophilic granuloma. Eur J Radiol 1994; 18: 205–209

[125] DeYoung BR, Unni KK. Langerhans' cell histiocytosis. In: Fletcher CDM, Unni KK, Mertens F, eds. World Health Organization Classification of Tumours. Pathology and Genetics of Tumours of Soft Tissue and Bone. Lyon, France: IARC Press; 2002:345–346

[126] Ghanem I, Tolo VT, D'Ambra P, Malogalowkin MH. Langerhans cell histiocytosis of bone in children and adolescents. J Pediatr Orthop 2003; 23: 124–130

[127] Hindman BW, Thomas RD, Young LW, Yu L. Langerhans cell histiocytosis: unusual skeletal manifestations observed in thirty-four cases. Skeletal Radiol 1998; 27: 177–181

[128] Meyers SP. Eosinophilic granuloma. In: MRI of Bone and Soft Tissue Tumors and Tumorlike Lesions. Stuttgart, Germany: Thieme; 2008:406–412

[129] Monroc M, Ducou le Pointe H, Haddad S, Josset P, Montagne JP. Soft tissue signal abnormality associated with eosinophilic granuloma: correlation of MR imaging with pathologic findings. Pediatr Radiol 1994; 24: 328–332

[130] Song YS, Lee IS, Yi JH, Cho KH, Kim K, Song JW. Radiologic findings of adult pelvis and appendicular skeletal Langerhans cell histiocytosis in nine patients. Skeletal Radiol 2011; 40: 1421–1426

[131] Stull MA, Kransdorf MJ, Devaney KO. Langerhans cell histiocytosis of bone. Radiographics 1992; 12: 801–823

[132] Yamamura S, Sato K, Sugiura H, et al. Prostaglandin levels of primary bone tumor tissues correlate with peritumoral edema demonstrated by magnetic resonance imaging. Cancer 1997; 79: 255–261

▸ Erdheim-Chester Disease

[133] Bancroft LW, Berquist TH. Erdheim-Chester disease: radiographic findings in five patients. Skeletal Radiol 1998; 27: 127–132

[134] Dion E, Graef C, Miquel A, et al. Bone involvement in Erdheim-Chester disease: imaging findings including periostitis and partial epiphyseal involvement. Radiology 2006; 238: 632–639

[135] Gottlieb R, Chen A. MR findings of Erdheim-Chester disease. J Comput Assist Tomogr 2002; 26: 257–261

[136] Kenn W, Eck M, Allolio B, et al. Erdheim-Chester disease: evidence for a disease entity different from Langerhans cell histiocytosis? Three cases with detailed radiological and immunohistochemical analysis. Hum Pathol 2000; 31: 734–739

[137] Kim NR, Ko YH, Choe YH, Lee HG, Huh B, Ahn GH. Erdheim-Chester disease with extensive marrow necrosis: a case report and literature review. Int J Surg Pathol 2001; 9: 73–79

[138] Kushihashi T, Munechika H, Sekimizu M, Fujimaki E. Erdheim-Chester disease involving bilateral lower extremities: MR features. AJR Am J Roentgenol 2000; 174: 875–876

[139] Meyers SP. Erdheim-Chester disease. In: MRI of Bone and Soft Tissue Tumors and Tumorlike Lesions. Stuttgart, Germany: Thieme; 2008:413–415

[140] Murray D, Marshall M, England E, Mander J, Chakera TMH. Erdheim-chester disease. Clin Radiol 2001; 56: 481–484

▶ Ewing Sarcoma

[141] Dyke JP, Panicek DM, Healey JH, et al. Osteogenic and Ewing sarcomas: estimation of necrotic fraction during induction chemotherapy with dynamic contrast-enhanced MR imaging. Radiology 2003; 228: 271–278

[142] Kaste SC. Imaging pediatric bone sarcomas. Radiol Clin North Am 2011; 49: 749–765, vi–vii

[143] Meyers SP. Ewing's sarcoma. In: MRI of Bone and Soft Tissue Tumors and Tumorlike Lesions. Stuttgart, Germany: Thieme; 2008:416–422

[144] Miller SL, Hoffer FA, Reddick WE, et al. Tumor volume or dynamic contrast-enhanced MRI for prediction of clinical outcome of Ewing sarcoma family of tumors. Pediatr Radiol 2001; 31: 518–523

[145] Saifuddin A, Whelan J, Pringle JA, Cannon SR. Malignant round cell tumours of bone: atypical clinical and imaging features. Skeletal Radiol 2000; 29: 646–651

[146] Ushigome S, Machinami R, Sorensen PH. Ewing'sarcoma/primitive neuroectodermal tumour (PNET). In: Fletcher CDM, Unni KK, Mertens F, eds. World Health Organization Classification of Tumours. Pathology and Genetics of Tumours of Soft Tissue and Bone. Lyon, France: IARC Press; 2002:298–300

[147] van der Woude HJ, Bloem JL, Verstraete KL, Taminiau AH, Nooy MA, Hogendoorn PC. Osteosarcoma and Ewing's sarcoma after neoadjuvant chemotherapy: value of dynamic MR imaging in detecting viable tumor before surgery. AJR Am J Roentgenol 1995; 165: 593–598

[148] van der Woude HJ, Bloem JL, Hogendoorn PC. Preoperative evaluation and monitoring chemotherapy in patients with high-grade osteogenic and Ewing's sarcoma: review of current imaging modalities. Skeletal Radiol 1998; 27: 57–71

▶ Extramedullary Hematopoiesis

[149] Dibbern DA, Loevner LA, Lieberman AP, Salhany KE, Freese A, Marcotte PJ. MR of thoracic cord compression caused by epidural extramedullary hematopoiesis in myelodysplastic syndrome. AJNR Am J Neuroradiol 1997; 18: 363–366

[150] Niggemann P, Krings T, Hans F, Thron A. Fifteen-year follow-up of a patient with beta thalassaemia and extramedullary haematopoietic tissue compressing the spinal cord. Neuroradiology 2005; 47: 263–266

[151] Rajiah P, Hayashi R, Bauer TW, Sundaram M. Extramedullary hematopoiesis in unusual locations in hematologically compromised and noncompromised patients. Skeletal Radiol 2011; 40: 947–953

[152] Tan TC, Tsao J, Cheung FC. Extramedullary haemopoiesis in thalassemia intermedia presenting as paraplegia. J Clin Neurosci 2002; 9: 721–725

▶ Fibrosarcoma

[153] Christensen DR, Ramsamooj R, Gilbert TJ. Sclerosing epithelioid fibrosarcoma: short T2 on MR imaging. Skeletal Radiol 1997; 26: 619–621

[154] Coffin CM, Fletcher JA. Infantile fibrosarcoma. In: Fletcher CDM, Unni KK, Mertens F, eds. World Health Organization Classification of Tumours. Pathology and Genetics of Tumours of Soft Tissue and Bone. Lyon, France: IARC Press; 2002:98–100

[155] Eich GF, Hoeffel JC, Tschäppeler H, Gassner I, Willi UV. Fibrous tumours in children: imaging features of a heterogeneous group of disorders. Pediatr Radiol 1998; 28: 500–509

[156] Fisher C, van den Berg E, Molenaar WM. Adult fibrosarcoma. In: Fletcher CDM, Unni KK, Mertens F, eds. World Health Organization Classification of Tumours. Pathology and Genetics of Tumours of Soft Tissue and Bone. Lyon, France: IARC Press; 2002:100–101

[157] Folpe A, van den Berg E, Molenaar WM. Low grade fibromyxoid sarcoma. In: Fletcher CDM, Unni KK, Mertens F, eds. World Health Organization Classification of Tumours. Pathology and Genetics of Tumours of Soft Tissue and Bone. Lyon, France: IARC Press; 2002:104–105

[158] Kahn LB, Vigorita V. Fibrosarcoma of bone. In: Fletcher CDM, Unni KK, Mertens F, eds. World Health Organization Classification of Tumours. Pathology and Genetics of Tumours of Soft Tissue and Bone. Lyon, France: IARC Press; 2002:289–290

[159] Meis-Kindblom JM, Kindblom LG, van den Berg E, Molenaar WM. Sclerosing epithelioid fibrosarcoma. In: Fletcher CDM, Unni KK, Mertens F, eds. World Health Organization Classification of Tumours. Pathology and Genetics of Tumours of Soft Tissue and Bone. Lyon, France: IARC Press; 2002:106–107

[160] Mentzel T, van den Berg E, Molenaar WM. Myxofibrosarcoma. In: Fletcher CDM, Unni KK, Mertens F, eds. World Health Organization Classification of Tumours. Pathology and Genetics of Tumours of Soft Tissue and Bone. Lyon, France: IARC Press; 2002:102–103

[161] Meyers SP. Fibrosarcoma. In: MRI of Bone and Soft Tissue Tumors and Tumorlike Lesions. Stuttgart, Germany: Thieme; 2008:433–437

▶ Fibrous Cortical Defect and NonossifyingFibroma

[162] Biermann JS. Common benign lesions of bone in children and adolescents. J Pediatr Orthop 2002; 22: 268–273

[163] Jee WH, Choe BY, Kang HS, et al. Nonossifying fibroma: characteristics at MR imaging with pathologic correlation. Radiology 1998; 209: 197–202

[164] Kyriakos M. Benign fibrous histicytoma of bone. In: Fletcher CDM, Unni KK, Mertens F, eds. World Health Organization Classification of Tumours. Pathology and Genetics of Tumours of Soft Tissue and Bone. Lyon, France: IARC Press; 2002:292–293

[165] Meyers SP. Fibrous cortical defect and non-ossifying fibroma. In: MRI of Bone and Soft Tissue Tumors and Tumorlike Lesions. Stuttgart, Germany: Thieme; 2008:438–448

[166] Suh JS, Cho JH, Shin KH, et al. MR appearance of distal femoral cortical irregularity (cortical desmoid). J Comput Assist Tomogr 1996; 20: 328–332

▶ Fibrous Dysplasia

[167] Chong VF, Khoo JB, Fan YF. Fibrous dysplasia involving the base of the skull. AJR Am J Roentgenol 2002; 178: 717–720

[168] Cohen MM, Siegal GP. McCune Albright syndrome. In: Fletcher CDM, Unni KK, Mertens F, eds. World Health Organization Classification of Tumours. Pathology and Genetics of Tumours of Soft Tissue and Bone. Lyon, France: IARC Press; 2002:357–359

[169] DiCaprio MR, Enneking WF. Fibrous dysplasia: pathophysiology, evaluation, and treatment. J Bone Joint Surg Am 2005; 87: 1848–1864

[170] Fitzpatrick KA, Taljanovic MS, Speer DP, et al. Imaging findings of fibrous dysplasia with histopathologic and intraoperative correlation. AJR Am J Roentgenol 2004; 182: 1389–1398

[171] Iwasko N, Steinbach LS, Disler D, et al. Imaging findings in Mazabraud's syndrome: seven new cases. Skeletal Radiol 2002; 31: 81–87

[172] Jee WH, Choi KH, Choe BY, Park JM, Shinn KS. Fibrous dysplasia: MR imaging characteristics with radiopathologic correlation. AJR Am J Roentgenol 1996; 167: 1523–1527

[173] Kaushik S, Smoker WRK, Frable WJ. Malignant transformation of fibrous dysplasia into chondroblastic osteosarcoma. Skeletal Radiol 2002; 31: 103–106

[174] Kransdorf MJ, Moser RP, Gilkey FW. Fibrous dysplasia. Radiographics 1990; 10: 519–537

[175] Leet AI, Magur E, Lee JS, Wientroub S, Robey PG, Collins MT. Fibrous dysplasia in the spine: prevalence of lesions and association with scoliosis. J Bone Joint Surg Am 2004; 86-A: 531–537

[176] Meyers SP. Fibrous dysplasia. In: MRI of Bone and Soft Tissue Tumors and Tumorlike Lesions. Stuttgart, Germany: Thieme; 2008:449–455

[177] Shah ZK, Peh WCG, Koh WL, Shek TWH. Magnetic resonance imaging appearances of fibrous dysplasia. Br J Radiol 2005; 78: 1104–1115

[178] Siegal G, Dal Cin P, Araujo ES. Fibrous dysplasia. In: Fletcher CDM, Unni KK, Mertens F, eds. World Health Organization Classification of Tumours. Pathology and Genetics of Tumours of Soft Tissue and Bone. Lyon, France: IARC Press; 2002:341–342

▶ Fluorosis

[179] Haettich B, Lebreton C, Prier A, Kaplan G. Magnetic resonance imaging of fluorosis and stress fractures due to fluoride [in French] Rev Rhum Mal Osteoartic 1991; 58: 803–808

[180] Muthukumar N. Ossification of the ligamentum flavum as a result of fluorosis causing myelopathy: report of two cases. Neurosurgery 2005; 56: E622–, discussion E622

[181] Reddy DR, Srikanth RD, Misra M. Fluorosis. Surg Neurol 1998; 49: 635–636

▶ Focal Fibrocartilaginous Dysplasia

[182] Bakman M, Monu JU. Focal fibrocartilaginous dysplasia (FFCD). Pediatr Radiol 2007; 37: 107

[183] Choi IH, Kim CJ, Cho TJ, et al. Focal fibrocartilaginous dysplasia of long bones: report of eight additional cases and literature review. J Pediatr Orthop 2000; 20: 421–427

[184] Kim CJ, Choi IH, Cho TJ, Chung CY, Chi JG. The histological spectrum of subperiosteal fibrocartilaginous pseudotumor of long bone (focal fibrocartilaginous dysplasia). Pathol Int 1999; 49: 1000–1006

▶ Fracture

[185] Ahovuo JA, Kiuru MJ, Visuri T. Fatigue stress fractures of the sacrum: diagnosis with MR imaging. Eur Radiol 2004; 14: 500–505

[186] Berger FH, de Jonge MC, Maas M. Stress fractures in the lower extremity:the importance of increasing awareness amongst radiologists. Eur J Radiol 2007; 62: 16–26

[187] Grangier C, Garcia J, Howarth NR, May M, Rossier P. Role of MRI in the diagnosis of insufficiency fractures of the sacrum and acetabular roof. Skeletal Radiol 1997; 26: 517–524

[188] Meyers SP, Wiener SN. Magnetic resonance imaging features of fractures using the short tau inversion recovery (STIR) sequence: correlation with radiographic findings. Skeletal Radiol 1991; 20: 499–507

▶ Gaucher Disease

[189] Maas M, Poll LW, Terk MR. Imaging and quantifying skeletal involvement in Gaucher disease. Br J Radiol 2002; 75 Suppl 1: A13–A24

[190] Poll LW, Koch JA, vom Dahl S, et al. Magnetic resonance imaging of bone marrow changes in Gaucher disease during enzyme replacement therapy: first German long-term results. Skeletal Radiol 2001; 30: 496–503

[191] Roca M, Mota J, Alfonso P, Pocoví M, Giraldo P. S-MRI score: a simple method for assessing bone marrow involvement in Gaucher disease. Eur J Radiol 2007; 62: 132–137

[192] Wenstrup RJ, Roca-Espiau M, Weinreb NJ, Bembi B. Skeletal aspects of Gaucher disease: a review. Br J Radiol 2002; 75 Suppl 1: A2–A12

▶ Ganglia

[193] Abdelwahab IF, Kenan S, Hermann G, Klein MJ, Lewis MM. Periosteal ganglia: CT and MR imaging features. Radiology 1993; 188: 245–248

[194] Bisset GS 3rd. MR imaging of soft-tissue masses in children. Magn Reson Imaging Clin North Am 1996; 4(4): 697–719

[195] Blanco JF, De Pedro JA, Paniagua JC. Periosteal ganglion in a child. Arch Orthop Trauma Surg 2003; 123: 115–117

[196] Forest M. Ganglion and epidermoid cyst. In: Forest M, Tomeno B, Vanel D. Orthopedic Surgical Pathology: Diagnosis of Tumors and Pseudotumoral Lesions of Bone and Joints. New York, NY: Churchill Livingstone; 1998: 547–553

▶ Geodes/Osteoarthritic Cysts

[197] Meyers SP. Geodes. In: MRI of Bone and Soft Tissue Tumors and Tumorlike Lesions. Stuttgart, Germany: Thieme; 2008: 456–461

[198] Resnick D. Degenerative disease of extraspinal locations. In: Diagnosis of Bone and Joint Disorders. 4th ed. Philadelphia, PA: WB Saunders; 2002: 1271–1381

[199] Unni KK. Conditions that commonly simulate primary neoplasms of bone. In: Dahlin's Bone Tumors: General Aspects and Data on 11,087 Cases. 5th ed. Philadelphia, PA: Lippincott-Raven; 1996: 367–376

▶ Giant Cell Tumor of Bone

[200] Aoki J, Tanikawa H, Ishii K, et al. MR findings indicative of hemosiderin in giant-cell tumor of bone: frequency, cause, and diagnostic significance. AJR Am J Roentgenol 1996; 166: 145–148

[201] Bullough PG, Bansal M. Malignancy in giant cell tumour. In: Fletcher CDM, Unni KK, Mertens F, eds. World Health Organization Classification of Tumours. Pathology and Genetics of Tumours of Soft Tissue and Bone. Lyon, France: IARC Press; 2002:313

[202] Kransdorf MJ, Sweet DE, Buetow PC, Giudici MA, Moser RP. Giant cell tumor in skeletally immature patients. Radiology 1992; 184: 233–237

[203] Manaster BJ, Doyle AJ. Giant cell tumors of bone. Radiol Clin North Am 1993; 31: 299–323

[204] McEnery KW, Raymond AK. Giant cell tumor of the fourth metacarpal. AJR Am J Roentgenol 1999; 172: 1092

[205] Meyers SP. Giant cell tumor of bone. In: MRI of Bone and Soft Tissue Tumors and Tumorlike Lesions. Stuttgart, Germany: Thieme; 2008: 462–468

[206] Meyers SP, Yaw K, Devaney K. Giant cell tumor of the thoracic spine: MR appearance. AJNR Am J Neuroradiol 1994; 15: 962–964

[207] Murphey MD, Nomikos GC, Flemming DJ, Gannon FH, Temple HT, Kransdorf MJ. From the archives of AFIP. Imaging of giant cell tumor and giant cell reparative granuloma of bone: radiologic-pathologic correlation. Radiographics 2001; 21: 1283–1309

[208] Reid R, Banerjee SS. Sciot. Giant cell tumour. In: Fletcher CDM, Unni KK, Mertens F, eds. World Health Organization Classification of Tumours. Pathology and Genetics of Tumours of Soft Tissue and Bone. Lyon, France: IARC Press; 2002: 310–312

[209] Stacy GS, Peabody TD, Dixon LB. Mimics on radiography of giant cell tumor of bone. AJR Am J Roentgenol 2003; 181: 1583–1589

[210] Yamamura S, Sato K, Sugiura H, et al. Prostaglandin levels of primary bone tumor tissues correlate with peritumoral edema demonstrated by magnetic resonance imaging. Cancer 1997; 79: 255–261

[211] Zhen W, Yaotian H, Songjian L, Ge L, Qingliang W. Giant-cell tumour of bone: the long-term results of treatment by curettage and bone graft. J Bone Joint Surg Br 2004; 86: 212–216

▶ Giant Cell Tumor of the Tendon Sheath and/or Soft Tissue

[212] Al-Qattan MM. Giant cell tumours of tendon sheath: classification and recurrence rate. J Hand Surg [Br] 2001; 26: 72–75

[213] Gibbons CL, Khwaja HA, Cole AS, Cooke PH, Athanasou NA. Giant-cell tumour of the tendon sheath in the foot and ankle. J Bone Joint Surg Br 2002; 84: 1000–1003

[214] Huang GS, Lee CH, Chan WP, Chen CY, Yu JS, Resnick D. Localized nodular synovitis of the knee: MR imaging appearance and clinical correlates in 21 patients. AJR Am J Roentgenol 2003; 181: 539–543

[215] Jelinek JS, Kransdorf MJ, Shmookler BM, Aboulafia AA, Malawer MM. Giant cell tumor of the tendon sheath: MR findings in nine cases. AJR Am J Roentgenol 1994; 162: 919–922

[216] Kitagawa Y, Ito H, Amano Y, Sawaizumi T, Takeuchi T. MR imaging for preoperative diagnosis and assessment of local tumor extent on localized giant cell tumor of tendon sheath. Skeletal Radiol 2003; 32: 633–638

[217] Llauger J, Palmer J, Rosón N, Cremades R, Bagué S. Pigmented villonodular synovitis and giant cell tumors of the tendon sheath: radiologic and pathologic features. AJR Am J Roentgenol 1999; 172: 1087–1091

[218] Ly JQ, Carlson CL, LaGatta LM, Beall DP. Giant cell tumor of the peroneus tendon sheath. AJR Am J Roentgenol 2003; 180: 1442

[219] Meyers SP. Giant cell tumor of the tendon sheath and/or soft tissue. In: MRI of Bone and Soft Tissue Tumors and Tumorlike Lesions. Stuttgart, Germany: Thieme; 2008:469–475

[220] Monaghan H, Salter DM, Al-Nafussi A. Giant cell tumour of tendon sheath (localised nodular tenosynovitis): clinicopathological features of 71 cases. J Clin Pathol 2001; 54: 404–407

[221] Somerhausen N, Cin PD. Giant cell tumor of the tendon sheath. In: Fletcher CDM, Unni KK, Mertens F, eds. World Health Organization Classification of Tumours. Pathology and Genetics of Tumours of Soft Tissue and Bone. Lyon, France: IARC Press; 2002:110–111

[222] Somerhausen N, Cin PD. Diffuse-type giant cell tumor of the tendon sheath. In: Fletcher CDM, Unni KK, Mertens F, eds. World Health Organization Classification of Tumours. Pathology and Genetics of Tumours of Soft Tissue and Bone. Lyon, France: IARC Press; 2002: 112–114

[223] Wu NL, Hsiao PF, Chen BF, Chen HC, Su HY. Malignant giant cell tumor of the tendon sheath. Int J Dermatol 2004; 43: 54–57

▶ Glomus Tumor

[224] Baek HJ, Lee SJ, Cho KH, et al. Subungual tumors: clinicopathologic correlation with US and MR imaging findings. Radiographics 2010; 30: 1621–1636

[225] Bhaskaranand K, Navadgi BC. Glomus tumour of the hand. J Hand Surg [Br] 2002; 27: 229–231

[226] Boudghene FP, Gouny P, Tassart M, Callard P, Le Breton C, Vayssairat M. Subungual glomus tumor: combined use of MRI and three-dimensional contrast MR angiography. J Magn Reson Imaging 1998; 8: 1326–1328

[227] Dalrymple NC, Hayes J, Bessinger VJ, Wolfe SW, Katz LD. MRI of multiple glomus tumors of the finger. Skeletal Radiol 1997; 26: 664–666

[228] Drapé JL, Idy-Peretti I, Goettmann S, et al. Subungual glomus tumors: evaluation with MR imaging. Radiology 1995; 195: 507–515

[229] Folpe AL. Glomus tumours. In: Fletcher CDM, Unni KK, Mertens F, eds. World Health Organization Classification of Tumours. Pathology and Genetics of Tumours of Soft Tissue and Bone. Lyon, France: IARC Press; 2002:136–137

[230] Meyers SP. Glomus tumor. In: MRI of Bone and Soft Tissue Tumors and Tumorlike Lesions. Stuttgart, Germany: Thieme; 2008:476–478

[231] Opdenakker G, Gelin G, Palmers Y. MR imaging of a subungual glomus tumor. AJR Am J Roentgenol 1999; 172: 250–251

[232] Perks FJ, Beggs I, Lawson GM, Davie R. Juxtacortical glomus tumor of the distal femur adjacent to the popliteal fossa. AJR Am J Roentgenol 2003; 181: 1590–1592

[233] Theumann NH, Goettmann S, Le Viet D, et al. Recurrent glomus tumors of fingertips: MR imaging evaluation. Radiology 2002; 223: 143–151

[234] Tomak Y, Akcay I, Dabak N, Eroglu L. Subungual glomus tumours of the hand: diagnosis and treatment of 14 cases. Scand J Plast Reconstr Surg Hand Surg 2003; 37: 121–124

▶ Glycogen Storage Disease

[235] Scherer A, Engelbrecht V, Neises G, et al. MR imaging of bone marrow in glycogen storage disease type IB in children and young adults. AJR Am J Roentgenol 2001; 177: 421–425

▶ Gout

[236] Liu SZ, Yeh LR, Chou YJ, Chen CKH, Pan HB. Isolated intraosseous gout in hallux sesamoid mimicking a bone tumor in a teenaged patient. Skeletal Radiol 2003; 32: 647–650

[237] Meyers SP. Gout. In: MRI of Bone and Soft Tissue Tumors and Tumorlike Lesions. Stuttgart, Germany: Thieme; 2008: 479–483

[238] Monu JUV, Pope TL. Gout: a clinical and radiologic review. Radiol Clin North Am 2004; 42: 169–184

[239] Yu JS, Chung C, Recht M, Dailiana T, Jurdi R. MR imaging of tophaceous gout. AJR Am J Roentgenol 1997; 168: 523–527

▶ Granulocyte/Macrophage Colony Stimulating Factor

[240] Altehoefer C, Bertz H, Ghanem NA, Langer M. Extent and time course of morphological changes of bone marrow induced by granulocyte-colony

stimulating factor as assessed by magnetic resonance imaging of healthy blood stem cell donors. J Magn Reson Imaging 2001; 14: 141–146

[241] Chabanova E, Johnsen HE, Knudsen LM, et al. Magnetic resonance investigation of bone marrow following priming and stem cell mobilization. J Magn Reson Imaging 2006; 24: 1364–1370

[242] Ciray I, Lindman H, Aström GKO, Wanders A, Bergh J, Ahlström HK. Effect of granulocyte colony-stimulating factor (G-CSF)-supported chemotherapy on MR imaging of normal red bone marrow in breast cancer patients with focal bone metastases. Acta Radiol 2003; 44: 472–484

[243] Hartman RP, Sundaram M, Okuno SH, Sim FH. Effect of granulocyte-stimulating factors on marrow of adult patients with musculoskeletal malignancies: incidence and MRI findings. AJR Am J Roentgenol 2004; 183: 645–653

▸ Hemangioendothelioma

[244] Boutin RD, Spaeth HJ, Mangalik A, Sell JJ. Epithelioid hemangioendothelioma of bone. Skeletal Radiol 1996; 25: 391–395

[245] Brennan JW, Midha R, Ang LC, Perez-Ordonez B. Epithelioid hemangioendothelioma of the spine presenting as cervical myelopathy: case report. Neurosurgery 2001; 48: 1166–1169

[246] Calonje E. Retiform haemangioendothelioma. In: Fletcher CDM, Unni KK, Mertens F, eds. World Health Organization Classification of Tumours. Pathology and Genetics of Tumours of Soft Tissue and Bone. Lyon, France: IARC Press; 2002:165–166

[247] Calonje E. Papillary intralymphatic angioendothelioma. In: Fletcher CDM, Unni KK, Mertens F, eds. World Health Organization Classification of Tumours. Pathology and Genetics of Tumours of Soft Tissue and Bone. Lyon, France: IARC Press; 2002:167

[248] Larochelle O, Périgny M, Lagacé R, Dion N, Giguère C. Best cases from the AFIP: epithelioid hemangioendothelioma of bone. Radiographics 2006; 26: 265–270

[249] Meyers SP. Hemangioendothelioma. In: MRI of Bone and Soft Tissue Tumors and Tumorlike Lesions. Stuttgart, Germany: Thieme; 2008:484–490

[250] Rubin BP. Composite haemangioendothelioma. In: Fletcher CDM, Unni KK, Mertens F, eds. World Health Organization Classification of Tumours. Pathology and Genetics of Tumours of Soft Tissue and Bone. Lyon, France: IARC Press; 2002:168–169

[251] Tsang WYW. Kaposiform haemangioendothelioma. In: Fletcher CDM, Unni KK, Mertens F, eds. World Health Organization Classification of Tumours. Pathology and Genetics of Tumours of Soft Tissue and Bone. Lyon, France: IARC Press; 2002:163–164

[252] Weiss SW, Bridge JA. Epithelioid haemangioendothelioma. In: Fletcher CDM, Unni KK, Mertens F, eds. World Health Organization Classification of Tumours. Pathology and Genetics of Tumours of Soft Tissue and Bone. Lyon, France: IARC Press; 2002:173–174

[253] Wenger DE, Wold LE. Malignant vascular lesions of bone: radiologic and pathologic features. Skeletal Radiol 2000; 29: 619–631

▸ Hemangioma

[254] Adler CP, Wold L. Haemangioma and related lesions. In: Fletcher CDM, Unni KK, Mertens F, eds. World Health Organization Classification of Tumours. Pathology and Genetics of Tumours of Soft Tissue and Bone. Lyon, France: IARC Press; 2002:320–323

[255] Calonje E. Haemangiomas. In: Fletcher CDM, Unni KK, Mertens F, eds. World Health Organization Classification of Tumours. Pathology and Genetics of Tumours of Soft Tissue and Bone. Lyon, France: IARC Press; 2002:156–158

[256] Fetsch JF. Epithelioid haemangioma. In: Fletcher CDM, Unni KK, Mertens F, eds. World Health Organization Classification of Tumours. Pathology and Genetics of Tumours of Soft Tissue and Bone. Lyon, France: IARC Press; 2002:159–160

[257] Meyers SP. Hemangiomas. In: MRI of Bone and Soft Tissue Tumors and Tumorlike Lesions. Stuttgart, Germany: Thieme; 2008:491–501

[258] Yochum TR, Lile RL, Schultz GD, Mick TJ, Brown CW. Acquired spinal stenosis secondary to an expanding thoracic vertebral hemangioma. Spine 1993; 18: 299–305

▸ Hemangiopericytoma

[259] Gengler C, Guillou L. Solitary fibrous tumour and haemangiopericytoma: evolution of a concept. Histopathology 2006; 48: 63–74

[260] Guillou L, Fletcher JA, Fletcher CDM, Mandahl N. Extrapleural solitary fibrous tumour and haemangiopericytoma. In: Fletcher CDM, Unni KK, Mertens F, eds. World Health Organization Classification of Tumours. Pathology and Genetics of Tumours of Soft Tissue and Bone. Lyon, France: IARC Press; 2002:86–90

[261] Juan CJ, Huang GS, Hsueh CJ, et al. Primary hemangiopericytoma of the tibia: MR and angiographic correlation. Skeletal Radiol 2000; 29: 49–53

[262] Meyers SP. Hemangiopericytoma. In: MRI of Bone and Soft Tissue Tumors and Tumorlike Lesions. Stuttgart, Germany: Thieme; 2008:502–506

[263] Rodriguez-Galindo C, Ramsey K, Jenkins JJ, et al. Hemangiopericytoma in children and infants. Cancer 2000; 88: 198–204

▸ Hematologic Disorders

[264] Lorand-Metze I, Santiago GF, Lima CSP, Zanardi VA, Torriani M. Magnetic resonance imaging of femoral marrow cellularity in hypocellular haemopoietic disorders. Clin Radiol 2001; 56: 107–110

[265] Loevner LA, Tobey JD, Yousem DM, Sonners AI, Hsu WC. MR imaging characteristics of cranial bone marrow in adult patients with underlying systemic disorders compared with healthy control subjects. AJNR Am J Neuroradiol 2002; 23: 248–254

[266] Tyler PA, Madani G, Chaudhuri R, Wilson LF, Dick EA. The radiological appearances of thalassaemia. Clin Radiol 2006; 61: 40–52

▸ Hematopoietic Disorders

[267] Dibbern DA, Loevner LA, Lieberman AP, Salhany KE, Freese A, Marcotte PJ. MR of thoracic cord compression caused by epidural extramedullary hematopoiesis in myelodysplastic syndrome. AJNR Am J Neuroradiol 1997; 18: 363–366

[268] Levin TL, Sheth SS, Hurlet A, et al. MR marrow signs of iron overload in transfusion-dependent patients with sickle cell disease. Pediatr Radiol 1995; 25: 614–619

[269] Niggemann P, Krings T, Hans F, Thron A. Fifteen-year follow-up of a patient with beta thalassaemia and extramedullary haematopoietic tissue compressing the spinal cord. Neuroradiology 2005; 47: 263–266

[270] Salehi SA, Koski T, Ondra SL. Spinal cord compression in beta-thalassemia: case report and review of the literature. Spinal Cord 2004; 42: 117–123

[271] States LJ. Imaging of metabolic bone disease and marrow disorders in children. Radiol Clin North Am 2001; 39: 749–772

▸ Hemochromatosis/Iron Overload

[272] Emy PY, Levin TL, Sheth SS, Ruzal-Shapiro C, Garvin J, Berdon WE. Iron overload in reticuloendothelial systems of pediatric oncology patients who have undergone transfusions: MR observations. AJR Am J Roentgenol 1997; 168: 1011–1015

[273] Kornreich L, Horev G, Yaniv I, Stein J, Grunebaum M, Zaizov R. Iron overload following bone marrow transplantation in children: MR findings. Pediatr Radiol 1997; 27: 869–872

[274] Levin TL, Sheth SS, Hurlet A, et al. MR marrow signs of iron overload in transfusion-dependent patients with sickle cell disease. Pediatr Radiol 1995; 25: 614–619

▸ Hypertrophic Osteoarthropathy–Primary

[275] Araki Y, Tsukaguchi I, Nakamura H. Pachydermoperiostosis involving the skull and spine: MR findings. AJR Am J Roentgenol 1993; 160: 664–665

[276] Capelastegui A, Astigarraga E, García-Iturraspe C. MR findings in pulmonary hypertrophic osteoarthropathy. Clin Radiol 2000; 55: 72–75

[277] Demirpolat G, Sener RN, Stun EE. MR imaging of pachydermoperiostosis. J Neuroradiol 1999; 26: 61–63

[278] Loredo R, Pathria MN, Salonen D, Resnick D. Magnetic resonance imaging in pachydermoperiostosis. Clin Imaging 1996; 20: 212–218

[279] Resnick D. Enostosis, hyperostosis, and periostitis. In: Resnick D, Draud LA,. Diagnosis of Bone and Joint Disorders.Vol 3. 4th ed.Philadelphia, PA: WBSaunders; 2002:4870–4919

▸ Hypertrophic Osteoarthropathy–Secondary

[280] Capelastegui A, Astigarraga E, García-Iturraspe C. MR findings in pulmonary hypertrophic osteoarthropathy. Clin Radiol 2000; 55: 72–75

[281] Resnick D. Enostosis, hyperostosis, and periostitis. In: Resnick D, Draud LA. Diagnosis of Bone and Joint Disorders.Vol 3. 4th ed.Philadelphia, PA: WBSaunders; 2002:4870–4919

[282] Sainani NI, Lawande MA, Parikh VP, Pungavkar SA, Patkar DP, Sase KS. MRI diagnosis of hypertrophic osteoarthropathy from a remote childhood malignancy. Skeletal Radiol 2007; 36 Suppl 1: S63–S66

[283] Varan A, Kutluk T, Demirkazik FB, Akyüz C, Büyükpamukçu M. Hypertrophic osteoarthropathy in a child with nasopharyngeal carcinoma. Pediatr Radiol 2000; 30: 570–572

▸ Hypervitaminosis A and D/Hypovitaminosis

[284] Lips P. Hypervitaminosis A and fractures. N Engl J Med 2003; 348: 347–349

[285] Romero JB, Schreiber A, Von Hochstetter AR, Wagenhauser FJ, Michel BA, Theiler R. Hyperostotic and destructive osteoarthritis in a patient with vitamin A intoxication syndrome: a case report. Bull Hosp Jt Dis 1996; 54: 169–174

[286] Jiang YB, Wang YZ, Zhao J, et al. Bone remodeling in hypervitaminosis D3. Radiologic-microangiographic-pathologic correlations. Invest Radiol 1991; 26: 213–219

[287] Resnick D. Hypervitaminosis and hypovitaminosis In: Resnick D, Draud LA. Diagnosis of Bone and Joint Disorders.Vol 3. 4th ed.Philadelphia, PA: WBSaunders; 2002:3456–3464

▸ Hypoparathyroidism, Pseudo-, Pseudo-pseudo-hypoparathyroidism

[288] Koch CA. Rapid increase in bone mineral density in a child with osteoporosis and autoimmune hypoparathyroidism treated with PTH 1–34 [Retraction in Exp Clin Endocrinol Diabetes 2002;110(2):100]. Exp Clin Endocrinol Diabetes 2001; 109: 350–354

[289] Rastogi R, Beauchamp NJ, Ladenson PW. Calcification of the basal ganglia in chronic hypoparathyroidism. J Clin Endocrinol Metab 2003; 88: 1476–1477

[290] Resnick D. Parathyroid disorders and renal osteodystrophy. In: Resnick D, Draud LA. Diagnosis of Bone and Joint Disorders. Vol 3. 4th ed.Philadelphia, PA: WBSaunders; 2002:2043–2111

[291] Xiong L, Zeng QY, Jinkins JR. CT and MRI characteristics of ossification of the ligamenta flava in the thoracic spine. Eur Radiol 2001; 11: 1798–1802

[292] Yamamoto Y, Noto Y, Saito M, Ichizen H, Kida H. Spinal cord compression by heterotopic ossification associated with pseudohypoparathyroidism. J Int Med Res 1997; 25: 364–368

▸ Infantile Cortical Hyperostosis (Caffey Disease)

[293] Katz DS, Eller DJ, Bergman G, Blankenberg FG. Caffey's disease of the scapula: CT and MR findings. AJR Am J Roentgenol 1997; 168: 286–287

[294] Resnick D. Enostosis, hyperostosis, and periostitis. In: Resnick D, Draud LA;. Diagnosis of Bone and Joint Disorders.Vol 3. 4th ed.Philadelphia, PA: WBSaunders; 2002:4870–4919

[295] Saatci I, Brown JJ, McAlister WH. MR findings in a patient with Caffey's disease. Pediatr Radiol 1996; 26: 68–70

▸ Inherited Anemias

[296] Aydingöz U, Oto A, Cila A. Spinal cord compression due to epidural extramedullary haematopoiesis in thalassaemia: MRI. Neuroradiology 1997; 39: 870–872

[297] Lorand-Metze I, Santiago GF, Lima CSP, Zanardi VA, Torriani M. Magnetic resonance imaging of femoral marrow cellularity in hypocellular haemopoietic disorders. Clin Radiol 2001; 56: 107–110

[298] Niggemann P, Krings T, Hans F, Thron A. Fifteen-year follow-up of a patient with beta thalassaemia and extramedullary haematopoietic tissue compressing the spinal cord. Neuroradiology 2005; 47: 263–266

[299] Salehi SA, Koski T, Ondra SL. Spinal cord compression in beta-thalassemia: case report and review of the literature. Spinal Cord 2004; 42: 117–123

[300] States LJ. Imaging of metabolic bone disease and marrow disorders in children. Radiol Clin North Am 2001; 39: 749–772

[301] Tan TC, Tsao J, Cheung FC. Extramedullary haemopoiesis in thalassemia intermedia presenting as paraplegia. J Clin Neurosci 2002; 9: 721–725

[302] Tyler PA, Madani G, Chaudhuri R, Wilson LF, Dick EA. The radiological appearances of thalassaemia. Clin Radiol 2006; 61: 40–52

▸ Leiomyoma

[303] Hashimoto H, Quade B. Angioleiomyoma. In: Fletcher CDM, Unni KK, Mertens F, eds. World Health Organization Classification of Tumours. Pathology and Genetics of Tumours of Soft Tissue and Bone. Lyon, France: IARC Press; 2002:128–129

[304] McCarthy E. Leiomyoma of bone. In: Fletcher CDM, Unni KK, Mertens F, eds. World Health Organization Classification of Tumours. Pathology and Genetics of Tumours of Soft Tissue and Bone. Lyon, France: IARC Press; 2002:326

[305] Meyers SP. Leiomyoma. In: MRI of Bone and Soft Tissue Tumors and Tumorlike Lesions. Stuttgart, Germany: Thieme; 2008:521–524

▸ Leiomyosarcoma

[306] Evans HL, Shipley J. Leiomyosarcoma. In: Fletcher CDM, Unni KK, Mertens F, eds. World Health Organization Classification of Tumours. Pathology and Genetics of Tumours of Soft Tissue and Bone. Lyon, France: IARC Press; 2002:131–134

[307] McCarthy E. Leiomyosarcoma of bone. In: Fletcher CDM, Unni KK, Mertens F, eds. World Health Organization Classification of Tumours. Pathology and Genetics of Tumours of Soft Tissue and Bone. Lyon, France: IARC Press; 2002:327

[308] Meyers SP. Leiomyosarcoma. In: MRI of Bone and Soft Tissue Tumors and Tumorlike Lesions. Stuttgart, Germany: Thieme; 2008:525–530

▸ Leukemia

[309] Bollow M, Knauf W, Korfel A, et al. Initial experience with dynamic MR imaging in evaluation of normal bone marrow versus malignant bone marrow infiltrations in humans. J Magn Reson Imaging 1997; 7: 241–250

[310] Hernandez RJ, Teo ELHJ. Diffuse marrow disorders in children. Magn Reson Imaging Clin N Am 1998; 6: 605–626

[311] Kraemer M, Weissinger F, Kraus R, Beer M, Kunzmann V, Wilhelm M. Aseptic necrosis of both femoral heads as first symptom of chronic myelogenous leukemia. Ann Hematol 2003; 82: 44–46

[312] Lal A, Tallman MS, Soble MB, Golubovich I, Peterson L. Hairy cell leukemia presenting as localized skeletal involvement. Leuk Lymphoma 2002; 43: 2207–2211

[313] Lecouvet FE, Vande Berg BC, Michaux L, et al. Early chronic lymphocytic leukemia: prognostic value of quantitative bone marrow MR imaging findings and correlation with hematologic variables. Radiology 1997; 204: 813–818

[314] Leone J, Vilque JP, Pignon B, et al. Avascular necrosis of the femoral head as a complication of chronic myelogenous leukaemia. Skeletal Radiol 1996; 25: 696–698

[315] Meyers SP. Leukemia. In: MRI of Bone and Soft Tissue Tumors and Tumorlike Lesions. Stuttgart, Germany: Thieme; 2008:531–539

[316] Moulopoulos LA, Dimopoulos MA. Magnetic resonance imaging of the bone marrow in hematologic malignancies. Blood 1997; 90: 2127–2147

[317] States LJ. Imaging of metabolic bone disease and marrow disorders in children. Radiol Clin North Am 2001; 39: 749–772

[318] Takagi S, Tanaka O. The role of magnetic resonance imaging in the diagnosis and monitoring of myelodysplastic syndromes or leukemia. Leuk Lymphoma 1996; 23: 443–450

[319] Tardivon AA, Vanel D, Munck JN, Bosq J. Magnetic resonance imaging of the bone marrow in lymphomas and leukemias. Leuk Lymphoma 1997; 25: 55–68

[320] Vande Berg BC, Michaux L, Scheiff JM, et al. Sequential quantitative MR analysis of bone marrow: differences during treatment of lymphoid versus myeloid leukemia. Radiology 1996; 201: 519–523

▸ Lipoma

[321] Campbell RSD, Grainger AJ, Mangham DC, Beggs I, Teh J, Davies AM. Intraosseous lipoma: report of 35 new cases and a review of the literature. Skeletal Radiol 2003; 32: 209–222

[322] Chan LP, Gee R, Keogh C, Munk PL. Imaging features of fat necrosis. AJR Am J Roentgenol 2003; 181: 955–959

[323] Meyers SP. Lipoma, atypical lipoma, and hibernoma. In: MRI of Bone and Soft Tissue Tumors and Tumorlike Lesions. Stuttgart, Germany: Thieme; 2008: 543–553

[324] Nielsen GP, Mandahl N. Lipoma. In: Fletcher CDM, Unni KK, Mertens F, eds. World Health Organization Classification of Tumours. Pathology and Genetics of Tumours of Soft Tissue and Bone. Lyon, France: IARC Press; 2002:20–22

[325] Propeck T, Bullard MA, Lin J, Doi K, Martel W. Radiologic-pathologic correlation of intraosseous lipomas. AJR Am J Roentgenol 2000; 175: 673–678

▸ Liposarcoma

[326] Antonescu C, Ladanyl M. Myxoid liposarcoma. In: Fletcher CDM, Unni KK, Mertens F, eds. World Health Organization Classification of Tumours. Pathology and Genetics of Tumours of Soft Tissue and Bone. Lyon, France: IARC Press; 2002:40–43

[327] Dei Tos AP, Pedeutour F. Atypical lipomatous tumour/Well differentiated liposarcoma. In: Fletcher CDM, Unni KK, Mertens F, eds. World Health Organization Classification of Tumours. Pathology and Genetics of Tumours of Soft Tissue and Bone. Lyon, France: IARC Press; 2002: 35–37

[328] Dei Tos AP, Pedeutour F. Dedifferentiated liposarcoma. In: Fletcher CDM, Unni KK, Mertens F, eds. World Health Organization Classification of Tumours. Pathology and Genetics of Tumours of Soft Tissue and Bone. Lyon, France: IARC Press; 2002:38–39

[329] Meyers SP. Liposarcoma. In: MRI of Bone and Soft Tissue Tumors and Tumorlike Lesions. Stuttgart, Germany: Thieme; 2008: 554–562

▸ Liposclerosing Myxofibrous Tumor

[330] Kransdorf MJ, Murphey MD, Sweet DE. Liposclerosing myxofibrous tumor: a radiologic-pathologic-distinct fibro-osseous lesion of bone with a marked predilection for the intertrochanteric region of the femur. Radiology 1999; 212: 693–698

[331] Matsuba A, Ogose A, Tokunaga K, et al. Activating Gs alpha mutation at the Arg201 codon in liposclerosing myxofibrous tumor. Hum Pathol 2003; 34: 1204–1209

[332] Meyers SP. Liposclerosing myxofibrous tumor. In: MRI of Bone and Soft Tissue Tumors and Tumorlike Lesions. Stuttgart, Germany: Thieme; 2008: 563–565

[333] Murphey MD, Carroll JF, Flemming DJ, Pope TL, Gannon FH, Kransdorf MJ. From the archives of the AFIP: benign musculoskeletal lipomatous lesions. Radiographics 2004; 24: 1433–1466

[334] Ragsdale BD. Polymorphic fibro-osseous lesions of bone: an almost site-specific diagnostic problem of the proximal femur. Hum Pathol 1993; 24: 505–512

▸ Low Grade Myofibroblastic Sarcoma

[335] San Miguel P, Fernández G, Ortiz-Rey JA, Larrauri P. Low-grade myofibroblastic sarcoma of the distal phalanx. J Hand Surg Am 2004; 29: 1160–1163

▸ Lymphoma

[336] Häussler MD, Fenstermacher MJ, Johnston DA, Harle TS. MRI of primary lymphoma of bone: cortical disorder as a criterion for differential diagnosis. J Magn Reson Imaging 1999; 9: 93–100

[337] Hicks DG, Gokan T, O'Keefe RJ, et al. Primary lymphoma of bone: correlation of magnetic resonance imaging features with cytokine production by tumor cells. Cancer 1995; 75: 973–980

[338] Krishnan A, Shirkhoda A, Tehranzadeh J, Armin AR, Irwin R, Les K. Primary bone lymphoma: radiographic-MR imaging correlation. Radiographics 2003; 23: 1371–1383, discussion 1384–1387

[339] Mengiardi B, Honegger H, Hodler J, Exner UG, Csherhati MD, Brühlmann W. Primary lymphoma of bone: MRI and CT characteristics during and after successful treatment. AJR Am J Roentgenol 2005; 184: 185–192

[340] Meyers SP. Lymphoma. In: MRI of Bone and Soft Tissue Tumors and Tumorlike Lesions. Stuttgart, Germany: Thieme; 2008:570–583

[341] Moulopoulos LA, Dimopoulos MA. Magnetic resonance imaging of the bone marrow in hematologic malignancies. Blood 1997; 90: 2127–2147

[342] Parker BR. Leukemia and lymphoma in childhood. Radiol Clin North Am 1997; 35: 1495–1516

[343] Varan A, Cila A, Büyükpamukçu M. Prognostic importance of magnetic resonance imaging in bone marrow involvement of Hodgkin disease. Med Pediatr Oncol 1999; 32: 267–271

[344] Zhang X, Chang CK, Song LX, Xu L, Wu LY, Li X. Primary lymphoma of bone: a case report and review of the literature. Med Oncol 2011; 28: 202–206

▸ Malignant Fibrous Histiocytoma, Myxfibrosarcoma

[345] Link TM, Haeussler MD, Poppek S, et al. Malignant fibrous histiocytoma of bone: conventional X-ray and MR imaging features. Skeletal Radiol 1998; 27: 552–558

[346] Meyers SP. Malignant Fibrous Histiocytoma. In: MRI of Bone and Soft Tissue Tumors and Tumorlike Lesions. Stuttgart, Germany: Thieme; 2008:584–593

[347] Steiner GC, Jundt G, Martignetti JA. Malignant fibous histiocytoma of bone. In: Fletcher CDM, Unni KK, Mertens F, eds. World Health Organization Classification of Tumours. Pathology and Genetics of Tumours of Soft Tissue and Bone. Lyon, France: IARC Press; 2002:294–296

▸ Marrow Hyperplasia from Exogenous Erythropoietin

[348] Djukanovic B-PL, Lezaic V, Stojanovic N, Marisavljevic D, Pavlovic-Kentera V. In vivo effects of recombinant human erythropoietin on bone marrow hematopoeisis in patients with chronic renal failure. Eur J Med Res 1998; 16: 564–570

[349] Horina JH, Schmid CR, Roob JM, et al. Bone marrow changes following treatment of renal anemia with erythropoietin. Kidney Int 1991; 40: 917–922

[350] Jensen KE, Stenver D, Jensen M, et al. Magnetic resonance imaging of the bone marrow following treatment with recombinant human erythropoietin in patients with end-stage renal disease. Int J Artif Organs 1990; 13: 477–481

▸ Mastocytosis

[351] Arias M, Villalba C, Requena I, Vázquez-Veiga H, Sesar A, Pereiro I. Acute spinal epidural hematoma and systemic mastocytosis. Spine 2004; 29: E161–E163

[352] Avila NA, Ling A, Metcalfe DD, Worobec AS. Mastocytosis: magnetic resonance imaging patterns of marrow disease. Skeletal Radiol 1998; 27: 119–126

[353] Boncoraglio GB, Brucato A, Carriero MR, et al. Systemic mastocytosis: a potential neurologic emergency. Neurology 2005; 65: 332–333

[354] Fritz J, Fishman EK, Carrino JA, Horger MS. Advanced imaging of skeletal manifestations of systemic mastocytosis. Skeletal Radiol 2012; 41: 887–897epub ahead of print

[355] Myers B, Grimley C, Jones SG, Clark D, Kerslake R. Skin, bone marrow and magnetic resonance imaging appearances in systemic mastocytosis. Br J Haematol 2003; 122: 876

[356] Roca M, Mota J, Giraldo P, García Erce JA. Systemic mastocytosis: MRI of bone marrow involvement. Eur Radiol 1999; 9: 1094–1097

[357] Siegel S, Sadler MA, Yook C, Chang V, Miller J. Systemic mastocytosis with involvement of the pelvis: a radiographic and clinicopathologic study—a case report. Clin Imaging 1999; 23: 245–248

[358] Valent P, Horny HP, Li CY, et al. Mastocytosis. In: Jaffe ES, Harris NL, Sein H, Vardiman JW, eds. World Health Organization Classification of Tumours. Pathology and Genetics of Tumours. Tumours of Haematopoietic and Lymphoid Tissues. Lyon, France: IARC Press; 2001:293–302

▸ Metastatic Lesions

[359] Algra PR, Heimans JJ, Valk J, Nauta JJ, Lachniet M, Van Kooten B. Do metastases in vertebrae begin in the body or the pedicles? Imaging study in 45 patients. AJR Am J Roentgenol 1992; 158: 1275–1279

[360] Baker LL, Goodman SB, Perkash I, Lane B, Enzmann DR. Benign versus pathologic compression fractures of vertebral bodies: assessment with conventional spin-echo, chemical-shift, and STIR MR imaging. Radiology 1990; 174: 495–502

[361] Kim SH, Smith SE, Mulligan ME. Hematopoietic tumors and metastases involving bone. Radiol Clin North Am 2011; 49: 1163–1183, vi

[362] Meyers SP. Metastatic lesions. In: MRI of Bone and Soft Tissue Tumors and Tumorlike Lesions. Stuttgart, Germany: Thieme; 2008:601–608

[363] Schweitzer ME, Levine C, Mitchell DG, Gannon FH, Gomella LG. Bull's-eyes and halos: useful MR discriminators of osseous metastases. Radiology 1993; 188: 249–252

[364] Wenaden AET, Szyszko TA, Saifuddin A. Imaging of periosteal reactions associated with focal lesions of bone. Clin Radiol 2005; 60: 439–456

▸ Multiple Myeloma

[365] Lecouvet FE, Vande Berg BC, Michaux L, et al. Stage III multiple myeloma: clinical and prognostic value of spinal bone marrow MR imaging. Radiology 1998; 209: 653–660

[366] Libshitz HI, Malthouse SR, Cunningham D, MacVicar AD, Husband JE. Multiple myeloma: appearance at MR imaging. Radiology 1992; 182: 833–837

[367] Meyers SP. Multiple myeloma. In: MRI of Bone and Soft Tissue Tumors and Tumorlike Lesions. Stuttgart, Germany: Thieme; 2008:611–617

[368] Moulopoulos LA, Dimopoulos MA. Magnetic resonance imaging of the bone marrow in hematologic malignancies. Blood 1997; 90: 2127–2147

[369] Moulopoulos LA, Varma DG, Dimopoulos MA, et al. Multiple myeloma: spinal MR imaging in patients with untreated newly diagnosed disease. Radiology 1992; 185: 833–840

[370] Pearce T, Philip S, Brown J, Koh DM, Burn PR. Bone metastases from prostate, breast and multiple myeloma: differences in lesion conspicuity at short-tau inversion recovery and diffusion-weighted MRI. Br J Radiol 2012; 85: 1102–1106

[371] Shaughnessy J. Primer on medical genomics, IX: Scientific and clinical applications of DNA microarrays—multiple myeloma as a disease model. Mayo Clin Proc 2003; 78: 1098–1109

[372] Tan E, Weiss BM, Mena E, Korde N, Choyke PL, Landgren O. Current and future imaging modalities for multiple myeloma and its precursor states. Leuk Lymphoma 2011; 52: 1630–1640

▸ Myelodysplastic Syndromes

[373] Kusumoto S, Jinnai I, Matsuda A, et al. Bone marrow patterns in patients with aplastic anaemia and myelodysplastic syndrome: observations with magnetic resonance imaging. Eur J Haematol 1997; 59: 155–161

[374] Moulopoulos LA, Dimopoulos MA. Magnetic resonance imaging of the bone marrow in hematologic malignancies. Blood 1997; 90: 2127–2147

[375] Olipitz W, Beham-Schmid C, Aigner R, Raith J, Linkesch W, Sill H. Acute myelofibrosis: multifocal bone marrow infiltration detected by scintigraphy and magnetic resonance imaging. Ann Hematol 2000; 79: 275–278

[376] Takagi S, Tanaka O, Origasa H, Miura Y. Prognostic significance of magnetic resonance imaging of femoral marrow in patients with myelodysplastic syndromes. J Clin Oncol 1999; 17: 277–283

[377] Vardiman JW. Myelodysplastic/myeloproliferative diseases: introduction. In: Jaffe ES, Harris NL, Sein H, Vardiman JW, eds. World Health Organization Classification of Tumours. Pathology and Genetics of Tumours. Tumours of Haematopoeitic and Lymphoid Tissues. Lyon, France: IARC Press; 2001:47–48

▸ Neurofibroma, Malignant Peripheral Nerve Sheath Tumor

[378] Khong PL, Goh WH, Wong VC, Fung CW, Ooi GC. MR imaging of spinal tumors in children with neurofibromatosis 1. AJR Am J Roentgenol 2003; 180: 413–417

[379] Meyers SP. Neurofibroma, malignant peripheral nerve sheath tumor. In: MRI of Bone and Soft Tissue Tumors and Tumorlike Lesions. Stuttgart, Germany: Thieme; 2008:633–641

[380] Von Deimling A, Foster R, Krone W. Neurofibromatosis type 1. In: Kleihues P, Cavenee WK, eds. World Health Organization Classification of Tumours. Pathology and Genetics of Tumours of the Nervous System. Lyon, France: IARC Press; 2000:216–218

[381] Woodruff JM, Kourea HP, Louis DN, Scheithauer BW. Neurofibroma. In: Kleihues P, Cavenee WK, eds. World Health Organization Classification of Tumours. Pathology and Genetics of Tumours of the Nervous System. Lyon, France: IARC Press; 2000:167–168

► Osteiitis Condensans

[382] Clarke DP, Higgins JN, Valentine AR, Black C. Magnetic resonance imaging of osteitis condensans ilii. Br J Rheumatol 1994; 33: 599–600

[383] Olivieri I, Ferri S, Barozzi L. Osteitis condensans ilii. Br J Rheumatol 1996; 35: 295–297

[384] Major NM, Helms CA. Pelvic stress injuries: the relationship between osteitis pubis (symphysis pubis stress injury) and sacroiliac abnormalities in athletes. Skeletal Radiol 1997; 26: 711–717

► Osteoblastoma

[385] Atesok KI, Alman BA, Schemitsch EH, Peyser A, Mankin H. Osteoid osteoma and osteoblastoma. J Am Acad Orthop Surg 2011; 19: 678–689

[386] Della Rocca C, Huvos AG. Osteoblastoma: varied histological presentations with a benign clinical course. An analysis of 55 cases. Am J Surg Pathol 1996; 20: 841–850

[387] James SLJ, Panicek DM, Davies AM. Bone marrow oedema associated with benign and malignant bone tumours. Eur J Radiol 2008; 67: 11–21

[388] Kroon HM, Schurmans J. Osteoblastoma: clinical and radiologic findings in 98 new cases. Radiology 1990; 175: 783–790

[389] Malcolm AJ, Schiller AL, Schneider-Stock R. Osteoblastoma. In: Fletcher CDM, Unni KK, Mertens F, eds. World Health Organization Classification of Tumours. Pathology and Genetics of Tumours of Soft Tissue and Bone. Lyon, France: IARC Press; 2002:262–263

[390] Meyers SP. Osteoblastoma. In: MRI of Bone and Soft Tissue Tumors and Tumorlike Lesions. Stuttgart, Germany: Thieme; 2008:668–673

[391] Papagelopoulos PJ, Galanis EC, Sim FH, Unni KK. Clinicopathologic features, diagnosis, and treatment of osteoblastoma. Orthopedics 1999; 22: 244–247, quiz 248–249

[392] Yamamura S, Sato K, Sugiura H, et al. Prostaglandin levels of primary bone tumor tissues correlate with peritumoral edema demonstrated by magnetic resonance imaging. Cancer 1997; 79: 255–261

► Osteochondritis Dissecans

[393] Kijowski R, De Smet AA. MRI findings of osteochondritis dissecans of the capitellum with surgical correlation. AJR Am J Roentgenol 2005; 185: 1453–1459

[394] O'Connor MA, Palaniappan M, Khan N, Bruce CE. Osteochondritis dissecans of the knee in children. A comparison of MRI and arthroscopic findings. J Bone Joint Surg Br 2002; 84: 258–262

[395] Sanders TG, Paruchuri NB, Zlatkin MB. MRI of osteochondral defects of the lateral femoral condyle: incidence and pattern of injury after transient lateral dislocation of the patella. AJR Am J Roentgenol 2006; 187: 1332–1337

[396] Schmid MR, Hodler J, Vienne P, Binkert CA, Zanetti M. Bone marrow abnormalities of foot and ankle: STIR versus T1-weighted contrast-enhanced fat-suppressed spin-echo MR imaging. Radiology 2002; 224: 463–469

► Osteochondroma

[397] Karasick D, Schweitzer ME, Eschelman DJ. Symptomatic osteochondromas: imaging features. AJR Am J Roentgenol 1997; 168: 1507–1512

[398] Kivioja A, Ervasti H, Kinnunen J, Kaitila I, Wolf M, Böhling T. Chondrosarcoma in a family with multiple hereditary exostoses. J Bone Joint Surg Br 2000; 82: 261–266

[399] Khurana J, Abdul-Karim F, Bovee JVMG. Osteochondroma. In: Fletcher CDM, Unni KK, Mertens F, eds. World Health Organization Classification of Tumours. Pathology and Genetics of Tumours of Soft Tissue and Bone. Lyon, France: IARC Press; 2002:234–236

[400] Lee KCY, Davies AM, Cassar-Pullicino VN. Imaging the complications of osteochondromas. Clin Radiol 2002; 57: 18–28

[401] Martin C, Munk PL, O'Connell JX, Lee MJ, Masri B, Wambeek N. Malignant degeneration of an osteochondroma with unusual intra-bursal invasion. Skeletal Radiol 1999; 28: 540–543

[402] Mehta M, White LM, Kna T, Kandel RA, Wunder JS, Bell RS. MR imaging of symptomatic osteochondromas with pathological correlation. Skeletal Radiol 1998; 27: 427–433

[403] Meyers SP. Osteochondroma. In: MRI of Bone and Soft Tissue Tumors and Tumorlike Lesions. Stuttgart, Germany: Thieme; 2008:645–653

[404] Murphey MD, Choi JJ, Kransdorf MJ, Flemming DJ, Gannon FH. Imaging of osteochondroma: variants and complications with radiologic-pathologic correlation. Radiographics 2000; 20: 1407–1434

[405] Pierz KA, Womer RB, Dormans JP. Pediatric bone tumors: osteosarcoma Ewing's sarcoma, and chondrosarcoma associated with multiple hereditary osteochondromatosis. J Pediatr Orthop 2001; 21: 412–418

[406] Sakamoto A, Tanaka K, Matsuda S, Harimaya K, Iwamoto Y. Vascular compression caused by solitary osteochondroma: useful diagnostic methods of magnetic resonance angiography and Doppler ultrasonography. J Orthop Sci 2002; 7: 439–443

[407] Uri DS, Dalinka MK, Kneeland JB. Muscle impingement: MR imaging of a painful complication of osteochondromas. Skeletal Radiol 1996; 25: 689–692

[408] Vanhoenacker FM, Van Hul W, Wuyts W, Willems PJ, De Schepper AM. Hereditary multiple exostoses: from genetics to clinical syndrome and complications. Eur J Radiol 2001; 40: 208–217

[409] Woertler K, Lindner N, Gosheger G, Brinkschmidt C, Heindel W. Osteochondroma: MR imaging of tumor-related complications. Eur Radiol 2000; 10: 832–840

► Osteofibrous Dysplasia

[410] Anderson MJ, Townsend DR, Johnston JO, Bohay DR. Osteofibrous dysplasia in the newborn. Report of a case. J Bone Joint Surg Am 1993; 75: 265–267

[411] Bloem JL, van der Heul RO, Schuttevaer HM, Kuipers D. Fibrous dysplasia vs adamantinoma of the tibia: differentiation based on discriminant analysis of clinical and plain film findings. AJR Am J Roentgenol 1991; 156: 1017–1023

[412] Dominguez R, Saucedo J, Fenstermacher M. MRI findings in osteofibrous dysplasia. Magn Reson Imaging 1989; 7: 567–570

[413] Hindman BW, Bell S, Russo T, Zuppan CW. Neonatal osteofibrous dysplasia: report of two cases. Pediatr Radiol 1996; 26: 303–306

[414] Kahn LB. Adamantinoma, osteofibrous dysplasia and differentiated adamantinoma. Skeletal Radiol 2003; 32: 245–258

[415] Khanna M, Delaney D, Tirabosco R, Saifuddin A. Osteofibrous dysplasia, osteofibrous dysplasia-like adamantinoma and adamantinoma: correlation of radiological imaging features with surgical histology and assessment of the use of radiology in contributing to needle biopsy diagnosis. Skeletal Radiol 2008; 37: 1077–1084

[416] Meyers SP. Osteofibrous dysplasia. In: MRI of Bone and Soft Tissue Tumors and Tumorlike Lesions. Stuttgart, Germany: Thieme; 2008:654–659

[417] Park YK, Unni KK, McLeod RA, Pritchard DJ. Osteofibrous dysplasia: clinicopathologic study of 80 cases. Hum Pathol 1993; 24: 1339–1347

[418] Sakamoto A, Oda Y, Iwamoto Y, Tsuneyoshi M. A comparative study of fibrous dysplasia and osteofibrous dysplasia with regard to expressions of c-fos and c-jun products and bone matrix proteins: a clinicopathologic review and immunohistochemical study of c-fos, c-jun, type I collagen, osteonectin, osteopontin, and osteocalcin. Hum Pathol 1999; 30: 1418–1426

[419] Sakamoto A, Oda Y, Oshiro Y, Tamiya S, Iwamoto Y, Tsuneyoshi M. Immunoexpression of neurofibromin, S-100 protein, and leu-7 and mutation analysis of the NF1 gene at codon 1423 in osteofibrous dysplasia. Hum Pathol 2001; 32: 1245–1251

[420] Vigorita VJ, Ghelman B, Hogendoorn PCW. Osteofibrous dysplasia. In: Fletcher CDM, Unni KK, Mertens F, eds. World Health Organization Classification of Tumours. Pathology and Genetics of Tumours of Soft Tissue and Bone. Lyon, France: IARC Press; 2002:343–344

► Osteoid Osteoma

[421] Assoun J, Richardi G, Railhac JJ, et al. Osteoid osteoma: MR imaging versus CT. Radiology 1994; 191: 217–223

[422] Chai JW, Hong SH, Choi JY, et al. Radiologic diagnosis of osteoid osteoma: from simple to challenging findings. Radiographics 2010; 30: 737–749

[423] Ebrahim FS, Jacobson JA, Lin J, Housner JA, Hayes CW, Resnick D. Intraarticular osteoid osteoma: sonographic findings in three patients with radiographic, CT, and MR imaging correlation. AJR Am J Roentgenol 2001; 177: 1391–1395

[424] Ehara S, Rosenthal DI, Aoki J, et al. Peritumoral edema in osteoid osteoma on magnetic resonance imaging. Skeletal Radiol 1999; 28: 265–270

[425] Iyer RS, Chapman T, Chew FS. Pediatric bone imaging: diagnostic imaging of osteoid osteoma. AJR Am J Roentgenol 2012; 198: 1039–1052

[426] Kayser F, Resnick D, Haghighi P, et al. Evidence of the subperiosteal origin of osteoid osteomas in tubular bones: analysis by CT and MR imaging. AJR Am J Roentgenol 1998; 170: 609–614

[427] Klein MJ, Parisien MV, Schneider-Stock R. Osteoid osteoma. In: Fletcher CDM, Unni KK, Mertens F, eds. World Health Organization Classification of Tumours. Pathology and Genetics of Tumours of Soft Tissue and Bone. Lyon, France: IARC Press; 2002:260–261

[428] Kransdorf MJ, Stull MA, Gilkey FW, Moser RP. Osteoid osteoma. Radiographics 1991; 11: 671–696

[429] Meyers SP. Osteoid Osteoma. In: MRI of Bone and Soft Tissue Tumors and Tumorlike Lesions. Stuttgart, Germany: Thieme; 2008:660–667

[430] Rosenthal DI, Hornicek FJ, Torriani M, Gebhardt MC, Mankin HJ. Osteoid osteoma: percutaneous treatment with radiofrequency energy. Radiology 2003; 229: 171–175

[431] Spouge AR, Thain LM. Osteoid osteoma: MR imaging revisited. Clin Imaging 2000; 24: 19–27

[432] Woods ER, Martel W, Mandell SH, Crabbe JP. Reactive soft-tissue mass associated with osteoid osteoma: correlation of MR imaging features with pathologic findings. Radiology 1993; 186: 221–225

▸ Osteoma, Enostoses/Bone Islands, Osteopoikilosis, and Melorheostosis

[433] Avrahami E, Even I. Osteoma of the inner table of the skull—CT diagnosis. Clin Radiol 2000; 55: 435–438

[434] Cerase A, Priolo F. Skeletal benign bone-forming lesions. Eur J Radiol 1998; 27 Suppl 1: S91–S97

[435] Chikuda H, Goto T, Ishida T, Iijima T, Nakamura K. Juxtacortical osteoma of the ulna. J Orthop Sci 2002; 7: 721–723

[436] Lambiase RE, Levine SM, Terek RM, Wyman JJ. Long bone surface osteomas: imaging features that may help avoid unnecessary biopsies. AJR Am J Roentgenol 1998; 171: 775–778

[437] Meyers SP. Osteoma, enostoses, osteopoikilosis, and melorheostosis. In: MRI of Bone and Soft Tissue Tumors and Tumorlike Lesions. Stuttgart, Germany: Thieme; 2008:674–678

[438] Motimaya A, Meyers SP. Melorheotosis involving the cervical and upper thoracic spine: radiographic, CT and MR imaging findings. AJNR Am J Neuroradiol 2006; 27: 1198–1200

[439] Peyser AB, Makley JT, Callewart CC, Brackett B, Carter JR, Abdul-Karim FW. Osteoma of the long bones and the spine. A study of eleven patients and a review of the literature. J Bone Joint Surg Am 1996; 78: 1172–1180

[440] Sundaram M, Falbo S, McDonald D, Janney C. Surface osteomas of the appendicular skeleton. AJR Am J Roentgenol 1996; 167: 1529–1533

▸ Osteomyelitis

[441] Chhem RK, Wang S, Jaovisidha S, et al. Imaging of fungal, viral, and parasitic musculoskeletal and spinal diseases. Radiol Clin North Am 2001; 39: 357–378

[442] De Vuyst D, Vanhoenacker F, Gielen J, Bernaerts A, De Schepper AM. Imaging features of musculoskeletal tuberculosis. Eur Radiol 2003; 13: 1809–1819

[443] Jaramillo D. Infection: musculoskeletal. Pediatr Radiol 2011; 41 Suppl 1: S127–S134

[444] Karchevsky M, Schweitzer ME, Morrison WB, Parellada JA. MRI findings of septic arthritis and associated osteomyelitis in adults. AJR Am J Roentgenol 2004; 182: 119–122

[445] Kleinman PK. A regional approach to osteomyelitis of the lower extremities in children. Radiol Clin North Am 2002; 40: 1033–1059

[446] Ledermann HP, Morrison WB, Schweitzer ME. MR image analysis of pedal osteomyelitis: distribution, patterns of spread, and frequency of associated ulceration and septic arthritis. Radiology 2002; 223: 747–755

[447] Ledermann HP, Morrison WB, Schweitzer ME. Pedal abscesses in patients suspected of having pedal osteomyelitis: analysis with MR imaging. Radiology 2002; 224: 649–655

[448] Marui T, Yamamoto T, Akisue T, et al. Subacute osteomyelitis of long bones: diagnostic usefulness of the "penumbra sign" on MRI. Clin Imaging 2002; 26: 314–318

[449] Meyers SP. Osteomyelitis. In: MRI of Bone and Soft Tissue Tumors and Tumorlike Lesions.Stuttgart, Germany: Thieme; 2008:679–692

[450] Moore SL, Rafii M. Imaging of musculoskeletal and spinal tuberculosis. Radiol Clin North Am 2001; 39: 329–342

[451] Oudjhane K, Azouz EM. Imaging of osteomyelitis in children. Radiol Clin North Am 2001; 39: 251–266

[452] Santiago Restrepo C, Giménez CR, McCarthy K. Imaging of osteomyelitis and musculoskeletal soft tissue infections: current concepts. Rheum Dis Clin North Am 2003; 29: 89–109

[453] Sharma P. MR features of tuberculous osteomyelitis. Skeletal Radiol 2003; 32: 279–285

[454] Struk DW, Munk PL, Lee MJ, Ho SG, Worsley DF. Imaging of soft tissue infections. Radiol Clin North Am 2001; 39: 277–303

▸ Osteopetrosis

[455] Curé JK, Key LL, Goltra DD, VanTassel P. Cranial MR imaging of osteopetrosis. AJNR Am J Neuroradiol 2000; 21: 1110–1115

[456] Elster AD, Theros EG, Key LL, Chen MYM. Cranial imaging in autosomal recessive osteopetrosis. Part I. Facial bones and calvarium. Radiology 1992; 183: 129–135

[457] Martin D, Chapman T. Infantile osteopetrosis on head CT. Pediatr Radiol 2009; 39: 308

[458] Tolar J, Teitelbaum SL, Orchard PJ. Osteopetrosis. N Engl J Med 2004; 351: 2839–2849

▸ Osteosarcoma

[459] Ayala AG, Czerniak B, Raymond AK, Knuutila S. Periosteal osteosarcoma. In: Fletcher CDM, Unni KK, Mertens F, eds. World Health Organization Classification of Tumours. Pathology and Genetics of Tumours of Soft Tissue and Bone. Lyon, France: IARC Press; 2002:282–283

[460] Fletcher BD. Imaging pediatric bone sarcomas: diagnosis and treatment-related issues. Radiol Clin North Am 1997; 35: 1477–1494

[461] Forest M. Secondary osteosarcomas. In: Fletcher CDM, Unni KK, Mertens F, eds. World Health Organization Classification of Tumours. Pathology and Genetics of Tumours of Soft Tissue and Bone. Lyon, France: IARC Press; 2002:277–278

[462] Futani H, Okayama A, Maruo S, Kinoshita G, Ishikura R. The role of imaging modalities in the diagnosis of primary dedifferentiated parosteal osteosarcoma. J Orthop Sci 2001; 6: 290–294

[463] Ilaslan H, Sundaram M, Unni KK, Shives TC. Primary vertebral osteosarcoma: imaging findings. Radiology 2004; 230: 697–702

[464] Inwards CY, Knuutila S. Low grade central osteosarcoma. In: Fletcher CDM, Unni KK, Mertens F, eds. World Health Organization Classification of Tumours. Pathology and Genetics of Tumours of Soft Tissue and Bone. Lyon, France: IARC Press; 2002:275–276

[465] Jelinek JS, Murphey MD, Kransdorf MJ, Shmookler BM, Malawer MM, Hur RC. Parosteal osteosarcoma: value of MR imaging and CT in the prediction of histologic grade. Radiology 1996; 201: 837–842

[466] Kalil R, Bridge JA. Small cell osteosarcoma. In: Fletcher CDM, Unni KK, Mertens F, eds. World Health Organization Classification of Tumours. Pathology and Genetics of Tumours of Soft Tissue and Bone. Lyon, France: IARC Press; 2002:273–274

[467] Kaste SC. Imaging pediatric bone sarcomas. Radiol Clin North Am 2011; 49: 749–765, vi–vii

[468] Logan PM, Mitchell MJ, Munk PL. Imaging of variant osteosarcomas with an emphasis on CT and MR imaging. AJR Am J Roentgenol 1998; 171: 1531–1537

[469] Matsuno T, Okada K, Knuutila S. Telangiectatic osteosarcoma. In: Fletcher CDM, Unni KK, Mertens F, eds. World Health Organization Classification of Tumours. Pathology and Genetics of Tumours of Soft Tissue and Bone. Lyon, France: IARC Press; 2002:271–272

[470] Meyers SP. Osteosarcoma. In: MRI of Bone and Soft Tissue Tumors and Tumorlike Lesions. Stuttgart, Germany: Thieme; 2008:693–712

[471] Murphey MD, wan Jaovisidha S, Temple HT, Gannon FH, Jelinek JS, Malawer MM. Telangiectatic osteosarcoma: radiologic-pathologic comparison. Radiology 2003; 229: 545–553

[472] Murphey MD, Robbin MR, McRae GA, Flemming DJ, Temple HT, Kransdorf MJ. The many faces of osteosarcoma. Radiographics 1997; 17: 1205–1231

[473] Murphey MD, Jelinek JS, Temple HT, Flemming DJ, Gannon FH. Imaging of periosteal osteosarcoma: radiologic-pathologic comparison. Radiology 2004; 233: 129–138

[474] Raymond AK, Ayala AG, Knuutila S. Conventional osteosarcoma. In: Fletcher CDM, Unni KK, Mertens F, eds. World Health Organization Classification of Tumours. Pathology and Genetics of Tumours of Soft Tissue and Bone. Lyon, France: IARC Press; 2002:264–270

[475] Reddick WE, Wang S, Xiong X, et al. Dynamic magnetic resonance imaging of regional contrast access as an additional prognostic factor in pediatric osteosarcoma. Cancer 2001; 91: 2230–2237

[476] Tsai JC, Dalinka MK, Fallon MD, Zlatkin MB, Kressel HY. Fluid-fluid level: a nonspecific finding in tumors of bone and soft tissue. Radiology 1990; 175: 779–782

[477] Unni KK, Knuutila S. Parosteal osteosarcoma. In:Fletcher CDM, Unni KK, Mertens F, eds.World Health Organization Classification of Tumours. Pathology and Genetics of Tumours of Soft Tissue and Bone. Lyon, France: IARC Press 2002;279–281

[478] Vanel D, Picci P, De Paolis M, Mercuri M. Radiological study of 12 high-grade surface osteosarcomas. Skeletal Radiol 2001; 30: 667–671

[479] Wold L, McCarthy E, Knuutila S. High grade surface osteosarcoma. Unni KK, Knuutila S. Parosteal osteosarcoma. In: Fletcher CDM, Unni KK, Mertens F, eds. World Health Organization Classification of Tumours. Pathology and Genetics of Tumours of Soft Tissue and Bone. Lyon, France: IARC Press; 2002:284–285

▸ Paget Disease

[480] Boutin RD, Spitz DJ, Newman JS, Lenchik L, Steinbach LS. Complications in Paget disease at MR imaging. Radiology 1998; 209: 641–651

[481] Forest M, De Pineux G. Knuutila. Secondary osteosarcomas. In: Fletcher CDM, Unni KK, Mertens F, eds. World Health Organization Classification of Tumours. Pathology and Genetics of Tumours of Soft Tissue and Bone. Lyon, France: IARC Press; 2002:277–278

[482] Meyers SP. Paget's disease. In: MRI of Bone and Soft Tissue Tumors and Tumorlike Lesions. Stuttgart, Germany: Thieme; 2008:713–720

[483] Sundaram M, Khanna G, El-Khoury GY. T1-weighted MR imaging for distinguishing large osteolysis of Paget's disease from sarcomatous degeneration. Skeletal Radiol 2001; 30: 378–383

[484] Whitten CR, Saifuddin A. MRI of Paget's disease of bone. Clin Radiol 2003; 58: 763–769

▸ Periosteal Reaction

[485] Nichols RE, Dixon LB. Radiographic analysis of solitary bone lesions. Radiol Clin North Am 2011; 49: 1095–1114, v

[486] Wenaden AET, Szyszko TA, Saifuddin A. Imaging of periosteal reactions associated with focal lesions of bone. Clin Radiol 2005; 60: 439–456

[487] Wyers MR. Evaluation of pediatric bone lesions. Pediatr Radiol 2010; 40: 468–473

▸ Pigmented Villonodular Synovitis (PVNS)

[488] Al-Nakshabandi NA, Ryan AG, Choudur H, et al. Pigmented villonodular synovitis. Clin Radiol 2004; 59: 414–420

[489] Meyers SP. Pigmented villonodular synovitis. In: MRI of Bone and Soft Tissue Tumors and Tumorlike Lesions. Stuttgart, Germany: Thieme; 2008:726–729

[490] Murphey MD, Rhee JH, Lewis RB, Fanburg-Smith JC, Flemming DJ, Walker EA. Pigmented villonodular synovitis: radiologic-pathologic correlation. Radiographics 2008; 28: 1493–1518

▸ Red Marrow Reconversion

[491] Barnewolt CE, Shapiro F, Jaramillo D. Normal gadolinium-enhanced MR images of the developing appendicular skeleton, I: Cartilaginous epiphysis and physis. AJR Am J Roentgenol 1997; 169: 183–189

[492] Dwek JR, Shapiro F, Laor T, Barnewolt CE, Jaramillo D. Normal gadolinium-enhanced MR images of the developing appendicular skeleton, II: Epiphyseal and metaphyseal marrow. AJR Am J Roentgenol 1997; 169: 191–196

[493] Moore SG, Dawson KL. Red and yellow marrow in the femur: age-related changes in appearance at MR imaging. Radiology 1990; 175: 219–223

[494] Ollivier L, Gerber S, Vanel D, Brisse H, Leclère J. Improving the interpretation of bone marrow imaging in cancer patients. Cancer Imaging 2006; 20: 194–198

[495] Waitches G, Zawin JK, Poznanski AK. Sequence and rate of bone marrow conversion in the femora of children as seen on MR imaging: are accepted standards accurate? AJR Am J Roentgenol 1994; 162: 1399–1406

▸ Reflex Sympathetic Dystrophy

[496] Bennett DS, Brookoff D. Complex regional pain syndromes (reflex sympathetic dystrophy and causalgia) and spinal cord stimulation. Pain Med 2006; 7 Suppl 1: S64–S96

[497] Crozier F, Champsaur P, Pham T, et al. Magnetic resonance imaging in reflex sympathetic dystrophy syndrome of the foot. Joint Bone Spine 2003; 70: 503–508

[498] Korompilias AV, Karantanas AH, Lykissas MG, Beris AE. Bone marrow edema syndrome. Skeletal Radiol 2009; 38: 425–436

[499] Lechevalier D, Banal F, Damiano J, Imbert I, Magnin J, Boyer B. Reflex sympathetic dystrophy of the foot: MRI with fat suppression is essential (letter with the drafting). Joint Bone Spine 2004; 71: 446–447, author reply 446–447

[500] Quisel A, Gill JM, Witherell P. Complex regional pain syndrome: which treatments show promise? J Fam Pract 2005; 54: 599–603

[501] Quisel A, Gill JM, Witherell P. Complex regional pain syndrome underdiagnosed. J Fam Pract 2005; 54: 524–532

[502] Sintzoff S, Sintzoff S, Stallenberg B, Matos C. Imaging in reflex sympathetic dystrophy. Hand Clin 1997; 13: 431–442

▸ Renal Osteodystrophy–Secondary Hyperparathyroidism, Primary Hyperparathyroidism, Brown Tumor

[503] Al-Gahtany M, Cusimano M, Singer W, Bilbao J, Kovacs K, Marotta T. Brown tumors of the skull base. Case report and review of the literature. J Neurosurg 2003; 98: 417–420

[504] Davies AM, Evans N, Mangham DC, Grimer RJ. MR imaging of brown tumour with fluid-fluid levels: a report of three cases. Eur Radiol 2001; 11: 1445–1449

[505] Hong WS, Sung MS, Chun KA, et al. Emphasis on the MR imaging findings of brown tumor: a report of five cases. Skeletal Radiol 2011; 40: 205–213

[506] Jevtic V. Imaging of renal osteodystrophy. Eur J Radiol 2003; 46: 85–95

[507] Murphey MD, Sartoris DJ, Quale JL, Pathria MN, Martin NL. Musculoskeletal manifestations of chronic renal insufficiency. Radiographics 1993; 13: 357–379

[508] Mustonen AOT, Kiuru MJ, Stahls A, Bohling T, Kivioja A, Koskinen SK. Radicular lower extremity pain as the first symptom of primary hyperparathyroidism. Skeletal Radiol 2004; 33: 467–472

▸ Rhabdomyosarcoma

[509] Lucas DR, Ryan JR, Zalupski MM, Gross ML, Ravindranath Y, Ortman B. Primary embryonal rhabdomyosarcoma of long bone. Case report and review of the literature. Am J Surg Pathol 1996; 20: 239–244

[510] Meyers SP. Rhabdomyosarcoma. In: MRI of Bone and Soft Tissue Tumors and Tumorlike Lesions. Stuttgart, Germany: Thieme; 2008:732–737

▸ Rheumatoid Arthritis

[511] Boutry N, Lardé A, Lapègue F, Solau-Gervais E, Flipo RM, Cotten A. Magnetic resonance imaging appearance of the hands and feet in patients with early rheumatoid arthritis. J Rheumatol 2003; 30: 671–679

[512] Goldbach-Mansky R, Mahadevan V, Yao L, Lipsky PE. The evaluation of bone damage in rheumatoid arthritis with magnetic resonance imaging. Clin Exp Rheumatol 2003; 21 Suppl 31: S50–S53

[513] Meyers SP. Rheumatoid arthritis. In: MRI of Bone and Soft Tissue Tumors and Tumorlike Lesions. Stuttgart, Germany: Thieme; 2008:738–743

[514] Østergaard M, Hansen M, Stoltenberg M, et al. New radiographic bone erosions in the wrists of patients with rheumatoid arthritis are detectable with magnetic resonance imaging a median of two years earlier. Arthritis Rheum 2003; 48: 2128–2131

▸ Sarcoid

[515] Fisher AJ, Gilula LA, Kyriakos M, Holzaepfel CD. MR imaging changes of lumbar vertebral sarcoidosis. AJR Am J Roentgenol 1999; 173: 354–356

[516] Franco M, Passeron C, Tieulie N, Verdier JF, Benisvy D. Long-term radiographic follow-up in a patient with osteosclerotic sarcoidosis of the spine and pelvis. Rev Rhum Engl Ed 1998;65(10):586–590

[517] Jelinek JS, Mark AS, Barth WF. Sclerotic lesions of the cervical spine in sarcoidosis. Skeletal Radiol 1998; 27: 702–704

[518] Meyers SP. Sarcoid. In: MRI of Bone and Soft Tissue Tumors and Tumorlike Lesions. Stuttgart, Germany: Thieme; 2008:744–746

[519] Moore SL, Teirstein AE. Musculoskeletal sarcoidosis: spectrum of appearances at MR imaging. Radiographics 2003; 23: 1389–1399

[520] Poyanli A, Poyanli O, Sencer S, Akan K, Sayrak H, Acunaş B. Vertebral sarcoidosis: imaging findings. Eur Radiol 2000; 10: 92–94

[521] Rúa-Figueroa I, Gantes MA, Erausquin C, Mhaidli H, Montesdeoca A. Vertebral sarcoidosis: clinical and imaging findings. Semin Arthritis Rheum 2002; 31: 346–352

[522] Valencia MP, Deaver PM, Mammarappallil MC. Sarcoidosis of the thoracic and lumbar vertebrae, mimicking metastasis or multifocal osteomyelitis by MRI: case report. Clin Imaging 2009; 33: 478–481

▸ Schwannoma

[523] Meyers SP. Schwannoma. In: MRI of Bone and Soft Tissue Tumors and Tumorlike Lesions. Stuttgart, Germany: Thieme; 2008:747–752

[524] Mutema GK, Sorger J. Intraosseous schwannoma of the humerus. Skeletal Radiol 2002; 31: 419–421

[525] Woodruff JM, Kourea HP, Louis DN, Scheithauer BW. Schwannoma. In: Kleihues P, Cavenee WK, eds. World Health Organization Classification of Tumours. Pathology and Genetics of Tumours of the Nervous System. Lyon, France: IARC Press; 2000:164–166

▸ Serous Atrophy of Marrow

[526] Kuwashima S, Nishimura G, Yamato M, Fujioka M. Magnetic resonance imaging of clival marrow in patients with anorexia nervosa. Acta Paediatr Jpn 1996; 38: 114–117

[527] Okamoto K, Ito J, Ishikawa K, Sakai K, Tokiguchi S. Change in signal intensity on MRI of fat in the head of markedly emaciated patients. Neuroradiology 2001; 43: 134–138

[528] Vande Berg BC, Malghem J, Devuyst O, Maldague BE, Lambert MJ. Anorexia nervosa: correlation between MR appearance of bone marrow and severity of disease. Radiology 1994; 193: 859–864

[529] Vande Berg BC, Malghem J, Lecouvet FE, Lambert M, Maldague BE. Distribution of serouslike bone marrow changes in the lower limbs of patients with anorexia nervosa: predominant involvement of the distal extremities. AJR Am J Roentgenol 1996; 166: 621–625

▸ Sickle Cell Disease with Extramedullary Hematopoiesis

[530] Castelli R, Graziadei G, Karimi M, Cappellini MD. Intrathoracic masses due to extramedullary hematopoiesis. Am J Med Sci 2004; 328: 299–303

[531] Collins WO, Younis RT, Garcia MT. Extramedullary hematopoiesis of the paranasal sinuses in sickle cell disease. Otolaryngol Head Neck Surg 2005; 132: 954–956

▸ Stress Fracture

[532] Ahovuo JA, Kiuru MJ, Visuri T. Fatigue stress fractures of the sacrum: diagnosis with MR imaging. Eur Radiol 2004; 14: 500–505

[533] Berger FH, de Jonge MC, Maas M. Stress fractures in the lower extremity. The importance of increasing awareness amongst radiologists. Eur J Radiol 2007; 62: 16–26

[534] Grangier C, Garcia J, Howarth NR, May M, Rossier P. Role of MRI in the diagnosis of insufficiency fractures of the sacrum and acetabular roof. Skeletal Radiol 1997; 26: 517–524

[535] Meyers SP, Wiener SN. Magnetic resonance imaging features of fractures using the short tau inversion recovery (STIR) sequence: correlation with radiographic findings. Skeletal Radiol 1991; 20: 499–507

▸ Syndromes of Hyperostosis, Osteitis, and Skin Lesions (SAPHO Syndrome)

[536] Boutin RD, Resnick D. The SAPHO syndrome: an evolving concept for unifying several idiopathic disorders of bone and skin. AJR Am J Roentgenol 1998; 170: 585–591

[537] Davies AM, Marino AJ, Evans N, Grimer RJ, Deshmukh N, Mangham DC. SAPHO syndrome: 20-year follow-up. Skeletal Radiol 1999; 28: 159–162

[538] Kirchhoff T, Merkesdal S, Rosenthal H, et al. Diagnostic management of patients with SAPHO syndrome: use of MR imaging to guide bone biopsy at CT for microbiological and histological work-up. Eur Radiol 2003; 13: 2304–2308

[539] Resnick D. Enostosis, hyperostosis, and periostitis. In: Resnick D, Daud LA. Diagnosis of Bone and Joint Disorders. Vol 3. 4th ed.Philadelphia, PA: WBSaunders; 2002:4870–4919

▸ Synovial Cyst

[540] Meyers SP. Synovial cyst. In: MRI of Bone and Soft Tissue Tumors and Tumorlike Lesions. Stuttgart, Germany: Thieme; 2008:758–761

[541] Tschirch FT, Schmid MR, Pfirrmann CW, Romero J, Hodler J, Zanetti M. Prevalence and size of meniscal cysts, ganglionic cysts, synovial cysts of the popliteal space, fluid-filled bursae, and other fluid collections in asymptomatic knees on MR imaging. AJR Am J Roentgenol 2003; 180: 1431–1436

▸ Thyroid Acropachy

[542] Fatourechi V, Ahmed DDF, Schwartz KM. Thyroid acropachy: report of 40 patients treated at a single institution in a 26-year period. J Clin Endocrinol Metab 2002; 87: 5435–5441

[543] Vanhoenacker FM, Pelckmans MC, De Beuckeleer LH, Colpaert CG, De Schepper AM. Thyroid acropachy: correlation of imaging and pathology. Eur Radiol 2001; 11: 1058–1062

▸ Transient Bone Marrow Edema

[544] Balakrishnan A, Schemitsch EH, Pearce D, McKee MD. Distinguishing transient osteoporosis of the hip from avascular necrosis. Can J Surg 2003; 46: 187–192

[545] Korompilias AV, Karantanas AH, Lykissas MG, Beris AE. Bone marrow edema syndrome. Skeletal Radiol 2009; 38: 425–436

[546] Malizos KN, Zibis AH, Dailiana Z, Hantes M, Karachalios T, Karantanas AH. MR imaging findings in transient osteoporosis of the hip [Erratum: Corrected in Eur J Radiol 2005;53(2):322. Karahalios, Theophilos corrected to Karachalios, Theophilos]. Eur J Radiol 2004; 50: 238–244

[547] Toms AP, Marshall TJ, Becker E, Donell ST, Lobo-Mueller EM, Barker T. Regional migratory osteoporosis: a review illustrated by five cases. Clin Radiol 2005; 60: 425–438

[548] Yamamoto T, Kubo T, Hirasawa Y, Noguchi Y, Iwamoto Y, Sueishi K. A clinicopathologic study of transient osteoporosis of the hip. Skeletal Radiol 1999; 28: 621–627

▸ Waldenström Macroglobulinemia

[549] Berger F, Isaacson PG, Piris MA, Harris NL. Lymphoplamacytic lymphoma/ Waldenstrom macroglobulinema. In: Jaffe ES, Harris NL, Sein H, Vardiman JW, eds. World Health Organization Classification of Tumours. Pathology and Genetics of Tumours. Tumours of Haematopoeitic and Lymphoid Tissues. Lyon, France: IARC Press; 2001:132–134

[550] Moulopoulos LA, Dimopoulos MA. Magnetic resonance imaging of the bone marrow in hematologic malignancies. Blood 1997; 90: 2127–2147

Chapter 11

Lesions within Joints

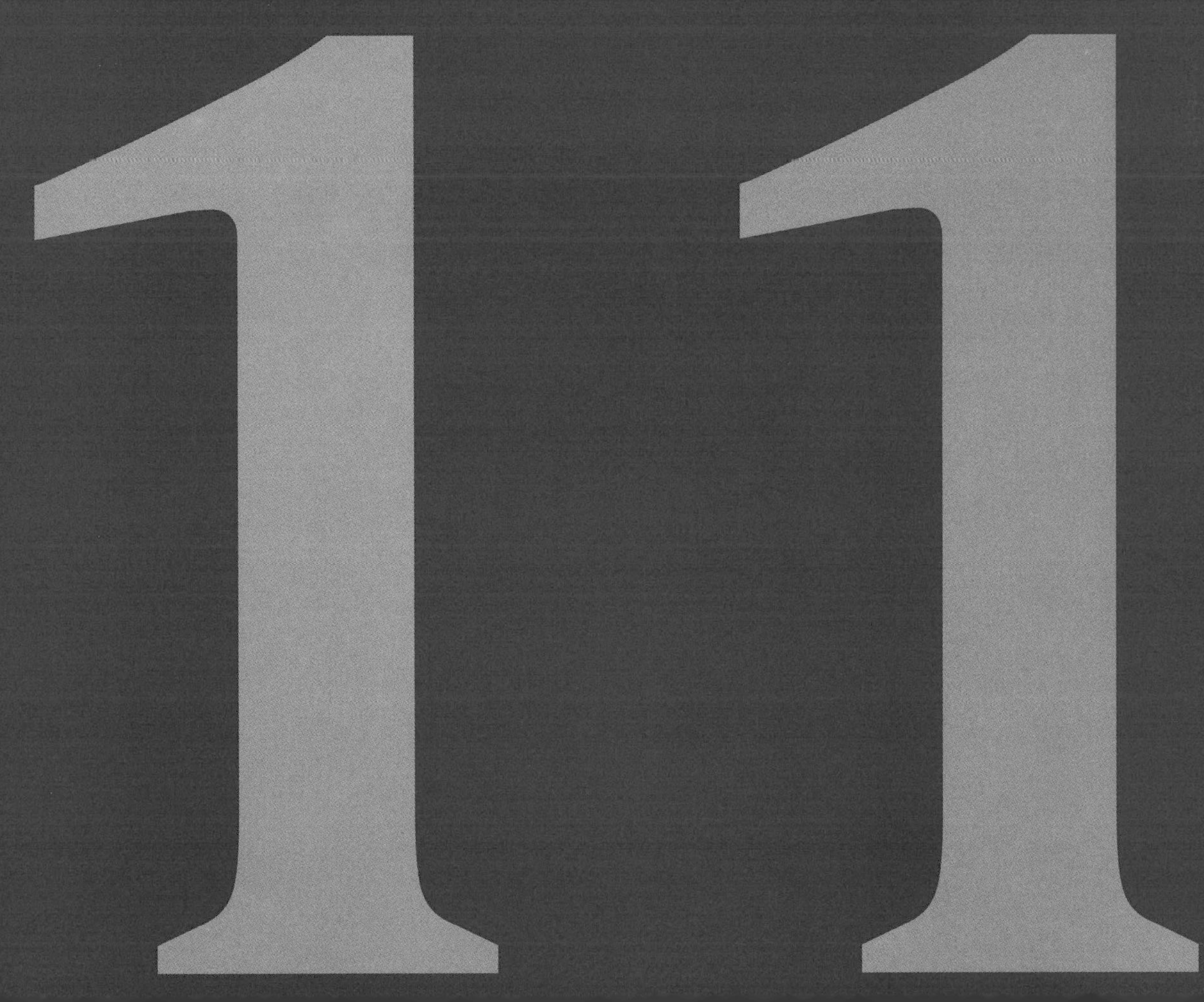

11 Lesions within Joints

Steven P. Meyers

11.1 Tumors and Tumor-Like Lesions within Joints

- Nonmalignant
  - Synovial osteochondroma/osteochondromatosis
  - Synovial chondroma/chondromatosis
  - Pigmented villonodular synovitis (PVNS)
  - Nodular synovitis (also referred to as giant cell tumors of the tendon sheath and soft tissue)
  - Ganglia
  - Meniscal cyst
  - Paralabral cyst
  - Rheumatoid arthritis
  - Juvenile idiopathic arthritis
  - Transient toxic synovitis of the hip
  - Psoriatic arthritis
  - Gout/tophi
  - Calcium pyrophosphate dihydrate (CPPD) deposition disease
  - Eosinophilic granuloma
  - Infectious synovitis
  - Fracture and hemarthrosis
  - Osteochondritis dissecans
  - Synovial hemangioma
  - Lipoma arborescens
  - Intra-articular lipoma
  - Intraosseous giant cell tumor with joint extension
  - Chondroblastoma
  - Osteoid osteoma
  - Osteoblastoma
  - Osteochondroma
- Malignant
  - Intra-articular extension from intraosseous metastatic tumor
  - Intra-articular extension from myeloma
  - Intra-articular extension from lymphoma involving bone
  - Intra-articular extension from leukemia
  - Intra-articular extension from primary malignant bone tumors
  - Synovial chondrosarcoma

Table 11.1 Tumors and tumor-like lesions within joints

Tumor or tumor-like lesion	MRI findings	Comments
Nonmalignant		
Synovial osteochondroma/ osteochondromatosis (▶ Fig. 11.1; ▶ Fig. 11.2)	Magnetic resonance imaging (MRI) features of osteochondromatosis are dependent on the relative proportions of cartilage, calcified cartilage, and mineralized osseous tissue within the lesions. Calcifications result in low signal on T1-weighted imaging (T1WI), proton density–weighted imaging (PDWI), T2-weighted imaging (T2WI), and fat-suppressed (FS) T2WI. Lesions with extensive calcification can have signal voids. Mature ossifications can have peripheral low signal on T1WI and T2WI surrounding a central region with fat signal. Noncalcified portions of the lesions can have low to intermediate signal on T1WI, intermediate signal on PDWI, and slightly high to high signal on T2WI and FS T2WI. Lesions can show irregular, thin-peripheral and/or septal enhancement.	Primary synovial ostechondromatosis is a benign disorder that results from cartilaginous and osseous metaplastic proliferation in the synovium of joints. The osteocartilaginous nodules can become detached forming intra-articular loose bodies. Secondary synovial osteochondromatosis occurs from avulsion of osteochondral fragments into the joint forming loose bodies, which can enlarge via nutrient supply from synovial fluid.

(continued on page 568)

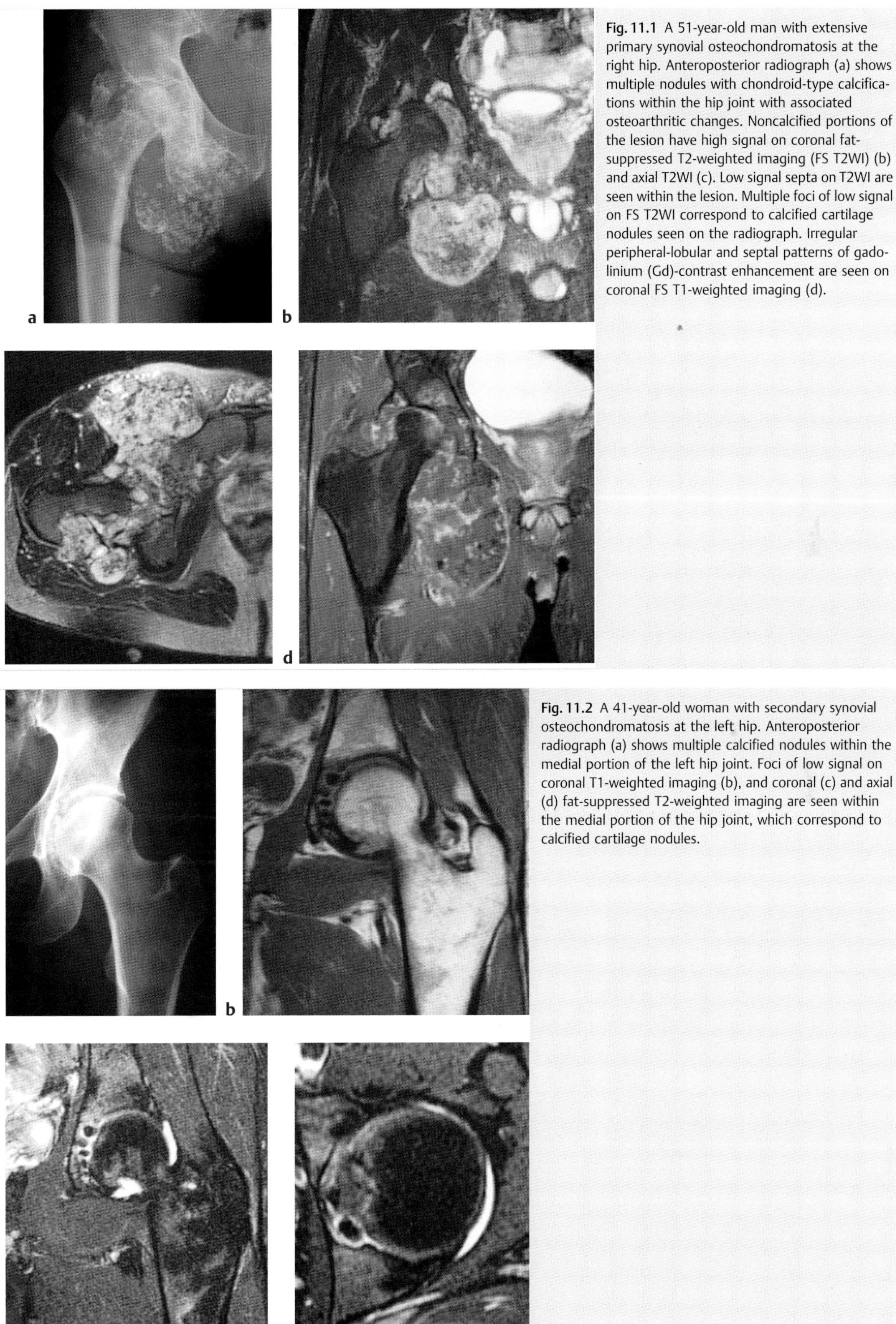

Fig. 11.1 A 51-year-old man with extensive primary synovial osteochondromatosis at the right hip. Anteroposterior radiograph (a) shows multiple nodules with chondroid-type calcifications within the hip joint with associated osteoarthritic changes. Noncalcified portions of the lesion have high signal on coronal fat-suppressed T2-weighted imaging (FS T2WI) (b) and axial T2WI (c). Low signal septa on T2WI are seen within the lesion. Multiple foci of low signal on FS T2WI correspond to calcified cartilage nodules seen on the radiograph. Irregular peripheral-lobular and septal patterns of gadolinium (Gd)-contrast enhancement are seen on coronal FS T1-weighted imaging (d).

Fig. 11.2 A 41-year-old woman with secondary synovial osteochondromatosis at the left hip. Anteroposterior radiograph (a) shows multiple calcified nodules within the medial portion of the left hip joint. Foci of low signal on coronal T1-weighted imaging (b), and coronal (c) and axial (d) fat-suppressed T2-weighted imaging are seen within the medial portion of the hip joint, which correspond to calcified cartilage nodules.

Table 11.1 (Cont.) Tumors and tumor-like lesions within joints

Tumor or tumor-like lesion	MRI findings	Comments
Synovial chondroma/ chondromatosis (▶ Fig. 11.3; ▶ Fig. 11.4)	Synovial chondromas are typically radiolucent and have low to intermediate signal on T1WI (i.e., iso- or hyperintense relative to muscle), intermediate signal on PDWI, and slightly high to high signal on T2WI and FS T2WI. Low signal septae on T2WI can be seen within the lesions. Synovial chondromas can show irregular, thin-peripheral, and/or septal gadolinium-contrast (Gd-contrast) enhancement.	Primary synovial chondromatosis accounts for < 1% of benign soft-tissue tumors and is a benign disorder that results from cartilaginous metaplastic proliferation in synovium of joints. It usually occurs in patients from 25 to 65 years, mean = 44 years. The cartilaginous nodules can become detached, forming intra-articular loose bodies. Metaplasia of connective tissue into cartilage can also occur in bursae and in tendon sheaths. Secondary synovial chondromatosis occurs from avulsion of hyaline cartilage into the joint, forming loose bodies that can enlarge via nutrient supply from synovial fluid.
Pigmented villonodular synovitis (PVNS) (▶ Fig. 11.5)	Often appears as irregular, multinodular, and/or diffuse thickening of synovium. Occasionally occurs as single nodular intra-articular lesions. Lesions often have low or low-intermediate signal on T1WI, PDWI, and T2WI. Areas of low signal on T2WI and T2*WI are secondary to hemosiderin in PVNS. Areas of slightly-high to high signal on T2WI and FS T2WI can also occur from edema and/or inflammatory reaction. Joint effusions are usually present, rarely with fluid/fluid levels. PVNS can show Gd-contrast enhancement in irregular heterogeneous and/or homogeneous patterns.	Benign intra-articular lesions of proliferative synovium (tendon sheaths, joints, and bursae) containing zones of recent or remote hemorrhage. PVNS has similar histopathological features with giant cell tumors of the tendon sheath/nodular synovitis; although PVNS lesions have frondlike or villous growth patterns and contain large amounts of hemosiderin. Accounts for < 1% of benign and all soft-tissue tumors. Patients range in age from 9 to 74 years (mean = 38 years, median age = 32 years).

(continued on page 570)

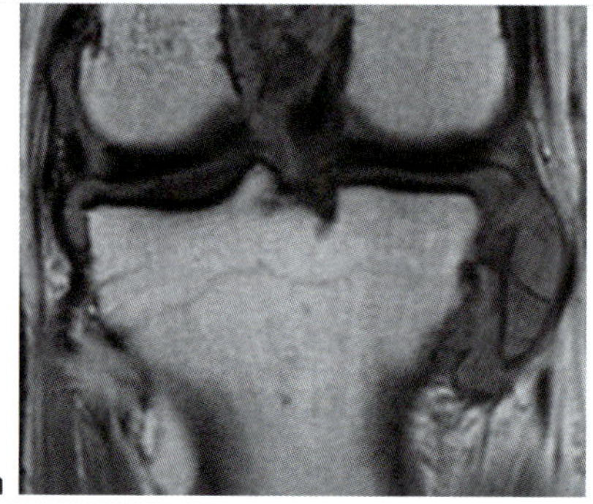
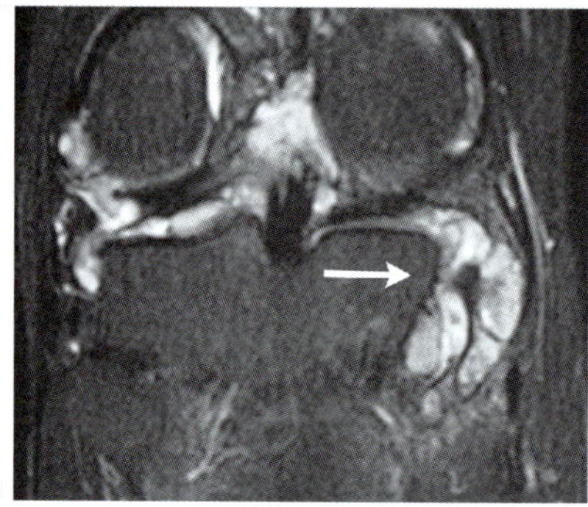
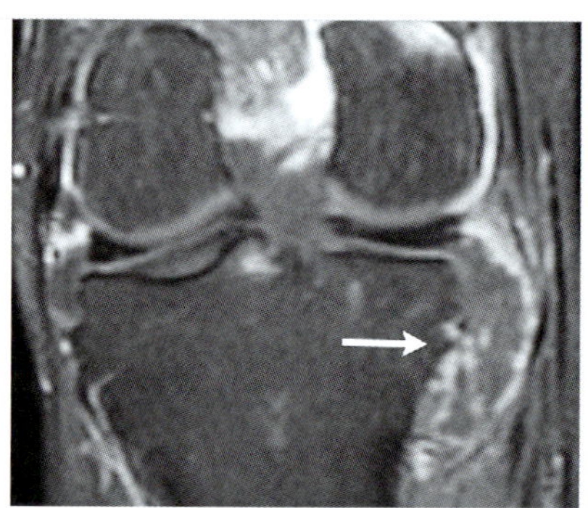

Fig. 11.3 A 37-year-old woman with primary synovial chondromatosis at the knee. Multiple lobulated zones are seen that have intermediate signal on coronal proton density–weighted imaging (PDWI) (a) and high signal (arrow) on coronal fat-suppressed (FS) T2-weighted imaging (b). The lobules have thin margins of low signal. The lesions show irregular peripheral-lobular and septal patterns of Gd-contrast enhancement (arrow) on coronal FS T1-weighted imaging (c). No mineralized zones were seen on radiographs (not shown).

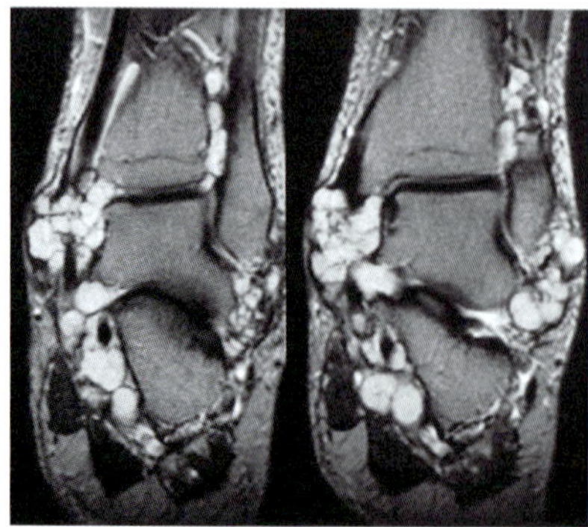
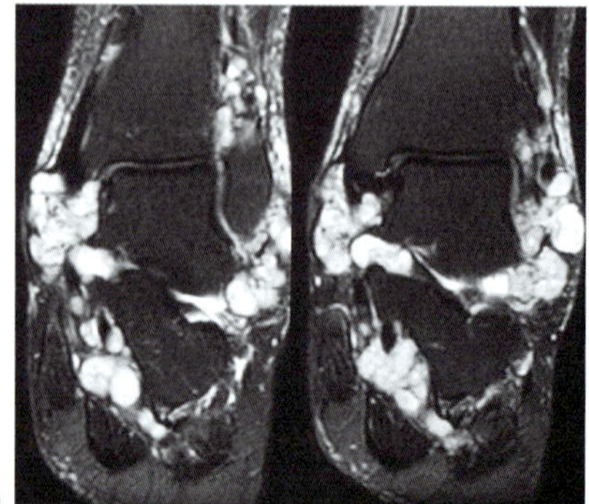
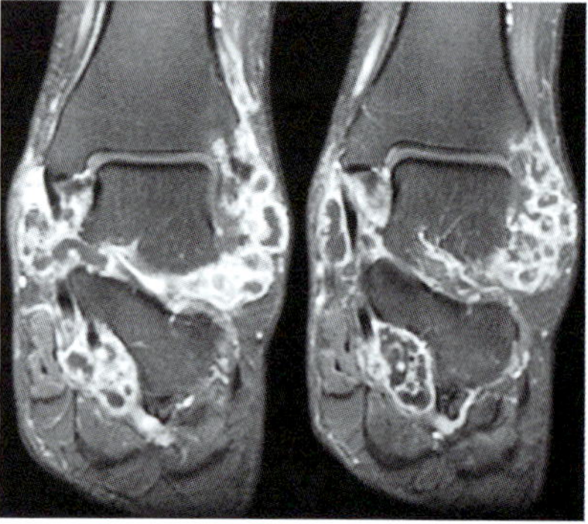

Fig. 11.4 A 57-year-old man with primary synovial chondromatosis at the ankle. Multiple lobulated zones are seen at the ankle joint and tendon sheaths that have high signal on coronal T2-weighted imaging (T2WI) (a) and coronal fat-suppressed (FS) T2WI (b). The lobules have thin margins of low signal on T2WI and FS T2WI. The lesion shows irregular peripheral-lobular and septal patterns of Gd-contrast enhancement on coronal FS T1-weighted imaging (c). No mineralized zones were seen on radiographs (not shown).

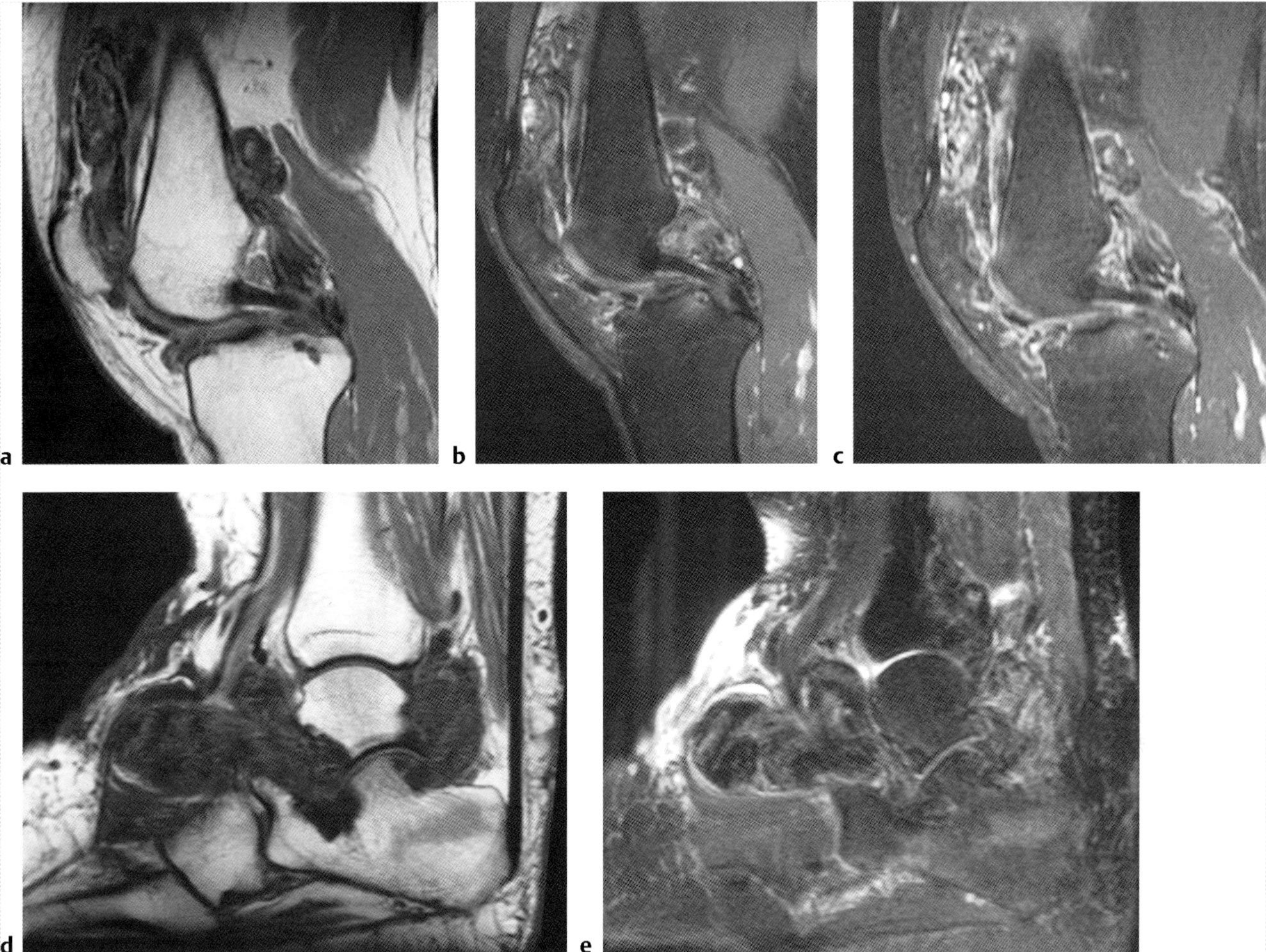

Fig. 11.5 A 36-year-old woman with pigmented villonodular synovitis (PVNS) involving the knee. Poorly defined and ovoid zones with heterogeneous intermediate and low signal on sagittal T1-weighted imaging (T1WI) (a), and heterogeneous intermediate, slightly high and low signal on sagittal fat-suppressed T2-weighted imaging (FS T2WI) (b) are seen in the anterior and posterior portions of the knee joint. Heterogeneous gadolinium-contrast enhancement of the lesions is seen on sagittal FS T1WI (c). A 53-year-old woman with PVNS involving the ankle and foot at the talocalcaneal and tibiotalar joints. Multiple lobulated zones with low and intermediate signal on sagittal T1WI (d), and low, intermediate, and high signal on sagittal FS T2WI (e) are seen in the ankle joint associated with osseous erosions.

Table 11.1 (Cont.) Tumors and tumor-like lesions within joints

Tumor or tumor-like lesion	MRI findings	Comments
Nodular synovitis (also referred to as giant cell tumors of the tendon sheath and soft tissue) (▶ Fig. 11.6)	Lesions can be ovoid or multilobulated and usually have low-intermediate or intermediate signal on T1WI and PDWI that is often similar to or less than muscle. On T2WI and FS T2WI, lesions can have mixed intermediate and/or high signal. Small zones of low signal on T2WI can represent small sites of hemosiderin deposition. Lesions often show Gd-contrast enhancement in either or homogeneous or heterogeneous pattern. Erosions of adjacent bone can be seen with some lesions.	Benign proliferative lesions of synovium (tendon sheaths, joints, and bursae). Can occur as localized nodular lesions attached to tendon sheaths outside of joints (hands, feet) or within joints (infrapatellar portion of knee joint); or as a diffuse form near/outside of large joints such as the knee and ankles. PVNS has histopathological features that are similar to nodular synovitis; although PVNS only occurs in joints and differs in that there are frondlike or villous growth patterns and they contain large amounts of hemosiderin. Nodular synovitis accounts for 4% of benign soft-tissue tumors and 2% of all soft-tissue tumors. It occurs in patients 6 to 71 years, mean = 39 to 46 years, peak ages in third to fourth decades.
Ganglia (▶ Fig. 11.7)	Lobulated structures with high signal on T2WI, no Gd-contrast enhancement.	Cystlike structure next to or within a joint, or adjacent to labral cartilage. Ganglia lack a synovial lining and contain hyaluronic acid and other mucopolysaccharides. They result from myxoid degeneration of connective tissue.
Meniscal cyst (▶ Fig. 11.8)	Circumscribed lobulated structure with high signal on T2WI, which is adjacent to or extends into a torn meniscus and lacks central Gd-contrast enhancement.	Pseudocyst-like structures without an endothelial lining that are typically within or adjacent to a torn or degenerated meniscus. Surgical treatment often occurs when the meniscal tear extends to the articular surface.

(continued on page 572)

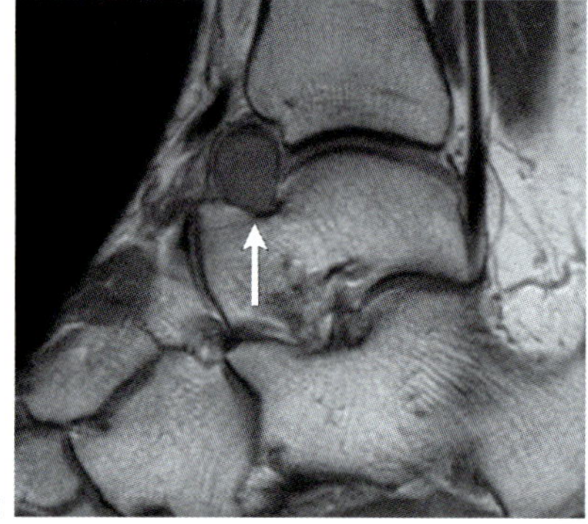

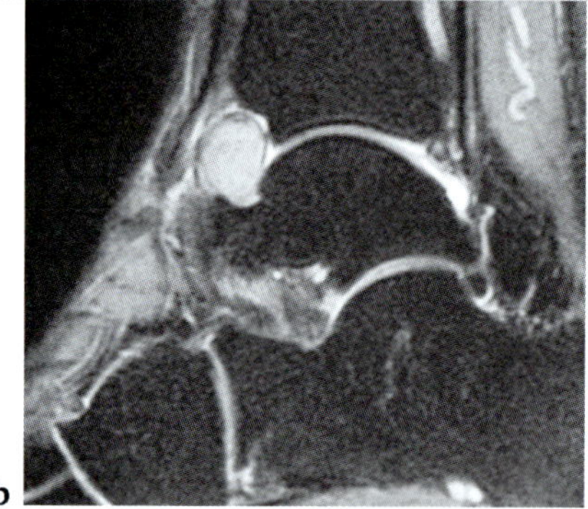

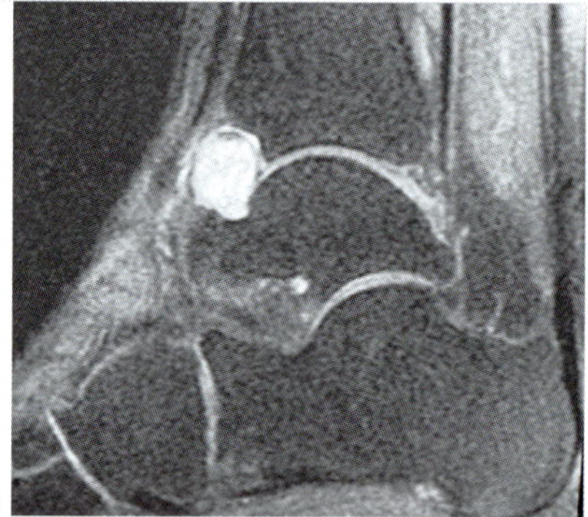

Fig. 11.6 A 68-year-old woman with a giant cell tumor of the tendon sheath/nodular synovitis at the ankle. An ovoid lesion with well-defined margins (arrow) is seen, which has mostly intermediate signal on sagittal T1-weighted imaging (T1WI) (a) and high signal on sagittal fat-suppressed T2-weighted imaging (FS T2WI) (b). The lesion shows prominent Gd-contrast enhancement on sagittal FS T1WI (c).

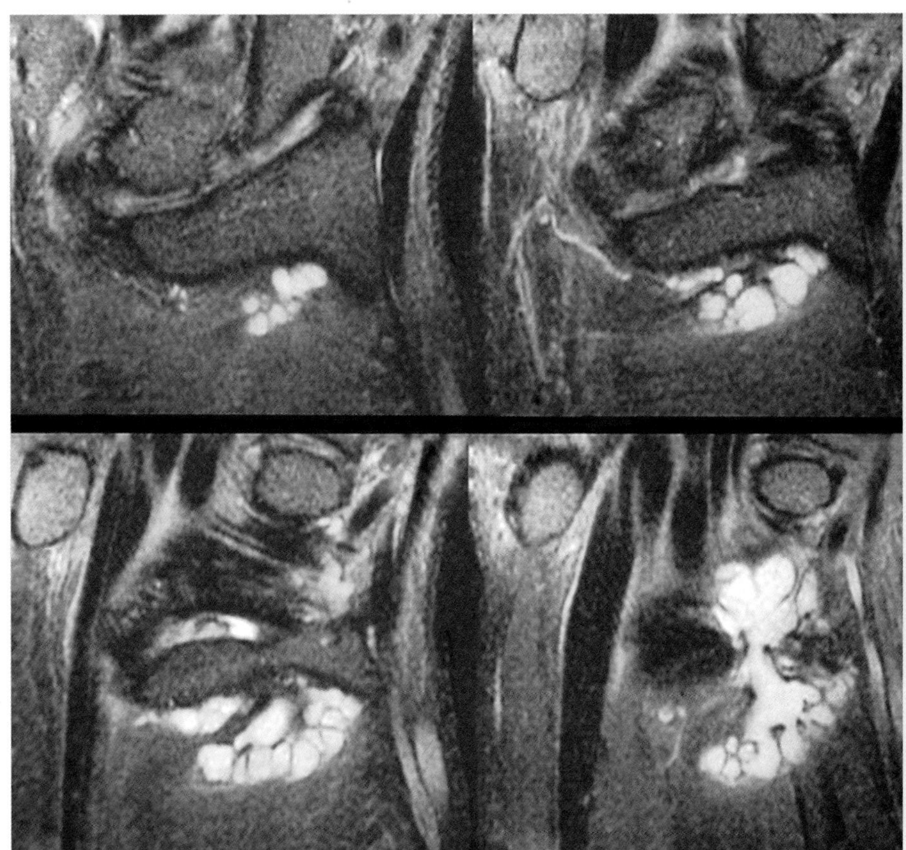

Fig. 11.7 A multilobulated ganglion cyst is seen at the wrist, which has high signal on coronal T2-weighted imaging.

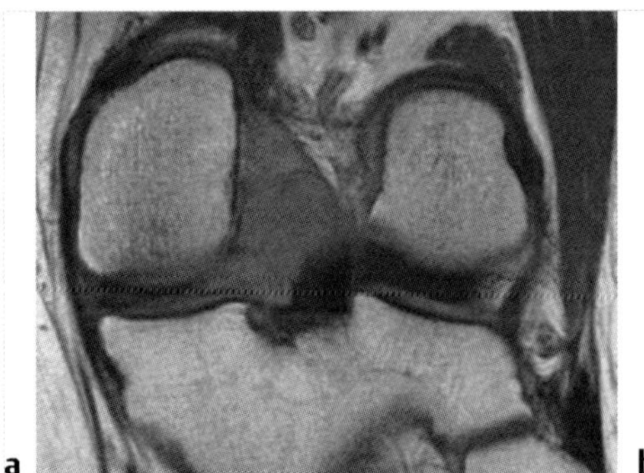

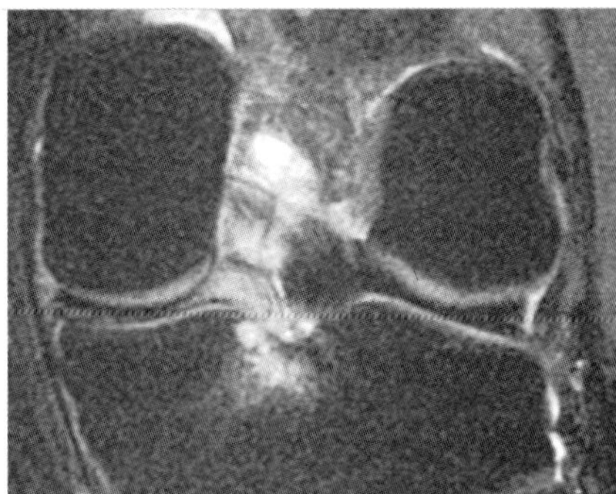

Fig. 11.8 Intra-articular meniscal cyst is seen adjacent to a tear of the inner portion of the medial meniscus. The meniscal cyst has intermediate signal on coronal proton density–weighted imaging (a) and high signal on fat-suppressed T2-weighted imaging (b).

Table 11.1 (Cont.) Tumors and tumor-like lesions within joints

Tumor or tumor-like lesion	MRI findings	Comments
Paralabral cyst (▶ Fig. 11.9)	Lobulated structures with high signal on T2WI, no Gd-contrast enhancement.	Cysts lined by synovium (synovial cyst) resulting from extrusion of joint fluid through a labroscapular defect. Pseudocysts (ganglia) can appear in similar location and have similar MRI features as synovial cysts. Ganglia lack synovial lining and result from myxoid degeneration of connective tissue.

(continued on page 574)

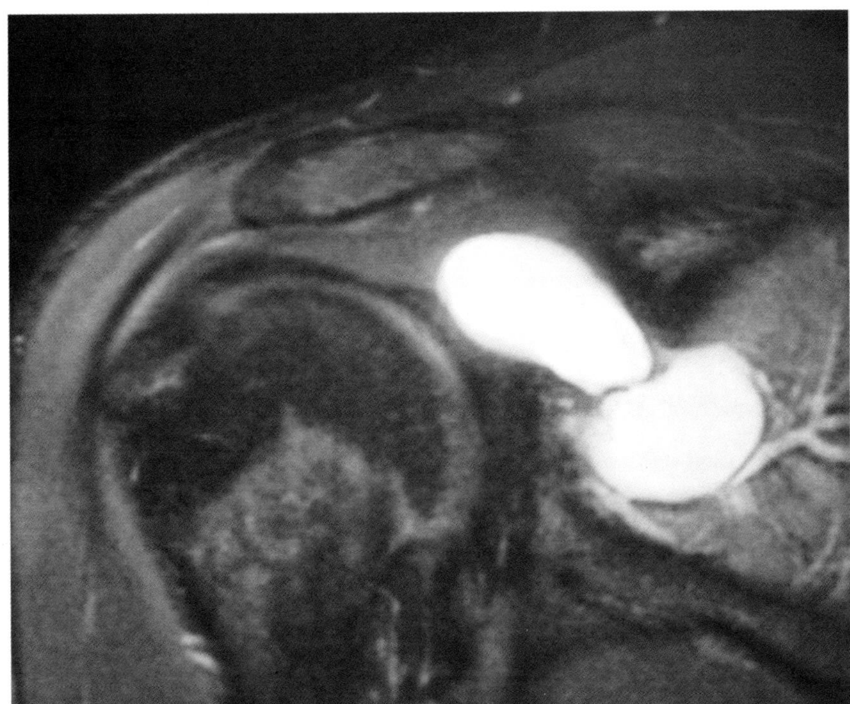

Fig. 11.9 Paralabral cyst adjacent to the glenoid labrum has high signal on fat-suppressed T2-weighted imaging.

Table 11.1 (Cont.) Tumors and tumor-like lesions within joints

Tumor or tumor-like lesion	MRI findings	Comments
Rheumatoid arthritis (▶ Fig. 11.10; ▶ Fig. 11.11; ▶ Fig. 11.12)	Hypertrophied synovium seen with rheumatoid arthritis can be diffuse, nodular, and/or villous, and usually has low to intermediate or intermediate signal on T1WI and PDWI. On T2WI, hypertrophied synovium can have low to intermediate, intermediate, and/or slightly high to high signal that is typically lower than joint fluid Signal heterogeneity of hypertrophied synovium on T2WI can result from variable amounts of fibrin, hemosiderin, and fibrosis. Chronic fibrotic nonvascular synovium usually has low signal on T1WI and T2WI. Hypertrophied synovium can show prominent homogeneous or variable heterogeneous Gd-contrast enhancement. Joint effusions can be seen. Zones of erosion and/or destruction of hyaline cartilage and subchondral bone, meniscal damage; bursal and joint fluid collections containing "rice bodies," other extra-articular cysts; intraosseous cystic-like areas, joint effusion, and rheumatoid nodules can eventually occur.	Chronic multisystem disease of unknown etiology with persistent inflammatory synovitis involving peripheral joints in a symmetric distribution. Hypertrophy and hyperplasia of synovial cells occurs in association with neovascularization, thrombosis, edema, with collections of B cells, antibody-producing plasma cells (rheumatoid factor and polyclonal immunoglobulins), and perivascular mononuclear T cells (CD4 +, CD8 +). T cells produce interleukins 2, 6, and 10; interferon gamma granulocyte-macrophage colony stimulating factor, and tumor necrosis factor alpha. Activated macrophages produce interleukins 1, 6, 7, 10 as well as interferon gamma; granulocyte-macrophage colony stimulating factor, and tumor necrosis factor alpha. These immune modulators (also referred to as cytokines and chemokines) are responsible for the inflammatory synovial pathology associated with rheumatoid arthritis. Activated fibroblasts producing collagenase, proteases, and cathepsins are present in the synovial lining and subsynovial tissue at the bone–cartilage interface where progressive cartilage degradation occurs leading to joint dysfunction. Affects approximately 1% of the world population. Eighty percent of adult patients present between the ages of 35 and 50 years. In patients with juvenile rheumatoid arthritis (now referred to as juvenile idiopathic arthritis), patients range from 5 to 16 years, mean = 10.2 years.

(continued on page 576)

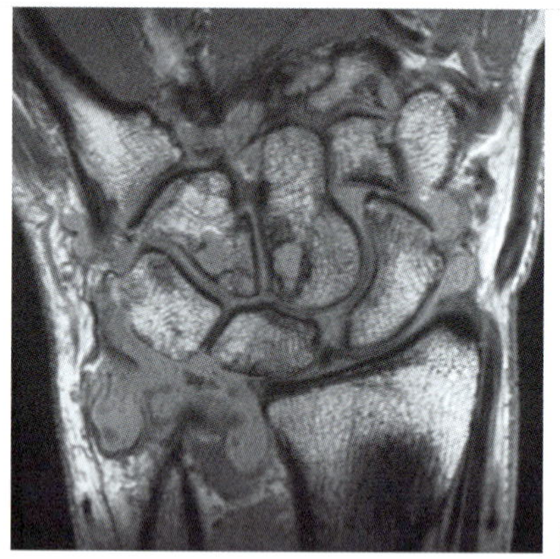

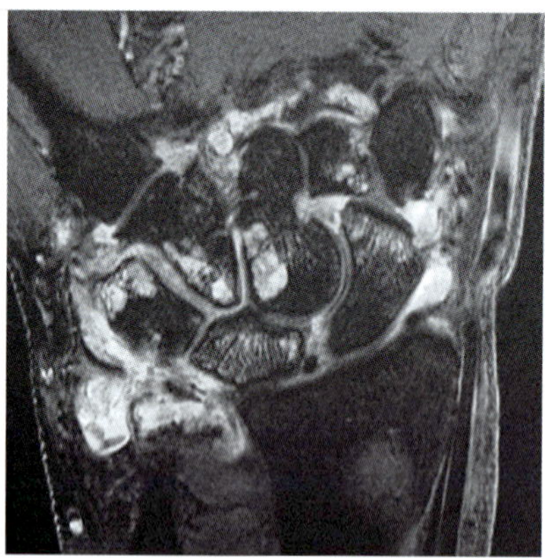

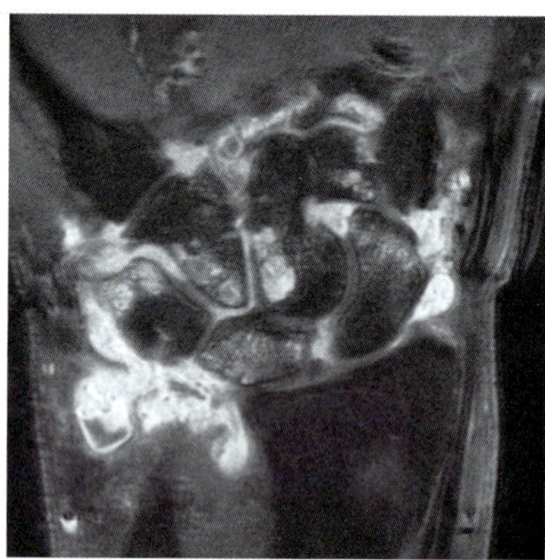

Fig. 11.10 A 62-year-old man with rheumatoid arthritis. Extensive multifocal synovial proliferation/pannus and joint fluid are present in the radial-ulnar, carpal, and carpal-metacarpal joints with intraosseous extension as seen on coronal proton density–weighted imaging (a). The pannus has heterogeneous intermediate to slightly high signal on fat-suppressed (FS) T2-weighted imaging (b) and shows Gd-contrast enhancement on FS T1-weighted imaging (c).

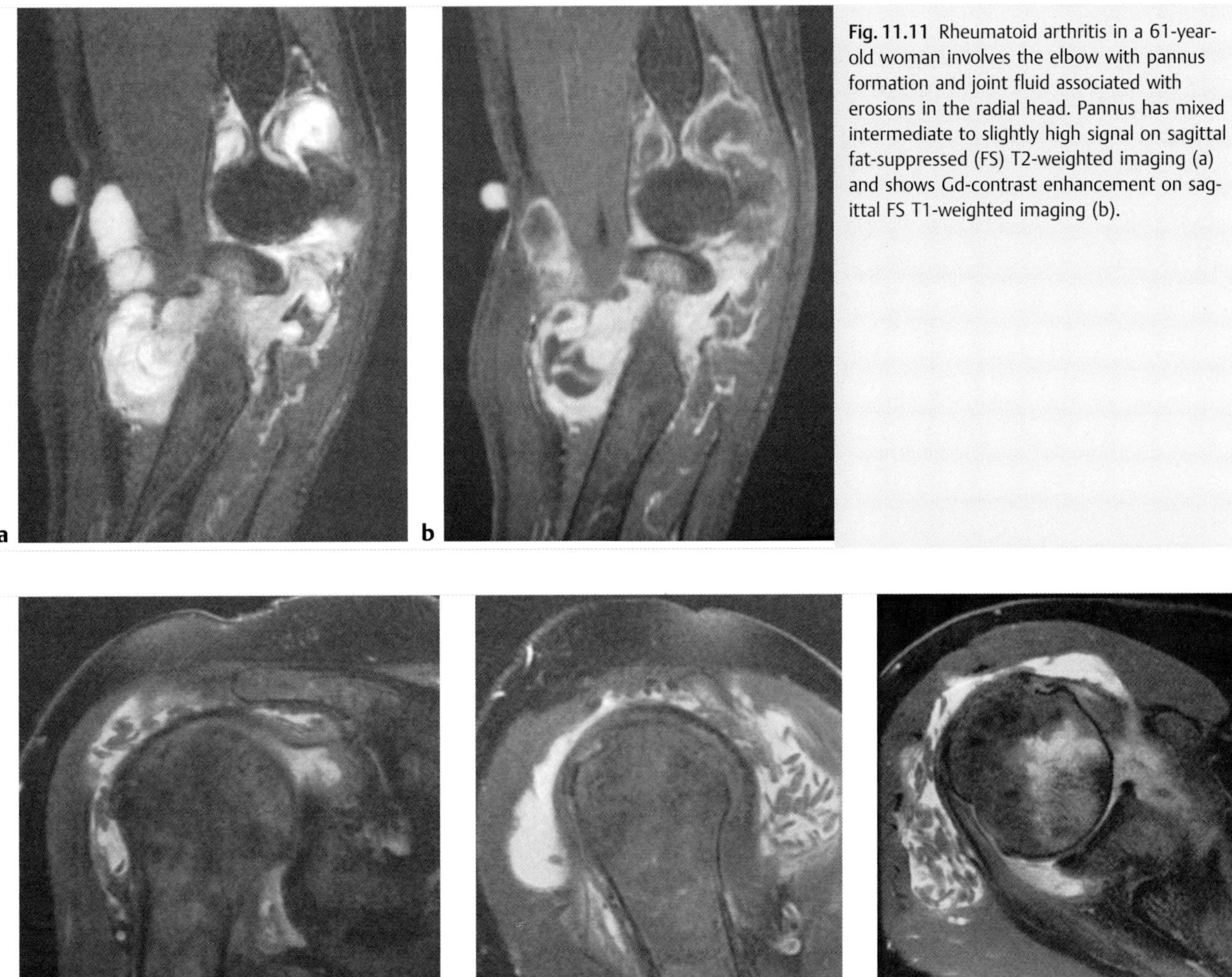

Fig. 11.11 Rheumatoid arthritis in a 61-year-old woman involves the elbow with pannus formation and joint fluid associated with erosions in the radial head. Pannus has mixed intermediate to slightly high signal on sagittal fat-suppressed (FS) T2-weighted imaging (a) and shows Gd-contrast enhancement on sagittal FS T1-weighted imaging (b).

Fig. 11.12 A 69-year-old woman with rheumatoid arthritis involving the glenohumeral joint and bursa of the shoulder with hypertrophied synovium appearing as "rice bodies." The ovoid and spheroid zones of synovial proliferation have intermediate signal on coronal (a), sagittal (b), and axial (c) fat-suppressed T2 weighted imaging and are located within a large effusion in the subdeltoid bursa.

Table 11.1 (Cont.) Tumors and tumor-like lesions within joints

Tumor or tumor-like lesion	MRI findings	Comments
Juvenile idiopathic arthritis (▶ Fig. 11.13)	Moderate to large joint effusion (usually in suprapatellar bursa), Synovial thickening > 3 mm; Involved synovium can have low-intermediate signal on T1WI; intermediate or mixed intermediate, slightly high to high signal on T2WI, ± zones of low signal on T2WI from hemosiderin/fibrin; typical Gd-contrast enhancement of thickened synovium. Quantitative assessment of dynamic contrast enhancement can correlate with disease activity and response to treatment.	Most common noninfectious inflammatory arthritis in children, prevalence 16 to 150/100,000; usually begins in children < 16 years, persists for at least 6 weeks. Rheumatoid factor positive in only 5 to 10%. Synovial proliferation occurs containing inflammatory cells associated with increased secretion of synovial fluid and eventual pannus formation. Can result in articular and bone erosion leading to joint dysfunction and disability. Often involves the knee. Oligoarticular form (50 to 60%) involves less than five joints in the first 6 months; Systemic type (10 to 20%) involves > 5 joints and is associated with fever, myalgias, adenopathy, hepatosplenomegaly, and serositis. Can be treated with nonsteroidal anti-inflammatory drugs, methotrexate, systemic corticosteroids, biologic therapy.
Transient toxic synovitis of the hip (▶ Fig. 11.14)	Small joint effusion associated with mild thickening of Gd-contrast enhancing synovium. Usually, no signal alteration or Gd-contrast enhancement of adjacent bone marrow in toxic synovitis (unlike that commonly seen with pyogenic synovitis).	Noninfectious reactive synovitis in children, most common cause of acute hip pain in children 3 to 10 years, autoimmune etiology, which may be related to viral infection or other respiratory illness 2 to 3 weeks earlier. Nonspecific inflammation and hypertrophy of synovium are seen associated with a small joint effusion. Diagnosis of exclusion, fluid from joint aspiration lacks increased white blood cells (WBC). Symptoms usually resolve after 2 weeks. Treatment includes rest and anti-inflammatory medications.
Psoriatic arthritis (▶ Fig. 11.15)	Radiographs show marginal bone erosions that progress centrally, joint space narrowing, periarticular new bone formation. MRI shows Gd-contrast enhancing hypertrophied synovium, joint fluid, inflammatory changes involving bone marrow, and periarticular soft tissues. Enthesitis and tenosynovitis are also seen with MRI. The MRI findings may be seen prior to radiographic findings.	Chronic inflammatory arthritis that occurs in 14% of patients with psoriasis. Persistent synovial inflammation can lead to progressive joint damage, osseous erosions, bone marrow edema, and inflammation. Inflammation can also occur in tendon sheaths and periarticular soft tissues. Most frequent location is the hand, with arthritis asymmetrically involving metacarpophalangeal joints, proximal and distal interphalangeal joints. Also involves the feet and axial skeleton. Enthesitis and dactlytitis also occur.

(continued on page 578)

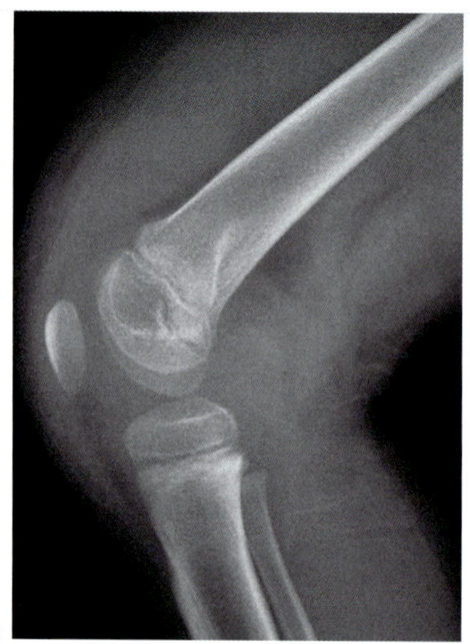

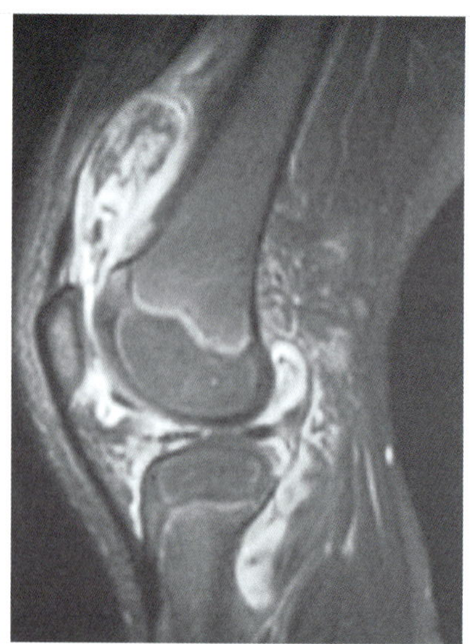

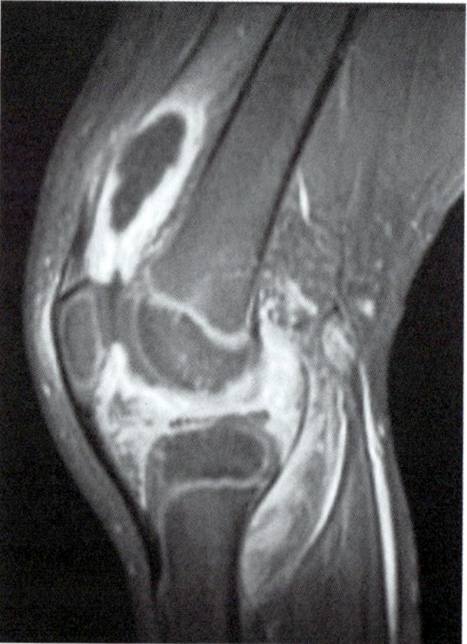

Fig. 11.13 Juvenile idiopathic arthritis in a 4-year-old girl. A moderate to large joint effusion is seen on lateral radiograph (a). Synovial thickening with mixed low, intermediate, and high signal is seen on sagittal fat-suppressed (FS) T2-weighted imaging (b), which shows Gd-contrast enhancement on sagittal FS T1-weighted imaging (c).

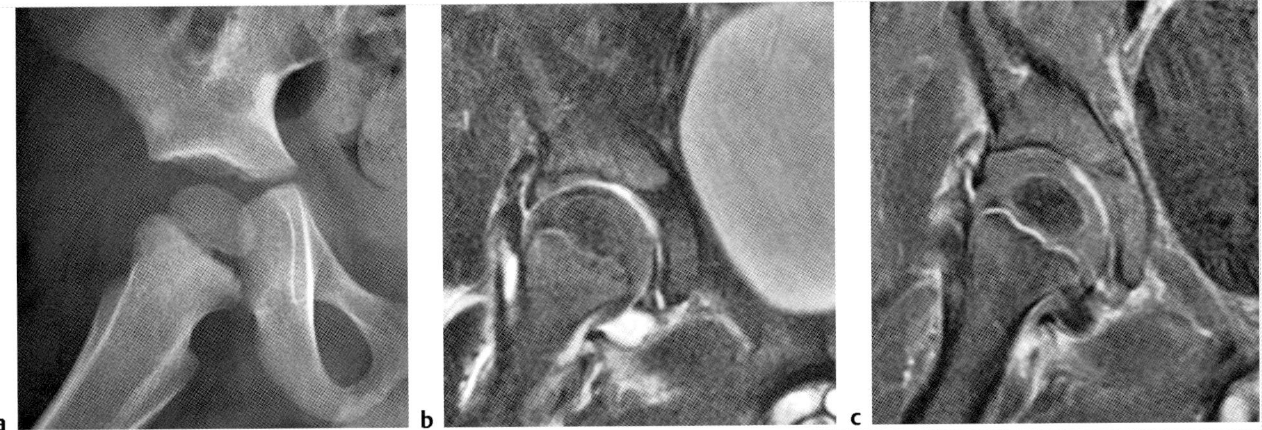

Fig. 11.14 Transient toxic synovitis in a 3-year-old boy. Radiograph shows a slightly widened hip joint (a). Coronal fat-suppressed (FS) T2-weighted imaging (b) shows a joint effusion without abnormal signal in the femoral marrow. Coronal FS T1-weighted imaging shows peripheral Gd-contrast enhancement involving the inflammed synovial membrane.

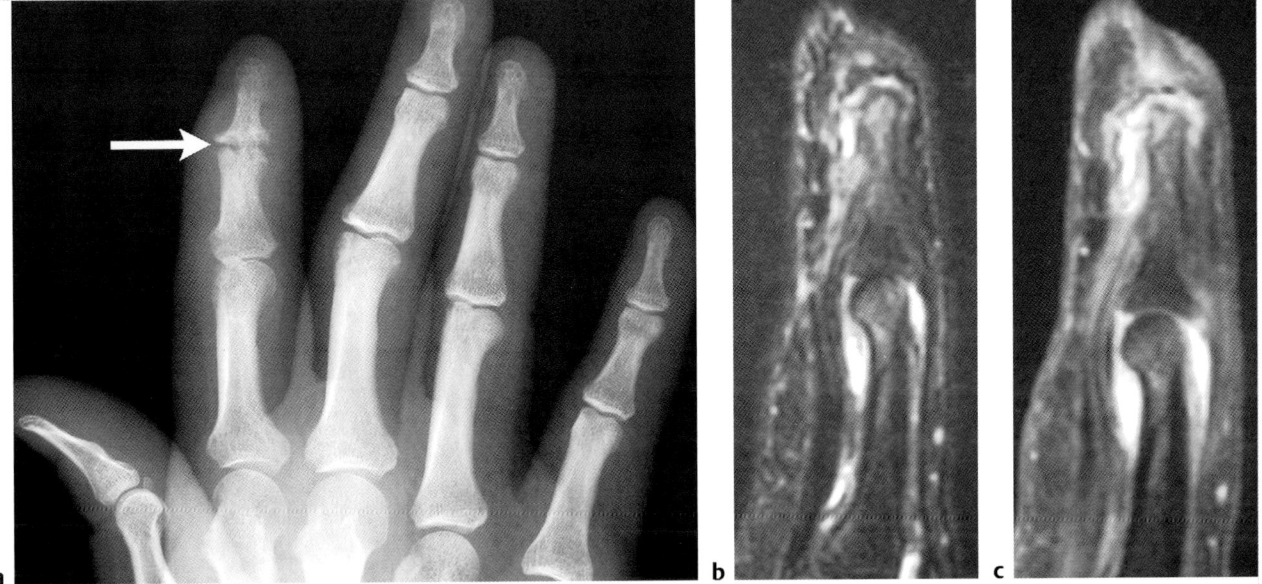

Fig. 11.15 Psoriatic arthritis involving the hand in a 37-year-old man. Radiograph shows soft tissue swelling involving the second finger with distal interphalangeal joint space narrowing and marginal erosions (arrow) (a). Synovial thickening is seen in the middle and distal interphalangeal joints, which has high signal on fat-suppressed (FS) T2-weighted imaging (b) and shows prominent Gd-contrast enhancement on sagittal FS T1-weighted imaging (c). Poorly defined zones with high signal and Gd-contrast enhancement are seen in the marrow and periarticular soft tissues.

Table 11.1 (Cont.) Tumors and tumor-like lesions within joints

Tumor or tumor-like lesion	MRI findings	Comments
Gout/tophi (▶ Fig. 11.16)	Tophi have variable sizes and shapes and often have low-intermediate signal on T1WI, FS T2WI, and T2WI. Zones of high signal on T2WI can be seen secondary to regions with increased hydration and proteinaceous zones associated with the deposits of urate crystals. Erosions of bone, synovial pannus, joint effusion, bone marrow, and soft-tissue edema can be seen with MRI. Tophi may be associated with heterogeneous, diffuse, or peripheral/marginal Gd-contrast enhancement patterns. Contrast enhancement seen with tophi is likely secondary to the hypervascular granulation tissue and reactive inflammatory cells in the synovium and/or adjacent soft tissues.	Inflammatory disease involving synovium resulting from deposition of monosodium urate crystals when serum urate levels exceed its solubility (7 mg/dL in men and 6 mg/dL in women) in various tissues and body fluids. Can be a primary disorder (inherited metabolic defects in purine metabolism or abnormal renal tubular secretion of urate) or secondary disorder (medications (thiazide diuretics, alcohol, salicylates, cyclosporin) that results from diminished renal excretion of uric acid salts, or from increased metabolic turnover of nucleic acids associated with malignancy; chemotherapy; or endocrine, vascular, or myeloproliferative diseases. Prevalence of gout ranges from 0.5 to 2.8% of men and from 0.1 to 0.6% of women in the United States. Accounts for 5% of arthritis cases. Usually occurs in middle-aged and elderly patients.
Calcium Pyrophosphate Dihydrate (CPPD) Deposition Disease (▶ Fig. 11.17)	Radiographs and CT show chondrocalicinosis, which is typically difficult to visualize with MRI except at the C1-odontoid articulation. At C1–2, hypertophy of synovium may occur which can have low-intermediate signal on T1WI and T2WI. Small zones of low signal may correspond to calcifications seen with CT.	CPPD disease is a common disorder usually seen in older adults in which there is deposition of CPPD crystals resulting in calcifications of hyaline and fibrocartilage, and is associated with cartilage degeneration, subchondral cysts and osteophyte formation. Symptomatic CPPD is referred to as pseudogout because of overlapping clinical features. Usually occurs in the knee, hip, shoulder, elbow, and wrist, and occasionally at the odontoid-C1 articulation.
Eosinophilic granuloma (▶ Fig. 11.18)	Intramedullary lesion associated with trabecular and cortical bone destruction.Typically has low-intermediate signal on T1WI and PDWI and heterogeneous slightly high to high signal on T2WI. Poorly defined zones of high signal on T2WI are usually seen in the marrow peripheral to the lesions secondary to inflammatory changes. Extension of lesions from the marrow into adjacent soft tissues through areas of cortical disruption are commonly seen as well as linear periosteal zones of high signal on T2WI. Lesions typically show prominent Gd-contrast enhancement in marrow and in extraosseous soft tissue portions of the lesions.	Benign tumor-like lesions consisting of Langerhans cells (histiocytes), and variable amounts of lymphocytes, polymorphonuclear cells, and eosinophils. Account for 1% of primary bone lesions and 8% of tumor-like lesions. Occur in patients with median age = 10 years, average = 13.5 years, peak incidence is between 5 and 10 years; 80 to 85% occur in patients less than 30 years.

(continued on page 580)

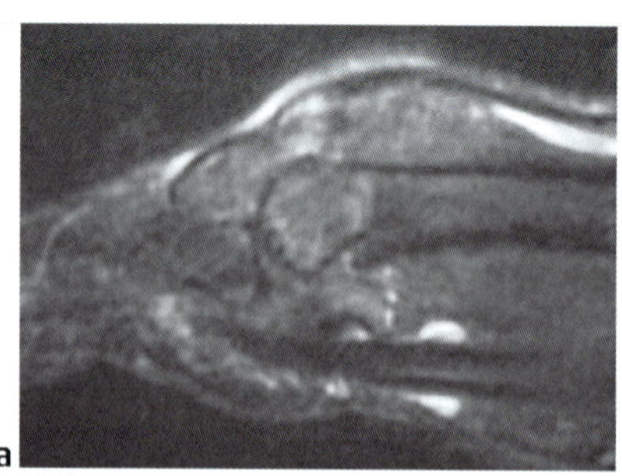
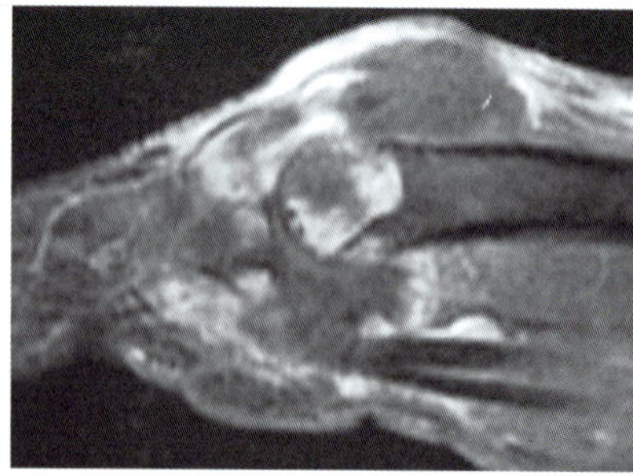

Fig. 11.16 A 53-year-old man with gout involving a metatarsal-phalangeal joint. Bone erosions are seen associated with soft tissue lesions (tophus) with heterogeneous intermediate and slightly high signal on fat-suppressed (FS) T2-weighted imaging (a). Only peripheral irregular gadolinium-contrast enhancement is seen with the intraosseous and extraosseous gout lesions on sagittal FS T1-weighted imaging (b).

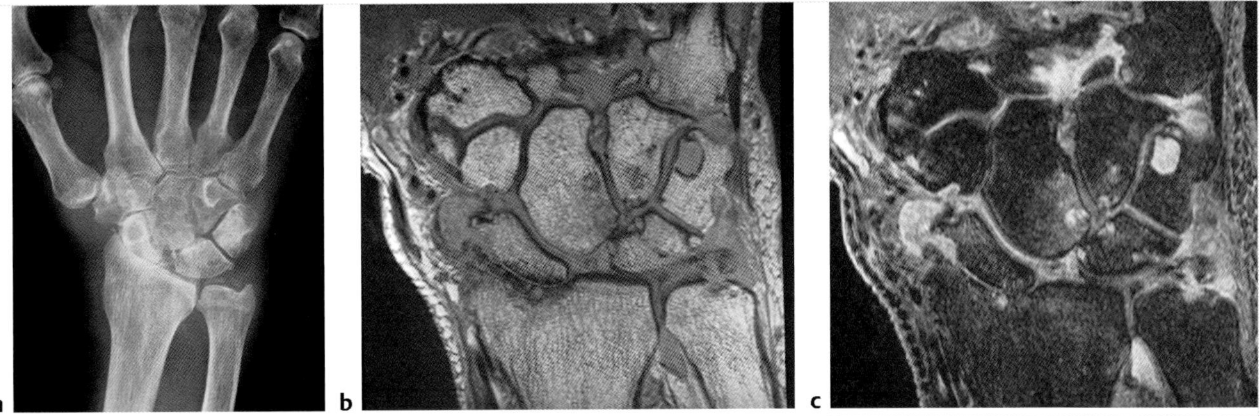

Fig. 11.17 An 85-year-old man with calcium pyrophosphate dihydrate (CPPD) deposition at the wrist with chondrocalcinosis, and multiple osseous erosions (a). Multifocal synovial proliferation and joint fluid are present in the radial-ulnar, carpal, and carpal-metacarpal joints with intraosseous extension as seen on coronal proton density–weighted imaging (b). Thickened synovium has heterogeneous intermediate to slightly high signal on fat-suppressed T2-weighted imaging (c).

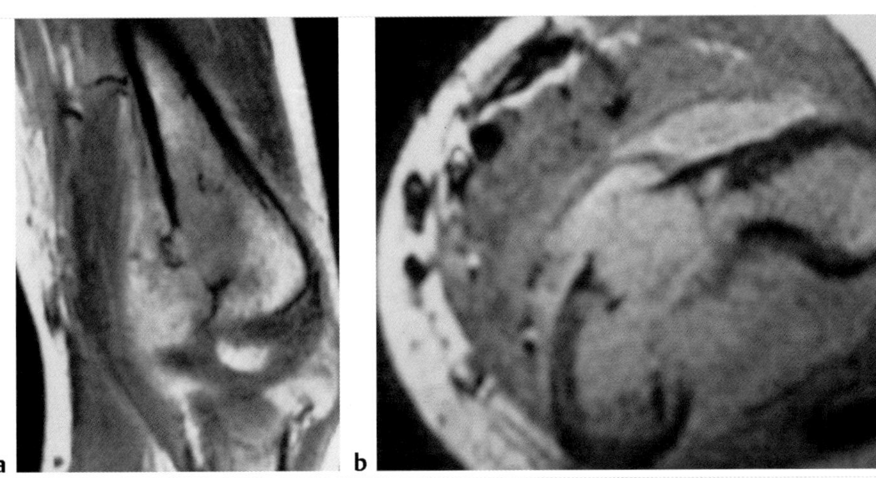

Fig. 11.18 A 5-year-old boy with an eosinophilic granuloma involving the distal humerus. The lesion in the marrow is associated with cortical destruction and extraosseous extension into the adjacent soft tissues (arrow) as seen on sagittal Gd-contrast enhanced T1-weighted imaging (a) and axial proton density–weighted imaging (b).

Table 11.1 (Cont.) Tumors and tumor-like lesions within joints

Tumor or tumor-like lesion	MRI findings	Comments
Infectious synovitis (▶ Fig. 11.19)	Pyogenic and nonpyogenic infectious synovitis: joint effusion, Gd-contrast enhancement of thickened synovium. With pyogenic synovitis, bone and cartilage erosion and destruction can progress rapidly with associated osteomyelitis. Abnormal high signal on FS T2WI and Gd-contrast enhancement are often seen in the bone marrow adjacent to the infected joint.	Can be pyogenic or nonpyogenic. Pyogenic arthritis resulting from bacterial infection (often *Stapylococcus aureus*) usually occurs in children (2 to 3 years, peak age) and frequently involves the lower extremities (75%; hip > knee > ankle > elbow). Associated with fever, localized pain, erythema, edema, limp, and lack of weight bearing. Tuberculous arthritis is a nonpyogenic cause of synovitis Early MRI features of pyogenic synovitis may overlap those of toxic synovitis. The presence of all four of the following is highly predictive for septic arthritis versus transient synovitis: erythrocyte sedimentation rate (ESR) > 40 mm/h; WBC > 12,000 cells per cubic cm; pain; and non–weight-bearing). Tuberculous synovitis usually has a more indolent course than pyogenic synovitis.
Fracture and hemarthrosis (▶ Fig. 11.20; ▶ Fig. 11.21)	Fluid-fluid levels and debris can be seen with zones of mixed low, intermediate, and/or high signal on T1WI and T2WI within joints.	Fractures involving articular surfaces of bone can result in loose osteochondral fragments, marrow fat, hemorrhage, and inflammatory reaction within joints.
Osteochondritis dissecans (▶ Fig. 11.22)	Subchondral lesions in marrow ranging from 1 to 3 cm with low-intermediate signal on T1WI and T2WI. Small irregular zones with slightly high to high signal may be seen with FS T2WI. A linear zone with high signal on T2WI along the margins can represent tracking of synovial fluid from a defect in the overlying hyaline cartilage and is associated with an increased risk of fragmentation and separation.	Osteochondrosis in which there is localized necrosis followed by reossification and healing unless there is osteochondral fragmentation and separation. Lesions commonly occur at the lateral surface of the medial femoral condyle, as well as the capitellum, talar dome, and femoral head.

(continued on page 582)

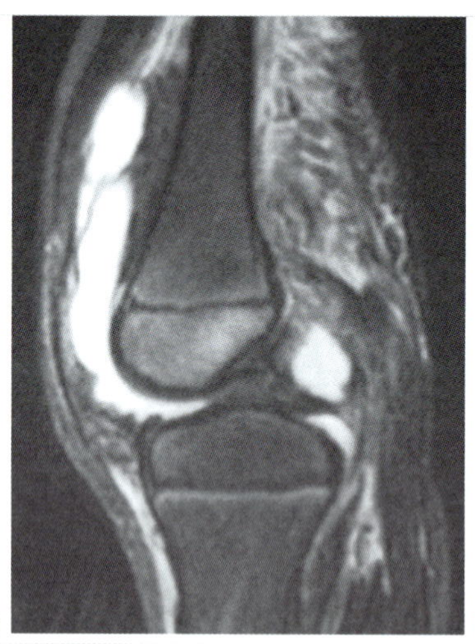
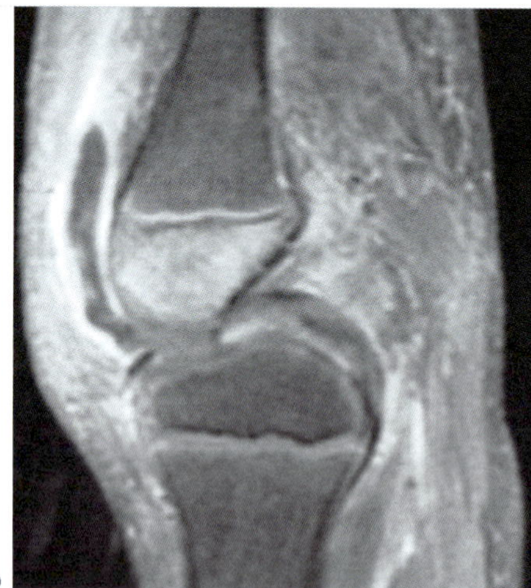

Fig. 11.19 Pyogenic infectious synovitis in an 11-year-old boy. Joint fluid is seen on sagittal fat-suppressed T2-weighted imaging (FS T2WI) (a). Gadolinium-contrast enhancing thickened synovium is seen on sagittal FS T1-weighted imaging. (b) A poorly defined zone with abnormal increased signal on FS T2WI and Gd-contrast enhancement is seen in the marrow of the distal femur representing osteomyelitis.

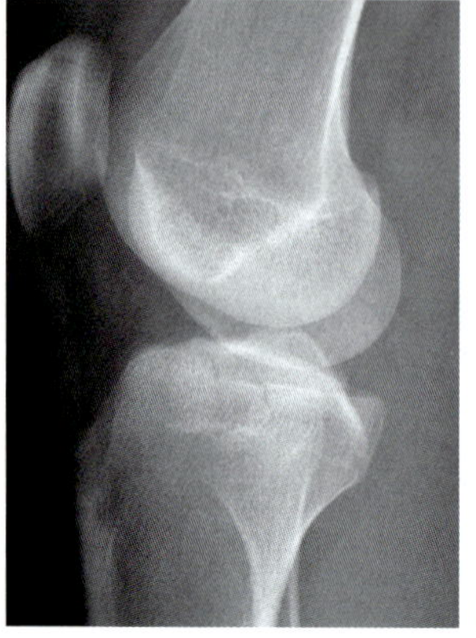
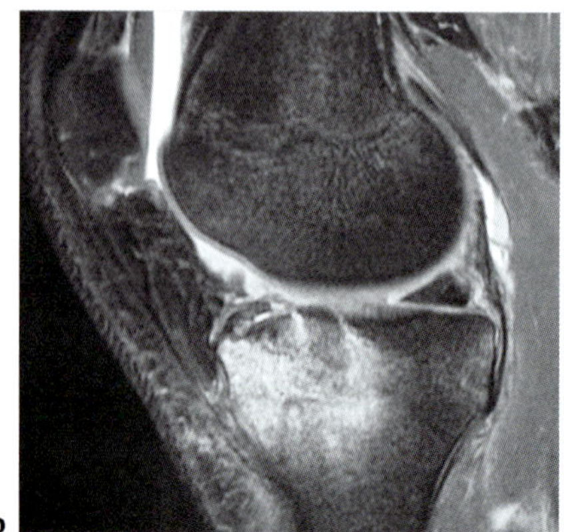
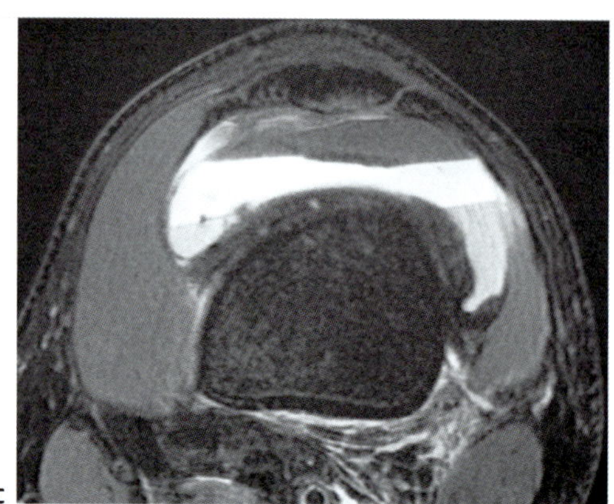

Fig. 11.20 Traumatic fracture of the lateral tibial plateau as seen on lateral radiograph (a). Poorly defined zones of high signal are seen in the marrow extending to the joint on sagittal T2-weighted imaging (T2WI) (b). Also seen is a layering lipohemarthrosis on axial fat-suppressed (FS) T2WI (c). *(continued)*

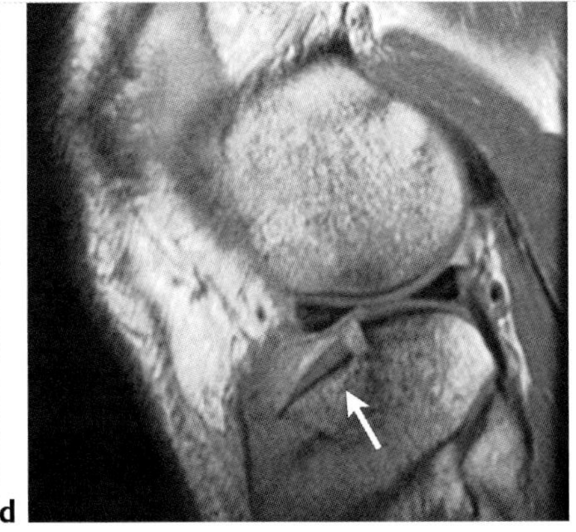

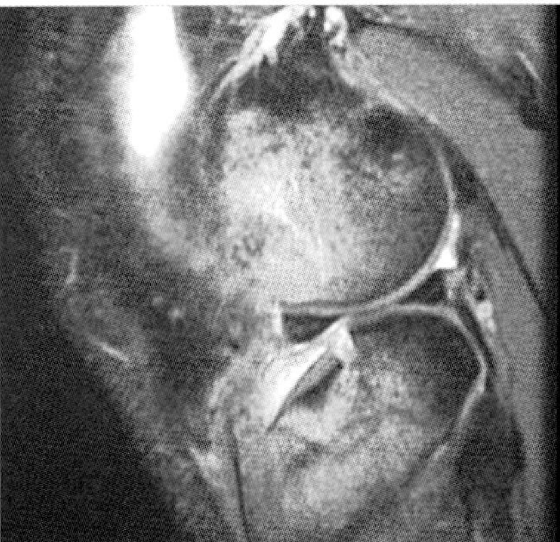

Fig. 11.20 (*continued*) Traumatic fracture of the tibia in another patient with an impacted fracture fragment (arrow) and poorly defined zones of low-intermediate signal in the marrow on sagittal proton density–weighted imaging (d) and high signal on sagittal FS T2WI (e).

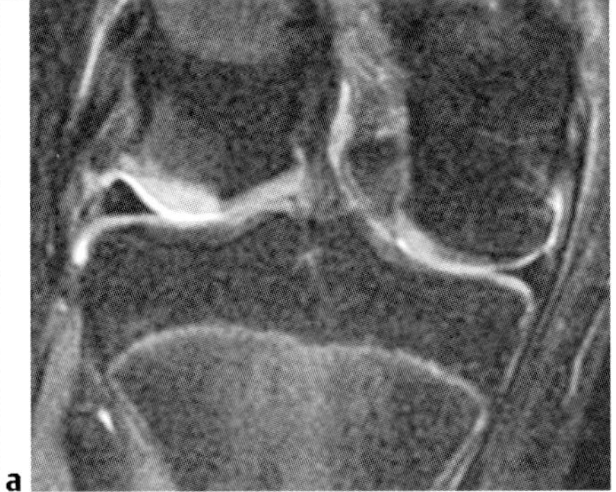

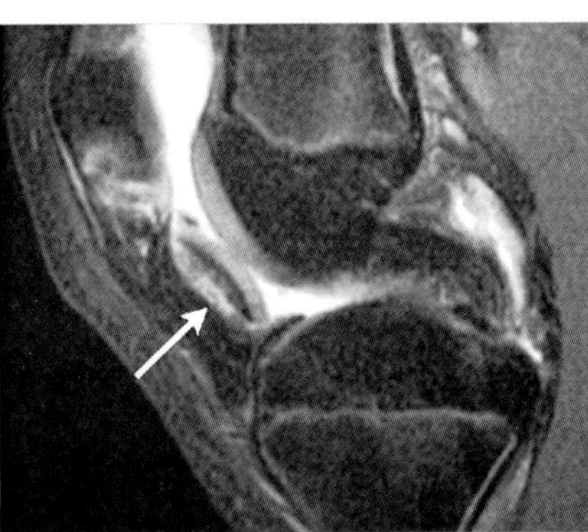

Fig. 11.21 A traumatic osteochondral fracture is seen involving the lateral femoral condyle where there is a high signal defect on coronal fat-suppressed T2-weighted imaging (FS T2WI) (a). An osteochondral fragment (arrow) is seen anterior to the distal femur within a joint effusion on sagittal FS T2WI (b).

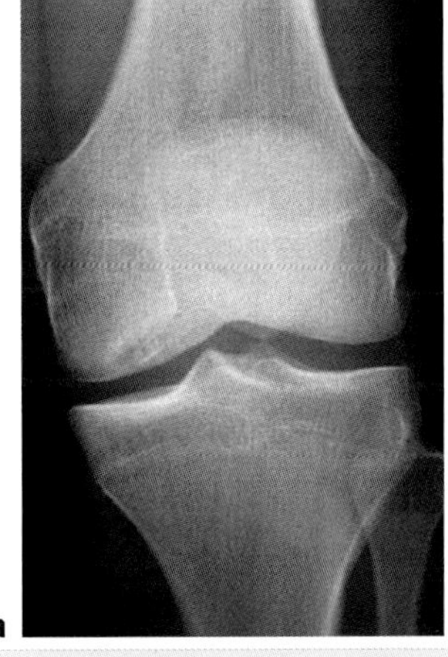

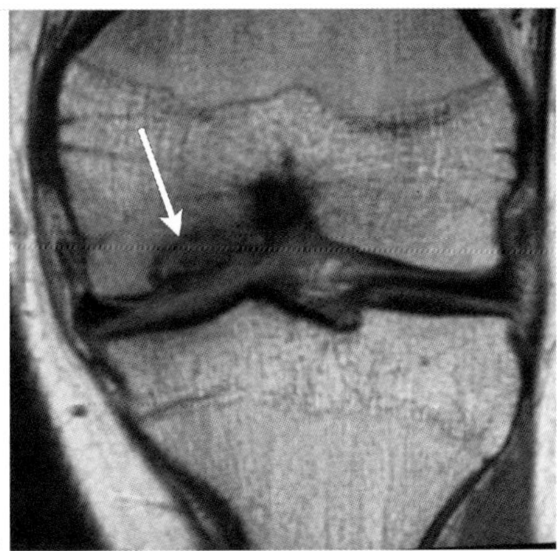

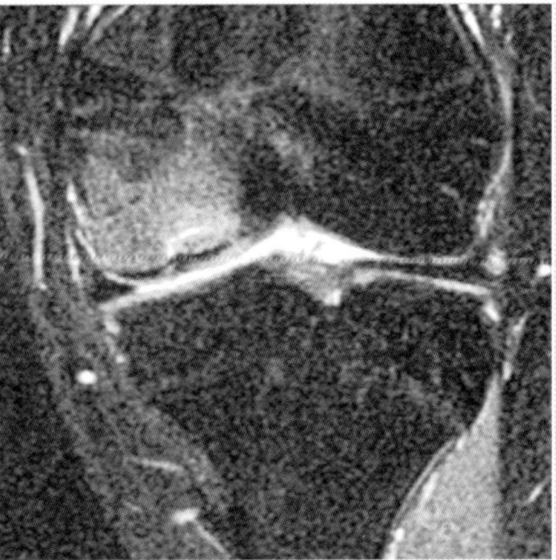

Fig. 11.22 Osteochondritis dissecans. A radiolucent zone is seen at the lateral aspect of the medial femoral condyle (a), which has mixed low and intermediate signal (arrow) on coronal T1-weighted imaging (b). A poorly defined zone with high signal is seen in the marrow on fat-suppressed T2-weighted imaging (c), as well as a joint effusion. Sites of discontinuity are seen involving the hyaline cartilage and subchondral bone.

Table 11.1 (Cont.) Tumors and tumor-like lesions within joints

Tumor or tumor-like lesion	MRI findings	Comments
Synovial hemangioma (▶ Fig. 11.23)	Lesions can have well-circumscribed margins with or without lobulations. Usually have low-intermediate signal or heterogeneous low-intermediate and high signal on T1WI and PDWI. The high signal zones on T1WI and PDWI can range from thin linear zones to thick irregular zones, and are most often secondary to fat and occasionally from slow-flowing blood within these lesions. On T2WI, hemangiomas usually have distinct margins with or without lobulations, and slightly high to high signal. On FS T2WI, hemangiomas typically have high signal except for zones of fat within the lesions. Lesions usually show prominent Gd-contrast enhancement. Prominent adjacent veins may be seen.	Benign hamartomatous lesions consisting of capillary, cavernous, and/or malformed venous vessels with varying amounts of mature adipose tissue.
Lipoma arborescens (▶ Fig. 11.24)	Appears as multiple nodular or frondlike deposits with fat signal within hypertrophied synovium, often associated with a joint effusion.	Disorder with multiple villous or frondlike zones of fatty deposition in synovium within a joint, tendon sheath, and/or bursa. Most frequently involves the knee. May be idiopathic or occur in the setting of degenerative arthritis, collagen vascular disorders, or trauma. Occurs in patients 9 to 66 years.
Intra-articular lipoma (▶ Fig. 11.25)	Lesions usually have circumscribed margins and have MRI signal comparable to subcutaneous fat on T1WI, PDWI, T2WI, and FS T2WI. Often do not show Gd-contrast enhancement except for minimal to mild enhancement along the thin nonfatty septa.	Common benign hamartomas composed of mature white adipose tissue without cellular atypia. Most common soft-tissue tumor, representing 10% of all soft-tissue tumors and 16% of benign soft-tissue tumors.

(continued on page 584)

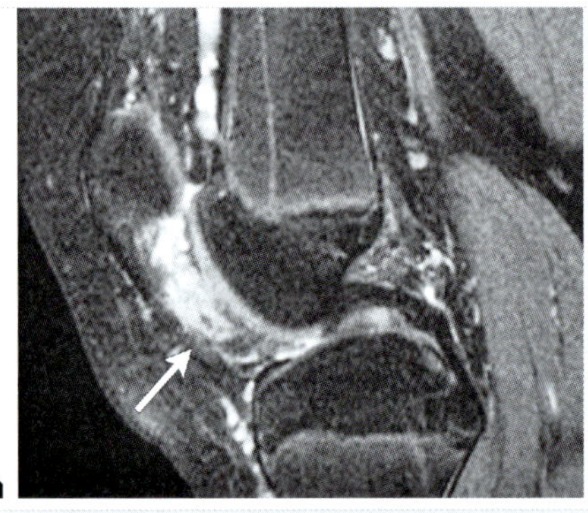

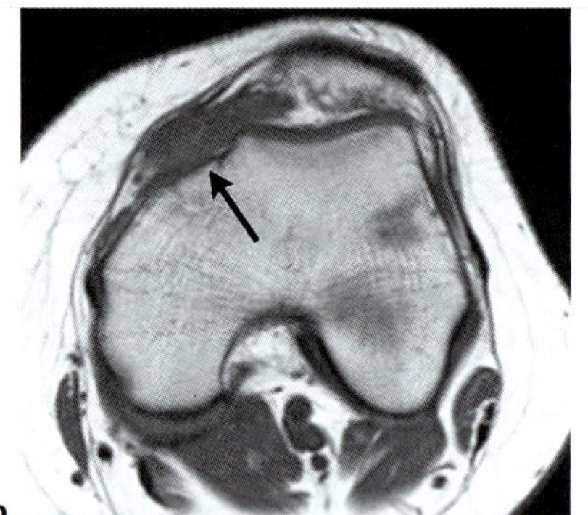

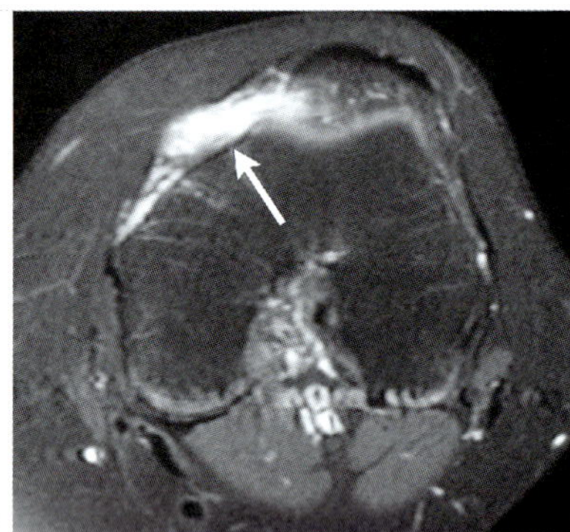

Fig. 11.23 A 13-year-old girl with a synovial hemangioma in the knee. The lesion (arrow) has high signal on sagittal fat-suppressed (FS) T2-weighted imaging (a). Multiple enlarged veins are seen adjacent to the hemangioma. The hemangioma (arrow) has intermediate signal on axial T1-weighted imaging (T1WI) (b), and shows prominent Gd-contrast enhancement (arrow) on axial FS T1WI (c).

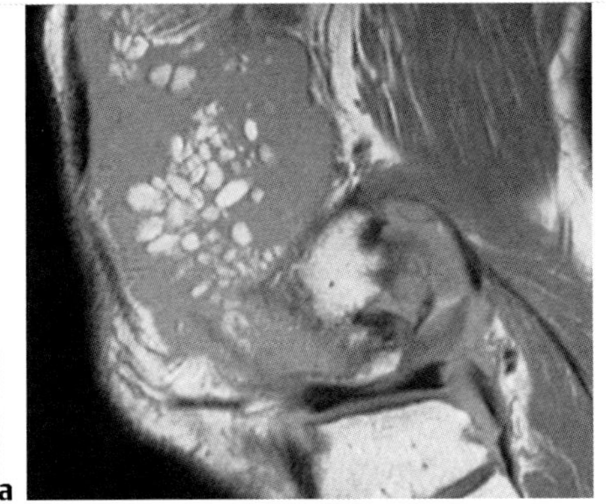
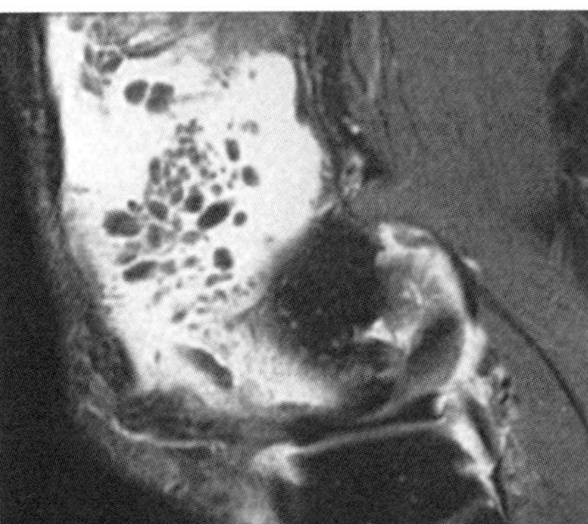

Fig. 11.24 A 37-year-old man with lipoma arborescens at the knee. Multiple nodular and frondlike/villous deposits with fat signal are seen within hypertrophied synovium on sagittal proton density–weighted imaging (a). The fat signal is suppressed on sagittal fat-suppressed T2-weighted imaging (b). The hypertrophied fatty synovium is seen within a large joint effusion.

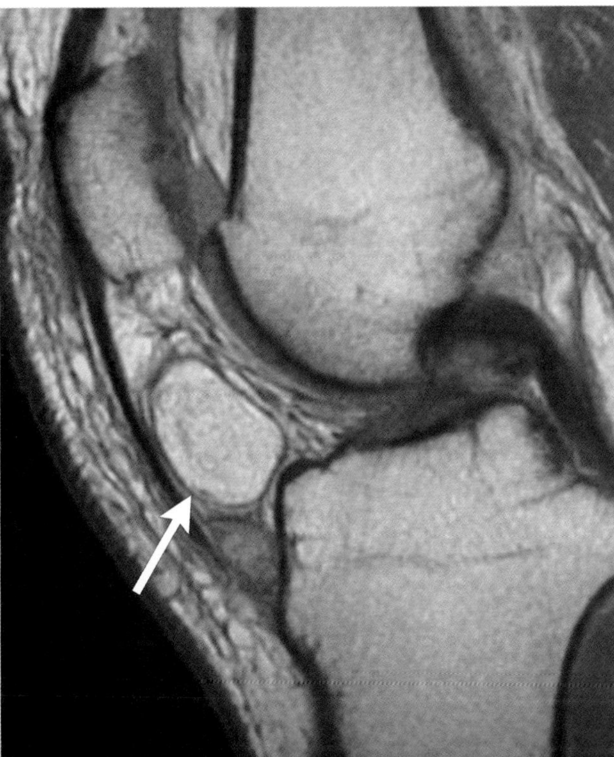

Fig. 11.25 A 56-year-old man with a lipoma in the Hoffa fat pad, which has high signal on sagittal T1-weighted imaging (arrow).

Table 11.1 (Cont.) Tumors and tumor-like lesions within joints

Tumor or tumor-like lesion	MRI findings	Comments
Intraosseous giant cell tumor with joint extension (▶ Fig. 11.26)	Intraosseous lesions near the ends of long bones, which often have low to intermediate signal on T1WI and PDWI, intermediate to high signal on T2WI, and high signal on FS PDWI and FS T2WI. Aneurysmal bone cysts can be seen in 14% of giant cell tumors, resulting in cystic zones with variable signal and fluid-fluid levels. Lesions frequently have areas of cortical destruction with extraosseous extension including into joints. Tumors show mild to prominent Gd-contrast enhancement.	Aggressive bone tumors composed of neoplastic ovoid mononuclear cells and scattered multinucleated osteoclast-like giant cells. Account for approximately 5 to 9.5% of all bone tumors and up to 23% of benign bone tumors. Malignant giant cell tumors account for 5.8% of all giant cell tumors. Occurs in patients age 4 to 81 years, median = 30 years, mean = 33 years.
Chondroblastoma (▶ Fig. 11.27)	Lesions typically involve the physeal plate, adjacent epiphysis, and metaphysis. Lesions often have fine lobular margins and typically have low-intermediate heterogeneous signal on T1WI and mixed low, intermediate, and/or high signal on T2WI. Areas of low signal on T2WI are secondary to chondroid matrix mineralization and/or hemosiderin. Lesions can show marginal or septal Gd-contrast enhancement patterns. Cortical disruption and extraosseous extension into joints is uncommon, although reactive synovitis and joint effusion commonly occur. Perilesional zones with high signal on T2WI and Gd-contrast enhancement are commonly seen in bone marrow as well as periosteal location indicating reactive hyperemia and/or edema.	Benign cartilaginous tumors with chondroblast-like cells and areas of chondroid matrix formation usually involving the epiphysis. Usually present before cessation of endochondral bone growth. Account for 5 to 9% of benign bone lesions, 1 to 3% of all bone lesions. Occurs in patients with median age = 17 years, mean age = 16 years for lesions in long bones, mean age = 28 years in other bones.
Osteoid osteoma (▶ Fig. 11.28)	Typically shows dense fusiform thickening of the cortex, which has low signal on T1WI, PDWI, T2WI, and FS T2WI. Within the thickened cortex, a spheroid or ovoid zone (nidus) measuring less than 1.5 cm is seen in the region of the original external surface of bone cortex. The nidus can have irregular, distinct, or indistinct margins relative to the adjacent region of cortical thickening. The nidus can have low-intermediate signal on T1WI and PDWI, and low-intermediate or high signal on T2WI and FS T2WI. Calcifications in the nidus can be seen as low signal on T2WI. After Gd-contrast administration, variable degrees of enhancement are seen at the nidus. Intra-articular lesions typically have associated reactive synovitis and joint effusion.	Benign osteoblastic lesion consisting of a circumscribed nidus less than 1.5 cm, and usually surrounded by reactive bone formation. These lesions are usually painful and have limited growth potential. Osteoid osteoma accounts for 11 to 13% of primary benign bone tumors. Occurs in patients age 6 to 30 years, median = 17 years. Approximately 75% occur in patients less than 25 years.
Osteoblastoma (▶ Fig. 11.29)	Expansile lesion often greater than 1.5 cm in diameter with low-intermediate signal on T1WI and intermediate-high signal on T2WI and FS T2WI, usually show Gd-contrast enhancement. Lesions usually have poorly defined zones with high signal on T2WI and FS T2WI and Gd-contrast enhancement in the marrow (edema, inflammation) beyond the zone of sclerosis or in adjacent soft tissues from prostaglandin synthesis by these lesions.	Rare benign bone-forming neoplasm (2% of bone tumors) usually occurs in patients age 6 to 30 years, median = 15 years. Histologically related to osteoid osteomas.

(continued on page 586)

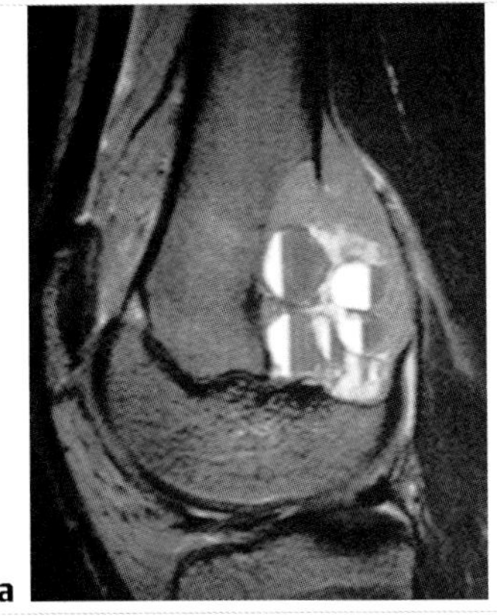
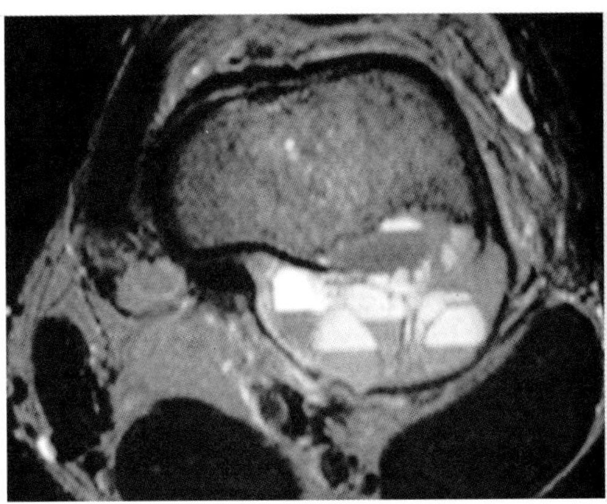

Fig. 11.26 A 17-year-old boy with a giant cell tumor involving the distal metaphyseal portion of the femur associated with a secondary aneurysmal bone cyst. The tumor has mixed intermediate and high signal on sagittal (a) and axial (b) T2-weighted imaging. Multiple fluid-fluid levels are seen at the aneurysmal cyst associated with the tumor within bone and at the extraosseous portion, which extends through disrupted cortex dorsally into the knee joint.

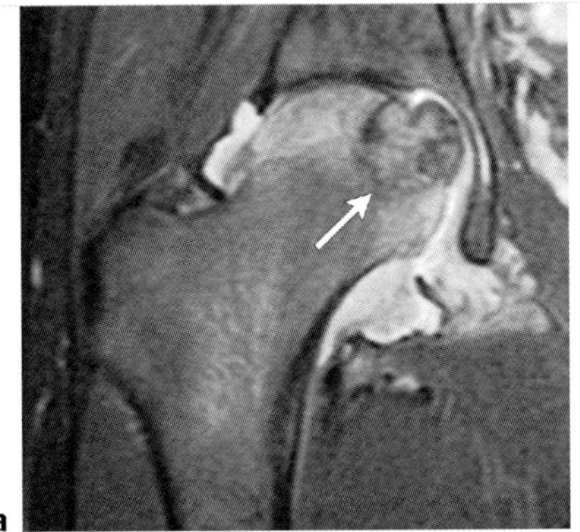
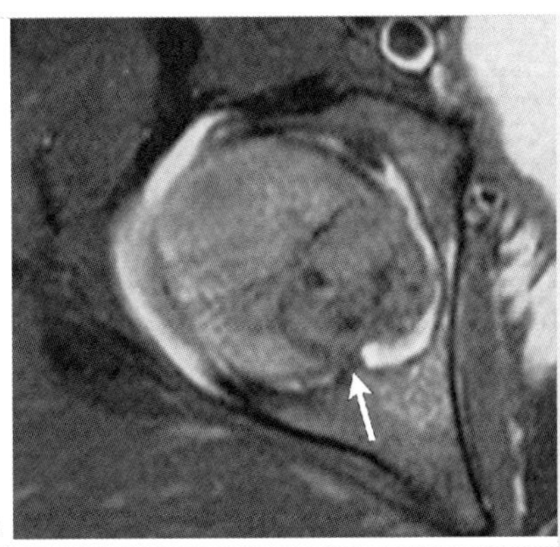

Fig. 11.27 A 17-year-old boy with chondroblastoma in the proximal femur. The lesion is located mostly in the epiphysis but also involves the physeal plate and a small portion of the metaphysis. The lesion has expanded and thinned the medial margin of the femoral head with resultant extension into the hip joint. The lesion has slightly lobulated margins and has heterogeneous slightly high signal on coronal (a) and axial (b) fat-suppressed T2-weighted imaging as well as in the adjacent marrow (arrows). A joint effusion is also present.

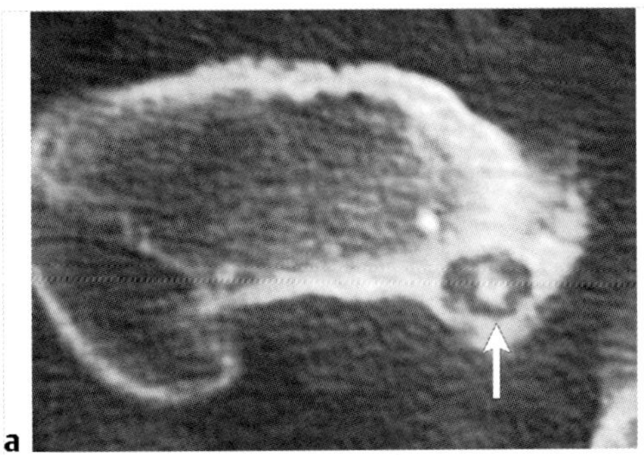
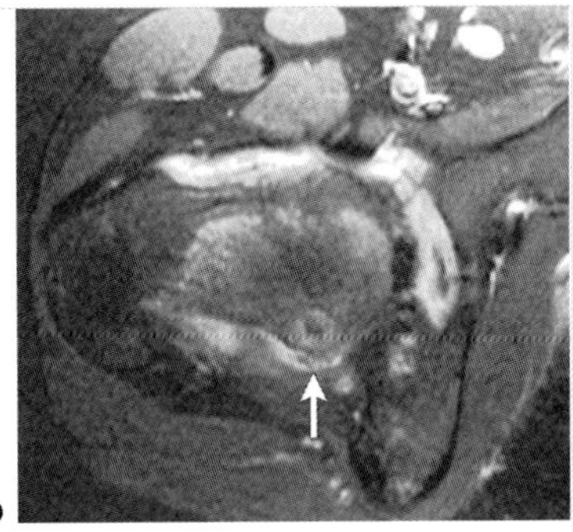

Fig. 11.28 Osteoid osteoma involving the intra-articular portion of the proximal femur in a 17-year-old girl. Computed tomographic image shows a lucent nidus (arrow) within thickened cortical bone and medullary sclerosis (a). The nidus (arrow) shows Gd-contrast enhancement on axial fat-suppressed T1-weighted imaging (b). Poorly defined zones with Gd-contrast enhancement are seen in the marrow adjacent to the nidus, as well as Gd-enhancing synovium peripheral to fluid in the hip joint.

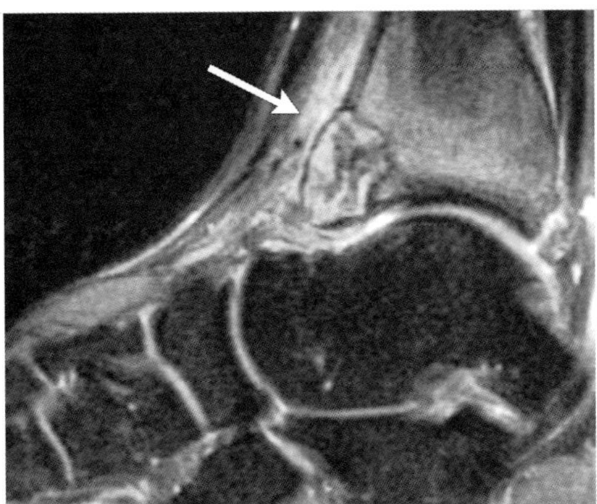
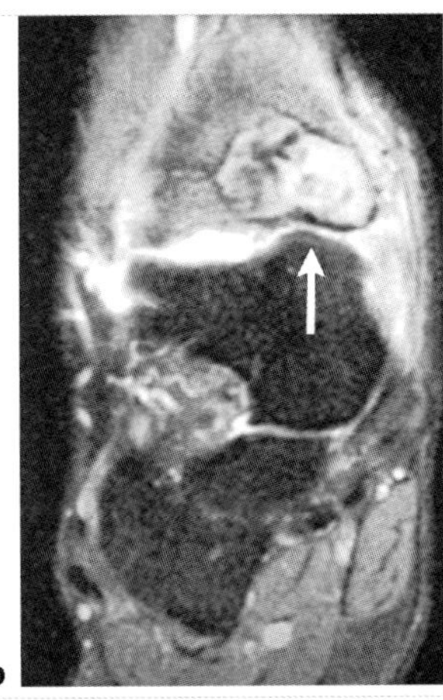

Fig. 11.29 A 24-year-old man with an osteoblastoma involving the distal tibia, which has heterogeneous high and low signal on sagittal (a) and coronal (b) fat-suppressed T2-weighted imaging (arrows). A thin rim of low signal is seen at the periphery of the tumor and at the border with medullary bone. The tumor causes expansion and irregular thinning of the anterior cortical margin of the distal tibia. The lesion is associated with poorly defined zones of high signal in the adjacent marrow and extraosseous soft tissues as well as in the joint fluid associated with synovial inflammation.

Table 11.1 (Cont.) Tumors and tumor-like lesions within joints

Tumor or tumor-like lesion	MRI findings	Comments
Osteochondroma (▶ Fig. 11.30)	Circumscribed protruding lesion arising from outer cortex with a central zone with intermediate signal on T1WI and T2WI similar to marrow surrounded by a peripheral zone of low signal on T1 W and T2 W images. A cartilaginous cap is usually present in children and young adults. Increased malignant potential when cartilaginous cap is > 2 cm thick.	Benign cartilaginous tumors arising from defect at periphery of growth plate during bone formation with resultant bone outgrowth covered by a cartilaginous cap. Usually benign lesions unless associated with pain and increasing size of cartilaginous cap. Osteochondromas are common lesions, accounting for 14 to 35% of primary bone tumors. Occur with median age of 20 years; up to 75% percent of patients are less than 20 years.
Malignant		
Intra-articular extension from intraosseous metastatic tumor	Intramedullary lesions with low-intermediate signal on T1WI; low-intermediate to slightly high signal on PDWI; slightly high to high signal on T2WI and FS T2WI. Sclerotic lesions often have low signal on T1WI and mixed low, intermediate, and/or high signal on T2WI. Tumors frequently cause cortical destruction with extension into the extraosseous soft tissues including joints. Most lesions show Gd-contrast enhancement.	Proliferating neoplastic cells that are located in sites or organs separated or distant from their origins. Intraosseous metastatic lesions can have associated bone destruction and extraosseous extension, including into joints.
Intra-articular extension from myeloma (▶ Fig. 11.31)	Multiple or single intramedullary zones with low-intermediate signal on T1WI and PDWI; intermediate, slightly high, to high signal on T2WI; and slightly high to high signal on FS T2WI. Intramedullary lesions and corresponding signal abnormalities may be diffuse, focal with poorly defined or distinct margins, and/or in an extensive variegated pattern. Lesions usually show Gd-contrast enhancement. Tumors frequently cause cortical destruction with extension into the extraosseous soft tissues, including joints.	Malignant tumors composed of proliferating antibody-secreting plasma cells derived from single clones within bone marrow. Plasma cells normally account for less than 5% of the cells in bone marrow. Most common primary neoplasm of bone in adults, accounts for 44% of primary malignant bone tumors and 34% of all primary bone tumors. Occurs in patients age 16 to 80, median = 60 years. Most patients are older than 40 years.
Intra-articular extension from lymphoma involving bone (▶ Fig. 11.32)	Multiple or single intramedullary zones with low-intermediate signal on T1WI and PDWI; intermediate, slightly high, to high signal on T2WI; and slightly high to high signal on FS T2WI. Intramedullary lesions and corresponding signal abnormalities may be diffuse, focal with poorly defined or distinct margins, and/or in an extensive variegated pattern. Lesions usually show Gd-contrast enhancement. Tumors frequently cause cortical destruction with extension into the extraosseous soft tissues, including joints.	Lymphoma represents a group of lymphoid tumors whose neoplastic cells typically arise within lymphoid tissue (lymph nodes and reticuloendothelial organs). Unlike leukemia, lymphoma usually arises as discrete masses. Almost all primary lymphomas of bone are B cell non-Hodgkin lymphomas (NHLs). NHL frequently originates at extranodal sites and spreads in an unpredictable pattern.
Intra-articular extension from leukemia	Leukemic infiltration in marrow can appear as diffuse or poorly defined zones of low-intermediate signal on T1WI and PDWI, intermediate-slightly high to high signal on FS T2WI. Focal or geographic regions with similar signal alteration can also be seen. After Gd-contrast administration, leukemia can show Gd-contrast enhancement on T1WI and FS T1WI. Note should be made that Gd-contrast enhancement may be seen in normal vertebral marrow in children less than 7 years. Tumors can cause cortical destruction with extension into the extraosseous soft tissues, including joints.	Lymphoid neoplasms that have widespread involvement of the bone marrow as well as tumor cells in peripheral blood. Acute lymphoblastic leukemia (ALL) is the most frequent type in children and adolescents. In adults, chronic lymphocytic leukemia (CLL) is the most common type. Myelogenous leukemias represent neoplasms derived from abnormal myeloid progenitor cells that, if normal, would form erythrocytes, monocytes, granulocytes, and platelets. Acute myelogenous leukemia (AML) usually occurs in adolescents and young adults and accounts for approximately 20% of childhood leukemia. Chronic myelogenous leukemia (CML) occurs in adults older than 25 years.

(continued on page 588)

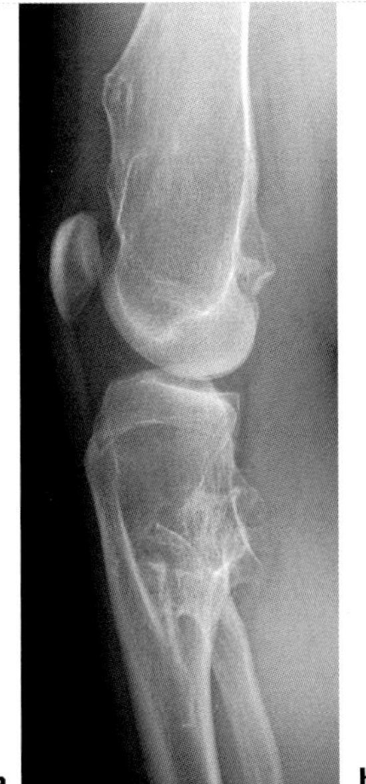

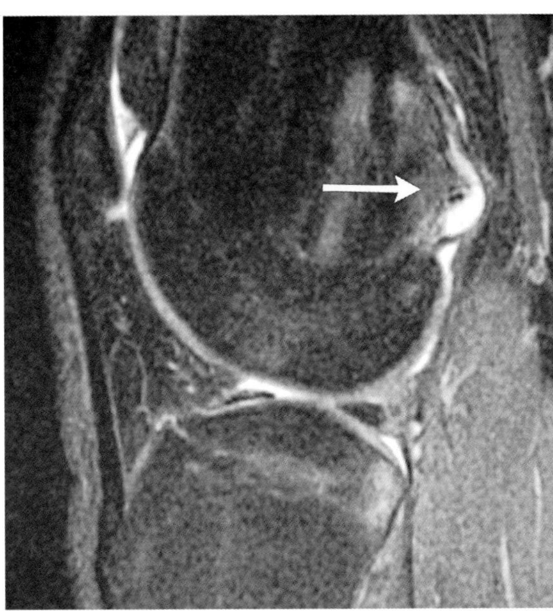

Fig. 11.30 Patient with multiple exostoses including osteochondromas at the distal dorsal femur and proximal dorsal surface of the tibia as seen on lateral radiograph (a). The osteochondroma at the dorsal femur has a thin cartilaginous cap with high signal (arrow) on sagittal fat-suppressed T2-weighted imaging (b).

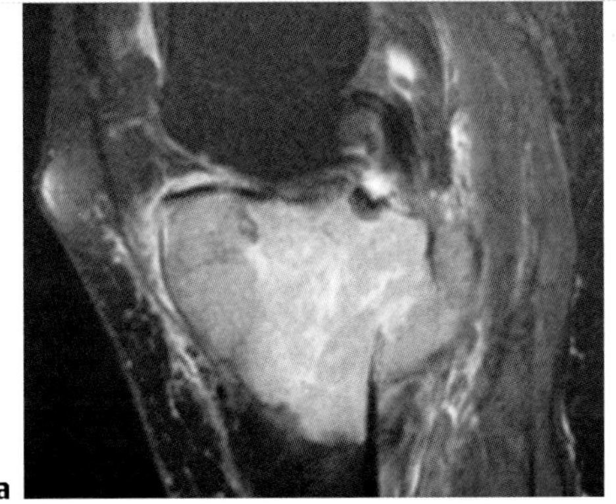

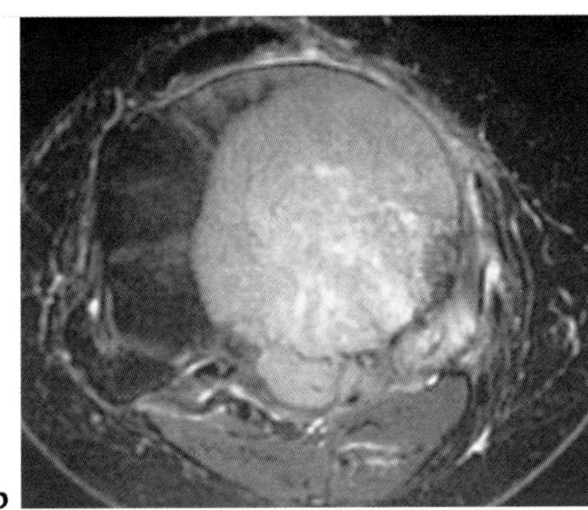

Fig. 11.31 A 77-year-old woman with myeloma involving the marrow of the proximal tibia associated with cortical destruction and extraosseous extension including the knee joint. The tumor has high signal on sagittal (a) and axial (b) fat-suppressed T2-weighted imaging.

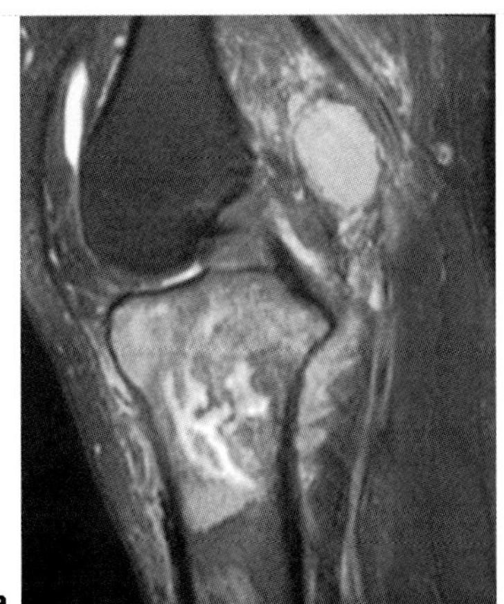

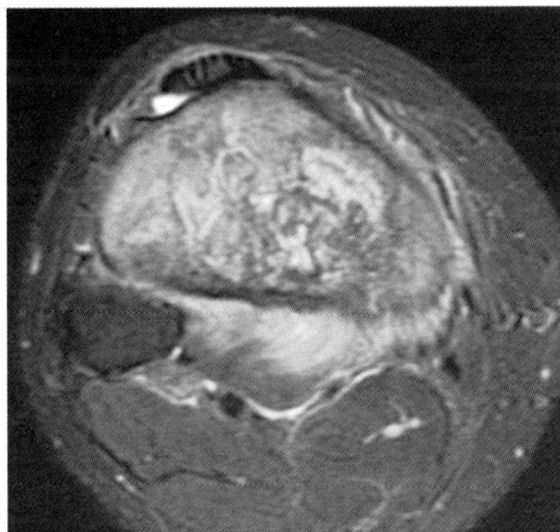

Fig. 11.32 A 32-year-old woman with large B cell non-Hodgkin lymphoma involving the marrow of the proximal tibia associated with cortical destruction and extraosseous extension into the knee joint. The lymphoma has heterogeneous high signal on sagittal (a) and axial (b) fat-suppressed T2-weighted imaging. A nodular lymphoma lesion is also seen dorsal to the posterior cruciate ligament.

Table 11.1 (Cont.) Tumors and tumor-like lesions within joints

Tumor or tumor-like lesion	MRI findings	Comments
Intra-articular extension from primary malignant bone tumors (▶ Fig. 11.33; ▶ Fig. 11.34)	Intramedullary zones with low-intermediate signal on T1WI; intermediate, slightly high, to high signal on T2WI; and slightly high to high signal on FS T2WI. Lesions usually show Gd-contrast enhancement. Tumors frequently cause cortical destruction with extension into the extraosseous soft tissues, including joints.	Primary sarcomas involving bone (osteosarcoma, chondrosarcoma, fibrosarcoma, etc.) can cause cortical destruction with extraosseous extension of tumor, including into joints.
Synovial chondrosarcoma	Lesions usually have low-intermediate signal on T1WI and heterogeneous predominantly high signal on T2WI. Zones of low signal on T2WI are related to the presence and degree of matrix mineralization and/or fibrous tissue. Lesions often have lobulated margins, with or without internal septations. Tumors usually show contrast-enhancement in patterns ranging from lobulated peripheral and/or septal, or homogeneous versus heterogeneous depending on the degree of matrix mineralization and/or necrosis.	Chondrosarcomas rarely arise within synovium.

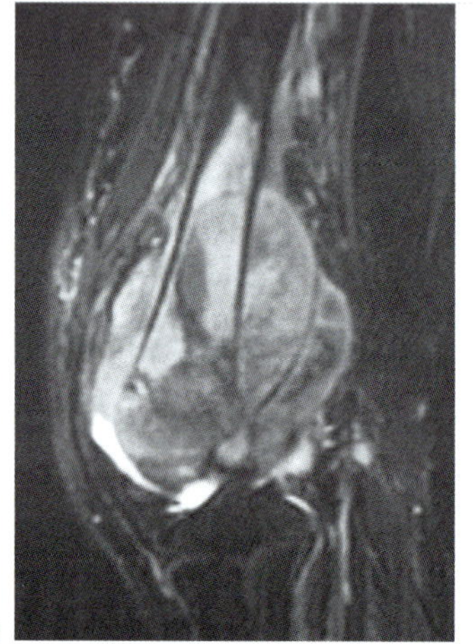

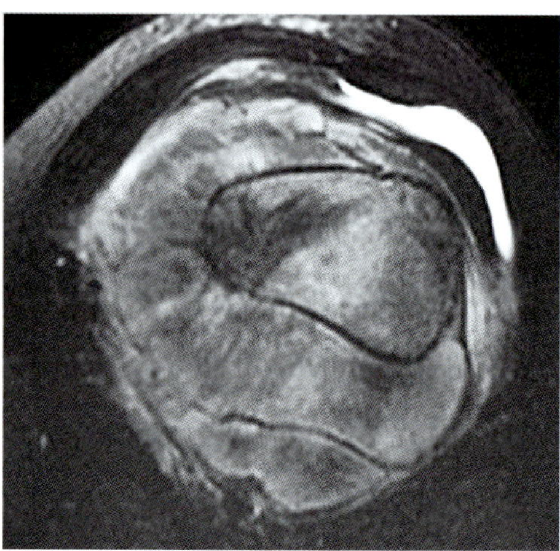

Fig. 11.33 Primary osteosarcoma in the distal metaphysis and epiphysis of the femur, which extends from the marrow into adjacent extraosseous tissues and knee joint via multiple zones of cortical disruption. The intramedullary and extraosseous tumor has heterogeneous slightly high, intermediate, and low signal on sagittal (a) and axial (b) fat-suppressed T2-weighted imaging. Irregular amorphous, divergent, and perpendicular bands and strands of low signal are seen in the extraosseous tumor representing tumor-induced bone formation/periosteal reaction. A thin, slightly irregular zone of low signal is seen at portions of the peripheral border of the extraosseous tumor representing a partially intact elevated periosteum.

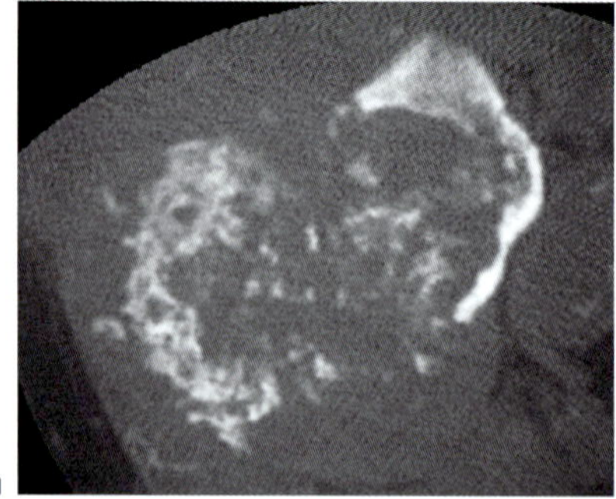

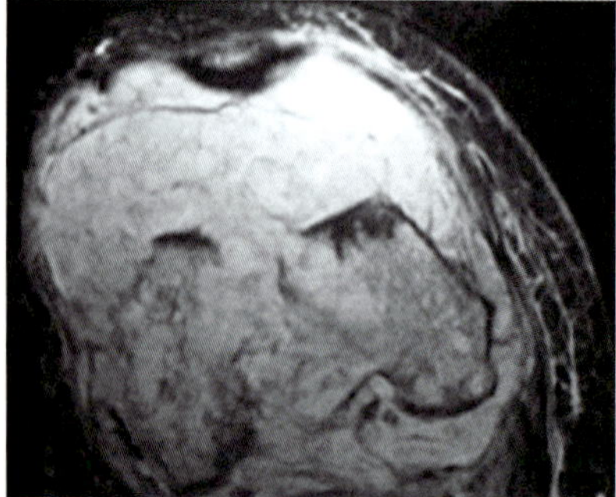

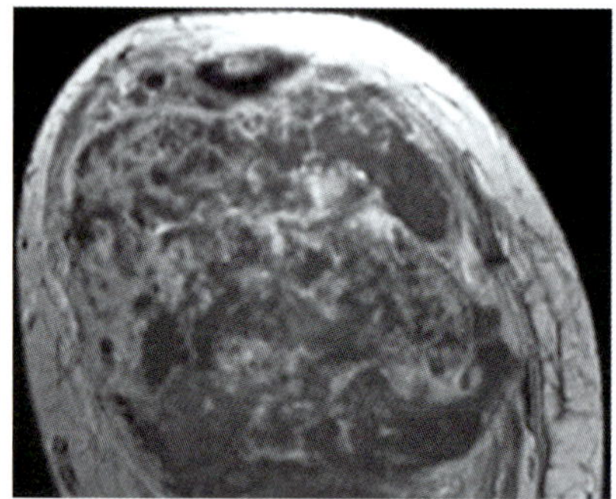

Fig. 11.34 A 60-year-old woman with a dedifferentiated chondrosarcoma involving the distal femur. Axial computed tomographic image (a) shows a destructive intraosseous lesion with chondroid matrix mineralization associated with cortical bone destruction. The tumor has heterogeneous high signal on axial fat-suppressed T2-weighted imaging (b). Tumor extension from the marrow into the knee joint and adjacent soft tissues is seen through sites of cortical bone destruction. The lesion shows irregular heterogeneous Gd-contrast enhancement on axial T1-weighted imaging (c).

11.2 Suggested Reading: Lesions within Joints

▶ Calcific Tendinitis

[1] Flemming DJ, Murphey MD, Shekitka KM, Temple HT, Jelinek JJ, Kransdorf MJ. Osseous involvement in calcific tendinitis: a retrospective review of 50 cases. AJR Am J Roentgenol 2003; 181: 965–972

[2] Porcellini G, Paladini P, Campi F, Pegreffi F. Osteolytic lesion of greater tuberosity in calcific tendinis of the shoulder. J Shoulder Elbow Surg 2009; 18: 210–215

▶ Calcium Pyrophosphate Deposition Disease

[3] Abreu M, Johnson K, Chung CB, et al. Calcification in calcium pyrophosphate dihydrate (CPPD) crystalline deposits in the knee: anatomic, radiographic, MR imaging, and histologic study in cadavers. Skeletal Radiol 2004; 33: 392–398

[4] Lin SH, Hsieh ET, Wu TY, Chang CW. Cervical myelopathy induced by pseudogout in ligamentum flavum and retro-odontoid mass: a case report. Spinal Cord 2006; 44: 692–694

[5] Mahmud T, Basu D, Dyson PHP. Crystal arthropathy of the lumbar spine: a series of six cases and a review of the literature. J Bone Joint Surg Br 2005; 87: 513–517

▶ Chondrosarcoma

[6] Taconis WK, van der Heul RO, Taminiau AM. Synovial chondrosarcoma: report of a case and review of the literature. Skeletal Radiol 1997; 26: 682–685

▶ Giant Cell Tumor (Nodular Synovitis) of the Tendon Sheath and/or Soft Tissue

[7] Al-Qattan MM. Giant cell tumours of tendon sheath: classification and recurrence rate. J Hand Surg [Br] 2001; 26: 72–75

[8] Gibbons CL, Khwaja HA, Cole AS, Cooke PH, Athanasou NA. Giant-cell tumour of the tendon sheath in the foot and ankle. J Bone Joint Surg Br 2002; 84: 1000–1003

[9] Huang GS, Lee CH, Chan WP, Chen CY, Yu JS, Resnick D. Localized nodular synovitis of the knee: MR imaging appearance and clinical correlates in 21 patients. AJR Am J Roentgenol 2003; 181: 539–543

[10] Jelinek JS, Kransdorf MJ, Shmookler BM, Aboulafia AA, Malawer MM. Giant cell tumor of the tendon sheath: MR findings in nine cases. AJR Am J Roentgenol 1994; 162: 919–922

[11] Kitagawa Y, Ito H, Amano Y, Sawaizumi T, Takeuchi T. MR imaging for preoperative diagnosis and assessment of local tumor extent on localized giant cell tumor of tendon sheath. Skeletal Radiol 2003; 32: 633–638

[12] Llauger J, Palmer J, Rosón N, Cremades R, Bagué S. Pigmented villonodular synovitis and giant cell tumors of the tendon sheath: radiologic and pathologic features. AJR Am J Roentgenol 1999; 172: 1087–1091

[13] Ly JQ, Carlson CL, LaGatta LM, Beall DP. Giant cell tumor of the peroneus tendon sheath. AJR Am J Roentgenol 2003; 180: 1442

[14] Meyers SP. Giant cell tumor of the tendon sheath and/or soft tissue. In: MRI of Bone and Soft Tissue Tumors and Tumorlike Lesions. Stuttgart, Germany: Thieme; 2008:469–475

[15] Monaghan H, Salter DM, Al-Nafussi A. Giant cell tumour of tendon sheath (localised nodular tenosynovitis): clinicopathological features of 71 cases. J Clin Pathol 2001; 54: 404–407

[16] Somerhausen N, Cin PD. Giant cell tumor of the tendon sheath. In: Fletcher CDM, Unni KK, Mertens F, eds. World Health Organization Classification of Tumours. Pathology and Genetics of Tumours of Soft Tissue and Bone. Lyon, France: IARC Press; 2002:110–111

[17] Somerhausen N, Cin PD. Diffuse-type giant cell tumor of the tendon sheath. In: Fletcher CDM, Unni KK, Mertens F, eds. World Health Organization Classification of Tumours. Pathology and Genetics of Tumours of Soft Tissue and Bone. IARC Press; 2002:112–114

[18] Wu NL, Hsiao PF, Chen BF, Chen HC, Su HY. Malignant giant cell tumor of the tendon sheath. Int J Dermatol 2004; 43: 54–57

▶ Gout

[19] Chen CK, Chung CB, Yeh LR, et al. Carpal tunnel syndrome caused by tophaceous gout: CT and MR imaging features in 20 patients. AJR Am J Roentgenol 2000; 175: 655–659

[20] Chen CK, Yeh LR, Pan HB, et al. Intra-articular gouty tophi of the knee: CT and MR imaging in 12 patients. Skeletal Radiol 1999; 28: 75–80

[21] Liu SZ, Yeh LR, Chou YJ, Chen CKH, Pan HB. Isolated intraosseous gout in hallux sesamoid mimicking a bone tumor in a teenaged patient. Skeletal Radiol 2003; 32: 647–650

[22] Meyers SP. Gout. In: MRI of Bone and Soft Tissue Tumors and Tumorlike Lesions Stuttgart, Germany: Thieme; 2008:479–483

[23] Monu JUV, Pope TL. Gout: a clinical and radiologic review. Radiol Clin North Am 2004; 42: 169–184

[24] Yu JS, Chung C, Recht M, Dailiana T, Jurdi R. MR imaging of tophaceous gout. AJR Am J Roentgenol 1997; 168: 523–527

▶ Hemangioma

[25] Adler CP, Wold L. Haemangioma and related lesions. In: Fletcher CDM, Unni KK, Mertens F, eds. World Health Organization Classification of Tumours. Pathology and Genetics of Tumours of Soft Tissue and Bone. Lyon, France: IARC Press; 2002:320–323

[26] Calonje E. Haemangiomas. In: Fletcher CDM, Unni KK, Mertens F, eds. World Health Organization Classification of Tumours. Pathology and Genetics of Tumours of Soft Tissue and Bone. Lyon, France: IARC Press; 2002:156–158

[27] Fayad LM, Hazirolan T, Bluemke D, Mitchell S. Vascular malformations in the extremities: emphasis on MR imaging features that guide treatment options [Erratum in Skeletal Radiol 2006;35(12):964. Fayad, Laura corrected t Fayad Laura M]. Skeletal Radiol 2006; 35: 127–137

[28] Meyers SP. Hemangiomas. In: MRI of Bone and Soft Tissue Tumors and Tumorlike Lesions. Stuttgart, Germany: Thieme; 2008:491–501

▶ Hematoma, Morel-Lavallée Lesion, Hemophilic Pseudotumor

[29] Bush CH. The magnetic resonance imaging of musculoskeletal hemorrhage. Skeletal Radiol 2000; 29: 1–9

[30] Jaovisidha S, Ryu KN, Hodler J, Schweitzer ME, Sartoris DJ, Resnick D. Hemophilic pseudotumor: spectrum of MR findings. Skeletal Radiol 1997; 26: 468–474

[31] Jelinek J, Kransdorf MJ. MR imaging of soft-tissue masses. Mass-like lesions that simulate neoplasms. Magn Reson Imaging Clin N Am 1995; 3: 727–741

[32] Meyers SP. Hematoma, Morel-Lavallee lesion, hemophilic pseudotumor. In: MRI of Bone and Soft Tissue Tumors and Tumorlike Lesions. Stuttgart, Germany: Thieme;2008:507–511

▶ Juvenile Idiopathic Arthritis

[33] Damasio MB, Malattia C, Martini A, Tomà P. Synovial and inflammatory diseases in childhood: role of new imaging modalities in the assessment of patients with juvenile idiopathic arthritis. Pediatr Radiol 2010; 40: 985–998

[34] Gylys-Morin VM, Graham TB, Blebea JS, et al. Knee in early juvenile rheumatoid arthritis: MR imaging findings. Radiology 2001; 220: 696–706

[35] Johnson K. Imaging of juvenile idiopathic arthritis. Pediatr Radiol 2006; 36: 743–758

[36] Kan JH, Graham TB. Combined pre-injection wrist and ankle MRI protocol and steroid joint injections in juvenile idiopathic arthritis. Pediatr Radiol 2011; 41: 1326–1332

[37] Kan JH, Hernanz-Schulman M, Damon BM, Yu C, Connolly SA. MRI features of three paediatric intra-articular synovial lesions: a comparative study. Clin Radiol 2008; 63: 805–812

[38] Kim HK, Zbojniewicz AM, Merrow AC, Cheon JE, Kim IO, Emery KH. MR findings of synovial disease in children and young adults: Part 1. Pediatr Radiol 2011; 41: 495–511, quiz 545–546

[39] Kim HK, Zbojniewicz AM, Merrow AC, Cheon JE, Kim IO, Emery KH. MR findings of synovial disease in children and young adults: Part 2. Pediatr Radiol 2011; 41: 512–524

[40] Malattia C, Damasio MB, Pistorio A, et al. Development and preliminary validation of a paediatric-targeted MRI scoring system for the assessment of disease activity and damage in juvenile idiopathic arthritis. Ann Rheum Dis 2011; 70: 440–446

[41] Southwood T. Juvenile idiopathic arthritis: clinically relevant imaging in diagnosis and monitoring. Pediatr Radiol 2008; 38 Suppl 3: S395–S402

▶ Intra-articular Lipoma

[42] Meyers SP. Lipoma, atypical lipoma, and hibernoma. In: MRI of Bone and Soft Tissue Tumors and Tumorlike Lesions. Stuttgart, Germany: Thieme; 2008: 543–553

[43] Murphey MD, Carroll JF, Flemming DJ, Pope TL, Gannon FH, Kransdorf MJ. From the archives of the AFIP: benign musculoskeletal lipomatous lesions. Radiographics 2004; 24: 1433–1466

[44] Nielsen GP, Mandahl N. Lipoma. In: Fletcher CDM, Unni KK, Mertens F, eds. World Health Organization Classification of Tumours. Pathology and Genetics of Tumours of Soft Tissue and Bone. Lyon, France: IARC Press; 2002:20–22

[45] Roberts CC, Liu PT, Colby TV. Encapsulated versus nonencapsulated superficial fatty masses: a proposed MR imaging classification. AJR Am J Roentgenol 2003; 180: 1419–1422

▸ Osteochondritis Dissecans

[46] Kijowski R, De Smet AA. MRI findings of osteochondritis dissecans of the capitellum with surgical correlation. AJR Am J Roentgenol 2005; 185: 1453–1459

[47] O'Connor MA, Palaniappan M, Khan N, Bruce CE. Osteochondritis dissecans of the knee in children. A comparison of MRI and arthroscopic findings. J Bone Joint Surg Br 2002; 84: 258–262

[48] Sanders TG, Paruchuri NB, Zlatkin MB. MRI of osteochondral defects of the lateral femoral condyle: incidence and pattern of injury after transient lateral dislocation of the patella. AJR Am J Roentgenol 2006; 187: 1332–1337

[49] Schmid MR, Hodler J, Vienne P, Binkert CA, Zanetti M. Bone marrow abnormalities of foot and ankle: STIR versus T1-weighted contrast-enhanced fat-suppressed spin-echo MR imaging. Radiology 2002; 224: 463–469

▸ Osteomyelitis/Septic Arthritis

[50] Karchevsky M, Schweitzer ME, Morrison WB, Parellada JA. MRI findings of septic arthritis and associated osteomyelitis in adults. AJR Am J Roentgenol 2004; 182: 119–122

[51] Ledermann HP, Morrison WB, Schweitzer ME. MR image analysis of pedal osteomyelitis: distribution, patterns of spread, and frequency of associated ulceration and septic arthritis. Radiology 2002; 223: 747–755

[52] Meyers SP. Osteomyelitis. In: MRI of Bone and Soft Tissue Tumors and Tumorlike Lesions.Stuttgart, Germany: Thieme; 2008:679–692

▸ Pigmented Villonodular Synovitis (PVNS)

[53] Al-Nakshabandi NA, Ryan AG, Choudur H, et al. Pigmented villonodular synovitis. Clin Radiol 2004; 59: 414–420

[54] De St. Aubain Somerhausen N, Dal Cin P. Diffuse-type giant cell tumor. In: Fletcher CDM, Unni KK, Mertens F, eds. World Health Organization Classification of Tumours. Pathology and Genetics of Tumours of Soft Tissue and Bone. Lyon, France: IARC Press; 2002:112–114

[55] Llauger J, Palmer J, Rosón N, Cremades R, Bagué S. Pigmented villonodular synovitis and giant cell tumors of the tendon sheath: radiologic and pathologic features. AJR Am J Roentgenol 1999; 172: 1087–1091

[56] Meyers SP. Pigmented villonodular synovitis. In: MRI of Bone and Soft Tissue Tumors and Tumorlike Lesions. Stuttgart, Germany: Thieme; 2008:726–729

[57] Murphey MD, Rhee JH, Lewis RB, Fanburg-Smith JC, Flemming DJ, Walker EA. Pigmented villonodular synovitis: radiologic-pathologic correlation. Radiographics 2008; 28: 1493–1518

▸ Rheumatoid Arthritis

[58] Boutry N, Lardé A, Lapègue F, Solau-Gervais E, Flipo RM, Cotten A. Magnetic resonance imaging appearance of the hands and feet in patients with early rheumatoid arthritis. J Rheumatol 2003; 30: 671–679

[59] Cimmino MA, Innocenti S, Livrone F, Magnaguagno F, Silvestri E, Garlaschi G. Dynamic gadolinium-enhanced magnetic resonance imaging of the wrist in patients with rheumatoid arthritis can discriminate active from inactive disease. Arthritis Rheum 2003; 48: 1207–1213

[60] Goldbach-Mansky R, Mahadevan V, Yao L, Lipsky PE. The evaluation of bone damage in rheumatoid arthritis with magnetic resonance imaging. Clin Exp Rheumatol 2003; 21 Suppl 31: S50–S53

[61] Meyers SP. Rheumatoid arthritis. In: MRI of Bone and Soft Tissue Tumors and Tumorlike Lesions.Stuttgart, Germany: Thieme; 2008:738–743

[62] Moran M, Fang C, Paul A. Rheumatoid arthritis presenting as an invasive soft-tissue tumour. Arch Orthop Trauma Surg 2002; 122: 538–540

[63] Narváez JA, Narváez J, Roca Y, Aguilera C. MR imaging assessment of clinical problems in rheumatoid arthritis. Eur Radiol 2002; 12: 1819–1828

[64] Østergaard M, Hansen M, Stoltenberg M, et al. New radiographic bone erosions in the wrists of patients with rheumatoid arthritis are detectable with magnetic resonance imaging a median of two years earlier. Arthritis Rheum 2003; 48: 2128–2131

[65] Taouli B, Zaim S, Peterfy CG, et al. Rheumatoid arthritis of the hand and wrist: comparison of three imaging techniques. AJR Am J Roentgenol 2004; 182: 937–943

▸ Scleroderma, Systemic Sclerosis

[66] Madani G, Katz RD, Haddock JA, Denton CP, Bell JR. The role of radiology in the management of systemic sclerosis. Clin Radiol 2008; 63: 959–967

[67] Schanz S, Fiẹrlbeck G, Ulmer A, et al. Localized scleroderma: MR findings and clinical features. Radiology 2011; 260: 817–824

[68] Schanz S, Henes J, Ulmer A, et al. Magnetic resonance imaging findings in patients with systemic scleroderma and musculoskeletal symptoms. Eur Radiol 2013; 23: 212–221

▸ Synovial Chondromatosis and Synovial Osteochondromatosis

[69] Crotty JM, Monu JU, Pope TL. Synovial osteochondromatosis. Radiol Clin North Am 1996; 34: 327–342, xi

[70] Kim SH, Hong SJ, Park JS, et al. Idiopathic synovial osteochondromatosis of the hip: radiographic and MR appearances in 15 patients. Korean J Radiol 2002; 3: 254–259

[71] Kramer J, Recht M, Deely DM, et al. MR appearance of idiopathic synovial osteochondromatosis. J Comput Assist Tomogr 1993; 17: 772–776

[72] McKenzie G, Raby N, Ritchie D. A pictorial review of primary synovial osteochondromatosis. Eur Radiol 2008; 18: 2662–2669

[73] Meyers SP. Synovial chondromatosis and synovial osteochondromatosis. In: MRI of Bone and Soft Tissue Tumors and Tumorlike Lesions. Stuttgart, Germany: Thieme; 2008:753–757

[74] Miller MV, King A, Mertens F. Synovial chondromatosis. In: Fletcher CDM, Unni KK, Mertens F, eds. World Health Organization Classification of Tumours. Pathology and Genetics of Tumours of Soft Tissue and Bone. Lyon, France: IARC Press; 2002:246

[75] Murphey MD, Vidal JA, Fanburg-Smith JC, Gajewski DA. Imaging of synovial chondromatosis with radiologic-pathologic correlation. Radiographics 2007; 27: 1465–1488

[76] Narváez JA, Narváez J, Ortega R, De Lama E, Roca Y, Vidal N. Hypointense synovial lesions on T2-weighted images: differential diagnosis with pathologic correlation. AJR Am J Roentgenol 2003; 181: 761–769

▸ Transient Toxic Synovitis

[77] McCarthy JJ, Noonan KJ. Toxic synovitis. Skeletal Radiol 2008; 37: 963–965

Chapter 12

Lesions Involving the Soft Tissues

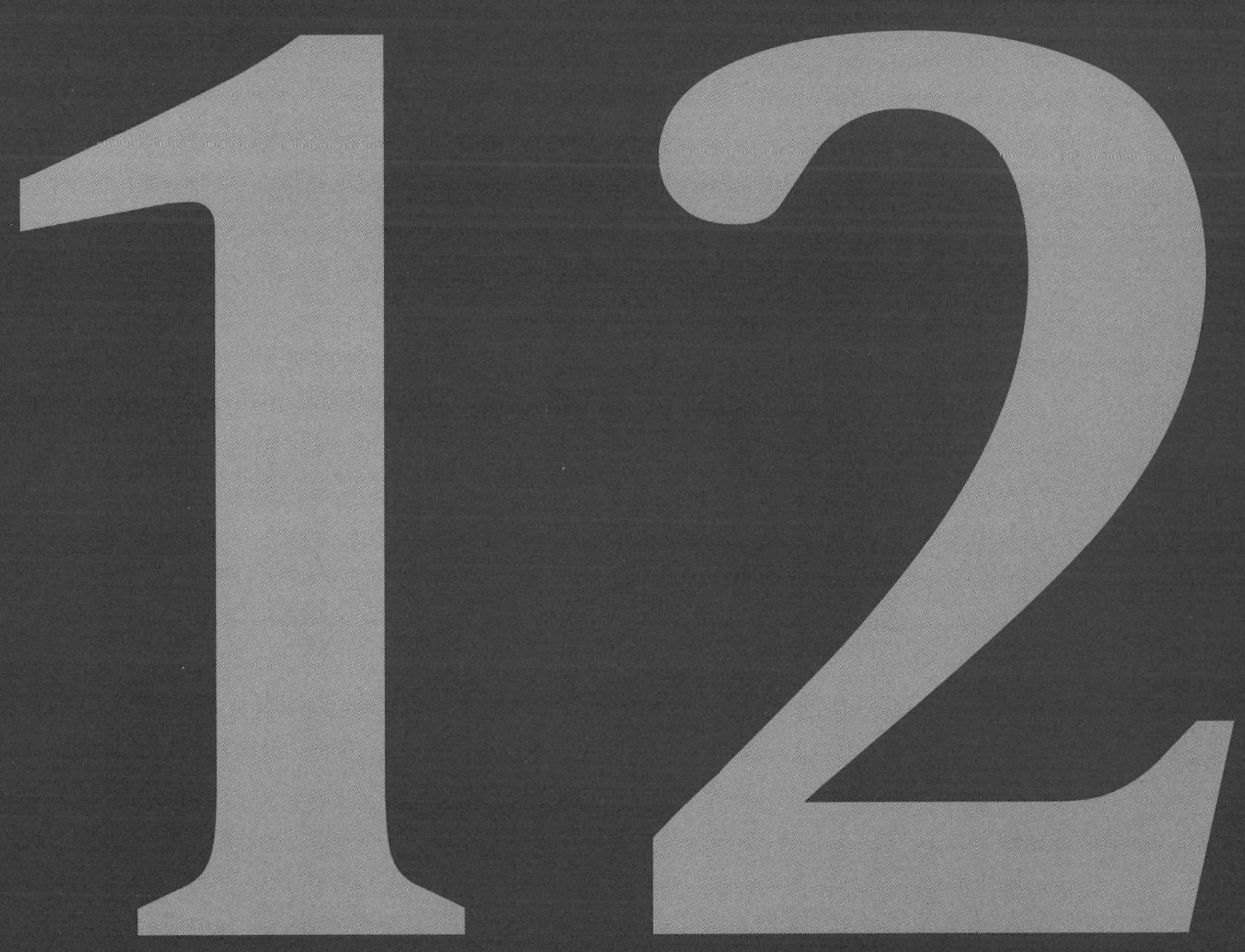

12 Lesions Involving the Soft Tissues

Steven P. Meyers

12.1 Nonmalignant Tumors and Tumor-Like Lesions Involving the Soft Tissues of the Extremities

- Lipoma
- Lipomatosis
- Atypical lipoma
- Hibernoma
- Lipoblastoma
- Hemangioma
- Angiomatosis/hemangiomatosis
- Muscle infarction with fat replacement
- Idiopathic and diabetic skeletal muscle necrosis
- Denervation of muscle
- Lymphangioma
- Nodular faciitis
- Nerve sheath tumor (schwannoma, neurofibroma)
- Neurothekeoma
- Granular cell tumor
- Traumatic neuroma
- Morton neuroma
- Lipoma of nerve (fibrolipomatosis hamartoma)
- Leiomyoma
- Solitary fibrous tumor
- Desmoid tumor/fibromatosis
- Myxoma
- Ganglion cyst
- Hematoma/seroma
- Heterotopic ossification
- Tumoral calcinosis
- Giant cell tumor of the tendon sheath
- Fibroma of the tendon sheath
- Xanthoma
- Amyloid
- Epidermoid
- Elastofibroma
- Aneurysm
- Hypothenar hammer syndrome
- Abscess/myositis
- Cat scratch disease
- Parasitic infection
- Sarcoid
- Giant cell reaction to foreign body
- Granuloma annulare
- Gout
- Rheumatoid arthritis
- Dermatomyositis
- Scleroderma/systemic sclerosis

Table 12.1 Nonmalignant tumors and tumor-like lesions involving the soft tissues of the extremities

Tumor/tumor-like lesion	MRI findings	Comments
Lipoma (▶ Fig. 12.1)	Often have circumscribed margins and have magnetic resonance imaging (MRI) signal comparable to subcutaneous fat on T1-weighted imaging (T1WI), proton density–weighted imaging (PDWI), T2-weighted imaging (T2WI), and fat-suppressed (FS) T2WI. Often do not show gadolinium (Gd)-contrast enhancement except for minimal to mild enhancement along the thin, nonfatty septa.	Common benign hamartomas composed of mature white adipose tissue without cellular atypia. Most common soft tissue tumor, representing 10% of all soft tissue tumors and 16% of benign soft tissue tumors.
Lipomatosis (▶ Fig. 12.2)	Infiltrating adipose tissue or multiple lobules of fat can be seen in muscles, facial planes, and/or subcutaneous fat.	Diffuse proliferation of mature adipose tissue. Can occur as several types. The diffuse type typically involves the soft tissues of an extremity or trunk in children with or without associated osseous hypertrophy. Multiple symmetric lipomatosis (Madelung disease) usually occurs in the neck, trunk, and pelvis of adult men (peak incidence in the fifth decade. Shoulder girdle lipomatosis usually occurs in women and involves the muscles at one shoulder and adjacent chest wall. Adiposis dolorosa (Dercum disease) usually occurs in obese postmenopausal women who have multiple painful fatty lesions in the extremities or trunk.

(continued on page 594)

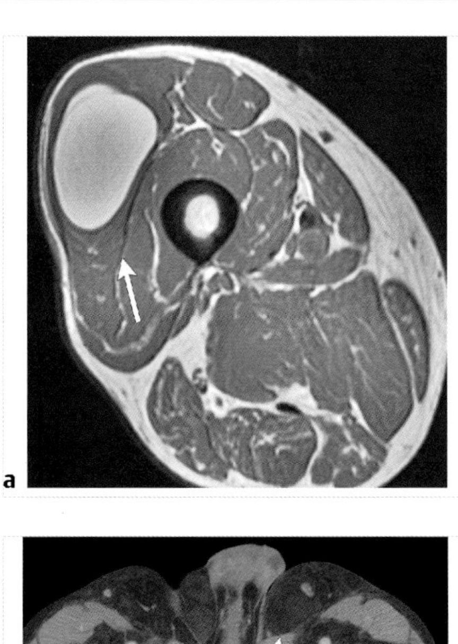

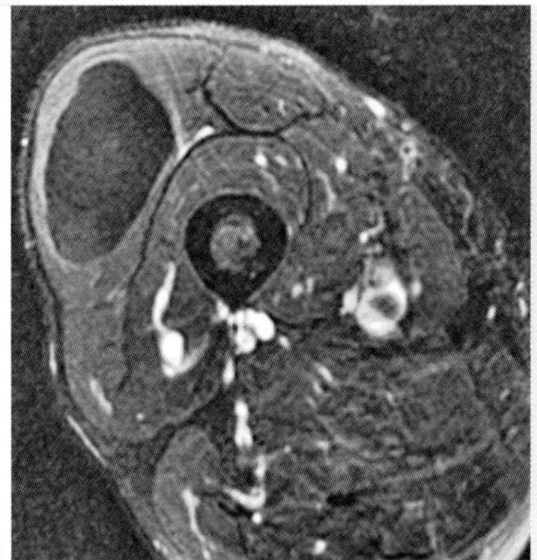

Fig. 12.1 A 71-year-old woman with an intramuscular lipoma in her thigh. The lipoma (arrow) has high signal on axial T1-weighted imaging (a). The fat signal of the lipoma is suppressed on axial fat-suppressed T2-weighted imaging (b).

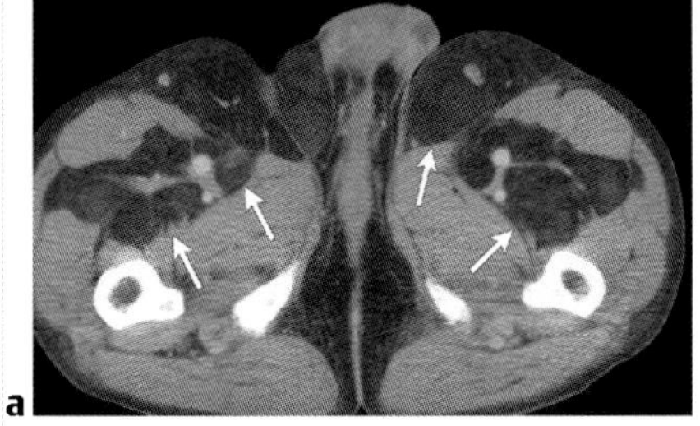

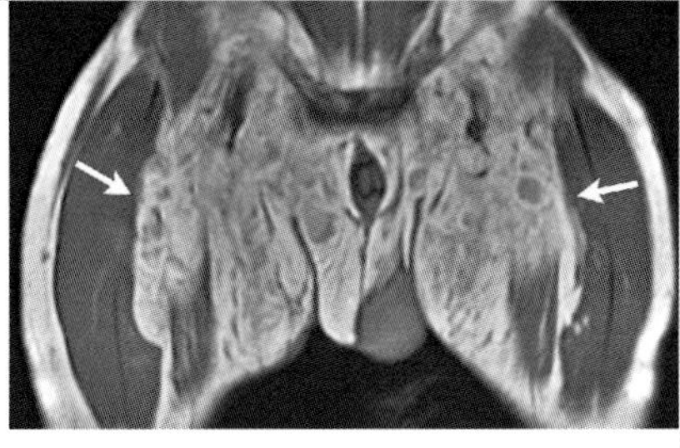

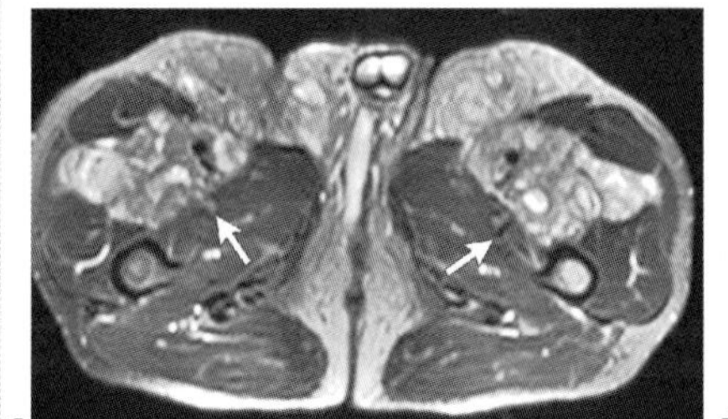

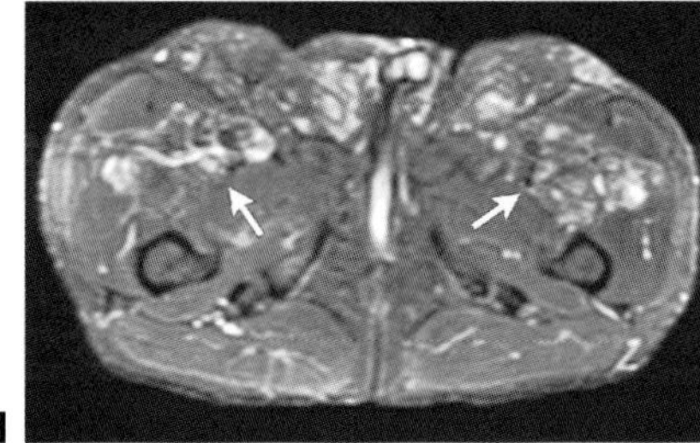

Fig. 12.2 A 42-year-old man with bilateral symmetric lipomatosis involving the inguinal regions, subcutaneous and intermuscular soft tissues of both proximal thighs. Multiple fatty lobules (arrows) are seen with thin peripheral nonfatty septa on axial computed tomographic image (a). Poorly defined zones with attenuation slightly higher than fat are also seen in the fatty lobules. On coronal T1-weighted imaging, the lesion has magnetic resonance imaging signal that is slightly lower than subcutaneous fat (arrows) and contains zones with mixed low-intermediate and intermediate signal (b). The lesion (arrows) contains zones with high signal on axial T2-weighted imaging (c) and axial fat-suppressed T2-weighted imaging (d).

Table 12.1 (Cont.) Nonmalignant tumors and tumor-like lesions involving the soft tissues of the extremities

Tumor/tumor-like lesion	MRI findings	Comments
Atypical lipoma (▶ Fig. 12.3)	Atypical lipomas may contain cystic/necrotic zones, calcifications, thick septa, and/or nodular zones, which may or may not show Gd-contrast enhancement. Most atypical lipomas contain more than 75% fat, whereas liposarcomas often have less than 75% fat. Distinguishing between atypical lipomas and low grade liposarcomas with MRI can be difficult and challenging.	Atypical lipomas account for up to 31% of lipomas. Lesions contain zones with osseous, chondroid, or fibrous metaplasia with myxoid changes. Atypical lipomas have been labeled as chondroid lipomas, osteolipomas, or benign mesenchymomas. Chondroid lipomas contain mature fat, lipoblasts, and chondroid matrix. Spindle cell and pleomorphic lipomas are variants that have varying proportions of mature fat cells, spindle cells, collagen, and multinucleated giant cells. Lipomas with high content of fibrous tissue content have been labeled as fibrolipomas.
Hibernoma (▶ Fig. 12.4)	Well-defined lesions that often have intermediate to high signal on T1WI (hypo- or isointense relative to subcutaneous fat), and slightly high signal on T2WI. Lesions can have slightly hyperintense signal relative to fat on FS T2WI and short TI inversion recovery (STIR). Internal septations and/or branching-serpentine slow-flow vascular channels may be seen on T1WI and T2WI. Lesions can show Gd-contrast enhancement within branching vascular channels.	Rare benign lesions derived from brown adipose tissue intermixed with white adipose tissue. Account for less than 2% of fatty tumors; occur in patients age 2 to over 75 years, mean = 32 to 38 years.
Lipoblastoma (▶ Fig. 12.5)	Lesions often have mixed low, intermediate, and high signal on T1WI, T2WI, and FS T2WI. Lesions often show heterogeneous Gd-contrast enhancement.	Rare benign mesenchymal tumors that contain embryonal fat. Account for less than 1% of benign soft tissue tumors. Patients are age < 1 year to 10 years, mean = 4 years.

(continued on page 596)

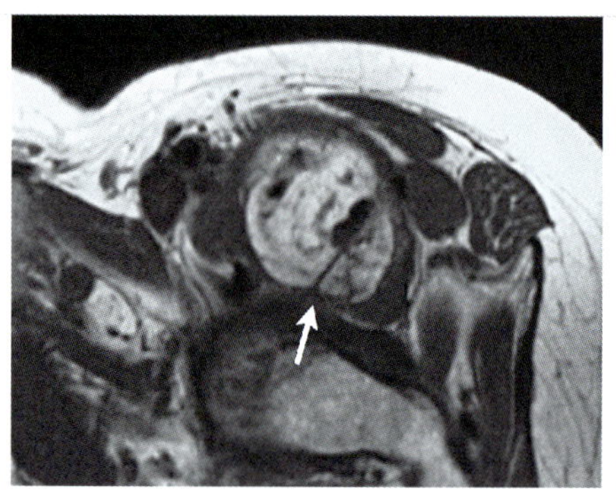

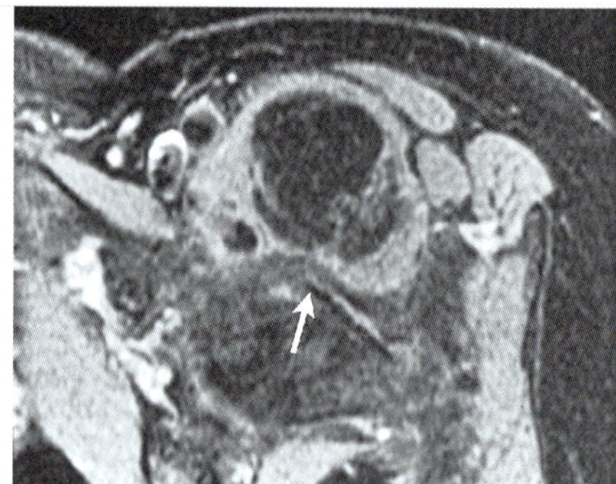

Fig. 12.3 A 55-year-old woman with an atypical lipoma/osteolipoma involving the iliopsoas muscle ventral to the proximal femur The lesion (arrow) contains mostly fat signal on axial T1-weighted imaging (a) as well curvilinear and small nodular zones of low signal. The signal of the fatty portions of the lesion is suppressed on axial fat-suppressed T2-weighted imaging (b), whereas several of the small, nonfatty portions show intermediate to high signal (arrow).

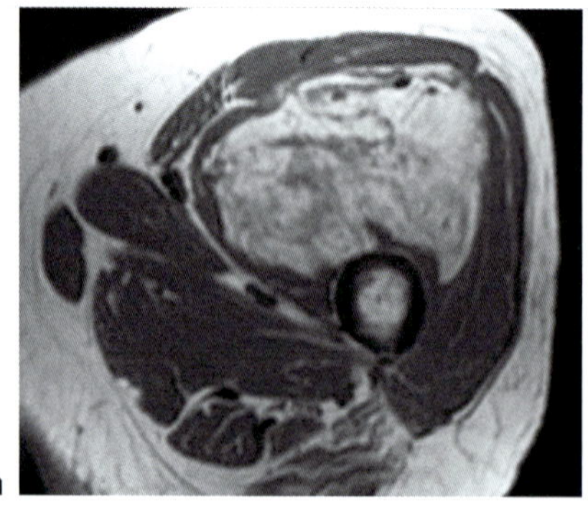

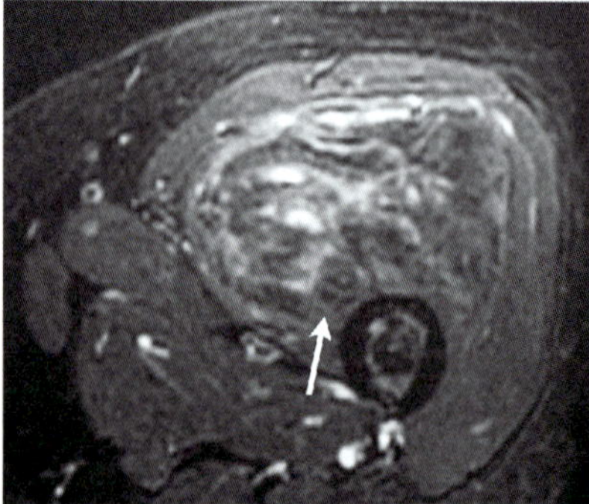

Fig. 12.4 A 71-year-old woman with a hibernoma involving the vastus muscles of the proximal thigh. The lesion has well-defined margins and contains mostly fat signal on axial T1-weighted imaging, which is slightly lower than subcutaneous fat (a) as well as curvilinear and small nodular zones of low signal. The signal of the fatty portions of the lesion is suppressed on axial fat-suppressed T2-weighted imaging (FS T2WI) (b), whereas nonfatty portions show intermediate to high signal on FS T2WI (arrow).

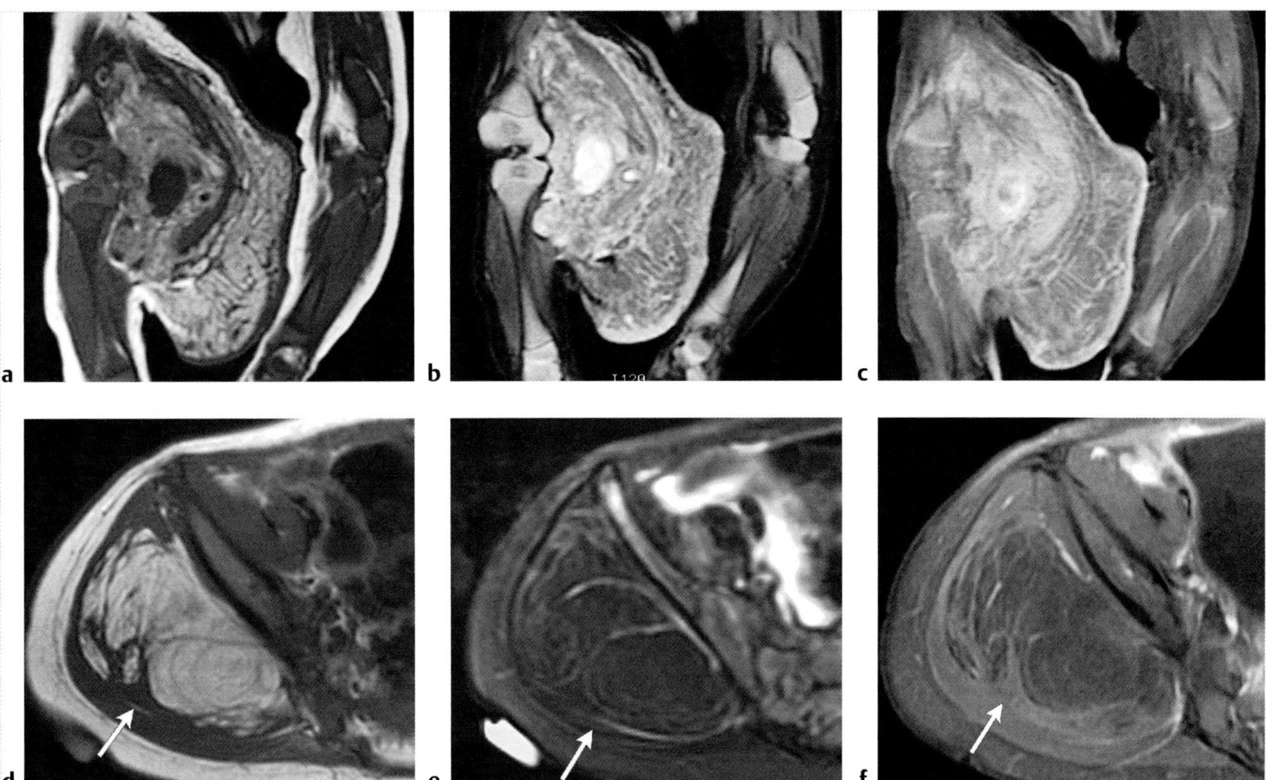

Fig. 12.5 A 3-month-old male with a large lipoblastoma involving the thigh. The lesion infiltrates adjacent muscles and subcutaneous tissues, and contains zones with magnetic resonance imaging signal approximating that of fat on coronal T1-weighted imaging (T1WI) (a). Many of the fatty zones have signal slightly lower than subcutaneous fat on T1WI as well as higher signal on coronal short TI inversion recovery (STIR) (b). The lesion shows heterogeneous gadolinium (Gd)-contrast enhancement on coronal fat-suppressed (FS) T1WI (c). A 1.5-year-old boy with a lipoblastoma (arrow) lateral to the iliac bone, which has signal mostly similar to fat and contains strands of intermediate signal on axial (d). The nonfatty strands within the lesion have slightly high signal on axial FS TWI (e) and show mild Gd-contrast enhancement on axial FS T1WI (arrow) (f).

Table 12.1 (Cont.) Nonmalignant tumors and tumor-like lesions involving the soft tissues of the extremities

Tumor/tumor-like lesion	MRI findings	Comments
Hemangioma (▶ Fig. 12.6)	Hemangiomas have circumscribed margins with or without lobulations and have low-intermediate signal or heterogeneous low-intermediate and high signal on T1WI and PDWI; and high signal on T2WI. On FS T2WI, hemangiomas typically have high signal except for zones of fat within the lesions. Zones of hemorrhage can sometimes be present in hemangiomas as well as phleboliths. Hemangiomas usually show prominent Gd-contrast enhancement.	Benign hamartomatous lesions of bone and soft tissues consisting of capillary, cavernous, and/or malformed venous vessels.
Angiomatosis/hemangiomatosis (▶ Fig. 12.7)	Multifocal, adjacent, and/or contiguous lesions involving different tissues crossing fascial planes. Lesion often have high signal on FS T2WI and show Gd-contrast enhancement.	Diffuse form of hemangiomas that can occur in soft tissue and/or bone, can occur over a large region (often up to 20 cm) and involve multiple tissue planes, and may contain lymphangiomatous portions. Contain mixtures of capillary and cavernous vessels with variable amounts of arteriovenous and adipose tissue. Considered benign (except for angiomatosis associated with Maffucci syndrome, which does have a malignant potential) and can recur after surgery.
Muscle infarct with fat replacement (▶ Fig. 12.8)	In the early phases of ischemia and infarction, poorly defined zones of increased signal on T2WI and FS T2WI can be seen in the involved muscles. Remote infarcts are seen as fatty replacement of muscle tissue.	Zones of ischemic injury and death involving muscle from trauma, corticosteroid treatment, chemotherapy, radiation treatment, diabetes, occlusive vascular disease, and collagen vascular and other autoimmune diseases.

(continued on page 598)

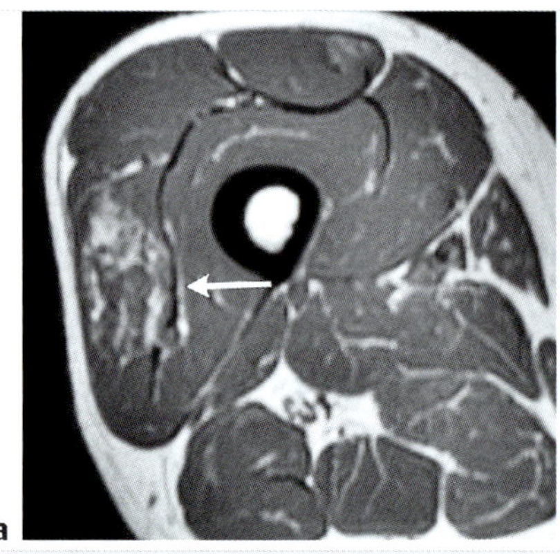

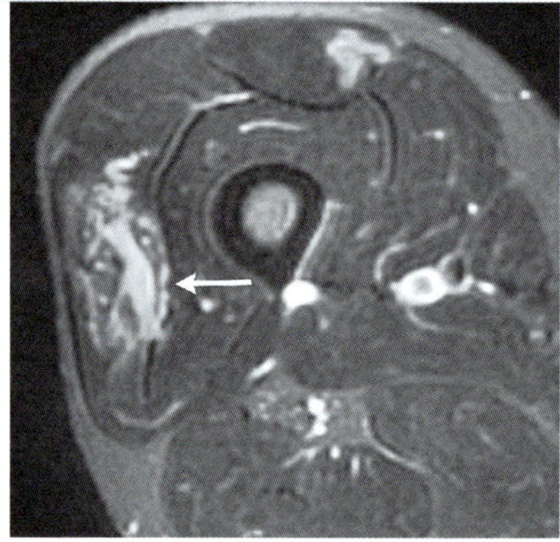

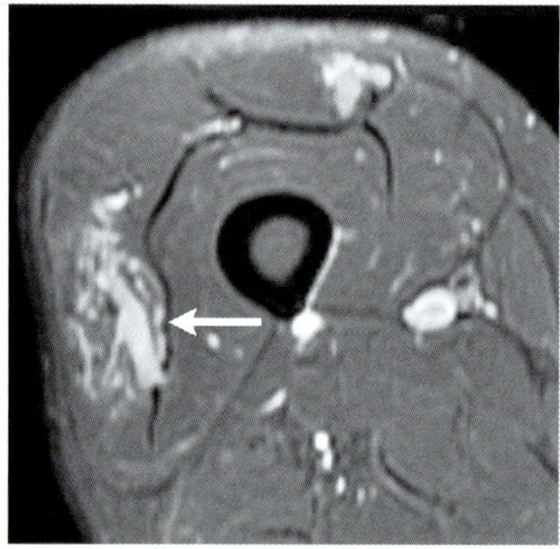

Fig. 12.6 A 57-year-old man with an intramuscular hemangioma in the thigh (arrow), which has mixed intermediate and high signal on axial T1-weighted imaging (T1WI) (a). The lesion has mostly high signal on axial fat-suppressed (FS) T2-weighted imaging (arrow) (b), and shows heterogeneous Gd-contrast enhancement in the lesion, which contains prominent veins on axial FS T1WI (arrow) (c).

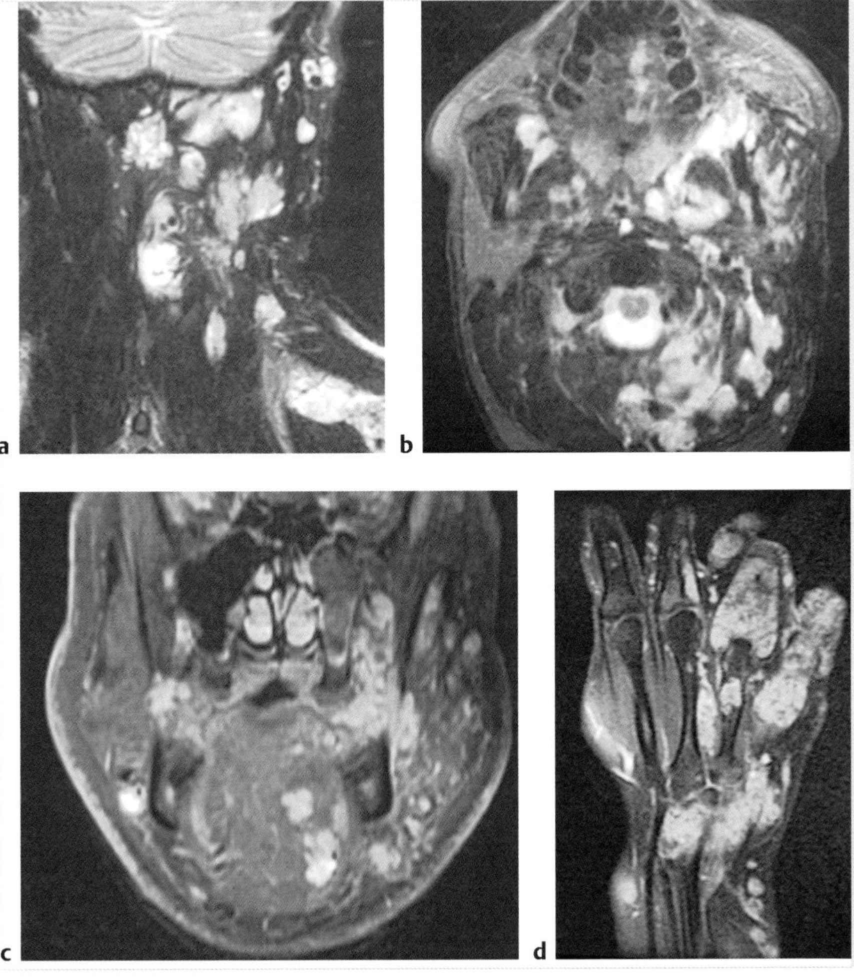

Fig. 12.7 A 22-year-old man with angiomatosis involving the soft tissues of the head and neck. The multifocal lesions involve multiple tissue planes and have high signal on coronal (a) and axial (b) fat-suppressed (FS) T2-weighted imaging, and show moderate gadolinium-contrast enhancement on coronal FS T1-weighted imaging (T1WI) (c). A 20-year-old woman with Maffucci syndrome with multiple contrast-enhancing enchondromas and hemangiomas involving the soft tissues of the hand on coronal FS T1WI (d).

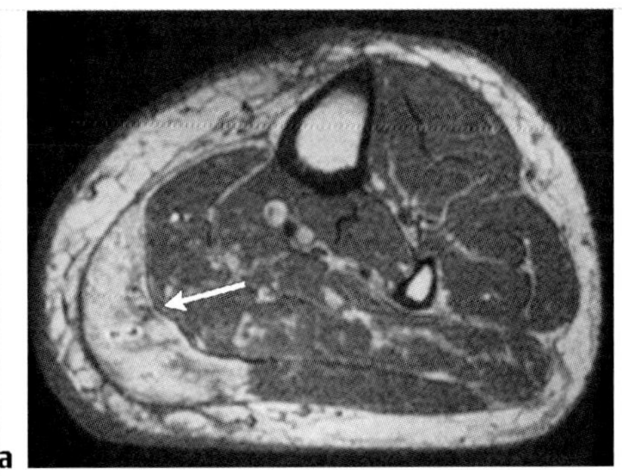

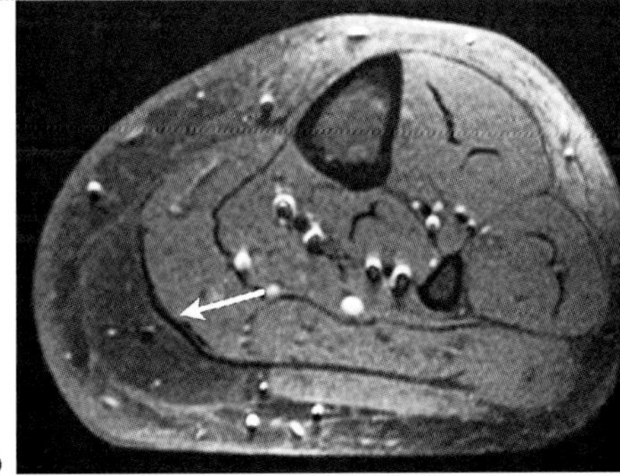

Fig. 12.8 A 60-year-old man with a remote infarct involving the medial gastrocnemius muscle. There is diffuse high signal on axial T1-weighted imaging (T1WI) (a) in the muscle (arrow) secondary to fatty atrophy resulting from the infarct, which has corresponding low signal on axial fat-suppressed T1WI (arrow) (b).

Table 12.1 (Cont.) Nonmalignant tumors and tumor-like lesions involving the soft tissues of the extremities

Tumor/tumor-like lesion	MRI findings	Comments
Idiopathic and diabetic skeletal muscle necrosis (▶ Fig. 12.9)	Swelling of muscle(s) with heterogeneous decreased signal on T1WI and heterogeneous slightly high to high signal on T2WI and FS T2WI. Poorly defined zones with high signal on FS T2WI are often seen in adjacent fascia and soft tissues. Lesions often show heterogeneous and variable Gd-contrast enhancement.	Necrosis of skeletal muscle, which can be associated with diabetes as well as alcoholism, or can be idiopathic. Lesion(s) present as rapidly evolving tender mass in skeletal muscle consisting of hemorrhagic necrosis, edema, and perivascular and endomysial lymphohistiocytic infiltrate. Occurs in the absence of trauma, infection (negative cultures), neoplastic disease, autoimmune myositis, or vasculitis. May be related to atheroemboli superimposed on diabetic small vessel disease. Most common in thigh muscles, 1.7:1 female to male ratio in patients ranging in age from 19 to 77 years, mean = 43 years. Creatine kinase can be three to four times the normal value, erythrocyte sedimentation rate (ESR) usually elevated. Treatment is typically conservative with supportive management consisting of analgesics, rest, and immobilization. Symptoms often resolve in 4 to 8 weeks.
Denervation of muscle (▶ Fig. 12.10)	In the early phases of denervation, within 15 days, involved muscles can have low signal on T1WI and slightly high to high signal on T2WI and FS T2WI without involvement of the adjacent fascia and subcutaneous fat. After 1 year, fatty replacement of the involved muscles with atrophy can be seen.	Early phases of denervation result in neurogenic edema. In chronic and complete muscle denervation, atrophy and fatty replacement of muscle typically occur after 1 year. Parsonage-Turner syndrome is one type of denervation that results in an acute painful shoulder from injury of the brachial plexus and damage to the suprascapular nerve (C5, C6) with involvement of the supraspinatus and/or infraspinatus muscles. Quadrilateral space syndrome results from damage or injury to the axillary nerve (C5, C6), which can affect the teres minor and deltoid muscles.
Lymphangioma (▶ Fig. 12.11)	Can be circumscribed lesions or occur in infiltrative pattern with extension within and between muscles. Often contain single or multiple cystic zones, which have predominantly low signal on T1WI and high signal on T2WI and FS T2WI. Fluid-fluid levels and zones with high signal on T1WI and variable signal on T2WI may result from cysts containing hemorrhage, high protein concentration, and/or necrotic debris. Septa between the cystic zones can vary in thickness and Gd-contrast enhancement, and usually have low signal on T1WI and low to intermediate signal on T2WI and FS T2WI. Nodular zones within the lesions can have variable degrees of Gd-contrast enhancement.	Benign vascular tumors that typically occur in soft tissue and only rarely in bone, which result from abnormal proliferation of lymphatic vessels. Lesions are composed of endothelium-lined lymphatic channels interspersed within connective tissue stroma. Account for less than 1% of benign soft tissue tumors and 5.6% of all benign lesions of infancy and childhood. Can occur in association with Turner syndrome and Proteus syndrome. Patients usually range in age from 1 to 50 years, mean = 19 years. Can be congenital, with approximately 50% present at birth. Approximately 85% are detected by age 2.

(continued on page 600)

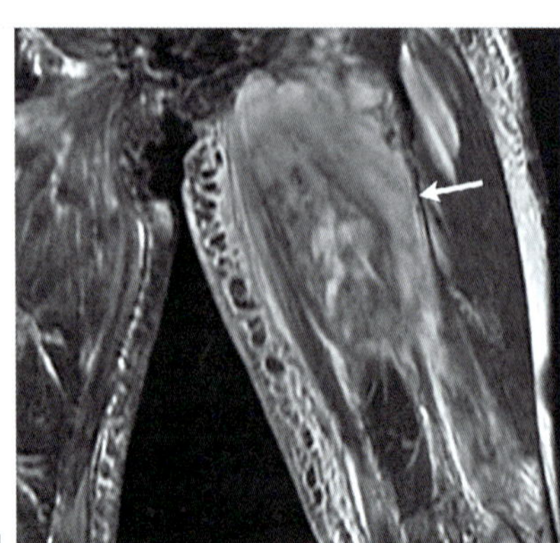

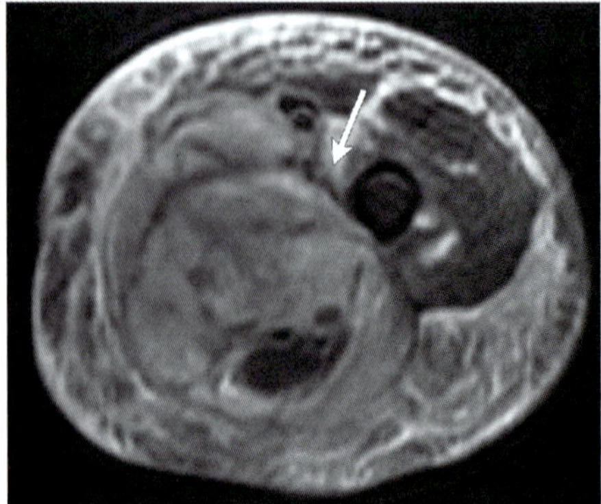

Fig. 12.9 A 55-year-old woman with diabetic myonecrosis involving the thigh. Coronal (a) and axial (b) fat-suppressed T2-weighted imaging shows irregular enlargement of the adductor muscles, which have abnormal heterogeneous slightly high to high signal (arrows). Poorly defined zones with high signal are also seen in the adjacent soft tissues.

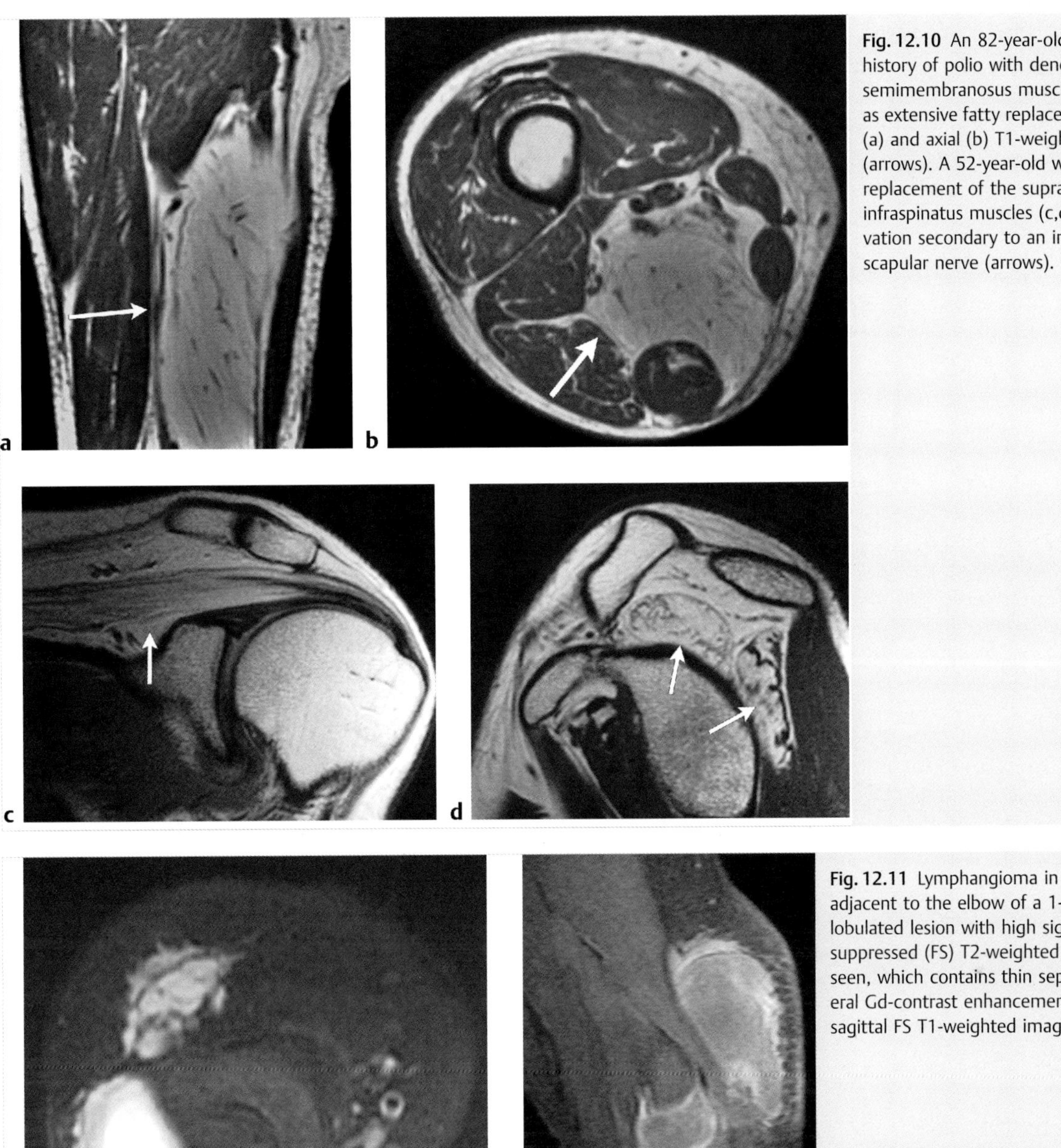

Fig. 12.10 An 82-year-old man with a history of polio with denervation of the semimembranosus muscle, which is seen as extensive fatty replacement on coronal (a) and axial (b) T1-weighted imaging (arrows). A 52-year-old woman with fatty replacement of the supraspinatus and infraspinatus muscles (c,d) from denervation secondary to an injured suprascapular nerve (arrows).

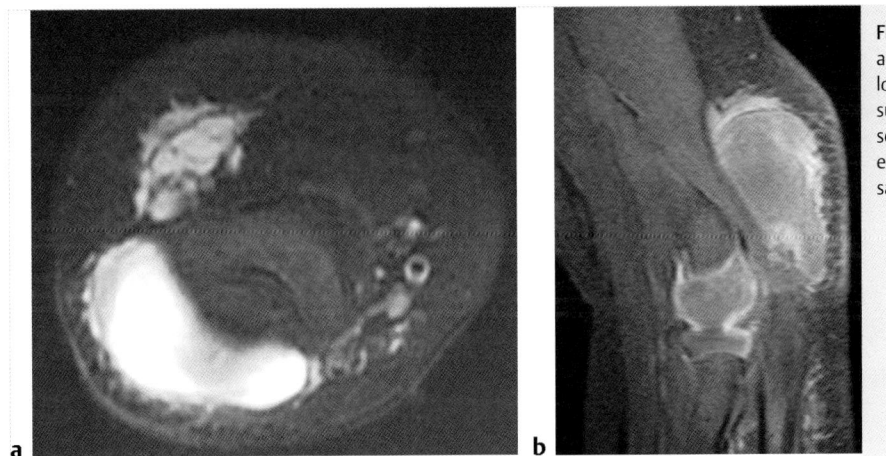

Fig. 12.11 Lymphangioma in the soft tissues adjacent to the elbow of a 1-year-old boy. A lobulated lesion with high signal on axial fat-suppressed (FS) T2-weighted imaging (a) is seen, which contains thin septa. Thin peripheral Gd-contrast enhancement is seen on sagittal FS T1-weighted imaging (b).

Table 12.1 (Cont.) Nonmalignant tumors and tumor-like lesions involving the soft tissues of the extremities

Tumor/tumor-like lesion	MRI findings	Comments
Nodular faciitis (▶ Fig. 12.12)	Lesions can have mildly irregular or stellate borders. Lesions usually have intermediate signal on T1WI and PDWI and homogeneous or mildly heterogeneous high signal on T2WI and FS T2WI. Surrounding edema is occasionally seen. Older lesions with high fibrous content may have intermediate signal on T2WI. Lesions can show homogeneous or peripheral rimlike patterns of Gd-contrast enhancement.	Benign reactive lesion consisting of proliferating fibroblasts, usually occurring in the subcutaneous tissue or muscle. Accounts for 11% of benign soft tissue tumors and 7% of all soft tissue tumors. Patients range from age 11 to 51 years, mean = 31 years.
Nerve sheath tumor (schwannoma, neurofibroma) (▶ Fig. 12.13; ▶ Fig. 12.14; ▶ Fig. 12.15)	*Localized neurofibromas and Schwannomas* are circumscribed ovoid or fusiform lesions with low-intermediate signal on T1WI, intermediate signal on PDWI, and intermediate to high signal on T2WI and FS T2WI. Lesions typically show moderate to prominent Gd-contrast enhancement. Multiple neurofibromas and schwannomas are frequently seen with neurofibromatosis 1 (NF1) and NF2, respectively. Neurofibromas can occur in various soft tissues. *Plexiform neurofibromas* appear as curvilinear and multinodular lesions involving multiple nerve branches and have low to intermediate signal on T1WI and intermediate, slightly high to high signal on T2WI and FS T2WI with or without bands or strands of low signal. Lesions usually show Gd-contrast enhancement.	Benign nerve sheath tumors include schwannomas and neurofibromas. Schwannomas are benign encapsulated tumors that contain differentiated neoplastic Schwann cells. Neurofibromas contain mixtures of Schwann cells, perineural-like cells, and interlacing fascicles of fibroblasts associated with abundant collagen. Unlike schwannomas, neurofibromas lack Antoni A and B regions and cannot be separated pathologically from the underlying nerve. Can be localized lesions or occur as diffuse or plexiform lesions. Multiple neurofibromas are typically seen with NF1. Multiple schwannomas are typically seen with NF2.
Neurothekeoma (▶ Fig. 12.16)	Occur as circumscribed lesions with low-intermediate signal on T1WI, high signal on T2WI, and heterogeneous Gd-contrast enhancement.	Neurothekeoma, also referred to as nerve sheath myxoma, is considered to be a neurofibroma with prominent myxoid matrix separated into lobules by fibrous connective tissue.
Granular cell tumor (▶ Fig. 12.17)	Tumors can have circumscribed and/or irregular margins and contain low-intermediate signal on T1WI and PDWI and slightly high to high signal on T2WI and FS T2WI. Tumors can also have low-intermediate signal on T2WI. Tumors can show prominent Gd-contrast enhancement.	Rare benign schwannian neoplasms that contain cells with diffuse granular cytoplasm and are immunoreactive to S-100 but not to HMB-45. Tumors are often located in the dermis/subcutis and occasionally within muscle. Occur more commonly in females compared with males, in adults over 30 years old.

(continued on page 602)

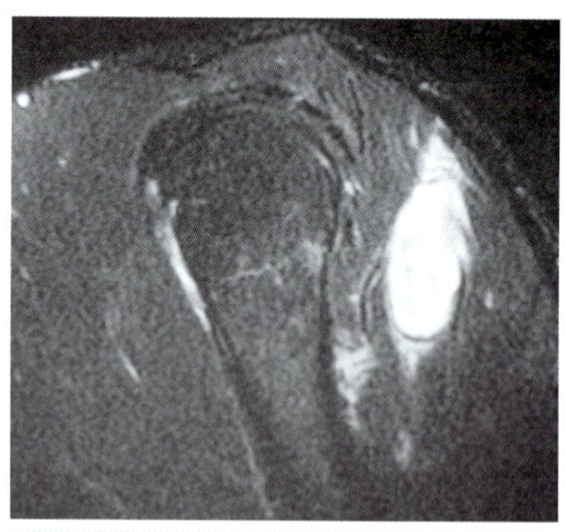
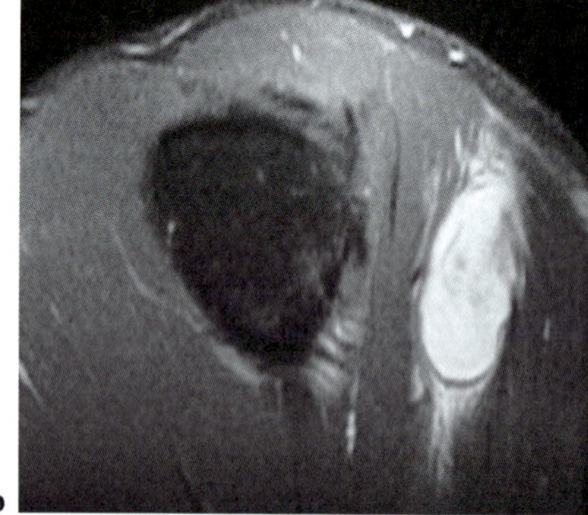

Fig. 12.12 A 43-year-old man with intramuscular nodular fasciitis involving the deltoid muscle at the left shoulder. The lesion has high signal on sagittal fat-suppressed (FS) T2-weighted imaging (a), which is surrounded by a thin rim of low signal and poorly defined zones of high signal in the adjacent soft tissues. The lesion shows prominent Gd-contrast enhancement on sagittal FS T1-weighted imaging (b).

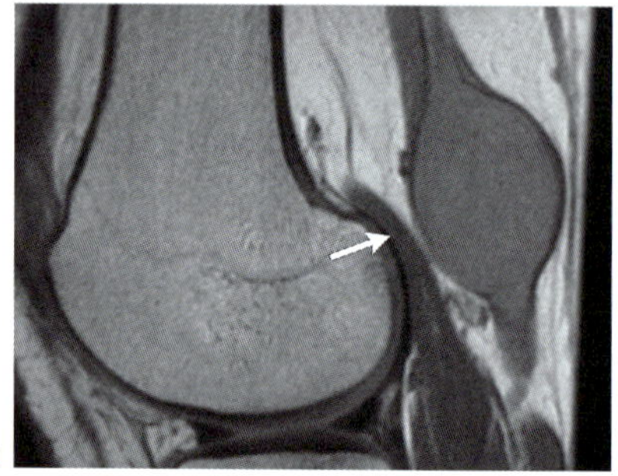
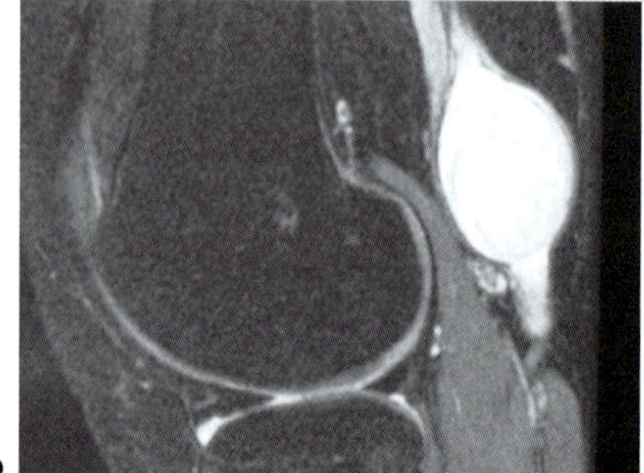
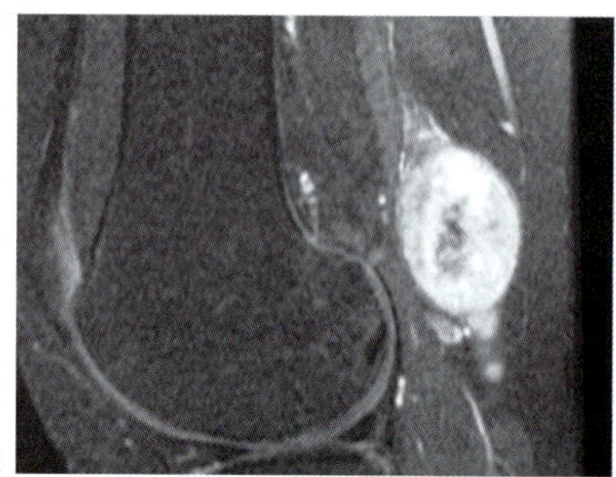

Fig. 12.13 A 17-year-old girl with a schwannoma (arrow) in the posterior soft tissues at the knee, which has intermediate signal on sagittal proton density–weighted imaging (a) and high signal on sagittal fat-suppressed (FS) T2-weighted imaging (b). The lesion shows heterogeneous Gd-contrast enhancement on sagittal FS T1-weighted imaging (c).

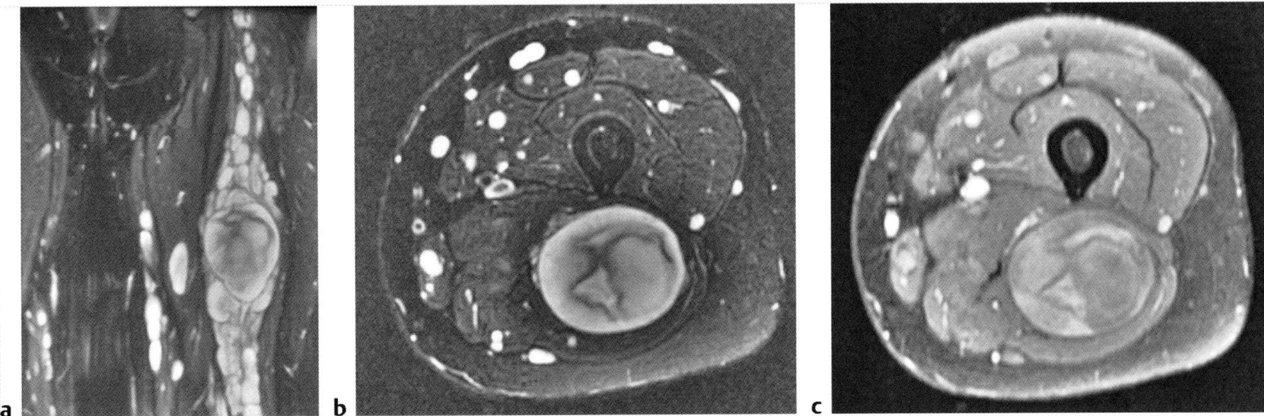

Fig. 12.14 A 23-year-old woman with neurofibromatosis 1 with multiple neurofibromas in the soft tissues on both thighs, which have high signal on coronal (a) and axial (b) fat-suppressed (FS) T2-weighted imaging. The lesions show Gd-contrast enhancement on axial FS T1-weighted imaging (c).

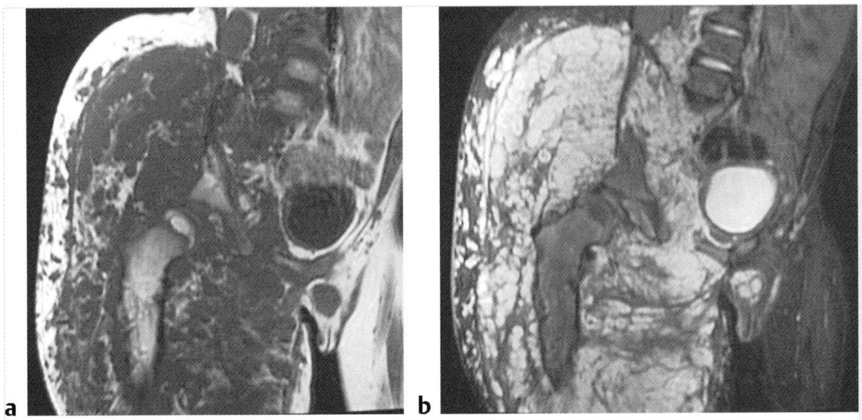

Fig. 12.15 A 7-year-old male with neurofibromatosis 1 and a large plexiform neurofibroma involving the right thigh. The tumor appears as curvilinear and multinodular zones with intermediate signal on coronal T1-weighted imaging (a), and heterogeneous high signal coronal fat-suppressed T2-weighted imaging (b).

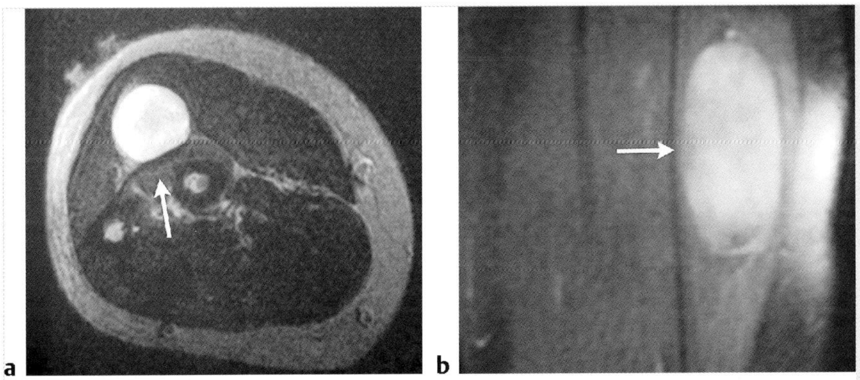

Fig. 12.16 A 38-year-old man with a neurothekeoma involving the flexor digitorum superficialis muscle of the proximal forearm. The lesion (arrows) has high signal on axial T2-weighted imaging (a) and shows moderate heterogeneous Gd-contrast enhancement on sagittal fat-suppressed T1-weighted imaging (b).

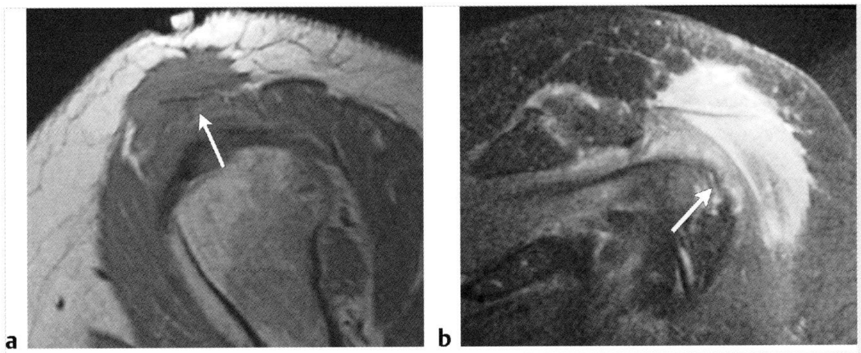

Fig. 12.17 A 56-year-old woman with a granular cell tumor involving the subcutaneous fat and superficial portion of the deltoid muscle. The tumor (arrows) has irregular margins and contains low-intermediate signal on sagittal proton density–weighted imaging (a). The tumor shows prominent Gd-contrast enhancement on coronal fat-suppressed T1-weighted imaging (b).

Table 12.1 (Cont.) Nonmalignant tumors and tumor-like lesions involving the soft tissues of the extremities

Tumor/tumor-like lesion	MRI findings	Comments
Traumatic neuroma (▶ Fig. 12.18)	Traumatic neuromas can appear as bulbous lesions at the end of a transected nerve (terminal neuroma) or as fusiform swelling of an intact nerve (spindle neuroma). Lesions often have low-intermediate signal on T1WI intermediate signal on PDWI, and mildly heterogeneous intermediate to high signal on T2WI and FS T2WI	Nonneoplastic lesions that result from complete or partial transection of nerves. The proximal end of the damaged or transected nerve undergoes a benign proliferative process that can be painful. Terminal neuromas are traumatic neuromas that result from transection or avulsion of nerves and occur 1 to 12 months after injury. Spindle neuromas are focal swelling of intact nerves damaged by chronic friction or irritation.
Morton neuroma (▶ Fig. 12.19)	Lesions located in the neurovascular bundle within the intermetatarsal space on the plantar side of the transverse metatarsal ligament. Appear as nodule with low-intermediate signal on T1WI and PDWI that is isointense or slightly hyperintense relative to muscle. Lesions often have low to intermediate signal on T2WI that is hypointense or isointense relative to fat. Lesions can have intermediate, slightly high, or high signal on FS T2WI. Lesions can show Gd-contrast enhancement, which is often more conspicuous with fat-suppression.	Nonneoplastic lesions that result from perineural fibrosis of a plantar digital nerve near the metatarsal head.
Lipoma of nerve (fibrolipomatosis hamartoma) (▶ Fig. 12.20)	Well-circumscribed fusiform-shaped lesions involving nerves. On T1WI, PDWI, and T2WI a network of cylindrical, longitudinally oriented, thin, curvilinear signal voids 1 to 3 mm in diameter is seen within a background of intermediate to high signal. This "coaxial cable" appearance is secondary to the combination of nerve fascicles with varying degrees of fatty infiltration, and epineural and perineural fibrosis. The degree of fatty proliferation varies among patients. Lesions may follow the branching patterns of nerves.	Rare benign lesions with varying degrees of fibrous and fatty (mature adipocytes) infiltration of the epineurium (nerve sheath) of peripheral nerves as well as within the interfascicular connective tissue (perinerium) of nerves.

(continued on page 604)

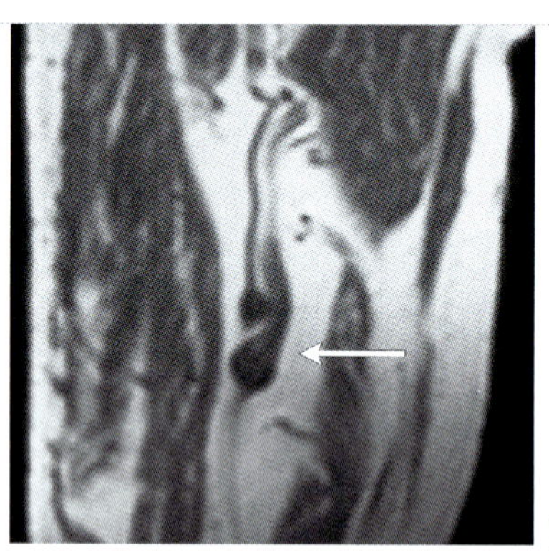
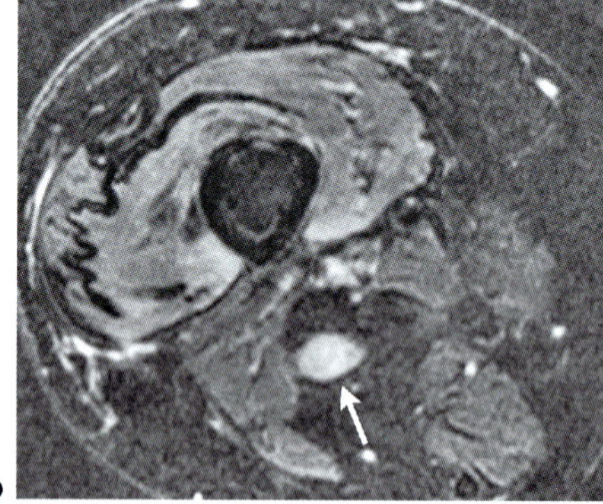
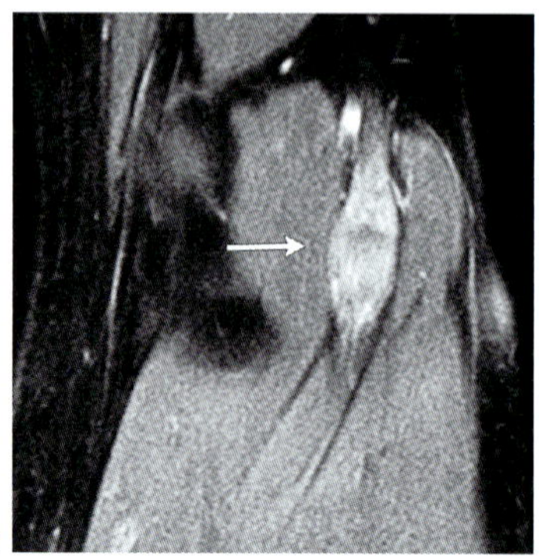
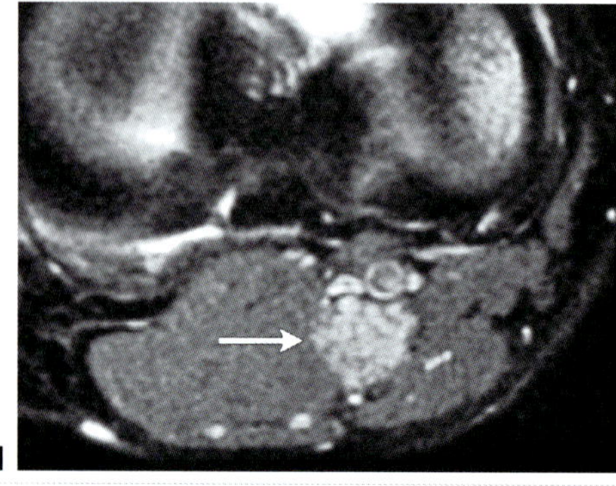

Fig. 12.18 A 33-year-old woman with a traumatic neuroma involving the sciatic nerve in the thigh after an amputation of the leg. The lesion (arrow) has bulbous-shaped ends, which have low-intermediate signal on sagittal T1-weighted imaging (a) and high signal on axial fat-suppressed T2-weighted imaging (FS T2WI) (b). A 35-year-old woman with a traumatic spindle neuroma posterior to the knee. The fusiform lesion (arrow) has heterogeneous mostly high signal on coronal (c) and axial (d) FS T2WI.

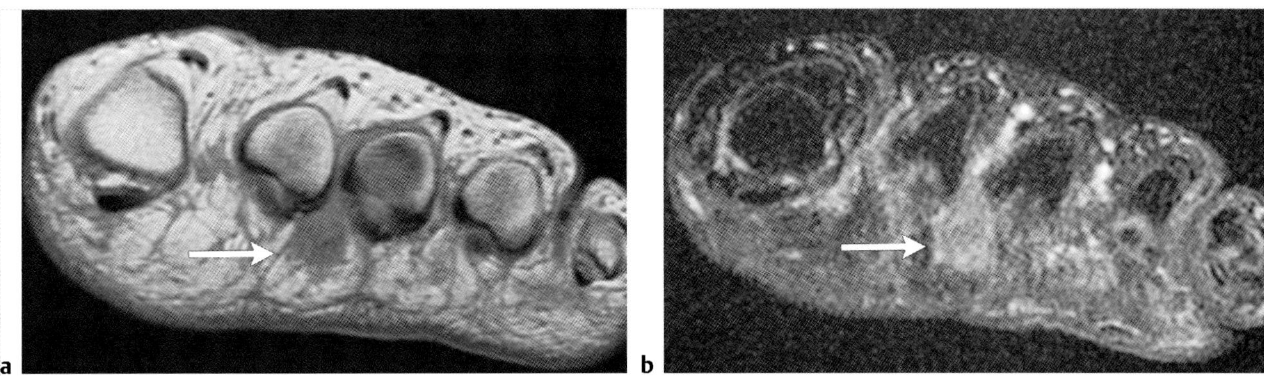

Fig. 12.19 Morton neuroma between the second and third digits in a 48-year-old woman. The nodular lesion (arrows) has intermediate signal on coronal proton density–weighted imaging (a) and intermediate to slightly high signal on coronal fat-suppressed T2-weighted imaging (b).

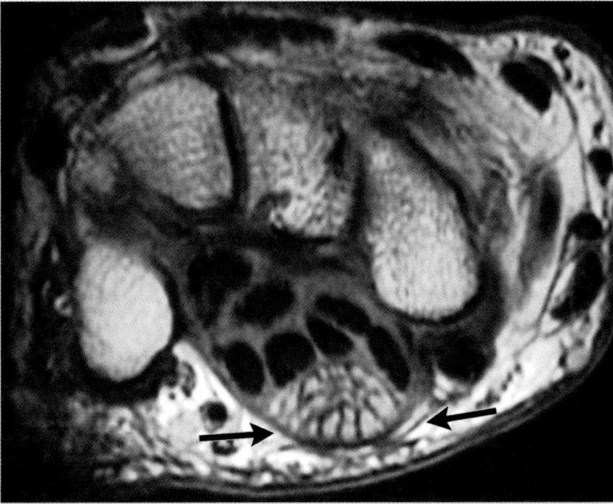

Fig. 12.20 A 59-year-old man with a fibrolipomatous hamartoma involving the median nerve at the wrist (arrows). Cylindrical longitudinally oriented thin curvilinear zones of low signal are seen within a background of intermediate to high signal on coronal proton density–weighted imaging.

Table 12.1 (Cont.) Nonmalignant tumors and tumor-like lesions involving the soft tissues of the extremities

Tumor/tumor-like lesion	MRI findings	Comments
Leiomyoma (▶ Fig. 12.21)	Lesions may have well defined or irregular margins and have low-intermediate signal on T1WI and intermediate to slightly high or high signal on T2WI and FS T2WI. Lesions usually show moderate to marked Gd-contrast enhancement.	Benign spindle cell tumors composed of mature smooth muscle bundles. Ninety-five percent of leiomyomas involve the female genitourinary tract, and 3% occur in the skin with the remainder in the gastrointestinal tract, bladder, and other sites. Curtaneous leiomyomas (leiomyoma cutis) arise from the pilar arrector muscles of the skin or from the network of muscle fibers in the deep dermis. Angioleiomyomas are tumors that contain mixtures of thick-walled vessels and smooth muscle cells.
Solitary fibrous tumor (SFT) (▶ Fig. 12.22)	SFTs often have circumscribed margins. Often have low to intermediate signal on T1WI and PDWI; low, intermediate, and/or slightly high signal on T2WI; and heterogeneous slightly high to high signal on FS T2WI. Usually show Gd-contrast enhancement.	Rare, benign, spindle-cell mesenchymal neoplasms that occur in a wide range of anatomical sites, including the extremities. Tumors typically show a hemangiopericytoma-like branching vascular pattern and resemble pleural SFTs. Account for less than 2% of soft tissue tumors. Median patient age from 50 to 60 years.
Desmoid tumor/fibromatosis (▶ Fig. 12.23; ▶ Fig. 12.24)	Lesions can have distinct and/or poorly defined margins, homogeneous or heterogeneous low-intermediate signal on T1WI, and variable intermediate-high signal on T2WI, ± zones of low signal. Myxoid zones in the lesions can have high signal on T2WI. Tumors with high cellularity tend to show higher signal on T2WI than lesions with larger proportions of collagen. Lesions show variable degrees and patterns (heterogeneous vs homogenous) of Gd-contrast enhancement. Pattern or degree of Gd-contrast enhancement by desmoids does not enable prediction of rate of tumor recurrence.	Desmoid tumors or fibromatosis represent a group of soft tissue lesions composed of benign fibrous tissue with elongated or spindle-shaped cells adjacent to collagen. Lesions are categorized by location as superficial (palmar–Dupuytren contracture, plantar–Ledderhose disease, penile–Peyronie disease) or deep (extra-abdominal, abdominal, or intra-abdominal). Aggressive fibromatosis is a type that usually occurs in the deep soft tissues and consists of proliferation of fibrous tissue that infiltrates adjacent tissues. Aggressive fibromatosis has a greater tendency to locally recur after surgery compared with circumscribed desmoid tumors. Desmoid tumors can occur in association with Gardner syndrome and Turcot syndrome.

(continued on page 606)

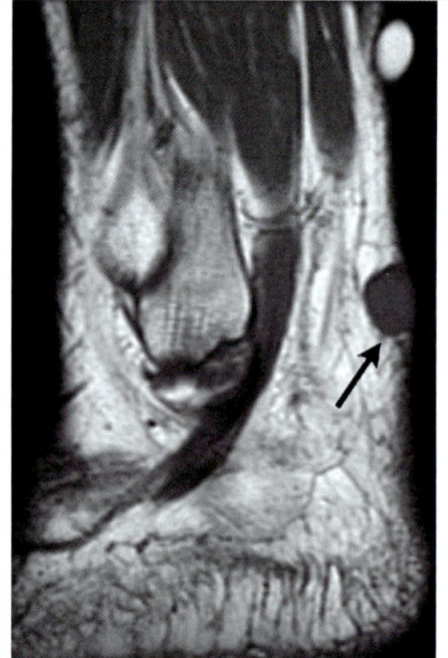

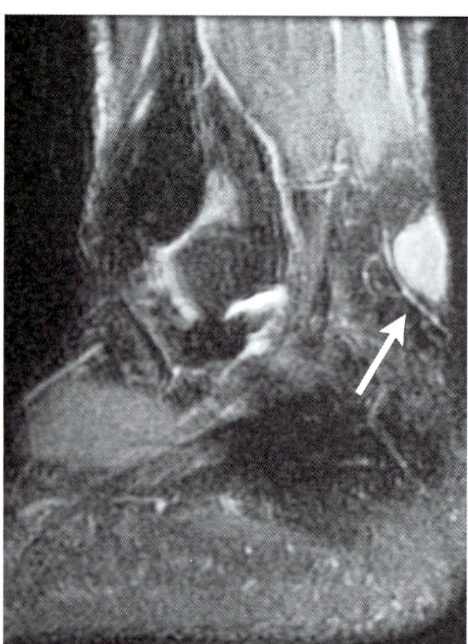

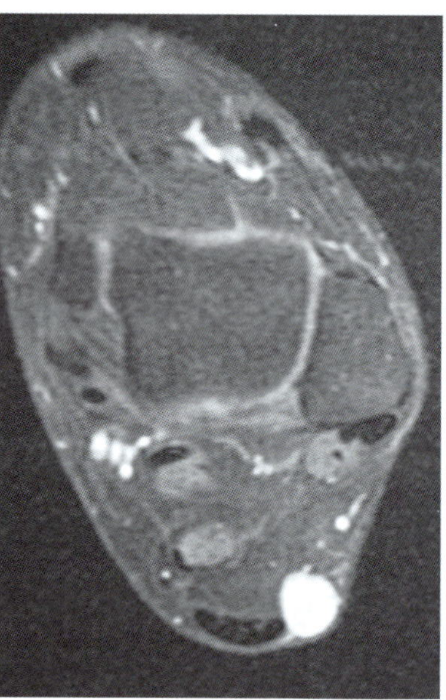

Fig. 12.21 A 60-year-old woman with a leiomyoma in the dorsal subcutaneous fat in the ankle region. The circumscribed lesion (arrows) has intermediate signal on sagittal T1-weighted imaging (T1WI) (a) and high signal on sagittal fat-suppressed (FS) T2-weighted imaging (b). The lesion shows prominent Gd-contrast enhancement on axial FS T1WI (c).

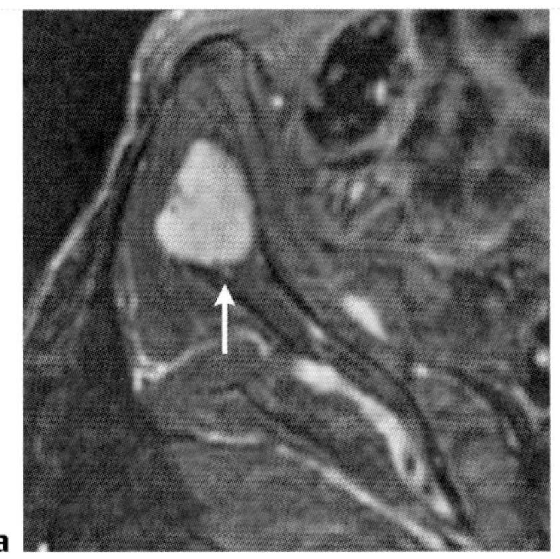
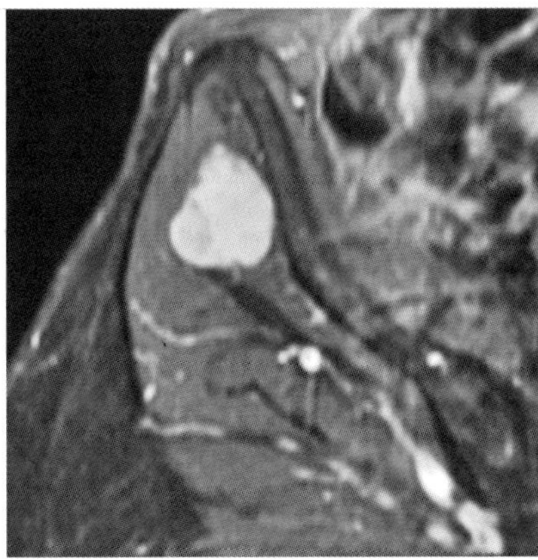

Fig. 12.22 An 81-year-old man with a solitary fibrous tumor involving the gluteus minimus muscle. The lesion (arrow) has circumscribed margins; high signal on axial fat-suppressed (FS) T2-weighted imaging (a), and shows Gd-contrast enhancement on axial FS T1-weighted imaging (b).

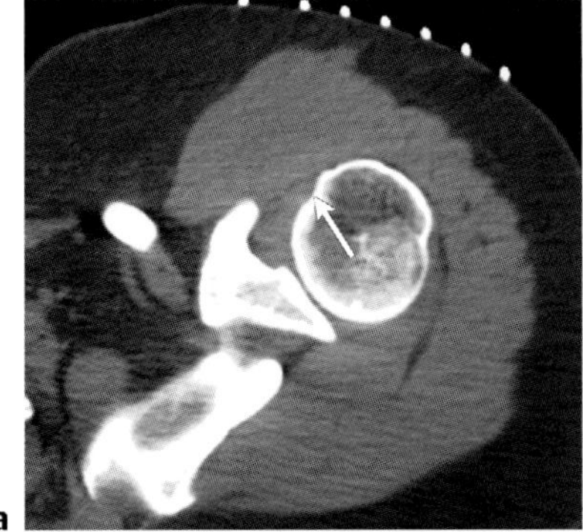
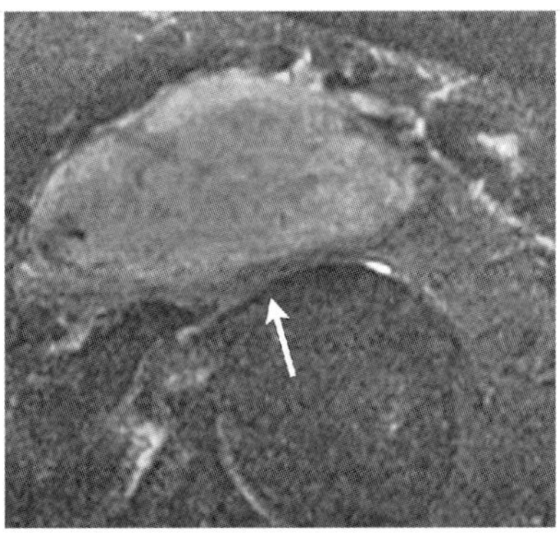
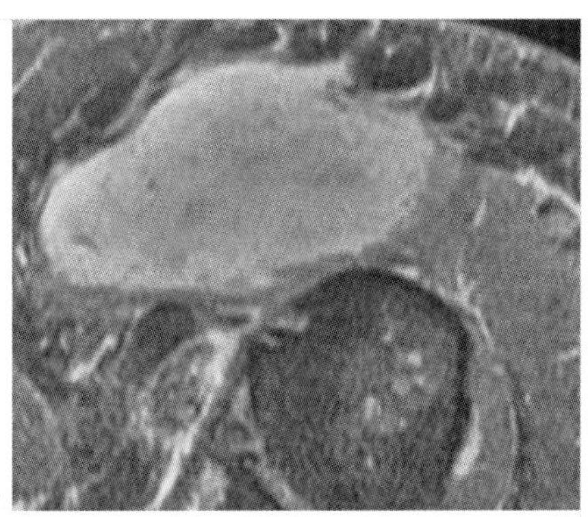

Fig. 12.23 A 42-year-old woman with a desmoid tumor involving the soft tissues at the shoulder. The lesion (arrows) has intermediate attenuation on axial computed tomographic (a) and slightly high signal on axial fat-suppressed (FS) T2-weighted imaging (b). The lesion shows Gd-contrast enhancement on axial FS T1-weighted imaging (c).

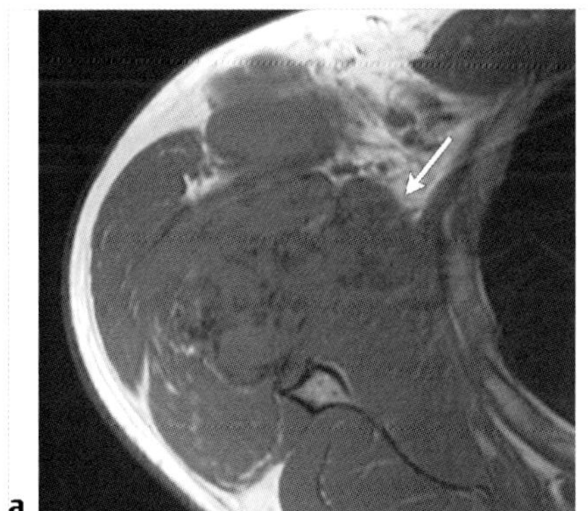
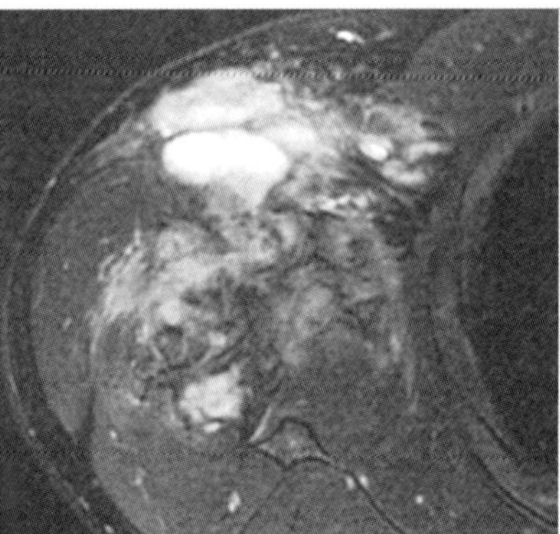
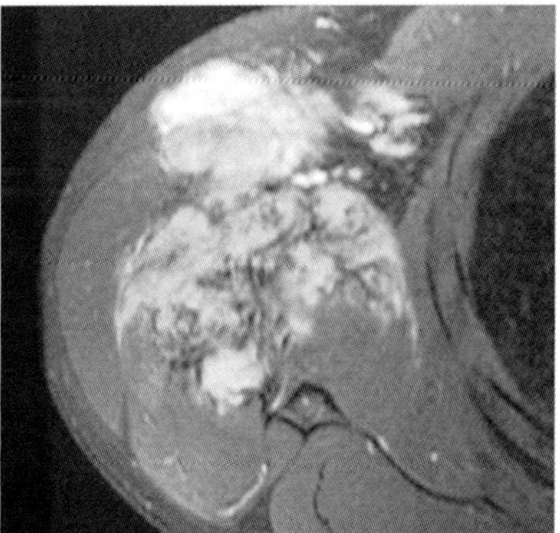

Fig. 12.24 A 32-year-old man with aggressive fibromatosis involving the soft tissues in the right axilla. Magnetic resonance imaging shows a lobulated lesion with indistinct margins, which has intermediate signal with small low signal zones on axial T1-weighted imaging (T1WI) (a), and slightly high and high signal on axial fat-suppressed (FS) T2-weighted imaging (b). Foci and thin curvilinear zones of low signal are also seen. The lesion shows prominent heterogeneous Gd-contrast enhancement on axial FS T1WI (c).

Table 12.1 (Cont.) Nonmalignant tumors and tumor-like lesions involving the soft tissues of the extremities

Tumor/tumor-like lesion	MRI findings	Comments
Myxoma (▶ Fig. 12.25)	Lesions usually have low or low-intermediate signal on T1WI and PDWI; and high signal on T2WI and FS T2WI. Myxomas can have heterogeneous mild or moderate degrees of enhancement in noncystic portions.	Benign lesions that contain fibroblasts (spindle cells) and abundant mucoid material (glycosaminoglycans, other mucopolysaccharides). Account for 3% of benign soft tissue tumors/lesions and 2% of all soft tissue tumors/lesions. Occur in adults age 24 to 74 years, average = 52 years.
Ganglion cyst (▶ Fig. 12.26)	Ganglia are sharply defined lesions with low signal on T1WI, low-intermediate signal on PDWI, and homogeneous high signal on T2WI. Some ganglia may have intermediate signal on T1WI secondary to elevated proteinaceous or fibrous content. Low signal septa on T2WI can be seen. Peripheral rimlike Gd-contrast enhancement can be seen as well as complete lack of enhancement.	Ganglia are juxta-articular benign myxoid lesions that arise from degeneration of periarticular connective tissue, prior trauma, or prior inflammation. Ganglia may be derived from tendons, tendon sheaths, joint capsules, bursae, or ligaments.

(continued on page 608)

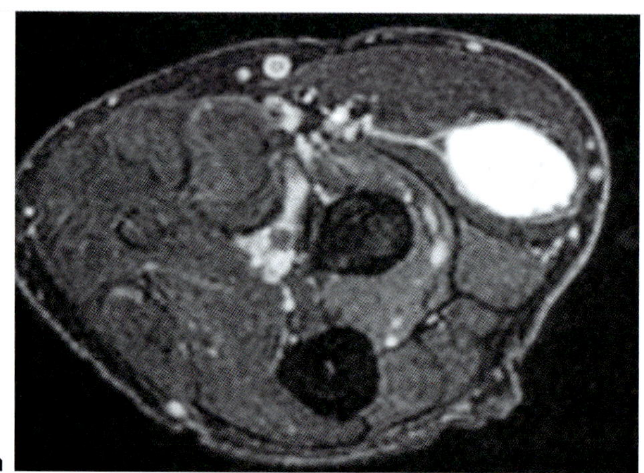

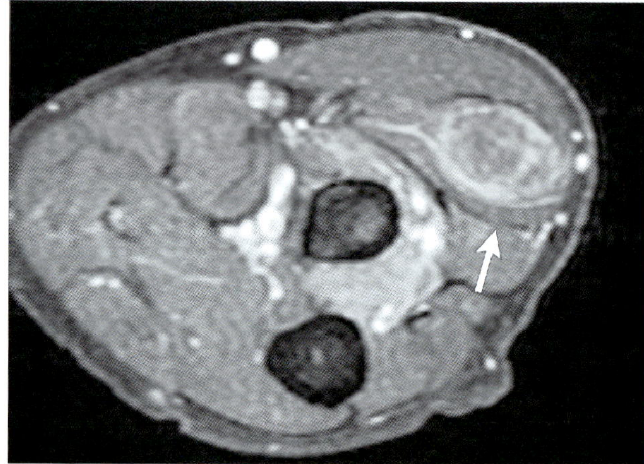

Fig. 12.25 A 77-year-old man with an intramuscular myxoma involving the extensor carpi radialis longus and brevis muscles of the proximal forearm. The lesion has high signal on axial fat-suppressed (FS) T2-weighted imaging (a) and shows mild irregular Gd-contrast enhancement on axial FS T1-weighted imaging (arrow) (b).

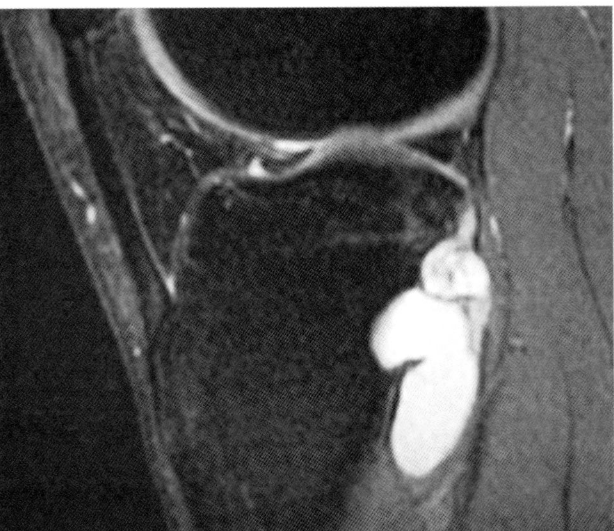

Fig. 12.26 Periosteal ganglion along the posterolateral proximal tibia of a 30-year-old man. The lesion has sharply defined margins and has high signal on sagittal fat-suppressed T2-weighted imaging. The lesion causes erosion and concave deformity of the tibial cortex.

Table 12.1 (Cont.) Nonmalignant tumors and tumor-like lesions involving the soft tissues of the extremities

Tumor/tumor-like lesion	MRI findings	Comments
Hematoma/seroma (▶ Fig. 12.27; ▶ Fig. 12.28)	Acute hematomas (<3 to 7 days) have mostly intermediate signal similar to muscle on T1WI; and mixed low-intermediate and/or high signal relative to muscle on PDWI, T2WI, and FS T2WI. Poorly defined zones of high signal on PDWI, T2WI, and FS T2WI may also be seen peripheral to the hematoma, representing adjacent edema. Subacute hematomas (1 week to 3 months) have high and/or intermediate signal on T1WI, and high signal on FS T1WI, PDWI, T2WI, and FS T2WI. Peripheral and central zones of low signal on PDWI, T2WI, and FS T2WI can be seen in mid to late subacute hematomas secondary to the presence of hemosiderin from breakdown of blood cells and oxidation/metabolism of hemoglobin. Mild peripheral Gd-contrast can be seen. Chronic hematomas (>3 months) usually have high signal on T1WI, PDWI, T2WI, and FS T2WI. A thick peripheral rim of low signal on T2WI from hemosiderin is often seen with chronic hematomas. Chronic hematomas often evolve eventually into zones with low-intermediate signal on T1WI and T2WI secondary to fibrosis and residual hemosiderin.	Hematomas are extravascular collections of red and white blood cells, which can result from trauma, surgery, coagulopathy (hemophilia, thrombocytopenia, medications/Coumadin/heparin, and sepsis). An acute hematoma is defined as one less than a few days in age. A subacute hematoma has a duration of 1 week to 3 months, and chronic hematomas are older than 3 months. One form of chronic hematoma is the Morel-Lavallée lesion, which refers to an encapsulated lesion in the subcutaneous fat containing proteinaceous fluid from episodes of rebleeding caused by traumatic separaration of the subcutaneous fibrofatty tissue from adjacent vascularized fascia. Hemophilic pseudotumors are chronic, slow-growing, encapsulated cystic lesions in bone or soft tissues secondary to recurrent hemorrhage that occur in 1 to 2% of patients with hemophilia.

(continued on page 610)

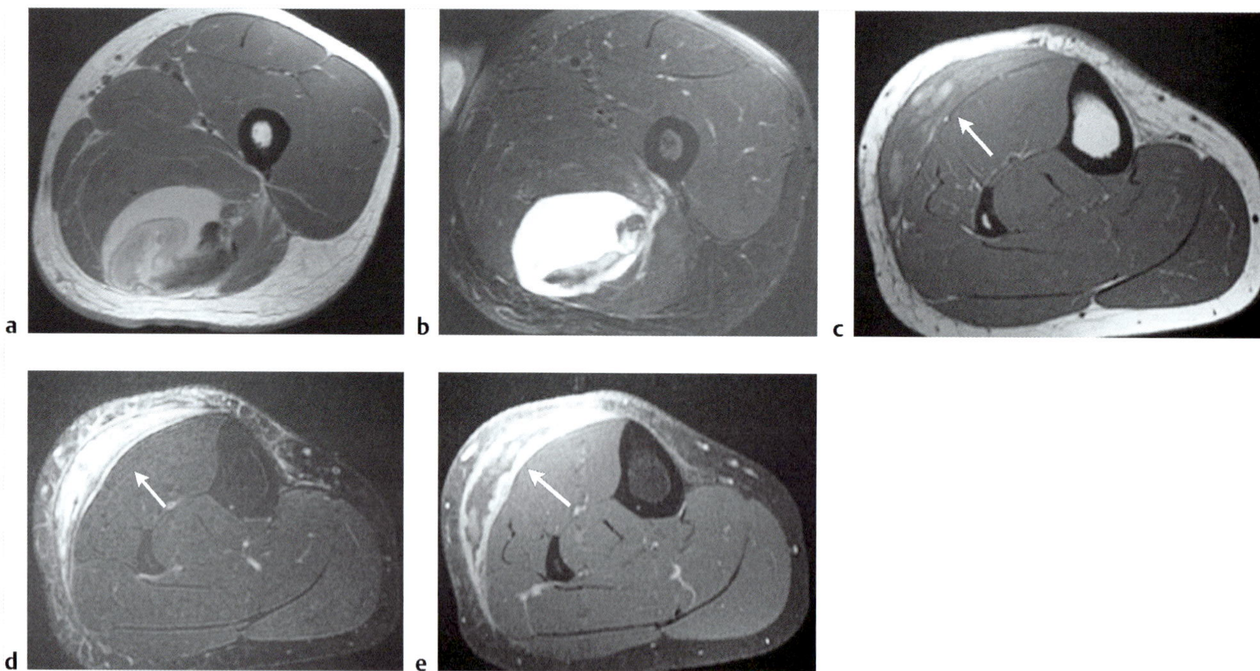

Fig. 12.27 Subacute intramuscular hematoma involving the semitendinosus muscle in the upper thigh. The hematoma has heterogeneous slightly high, intermediate, and low signal on axial proton density–weighted imaging (a) and heterogeneous high, slightly high, and low signal on axial fat-suppressed T2-weighted imaging (FS T2WI) (b). A 14-year-old girl with a subacute hematoma (arrows) in the subcutaneous fat of the medial leg, which has mostly intermediate signal and irregular zones of high signal on axial T1-weighted imaging (T1WI) (c) and heterogeneous high and slightly high signal on axial FS T2WI (d). The hematoma has intermediate signal centrally and shows irregular peripheral zones of Gd-contrast enhancement on axial FS T1WI (e).

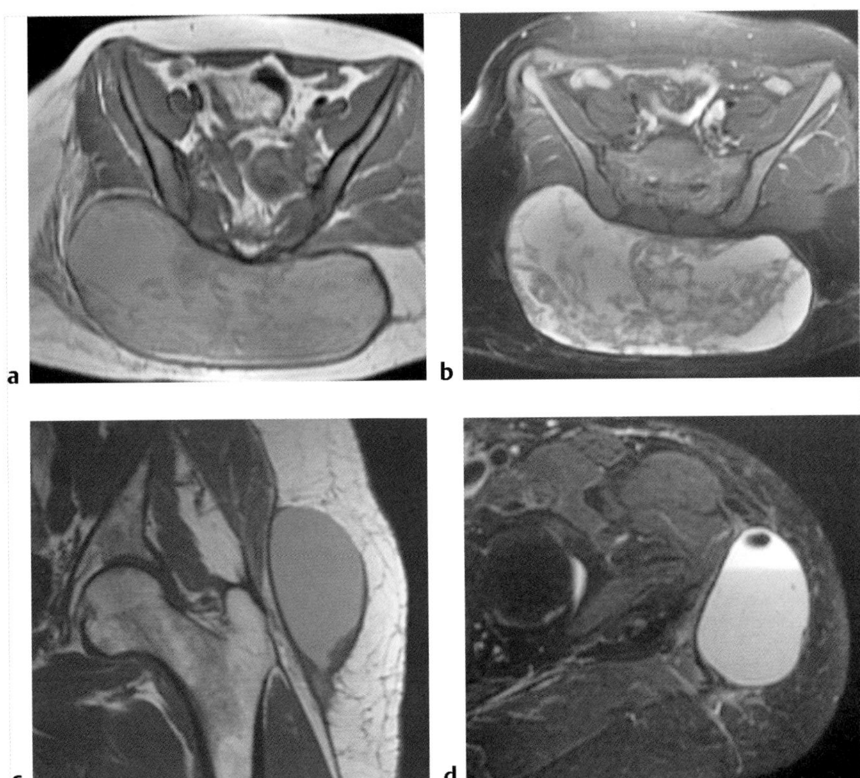

Fig. 12.28 A 32-year-old woman with a chronic hematoma in the subcutaneous fat posterior to the sacrum, also referred to as a Morel-Lavallée lesion. The hematoma has intermediate signal on axial proton density–weighted imaging (a), which is slightly hyperintense to muscle, and heterogeneous mostly high signal on axial fat-suppressed T2-weighted imaging (FS T2WI) (b). The hematoma contains debris and is surrounded by a rim of low signal. A 71-year-old woman with a chronic hematoma in the subcutaneous fat of the upper thigh (Morel-Lavallée lesion), which has intermediate signal on coronal T1-weighted imaging (c) and heterogeneous mostly high signal on axial FS T2WI (d). The hematoma contains debris and a fluid-fluid level and is surrounded by a rim of low signal.

Table 12.1 (Cont.) Nonmalignant tumors and tumor-like lesions involving the soft tissues of the extremities

Tumor/tumor-like lesion	MRI findings	Comments
Heterotopic ossification (▶ Fig. 12.29)	MRI features vary depending on the age, location, and degree of mineralization/ossification. Lesions less than 2 weeks have localized mass effect with poorly defined margins, heterogeneous low-intermediate or slightly high signal on T1WI, and heterogeneous slightly high to high signal on T2WI and FS T2WI. Poorly defined zones of high signal on T2WI may be seen in the adjacent soft tissues. After 2 weeks, curvilinear and/or amorphous zones of low signal on T2WI and FS T2WI can be seen at the peripheral portions of the subacute lesions resulting from mineralization/ossification. Subsequent progressive centripetal mineralization/ossification appears as irregular zones of low signal on T2WI with heterogeneous Gd-contrast enhancement. Old lesions have well-defined margins, and variable low signal on T1WI, PDWI, and T2WI depending on the degree of mineralization/ossification, fibrosis, and hemosiderin deposition. Zones of high signal on T1WI and T2WI may occur from fatty marrow metaplasia. Gd-contrast enhancement in old mature lesions is often minimal or absent.	Heterotopic ossification or myositis ossificans are nonneoplastic reparative extraosseous lesions that are composed of reactive hypercellular fibrous tissue, cartilage, and/or bone. These lesions can arise secondary to trauma (myositis ossificans circumscripta, ossifying hematoma), although they may also occur without a history of prior injury (pseudomalignant osseous tumor of the soft tissues).
Tumoral calcinosis (▶ Fig. 12.30)	Radiographs and computed tomography show lobular and/or multiloculated opacities, which may contain radiolucent strands secondary to fibrous septae and calcium fluid levels. Erosion of bone adjacent to the tumoral calcinosis can occur. Lesions have variable signal on MRI with mixed low and intermediate signal on T1WI, and mixed low, intermediate, and/or high signal on T2WI. Gd-contrast may occur in septae or surrounding the lesions secondary to inflammatory reaction.	Rare metabolic disorder related to abnormal phosphate metabolism with elevated levels of 1,25-dihydroxyvitamin D resulting in hyperphosphatemia with precipitation of calcium salts in juxta-articular soft tissues. Common locations include the soft tissues near bursae at the hips, shoulders, elbows, buttocks, and scapula. Can be hereditary in up to 33% as autosomal dominant with variable penetrance. Lesions consist of deposits of hydroxyapatite with or without fibrous septae, macrophages and chronic inflammatory cells, and multinucleated giant cells.

(continued on page 612)

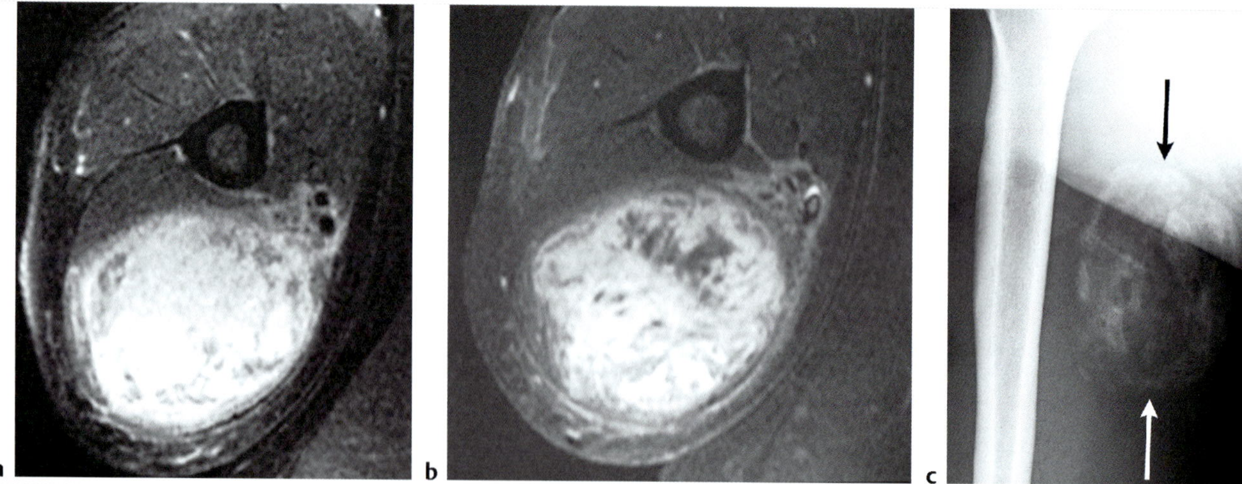

Fig. 12.29 A 19-year-old man with myositis ossificans involving the triceps brachii muscle of the upper arm, which has heterogeneous high signal on axial fat-suppressed (FS) T2-weighted imaging (a). The lesion shows prominent slightly heterogeneous Gd-contrast enhancement on axial FS T1-weighted imaging (b). Poorly defined zones of Gd-contrast enhancement are also seen in the soft tissues adjacent to the nodular mass-like portion of the lesion. A radiograph (c) obtained 10 days after the magnetic resonance imaging examination shows predominantly peripheral mineralization at the lesion (arrows).

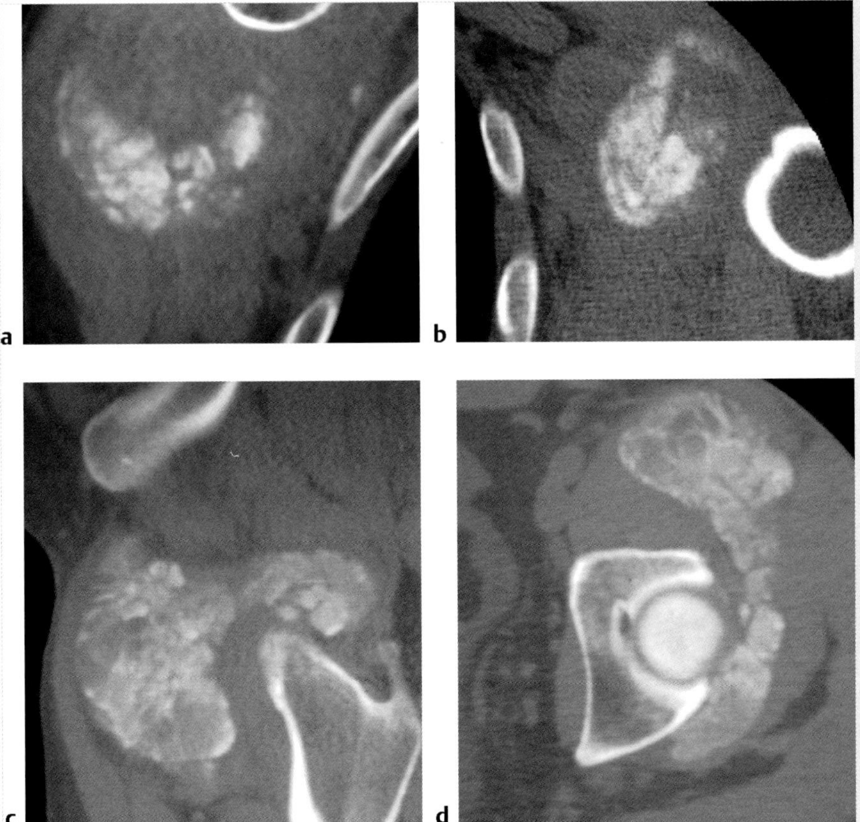

Fig. 12.30 Oblique coronal (a) and axial (b) computed tomographic images show amorphous opacities in the soft tissues at the shoulder and axillary region from tumoral calcinosis in a 76-year-old man. A 34-year-old man (c,d) with tumoral calcinosis adjacent to the hip.

Table 12.1 (Cont.) Nonmalignant tumors and tumor-like lesions involving the soft tissues of the extremities

Tumor/tumor-like lesion	MRI findings	Comments
Giant cell tumor of the tendon sheath (nodular synovitis) (▶ Fig. 12.31)	Lesions usually have well-defined margins and are often adjacent to a tendon/tendon sheath. Lesions have low-intermediate or intermediate signal on T1WI and PDWI, and mixed low, intermediate, and/or high signal on T2WI and FS T2WI. Zones of low signal on T2WI often correspond to sites of hemosiderin deposition. Lesions often show Gd-contrast enhancement in either a homogeneous or a heterogeneous pattern.	Giant cell tumors of the tendon sheath and pigmented villonodular synovitis represent benign proliferative lesions of synovium (tendon sheaths, joints, and bursae). Giant cell tumors of the tendon sheaths can occur as localized nodular lesions attached to tendon sheaths outside of joints (hands, feet) or within joints (infrapatellar portion of knee joint), or as a diffuse form near/outside of large joints such as the knees and ankles.
Fibroma of the tendon sheath (▶ Fig. 12.32)	Lesions are ovoid or fusiform and well circumscribed, and are located adjacent to tendons of the fingers, hands, wrists, feet, and other locations. Lesions usually have low-intermediate signal on T1WI. On T2WI, lesions can have a slightly heterogeneous low-intermediate signal in half, intermediate signal in a third, or mixed low and intermediate signal and/or high signal in the remainder. Lesions can show diffuse or peripheral Gd-contrast enhancement.	Fibromas of the tendon sheath are benign, small fibrous nodules involving tendons and tendon sheaths of the fingers, hands, wrists, or feet.
Xanthoma (▶ Fig. 12.33)	Xanthomas in tendons often appear as zones of fusiform-enlargement with diffuse heterogeneous signal. Xanthomas usually contain multiple longitudinally oriented linear zones or striations with intermediate signal on T1WI and PDWI, and intermediate to slightly high signal on T2WI and FS T2WI interspersed among bands of low signal within the enlarged tendons. On axial images, xanthomas often have a stippled or reticulated pattern on T1WI and T2WI resulting from collagen bundles with low signal surrounded by higher signal from lipid deposits, foamy histiocytes, and inflammatory reaction.	Xanthomas are localized accumulations of lipids within normal structures such as tendons, skin, and bone. Considered reactive lesions and are not true neoplasms. Often occur in the setting of types I, II, and III hyper-lipoproteinemia.

(continued on page 614)

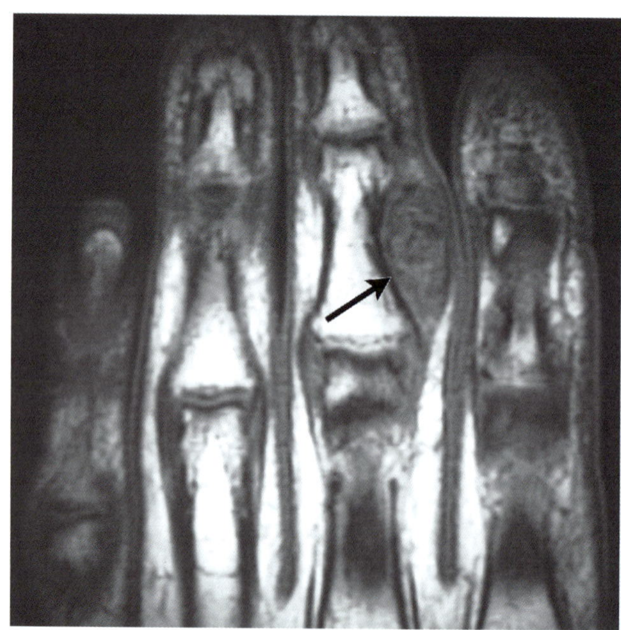

Fig. 12.31 A 28-year-old man with a giant cell tumor of the tendon sheath involving a finger. An ovoid lesion with well-defined margins is seen adjacent to a flexor tendon sheath and middle phalanx (arrow). The lesion has low-intermediate signal on coronal T1-weighted imaging (a). *(continued)*

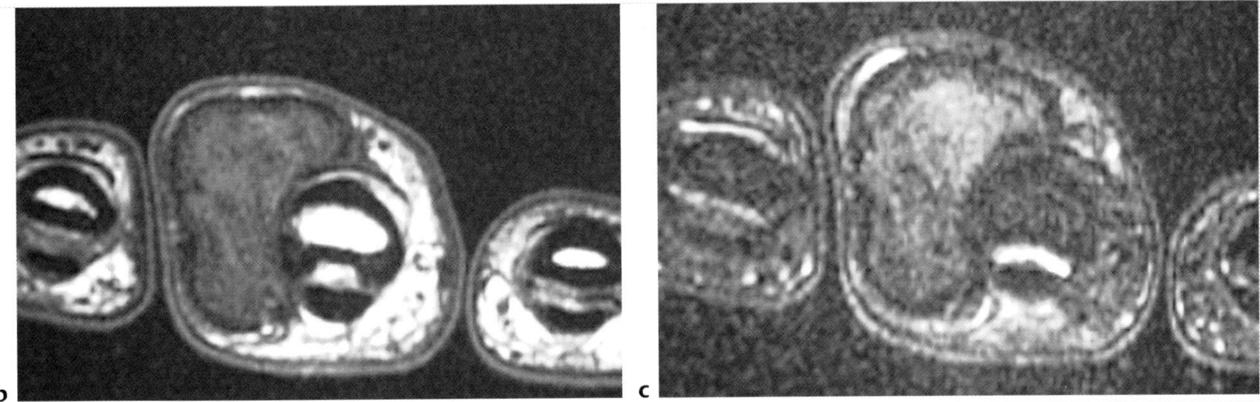

Fig. 12.31 (*continued*) The lesion has low-intermediate signal on axial T1-weighted imaging (b), and mixed low, intermediate, and and slightly high signal on axial fat-suppressed T2-weighted imaging (c).

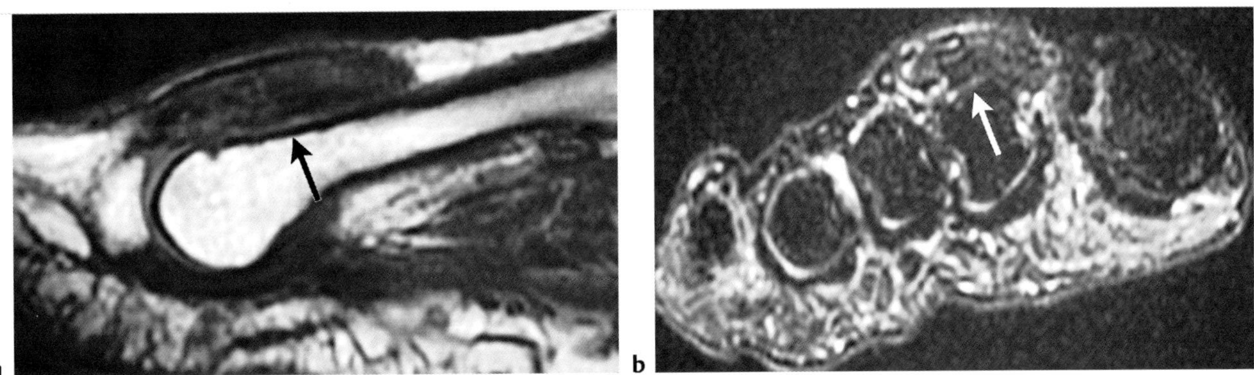

Fig. 12.32 A 63-year-old woman with a fibroma involving an extensor tendon sheath in the foot. The lesion has a fusiform shape with well-circumscribed margins (arrows) and has zones of low and intermediate signal on sagittal T1-weighted imaging (a) as well as on axial fat-suppressed T2-weighted imaging (b).

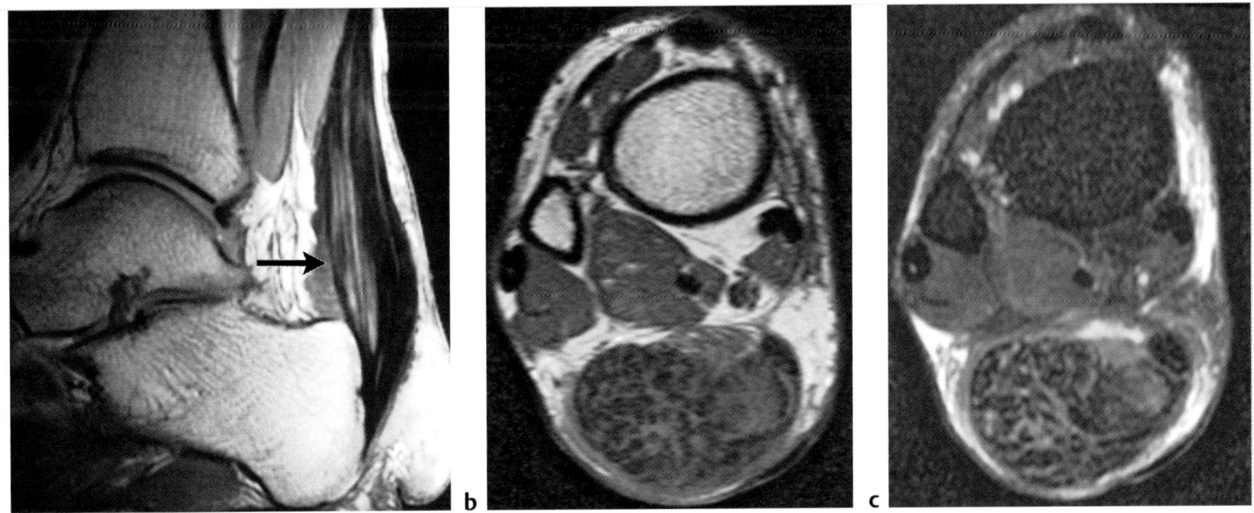

Fig. 12.33 Xanthoma involving the Achilles tendon in a 33-year-old woman with hypercholesterolemia. Fusiform enlargement of the tendon is seen (arrow), within which low signal tendon fibers are separated by amorphous zones with intermediate to slightly high signal on sagittal T2-weighted imaging (T2WI) (a), and intermediate signal on axial T1-weighted imaging (b) and axial fat-suppressed T2WI (c).

Table 12.1 (Cont.) Nonmalignant tumors and tumor-like lesions involving the soft tissues of the extremities

Tumor/tumor-like lesion	MRI findings	Comments
Amyloid (▶ Fig. 12.34)	Lesions in soft tissue can have low-intermediate signal on T1WI, and intermediate to slightly high signal on T2WI. Lesions can show Gd-contrast enhancement.	Uncommon disease in which various tissues (including bone, muscle, tendons, tendon sheaths, ligaments, and synovium) are infiltrated with extracellular eosinophilic material composed of insoluble proteins with beta-pleated sheet configurations (amyloid protein). Amyloidomas are single sites of involvement. Amyloidosis can be a primary disorder associated with an immunologic dyscrasia or secondary to a chronic inflammatory disease.
Epidermoid (▶ Fig. 12.35)	Epidermoids are circumscribed lesions with or without lobulated margins, and usually have low signal or low-intermediate signal on T1WI, and high signal on T2WI and FS T2WI that may approximate cerebrospinal fluid. Lesions occasionally contain foci of high signal on T1WI. Epidermoids may show minimal peripheral Gd-contrast enhancement, but no enhancement is typically seen centrally.	Epidermoids are ectoderm-lined inclusion cysts that contain only squamous epithelium and keratin debris. Epidermoids often slowly enlarge but are not considered to be neoplasms.
Elastofibroma (▶ Fig. 12.36)	Lesions often range from 5 to 10 cm and frequently have a lenticular shape with or without well-defined margins. On T1WI and T2WI, lesions often have mostly intermediate signal that is isointense to muscle, as well as variable amounts of high signal from intralesional fatty deposits. After Gd-contrast administration, lesion usually shows variable degrees of enhancement often in a heterogeneous pattern.	Benign, slow-growing, fibroblastic, tumor-like lesions that contain large amounts of enlarged coarse elastic fibers. Typically occur in patients over age 50 and most are located between the lower scapula and chest wall. Considered fibroblastic pseudotumors that result from repetitive trauma or friction between the lower scapula and adjacent chest wall, or result from focal abnormal elastogenesis. Account for 0.3% of benign soft tissue tumors. Typically asymptomatic. Age ranges from 48 to 74 years, mean = 61 years, median = 70 years. Peak occurrence is in the seventh and eighth decades.
Aneurysm (▶ Fig. 12.37)	Saccular aneurysms are focal well-circumscribed structures contiguous with arteries. Signal voids are usually seen where there is fast blood flow in nonthrombosed portions of the aneurysms. Variable mixed signal on T1WI and T2WI can be seen in thrombosed portions of the aneurysms.	Aneurysms are focal or diffuse zones of arterial dilatation that are associated with wall abnormalities and increased risk of rupture. Focal aneurysms are also referred to as saccular aneurysms, which typically occur at arterial branch points. Giant aneurysms are saccular aneurysms that measure more than 2.5 cm in diameter.

(continued on page 616)

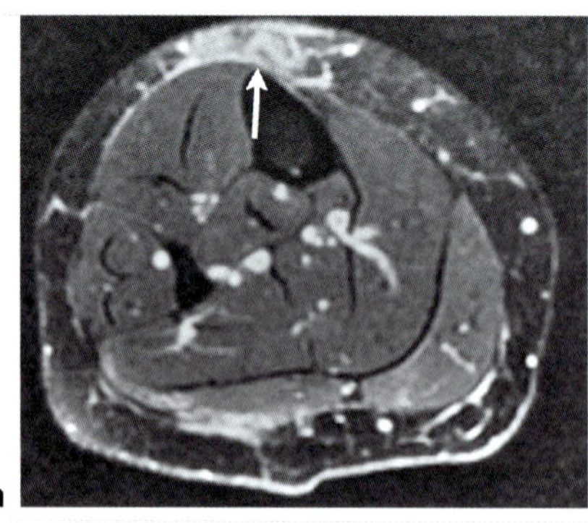

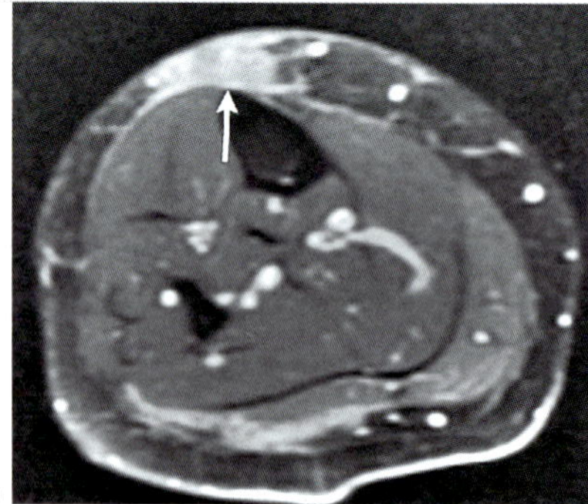

Fig. 12.34 A 55-year-old woman with amyloid in the subcutaneous fat (arrow) and within the lateral gastrocnemius muscle. The lesions have slightly irregular margins and have high signal on axial fat-suppressed (FS) T2-weighted imaging (a) and show Gd-contrast enhancement on axial FS T1-weighted imaging (b).

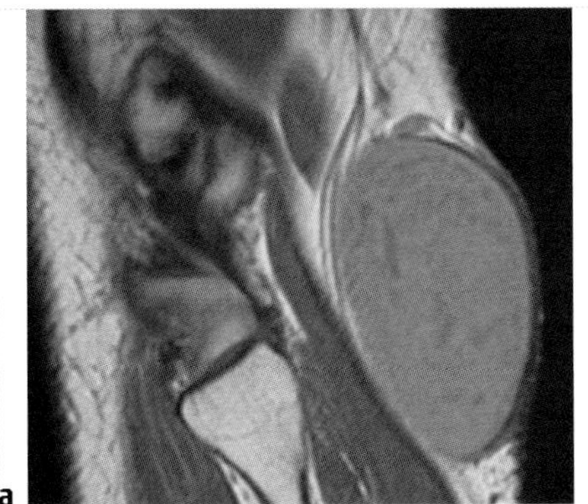
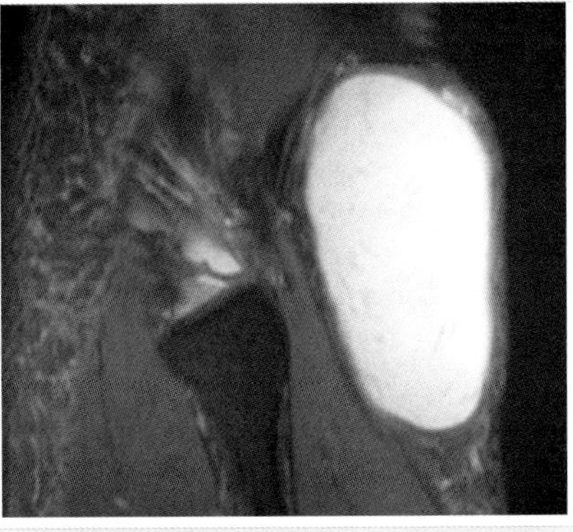
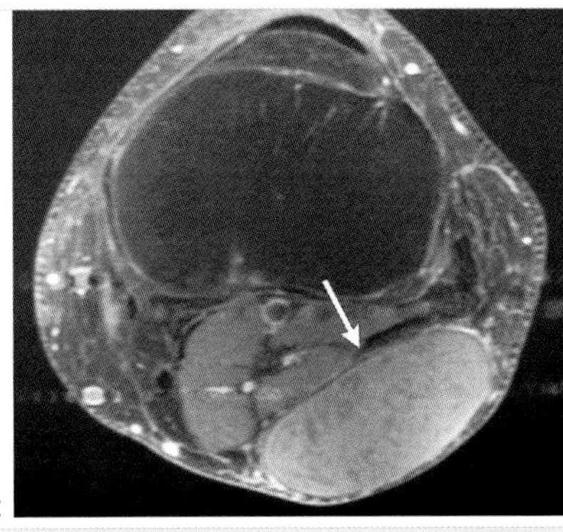

Fig. 12.35 A 47-year-old man with an epidermoid involving the posterior soft tissues at the knee. The lesion has intermediate signal on sagittal proton density–weighted imaging (a) and high signal on sagittal fat-suppressed (FS) T2-weighted imaging (b). The lesion (arrow) shows no Gd-contrast enhancement on axial FS T1-weighted imaging (c).

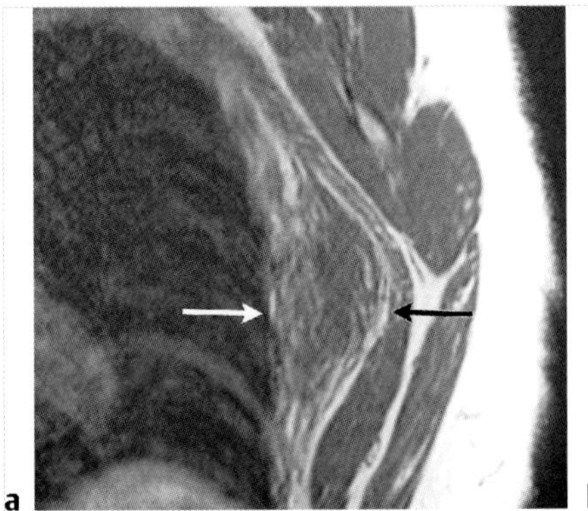
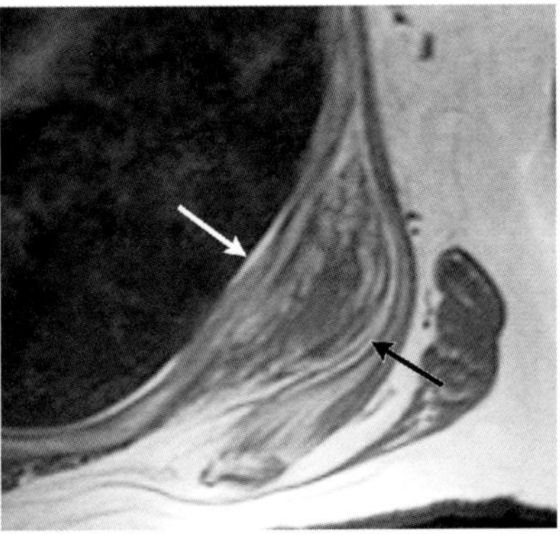
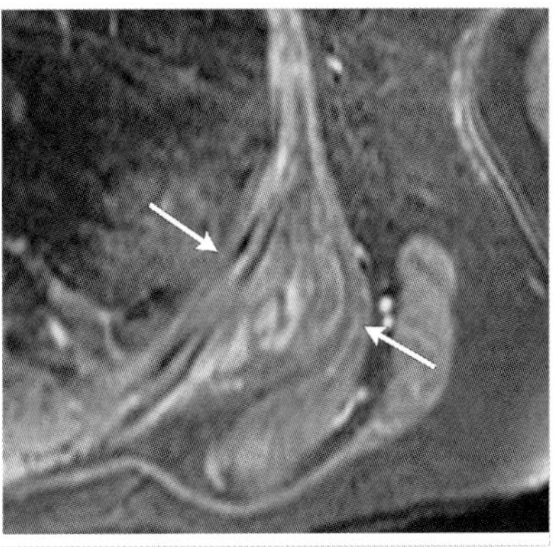

Fig. 12.36 Elastofibroma located between the lower scapula and chest wall in a 68-year-old woman. Coronal (a) and axial (b) T1-weighted imaging (T1WI) shows a lens-shaped lesion that has mixed intermediate and high signal (arrows). The high signal results from fat components within the lesion. The lesion (arrows) shows a heterogeneous pattern of Gd-contrast enhancement on axial fat-suppressed T1WI (c).

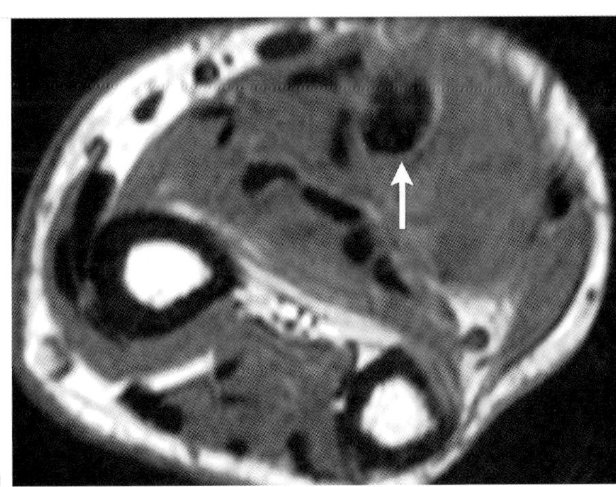
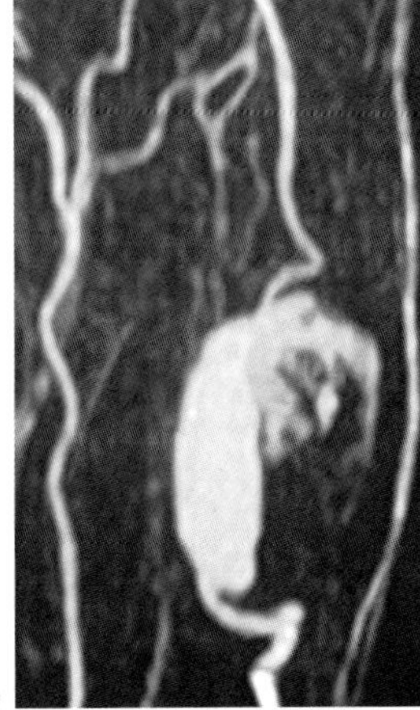

Fig. 12.37 A large aneurysm of the ulnar artery is seen (arrow), which has a flow void on axial T1-weighted imaging (a) representing a patent channel that is adjacent to thrombus, which has intermediate signal. The aneurysm is seen on three-dimensional time of flight magnetic resonance angiography (b).

Table 12.1 (Cont.) Nonmalignant tumors and tumor-like lesions involving the soft tissues of the extremities

Tumor/tumor-like lesion	MRI findings	Comments
Hypothenar hammer syndrome (▶ Fig. 12.38)	Thrombosis of the distal ulnar artery can be seen as a lack of intraluminal signal void. The thrombosed vessel can have intermediate to high signal on T1WI, and heterogeneous high signal on FS T2WI.	Thrombosis of the superficial branch of the distal ulnar artery can occur from trauma as it travels along the hypothenar muscles after exiting from the Guyon canal. Emboli into the superficial palmar arch can result in symptoms.
Abscess/myositis (▶ Fig. 12.39)	Deep infections and myositis typically show poorly defined zones of decreased signal on T1WI, and slightly high to high signal on T2WI and FS T2WI with corresponding Gd-contrast enhancement. Progression to abscess formation occurs with circumscribed zones that have low signal on T1WI and high signal on T2WI (with or without an air-fluid level) that is surrounded by a rim of low signal on T2WI. Rimlike Gd-contrast enhancement is usually seen. Peripherally, a poorly defined zone of high signal may be seen secondary to edema and/or inflammation.	Infection of muscles (myositis) and deep soft tissues from bacteria, fungi, or mycobacteria can eventually progress to liquefaction with necrosis (abscess formation) enclosed by a pseudocapsule surrounded by zones of edema and inflammatory reaction.
Cat scratch disease (▶ Fig. 12.40)	Single or multiple enlarged lymph nodes are often seen, as well as localized granulomatous lesions. Lesions often occur in the epitrochlear and axillary regions and have low-intermediate signal on T1WI and intermediate to high signal on T2WI. Lesions can have irregular margins with peripheral edematous changes. Lesions can show Gd-contrast enhancement.	Infection by the gram-negative bacillus *Bartonella henselae* can result in self-limited regional adenitis. This infection usually occurs in patients less than 30 years of age and is often related to contact with cats.
Parasitic infection (▶ Fig. 12.41)	Parasitic infections can vary from cystic-appearing lesions to poorly marginated or circumscribed solid lesions depending on the infectious organism and stage of its life cycle.	Parasitic infections can occur in soft tissues in endemic regions or in immunocompromised patients.

(continued on page 618)

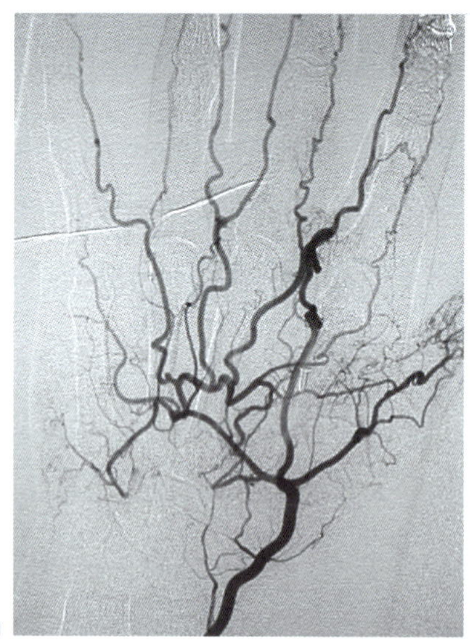
a

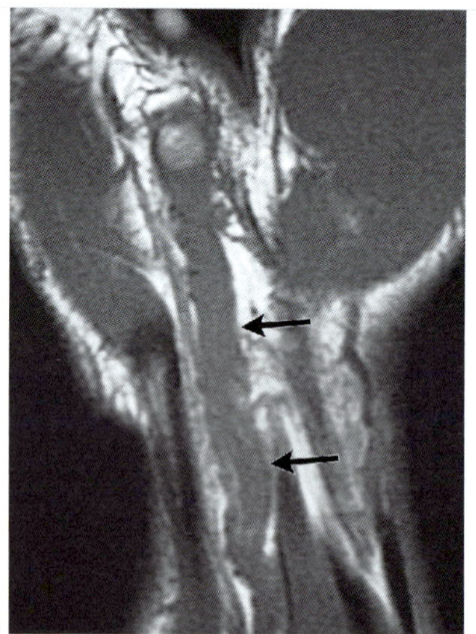
b

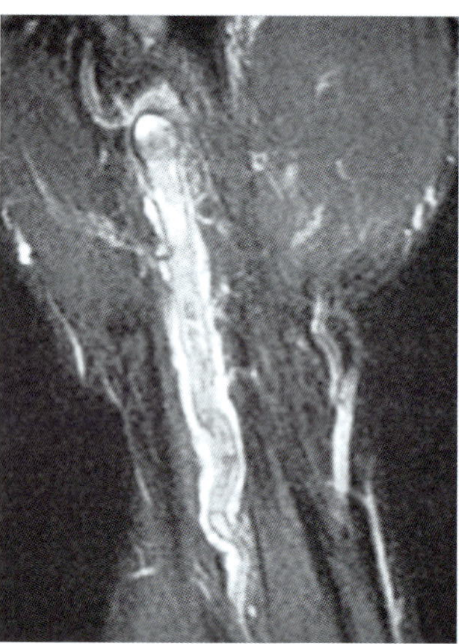
c

Fig. 12.38 Hypothenar hammer injury in a 46-year-old man resulting in thrombosis of the ulnar artery. Arteriogram (a) shows occlusion of the ulnar artery and patency of the radial artery. The occluded ulnar artery (arrows) contains intermediate and high signal on coronal T1-weighted imaging (b) and heterogeneous mostly high signal on coronal fat-suppressed T2-weighted imaging (c).

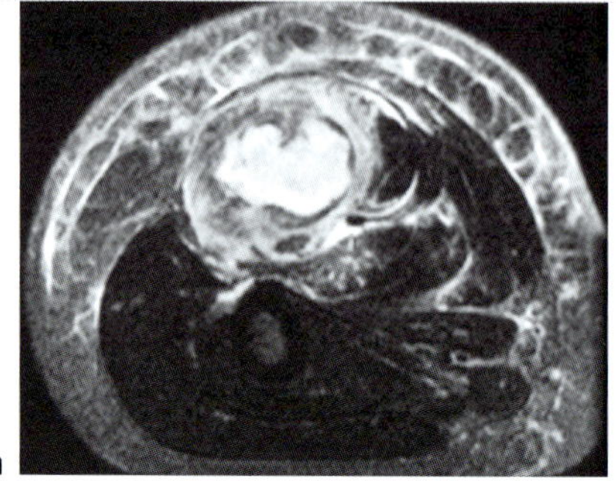
a

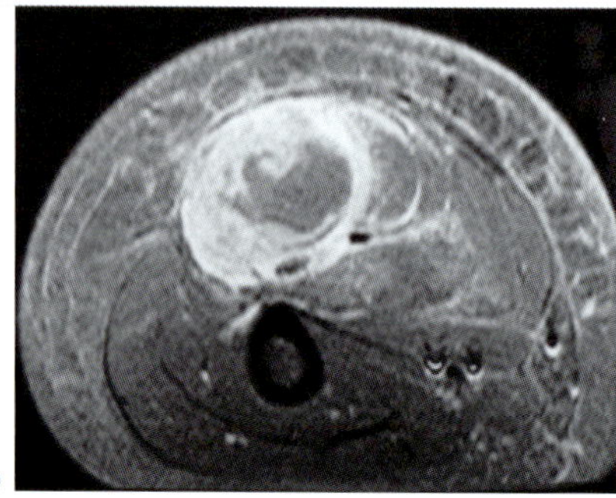
b

Fig. 12.39 A 15-year-old male with myositis and abscess involving the anterior thigh muscles as seen as a poorly defined zone with slightly high to high signal surrounding a circumscribed central zone (abscess) with high signal on axial T2-weighted imaging (a). Irregular peripheral Gd-contrast enhancement is seen in the soft tissues surrounding the abscess on axial fat-suppressed T1-weighted imaging (b).

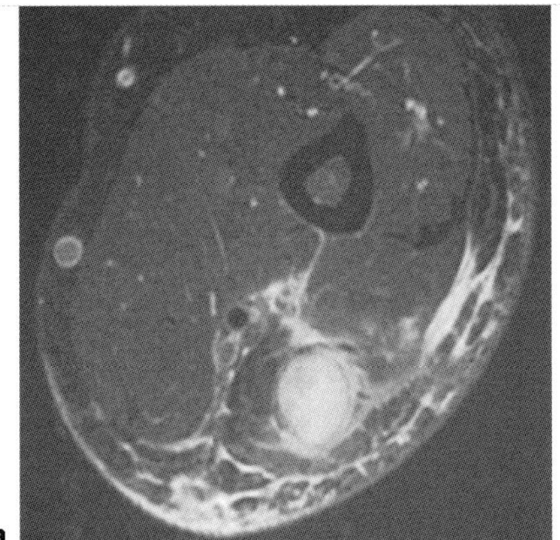

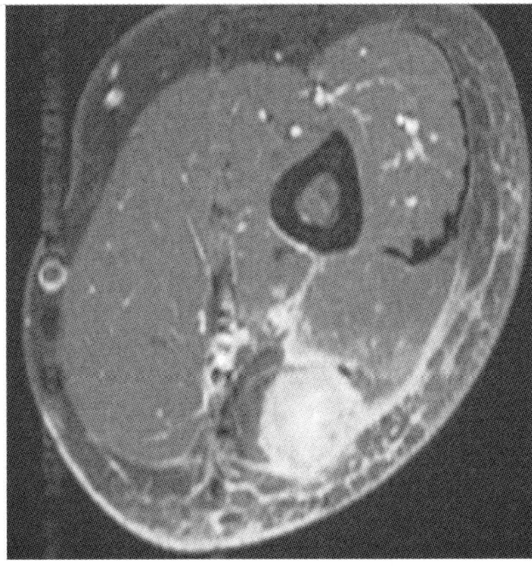

Fig. 12.40 A 45-year-old man with cat scratch disease with a granuloma involving a lymph node in the distal arm. The nodular lesion has slightly high to high signal on axial fat-suppressed (FS) T2-weighted imaging (a) and shows Gd-contrast enhancement on axial FS T1-weighted imaging (b). Irregular linear zones of inflammatory reaction are seen in the soft tissues peripheral to the nodular lesion.

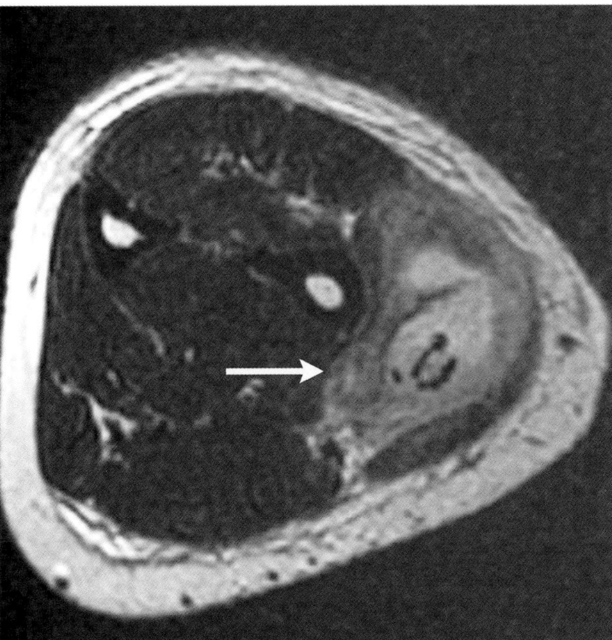

Fig. 12.41 A 34-year-old woman with intramuscular infection from cystercercosis in the forearm. A curvilinear zone with low signal representing the senescent parasite is surrounded by an abscess and solid inflammatory reaction with slightly high signal and high signal on axial T2-weighted imaging (arrow).

Table 12.1 (Cont.) Nonmalignant tumors and tumor-like lesions involving the soft tissues of the extremities

Tumor/tumor-like lesion	MRI findings	Comments
Sarcoid (▶ Fig. 12.42)	Sarcoid granulomas can also occur in subcutaneous fat and may be associated with superficial adenopathy. Lesions are often nodular with low to intermediate signal on T1WI and intermediate to high signal on T2WI. Lesions usually show Gd-contrast enhancement. Sarcoid can also involve muscles as discrete lesions.	Chronic systemic granulomatous disease of unknown etiology in which noncaseating granulomas occur in various tissues and organs. Common sites of involvement include the lungs, lymph nodes, liver, spleen, skin, and eyes.
Giant cell reaction to foreign body	Lesions usually occur in soft tissue and often have low-intermediate signal on T1WI and low, intermediate, and/or high signal on T2WI. Lesions can show Gd-contrast enhancement. Sites of bone erosion or destruction may be seen, particularly with penetrating trauma. The MRI signal of the foreign body varies based on its composition.	Reactive granulomatous lesions can form adjacent to foreign bodies and may simulate neoplasm.
Granuloma annulare (▶ Fig. 12.43)	Poorly defined subcutaneous lesion with intermediate signal on T1WI, heterogeneous intermediate to slightly high signal on T2WI, and high signal on FS T2WI. Usually shows Gd-contrast enhancement.	Benign inflammatory disorder that can involve the epidermis, dermis, and subcutaneous fat. Often occurs in children and young adults. Lesions can occur as localized, generalized, or subcutaneous forms. The localized type can appear as one or more lesions. The generalized type has a slightly wider distribution than the localized type. The subcutaneous type often affects children between 2 and 5 years.

(continued on page 620)

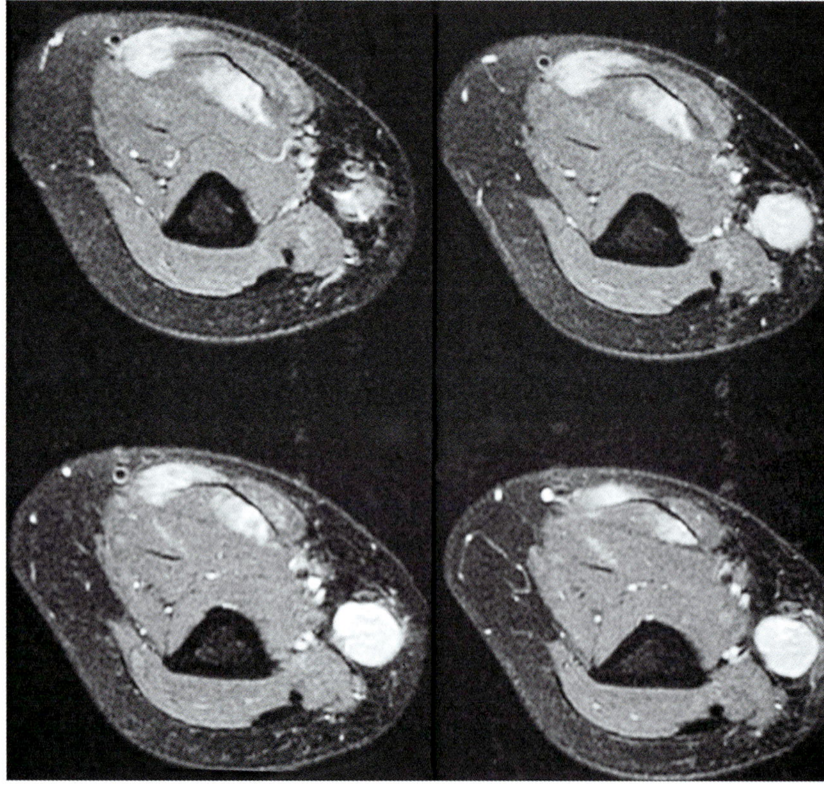

Fig. 12.42 A 49-year-old woman with sarcoid granulomas in the subcutaneous fat and within the biceps brachii muscle at the distal arm. The intramuscular lesions have slightly irregular margins and have high signal on axial fat-suppressed T2-weighted imaging.

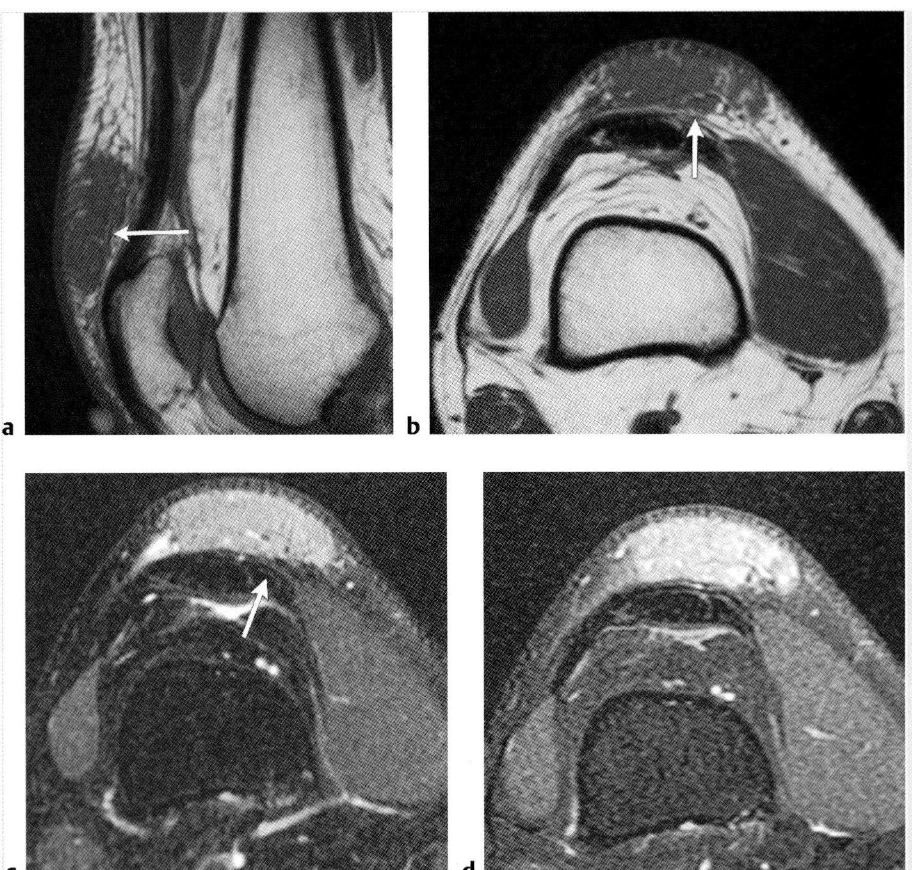

Fig. 12.43 An irregularly marginated subcutaneous lesion (granuloma annulare) (arrows) is seen, which has intermediate signal on sagittal (a) and axial (b) T1-weighted imaging (T1WI) and slightly high to high signal on axial fat-suppressed (FS) T2-weighted imaging (c). The lesion shows Gd-contrast enhancement on axial FS T1WI (d).

Table 12.1 (Cont.) Nonmalignant tumors and tumor-like lesions involving the soft tissues of the extremities

Tumor/tumor-like lesion	MRI findings	Comments
Gout (▶ Fig. 12.44)	Tophi have variable sizes and shapes and have low-intermediate signal on T1WI, FS T2WI, and T2WI. Zones of high signal on T2WI can also be seen in tophi. Erosions of bone, synovial pannus, joint effusion, bone marrow and soft tissue edema can be seen with MRI. Tophi may show heterogeneous, diffuse, or peripheral/marginal Gd-contrast enhancement patterns.	Gout is an inflammatory disease involving synovium resulting from deposition of monosodium urate crystals and occurs when the serum urate level exceeds its solubility in various tissues and body fluid.
Rheumatoid arthritis (▶ Fig. 12.45)	MRI can show diffuse and/or localized zones of synovial hypertrophy; soft tissue swelling; zones of erosion and/or destruction of hyaline cartilage, meniscal damage, subchondral bone, tendons, ligaments; bursal fluid collections containing "rice bodies," other extra-articular cysts; intraosseous cystic-like areas, joint effusion, and rheumatoid nodules. With tendon and ligament involvement, abnormal increased signal is seen on PDWI and T2WI. Tendons and ligaments may be thickened from partial tearing or thinned. Tenosynovitis is usually seen with fluid and hypertrophied synovium within tendon sheaths.	Chronic multisystem disease of unknown etiology in which there is a persistent inflammatory synovitis that typically involves peripheral joints in a symmetric distribution. The inflammatory synovitis can result in progressive destruction of cartilage and bone leading to joint dysfunction.
Dermatomyositis (▶ Fig. 12.46)	In acute and subacute phases, poorly defined zones of high signal on T2WI are seen in muscles, subcutaneous fat, and fascia secondary to ischemic or infarcted muscle secondary to vasculitis. Zones of low signal on T2WI can result from calcifications seen on radiographs and computed tomographic scans. Milk of calcium collections have variable signal on T1WI and T2WI depending on the relative proportions of fluid and fluid-calcium levels. Poorly defined zones of Gd-contrast enhancement can be seen in muscles, fascia, and/or subcutaneous fat if there is active inflammation and/or ischemia-infarction. Muscle atrophy with fatty infiltration can be seen in the chronic phases.	Nonsuppurative autoimmune systemic vasculopathy involving muscle fibers, skin, and blood vessels. Can be associated with other connective tissue diseases such as scleroderma and mixed connective tissue disease. Incidence: 2 to 8 per million; prevalence: 4 to 60 per million. Juvenile dermatomyositis occurs in children between 2 and 15 years of age. Adult dermatomyositis occurs with peak incidence in the fifth decade.

(continued on page 622)

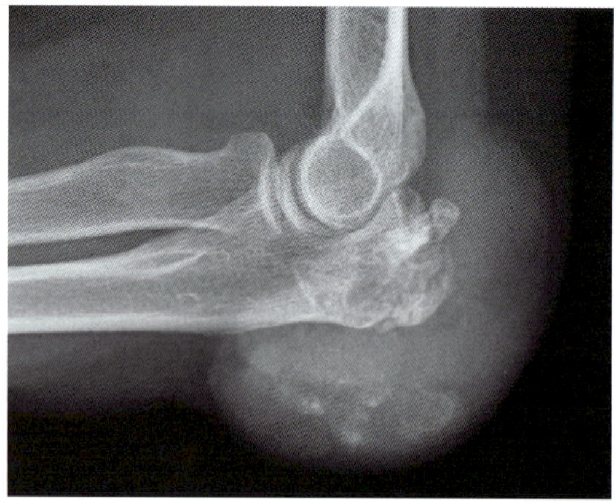

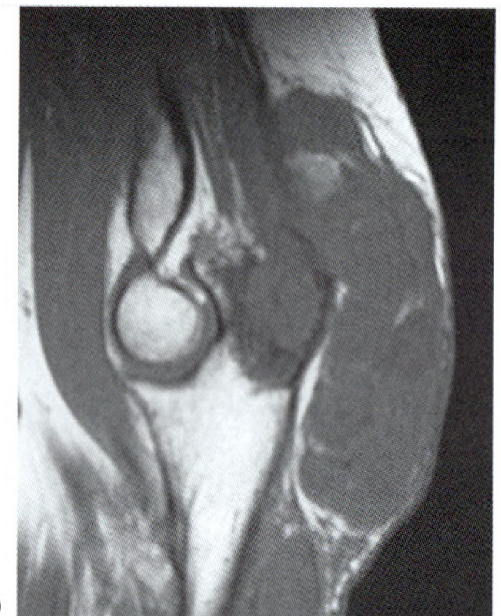

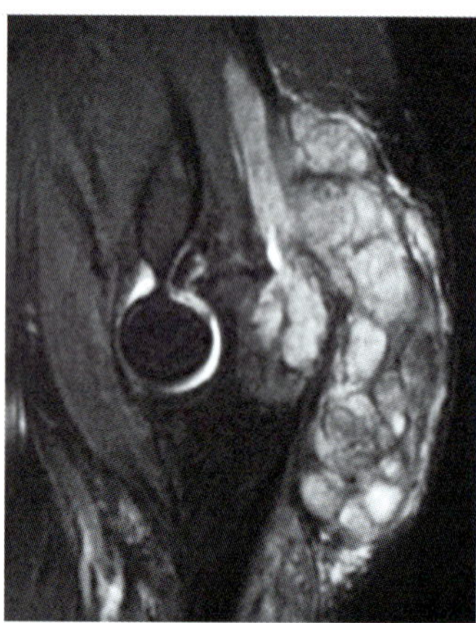

Fig. 12.44 A 57-year-old woman with gout and a large tophus containing several calcifications in the superificial soft tissues at the elbow associated bone erosion as seen on a lateral radiograph (a). The tophus has intermediate signal on sagittal T1-weighted imaging (b) and mixed high, slightly high, intermediate, and low signal on sagittal fat-suppressed T2-weighted imaging (c).

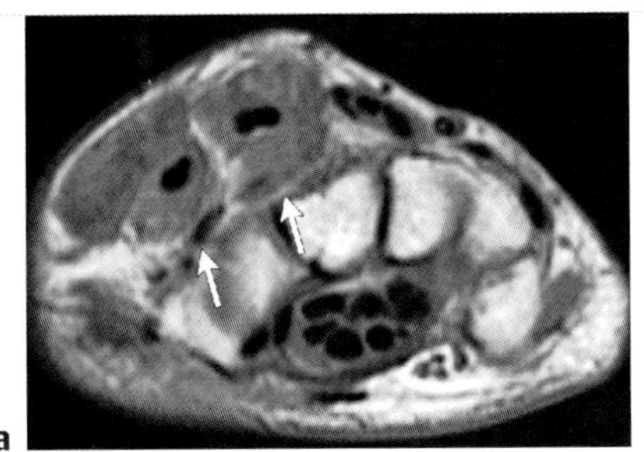
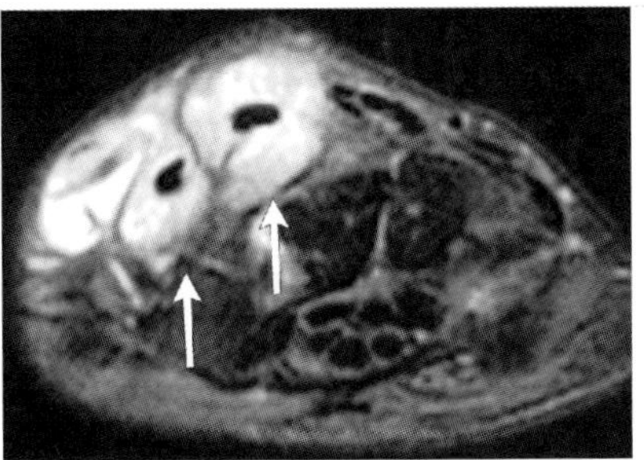
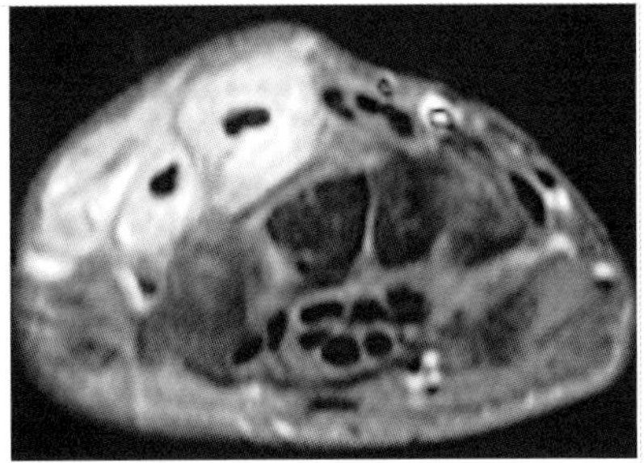

Fig. 12.45 A 48-year-old woman with rheumatoid arthritis. Hypertrophied synovium (pannus) is seen in the tendon sheaths of the extensor carpi radialis brevis and longus tendons (arrows). The pannus has intermediate signal on axial T1-weighted imaging (T1WI) (a) and heterogeneous intermediate to high signal on axial fat-suppressed (FS) T2-weighted imaging (b). The pannus shows prominent Gd-contrast enhancement on axial FS T1WI (c).

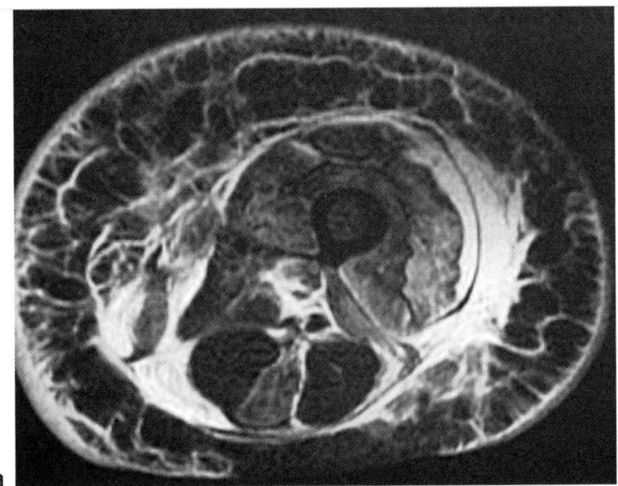
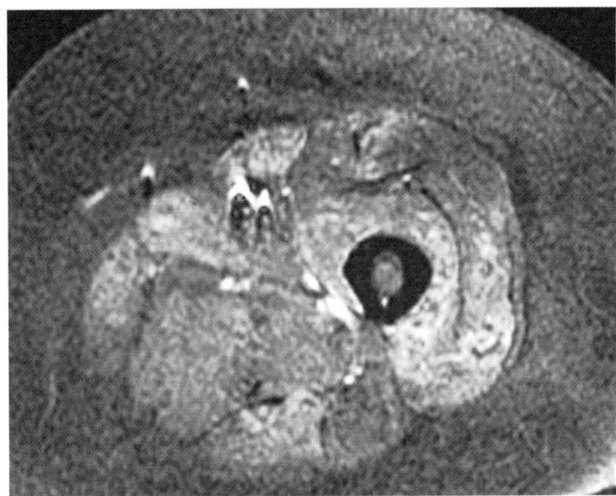

Fig. 12.46 A 78-year-old woman with dermatomyositis involving the thigh. Poorly defined zones of abnormal high signal on fat-suppressed T2-weighted imaging (FS T2WI) (a) and abnormal gadolinium-contrast enhancement on FS T1-weighted imaging (b) are seen in the thigh muscles secondary to active inflammation. Zones of abnormal high signal on axial FS T2WI are also seen in the subcutaneous fat.

Table 12.1 (Cont.) Nonmalignant tumors and tumor-like lesions involving the soft tissues of the extremities

Tumor/tumor-like lesion	MRI findings	Comments
Scleroderma/systemic sclerosis (▶ Fig. 12.47)	Irregular zones with abnormal high signal on T2WI and Gd-contrast enhancement are usually seen involving muscle fascia and adjacent muscles, subcutaneous fatty tissue septa. Gd-contrast of thickened synovium in joints and tendon sheaths has also been reported.	Severe connective tissue disorder with inflammation and microvascular alterations resulting in progressive deposition of collagen bundles in muscle fascia, subcutaneous fatty tissue septa, and articular synovium. Can also involve the lungs, heart, and peripheral arteries. Median age = 46 years. Often have antibodies to antinuclear antibody (ANA), SCL-70, and have elevated serum creatine kinase and C-reactive protein. Patients usually present with joint pain. A subgroup has additional features of calcinosis, Raynaud phenomenon, esophageal dysmotility, and telangiectasis (CREST syndrome). A localized form of scleroderma is referred to as linear morphea, which is not associated with Raynaud phenomenon, involvement of internal organs, or digital sclerosis.

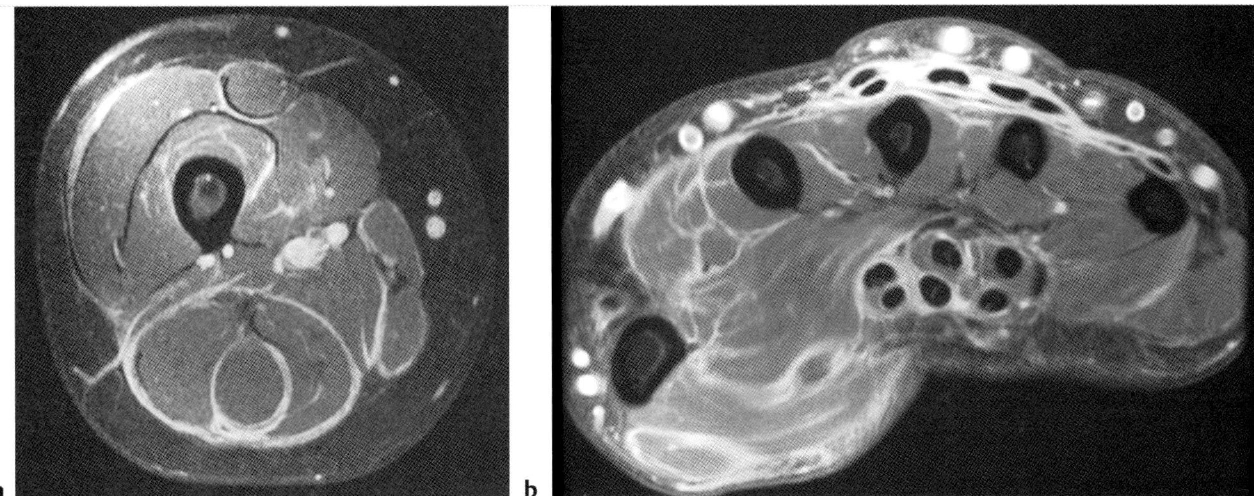

Fig. 12.47 An 18-year-old woman with systemic sclerosis (scleroderma). Axial fat-suppressed T1-weighted imaging shows abnormal gadolinium-contrast enhancement involving the intermuscular fascia of the thigh (a) and hand (b). Abnormal Gd-contrast enhancement is also seen involving the inflamed synovium of the extensor and flexor tendon sheaths of the hand.

12.2 Malignant Tumors Involving the Musculoskeletal Soft Tissues

- Malignant fibrous histiocytoma (MFH)/undifferentiated pleomorphic sarcoma
- Fibrosarcoma/myxofibrosarcoma
- Low grade myofibroblastic sarcoma
- Well-differentiated liposarcoma
- Myxoid liposarcoma
- Myxoid-round cell liposarcoma
- Pleopmorphic liposarcoma
- Dedifferentiated liposarcoma
- Metastatic disease
- Myeloma
- Lymphoma
- Leukemia
- Synovial cell sarcoma
- Malignant peripheral nerve sheath tumor (MPNST)
- Clear cell sarcoma (melanoma of soft parts)
- Leiomyosarcoma
- Rhabdomyosarcoma
- Hemangioendothelioma
- Hemangiopericytoma
- Angiosarcoma
- Extraosseous osteosarcoma
- Extraosseous Ewing sarcoma
- Extraosseous chondrosarcoma
- Malignant giant cell tumor of soft tissues
- Dermatofibrosarcoma (DFS)/dermatofibrosarcoma protuberans (DFSP)

Table 12.2 Malignant tumors involving the musculoskeletal soft tissues

Tumor	MRI findings	Comments
Malignant fibrous histiocytoma (MFH)/ undifferentiated pleomorphic sarcoma (▶ Fig. 12.48)	Tumors have poorly defined and/or circumscribed margins, and often have low-intermediate signal on T1-weighted imaging (T1WI) and heterogeneous intermediate-high signal on T2-weighted imaging (T2WI) and fat-suppressed (FS) T2WI. Tumors show heterogeneous often prominent gadolinium (Gd)-contrast enhancement.	Malignant tumors involving soft tissue and rarely bone, which are presumed to derive from undifferentiated mesenchymal cells. The World Health Organization now uses the term of undifferentiated pleomorphic sarcoma for MFH.

(continued on page 626)

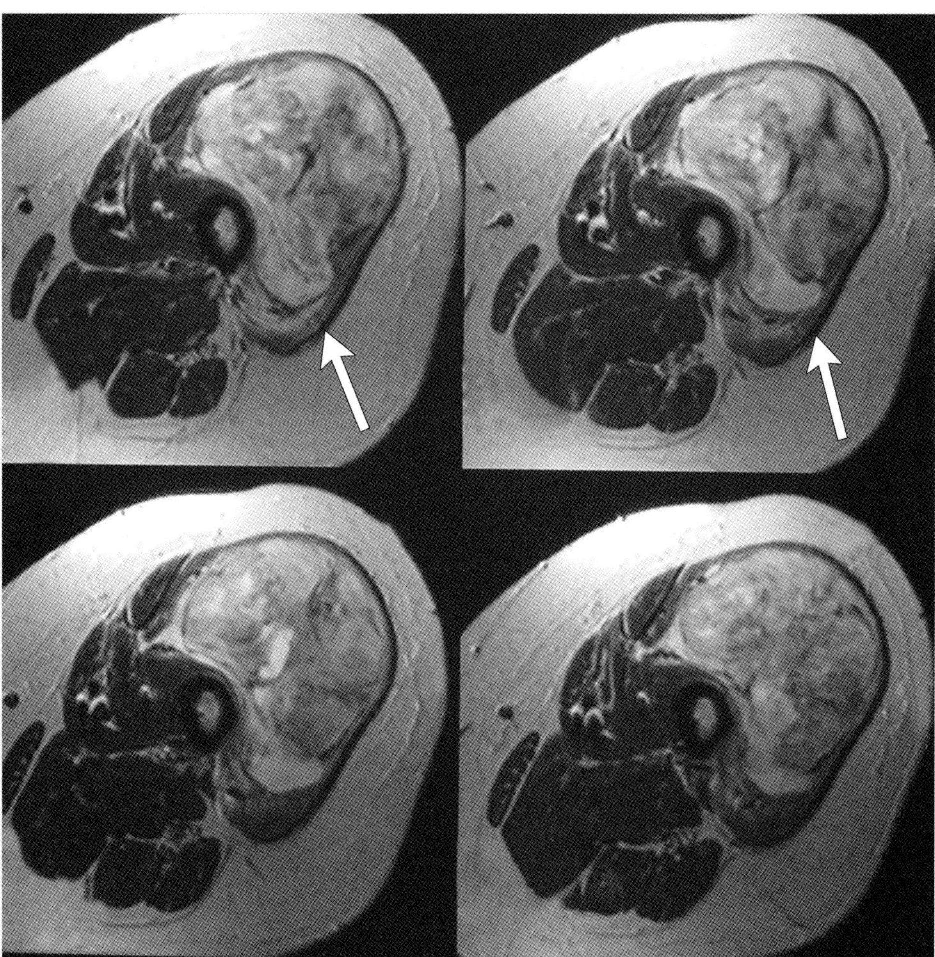

Fig. 12.48 A 66-year-old woman with a malignant fibrous histiocytoma involving the vastus lateralis muscle of the proximal thigh. The tumor (arrows) has heterogeneous slightly high and high signal on axial T2-weighted imaging.

Table 12.2 (Cont.) Malignant tumors involving the musculoskeletal soft tissues

Tumor	MRI findings	Comments
Fibrosarcoma/myxofibrosarcoma (▶ Fig. 12.49; ▶ Fig. 12.50; ▶ Fig. 12.51)	Tumors can have slightly irregular margins, with or without associated destruction and invasion of adjacent bone. *High grade fibrosarcomas* may have an infiltrative pattern with respect to adjacent soft tissues. Lesions usually have low-intermediate signal on T1WI, intermediate to slightly high signal on proton density–weighted imaging (PDWI), and heterogeneous intermediate-high signal on T2WI. Margins of lesions may be indistinct on T2WI for high grade lesions. Zones with high signal on T2WI can be seen in myxoid regions of *myxofibrosarcoma*. For *sclerosing epithelioid fibrosarcoma*, zones of low signal on T1WI and T2WI can be seen from regions of decreased cellularity and dense collagen deposition in these neoplasms. Tumors usually show heterogeneous Gd-contrast enhancement. Enhancing margins may be indistinct for high grade lesions.	Uncommon malignant tumors consisting of bundles of fibroblasts/spindle cells with varying proportions of collagen, lacking other tissue-differentiating features such as tumor bone, osteoid, or cartilage. Infantile fibrosarcoma accounts for < 1% of malignant soft tissue tumors and 12% of soft tissue and occurs in young patients, mean age = 2 years. Adult fibrosarcomas account for 4% of malignant soft tissue tumors, mean age = 41 years. Variants of fibrosarcoma include myxofibrosarcoma, low grade fibromyxoid sarcoma, and sclerosing epithelioid fibrosarcoma.
Low grade myofibroblastic sarcoma (▶ Fig. 12.52)	Tumors can have poorly defined and/or circumscribed margins, and often have low-intermediate signal on T1WI and heterogeneous intermediate-high signal on T2WI and FS T2WI. Tumors usually show Gd-contrast enhancement.	Distinct atypical myofibroblastic tumor with fibromatosis-like features, composed of spindle-shaped tumor cells in fascicles or storiform patterns, occurs in adults and children. Can have aggressive growth when necrosis and increased cell proliferation are present.

(continued on page 628)

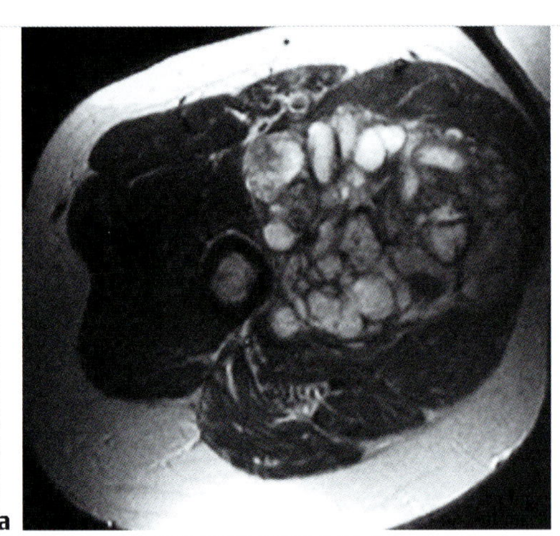

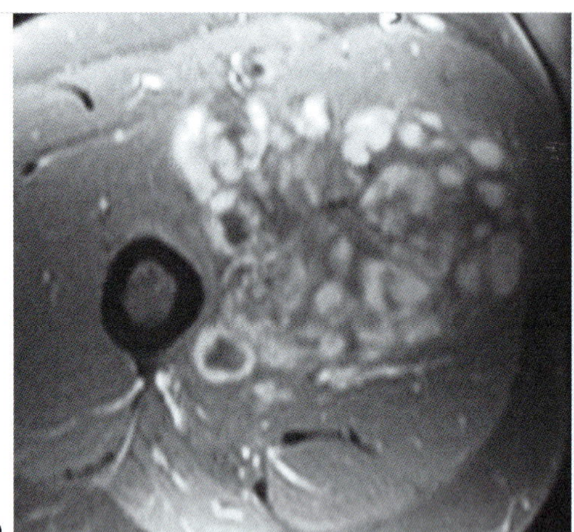

Fig. 12.49 A 37-year-old man with a myxofibrosarcoma involving the adductor muscles in the proximal thigh that has mixed zones of low, intermediate, and high signal on axial T2-weighted imaging (a). The tumor shows prominent heterogeneous Gd-contrast enhancement on axial fat-suppressed T1-weighted imaging (b).

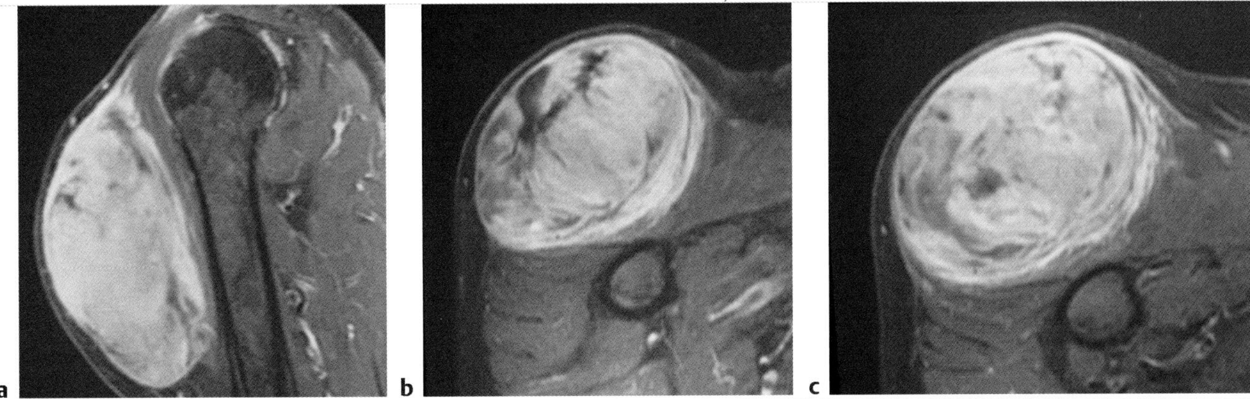

Fig. 12.50 An 82-year-old man with a low grade myxofibrosarcoma involving the soft tissues anterior to the proximal humerus. The tumor shows prominent, slightly heterogeneous Gd-contrast enhancement on sagittal (a) and axial (b) fat-suppressed (FS) T1-weighted imaging, and has slightly heterogeneous high signal on axial FS T2-weighted imaging (c). The tumor has circumscribed margins with the superficial soft tissue but indistinct margins with the muscles deep to the lesion consistent with invasion.

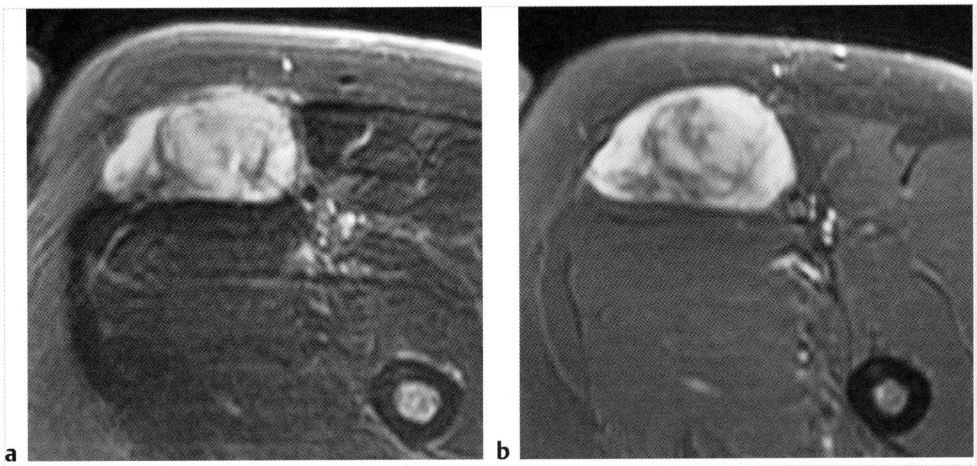

Fig. 12.51 A low-grade fibromyxoid sarcoma in the anterior medial thigh muscle in a 37-year-old man has heterogeneous, mostly high signal on axial fat-suppressed (FS) T2-weighted imaging (a) and shows heterogeneous Gd-contrast enhancement on axial FS T1-weighted imaging (b).

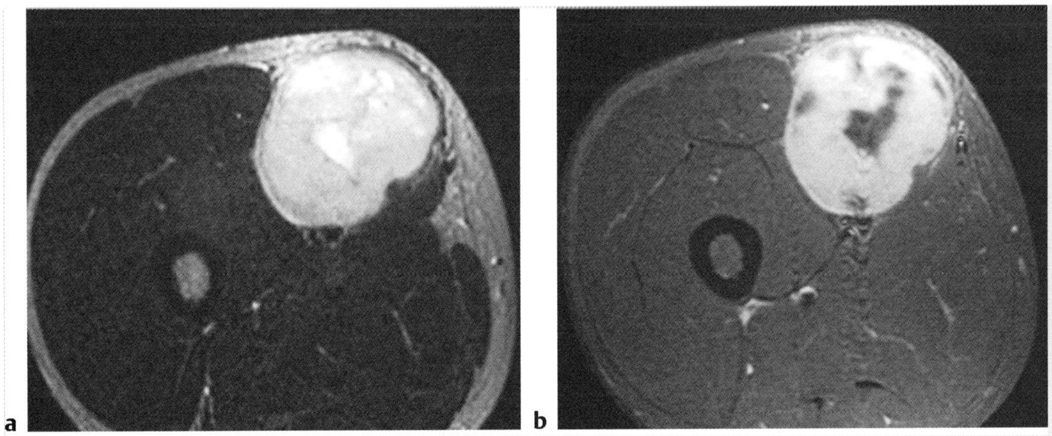

Fig. 12.52 A low-grade myofibroblastic sarcoma in the lateral anterior thigh muscle of a 13-year-old boy has heterogeneous, mostly high signal on axial T2-weighted imaging (a) and shows heterogeneous Gd-contrast enhancement on axial fat-suppressed T1-weighted imaging (b).

Table 12.2 (Cont.) Malignant tumors involving the musculoskeletal soft tissues

Tumor	MRI findings	Comments
Well-differentiated liposarcoma (▶ Fig. 12.53)	Tumors contain up to 75% overall fat signal, and contain thick nonadipose septae, and/or nodular nonadipose zones. The nonadipose zones can have low-intermediate signal on T1WI and PDWI, and low, intermediate, and/or high signal on T2WI. Nonadipose tumor portions show variable degrees of Gd-contrast enhancement.	Malignant mesenchymal tumors containing portions showing differentiation into adipose tissue. Compared with benign lipomas, these tumors have thicker and more numerous fibrous and/or nonfatty septae containing fibroblastic spindle cells, atypical cells, and vacuolated lipoblasts surrounding various-sized lobules of fat. Fat cells have nuclear atypia, and hyperchromatic stromal cells are seen in fibrous septa. Account for 40 to 54% of liposarcomas. Occurs in patients age 39 to 77 years, mean = 50 years.
Myxoid liposarcoma (▶ Fig. 12.54)	Tumors usually have mostly low signal on T1WI and may contain small zones of high fat signal in lacy, amorphous, and/or linear configurations. Most myxoid liposarcomas contain less than 26% fat. Some myxoid liposarcomas do not contain fatty zones. Tumors can have heterogeneous or homogeneous high signal on PDWI and T2WI, and some have a multiloculated pattern. Low signal septa may be present on T2WI. Tumors usually show Gd-contrast enhancement in varying degrees and patterns, or rarely none at all.	Composed of proliferating stellate and/or fusiform neoplastic lipoblasts in varying stages of differentiation, signet cells containing lipids, variable myxoid matrix, and plexiform capillary network. Mitotic activity is usually low. Osseous, cartilaginous, and/or leiomyomatous metaplasia may occur in these tumors. Fat content in these myxoid liposarcomas is usually less than 10 to 25% of tumor volume. Account for 23% of liposarcomas. Occurs in patients age 18 to 67 years, mean = 42 years. Associated with chromosomal translocation t(12;16) (q13;p11), which also occurs in myxoid-round cell liposarcomas.

(continued on page 630)

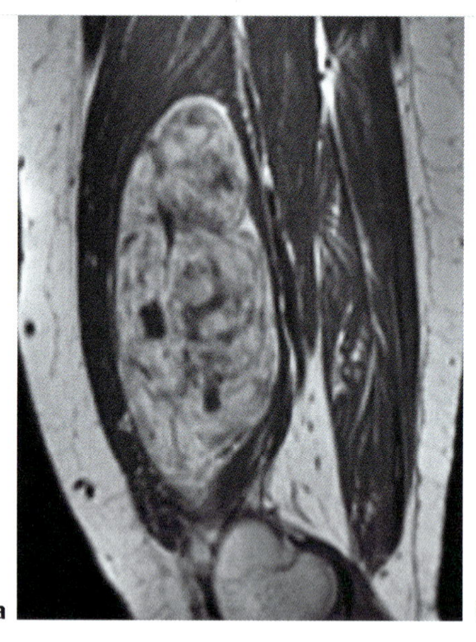
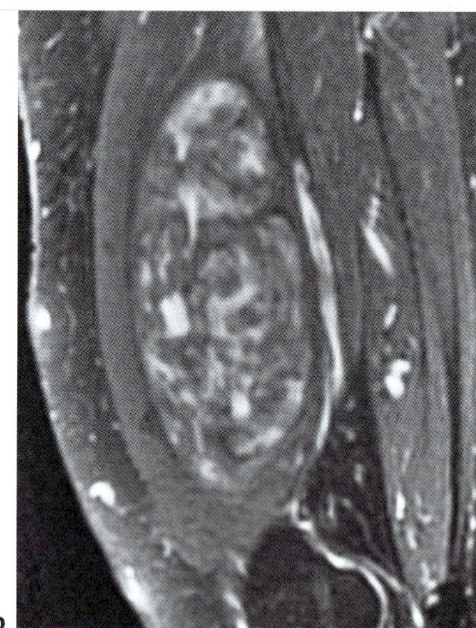
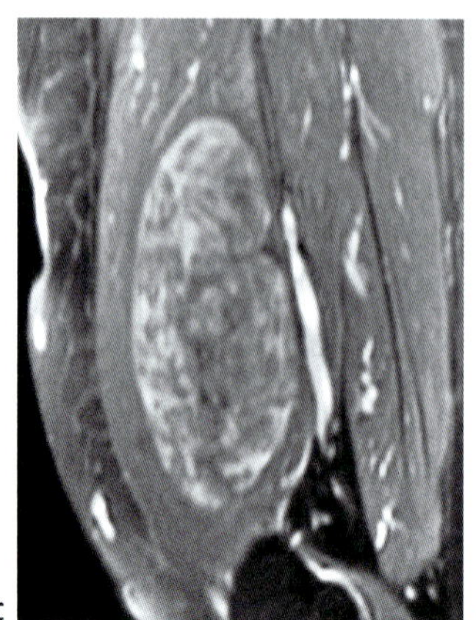
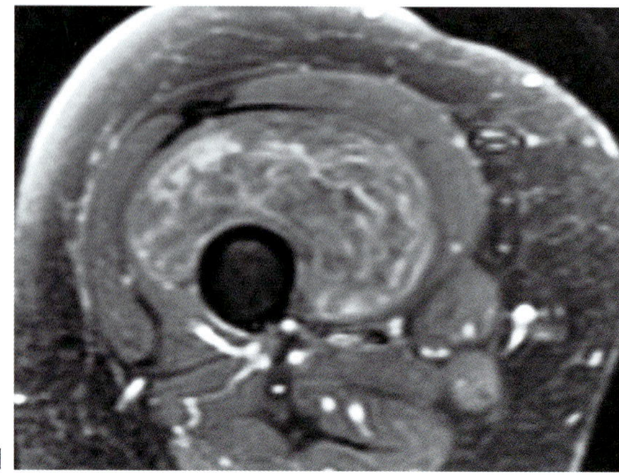

Fig. 12.53 A 67-year-old woman with a well-differentiated low grade liposarcoma involving the vastus intermedius muscle of the thigh. The tumor has high fat signal on sagittal T1-weighted imaging (T1WI) (a) as well as zones with low-intermediate signal. The nonfatty portions of the tumor have slightly high and high signal on fat-suppressed (FS) T2-weighted imaging (b) and show Gd-contrast enhancement on sagittal (c) and axial (d) FS T1WI.

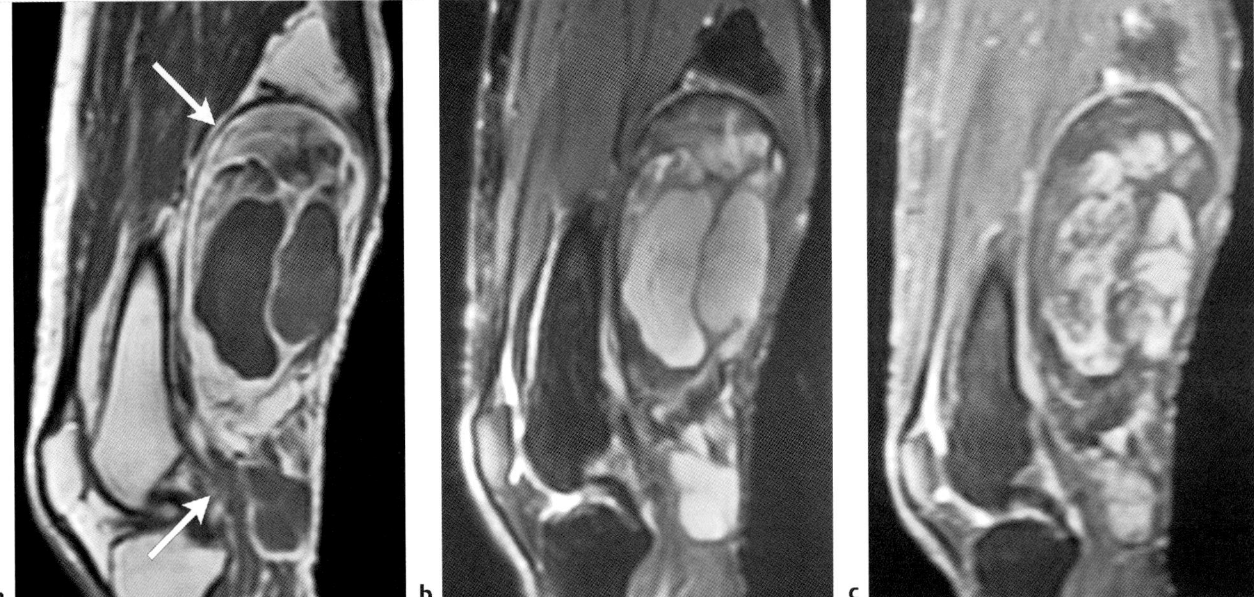

Fig. 12.54 A 68-year-old woman with a myxoid liposarcoma involving the posterior distal thigh. This tumor (arrows) has circumscribed margins and contains both high and low-intermediate signal on sagittal T1-weighted imaging (T1WI) (a). Some of the zones with high signal on T1WI secondary to fat are suppressed on sagittal fat-suppressed (FS) T2-weighted imaging (b), whereas most of the tumor has high signal from the myxoid components. The tumor shows heterogeneous Gd-contrast enhancement on sagittal FS T1WI (c).

Table 12.2 (Cont.) Malignant tumors involving the musculoskeletal soft tissues

Tumor	MRI findings	Comments
Myxoid-round cell liposarcoma (▶ Fig. 12.55)	Tumors can have relatively well defined margins (72%) or poorly defined margins (28%), and have heterogeneous/mixed low, intermediate, and/or high signal on T1WI, PDWI, and T2WI. Most round cell liposarcomas contain less than 26% fat. Tumors usually show prominent Gd-contrast enhancement (61%) in a heterogeneous pattern that may be globular or nodular.	Contain round small neoplastic cells with single naked round or slightly oval nuclei, scarce cytoplasm containing vacuoles with minimal intracellular lipid. Tumor cells have low mitotic activity and occur within a myxoid matrix. Have been considered to represent poorly differentiated myxoid liposarcomas. Account for 6% of liposarcomas. Occurs in patients age 30 to 64 years, mean = 43 years.
Pleomorphic liposarcoma (▶ Fig. 12.56)	Tumors often have relatively well defined margins and have heterogeneous/mixed low, intermediate, and/or high signal on T1WI, PDWI, and T2WI. Less than 26% of the tumor volumes have fat signal. Tumors usually show prominent Gd-contrast enhancement in a heterogeneous pattern.	Tumors contain lipogenic and nonlipogenic zones, which have features similar to malignant fibrous histiocytoma, round cell liposarcoma, and/or epithelioid carcinoma. Tumors have prominent cellular pleomorphism with malignant pleomorphic lipoblasts, pleomorphic spindle cells, and occasional giant cells. Mitoses are common. Variable degrees of necrosis are seen. Most tumors have infiltrative borders microscopically. Account for 5 to 7% of liposarcomas. Occurs in patients age 41 to 78 years, mean = 60 years.
Dedifferentiated liposarcoma (▶ Fig. 12.57)	Tumors can contain portions with features of a well-differentiated liposarcoma as well as a focal nonlipomatous mass. Frequently occur in the retroperitoneum and can be large (mean = 19.3 cm). Tumors can have circumscribed and/or irregular/poorly defined margins. Tumors often have heterogeneous/mixed low, intermediate, and/or high signal on T1WI, PDWI, and T2WI. Hemorrhage and necrosis can be seen in the nonlipomatous portions. Tumors often show prominent Gd-contrast enhancement in nonlipomatous portions in a heterogeneous or homogeneous pattern.	Occur most frequently in the retroperitoneum and often contain both well-differentiated and poorly differentiated zones. The poorly differentiated component is usually a high grade sarcoma. Account for 10% of liposarcomas. Occurs in patients age 42 to 78 years, mean = 63 years.

(continued on page 632)

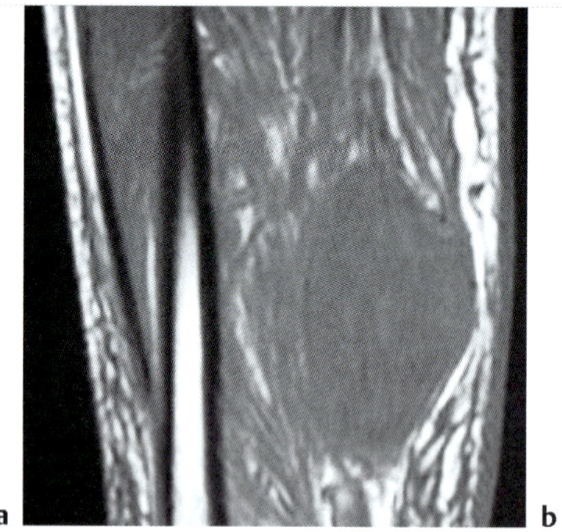
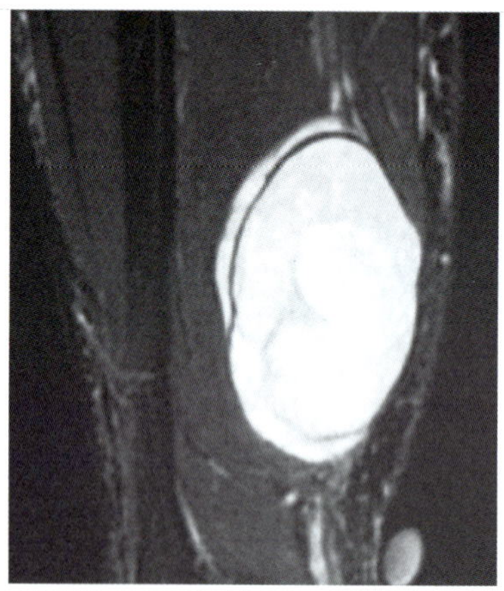
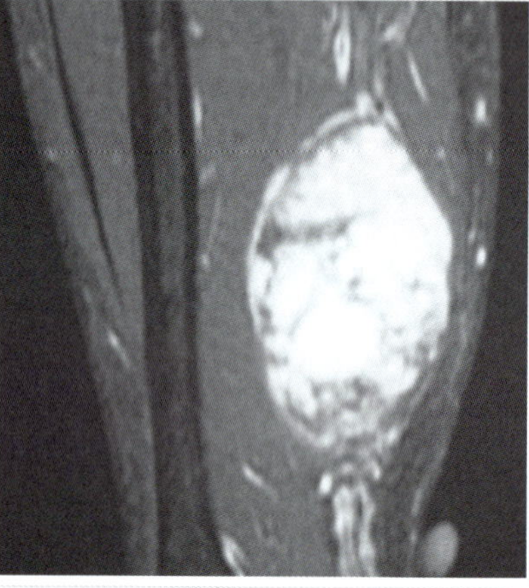

Fig. 12.55 Myxoid-round cell liposarcoma involving the posterior thigh muscles in a 49-year-old man has intermediate signal on sagittal T1-weighted imaging (T1WI) (a), mostly high signal on sagittal fat-suppressed (FS) T2-weighted imaging (b), and shows Gd-contrast enhancement on sagittal FS T1WI (c).

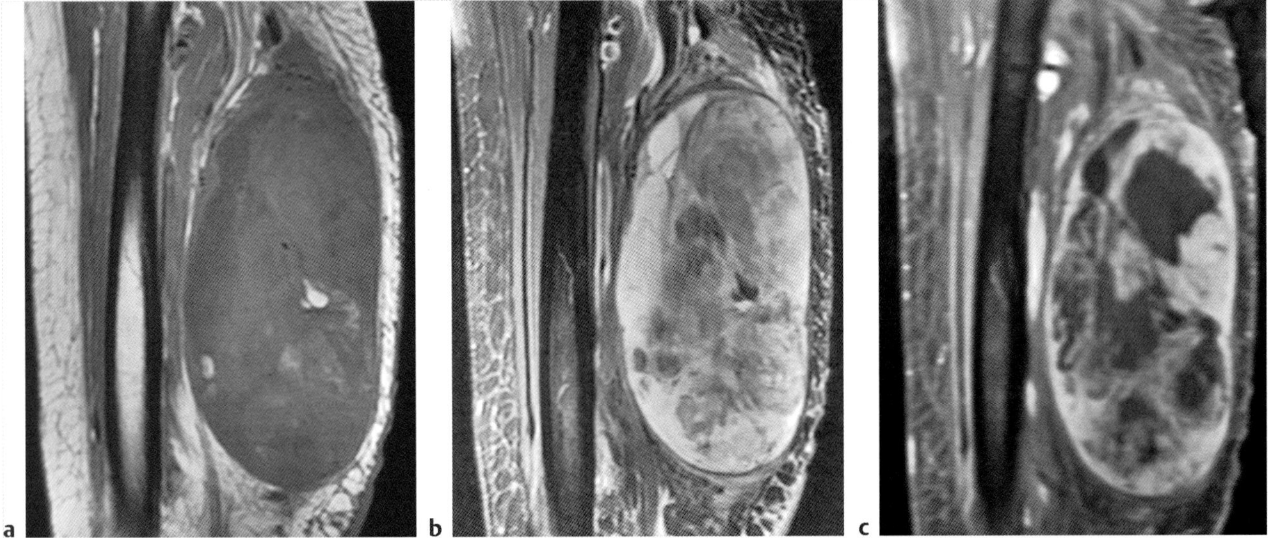

Fig. 12.56 An 83-year-old woman with a large, high grade pleomorphic liposarcoma involving the posterior left thigh. The tumor has heterogeneous intermediate signal and small zones with high signal on sagittal T1-weighted imaging (T1WI) (a), heterogeneous high, intermediate, and low signal on sagittal fat-suppressed (FS) T2-weighted imaging (b), and shows heterogeneous Gd-contrast enhancement on sagittal FS T1WI (c).

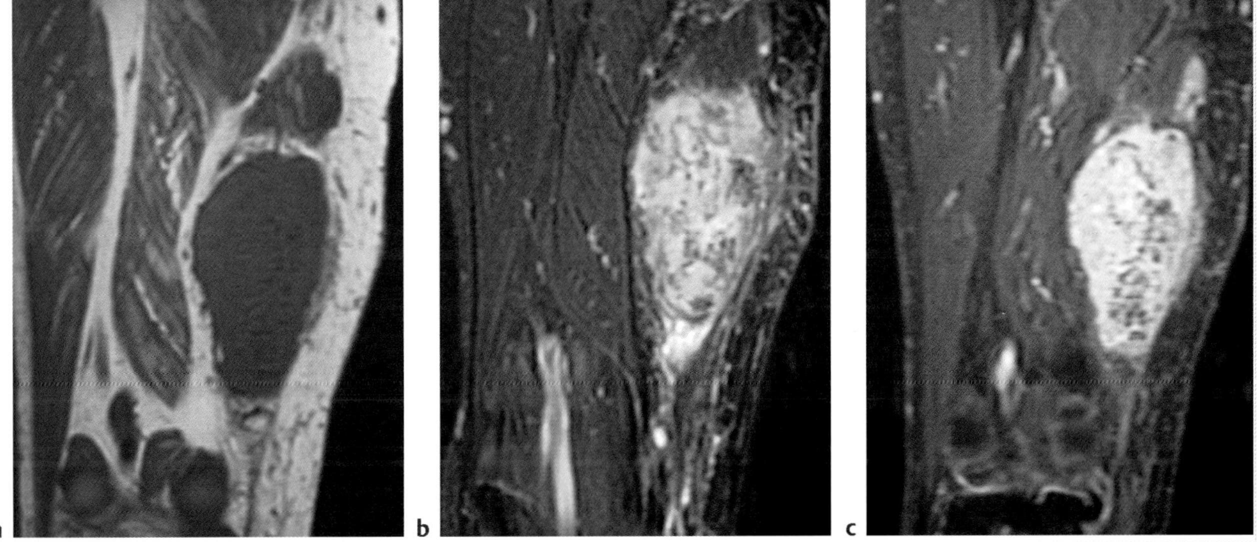

Fig. 12.57 A 71-year-old woman with a dedifferentiated liposarcoma in the distal thigh. A mass lesion is seen involving the soft tissues of the medial thigh, which has irregular margins and has intermediate signal on coronal T1-weighted imaging (T1WI) (a), heterogeneous mostly high signal on coronal fat-suppressed (FS) T2-weighted imaging (b), and shows heterogeneous Gd-contrast enhancement on coronal FS T1WI (c).

Table 12.2 (Cont.) Malignant tumors involving the musculoskeletal soft tissues

Tumor	MRI findings	Comments
Metastatic disease (▶ Fig. 12.58)	Tumors can occur as lymphadenopathy or as focal lesions. Lesions have low-intermediate signal on T1WI and intermediate to slightly high signal or high signal on T2WI and FS T2WI. Variability in MRI signal characteristics may be related to differing histological features of the metastatic lesions. Tumors can show variable degrees of Gd-contrast enhancement.	Metastatic lesions are proliferating neoplastic cells that are located in sites or organs separated or distant from their origins.
Myeloma (▶ Fig. 12.59)	Lesions usually have low-intermediate signal on T1WI, slightly high to high signal on T2WI, and high signal on FS T2WI. Extraosseous tumors can occur from extension from intraosseous lesions, or primarily within the soft tissues. Lesions may have poorly defined or distinct margins. Most lesions show Gd-contrast enhancement. Zones of high signal on T2WI peripheral to the Gd-contrast enhancing portion of the lesion may represent zones of tumor invasion or perilesional edema.	Malignant tumors composed of proliferating antibody-secreting plasma cells derived from single clones. Usually occur in bone and occasionally in soft tissue.
Lymphoma (▶ Fig. 12.60)	Lymphadenopathy from Hodgkin lymphoma (HL) and lesions of non-Hodgkin lymphoma (NHL) have low-intermediate signal on T1WI and intermediate to slightly high signal on T2WI. Variability in MRI signal may be related to differing histological features (such as the degree of fibrosis) for the subtypes of HL. After Gd-contrast administration, HL and NHL can show variable Gd-contrast enhancement.	Lymphomas are tumors in which neoplastic cells arise within lymphoid tissue. HL usually occurs in lymph nodes and spreads along nodal chains, whereas NHL frequently originates at extranodal sites and spreads in an unpredictable pattern. Mycosis fungoides is a T cell lymphoma that involves the skin.

(continued on page 634)

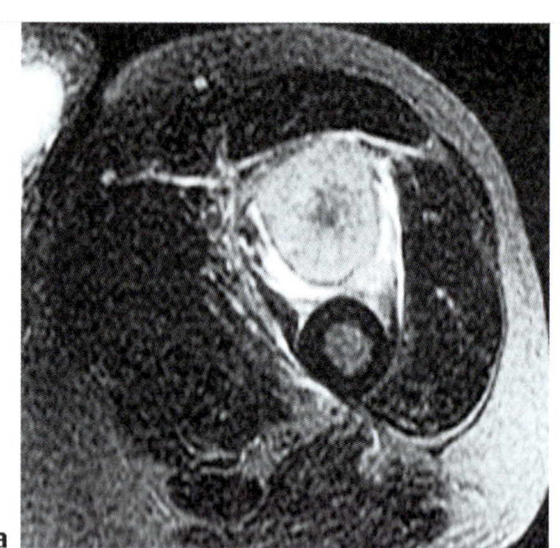
a

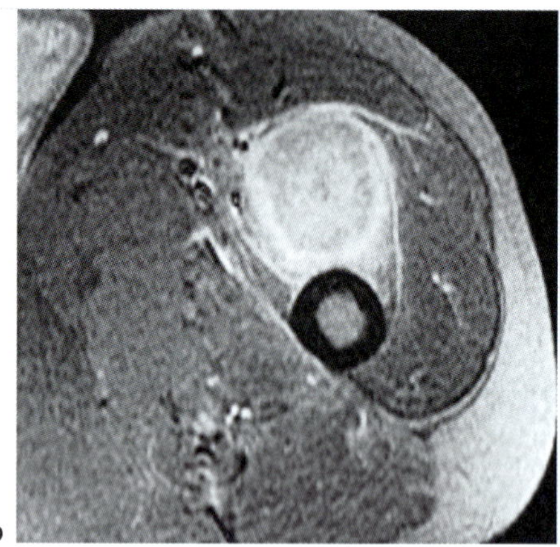
b

Fig. 12.58 A 51-year-old man with a metastatic lesion from lung carcinoma involving the vastus intermedius muscle of the upper thigh, which has high signal on axial fat-suppressed (FS) T2-weighted imaging (a). The tumor shows Gd-contrast enhancement on axial FS T1-weighted imaging (b).

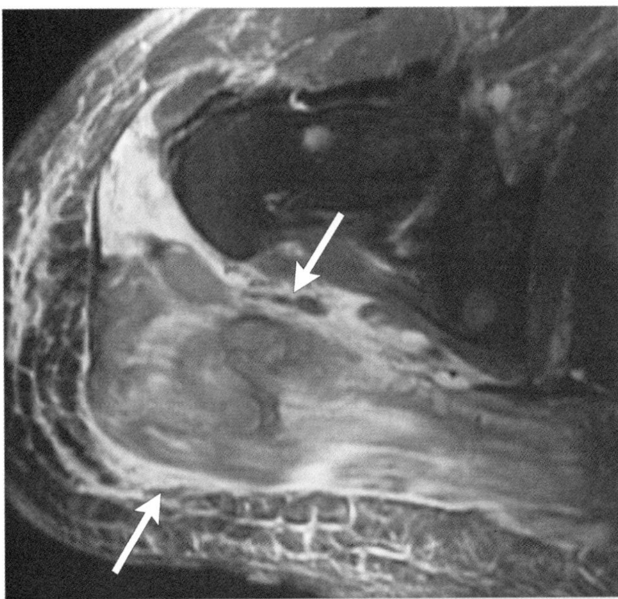

Fig. 12.59 Myeloma with poorly defined high signal on fat-suppressed T2-weighted imaging involving the muscles posterior to the right hip in a 77-year-old man (arrows).

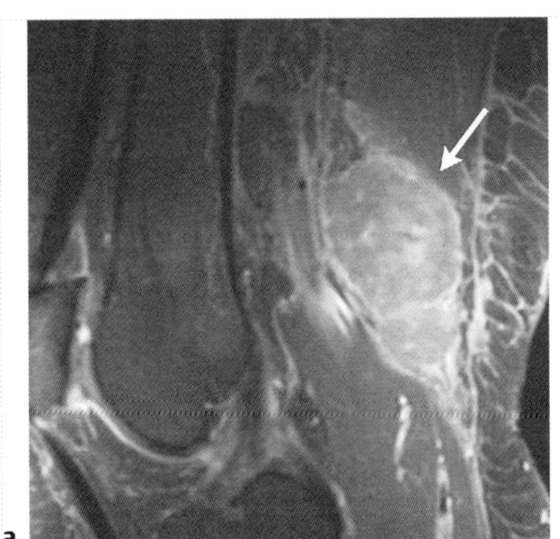

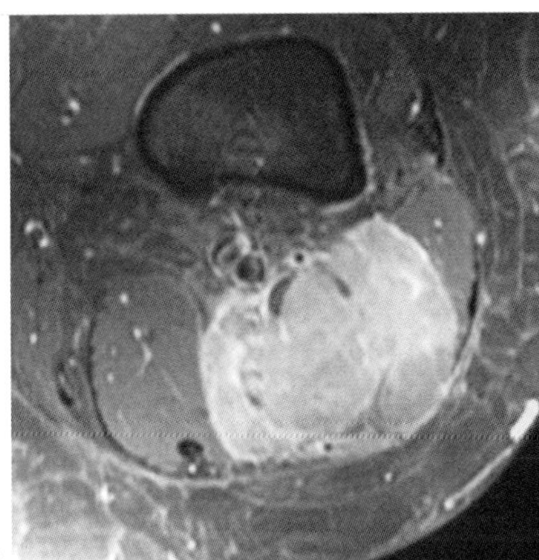

Fig. 12.60 A 51-year-old woman with large B cell non–Hodgkin lymphoma (arrow) involving the posterior soft tissues at the distal thigh, which shows slightly heterogeneous Gd-contrast enhancement on sagittal (a) and axial (b) fat-suppressed T1-weighted imaging.

Table 12.2 (Cont.) Malignant tumors involving the musculoskeletal soft tissues

Tumor	MRI findings	Comments
Leukemia (▶ Fig. 12.61)	Single or multiple well-circumscribed or poorly defined infiltrative lesions involving marrow; low-intermediate signal on T1WI and occasionally in soft tissue, intermediate-high signal on T2WI and FS T2WI, often shows Gd-contrast enhancement, ± cortical bone destruction and extraosseous extension.	Malignant lymphoid neoplasms with involvement of bone marrow with tumor cells also in peripheral blood.
Synovial cell sarcoma (▶ Fig. 12.62)	Tumors are often ovoid and/or lobulated lesions, which often have low-intermediate signal on T1WI, and heterogeneous signal (various combinations of intermediate, slightly high, high, and/or low signal) on T2WI. Multiloculated cystic zones are present in 77%. Calcifications may occur in up to 30%. Tumors show various patterns of Gd-contrast enhancement.	Mesenchymal tumors composed of spindle cells and cells with varying degrees of epithelial differentiation. Account for 5% of primary malignant soft tissue tumors. Occurs in patients 14 to 58 years, mean age = 32 years. More than 90% of synovial sarcomas have a chromosomal translocation, t(X;18) (p11;q11).
Malignant peripheral nerve sheath tumor (MPNST) (▶ Fig. 12.63)	These lesions usually have heterogeneous signal on T1WI and T2WI as well as heterogeneous Gd-contrast enhancement because of necrosis and hemorrhage. Some MPNSTs are similar in appearance to benign nerve sheath tumors.	MPNSTs are malignant tumors of the peripheral nerve sheath that contain mixtures of packed hyperchromatic spindle cells with elongated nuclei and slightly eosinophilic cytoplasm, mitotic figures, and zones of necrosis. Approximately 50% of MPNSTs occur in patients with neurofibromatosis 1 (NF1), followed by de novo evolution from peripheral nerves. MPNSTs infrequently arise from schwannomas, gangioneuroblastomas/ganglioneuromas, and pheochromocytomas.

(continued on page 636)

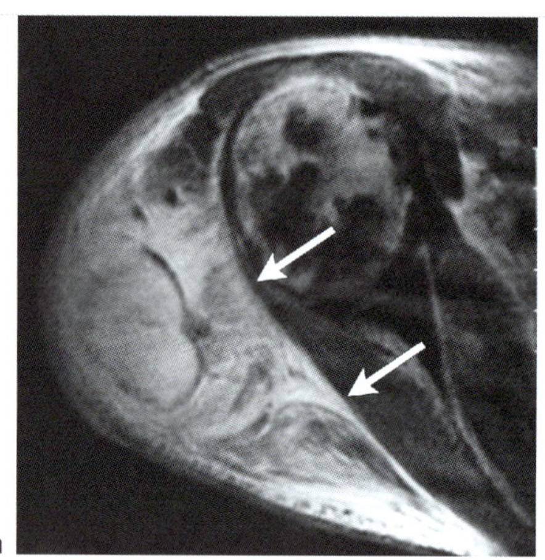

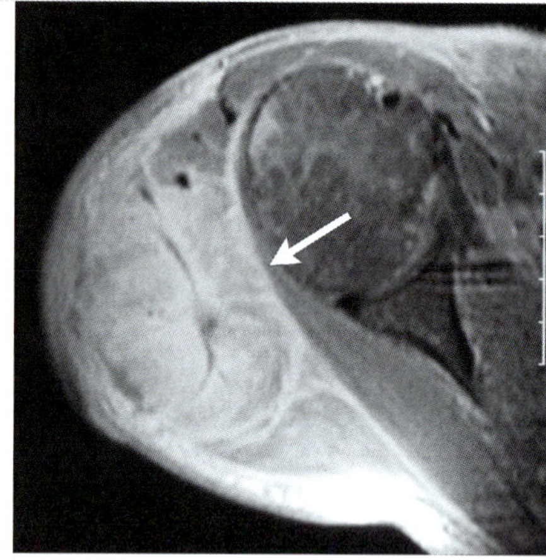

Fig. 12.61 A 69-year-old man with acute myelogenous leukemia involving the soft tissues at the right shoulder and marrow of the right humerus. Leukemic involvement in the soft tissues (arrows) has poorly defined margins, heterogeneous slightly high and high signal on axial fat-suppressed T2-weighted imaging (FS T2WI) (a) and Gd-contrast enhancement on axial FS T1-weighted imaging (b). Leukemic tissue in the marrow of the humerus has heterogeneous slightly-high signal on axial FS T2WI. The leukemic tissue in marrow shows minimal Gd-contrast enhancement, whereas the leukemic involvement in the extraosseous soft tissues shows prominent Gd-contrast enhancement.

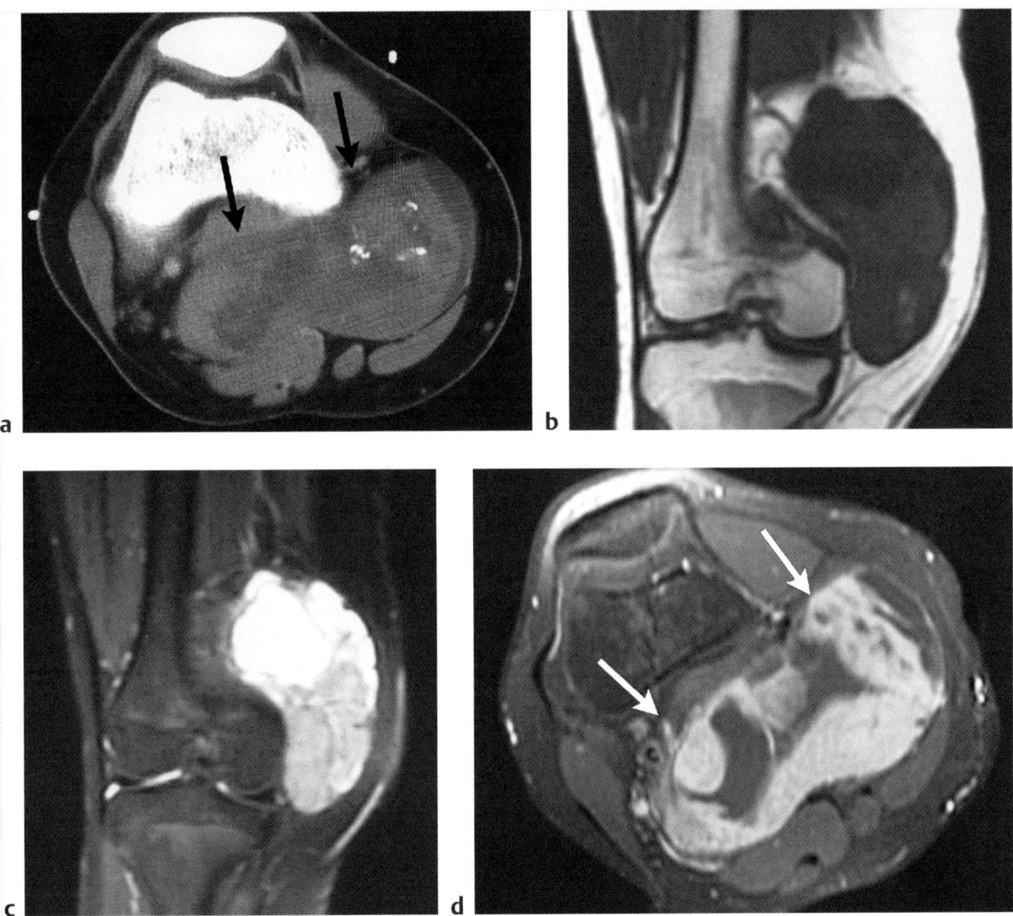

Fig. 12.62 A 15-year-old boy with a synovial sarcoma involving the dorsal soft tissues at the knee deep to the sartorius, gracilis, and semimembranosus muscles. Axial computed tomographic image (a) shows the tumor to have intermediate attenuation as well as irregular calcifications and cystic-like zones (arrows). The tumor has slightly lobulated margins, and has intermediate and slightly low signal on coronal T1-weighted imaging (T1WI) (b) as well as a small zone of high signal from hemorrhage. The tumor has heterogeneous slightly high and high signal on coronal fat-suppressed (FS) T2-weighted imaging (c). The tumor (arrows) shows heterogeneous Gd-contrast enhancement on axial FS T1WI (d).

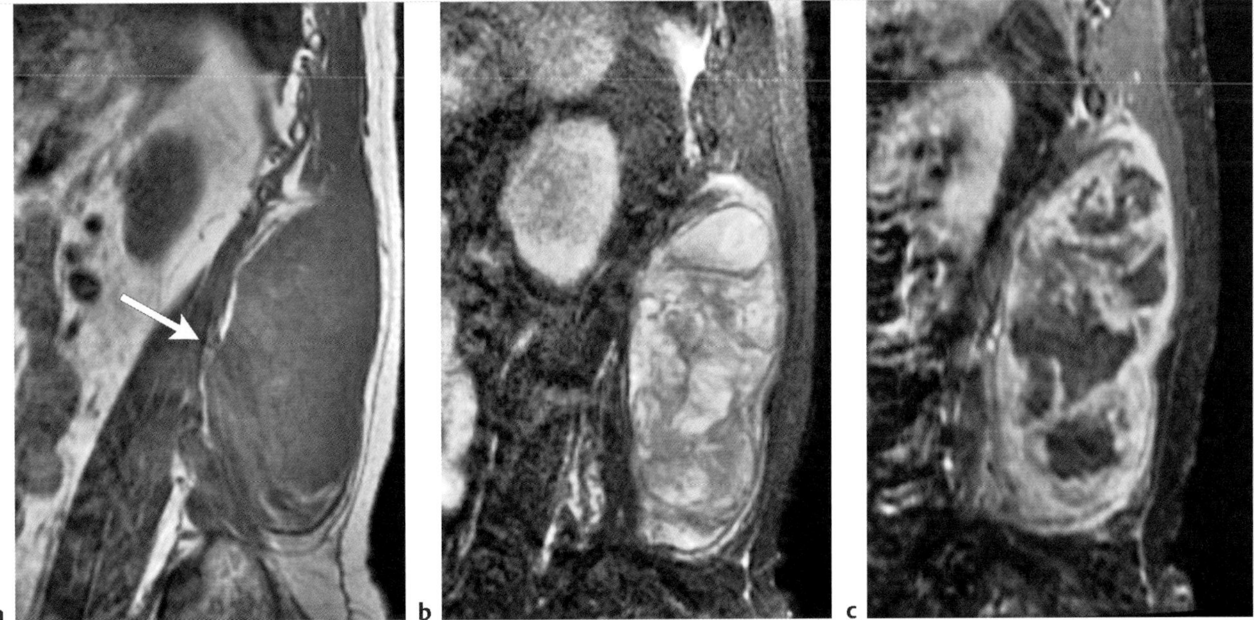

Fig. 12.63 Malignant peripheral nerve sheath tumor in the posterior paraspinal soft tissues of a 51-year-old man. The tumor (arrow) has heterogeneous mostly intermediate signal on sagittal T1-weighted imaging (T1WI) as well as small zones with slightly high and high signal (a), mixed high, low, and intermediate signal on sagittal fat-suppressed (FS) T2-weighted imaging (b). The tumor shows heterogeneous irregular Gd-contrast enhancement on sagittal FS T1WI (c).

Table 12.2 (Cont.) Malignant tumors involving the musculoskeletal soft tissues

Tumor	MRI findings	Comments
Clear cell sarcoma (melanoma of soft parts) (▶ Fig. 12.64)	Tumors can have well-defined or irregular margins and usually have low-intermediate signal on T1WI and intermediate to slightly high or high signal on T2WI and FS T2WI. Tumors usually show Gd-contrast enhancement. Erosion into bone can occur.	Rare malignant tumors with melanocytic differentiation (immunoreactive to S100 protein, HMB45) that occur in patients between 10 and 50 years of age. Usually occurs in the deep soft tissues involving aponeuroses and tendons.
Leiomyosarcoma (▶ Fig. 12.65)	Lesions may have well-defined or irregular margins and often have intermediate signal on T1WI and PDWI that can be hyperintense relative to muscle, and intermediate to slightly high or high signal on T2WI and FS T2WI. Large lesions often have zones of necrosis or cystic change, which have low signal on T1WI and high signal on T2WI. Solid portions of the lesions usually show Gd-contrast enhancement.	Malignant mesodermal tumors associated with smooth muscle differentiation that can arise de novo or occur after radiation treatment. Tumors are usually composed of interleaved bundles or fascicles of plump spindle cells containing fusiform or cigar-shaped nuclei, frequent paranuclear vacuoles, and eosinophilic cytoplasm associated with a myxoid or collagenized stroma. Tumors are often immunoreactive to smooth muscle actin (SMA), desmin, and h-caldesmon. Account for 8% of primary malignant soft tissue tumors and 3% of all primary soft tissue tumors. Patients range in age from 35 to 79 years, mean = 58 years.
Rhabdomyosarcoma (▶ Fig. 12.66)	Tumors can have circumscribed and/or poorly defined margins, and typically have low-intermediate signal on T1WI and heterogeneous signal (various combinations of intermediate, slightly high, and/or high signal) on T2WI and FS T2WI. Tumors show variable degrees of Gd-contrast enhancement.	Malignant mesenchymal tumors with rhabdomyoblastic differentiation that occur primarily in soft tissue. Account for 2% of primary malignant soft tissue tumors and < 1% of all primary soft tissue tumors. Account for 19% of soft tissue sarcomas in children.
Hemangioendothelioma (▶ Fig. 12.67)	Tumors have lobulated well-defined or irregular margins, and have intermediate signal on T1WI and heterogeneous predominantly high signal on T2WI with or without internal low signal septations. Flow voids may be seen with the lesions. Tumors show heterogeneous Gd-contrast enhancement.	Low-grade malignant neoplasms composed of vasoformative/endothelial elements that occur in soft tissues and bone. These tumors are locally aggressive and rarely metastasize, compared with the high-grade endothelial tumors such as angiosarcoma. Account for < 1% of malignant and all soft tissue tumors. Patients range in age from 17 to 60 years, mean = 40 years.

(continued on page 638)

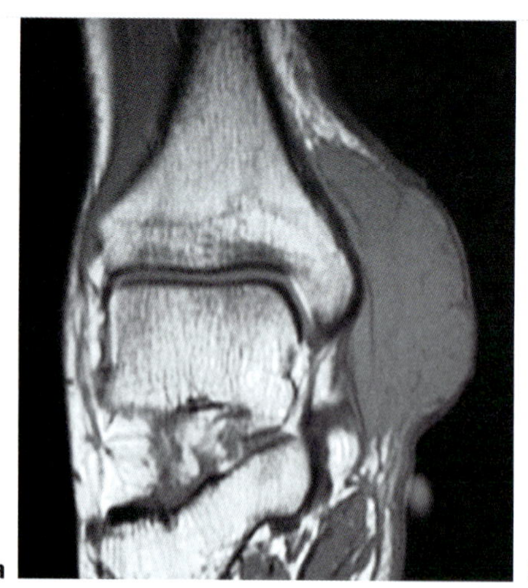

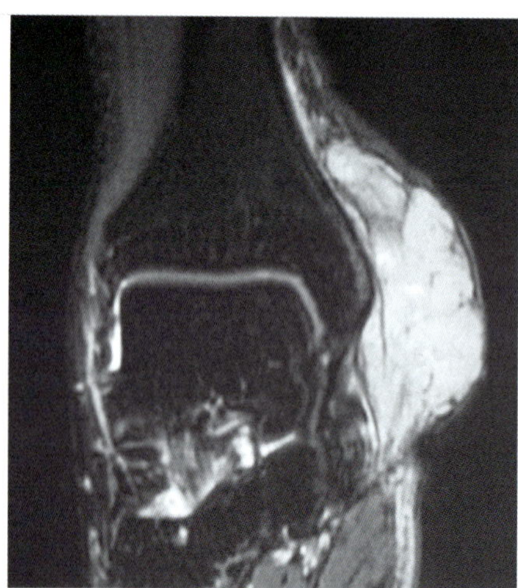

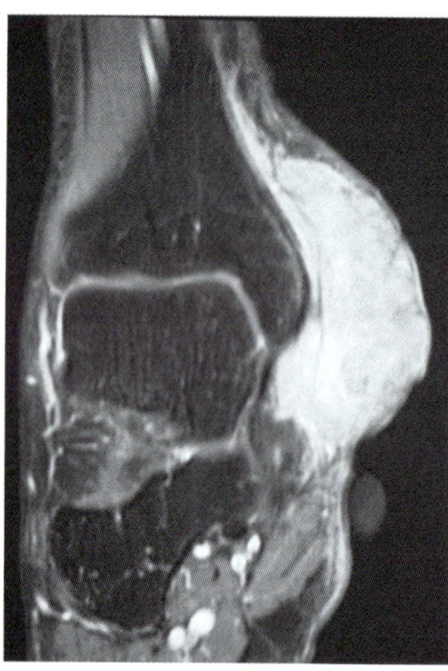

Fig. 12.64 A 32-year-old man with clear cell sarcoma (also referred to as melanoma of soft parts) involving the medial soft tissues at the ankle. The tumor has intermediate signal on coronal T1-weighted imaging (T1WI) (a) and high signal on coronal fat-suppressed (FS) T2-weighted imaging (b). The tumor shows prominent Gd-contrast enhancement on coronal FS T1WI (c).

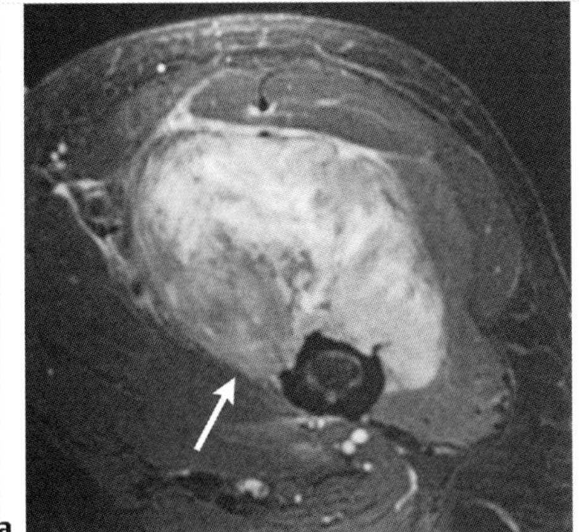

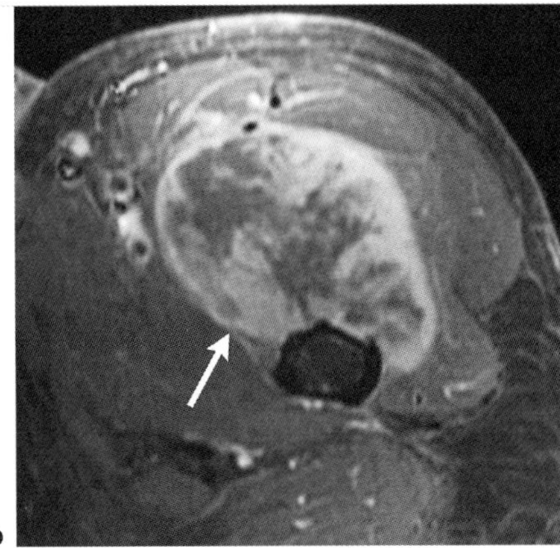

Fig. 12.65 A 55-year-old man with a leiomyosarcoma involving the muscles of the thigh (arrow), which has heterogeneous mostly high and slightly high signal on axial fat-suppressed (FS) T2-weighted imaging (a) as well as small zones of low signal. The tumor (arrow) shows Gd-contrast enhancement except at several sites of necrosis on axial FS T1-weighted imaging (b). Erosion of the outer cortical margin of the femur by the tumor is present.

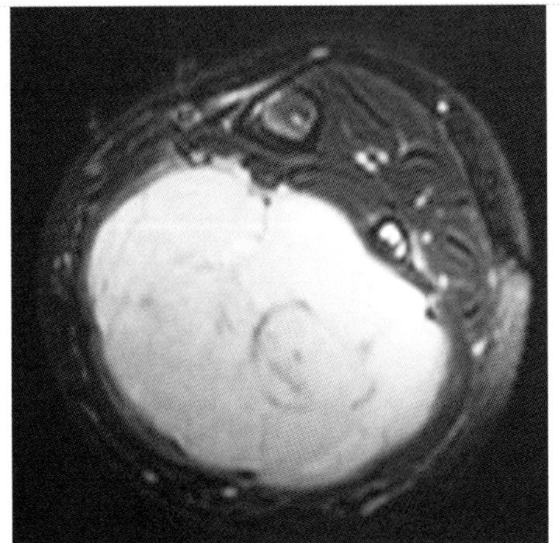

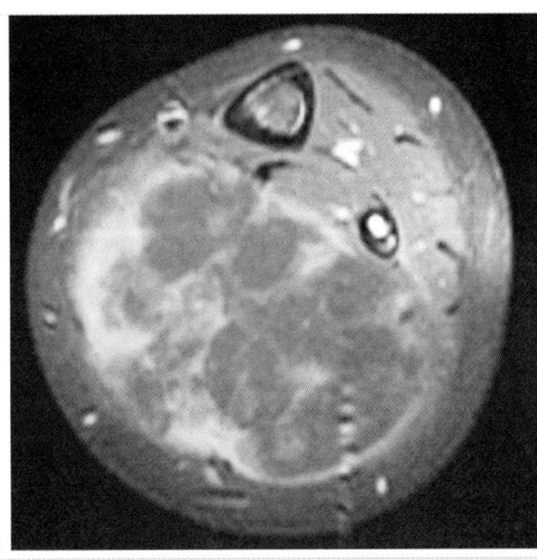

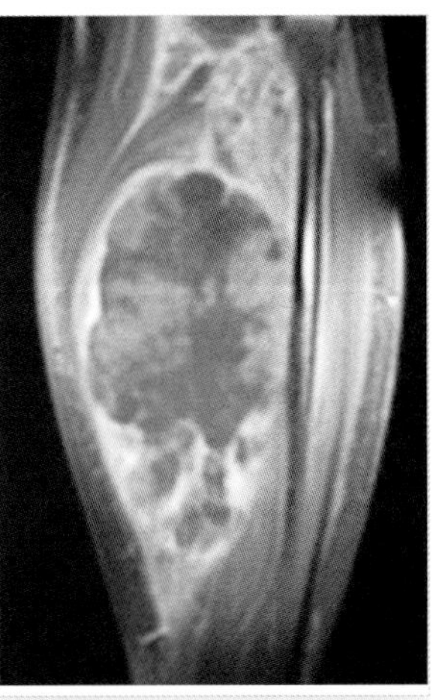

Fig. 12.66 A 2.5-year-old girl with an embryonal rhabdomyosarcoma involving the posterior calf. The tumor has mostly high signal with strands of low signal on axial fat-suppressed (FS) T2-weighted imaging (a). The tumor shows heterogeneous irregular peripheral and central Gd-contrast enhancement on axial (b) and sagittal (c) FS T1-weighted imaging. The tumor is associated with signal alteration of the adjacent fibula.

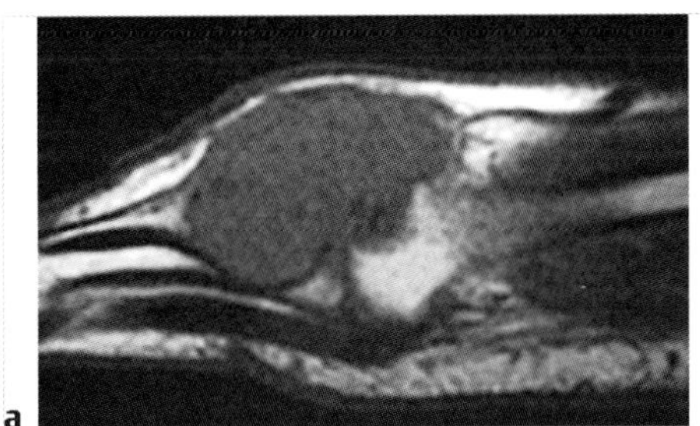

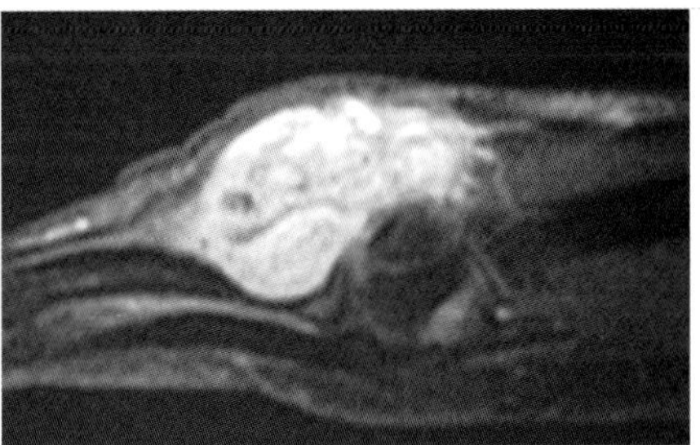

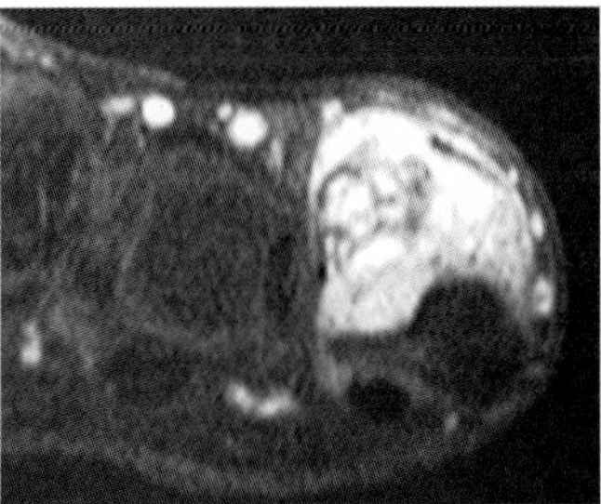

Fig. 12.67 A 36-year-old man with a hemangioendothelioma involving the dorsal soft tissues of the foot, which has intermediate signal on sagittal T1-weighted imaging (T1WI) (a), high signal on sagittal fat-suppressed (FS) T2-weighted imaging (b), and shows prominent Gd-contrast enhancement on coronal FS T1WI (c).

Table 12.2 (Cont.) Malignant tumors involving the musculoskeletal soft tissues

Tumor	MRI findings	Comments
Hemangiopericytoma (▶ Fig. 12.68)	Usually have well-defined margins, often have low-intermediate signal on T1WI, intermediate or slightly high-high signal on T2WI, and heterogeneous high signal on FS T2WI. On T2WI, lesions may contain tubular signal voids centrally or peripherally, likely representing tumor vessels. Can contain hemorrhagic zones with corresponding MR signal alteration. Typically show Gd-contrast enhancement.	Rare malignant tumors of presumed pericytic origin that contain variously shaped pericytic cells (oval, round, spindle-like) and adjacent irregular branching vascular spaces lined by endothelial cells. Usually occur in soft tissues and less frequently in bone. Account for < 1% of primary tumors in the soft tissues. Most tumors (90 to 95%) occur in adults, and 5 to 10% occur in children.
Angiosarcoma (▶ Fig. 12.69; ▶ Fig. 12.70)	Tumors have low-intermediate signal on T1WI, mixed low, intermediate, and/or high signal on T2WI, and show prominent Gd-contrast enhancement in a homogeneous or heterogeneous pattern.	Malignant tumors composed of neoplastic blood vessels in bone and/or soft tissues. These tumors can be associated with Paget disease, radiation treatment, bone infarcts, knee and hip prostheses, synthetic vessel grafts, prior trauma or surgery, osteomyelitis, and hereditary disorders (NF1, Maffucci syndrome, achondroplasia). Represent < 1% of malignant bone tumors; account for 2% of malignant soft tissue tumors. Patients range in age from 5 to 97 years, mean = 49 years. Superficial/cutaneous angiosarcomas can occur in the setting of lymphedema secondary to mastectomy and/or lymph node dissection (Stewart-Treves syndrome).
Extraosseous osteosarcoma (▶ Fig. 12.71)	Tumors have irregular poorly defined or slightly well circumscribed margins and heterogeneous signal on most MRI pulse sequences. Various combinations of low, intermediate, and/or high signal on T1WI, T2WI, and FS T2WI can be seen, depending on the presence and extent of hemorrhage and/or necrosis within the lesions. On T2WI and FS T2WI, tumors often have heterogeneous predominantly high signal. Fluid-fluid levels may be present at sites of hemorrhage or necrosis. Peripheral nonenhancing high signal on T2WI may be present and represent zones of edema and/or tumor invasion within adjacent tissues. Tumors often show heterogeneous patterns of Gd-contrast enhancement.	Malignant tumor composed of proliferating neoplastic spindle cells that produce osteoid and/or immature tumoral bone. Osteosarcoma most commonly occurs within bone and less frequently on the external surface of bone. Rarely, osteogenic sarcomas can also occur as extraskeletal primary lesions in the soft tissues.

(continued on page 640)

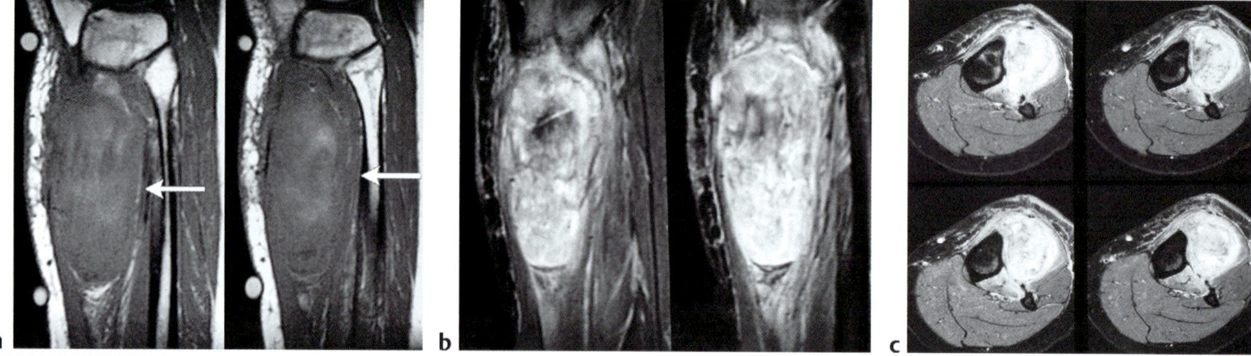

Fig. 12.68 A 29-year-old woman with a hemangiopericytoma involving the tibialis anterior, tibialis posterior, extensor digitorum longus, and popliteus muscles. The tumor (arrows) has mostly intermediate signal on sagittal T1-weighted imaging (a) as well as several zones of high signal at sites of hemorrhage. The tumor has mostly high signal on sagittal (b) and axial (c) fat-suppressed T2-weighted imaging as well as foci and curvilinear zones of low signal.

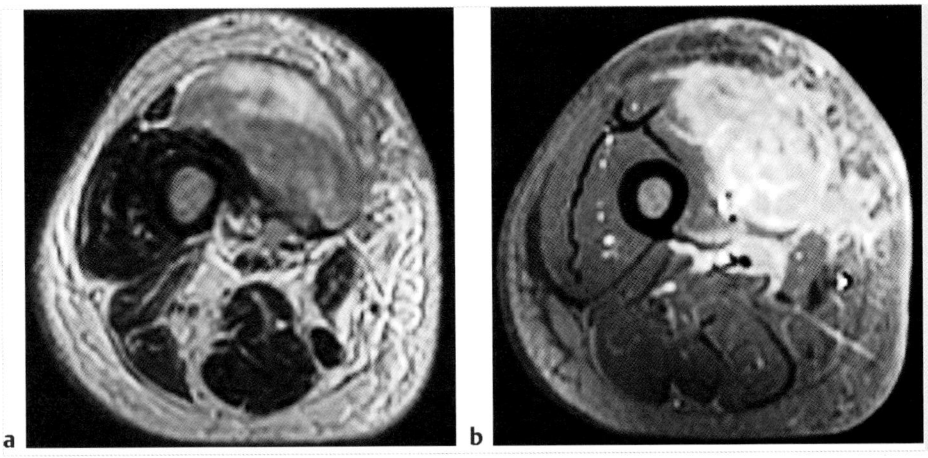

Fig. 12.69 A 74-year-old man with an angiosarcoma in the medial anterior thigh involving the vastus medialis muscle. The tumor has mixed low, intermediate, and high signal on axial T2-weighted imaging (a), and shows prominent Gd-contrast enhancement on fat-suppressed T1-weighted imaging (b).

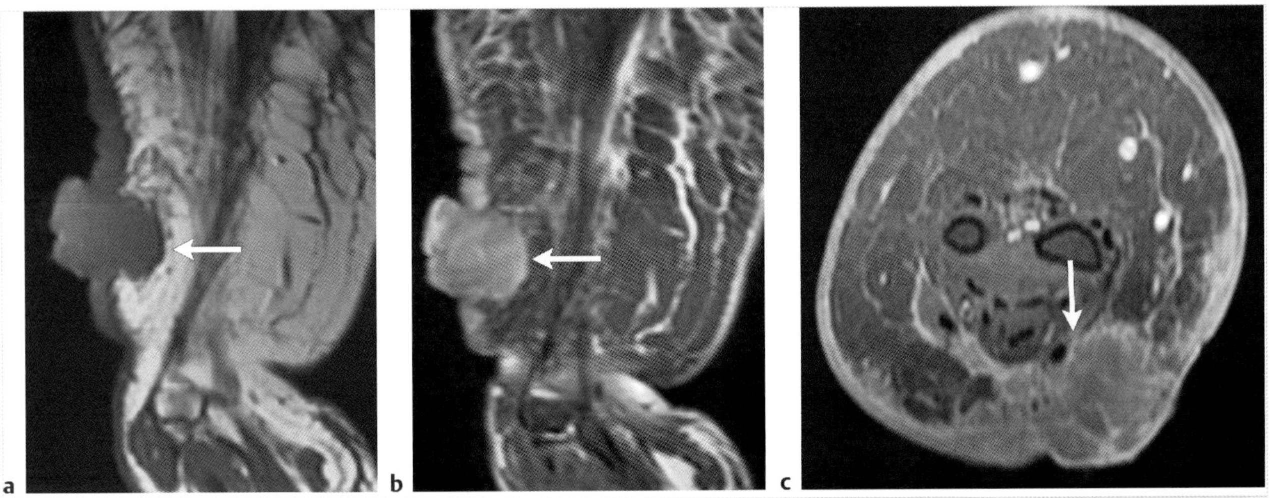

Fig. 12.70 A 53-year-old woman with a history of radiation treatment for breast cancer after mastectomy and lymph node dissection with subsequent development of an angiosarcoma associated with chronic lymphedema involving the upper extremity (Stewart-Treves syndrome). The tumor (arrows) has intermediate signal on sagittal T1-weighted imaging (a), slightly high signal on sagittal fat-suppressed (FS) T2-weighted imaging (b), and shows Gd-contrast enhancement on axial FS T1WI (c).

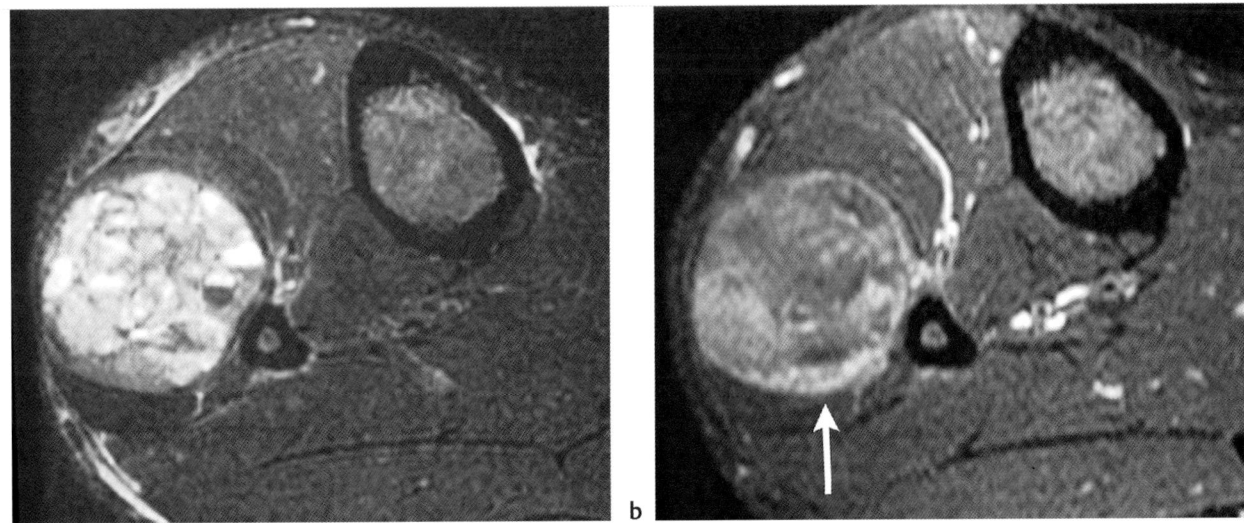

Fig. 12.71 A 32-year-old man with an extraosseous osteosarcoma involving the extensor digitorum longus muscle and peroneus longus and brevis muscles of the proximal lateral leg, which has heterogeneous mostly high signal on axial fat-suppressed (FS) T2-weighted imaging (a) as well as septa with low signal and fluid-fluid levels with high and low signal. Fluid-fluid levels represent sites of hemorrhage within the tumor. The tumor (arrow) shows heterogeneous Gd-contrast enhancement on axial FS T1-weighted imaging (b).

Table 12.2 (Cont.) Malignant tumors involving the musculoskeletal soft tissues

Tumor	MRI findings	Comments
Extraosseous Ewing sarcoma (▶ Fig. 12.72)	Tumors usually have low-intermediate signal on T1WI and heterogeneous slightly high to high signal on T2WI and FS T2W. Tumors often show prominent irregular Gd-contrast enhancement.	Malignant primitive tumors of bone and occasionally soft tissue that are composed of undifferentiated small cells with round nuclei.
Extraosseous chondrosarcoma (▶ Fig. 12.73)	Tumors have low-intermediate signal on T1WI, intermediate signal on PDWI, and heterogeneous intermediate-high or slightly high signal on T2WI. Foci of low signal on T1WI and T2WI can be seen secondary to chondroid matrix mineralization. Lesions typically show heterogeneous Gd-contrast enhancement.	Malignant tumors containing cartilage formed within sarcomatous stroma, with or without areas of calcification/ mineralization, myxoid material, and/or ossification.
Malignant giant cell tumor of soft tissues (▶ Fig. 12.74)	Lesions have lobular margins and usually have low-intermediate or intermediate signal on T1WI and PDWI that is often similar to or less than muscle. On T2WI and FS T2WI, lesions can have mixed intermediate and/or high signal. Small zones of low signal on T2WI often correspond to small sites of hemosiderin deposition. Lesions often show Gd-contrast enhancement in either homogeneous or heterogeneous pattern. Erosions of adjacent bone can be seen with some lesions.	Rare lesions that consist of synovial proliferation with fibrous collagenous tissue, varying amounts of scattered multinucleated giant cells, foamy macrophages, xanthoma cells, round-polygonal and/or spindle-shaped mononuclear cells, and malignant sarcomatous zones containing giant cells with bizarre nuclei, and pleomorphic spindle cells with nuclear atypia and mitoses.

(continued on page 642)

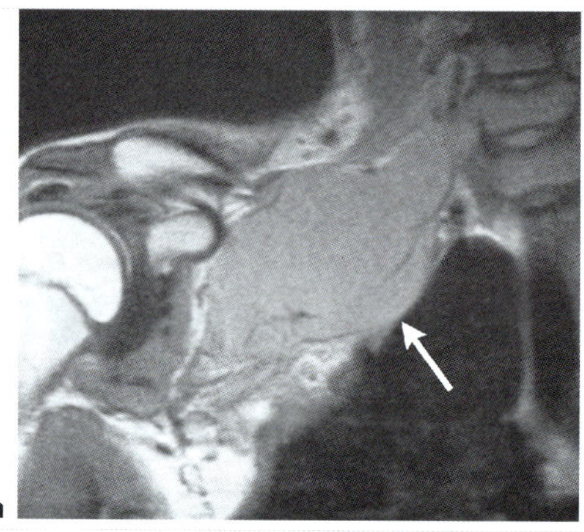
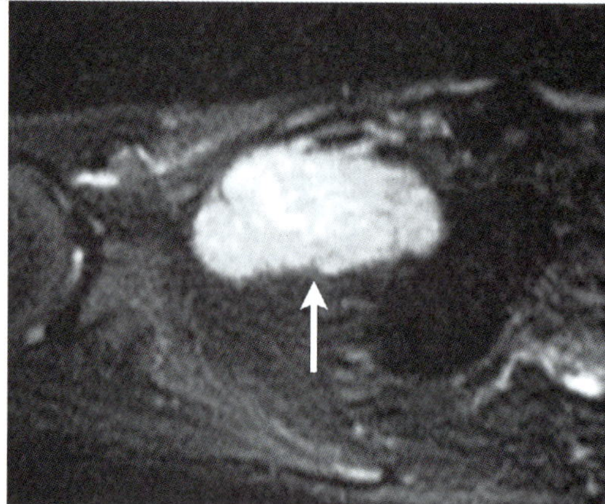

Fig. 12.72 An 11-year-old female with an extraosseous Ewing sarcoma in the soft tissues adjacent to the right clavicle. The tumor (arrows) has intermediate signal on coronal proton density–weighted imaging (a), and high signal on axial fat-suppressed T2-weighted imaging (b).

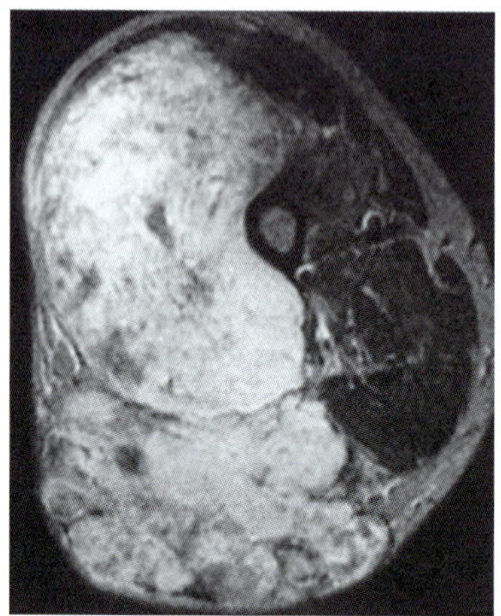
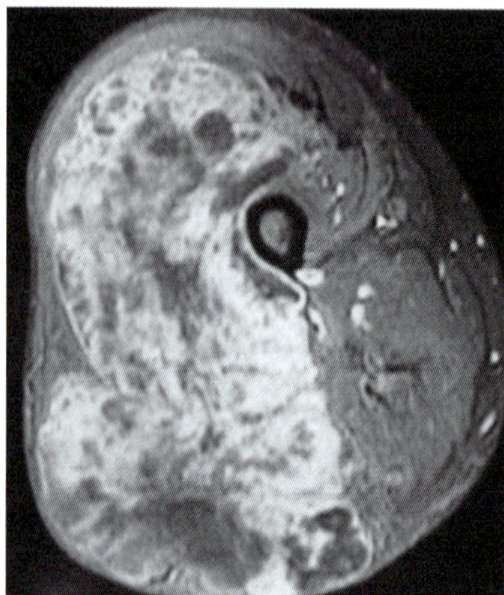

Fig. 12.73 A 65-year-old man with an extraosseous myxoid chondrosarcoma in the distal thigh, which has circumscribed margins and contains heterogeneous mostly high signal with small foci of low signal on axial T2-weighted imaging (a). The lesion shows prominent irregular heterogeneous Gd-contrast enhancement on axial fat-suppressed T1-weighted imaging (b).

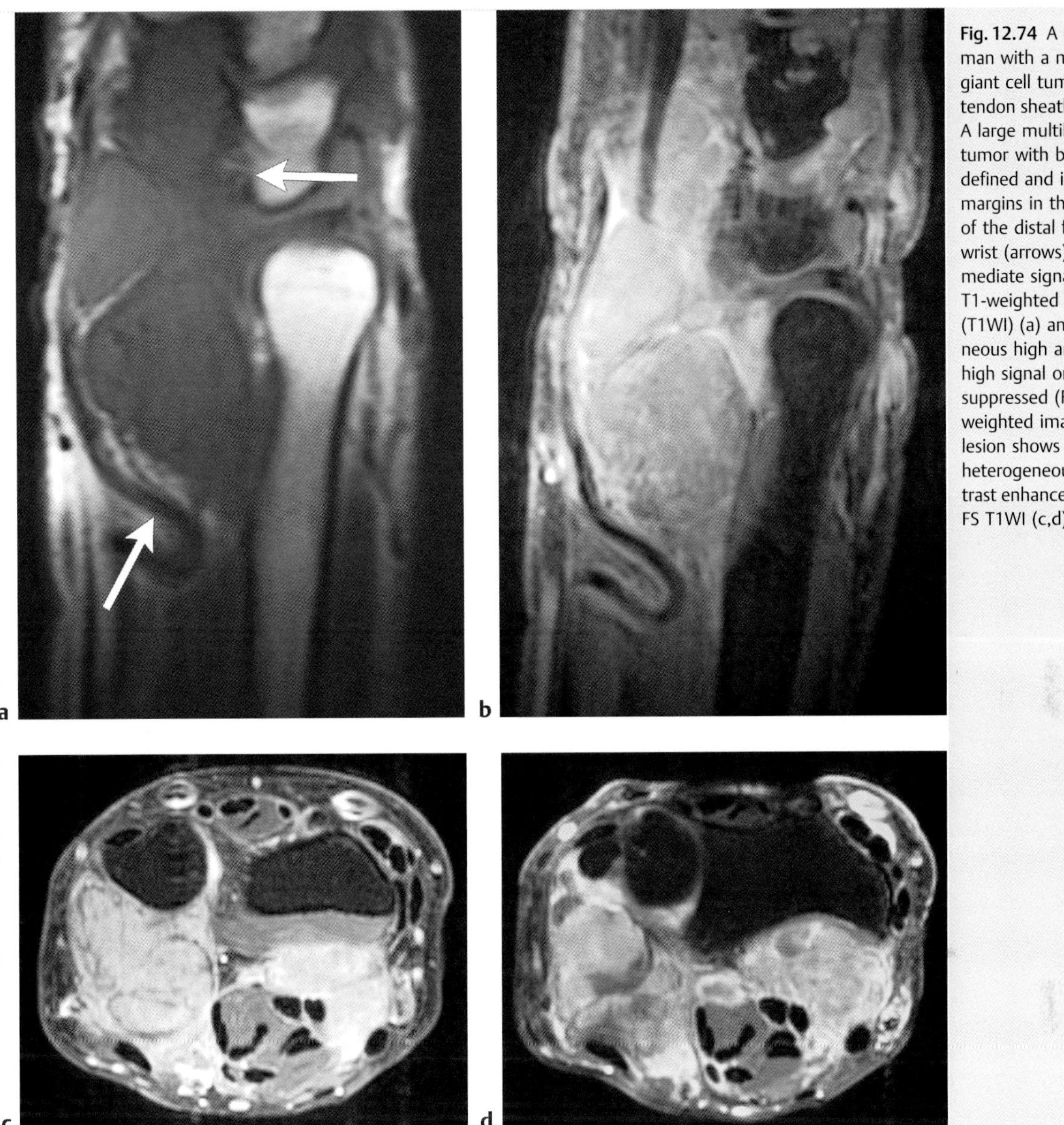

Fig. 12.74 A 60-year-old man with a malignant giant cell tumor of the tendon sheath at the wrist. A large multilobulated tumor with both well-defined and indistinct margins in the soft tissues of the distal forearm and wrist (arrows) has intermediate signal on sagittal T1-weighted imaging (T1WI) (a) and heterogeneous high and slightly-high signal on sagittal fat-suppressed (FS) T2-weighted imaging (b). The lesion shows prominent heterogeneous Gd-contrast enhancement on axial FS T1WI (c,d).

Table 12.2 (Cont.) Malignant tumors involving the musculoskeletal soft tissues

Tumor	MRI findings	Comments
Dermatofibrosarcoma (DFS), dermatofibro-sarcoma protuberans (DFSP) (▶ Fig. 12.75)	DFSs are small lesions with circumscribed and/or poorly defined margins involving the skin and/or subcutaneous adipose tissue. Tumors can have low-intermediate signal on T1WI and intermediate to high signal on T2WI and FS T2WI. DFSs show variable degrees of Gd-contrast enhancement. DFSPs are usually circumscribed lesions in the skin and subcutaneous adipose tissues that can measure up to 25 cm. Ten percent of DFSPs have poorly defined margins. DFSP tumors have low-intermediate signal on T1WI, intermediate, slightly high, and/or high signal on T2WI. DFSPs show heterogeneous or homogeneous Gd-contrast enhancement.	DFSs and DFSPs are dermal tumors containing fibroblastic cells with spindle-shaped nuclei. DFSP is associated with the chromosomal translocation t(17:22), which involves fusion of the *COL1A1* and *PDGF-beta* genes (6). The *COL1A1* is a collagen type 1-alpha-1 gene and *PDGFbeta* is a platelet-derived growth factor beta gene. These tumors account for approximately 6% of primary malignant soft tissue tumors and 2% of all primary soft tissue tumors. Age at presentation: 19 to 60 years, mean = 38 years. Tumors involve the dermis and are located above the investing fascia. DFSP extends from 8 to 60 mm, mean = 17 mm, deep to the skin margin. Approximately 30% may extend into or involve soft tissue deep to the superficial fascia. Trunk > head and neck > proximal limb girdle > lower extremity > hip and buttocks > foot and ankle > upper extremity > hand and wrist.

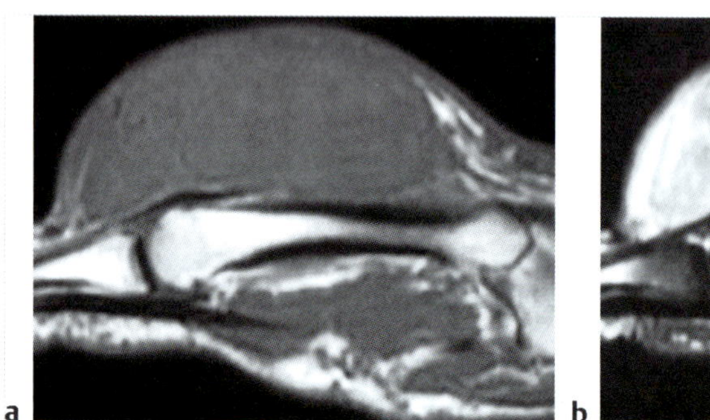

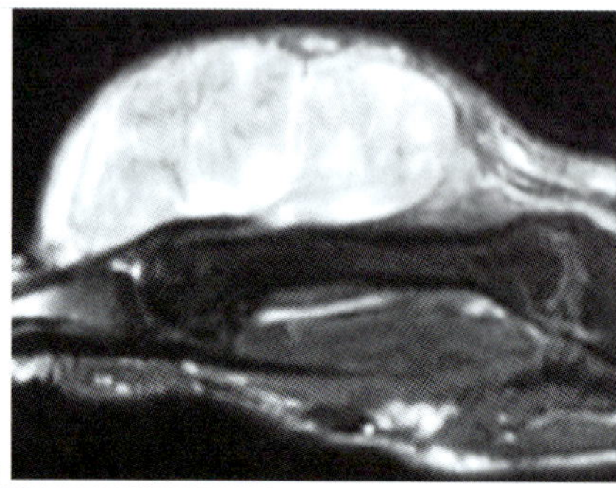

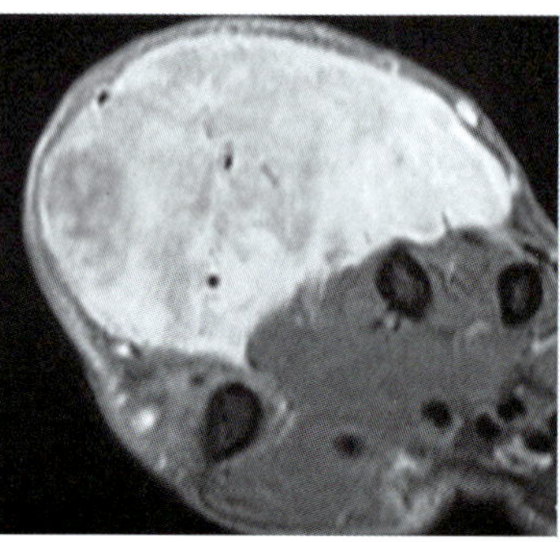

Fig. 12.75 A 52-year-old man with a dermatofibrosarcoma protuberans at the dorsal aspect of the hand involving the skin and subcutaneous fat. The tumor has intermediate signal on sagittal T1-weighted imaging (T1WI) (a) and heterogeneous mostly high signal on sagittal fat-suppressed (FS) T2-weighted imaging (b). The tumor shows prominent heterogeneous Gd-contrast enhancement on axial FS T1WI (c).

12.3 Suggested Reading: Lesions Involving the Soft Tissues

▶ Amyloid

[1] Bardin RL, Barnes CE, Stanton CA, Geisinger KR. Soft tissue amyloidoma of the extremities: a case report and review of the literature. Arch Pathol Lab Med 2004; 128: 1270–1273

[2] Escobedo EM, Hunter JC, Zink-Brody GC, Andress DL. Magnetic resonance imaging of dialysis-related amyloidosis of the shoulder and hip. Skeletal Radiol 1996; 25: 41–48

[3] Maheshwari AV, Muro-Cacho CA, Kransdorf MJ, Temple HT. Soft-tissue amyloidoma of the extremities: a case report and review of literature. Skeletal Radiol 2009; 38: 287–292

[4] Pasternak S, Wright BA, Walsh N. Soft tissue amyloidoma of the extremities: report of a case and review of the literature. Am J Dermatopathol 2007; 29: 152–155

▶ Angiosarcoma

[5] Abdelwahab IF, Klein MJ, Hermann G, Springfield D. Angiosarcomas associated with bone infarcts. Skeletal Radiol 1998; 27: 546–551

[6] Chopra S, Ors F, Bergin D. MRI of angiosarcoma associated with chronic lymphoedema: Stewart Treves syndrome. Br J Radiol 2007; 80: e310–e313

[7] Meis-Kindblom JM, Kindblom LG. Angiosarcoma of soft tissue: a study of 80 cases. Am J Surg Pathol 1998; 22: 683–697

[8] Meyers SP. Angiosarcoma. In: MRI of Bone and Soft Tissue Tumors and Tumorlike Lesions. Stuttgart, Germany: Thieme; 2008:344–346

[9] Roessner A, Boehling T. Angiosarcoma. In: Fletcher CDM, Unni KK, Mertens F, eds. World Health Organization Classification of Tumours. Pathology and Genetics of Tumours of Soft Tissue and Bone. Lyon, France: IARC Press; 2002:322–323

[10] Weiss SW, Lasota J, Miettinen MM. Angiosarcoma of soft tissue. In: Fletcher CDM, Unni KK, Mertens F, eds. World Health Organization Classification of Tumours. Pathology and Genetics of Tumours of Soft Tissue and Bone. Lyon, France: IARC Press; 2002:175–177

[11] Schindera ST, Streit M, Kaelin U, Stauffer E, Steinbach L, Anderson SE. Stewart-Treves syndrome: MR imaging of a postmastectomy upper-limb chronic lymphedema with angiosarcoma. Skeletal Radiol 2005; 34: 156–160

[12] Shon W, Ida CM, Boland-Froemming JM, Rose PS, Folpe A. Cutaneous angiosarcoma arising in massive localized lymphedema of the morbidly obese: a report of five cases and review of the literature. J Cutan Pathol 2011; 38: 560–564

▶ Calcific Tendinitis

[13] Flemming DJ, Murphey MD, Shekitka KM, Temple HT, Jelinek JJ, Kransdorf MJ. Osseous involvement in calcific tendinitis: a retrospective review of 50 cases. AJR Am J Roentgenol 2003; 181: 965–972

[14] Porcellini G, Paladini P, Campi F, Pegreffi F. Osteolytic lesion of greater tuberosity in calcific tendinis of the shoulder. J Shoulder Elbow Surg 2009; 18: 210–215

▶ Cat Scratch Disease

[15] Dong PR, Seeger LL, Yao L, Panosian CB, Johnson BL, Eckardt JJ. Uncomplicated cat-scratch disease: findings at CT, MR imaging, and radiography. Radiology 1995; 195: 837–839

[16] Gielen J, Wang XL, Vanhoenacker F, et al. Lymphadenopathy at the medial epitrochlear region in cat-scratch disease. Eur Radiol 2003; 13: 1363–1369

[17] Mele FM, Friedman M, Reznik AM. MR imaging of the knee: findings in cat-scratch disease. AJR Am J Roentgenol 1996; 166: 1232–1233

[18] Wang CW, Chang WC, Chao TK, Liu CC, Huang GS. Computed tomography and magnetic resonance imaging of cat-scratch disease: a report of two cases. Clin Imaging 2009; 33: 318–321

▶ Chondrosarcoma

[19] Bertoni F, Bacchini P, Hogendoorn PCW. Chondrosarcoma. In: Fletcher CDM, Unni KK, Mertens F, eds. World Health Organization Classification of Tumours. Pathology and Genetics of Tumours of Soft Tissue and Bone. Lyon, France: IARC Press; 2002:247–251

[20] Dei Tos AP, Wadden C, Fletcher CD. Extraskeletal myxoid chondrosarcoma: an immunohistochemical reappraisal of 39 cases. Appl Immunohistochem Mol Morphol 1997; 5: 73–77

[21] Johnson DBS, Breidahl W, Newman JS, Devaney K, Yahanda A. Extraskeletal mesenchymal chondrosarcoma of the rectus sheath. Skeletal Radiol 1997; 26: 501–504

[22] Lucas DR, Heim S. Extraskeletal myxoid chondrosarcoma. In: Fletcher CDM, Unni KK, Mertens F, eds. World Health Organization Classification of Tumours. Pathology and Genetics of Tumours of Soft Tissue and Bone. Lyon, France: IARC Press; 2002:213–214

[23] Meis-Kindblom JM, Bergh P, Gunterberg B, Kindblom LG. Extraskeletal myxoid chondrosarcoma: a reappraisal of its morphologic spectrum and prognostic factors based on 117 cases. Am J Surg Pathol 1999; 23: 636–650

[24] Meyers SP. Chondrosarcoma. In: MRI of Bone and Soft Tissue Tumors and Tumorlike Lesions. Stuttgart, Germany: Thieme; 2008:368–378

[25] Nakashima Y, Park YK, Sugano O. Mesenchymal chondrosarcoma. In: Fletcher CDM, Unni KK, Mertens F, eds. World Health Organization Classification of Tumours. Pathology and Genetics of Tumours of Soft Tissue and Bone. Lyon, France: IARC Press; 2002:255–256

[26] Taconis WK, van der Heul RO, Taminiau AMM. Synovial chondrosarcoma: report of a case and review of the literature. Skeletal Radiol 1997; 26: 682–685

▶ Clear Cell Sarcoma

[27] De Beuckeleer LH, De Schepper AM, Vandevenne JE, et al. MR imaging of clear cell sarcoma (malignant melanoma of the soft parts): a multicenter correlative MRI-pathology study of 21 cases and literature review. Skeletal Radiol 2000; 29: 187–195

[28] Malchau SS, Hayden J, Hornicek F, Mankin HJ. Clear cell sarcoma of soft tissues. J Surg Oncol 2007; 95: 519–522

[29] Walker EA, Salesky JS, Fenton ME, Murphey MD. Magnetic resonance imaging of malignant soft tissue neoplasms in the adult. Radiol Clin North Am 2011; 49: 1219–1234, vi

▶ Denervation of Muscle

[30] Bredella MA, Tirman PFJ, Fritz RC, Wischer TK, Stork A, Genant HK. Denervation syndromes of the shoulder girdle: MR imaging with electrophysiologic correlation. Skeletal Radiol 1999; 28: 567–572

[31] Cothran RL, Helms C. Quadrilateral space syndrome: incidence of imaging findings in a population referred for MRI of the shoulder. AJR Am J Roentgenol 2005; 184: 989–992

[32] Kim SJ, Choi JY, Huh YM, et al. Role of magnetic resonance imaging in entrapment and compressive neuropathy—what, where, and how to see the peripheral nerves on the musculoskeletal magnetic resonance image: part 2. Upper extremity. Eur Radiol 2007; 17: 509–522

[33] Kim SJ, Hong SH, Jun WS, et al. MR imaging mapping of skeletal muscle denervation in entrapment and compressive neuropathies. Radiographics 2011; 31: 319–332

[34] Linda DD, Harish S, Stewart BG, Finlay K, Parasu N, Rebello RP. Multimodality imaging of peripheral neuropathies of the upper limb and brachial plexus. Radiographics 2010; 30: 1373–1400

[35] Petchprapa CN, Rosenberg ZS, Sconfienza LM, Cavalcanti CF, Vieira RL, Zember JS. MR imaging of entrapment neuropathies of the lower extremity, I: The pelvis and hip. Radiographics 2010; 30: 983–1000

▶ Dermatofibrosarcoma and Dermatofibrosarcoma Protuberans

[36] Bowne WB, Antonescu CR, Leung DH, et al. Dermatofibrosarcoma protuberans: a clinicopathologic analysis of patients treated and followed at a single institution. Cancer 2000; 88: 2711–2720

[37] Khatri VP, Galante JM, Bold RJ, Schneider PD, Ramsamooj R, Goodnight JE. Dermatofibrosarcoma protuberans: reappraisal of wide local excision and impact of inadequate initial treatment. Ann Surg Oncol 2003; 10: 1118–1122

[38] Kransdorf MJ, Meis-Kindblom JM. Dermatofibrosarcoma protuberans: radiologic appearance. AJR Am J Roentgenol 1994; 163: 391–394

[39] Meyers SP. Dermatofibrosarcoma and dermatofibrosarcoma protuberans. In: MRI of Bone and Soft Tissue Tumors and Tumorlike Lesions. Stuttgart, Germany: Thieme; 2008: 383–385

[40] Riggs K, McGuigan KL, Morrison WB, Samie FH, Humphreys T. Role of magnetic resonance imaging in perioperative assessment of dermatofibrosarcoma protuberans. Dermatol Surg 2009; 35: 2036–2041

[41] Torreggiani WC, Al-Ismail K, Munk PL, Nicolaou S, O'Connell JX, Knowling MA. Dermatofibrosarcoma protuberans: MR imaging features. AJR Am J Roentgenol 2002; 178: 989–993

▶ Dermatomyositis

[42] Chan WP, Liu GC. MR imaging of primary skeletal muscle diseases in children. AJR Am J Roentgenol 2002; 179: 989–997

[43] Davis WR, Halls JE, Offiah AC, Pilkington C, Owens CM, Rosendahl K. Assessment of active inflammation in juvenile dermatomyositis: a novel magnetic resonance imaging-based scoring system. Rheumatology (Oxford) 2011; 50: 2237–2244

[44] Hanlon R, King S. Overview of the radiology of connective tissue disorders in children. Eur J Radiol 2000; 33: 74–84

[45] Hernandez RJ, Sullivan DB, Chenevert TL, Keim DR. MR imaging in children with dermatomyositis: musculoskeletal findings and correlation with clinical and laboratory findings. AJR Am J Roentgenol 1993; 161: 359–366

[46] Kimball AB, Summers RM, Turner M, et al. Magnetic resonance imaging detection of occult skin and subcutaneous abnormalities in juvenile dermatomyositis. Implications for diagnosis and therapy. Arthritis Rheum 2000; 43: 1866–1873

[47] Ladd PE, Emery KH, Salisbury SR, Laor T, Lovell DJ, Bove KE. Juvenile dermatomyositis: correlation of MRI at presentation with clinical outcome. AJR Am J Roentgenol 2011; 197: W153-: W15: 8

[48] Löfberg M, Liewendahl K, Lamminen A, Korhola O, Somer H. Antimyosin scintigraphy compared with magnetic resonance imaging in inflammatory myopathies. Arch Neurol 1998; 55: 987–993

[49] Mastaglia FL, Garle MJ, Phillips BA, Zilko PJ. Inflammatory myopathies: clinical, diagnostic and therapeutic aspects. Muscle Nerve 2003; 27: 407–425

[50] May DA, Disler DG, Jones EA, Balkissoon AA, Manaster BJ. Abnormal signal intensity in skeletal muscle at MR imaging: patterns, pearls, and pitfalls. Radiographics 2000; 20 Spec No: S295–S315

[51] Meyers SP. Dermatomyositis. In: MRI of Bone and Soft Tissue Tumors and Tumorlike Lesions. Stuttgart, Germany: Thieme; 2008:386–389

[52] Révelon G, Rahmouni A, Jazaerli N, et al. Acute swelling of the limbs: magnetic resonance pictorial review of fascial and muscle signal changes. Eur J Radiol 1999; 30: 11–21

[53] Samson C, Soulen RL, Gursel E. Milk of calcium fluid collections in juvenile dermatomyositis: MR characteristics. Pediatr Radiol 2000; 30: 28–29

▶ Dermoid and Epidermoid

[54] Meyers SP. Dermoid and epidermoid. In: MRI of Bone and Soft Tissue Tumors and Tumorlike Lesions. Stuttgart, Germany: Thieme; 2008:390–395

[55] Mhatre P, Hudgins PA, Hunter S. Dermoid cyst in the lumbosacral region: radiographic findings. AJR Am J Roentgenol 2000; 174: 874–875

[56] Smirniotopoulos JG, Chiechi MV. Teratomas, dermoids, and epidermoids of the head and neck. Radiographics 1995; 15: 1437–1455

[57] Timmer FA, Sluzewski M, Treskes M, van Rooij WJJ, Teepen JLJM, Wijnalda D. Chemical analysis of an epidermoid cyst with unusual CT and MR characteristics. AJNR Am J Neuroradiol 1998; 19: 1111–1112

▶ Desmoid Tumors

[58] Goldblum J, Fletcher JA. Superficial fibromatoses. In: Fletcher CDM, Unni KK, Mertens F, eds. World Health Organization Classification of Tumours. Pathology and Genetics of Tumours of Soft Tissue and Bone. Lyon, France: IARC Press; 2002:81–82

[59] Goldblum J, Fletcher JA. Desmoid-type fibromatoses. In: Fletcher CDM, Unni KK, Mertens F, eds. World Health Organization Classification of Tumours. Pathology and Genetics of Tumours of Soft Tissue and Bone. Lyon, France: IARC Press; 2002:83–84

[60] Kingston CA, Owens CM, Jeanes A, Malone M. Imaging of desmoid fibromatosis in pediatric patients. AJR Am J Roentgenol 2002; 178: 191–199

[61] Lee JC, Thomas JM, Phillips S, Fisher C, Moskovic E. Aggressive fibromatosis: MRI features with pathologic correlation. AJR Am J Roentgenol 2006; 186: 247–254

[62] Mahnken AH, Nolte-Ernsting CC, Wildberger JE, Wirtz DC, Günther RW. Cross-sectional imaging patterns of desmoplastic fibroma. Eur Radiol 2001; 11: 1105–1110

[63] Meyers SP. Desmoid tumors. In: MRI of Bone and Soft Tissue Tumors and Tumorlike Lesions. Stuttgart, Germany: Thieme; 2008:396–403

[64] O'Connell. Fibromatosis coli. In: Fletcher CDM, Unni KK, Mertens F, eds. World Health Organization Classification of Tumours. Pathology and Genetics of Tumours of Soft Tissue and Bone. Lyon, France: IARC Press; 2002:61–62

[65] Pignatti G, Barbanti-Bròdano G, Ferrari D, et al. Extraabdominal desmoid tumor. A study of 83 cases. Clin Orthop Relat Res 2000; 375: 207–213

[66] Spiegel DA, Dormans JP, Meyer JS, et al. Aggressive fibromatosis from infancy to adolescence. J Pediatr Orthop 1999; 19: 776–784

▶ Diabetic and Idiopathic Myonecrosis

[67] Bunch TJ, Birskovich LM, Eiken PW. Diabetic myonecrosis in a previously healthy woman and review of a 25-year Mayo Clinic experience. Endocr Pract 2002; 8: 343–346

[68] Kattapuram TM, Suri R, Rosol MS, Rosenberg AE, Kattapuram SV. Idiopathic and diabetic skeletal muscle necrosis: evaluation by magnetic resonance imaging. Skeletal Radiol 2005; 34: 203–209

[69] Kim SW, Kim SS. Myonecrosis of paralumbar spine muscle. Spine 2011; 36: E1162–E1165

[70] Rashidi A, Bahrani O. Diabetic myonecrosis of the thigh. J Clin Endocrinol Metab 2011; 96: 2310–2311

[71] Sahin I, Taskapan C, Taskapan H, et al. Diabetic muscle infarction: an unusual cause of muscle pain in a diabetic patient on hemodialysis. Int Urol Nephrol 2005; 37: 629–632

▶ Elastofibroma

[72] Hashimoto H, Bridge JA. Elastofibroma. In: Fletcher CDM, Unni KK, Mertens F, eds. World Health Organization Classification of Tumours. Pathology and Genetics of Tumours of Soft Tissue and Bone. Lyon, France: IARC Press; 2002:56–57

[73] Kransdorf MJ, Meis JM, Montgomery E. Elastofibroma: MR and CT appearance with radiologic-pathologic correlation. AJR Am J Roentgenol 1992; 159: 575–579

[74] Meyers SP. Elastofibroma. In: MRI of Bone and Soft Tissue Tumors and Tumorlike Lesions. Stuttgart, Germany: Thieme;:2008:404–405

[75] Naylor MF, Nascimento AG, Sherrick AD, McLeod RA. Elastofibroma dorsi: radiologic findings in 12 patients. AJR Am J Roentgenol 1996; 167: 683–687

[76] Parratt MT, Donaldson JR, Flanagan AM, et al. Elastofibroma dorsi: management, outcome and review of the literature. J Bone Joint Surg Br 2010; 92: 262–266

[77] Zembsch A, Schick S, Trattnig S, Walter J, Amann G, Ritschl P. Elastofibroma dorsi. Study of two cases and magnetic resonance imaging findings. Clin Orthop Relat Res 1999: 213–219

▶ Eosinophilic Granuloma/Langerhans Cell Histiocytosis

[78] Beltran J, Aparisi F, Bonmati LM, Rosenberg ZS, Present D, Steiner GC. Eosinophilic granuloma: MRI manifestations. Skeletal Radiol 1993; 22: 157–161

[79] Davies AM, Pikoulas C, Griffith J. MRI of eosinophilic granuloma. Eur J Radiol 1994; 18: 205–209

[80] DeYoung BR, Unni KK. Langerhans' cell histiocytosis. In: Fletcher CDM, Unni KK, Mertens F, eds. World Health Organization Classification of Tumours. Pathology and Genetics of Tumours of Soft Tissue and Bone. Lyon, France: IARC Press; 2002:345–346

[81] Hindman BW, Thomas RD, Young LW, Yu L. Langerhans cell histiocytosis: unusual skeletal manifestations observed in thirty-four cases. Skeletal Radiol 1998; 27: 177–181

[82] Meyers SP. Eosinophilic granuloma. In: MRI of Bone and Soft Tissue Tumors and Tumorlike Lesions. Stuttgart, Germany: Thieme; 2008:406–412

[83] Monroc M, Ducou le Pointe H, Haddad S, Josset P, Montagne JP. Soft tissue signal abnormality associated with eosinophilic granuloma: correlation of MR imaging with pathologic findings. Pediatr Radiol 1994; 24: 328–332

[84] Song YS, Lee IS, Yi JH, Cho KH, Kim K, Song JW. Radiologic findings of adult pelvis and appendicular skeletal Langerhans cell histiocytosis in nine patients. Skeletal Radiol 2011; 40: 1421–1426

[85] Yamamura S, Sato K, Sugiura H, et al. Prostaglandin levels of primary bone tumor tissues correlate with peritumoral edema demonstrated by magnetic resonance imaging. Cancer 1997; 79: 255–261

▶ Erdheim-Chester Disease

[86] Gottlieb R, Chen A. MR findings of Erdheim-Chester disease. J Comput Assist Tomogr 2002; 26: 257–261

[87] Kenn W, Eck M, Allolio B, et al. Erdheim-Chester disease: evidence for a disease entity different from Langerhans cell histiocytosis? Three cases with detailed radiological and immunohistochemical analysis. Hum Pathol 2000; 31: 734–739

[88] Kushihashi T, Munechika H, Sekimizu M, Fujimaki E. Erdheim-Chester disease involving bilateral lower extremities: MR features. AJR Am J Roentgenol 2000; 174: 875–876

[89] Meyers SP. Erdheim-Chester disease. In: MRI of Bone and Soft Tissue Tumors and Tumorlike Lesions. Stuttgart, Germany: Thieme; 2008:413–415

[90] Murray D, Marshall M, England E, Mander J, Chakera TMH. Erdheim-chester disease. Clin Radiol 2001; 56: 481–484

▶ Ewing Sarcoma

[91] Meyers SP. Ewing's Sarcoma. In: MRI of Bone and Soft Tissue Tumors and Tumorlike Lesions. Stuttgart, Germany: Thieme; 2008:416–422

[92] Ushigome S, Machinami R, Sorensen PH. Ewing's sarcoma/primitive neuroectodermal tumour (PNET). In: Fletcher CDM, Unni KK, Mertens F, eds. World Health Organization Classification of Tumours. Pathology and Genetics of Tumours of Soft Tissue and Bone. Lyon, France: IARC Press; 2002:298–300

▶ Extramedullary Hematopoiesis

[93] Dibbern DA, Loevner LA, Lieberman AP, Salhany KE, Freese A, Marcotte PJ. MR of thoracic cord compression caused by epidural extramedullary hematopoiesis in myelodysplastic syndrome. AJNR Am J Neuroradiol 1997; 18: 363–366

[94] Niggemann P, Krings T, Hans F, Thron A. Fifteen-year follow-up of a patient with beta thalassaemia and extramedullary haematopoietic tissue compressing the spinal cord. Neuroradiology 2005; 47: 263–266

[95] Rajiah P, Hayashi R, Bauer TW, Sundaram M. Extramedullary hematopoiesis in unusual locations in hematologically compromised and noncompromised patients. Skeletal Radiol 2011; 40: 947–953

[96] Tan TC, Tsao J, Cheung FC. Extramedullary haemopoiesis in thalassemia intermedia presenting as paraplegia. J Clin Neurosci 2002; 9: 721–725

▸ Fibrolipomatous Hamartoma

[97] Cavallaro MC, Taylor JA, Gorman JD, Haghighi P, Resnick D. Imaging findings in a patient with fibrolipomatous hamartoma of the median nerve. AJR Am J Roentgenol 1993; 161: 837–838

[98] De Maeseneer M, Jaovisidha S, Lenchik L, et al. Fibrolipomatous hamartoma: MR imaging findings. Skeletal Radiol 1997; 26: 155–160

[99] Marom EM, Helms CA. Fibrolipomatous hamartoma: pathognomonic on MR imaging. Skeletal Radiol 1999; 28: 260–264

[100] Meyers SP. Fibrolipomatous hamartoma. In: MRI of Bone and Soft Tissue Tumors and Tumorlike Lesions. Stuttgart, Germany: Thieme; 2008:426–427

[101] Nielsen GP. Lipomatosis of nerve. In: Fletcher CDM, Unni KK, Mertens F, eds. World Health Organization Classification of Tumours. Pathology and Genetics of Tumours of Soft Tissue and Bone. Lyon, France: IARC Press; 2002:24–25

[102] Ogose A, Hotta T, Higuchi T, Katsumi N, Koda H, Umezu H. Fibrolipomatous hamartoma in the foot: magnetic resonance imaging and surgical treatment: a report of two cases. J Bone Joint Surg Am 2002; 84-A: 432–436

[103] Toms AP, Anastakis D, Bleakney RR, Marshall TJ. Lipofibromatous hamartoma of the upper extremity: a review of the radiologic findings for 15 patients. AJR Am J Roentgenol 2006; 186: 805–811

[104] Van Breuseghem I, Sciot R, Pans S, Geusens E, Brys P, De Wever I. Fibrolipomatous hamartoma in the foot: atypical MR imaging findings. Skeletal Radiol 2003; 32: 651–655

▸ Fibroma of the Tendon Sheath

[105] Bertolotto M, Rosenberg I, Parodi RC, et al. Case report: fibroma of tendon sheath in the distal forearm with associated median nerve neuropathy: US, CT and MR appearances. Clin Radiol 1996; 51: 370–372

[106] Farshid G, Bridge JA. Fibroma of the tendon sheath. In: Fletcher CDM, Unni KK, Mertens F, eds. World Health Organization Classification of Tumours. Pathology and Genetics of Tumours of Soft Tissue and Bone. Lyon, France: IARC Press; 2002:66

[107] Fox MG, Kransdorf MJ, Bancroft LW, Peterson JJ, Flemming DJ. MR imaging of fibroma of the tendon sheath. AJR Am J Roentgenol 2003; 180: 1449–1453

[108] McGrory JE, Rock MG. Fibroma of tendon sheath involving the patellar tendon. Am J Orthop 2000; 29: 465–467

[109] Meyers SP. Fibroma of the tendon sheath. In: MRI of Bone and Soft Tissue Tumors and Tumorlike Lesions. Stuttgart, Germany: Thieme; 2008:428–429

[110] Moretti VM, de la Cruz M, Lackman RD, Fox EJ. Fibroma of tendon sheath in the knee: a report of three cases and literature review. Knee 2010; 17: 306–309

▸ Fibrosarcoma

[111] Christensen DR, Ramsamooj R, Gilbert TJ. Sclerosing epithelioid fibrosarcoma: short T2 on MR imaging. Skeletal Radiol 1997; 26: 619–621

[112] Coffin CM, Fletcher JA. Infantile fibrosarcoma. In: Fletcher CDM, Unni KK, Mertens F, eds. World Health Organization Classification of Tumours. Pathology and Genetics of Tumours of Soft Tissue and Bone. Lyon, France: IARC Press; 2002:98–100

[113] Eich GF, Hoeffel JC, Tschäppeler H, Gassner I, Willi UV. Fibrous tumours in children: imaging features of a heterogeneous group of disorders. Pediatr Radiol 1998; 28: 500–509

[114] Fisher C, van den Berg E, Molenaar WM. Adult fibrosarcoma. In: Fletcher CDM, Unni KK, Mertens F, eds. World Health Organization Classification of Tumours. Pathology and Genetics of Tumours of Soft Tissue and Bone. Lyon, France: IARC Press; 2002:100–101

[115] Folpe A, van den Berg E, Molenaar WM. Low grade fibromyxoid sarcoma. In: Fletcher CDM, Unni KK, Mertens F, eds. World Health Organization Classification of Tumours. Pathology and Genetics of Tumours of Soft Tissue and Bone. Lyon, France: IARC Press; 2002:104–105

[116] Meis-Kindblom JM, Kindblom LG, van den Berg E, Molenaar WM. Sclerosing epithelioid fibrosarcoma. In: Fletcher CDM, Unni KK, Mertens F, eds. World Health Organization Classification of Tumours. Pathology and Genetics of Tumours of Soft Tissue and Bone. Lyon, France: IARC Press; 2002:106–107

[117] Mentzel T, van den Berg E, Molenaar WM. Myxofibrosarcoma. In: Fletcher CDM, Unni KK, Mertens F, eds. World Health Organization Classification of Tumours. Pathology and Genetics of Tumours of Soft Tissue and Bone. Lyon, France: IARC Press; 2002:102–103

[118] Meyers SP. Fibrosarcoma. In: MRI of Bone and Soft Tissue Tumors and Tumorlike Lesions. Stuttgart, Germany: Thieme; 2008:433–437

▸ Ganglia

[119] Abdelwahab IF, Kenan S, Hermann G, Klein MJ, Lewis MM. Periosteal ganglia: CT and MR imaging features. Radiology 1993; 188: 245–248

[120] Bisset GS. MR imaging of soft-tissue masses in children. MRI Clinics of North America 1996;697–719

[121] Blanco JF, De Pedro JA, Paniagua JC. Periosteal ganglion in a child. Arch Orthop Trauma Surg 2003; 123: 115–117

[122] Forest M. Ganglion and epidermoid cyst. In: Forest M, Tomeno B, Vanel D. Orthopedic Surgical Pathology: Diagnosis of Tumors and Pseudotumoral Lesions of Bone and Joints 1998:547–553

▸ Giant Cell Tumor of the Tendon Sheath and/or Soft Tissue

[123] Al-Qattan MM. Giant cell tumours of tendon sheath: classification and recurrence rate. J Hand Surg [Br] 2001; 26: 72–75

[124] Gibbons CL, Khwaja HA, Cole AS, Cooke PH, Athanasou NA. Giant-cell tumour of the tendon sheath in the foot and ankle. J Bone Joint Surg Br 2002; 84: 1000–1003

[125] Huang GS, Lee CH, Chan WP, Chen CY, Yu JS, Resnick D. Localized nodular synovitis of the knee: MR imaging appearance and clinical correlates in 21 patients. AJR Am J Roentgenol 2003; 181: 539–543

[126] Jelinek JS, Kransdorf MJ, Shmookler BM, Aboulafia AA, Malawer MM. Giant cell tumor of the tendon sheath: MR findings in nine cases. AJR Am J Roentgenol 1994; 162: 919–922

[127] Kitagawa Y, Ito H, Amano Y, Sawaizumi T, Takeuchi T. MR imaging for preoperative diagnosis and assessment of local tumor extent on localized giant cell tumor of tendon sheath. Skeletal Radiol 2003; 32: 633–638

[128] Llauger J, Palmer J, Rosón N, Cremades R, Bagué S. Pigmented villonodular synovitis and giant cell tumors of the tendon sheath: radiologic and pathologic features. AJR Am J Roentgenol 1999; 172: 1087–1091

[129] Ly JQ, Carlson CL, LaGatta LM, Beall DP. Giant cell tumor of the peroneus tendon sheath. AJR Am J Roentgenol 2003; 180: 1442

[130] Meyers SP. Giant cell tumor of the tendon sheath and/or soft tissue. In: MRI of Bone and Soft Tissue Tumors and Tumorlike Lesions. Stuttgart, Germany: Thieme; 2008:469–475

[131] Monaghan H, Salter DM, Al-Nafussi A. Giant cell tumour of tendon sheath (localised nodular tenosynovitis): clinicopathological features of 71 cases. J Clin Pathol 2001; 54: 404–407

[132] Somerhausen N, Cin PD. Giant cell tumor of the tendon sheath. In: Fletcher CDM, Unni KK, Mertens F, eds. World Health Organization Classification of Tumours. Pathology and Genetics of Tumours of Soft Tissue and Bone. Lyon, France: IARC Press; 2002:110–111

[133] Somerhausen N, Cin PD. Diffuse-type giant cell tumor of the tendon sheath. In: Fletcher CDM, Unni KK, Mertens F, eds. World Health Organization Classification of Tumours. Pathology and Genetics of Tumours of Soft Tissue and Bone. Lyon, France: IARC Press; 2002:112–114

[134] Wu NL, Hsiao PF, Chen BF, Chen HC, Su HY. Malignant giant cell tumor of the tendon sheath. Int J Dermatol 2004; 43: 54–57

▸ Glomus Tumor

[135] Baek HJ, Lee SJ, Cho KH, et al. Subungual tumors: clinicopathologic correlation with US and MR imaging findings. Radiographics 2010; 30: 1621–1636

[136] Bhaskaranand K, Navadgi BC. Glomus tumour of the hand. J Hand Surg [Br] 2002; 27: 229–231

[137] Boudghene FP, Gouny P, Tassart M, Callard P, Le Breton C, Vayssairat M. Subungual glomus tumor: combined use of MRI and three-dimensional contrast MR angiography. J Magn Reson Imaging 1998; 8: 1326–1328

[138] Dalrymple NC, Hayes J, Bessinger VJ, Wolfe SW, Katz LD. MRI of multiple glomus tumors of the finger. Skeletal Radiol 1997; 26: 664–666

[139] Drapé JL, Idy-Peretti I, Goettmann S, et al. Subungual glomus tumors: evaluation with MR imaging. Radiology 1995; 195: 507–515

[140] Folpe AL. Glomus tumours. In: Fletcher CDM, Unni KK, Mertens F, eds. World Health Organization Classification of Tumours. Pathology and Genetics of Tumours of Soft Tissue and Bone. Lyon, France: IARC Press; 2002:136–137

[141] Meyers SP. Glomus tumor. In: MRI of Bone and Soft Tissue Tumors and Tumorlike Lesions. Stuttgart, Germany: Thieme; 2008:476–478

[142] Opdenakker G, Gelin G, Palmers Y. MR imaging of a subungual glomus tumor. AJR Am J Roentgenol 1999; 172: 250–251

[143] Perks FJ, Beggs I, Lawson GM, Davie R. Juxtacortical glomus tumor of the distal femur adjacent to the popliteal fossa. AJR Am J Roentgenol 2003; 181: 1590–1592

[144] Theumann NH, Goettmann S, Le Viet D, et al. Recurrent glomus tumors of fingertips: MR imaging evaluation. Radiology 2002; 223: 143–151

[145] Tomak Y, Akcay I, Dabak N, Eroglu L. Subungual glomus tumours of the hand: diagnosis and treatment of 14 cases. Scand J Plast Reconstr Surg Hand Surg 2003; 37: 121–124

▶ Gout

[146] Meyers SP. Gout. In: MRI of Bone and Soft Tissue Tumors and Tumorlike Lesions. Stuttgart, Germany: Thieme; 2008:479–483

[147] Monu JUV, Pope TL. Gout: a clinical and radiologic review. Radiol Clin North Am 2004; 42: 169–184

[148] Yu JS, Chung C, Recht M, Dailiana T, Jurdi R. MR imaging of tophaceous gout. AJR Am J Roentgenol 1997; 168: 523–527

▶ Granular Cell Tumor

[149] Arai E, Nishida Y, Tsukushi S, Sugiura H, Ishiguro N. Intramuscular granular cell tumor in the lower extremities. Clin Orthop Relat Res 2010; 468: 1384–1389

[150] Blacksin MF, White LM, Hameed M, Kandel R, Patterson FR, Benevenia J. Granular cell tumor of the extremity: magnetic resonance imaging characteristics with pathologic correlation. Skeletal Radiol 2005; 34: 625–631

[151] Elkousy H, Harrelson J, Dodd L, Martinez S, Scully S. Granular cell tumors of the extremities. Clin Orthop Relat Res 2000; 380: 191–198

▶ Granuloma Annulare

[152] Bancroft LW, Perniciaro C, Berquist TH. Granuloma annulare: radiographic demonstration of progressive mutilating arthropathy with vanishing bones. Skeletal Radiol 1998; 27: 211–214

[153] Chung S, Frush DP, Prose NS, Shea CR, Laor T, Bisset GS. Subcutaneous granuloma annulare: MR imaging features in six children and literature review. Radiology 1999; 210: 845–849

[154] Kransdorf MJ, Murphey MD, Temple HT. Subcutaneous granuloma annulare: radiologic appearance. Skeletal Radiol 1998; 27: 266–270

[155] Shehan JM, El-Azhary RA. Magnetic resonance imaging features of subcutaneous granuloma annulare. Pediatr Dermatol 2005; 22: 377–378

▶ Hemangioendothelioma

[156] Calonje E. Retiform haemangioendothelioma. In: Fletcher CDM, Unni KK, Mertens F, eds. World Health Organization Classification of Tumours. Pathology and Genetics of Tumours of Soft Tissue and Bone. Lyon, France: IARC Press; 2002:165–166

[157] Calonje E. Papillary intralymphatic angioendothelioma. In: Fletcher CDM, Unni KK, Mertens F, eds. World Health Organization Classification of Tumours. Pathology and Genetics of Tumours of Soft Tissue and Bone. Lyon, France: IARC Press; 2002:167

[158] Cooper JG, Edwards SL, Holmes JD. Kaposiform haemangioendothelioma: case report and review of the literature. Br J Plast Surg 2002; 55: 163–165

[159] Ignacio EA, Palmer KM, Mathur SC, Schwartz AM, Olan WJ. Epithelioid hemangioendothelioma of the lower extremity. Radiographics 1999; 19: 531–537

[160] Meyers SP. Hemangioendothelioma. In: MRI of Bone and Soft Tissue Tumors and Tumorlike Lesions. Stuttgart, Germany: Thieme; 2008:484–490

[161] Rubin BP. Composite haemangioendothelioma. In: Fletcher CDM, Unni KK, Mertens F, eds. World Health Organization Classification of Tumours. Pathology and Genetics of Tumours of Soft Tissue and Bone. Lyon, France: IARC Press; 2002:168–169

[162] Tsang WYW. Kaposiform haemangioendothelioma. In: Fletcher CDM, Unni KK, Mertens F, eds. World Health Organization Classification of Tumours. Pathology and Genetics of Tumours of Soft Tissue and Bone. Lyon, France: IARC Press; 2002:163–164

[163] Weiss SW, Bridge JA. Epithelioid haemangioendothelioma. In: Fletcher CDM, Unni KK, Mertens F, eds. World Health Organization Classification of Tumours. Pathology and Genetics of Tumours of Soft Tissue and Bone. Lyon, France: IARC Press; 2002:173–174

▶ Hemangioma

[164] Adler CP, Wold L. Haemangioma and related lesions. In: Fletcher CDM, Unni KK, Mertens F, eds. World Health Organization Classification of Tumours. Pathology and Genetics of Tumours of Soft Tissue and Bone. Lyon, France: IARC Press; 2002:320–323

[165] Calonje E. Haemangiomas. In: Fletcher CDM, Unni KK, Mertens F, eds. World Health Organization Classification of Tumours. Pathology and Genetics of Tumours of Soft Tissue and Bone. Lyon, France: IARC Press; 2002:156–158

[166] Cohen EK, Kressel HY, Perosio T, et al. MR imaging of soft-tissue hemangiomas: correlation with pathologic findings. AJR Am J Roentgenol 1988; 150: 1079–1081

[167] Fayad LM, Hazirolan T, Bluemke D, Mitchell S. Vascular malformations in the extremities: emphasis on MR imaging features that guide treatment options [Erratum in Skeletal Radiol 2006;35(12):964. Fayad, Laura corrected t Fayad Laura M]. Skeletal Radiol 2006; 35: 127–137

[168] Fetsch JF. Epithelioid haemangioma. In: Fletcher CDM, Unni KK, Mertens F, eds. World Health Organization Classification of Tumours. Pathology and Genetics of Tumours of Soft Tissue and Bone. Lyon, France: IARC Press; 2002:159–160

[169] Laor T, Burrows PE. Congenital anomalies and vascular birthmarks of the lower extremities. Magn Reson Imaging Clin N Am 1998; 6: 497–519

[170] Meyers SP. Hemangiomas. In: MRI of Bone and Soft Tissue Tumors and Tumorlike Lesions. Stuttgart, Germany: Thieme; 2008:491–501

[171] Weiss SW. Angiomatosis. In: Fletcher CDM, Unni KK, Mertens F, eds. World Health Organization Classification of Tumours. Pathology and Genetics of Tumours of Soft Tissue and Bone. Lyon, France: IARC Press; 2002:161

▶ Hemangiopericytoma

[172] Gengler C, Guillou L. Solitary fibrous tumour and haemangiopericytoma: evolution of a concept. Histopathology 2006; 48: 63–74

[173] Guillou L, Fletcher JA, Fletcher CDM, Mandahl N. Extrapleural solitary fibrous tumour and haemangiopericytoma. In: Fletcher CDM, Unni KK, Mertens F, eds. World Health Organization Classification of Tumours. Pathology and Genetics of Tumours of Soft Tissue and Bone. Lyon, France: IARC Press; 2002:86–90

[174] Meyers SP. Hemangiopericytoma. In: MRI of Bone and Soft Tissue Tumors and Tumorlike Lesions. Stuttgart, Germany: Thieme; 2008:502–506

[175] Rodriguez-Galindo C, Ramsey K, Jenkins JJ, et al. Hemangiopericytoma in children and infants. Cancer 2000; 88: 198–204

▶ Hematoma, Morel-Lavallée Lesion, Hemophilic Pseudotumor

[176] Bush CH. The magnetic resonance imaging of musculoskeletal hemorrhage. Skeletal Radiol 2000; 29: 1–9

[177] Jaovisidha S, Ryu KN, Hodler J, Schweitzer ME, Sartoris DJ, Resnick D. Hemophilic pseudotumor: spectrum of MR findings. Skeletal Radiol 1997; 26: 468–474

[178] Jelinek J, Kransdorf MJ. MR imaging of soft-tissue masses. Mass-like lesions that simulate neoplasms. Magn Reson Imaging Clin N Am 1995; 3: 727–741

[179] Meyers SP. Hematoma, Morel-Lavallee Lesion, Hemophilic Pseudotumor. In: MRI of Bone and Soft Tissue Tumors and Tumorlike Lesions. Stuttgart, Germany: Thieme;2008:507–511

[180] Park JS, Ryu KN. Hemophilic pseudotumor involving the musculoskeletal system: spectrum of radiologic findings. AJR Am J Roentgenol 2004; 183: 55–61

[181] Rubin JI, Gomori JM, Grossman RI, Gefter WB, Kressel HY. High-field MR imaging of extracranial hematomas. AJR Am J Roentgenol 1987; 148: 813–817

▶ Hemophilic Pseudotumor

[182] Jaovisidha S, Ryu KN, Hodler J, Schweitzer ME, Sartoris DJ, Resnick D. Hemophilic pseudotumor: spectrum of MR findings. Skeletal Radiol 1997; 26: 468–474

[183] Park JS, Ryu KN. Hemophilic pseudotumor involving the musculoskeletal system: spectrum of radiologic findings. AJR Am J Roentgenol 2004; 183: 55–61

▶ Hypothenar Hammer Injury of the Ulnar Artery

[184] Blum AG, Zabel JP, Kohlmann R, et al. Pathologic conditions of the hypothenar eminence: evaluation with multidetector CT and MR imaging. Radiographics 2006; 26: 1021–1044

[185] Drape JL, Feydy A, Guerini H, et al. Vascular lesions of the hand. Eur J Radiol 2005; 56: 331–343

▶ Kimura Disease

[186] Choi JA, Lee GK, Kong KY, et al. Imaging findings of Kimura's disease in the soft tissue of the upper extremity. AJR Am J Roentgenol 2005; 184: 193–199

[187] Huang GS, Lee HS, Chiu YC, Yu CC, Chen CY. Kimura's disease of the elbows. Skeletal Radiol 2005; 34: 555–558

▶ Leiomyoma

[188] Hashimoto H, Quade B. Angioleiomyoma. In: Fletcher CDM, Unni KK, Mertens F, eds. World Health Organization Classification of Tumours. Pathology and Genetics of Tumours of soft Tissue and Bone. Lyon, France: IARC Press; 2002:128–129

[189] Hashimoto H, Quade B. Leiomyoma of deep soft tissue. In: Fletcher CDM, Unni KK, Mertens F, eds. World Health Organization Classification of Tumours. Pathology and Genetics of Tumours of Soft Tissue and Bone. Lyon, France: IARC Press; 2002:130

[190] Meyers SP. Leiomyoma. In: MRI of Bone and Soft Tissue Tumors and Tumorlike Lesions. Stuttgart, Germany: Thieme; 2008:521–524

[191] Miki Y, Abe S, Tokizaki T, Harasawa A, Imamura T, Matsushita T. Imaging characteristics of calcified leiomyoma of deep soft tissue. J Orthop Sci 2007; 12: 601–605

[192] Yoo HJ, Choi JA, Chung JH, et al. Angioleiomyoma in soft tissue of extremities: MRI findings. Am J Roentgenol 2009; 192: W291-: W29: 4

▶ Leiomyosarcoma

[193] Bush CH, Reith JD, Spanier SS. Mineralization in musculoskeletal leiomyosarcoma: radiologic-pathologic correlation. AJR Am J Roentgenol 2003; 180: 109–113

[194] Evans HL, Shipley J. Leiomyosarcoma. In: Fletcher CDM, Unni KK, Mertens F, eds. World Health Organization Classification of Tumours. Pathology and Genetics of Tumours of Soft Tissue and Bone. Lyon, France: IARC Press; 2002:131–134

[195] McCarthy E. Leiomyosarcoma of bone. In: Fletcher CDM, Unni KK, Mertens F, eds. World Health Organization Classification of Tumours. Pathology and Genetics of Tumours of Soft Tissue and Bone. Lyon, France: IARC Press; 2002:327

[196] Meyers SP. Leiomyosarcoma. In: MRI of Bone and Soft Tissue Tumors and Tumorlike Lesions. Stuttgart, Germany: Thieme; 2008:525–530

[197] van Vliet M, Kliffen M, Krestin GP, van Dijke CF. Soft tissue sarcomas at a glance: clinical, histological, and MR imaging features of malignant extremity soft tissue tumors. Eur Radiol 2009; 19: 1499–1511

▶ Lipoblastoma

[198] Collins MH, Chatten J. Lipoblastoma/lipoblastomatosis: a clinicopathologic study of 25 tumors. Am J Surg Pathol 1997; 21: 1131–1137

[199] Harrer J, Hammon G, Wagner T, Bolkenius M. Lipoblastoma and lipoblastomatosis: a report of two cases and review of the literature. Eur J Pediatr Surg 2001; 11: 342–349

[200] Meyers SP. Lipoblastoma. In: MRI of Bone and Soft Tissue Tumors and Tumorlike Lesions. Stuttgart, Germany: Thieme; 2008:540–542

[201] Mognato G, Cecchetto G, Carli M, et al. Is surgical treatment of lipoblastoma always necessary? J Pediatr Surg 2000; 35: 1511–1513

[202] Moholkar S, Sebire NJ, Roebuck DJ. Radiological-pathological correlation in lipoblastoma and lipoblastomatosis. Pediatr Radiol 2006; 36: 851–856

[203] Reiseter T, Nordshus T, Borthne A, Roald B, Naess P, Schistad O. Lipoblastoma: MRI appearances of a rare paediatric soft tissue tumour. Pediatr Radiol 1999; 29: 542–545

[204] Sciot R, Mandahl N. Lipoblastoma. In: Fletcher CDM, Unni KK, Mertens F, eds. World Health Organization Classification of Tumours. Pathology and Genetics of Tumours of Soft Tissue and Bone. Lyon, France: IARC Press; 2002:26–27

▶ Lipoma, Atypical Lipoma, and Hibernoma

[205] Anderson SE, Schwab C, Stauffer E, Banic A, Steinbach LS. Hibernoma: imaging characteristics of a rare benign soft tissue tumor. Skeletal Radiol 2001; 30: 590–595

[206] Chan LP, Gee R, Keogh C, Munk PL. Imaging features of fat necrosis. AJR Am J Roentgenol 2003; 181: 955–959

[207] Della Volpe C, Salazard B, Casanova D, Vacheret H, Bartoli JF, Magalon G. Hibernoma of the antero-lateral thigh. Br J Plast Surg 2005; 58: 859–861

[208] Furlong MA, Fanburg-Smith JC, Miettinen M. The morphologic spectrum of hibernoma: a clinicopathologic study of 170 cases. Am J Surg Pathol 2001; 25: 809–814

[209] Gaskin CM, Helms CA. Lipomas, lipoma variants, and well-differentiated liposarcomas (atypical lipomas): results of MRI evaluations of 126 consecutive fatty masses. AJR Am J Roentgenol 2004; 182: 733–739

[210] Hosono M, Kobayashi H, Fujimoto R, et al. Septum-like structures in lipoma and liposarcoma: MR imaging and pathologic correlation. Skeletal Radiol 1997; 26: 150–154

[211] Kallas KM, Vaughan L, Haghighi P, Resnick D. Hibernoma of the left axilla; a case report and review of MR imaging. Skeletal Radiol 2003; 32: 290–294

[212] Kindblom LG, Meis-Kindblom JM, Mandahl N. Chondroid lipoma. In: Fletcher CDM, Unni KK, Mertens F, eds. World Health Organization Classification of Tumours. Pathology and Genetics of Tumours of Soft Tissue and Bone. Lyon, France: IARC Press; 2002:30

[213] Kransdorf MJ, Bancroft LW, Peterson JJ, Murphey MD, Foster WC, Temple HT. Imaging of fatty tumors: distinction of lipoma and well-differentiated liposarcoma. Radiology 2002; 224: 99–104

[214] Logan PM, Janzen DL, O'Connell JX, Munk PL, Connell DG. Chondroid lipoma: MRI appearances with clinical and histologic correlation. Skeletal Radiol 1996; 25: 592–595

[215] Matsumoto K, Hukuda S, Ishizawa M, Chano T, Okabe H. MRI findings in intramuscular lipomas. Skeletal Radiol 1999; 28: 145–152

[216] Meyers SP. Lipoma, atypical lipoma, and hibernoma. In: MRI of Bone and Soft Tissue Tumors and Tumorlike Lesions. Stuttgart, Germany: Thieme; 2008:543–55

[217] Miettinen MM, Fanburg-Smith JC, Mandahl N. Hibernoma. In: Fletcher CDM, Unni KK, Mertens F, eds. World Health Organization Classification of Tumours. Pathology and Genetics of Tumours of Soft Tissue and Bone. Lyon, France: IARC Press; 2002:33–34

[218] Miettinen MM, Fanburg-Smith JC, Mandahl N. Spindle cell lipoma/pleomorphic lipoma. In: Fletcher CDM, Unni KK, Mertens F, eds. World Health Organization Classification of Tumours. Pathology and Genetics of Tumours of Soft Tissue and Bone. Lyon, France: IARC Press; 2002:31–32

[219] Murphey MD, Carroll JF, Flemming DJ, Pope TL, Gannon FH, Kransdorf MJ. From the archives of the AFIP: benign musculoskeletal lipomatous lesions. Radiographics 2004; 24: 1433–1466

[220] Nielsen GP, Mandahl N. Lipoma. In: Fletcher CDM, Unni KK, Mertens F, eds. World Health Organization Classification of Tumours. Pathology and Genetics of Tumours of Soft Tissue and Bone. Lyon, France: IARC Press; 2002:20–22

[221] Ohguri T, Aoki T, Hisaoka M, et al. Differential diagnosis of benign peripheral lipoma from well-differentiated liposarcoma on MR imaging: is comparison of margins and internal characteristics useful? AJR Am J Roentgenol 2003; 180: 1689–1694

[222] Propeck T, Bullard MA, Lin J, Doi K, Martel W. Radiologic-pathologic correlation of intraosseous lipomas. AJR Am J Roentgenol 2000; 175: 673–678

[223] Roberts CC, Liu PT, Colby TV. Encapsulated versus nonencapsulated superficial fatty masses: a proposed MR imaging classification. AJR Am J Roentgenol 2003; 180: 1419–1422

▶ Lipomatosis

[224] Amine B, Leguilchard F, Benhamou CL. Dercum's disease (adiposis dolorosa): a new case-report. Joint Bone Spine 2004; 71: 147–149

[225] Drevelegas A, Pilavaki M, Chourmouzi D. Lipomatous tumors of soft tissue: MR appearance with histological correlation. Eur J Radiol 2004; 50: 257–267

[226] Haloi AK, Ditchfield M, Penington A, Phillips R. Facial infiltrative lipomatosis. Pediatr Radiol 2006; 36: 1159–1162

[227] Murphey MD, Carroll JF, Flemming DJ, Pope TL, Gannon FH, Kransdorf MJ. From the archives of the AFIP: benign musculoskeletal lipomatous lesions. Radiographics 2004; 24: 1433–1466

[228] Torigian DA, Siegelman ES. CT findings of pelvic lipomatosis of nerve. AJR Am J Roentgenol 2005; 184 Suppl: S94–S96

▶ Liposarcoma

[229] Antonescu C, Ladanyl M. Myxoid liposarcoma. In: Fletcher CDM, Unni KK, Mertens F, eds. World Health Organization Classification of Tumours. Pathology and Genetics of Tumours of Soft Tissue and Bone. Lyon, France: IARC Press; 2002:40–43

[230] Arkun R, Memis A, Akalin T, Ustun EE, Sabah D, Kandiloglu G. Liposarcoma of soft tissue: MRI findings with pathologic correlation. Skeletal Radiol 1997; 26: 167–172

[231] Dei Tos AP, Pedeutour F. Atypical lipomatous tumour/well differentiated liposarcoma. In: Fletcher CDM, Unni KK, Mertens F, eds. World Health Organization Classification of Tumours. Pathology and Genetics of Tumours of Soft Tissue and Bone. Lyon, France: IARC Press; 2002:35–37

[232] Dei Tos AP, Pedeutour F. Dedifferentiated liposarcoma. In: Fletcher CDM, Unni KK, Mertens F, eds. World Health Organization Classification of Tumours. Pathology and Genetics of Tumours of Soft Tissue and Bone. Lyon, France: IARC Press; 2002:38–39

[233] Downes KA, Goldblum JR, Montgomery EA, Fisher C. Pleomorphic liposarcoma: a clinicopathologic analysis of 19 cases. Mod Pathol 2001; 14: 179–184

[234] Hosono M, Kobayashi H, Fujimoto R, et al. Septum-like structures in lipoma and liposarcoma: MR imaging and pathologic correlation. Skeletal Radiol 1997; 26: 150–154

[235] Kransdorf MJ, Bancroft LW, Peterson JJ, Murphey MD, Foster WC, Temple HT. Imaging of fatty tumors: distinction of lipoma and well-differentiated liposarcoma. Radiology 2002; 224: 99–104

[236] Mentzel T, Pedeutour F. Pleomorphic liposarcoma. In: Fletcher CDM, Unni KK, Mertens F, eds. World Health Organization Classification of Tumours. Pathology and Genetics of Tumours of Soft Tissue and Bone. Lyon, France: IARC Press; 2002:44–45

[237] Meyers SP. Liposarcoma. In: MRI of Bone and Soft Tissue Tumors and Tumorlike Lesions. Stuttgart, Germany: Thieme; 2008:554–562

[238] Murphey MD, Arcara LK, Fanburg-Smith J. From the archives of the AFIP: imaging of musculoskeletal liposarcoma with radiologic-pathologic correlation. Radiographics 2005; 25: 1371–1395
[239] Ohguri T, Aoki T, Hisaoka M, et al. Differential diagnosis of benign peripheral lipoma from well-differentiated liposarcoma on MR imaging: is comparison of margins and internal characteristics useful? AJR Am J Roentgenol 2003; 180: 1689–1694
[240] Peterson JJ, Kransdorf MJ, Bancroft LW, O'Connor MI. Malignant fatty tumors: classification, clinical course, imaging appearance and treatment. Skeletal Radiol 2003; 32: 493–503
[241] Sung MS, Kang HS, Suh JS, et al. Myxoid liposarcoma: appearance at MR imaging with histologic correlation. Radiographics 2000; 20: 1007–1019
[242] Tateishi U, Hasegawa T, Beppu Y, Kawai A, Satake M, Moriyama N. Prognostic significance of MRI findings in patients with myxoid-round cell liposarcoma. AJR Am J Roentgenol 2004; 182: 725–731

▸ Low Grade Myofibroblastic Sarcoma

[243] San Miguel P, Fernández G, Ortiz-Rey JA, Larrauri P. Low-grade myofibroblastic sarcoma of the distal phalanx. J Hand Surg Am 2004; 29: 1160–1163

▸ Lymphangioma

[244] Benham A. Lymphangiona. In: Fletcher CDM, Unni KK, Mertens F, eds. World Health Organization Classification of Tumours. Pathology and Genetics of Tumours of Soft Tissue and Bone. Lyon, France: IARC Press; 2002:162–163
[245] Meyers SP. Lymphangioma. In: MRI of Bone and Soft Tissue Tumors and Tumorlike Lesions. Stuttgart, Germany: Thieme; 2008:566–569
[246] Ng EH, Shah VS, Armstrong DC, Clarke HM. Cavernous lymphangioma. J Pediatr 2001; 138: 146–148
[247] Reinhardt MA, Nelson SC, Sencer SF, Bostrom BC, Kurachek SC, Nesbit ME. Treatment of childhood lymphangiomas with interferon-alpha. J Pediatr Hematol Oncol 1997; 19: 232–236
[248] Siegel MJ, Glazer HS, St Amour TE, Rosenthal DD. Lymphangiomas in children: MR imaging. Radiology 1989; 170: 467–470
[249] Wever DJ, Heeg M, Mooyaart EL. Cystic hygroma of the shoulder region. A case report. Clin Orthop Relat Res 1997; 338: 215–218
[250] Winterer JT, Laubenberger J, Berger W, et al. Radiologic findings in lymphangioma of the posterior tibial nerve. J Comput Assist Tomogr 1998; 22: 28–30

▸ Lymphoma

[251] Meyers SP. Lymphoma. In: MRI of Bone and Soft Tissue Tumors and Tumorlike Lesions. Stuttgart, Germany: Thieme; 2008:570–583

▸ Malignant Fibrous Histiocytoma, Myxfibrosarcoma

[252] Belal A, Kandil A, Allam A, et al. Malignant fibrous histiocytoma: a retrospective study of 109 cases. Am J Clin Oncol 2002; 25: 16–22
[253] Coindre JM. Inflammatory malignant fibrous histiocytoma/undifferentiated pleomorphic sarcoma with prominent inflammation. In: Fletcher CDM, Unni KK, Mertens F, eds. World Health Organization Classification of Tumours. Pathology and Genetics of Tumours of Soft Tissue and Bone. Lyon, France: IARC Press; 2002:125–126
[254] Daw NC, Billups CA, Pappo AS, et al. Malignant fibrous histiocytoma and other fibrohistiocytic tumors in pediatric patients: the St. Jude Children's Research Hospital experience. Cancer 2003; 97: 2839–2847
[255] Fletcher CD, Gustafson P, Rydholm A, Willén H, Akerman M. Clinicopathologic re-evaluation of 100 malignant fibrous histiocytomas: prognostic relevance of subclassification. J Clin Oncol 2001; 19: 3045–3050
[256] Fletcher CDM, van den Berg E, Molenaar WM. Pleomorphic malignant fibrous histiocytoma/undifferentiated high grade pleomorphic sarcoma. In: Fletcher CDM, Unni KK, Mertens F, eds. World Health Organization Classification of Tumours. Pathology and Genetics of Tumours of Soft Tissue and Bone. Lyon, France: IARC Press; 2002:120–122
[257] Fletcher CDM. Giant cell malignant fibrous histiocytoma/undifferentiated pleomorphic sarcoma with giant cells. In: Fletcher CDM, Unni KK, Mertens F, eds. World Health Organization Classification of Tumours. Pathology and Genetics of Tumours of Soft Tissue and Bone. Lyon, France: IARC Press; 2002:123–124
[258] Mentzel T, van den Berg E, Molenaar WM. Myxofibrosarcoma. In: Fletcher CDM, Unni KK, Mertens F, eds. World Health Organization Classification of Tumours. Pathology and Genetics of Tumours of Soft Tissue and Bone. Lyon, France: IARC Press; 2002:102–103
[259] Meyers SP. Malignant fibrous histiocytoma. In: MRI of Bone and Soft Tissue Tumors and Tumorlike Lesions. Stuttgart, Germany: Thieme; 2008:584–593

▸ Metastatic Lesions

[260] Meyers SP. Metastatic lesions. In: MRI of Bone and Soft Tissue Tumors and Tumorlike Lesions. Stuttgart, Germany: Thieme; 2008:601–608

▸ Morton Neuroma

[261] Ashman CJ, Klecker RJ, Yu JS. Forefoot pain involving the metatarsal region: differential diagnosis with MR imaging. Radiographics 2001; 21: 1425–1440
[262] Erickson SJ, Canale PB, Carrera GF, et al. Interdigital (Morton) neuroma: high-resolution MR imaging with a solenoid coil. Radiology 1991; 181: 833–836
[263] Llauger J, Palmer J, Monill JM, Franquet T, Bagué S, Rosón N. MR imaging of benign soft-tissue masses of the foot and ankle. Radiographics 1998; 18: 1481–1498
[264] Meyers SP. Morton Neuroma. In: MRI of Bone and Soft Tissue Tumors and Tumorlike Lesions. Stuttgart, Germany: Thieme; 2008:609–610
[265] Murphey MD, Smith WS, Smith SE, Kransdorf MJ, Temple HT. From the archives of the AFIP. Imaging of musculoskeletal neurogenic tumors: radiologic-pathologic correlation. Radiographics 1999; 19: 1253–1280
[266] Terk MR, Kwong PK, Suthar M, Horvath BC, Colletti PM. Morton neuroma: evaluation with MR imaging performed with contrast enhancement and fat suppression. Radiology 1993; 189: 239–241
[267] Walker EA, Fenton ME, Salesky JS, Murphey MD. Magnetic resonance imaging of benign soft tissue neoplasms in adults. Radiol Clin North Am 2011; 49: 1197–1217, vi
[268] Weishaupt D, Treiber K, Kundert HP, et al. Morton neuroma: MR imaging in prone, supine, and upright weight-bearing body positions. Radiology 2003; 226: 849–856
[269] Zanetti M, Strehle JK, Kundert HP, Zollinger H, Hodler J. Morton neuroma: effect of MR imaging findings on diagnostic thinking and therapeutic decisions. Radiology 1999; 213: 583–588

▸ Muscle Infarct

[270] Meyers SP. Bone and muscle infarct. In: MRI of Bone and Soft Tissue Tumors and Tumorlike Lesions. Stuttgart, Germany: Thieme; 2008:512–518

▸ Myositis/Pyomyositis

[271] Marath H, Yates M, Lee M, Dhatariya K. Pyomyositis. J Diabetes Complications 2011; 25: 346–348
[272] Mitsionis GI, Manoudis GN, Lykissas MG, et al. Pyomyositis in children: early diagnosis and treatment. J Pediatr Surg 2009; 44: 2173–2178
[273] Santiago Restrepo C, Giménez CR, McCarthy K. Imaging of osteomyelitis and musculoskeletal soft tissue infections: current concepts. Rheum Dis Clin North Am 2003; 29: 89–109
[274] Struk DW, Munk PL, Lee MJ, Ho SG, Worsley DF. Imaging of soft tissue infections. Radiol Clin North Am 2001; 39: 277–303
[275] Taksande A, Vilhekar K, Gupta S. Primary pyomyositis in a child. Int J Infect Dis 2009; 13: e149–e151

▸ Myositis Ossificans

[276] Ehara S, Shiraishi H, Abe M, Mizutani H. Reactive heterotopic ossification. Its patterns on MRI. Clin Imaging 1998; 22: 292–296
[277] Gindele A, Schwamborn D, Tsironis K, Benz-Bohm G. Myositis ossificans traumatica in young children: report of three cases and review of the literature. Pediatr Radiol 2000; 30: 451–459
[278] Kransdorf MJ, Meis JM, Jelinek JS. Myositis ossificans: MR appearance with radiologic-pathologic correlation. AJR Am J Roentgenol 1991; 157: 1243–1248
[279] May DA, Disler DG, Jones EA, Balkissoon AA, Manaster BJ. Abnormal signal intensity in skeletal muscle at MR imaging: patterns, pearls, and pitfalls. Radiographics 2000; 20 Suppl 1: S295–S315
[280] Meyers SP. Myositis Ossificans. In: MRI of Bone and Soft Tissue Tumors and Tumorlike Lesions. Stuttgart, Germany: Thieme; 2008:618–623
[281] Micheli A, Trapani S, Brizzi I, Campanacci D, Resti M, de Martino M. Myositis ossificans circumscripta: a paediatric case and review of the literature. Eur J Pediatr 2009; 168: 523–529
[282] Parikh J, Hyare H, Saifuddin A. The imaging features of post-traumatic myositis ossificans, with emphasis on MRI. Clin Radiol 2002; 57: 1058–1066
[283] Rosenberg AE. Myositis ossificans and fibroosseous pseudotumor of digits. In: Fletcher CDM, Unni KK, Mertens F, eds. World Health Organization Classification of Tumours. Pathology and Genetics of Tumours of Soft Tissue and Bone. Lyon, France: IARC Press; 2002:52–54
[284] Tyler P, Saifuddin A. The imaging of myositis ossificans. Semin Musculoskelet Radiol 2010; 14: 201–216

▸ Myxoma

[285] Luna A, Martinez S, Bossen E. Magnetic resonance imaging of intramuscular myxoma with histological comparison and a review of the literature. Skeletal Radiol 2005; 34: 19–28
[286] Ly JQ, Bau JL, Beall DP. Forearm intramuscular myxoma. AJR Am J Roentgenol 2003; 181: 960

[287] Meyers SP. Myxoma. In: MRI of Bone and Soft Tissue Tumors and Tumorlike Lesions. Stuttgart, Germany: Thieme; 2008:624–626

[288] Murphey MD, McRae GA, Fanburg-Smith JC, Temple HT, Levine AM, Aboulafia AJ. Imaging of soft-tissue myxoma with emphasis on CT and MR and comparison of radiologic and pathologic findings. Radiology 2002; 225: 215–224

[289] Nielsen G, Stenman G. Intramuscular myxoma. In: Fletcher CDM, Unni KK, Mertens F, eds. World Health Organization Classification of Tumours. Pathology and Genetics of Tumours of Soft Tissue and Bone. Lyon, France: IARC Press; 2002:186–187

[290] Sundaram M, McDonald DJ, Merenda G. Intramuscular myxoma: a rare but important association with fibrous dysplasia of bone. AJR Am J Roentgenol 1989; 153: 107–108

[291] Walker EA, Fenton ME, Salesky JS, Murphey MD. Magnetic resonance imaging of benign soft tissue neoplasms in adults. Radiol Clin North Am 2011; 49: 1197–1217, vi

▸ Neurofibroma, Malignant Peripheral Nerve Sheath Tumor

[292] Khong PL, Goh WH, Wong VC, Fung CW, Ooi GC. MR imaging of spinal tumors in children with neurofibromatosis 1. AJR Am J Roentgenol 2003; 180: 413–417

[293] Lin J, Martel W. Cross-sectional imaging of peripheral nerve sheath tumors: characteristic signs on CT, MR imaging, and sonography. AJR Am J Roentgenol 2001; 176: 75–82

[294] Mautner VF, Friedrich RE, von Deimling A, et al. Malignant peripheral nerve sheath tumours in neurofibromatosis type 1: MRI supports the diagnosis of malignant plexiform neurofibroma. Neuroradiology 2003; 45: 618–625

[295] Meyers SP. Neurofibroma, malignant peripheral nerve sheath tumor. In: MRI of Bone and Soft Tissue Tumors and Tumorlike Lesions. Stuttgart, Germany: Thieme; 2008:633–641

[296] Murphey MD, Smith WS, Smith SE, Kransdorf MJ, Temple HT. From the archives of the AFIP. Imaging of musculoskeletal neurogenic tumors: radiologic-pathologic correlation. Radiographics 1999; 19: 1253–1280

[297] O'Rourke HO, Meyers SP, Katzman PJ. Neurothekeoma in the upper extremity: magnetic resonance imaging and computed tomography findings. J Comput Assist Tomogr 2005; 29: 847–850

[298] Von Deimling A, Foster R, Krone W. Neurofibromatosis type 1. In: Kleihues P, Cavenee WK, eds. World Health Organization Classification of Tumours. Pathology and Genetics of Tumours of the Nervous System. Lyon, France: IARC Press; 2000:216–218

[299] Woodruff JM, Kourea HP, Louis DN, Scheithauer BW. Neurofibroma. In: Kleihues P, Cavenee WK, eds. World Health Organization Classification of Tumours. Pathology and Genetics of Tumours of the Nervous System. Lyon, France: IARC Press; 2000:167–168

[300] Woodruff JM, Kourea HP, Louis DN, Scheithauer BW. Malignant peripheral nerve sheath tumour (MPNST). In: Kleihues P, Cavenee WK, eds. World Health Organization Classification of Tumours. Pathology and Genetics of Tumours of the Nervous System. Lyon, France: IARC Press; 2000:172–171

▸ Nodular Fasciitis

[301] Bancroft LW, Peterson JJ, Kransdorf MJ, Nomikos GC, Murphey MD. Soft tissue tumors of the lower extremities. Radiol Clin North Am 2002; 40: 991–1011

[302] Dinauer PA, Brixey CJ, Moncur JT, Fanburg-Smith JC, Murphey MD. Pathologic and MR imaging features of benign fibrous soft-tissue tumors in adults. Radiographics 2007; 27: 173–187

[303] Evans H, Bridge JA. Nodular fasciitis. In: Fletcher CDM, Unni KK, Mertens F, eds. World Health Organization Classification of Tumours. Pathology and Genetics of Tumours of Soft Tissue and Bone. Lyon, France: IARC Press; 2002:48–49

[304] Jelinek J, Kransdorf MJ. MR imaging of soft-tissue masses. Mass-like lesions that simulate neoplasms. Magn Reson Imaging Clin N Am 1995; 3: 727–741

[305] Laffan EE, Ngan BY, Navarro OM. Pediatric soft-tissue tumors and pseudotumors: MR imaging features with pathologic correlation, II: Tumors of fibroblastic/myofibroblastic, so-called fibrohistiocytic, muscular, lymphomatous, neurogenic, hair matrix, and uncertain origin. Radiographics 2009; 29: e36

[306] Meyers SP. Nodular fasciitis. In: MRI of Bone and Soft Tissue Tumors and Tumorlike Lesions. Stuttgart, Germany: Thieme; 2008:423–425

▸ Pigmented Villonodular Synovitis (PVNS)

[307] Al-Nakshabandi NA, Ryan AG, Choudur H, et al. Pigmented villonodular synovitis. Clin Radiol 2004; 59: 414–420

[308] De St. Aubain Somerhausen N, Dal Cin P. Diffuse-type giant cell tumor. In: Fletcher CDM, Unni KK, Mertens F, eds. World Health Organization Classification of Tumours. Pathology and Genetics of Tumours of Soft Tissue and Bone. Lyon, France: IARC Press; 2002:112–114

[309] Llauger J, Palmer J, Rosón N, Cremades R, Bagué S. Pigmented villonodular synovitis and giant cell tumors of the tendon sheath: radiologic and pathologic features. AJR Am J Roentgenol 1999; 172: 1087–1091

[310] Meyers SP. Pigmented Villonodular Synovitis. In: MRI of Bone and Soft Tissue Tumors and Tumorlike Lesions. Stuttgart, Germany: Thieme; 2008:726–729

[311] Murphey MD, Rhee JH, Lewis RB, Fanburg-Smith JC, Flemming DJ, Walker EA. Pigmented villonodular synovitis: radiologic-pathologic correlation. Radiographics 2008; 28: 1493–1518

▸ Rhabdomyosarcoma

[312] Ferrari A, Dileo P, Casanova M, et al. Rhabdomyosarcoma in adults. A retrospective analysis of 171 patients treated at a single institution. Cancer 2003; 98: 571–580

[313] Furlong MA, Mentzel T, Fanburg-Smith JC. Pleomorphic rhabdomyosarcoma in adults: a clinicopathologic study of 38 cases with emphasis on morphologic variants and recent skeletal muscle-specific markers. Mod Pathol 2001; 14: 595–603

[314] Kim EE, Valenzuela RF, Kumar AJ, Raney RB, Eftekari F. Imaging and clinical spectrum of rhabdomyosarcoma in children. Clin Imaging 2000; 24: 257–262

[315] Lucas DR, Ryan JR, Zalupski MM, Gross ML, Ravindranath Y, Ortman B. Primary embryonal rhabdomyosarcoma of long bone. Case report and review of the literature. Am J Surg Pathol 1996; 20: 239–244

[316] McCarville MB, Spunt SL, Pappo AS. Rhabdomyosarcoma in pediatric patients: the good, the bad, and the unusual. AJR Am J Roentgenol 2001; 176: 1563–1569

[317] Meyers SP. Rhabdomyosarcoma. In: MRI of Bone and Soft Tissue Tumors and Tumorlike Lesions. Stuttgart, Germany: Thieme; 2008:732–737

[318] Montgomery E, Barr FG. Pleomorphic rhabdomyosarcoma. In: Fletcher CDM, Unni KK, Mertens F, eds. World Health Organization Classification of Tumours. Pathology and Genetics of Tumours of Soft Tissue and Bone. Lyon, France: IARC Press; 2002:153–154

[319] Navarro OM. Soft tissue masses in children. Radiol Clin North Am 2011; 49: 1235–1259, vi–vii

[320] Parham DM, Barr FG. Embryonal rhabdomyosarcoma. In: Fletcher CDM, Unni KK, Mertens F, eds. World Health Organization Classification of Tumours. Pathology and Genetics of Tumours of Soft Tissue and Bone. Lyon, France: IARC Press; 2002:146–149

[321] Parham DM, Barr FG. Alveolar rhabdomyosarcoma. In: Fletcher CDM, Unni KK, Mertens F, eds. World Health Organization Classification of Tumours. Pathology and Genetics of Tumours of Soft Tissue and Bone. Lyon, France: IARC Press; 2002:150–152

[322] Van Rijn RR, Wilde JC, Bras J, Oldenburger F, McHugh KM, Merks JH. Imaging findings in noncraniofacial childhood rhabdomyosarcoma. Pediatr Radiol 2008; 38: 617–634

▸ Rheumatoid Arthritis

[323] Boutry N, Lardé A, Lapègue F, Solau-Gervais E, Flipo RM, Cotten A. Magnetic resonance imaging appearance of the hands and feet in patients with early rheumatoid arthritis. J Rheumatol 2003; 30: 671–679

[324] Meyers SP. Rheumatoid arthritis. In: MRI of Bone and Soft Tissue Tumors and Tumorlike Lesions. Stuttgart, Germany: Thieme; 2008:738–743

[325] Moran M, Fang C, Paul A. Rheumatoid arthritis presenting as an invasive soft-tissue tumour. Arch Orthop Trauma Surg 2002; 122: 538–540

[326] Narváez JA, Narváez J, Roca Y, Aguilera C. MR imaging assessment of clinical problems in rheumatoid arthritis. Eur Radiol 2002; 12: 1819–1828

▸ Sarcoid

[327] Meyers SP. Sarcoid. In: MRI of Bone and Soft Tissue Tumors and Tumorlike Lesions. Stuttgart, Germany: Thieme; 2008:744–746

[328] Moore SL, Teirstein AE. Musculoskeletal sarcoidosis: spectrum of appearances at MR imaging. Radiographics 2003; 23: 1389–1399

▸ Schwannoma

[329] Kang HJ, Shin SJ, Kang ES. Schwannomas of the upper extremity. J Hand Surg [Br] 2000; 25: 604–607

[330] Lin J, Martel W. Cross-sectional imaging of peripheral nerve sheath tumors: characteristic signs on CT, MR imaging, and sonography. AJR Am J Roentgenol 2001; 176: 75–82

[331] Louis DN, Stemmer-Rachamimov AO, Wiestler OD. Neurofibromatosis type 2. In: Kleihues P, Cavenee WK eds. World Health Organization Classification of Tumours. Pathology and Genetics of Tumours of the Nervous System. Lyon, France: IARC Press; 2000:219–222

[332] Meyers SP. Schwannoma. In: MRI of Bone and Soft Tissue Tumors and Tumorlike Lesions. Stuttgart, Germany: Thieme; 2008:747–752

[333] Murphey MD, Smith WS, Smith SE, Kransdorf MJ, Temple HT. From the archives of the AFIP. Imaging of musculoskeletal neurogenic tumors: radiologic-pathologic correlation. Radiographics 1999; 19: 1253–1280

[334] Woodruff JM, Kourea HP, Louis DN, Scheithauer BW. Schwannoma. In: Kleihues P, Cavenee WK eds. World Health Organization Classification of Tumours. Pathology and Genetics of Tumours of the Nervous System. Lyon, France: IARC Press; 2000:164–166

▸ Scleroderma, Systemic Sclerosis

[335] Madani G, Katz RD, Haddock JA, Denton CP, Bell JR. The role of radiology in the management of systemic sclerosis. Clin Radiol 2008; 63: 959–967

[336] Schanz S, Fierlbeck G, Ulmer A, et al. Localized scleroderma: MR findings and clinical features. Radiology 2011; 260: 817–824

[337] Schanz S, Henes J, Ulmer A, et al. Magnetic resonance imaging findings in patients with systemic scleroderma and musculoskeletal symptoms. Eur Radiol 2013; 23: 212–221

▸ Sickle Cell Disease with Extramedullary Hematopoiesis

[338] Castelli R, Graziadei G, Karimi M, Cappellini MD. Intrathoracic masses due to extramedullary hematopoiesis. Am J Med Sci 2004; 328: 299–303

[339] Collins WO, Younis RT, Garcia MT. Extramedullary hematopoiesis of the paranasal sinuses in sickle cell disease. Otolaryngol Head Neck Surg 2005; 132: 954–956

▸ Solitary Fibrous Tumor

[340] Garcia-Bennett J, Olivé CS, Rivas A, Domínguez-Oronoz R, Huguet P. Soft tissue solitary fibrous tumor. Imaging findings in a series of nine cases. Skeletal Radiol 2012; 41: 1427–1433[Epub ahead of print]

[341] Gengler C, Guillou L. Solitary fibrous tumour and haemangiopericytoma: evolution of a concept. Histopathology 2006; 48: 63–74

[342] Gold JS, Antonescu CR, Hajdu C, et al. Clinicopathologic correlates of solitary fibrous tumors. Cancer 2002; 94: 1057–1068

[343] Guillou L, Fletcher JA, Fletcher CDM, Mandahl N. Extrapleural solitary fibrous tumour and hemngiopericytoma. In: Fletcher CDM, Unni KK, Mertens F, eds. World Health Organization Classification of Tumours. Pathology and Genetics of Tumours of Soft Tissue and Bone. IARC Press; 2002:86–90

[344] Meyers SP. Solitary fibrous tumor. In: MRI of Bone and Soft Tissue Tumors and Tumorlike Lesions. Stuttgart, Germany: Thieme; 2008:430–432

▸ Synovial Cyst

[345] De Maeseneer M, Debaere C, Desprechins B, Osteaux M. Popliteal cysts in children: prevalence, appearance and associated findings at MR imaging. Pediatr Radiol 1999; 29: 605–609

[346] Meyers SP. Synovial cyst. In: MRI of Bone and Soft Tissue Tumors and Tumorlike Lesions. Stuttgart, Germany: Thieme; 2008:758–761

[347] Torreggiani WC, Al-Ismail K, Munk PL, et al. The imaging spectrum of Baker's (Popliteal) cysts. Clin Radiol 2002; 57: 681–691

[348] Tschirch FT, Schmid MR, Pfirrmann CW, Romero J, Hodler J, Zanetti M. Prevalence and size of meniscal cysts, ganglionic cysts, synovial cysts of the popliteal space, fluid-filled bursae, and other fluid collections in asymptomatic knees on MR imaging. AJR Am J Roentgenol 2003; 180: 1431–1436

▸ Synovial Sarcoma

[349] Antonescu CR, Kawai A, Leung DH, et al. Strong association of SYT-SSX fusion type and morphologic epithelial differentiation in synovial sarcoma. Diagn Mol Pathol 2000; 9: 1–8

[350] Chan JA, McMenamin ME, Fletcher CDM. Synovial sarcoma in older patients: clinicopathological analysis of 32 cases with emphasis on unusual histological features. Histopathology 2003; 43: 72–83

[351] Coindre JM, Pelmus M, Hostein I, Lussan C, Bui BN, Guillou L. Should molecular testing be required for diagnosing synovial sarcoma? A prospective study of 204 cases. Cancer 2003; 98: 2700–2707

[352] Fisher C, de Bruijn DRH, van Kessel AG. Synovial sarcoma. In: Fletcher CDM, Unni KK, Mertens F, eds. World Health Organization Classification of Tumours. Pathology and Genetics of Tumours of Soft Tissue and Bone. Lyon, France: IARC Press; 2002:200–204

[353] Jones BC, Sundaram M, Kransdorf MJ. Synovial sarcoma: MR imaging findings in 34 patients. AJR Am J Roentgenol 1993; 161: 827–830

[354] Kawai A, Woodruff J, Healey JH, Brennan MF, Antonescu CR, Ladanyi M. SYT-SSX gene fusion as a determinant of morphology and prognosis in synovial sarcoma. N Engl J Med 1998; 338: 153–160

[355] Ladanyi M, Antonescu CR, Leung DH, et al. Impact of SYT-SSX fusion type on the clinical behavior of synovial sarcoma: a multi-institutional retrospective study of 243 patients. Cancer Res 2002; 62: 135–140

[356] Lewis JJ, Antonescu CR, Leung DH, et al. Synovial sarcoma: a multivariate analysis of prognostic factors in 112 patients with primary localized tumors of the extremity. J Clin Oncol 2000; 18: 2087–2094

[357] McCarville MB, Spunt SL, Skapek SX, Pappo AS. Synovial sarcoma in pediatric patients. AJR Am J Roentgenol 2002; 179: 797–801

[358] Meyers SP. Synovial sarcoma. In: MRI of Bone and Soft Tissue Tumors and Tumorlike Lesions. Stuttgart, Germany: Thieme; 2008:762–768

[359] Murphey MD, Gibson MS, Jennings BT, Crespo-Rodríguez AM, Fanburg-Smith JF, Gajewski DA. From the archives of the AFIP: Imaging of synovial sarcoma with radiologic-pathologic correlation. Radiographics 2006; 26: 1543–1565

[360] O'Sullivan PJ, Harris AC, Munk PL. Radiological features of synovial cell sarcoma. Br J Radiol 2008; 81: 346–356

[361] Valenzuela RF, Kim EE, Seo JG, Patel S, Yasko AW. A revisit of MRI analysis for synovial sarcoma. Clin Imaging 2000; 24: 231–235

[362] van Rijswijk CSP, Hogendoorn PCW, Taminiau AHM, Bloem JL. Synovial sarcoma: dynamic contrast-enhanced MR imaging features. Skeletal Radiol 2001; 30: 25–30

▸ Traumatic Neuroma

[363] Boutin RD, Pathria MN, Resnick D. Disorders in the stumps of amputee patients: MR imaging. AJR Am J Roentgenol 1998; 171: 497–501

[364] Meyers SP. Traumatic neuroma. In: MRI of Bone and Soft Tissue Tumors and Tumorlike Lesions. Stuttgart, Germany: Thieme; 2008:642–644

[365] Murphey MD, Smith WS, Smith SE, Kransdorf MJ, Temple HT. From the archives of the AFIP. Imaging of musculoskeletal neurogenic tumors: radiologic-pathologic correlation. Radiographics 1999; 19: 1253–1280

▸ Tumoral Calcinosis

[366] Martinez S, Vogler JB, Harrelson JM, Lyles KW. Imaging of tumoral calcinosis: new observations. Radiology 1990; 174: 215–222

[367] Olsen KM, Chew FS. Tumoral calcinosis: pearls, polemics, and alternative possibilities. Radiographics 2006; 26: 871–885

[368] Şenol U, Karaal K, Çevikol C, Dinçer A. MR imaging findings of recurrent tumoral calcinosis. Clin Imaging 2000; 24: 154–156

▸ Xanthoma

[369] Barkhof F, Verrips A, Wesseling P, et al. Cerebrotendinous xanthomatosis: the spectrum of imaging findings and the correlation with neuropathologic findings. Radiology 2000; 217: 869–876

[370] Dotti MT, Federico A, Signorini E, et al. Cerebrotendinous xanthomatosis (van Bogaert-Scherer-Epstein disease): CT and MR findings. AJNR Am J Neuroradiol 1994; 15: 1721–1726

[371] Kelman CG, Disler DG, Kremer JM, Jennings TA. Xanthomatous infiltration of ankle tendons. Skeletal Radiol 1997; 26: 256–259

[372] Meyers SP. Xanthoma. In: MRI of Bone and Soft Tissue Tumors and Tumorlike Lesions. Stuttgart, Germany: Thieme; 2008:773–774

[373] Smithard A, Lamyman MJ, McCarthy CL, Gibbons CLMH, Cooke PJ, Athanasou N. Cerebrotendinous xanthomatosis presenting with bilateral Achilles tendon xanthomata. Skeletal Radiol 2007; 36: 171–175

[374] Yamamoto T, Kawamoto T, Marui T, et al. Multimodality imaging features of primary xanthoma of the calcaneus. Skeletal Radiol 2003; 32: 367–370

Index

A

B

C

R

S

T

U

V

W

X